4th Edition

HARRISON'S™

ENDOCRINOLOGY

Derived from Harrison's Principles of Internal Medicine, 19th Edition

Editors

DENNIS L. KASPER, MD
William Ellery Channing Professor of Medicine, Professor of Microbiology and Immunobiology, Department of Microbiology and Immunobiology, Harvard Medical School; Division of Infectious Diseases, Brigham and Women's Hospital
Boston, Massachusetts

STEPHEN L. HAUSER, MD
Robert A. Fishman Distinguished Professor and Chairman, Department of Neurology, University of California, San Francisco
San Francisco, California

J. LARRY JAMESON, MD, PhD
Robert G. Dunlop Professor of Medicine;
Dean, Perelman School of Medicine at the University of Pennsylvania;
Executive Vice-President, University of Pennsylvania for the Health System, Philadelphia, Pennsylvania

ANTHONY S. FAUCI, MD
Chief, Laboratory of Immunoregulation; Director, National Institute of Allergy and Infectious Diseases, National Institutes of Health, Bethesda, Maryland

DAN L. LONGO, MD
Professor of Medicine, Harvard Medical School; Senior Physician, Brigham and Women's Hospital; Deputy Editor, *New England Journal of Medicine*, Boston, Massachusetts

JOSEPH LOSCALZO, MD, PhD
Hersey Professor of the Theory and Practice of Medicine, Harvard Medical School; Chairman, Department of Medicine, and Physician-in-Chief, Brigham and Women's Hospital, Boston, Massachusetts

4th Edition

HARRISON'S™ ENDOCRINOLOGY

EDITOR

J. Larry Jameson, MD, PhD
Robert G. Dunlop Professor of Medicine;
Dean, Perelman School of Medicine at the University of Pennsylvania;
Executive Vice-President, University of Pennsylvania for the
Health System, Philadelphia, Pennsylvania

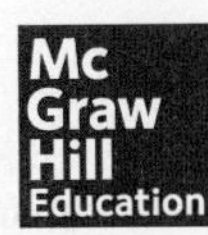

New York Chicago San Francisco Athens London Madrid Mexico City
Milan New Delhi Singapore Sydney Toronto

Harrison's Endocrinology, Fourth Edition

Dr. Fauci's work as an editor and author was performed outside the scope of his employment as a U.S. government employee. This work represents his personal and professional views and not necessarily those of the U.S. government.

1 2 3 4 5 6 7 8 9 DOW 21 20 19 18 17 16

ISBN 978-1-259-83572-8
MHID 1-259-83572-3

This book was set in Minion Pro by Cenveo® Publisher Services. The editors were James F. Shanahan and Kim J. Davis. The production supervisor was Catherine H. Saggese. Project management was provided by Sonam Arora of Cenveo® Publisher Services. The cover design was by Dreamit, Inc.

RR Donnelley was the printer and binder.

Library of Congress Cataloging-in-Publication Data

Names: Jameson, J. Larry, editor.
Title: Harrison's endocrinology / editor, J. Larry Jameson.
Other titles: Endocrinology
Description: Fourth edition. | New York: McGraw-Hill Education Medical, [2017] | Contained in: Harrison's principles of internal medicine. 19th ed. [2015]. | Includes index.
Identifiers: LCCN 2016006309 (print) | LCCN 2016007362 (ebook) | ISBN 9781259835728 (pbk. : alk. paper) | ISBN 1259835723 (pbk. : alk. paper) | ISBN 9781259835735 () | ISBN 1259835731 ()
Subjects: | MESH: Endocrine System Diseases | Metabolic Diseases
Classification: LCC RC648 (print) | LCC RC648 (ebook) | NLM WK 140 | DDC 616.4–dc23
LC record available at http://lccn.loc.gov/2016006309

CONTENTS

CONTRIBUTORS

Numbers in brackets refer to the chapter(s) written or co-written by the contributor.

John C. Achermann, MD, PhD, MB
Wellcome Trust Senior Research Fellow in Clinical Science, University College London; Professor of Paediatric Endocrinology, UCL Institute of Child Health, University College London, London, United Kingdom [10]

Wiebke Arlt, MD, DSc, FRCP, FMedSci
Professor of Medicine, Centre for Endocrinology, Diabetes and Metabolism, School of Clinical and Experimental Medicine, University of Birmingham; Consultant Endocrinologist, University Hospital Birmingham, Birmingham, United Kingdom [8]

Robert C. Basner, MD
Professor of Clinical Medicine, Division of Pulmonary, Allergy, and Critical Care Medicine, Columbia University College of Physicians and Surgeons, New York, New York [Appendix]

Shari S. Bassuk, ScD
Epidemiologist, Division of Preventive Medicine, Brigham and Women's Hospital, Boston, Massachusetts [16]

Shalender Bhasin, MBBS
Professor of Medicine, Harvard Medical School; Director, Research Program in Men's Health: Aging and Metabolism; Director, Boston Claude D. Pepper Older Americans Independence Center; Site Director, Harvard Catalyst Clinical Research Center at BWH, Brigham and Women's Hospital, Boston, Massachusetts [11]

George J. Bosl, MD
Professor of Medicine, Weill Cornell Medical College; Chair, Department of Medicine; Patrick M. Byrne Chair in Clinical Oncology, Memorial Sloan-Kettering Cancer Center, New York, New York [12]

F. Richard Bringhurst, MD
Associate Professor of Medicine, Harvard Medical School; Physician, Massachusetts General Hospital, Boston, Massachusetts [32]

Cynthia D. Brown, MD
Associate Professor of Clinical Medicine, Division of Pulmonary, Critical Care, Sleep and Occupational Medicine, Indiana University, Indianapolis, Indiana [Review and Self-Assessment]

Felicia Cosman, MD
Professor of Medicine, Columbia University College of Physicians and Surgeons, New York, New York [35]

Philip E. Cryer, MD
Professor of Medicine Emeritus, Washington University in St. Louis; Physician, Barnes-Jewish Hospital, St. Louis, Missouri [26]

Stephen N. Davis, MBBS, FRCP
Theodore E. Woodward Professor and Chairman of the Department of Medicine, University of Maryland School of Medicine; Physician-in-Chief, University of Maryland Medical Center, Baltimore, Maryland [26]

Marie B. Demay, MD
Professor of Medicine, Harvard Medical School; Physician, Massachusetts General Hospital, Boston, Massachusetts [32]

Robert H. Eckel, MD
Professor of Medicine, Division of Endocrinology, Metabolism and Diabetes, Division of Cardiology; Professor of Physiology and Biophysics, Charles A. Boettcher, II Chair in Atherosclerosis, University of Colorado School of Medicine, Anschutz Medical Campus, Director Lipid Clinic, University of Colorado Hospital, Aurora, Colorado [22]

David A. Ehrmann, MD
Professor, Department of Medicine, Section of Endocrinology, Diabetes, and Metabolism, The University of Chicago Pritzker School of Medicine, Chicago, Illinois [17]

Andrew J. Einstein, MD, PhD
Victoria and Esther Aboodi Assistant Professor of Medicine; Director, Cardiac CT Research; Co-Director, Cardiac CT and MRI, Department of Medicine, Cardiology Division, Department of Radiology, Columbia University College of Physicians and Surgeons, New York-Presbyterian Hospital, New York, New York [Appendix]

Murray J. Favus, MD
Professor of Medicine, Department of Medicine, Section of Endocrinology, Diabetes and Metabolism, Director Bone Program, University of Chicago Pritzker School of Medicine, Chicago, Illinois [36]

Darren R. Feldman, MD
Associate Professor in Medicine, Weill Cornell Medical Center; Assistant Attending, Genitourinary Oncology Service, Memorial Sloan-Kettering Cancer Center, New York, New York [12]

Jeffrey S. Flier, MD
Caroline Shields Walker Professor of Medicine and Dean, Harvard Medical School, Boston, Massachusetts [20]

Peter A. Gottlieb, MD
Professor of Pediatrics and Medicine, Barbara Davis Center, University of Colorado School of Medicine, Aurora, Colorado [30]

Janet E. Hall, MD, MSc
Professor of Medicine, Harvard Medical School and Associate Chief, Reproductive Endocrine Unit, Massachusetts General Hospital, Boston, Massachusetts [13–15]

Helen H. Hobbs, MD
Professor, Internal Medicine and Molecular Genetics, University of Texas Southwestern Medical Center; Investigator, Howard Hughes Medical Institute, Dallas, Texas [27]

Brian Houston, MD
Division of Cardiology, Department of Medicine, Johns Hopkins Hospital, Baltimore, Maryland [Review and Self-Assessment]

J. Larry Jameson
Robert G. Dunlop Professor of Medicine;
Dean, Perelman School of Medicine at the University of Pennsylvania;
Executive Vice-President, University of Pennsylvania for the Health System, Philadelphia, Pennsylvania [1–5, 7, 10, 11, 31]

Robert T. Jensen, MD
Chief, Cell Biology Section, National Institutes of Diabetes, Digestive and Kidney Diseases, National Institutes of Health, Bethesda, Maryland [28]

Harald Jüppner, MD
Professor of Pediatrics, Endocrine Unit and Pediatric Nephrology Unit, Massachusetts General Hospital, Boston, Massachusetts [34]

Sundeep Khosla, MD
Professor of Medicine and Physiology, College of Medicine, Mayo Clinic, Rochester, Minnesota [33]

Stephen M. Krane, MD
Persis, Cyrus and Marlow B. Harrison Distinguished Professor of Medicine, Harvard Medical School; Massachusetts General Hospital, Boston, Massachusetts [32]

Alexander Kratz, MD, MPH, PhD
Associate Professor of Clinical Pathology and Cell Biology, Columbia University College of Physicians and Surgeons; Director, Core Laboratory, Columbia University Medical Center and the New York Presbyterian Hospital; Director, the Allen Hospital Laboratory, New York, New York [Appendix]

Henry M. Kronenberg, MD
Professor of Medicine, Harvard Medical School; Chief, Endocrine Unit, Massachusetts General Hospital, Boston, Massachusetts [32]

Robert F. Kushner, MD, MS
Professor of Medicine, Northwestern University Feinberg School of Medicine, Chicago, Illinois [21]

Robert Lindsay, MD, PhD
Chief, Internal Medicine; Professor of Clinical Medicine, Helen Hayes Hospital, West Haverstraw, New York [35]

Dan L. Longo, MD
Professor of Medicine, Harvard Medical School; Senior Physician, Brigham and Women's Hospital; Deputy Editor, *New England Journal of Medicine,* Boston, Massachusetts [31]

Susan J. Mandel, MD, MPH
Professor of Medicine; Associate Chief, Division of Endocrinology, Diabetes and Metabolism, Perelman School of Medicine, University of Pennsylvania, Philadelphia, Pennsylvania [7]

JoAnn E. Manson, MD, DrPH
Professor of Medicine and the Elizabeth Fay Brigham Professor of Women's Health, Harvard Medical School; Chief, Division of Preventive Medicine, Brigham and Women's Hospital, Boston, Massachusetts [16]

Eleftheria Maratos-Flier, MD
Professor of Medicine, Harvard Medical School; Division of Endocrinology, Beth Israel Deaconess Medical Center, Boston, Massachusetts [20]

Kevin T. McVary, MD, FACS
Professor and Chairman, Division of Urology, Southern Illinois University School of Medicine, Springfield, Illinois [19]

Shlomo Melmed, MD
Senior Vice President and Dean of the Medical Faculty, Cedars-Sinai Medical Center, Los Angeles, California [3–5]

Robert J. Motzer, MD
Professor of Medicine, Joan and Sanford Weill College of Medicine of Cornell University D. Attending Physician, Genitourinary Oncology Service, Memorial Sloan-Kettering Cancer Center, New York, New York [12]

Hartmut P. H. Neumann, MD
Universitaet Freiburg, Medizinische Universitaetsklinik, Freiburg im Breisgau, Germany [9]

Michael A. Pesce, PhD
Professor Emeritus of Pathology and Cell Biology, Columbia University College of Physicians and Surgeons; Director, Biochemical Genetics Laboratory, Columbia University Medical Center, New York Presbyterian Hospital, New York, New York [Appendix]

John T. Potts, Jr., MD
Jackson Distinguished Professor of Clinical Medicine, Harvard Medical School; Physician-in-Chief and Director of Research Emeritus, Massachusetts General Hospital, Boston, Massachusetts [34]

Alvin C. Powers, MD
Joe C. Davis Chair in Biomedical Science; Professor of Medicine, Molecular Physiology and Biophysics; Director, Vanderbilt Diabetes Center; Chief, Division of Diabetes, Endocrinology, and Metabolism, Vanderbilt University School of Medicine, Nashville, Tennessee [23–25]

Daniel J. Rader, MD
Seymour Gray Professor of Molecular Medicine; Chair, Department of Genetics; Chief, Division of Translational Medicine and Human Genetics, Department of Medicine, Perelman School of Medicine at the University of Pennsylvania, Philadelphia, Pennsylvania [27]

Gary L. Robertson, MD
Emeritus Professor of Medicine, Northwestern University School of Medicine, Chicago, Illinois [6]

Michael V. Seiden, MD, PhD
Chief Medical Officer, McKesson Specialty Health, The Woodlands, Texas [18]

Rajesh V. Thakker, MD, FMedSci, FR
May Professor of Medicine, Academic Endocrine Unit, University of Oxford; O.C.D.E.M., Churchill Hospital, Headington, Oxford, United Kingdom [29]

Tamara J. Vokes, MD
Professor, Department of Medicine, Section of Endocrinology, University of Chicago, Chicago, Illinois [36]

Anthony P. Weetman, MD, DSc
University of Sheffield, School of Medicine Sheffield, Sheffield, United Kingdom [7]

Charles M. Wiener, MD
Vice President of Academic Affairs, Johns Hopkins Medicine International, Professor of Medicine and Physiology, Johns Hopkins School of Medicine, Baltimore, Maryland [Review and Self-Assessment]

PREFACE

Harrison's Principles of Internal Medicine has been a respected source of medical information for students, residents, internists, family physicians, and other health care providers for many decades. This book, *Harrison's Endocrinology*, now in its fourth edition, is a compilation of chapters related to the specialty of endocrinology, a field that includes some of the most commonly encountered diseases such as diabetes mellitus, obesity, thyroid disorders, and metabolic bone disease.

Our readers consistently note the practical value of the specialty sections of *Harrison's*. Specifically, these sections include a rigorous explanation of pathophysiology as a background for differential diagnosis and patient management. Our goal was to bring this information to readers in a more compact and usable form. Because the topic is more focused, it is possible to improve the presentation of the material by enlarging the text and the tables and providing clearly illustrated figures that elucidate challenging concepts. We have also included a Review and Self-Assessment section that includes questions and answers to provoke reflection and to provide additional teaching points.

The clinical manifestations of endocrine disorders can usually be explained by considering the physiologic role of hormones, which are either deficient or excessive. Thus, a thorough understanding of hormone action and principles of hormone feedback arms the clinician with a logical diagnostic approach and a conceptual framework for treating patients. The first chapter of the book, Approach to the Patient with Endocrine Disorders, provides this type of "systems" overview. Using numerous examples of translational research, this introduction links genetics, cell biology, and physiology with pathophysiology and treatment. The integration of pathophysiology with clinical management is a hallmark of *Harrison's*, and can be found throughout each of the subsequent disease-oriented chapters. The book is divided into six main sections that reflect the physiologic roots of endocrinology: (I) Introduction to Endocrinology; (II) Pituitary, Thyroid, and Adrenal Disorders; (III) Reproductive Endocrinology; (IV) Diabetes Mellitus, Obesity, Lipoprotein Metabolism; (V) Disorders Affecting Multiple Endocrine Systems; and (VI) Disorders of Bone and Calcium Metabolism.

While *Harrison's Endocrinology* is classic in its organization, readers will sense the impact of scientific advances as they explore the individual chapters in each section. In addition to the dramatic discoveries emanating from genetics and molecular biology, the introduction of an unprecedented number of new drugs, particularly for the management of diabetes, hypogonadism, and osteoporosis, is transforming the field of endocrinology. Numerous recent clinical studies involving common diseases like diabetes, obesity, hypothyroidism, hypogonadism, and osteoporosis provide powerful evidence for medical decision making and treatment. These rapid changes in endocrinology are exciting for new students of medicine and underscore the need for practicing physicians to continuously update their knowledge base and clinical skills.

Our access to information through web-based journals and databases is remarkably efficient, but also daunting, creating a need for books that synthesize concepts and highlight important facts. The preparation of these chapters is therefore a special craft that requires distillation of core information from the ever-expanding knowledge base. The editors are indebted to our authors, a group of internationally recognized authorities who are masters at providing a comprehensive overview while being able to distill a topic into a concise and interesting chapter. We are also indebted to our colleagues at McGraw-Hill. Jim Shanahan is a tireless champion for *Harrison's*, and these books were impeccably produced by Kim Davis.

We hope you find this book useful in your effort to achieve continuous learning on behalf of your patients.

J. Larry Jameson, MD, PhD

NOTICE

Medicine is an ever-changing science. As new research and clinical experience broaden our knowledge, changes in treatment and drug therapy are required. The authors and the publisher of this work have checked with sources believed to be reliable in their efforts to provide information that is complete and generally in accord with the standards accepted at the time of publication. However, in view of the possibility of human error or changes in medical sciences, neither the authors nor the publisher nor any other party who has been involved in the preparation or publication of this work warrants that the information contained herein is in every respect accurate or complete, and they disclaim all responsibility for any errors or omissions or for the results obtained from use of the information contained in this work. Readers are encouraged to confirm the information contained herein with other sources. For example and in particular, readers are advised to check the product information sheet included in the package of each drug they plan to administer to be certain that the information contained in this work is accurate and that changes have not been made in the recommended dose or in the contraindications for administration. This recommendation is of particular importance in connection with new or infrequently used drugs.

Review and self-assessment questions and answers were taken from Wiener CM, Brown CD, Houston B (eds). *Harrison's Self-Assessment and Board Review,* 19th ed. New York, McGraw-Hill, 2017, ISBN 978-1-259-64288-3 .

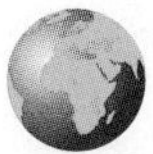
The global icons call greater attention to key epidemiologic and clinical differences in the practice of medicine throughout the world.

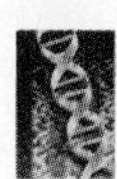
The genetic icons identify a clinical issue with an explicit genetic relationship.

SECTION I

INTRODUCTION TO ENDOCRINOLOGY

CHAPTER 1

APPROACH TO THE PATIENT WITH ENDOCRINE DISORDERS

J. Larry Jameson

The management of endocrine disorders requires a broad understanding of intermediary metabolism, reproductive physiology, bone metabolism, and growth. Accordingly, the practice of endocrinology is intimately linked to a conceptual framework for understanding hormone secretion, hormone action, and principles of feedback control **(Chap. 2)**. The endocrine system is evaluated primarily by measuring hormone concentrations, arming the clinician with valuable diagnostic information. Most disorders of the endocrine system are amenable to effective treatment once the correct diagnosis is determined. Endocrine deficiency disorders are treated with physiologic hormone replacement; hormone excess conditions, which usually are caused by benign glandular adenomas, are managed by removing tumors surgically or reducing hormone levels medically.

SCOPE OF ENDOCRINOLOGY

The specialty of endocrinology encompasses the study of glands and the hormones they produce. The term *endocrine* was coined by Starling to contrast the actions of hormones secreted internally (*endocrine*) with those secreted externally (*exocrine*) or into a lumen, such as the gastrointestinal tract. The term *hormone*, derived from a Greek phrase meaning "to set in motion," aptly describes the dynamic actions of hormones as they elicit cellular responses and regulate physiologic processes through feedback mechanisms.

Unlike many other specialties in medicine, it is not possible to define endocrinology strictly along anatomic lines. The classic endocrine glands—pituitary, thyroid, parathyroid, pancreatic islets, adrenals, and gonads—communicate broadly with other organs through the nervous system, hormones, cytokines, and growth factors. In addition to its traditional synaptic functions, the brain produces a vast array of peptide hormones, and this has led to the discipline of neuroendocrinology. Through the production of hypothalamic releasing factors, the central nervous system (CNS) exerts a major regulatory influence over pituitary hormone secretion **(Chap. 3)**. The peripheral nervous system stimulates the adrenal medulla. The immune and endocrine systems are also intimately intertwined. The adrenal hormone cortisol is a powerful immunosuppressant. Cytokines and interleukins (ILs) have profound effects on the functions of the pituitary, adrenal, thyroid, and gonads. Common endocrine diseases such as autoimmune thyroid disease and type 1 diabetes mellitus are caused by dysregulation of immune surveillance and tolerance. Less common diseases such as polyglandular failure, Addison's disease, and lymphocytic hypophysitis also have an immunologic basis.

The interdigitation of endocrinology with physiologic processes in other specialties sometimes blurs the role of hormones. For example, hormones play an important role in maintenance of blood pressure, intravascular volume, and peripheral resistance in the cardiovascular system. Vasoactive substances such as catecholamines, angiotensin II, endothelin, and nitric oxide are involved in dynamic changes of vascular tone in addition to their multiple roles in other tissues. The heart is the principal source of atrial natriuretic peptide, which acts in classic endocrine fashion to induce natriuresis at a distant target organ (the kidney). Erythropoietin, a traditional circulating hormone, is made in the kidney and stimulates erythropoiesis in bone marrow. The kidney is also integrally involved in the renin-angiotensin axis **(Chap. 8)** and is a primary target of several hormones, including parathyroid hormone (PTH), mineralocorticoids, and vasopressin. The gastrointestinal tract produces a surprising number of peptide hormones, such as cholecystokinin, ghrelin, gastrin, secretin, and vasoactive intestinal peptide, among many others. Carcinoid and islet tumors can secrete excessive amounts of these hormones, leading to specific clinical syndromes **(Chap. 28)**. Many of these gastrointestinal hormones are also produced in the CNS, where their functions are poorly understood. Adipose tissue produces leptin, which acts centrally to control appetite, along with adiponectin, resistin, and other hormones that regulate metabolism. As hormones such as inhibin, ghrelin, and leptin are discovered, they become integrated into the science and practice of medicine on the basis of their functional roles rather than their tissues of origin.

Characterization of hormone receptors frequently reveals unexpected relationships to factors in nonendocrine disciplines. The growth hormone (GH) and leptin receptors, for example, are members of the cytokine receptor family. The G protein–coupled receptors (GPCRs), which mediate the actions of many peptide hormones, are used in numerous physiologic processes, including vision, smell, and neurotransmission.

PATHOLOGIC MECHANISMS OF ENDOCRINE DISEASE

Endocrine diseases can be divided into three major types of conditions: (1) hormone excess, (2) hormone deficiency, and (3) hormone resistance (Table 1-1).

CAUSES OF HORMONE EXCESS

Syndromes of hormone excess can be caused by neoplastic growth of endocrine cells, autoimmune disorders, and excess hormone administration. Benign endocrine tumors, including parathyroid, pituitary, and adrenal adenomas, often retain the capacity to produce hormones, perhaps reflecting the fact that these

TABLE 1-1

CAUSES OF ENDOCRINE DYSFUNCTION

TYPE OF ENDOCRINE DISORDER	EXAMPLES
Hyperfunction	
Neoplastic	
Benign	Pituitary adenomas, hyperparathyroidism, autonomous thyroid or adrenal nodules, pheochromocytoma
Malignant	Adrenal cancer, medullary thyroid cancer, carcinoid
Ectopic	Ectopic ACTH, SIADH secretion
Multiple endocrine neoplasia (MEN)	MEN 1, MEN 2
Autoimmune	Graves' disease
Iatrogenic	Cushing's syndrome, hypoglycemia
Infectious/inflammatory	Subacute thyroiditis
Activating receptor mutations	LH, TSH, Ca^{2+}, PTH receptors, $G_s\alpha$
Hypofunction	
Autoimmune	Hashimoto's thyroiditis, type 1 diabetes mellitus, Addison's disease, polyglandular failure
Iatrogenic	Radiation-induced hypopituitarism, hypothyroidism, surgical
Infectious/inflammatory	Adrenal insufficiency, hypothalamic sarcoidosis
Hormone mutations	GH, LHβ, FSHβ, vasopressin
Enzyme defects	21-Hydroxylase deficiency
Developmental defects	Kallmann syndrome, Turner's syndrome, transcription factors
Nutritional/vitamin deficiency	Vitamin D deficiency, iodine deficiency
Hemorrhage/infarction	Sheehan's syndrome, adrenal insufficiency
Hormone Resistance	
Receptor mutations	
Membrane	GH, vasopressin, LH, FSH, ACTH, GnRH, GHRH, PTH, leptin, Ca^{2+}
Nuclear	AR, TR, VDR, ER, GR, PPARγ
Signaling pathway mutations	Albright's hereditary osteodystrophy
Postreceptor	Type 2 diabetes mellitus, leptin resistance

Abbreviations: ACTH, adrenocorticotropic hormone; AR, androgen receptor; ER, estrogen receptor; FSH, follicle-stimulating hormone; GHRH, growth hormone–releasing hormone; GnRH, gonadotropin-releasing hormone; GR, glucocorticoid receptor; LH, luteinizing hormone; PPAR, peroxisome proliferator activated receptor; PTH, parathyroid hormone; SIADH, syndrome of inappropriate antidiuretic hormone; TR, thyroid hormone receptor; TSH, thyroid-stimulating hormone; VDR, vitamin D receptor.

tumors are relatively well differentiated. Many endocrine tumors exhibit subtle defects in their "set points" for feedback regulation. For example, in Cushing's disease, impaired feedback inhibition of adrenocorticotropic hormone (ACTH) secretion is associated with autonomous function. However, the tumor cells are not completely resistant to feedback, as evidenced by ACTH suppression by higher doses of dexamethasone (e.g., high-dose dexamethasone test) (**Chap. 8**). Similar set point defects are also typical of parathyroid adenomas and autonomously functioning thyroid nodules.

The molecular basis of some endocrine tumors, such as the multiple endocrine neoplasia (MEN) syndromes (MEN 1, 2A, 2B), have provided important insights into tumorigenesis (**Chap. 29**). MEN 1 is characterized primarily by the triad of parathyroid, pancreatic islet, and pituitary tumors. MEN 2 predisposes to medullary thyroid carcinoma, pheochromocytoma, and hyperparathyroidism. The *MEN1* gene, located on chromosome 11q13, encodes a putative tumor-suppressor gene, menin. Analogous to the paradigm first described for retinoblastoma, the affected individual inherits a mutant copy of the *MEN1* gene, and tumorigenesis ensues after a somatic "second hit" leads to loss of function of the normal *MEN1* gene (through deletion or point mutations).

In contrast to inactivation of a tumor-suppressor gene, as occurs in MEN 1 and most other inherited cancer syndromes, MEN 2 is caused by activating mutations in a single allele. In this case, activating mutations of the *RET* protooncogene, which encodes a receptor tyrosine kinase, leads to thyroid C cell hyperplasia in childhood before the development of medullary thyroid carcinoma. Elucidation of this pathogenic mechanism has allowed early genetic screening for *RET* mutations in individuals at risk for MEN 2, permitting identification of those who may benefit from prophylactic thyroidectomy and biochemical screening for pheochromocytoma and hyperparathyroidism.

Mutations that activate hormone receptor signaling have been identified in several GPCRs. For example, activating mutations of the luteinizing hormone (LH) receptor cause a dominantly transmitted form of male-limited precocious puberty, reflecting premature stimulation of testosterone synthesis in Leydig cells (**Chap. 11**). Activating mutations in these GPCRs are located predominantly in the transmembrane domains and induce receptor coupling to $G_s\alpha$ even in the absence of hormone. Consequently, adenylate cyclase is activated, and cyclic adenosine monophosphate (AMP) levels increase in a manner that mimics hormone action. A similar phenomenon results from activating mutations in $G_s\alpha$. When these mutations occur early in development, they cause McCune-Albright syndrome. When they occur only in somatotropes, the activating $G_s\alpha$ mutations cause GH-secreting tumors and acromegaly (**Chap. 5**).

In autoimmune Graves' disease, antibody interactions with the thyroid-stimulating hormone (TSH) receptor mimic TSH action, leading to hormone overproduction (**Chap. 7**). Analogous to the effects of activating mutations of the TSH receptor, these stimulating autoantibodies induce conformational changes that release the receptor from a constrained state, thereby triggering receptor coupling to G proteins.

CAUSES OF HORMONE DEFICIENCY

Most examples of hormone deficiency states can be attributed to glandular destruction caused by autoimmunity, surgery, infection, inflammation, infarction, hemorrhage, or tumor infiltration (Table 1-1). Autoimmune damage to the thyroid gland (Hashimoto's thyroiditis) and pancreatic islet β cells (type 1 diabetes mellitus) is a prevalent cause of endocrine disease. Mutations in a number of hormones, hormone receptors, transcription factors, enzymes, and channels can also lead to hormone deficiencies.

HORMONE RESISTANCE

Most severe hormone resistance syndromes are due to inherited defects in membrane receptors, nuclear receptors, or the pathways that transduce receptor signals. These disorders are characterized by defective hormone action despite the presence of increased hormone levels. In complete androgen resistance, for example, mutations in the androgen receptor result in a female phenotypic appearance in genetic (XY) males, even though LH and testosterone levels are increased (**Chap. 29**). In addition to these relatively rare genetic disorders, more common acquired forms of functional hormone resistance include insulin resistance in type 2 diabetes mellitus, leptin resistance in obesity, and GH resistance in catabolic states. The pathogenesis of functional resistance involves receptor downregulation and postreceptor desensitization of signaling pathways; functional forms of resistance are generally reversible.

CLINICAL EVALUATION OF ENDOCRINE DISORDERS

Because most glands are relatively inaccessible, the physical examination usually focuses on the manifestations of hormone excess or deficiency as well as direct examination of palpable glands, such as the thyroid and gonads. For these reasons, it is important to evaluate patients in the context of their presenting symptoms, review of systems, family and social history, and exposure to medications that may affect the endocrine system. Astute clinical skills are required to detect subtle symptoms and signs suggestive of underlying endocrine disease. For example, a patient with Cushing's syndrome may manifest specific findings, such as central fat redistribution, striae, and proximal muscle weakness, in addition to features seen commonly in the general population, such as obesity, plethora, hypertension, and glucose intolerance. Similarly, the insidious onset of hypothyroidism—with mental slowing, fatigue, dry skin, and other features—can be difficult to distinguish from similar, nonspecific findings in the general population. Clinical judgment that is based on knowledge of disease prevalence and pathophysiology is required to decide when to embark on more extensive evaluation of these disorders. Laboratory testing plays an essential role in endocrinology by allowing quantitative assessment of hormone levels and dynamics. Radiologic imaging tests such as computed tomography (CT) scan, magnetic resonance imaging (MRI), thyroid scan, and ultrasound are also used for the diagnosis of endocrine disorders. However, these tests generally are employed only after a hormonal abnormality has been established by biochemical testing.

HORMONE MEASUREMENTS AND ENDOCRINE TESTING

Immunoassays are the most important diagnostic tool in endocrinology, as they allow sensitive, specific, and quantitative determination of steady-state and dynamic changes in hormone concentrations. Immunoassays use antibodies to detect specific hormones. For many peptide hormones, these measurements are now configured to use two different antibodies to increase binding affinity and specificity. There are many variations of these assays; a common format involves using one antibody to capture the antigen (hormone) onto an immobilized surface and a second antibody, coupled to a chemiluminescent (immunochemiluminescent assay [ICMA]) or radioactive (immunoradiometric assay [IRMA]) signal, to detect the antigen. These assays are sensitive enough to detect plasma hormone concentrations in the picomolar to nanomolar range, and they can readily distinguish structurally related proteins, such as PTH from PTH-related peptide (PTHrP). A variety of other techniques are used to measure specific hormones, including mass spectroscopy, various forms of chromatography, and enzymatic methods; bioassays are now rarely used.

Most hormone measurements are based on plasma or serum samples. However, urinary hormone determinations remain useful for the evaluation of some conditions. Urinary collections over 24 h provide an integrated assessment of the production of a hormone or metabolite, many of which vary during the day. It is important to assure complete collections of 24-h urine samples; simultaneous measurement of creatinine provides an internal control for the adequacy of collection and can be used to normalize some hormone measurements. A 24-h urine free cortisol measurement largely reflects the amount of unbound cortisol, thus providing a reasonable index of biologically available hormone. Other commonly used urine determinations include 17-hydroxycorticosteroids, 17-ketosteroids, vanillylmandelic acid, metanephrine, catecholamines, 5-hydroxyindoleacetic acid, and calcium.

The value of quantitative hormone measurements lies in their correct interpretation in a clinical context. The normal range for most hormones is relatively broad, often varying by a factor of two- to tenfold. The normal ranges for many hormones are sex- and age-specific. Thus, using the correct normative database is an essential part of interpreting hormone tests. The pulsatile nature of hormones and factors that can affect their secretion, such as sleep, meals, and medications, must also be considered. Cortisol values increase fivefold between midnight and dawn; reproductive hormone levels vary dramatically during the female menstrual cycle.

For many endocrine systems, much information can be gained from basal hormone testing, particularly when different components of an endocrine axis are assessed simultaneously. For example, low testosterone and elevated LH levels suggest a primary gonadal problem, whereas a hypothalamic-pituitary disorder is likely if both LH and testosterone are low. Because TSH is a sensitive indicator of thyroid function, it is generally recommended as a first-line test for thyroid disorders. An elevated TSH level is almost always the result of primary hypothyroidism, whereas a low TSH is most often caused by thyrotoxicosis. These predictions can be confirmed by determining the free thyroxine level. In the less common circumstance when free thyroxine and TSH are both low, it is important to consider secondary hypopituitarism caused by hypothalamic-pituitary disease. Elevated calcium and PTH levels suggest hyperparathyroidism, whereas PTH is suppressed in hypercalcemia caused by malignancy or granulomatous diseases. A suppressed ACTH in the setting of hypercortisolemia, or increased urine free cortisol, is seen with hyperfunctioning adrenal adenomas.

It is not uncommon, however, for baseline hormone levels associated with pathologic endocrine conditions to overlap with the normal range. In this circumstance, dynamic testing is useful to separate the two groups further. There are a multitude of dynamic endocrine tests, but all are based on principles of feedback regulation, and most responses can be rationalized based on principles that govern the regulation of endocrine axes. *Suppression tests* are used in the setting of suspected endocrine hyperfunction. An example is the dexamethasone suppression test used to evaluate Cushing's syndrome **(Chaps. 5 and 8)**. *Stimulation tests* generally are used to assess endocrine hypofunction. The ACTH stimulation test, for example, is used to assess the adrenal gland

TABLE 1-2

EXAMPLES OF PREVALENT ENDOCRINE AND METABOLIC DISORDERS IN THE ADULT

DISORDER	APPROX. PREVALENCE IN ADULTS[a]	SCREENING/TESTING RECOMMENDATIONS[b]	CHAPTER(S)
Obesity	34% BMI ≥30 68% BMI ≥25	Calculate BMI Measure waist circumference Exclude secondary causes Consider comorbid complications	**Chap. 21**
Type 2 diabetes mellitus	>7%	Beginning at age 45, screen every 3 years, or earlier in high-risk groups: Fasting plasma glucose (FPG) >126 mg/dL Random plasma glucose >200 mg/dL An elevated HbA1c Consider comorbid complications	**Chap. 23**
Hyperlipidemia	20–25%	Cholesterol screening at least every 5 years; more often in high-risk groups Lipoprotein analysis (LDL, HDL) for increased cholesterol, CAD, diabetes Consider secondary causes	**Chap. 27**
Metabolic syndrome	35%	Measure waist circumference, FPG, BP, lipids	**Chap. 22**
Hypothyroidism	5–10%, women 0.5–2%, men	TSH; confirm with free T_4 Screen women after age 35 and every 5 years thereafter	**Chap. 7**
Graves' disease	1–3%, women 0.1%, men	TSH, free T_4	**Chap. 7**
Thyroid nodules and neoplasia	2–5% palpable >25% by ultrasound	Physical examination of thyroid Fine-needle aspiration biopsy	**Chap. 7**
Osteoporosis	5–10%, women 2–5%, men	Bone mineral density measurements in women >65 years or in post-menopausal women or men at risk Exclude secondary causes	**Chap. 35**
Hyperparathyroidism	0.1–0.5%, women > men	Serum calcium PTH, if calcium is elevated Assess comorbid conditions	**Chap. 34**
Infertility	10%, couples	Investigate both members of couple Semen analysis in male Assess ovulatory cycles in female Specific tests as indicated	**Chaps. 11, 13**
Polycystic ovarian syndrome	5–10%, women	Free testosterone, DHEAS Consider comorbid conditions	**Chap. 13**
Hirsutism	5–10%	Free testosterone, DHEAS Exclude secondary causes Additional tests as indicated	**Chap. 17**
Menopause	Median age, 51	FSH	**Chap. 16**
Hyperprolactinemia	15% in women with amenorrhea or galactorrhea	PRL level MRI, if not medication-related	**Chap. 5**
Erectile dysfunction	10–25%	Careful history, PRL, testosterone Consider secondary causes (e.g., diabetes)	**Chap. 19**
Hypogonadism, male	1–2%	Testosterone, LH	**Chap. 11**
Gynecomastia	15%	Often, no tests are indicated Consider Klinefelter's syndrome Consider medications, hypogonadism, liver disease	**Chap. 11**
Klinefelter's syndrome	0.2%, men	Karyotype Testosterone	**Chap. 10**
Vitamin D deficiency	10%	Measure serum 25-OH vitamin D Consider secondary causes	**Chap. 32**
Turner's syndrome	0.03%, women	Karyotype Consider comorbid conditions	**Chap. 10**

[a]The prevalence of most disorders varies among ethnic groups and with aging. Data based primarily on U.S. population.

[b]See individual chapters for additional information on evaluation and treatment. Early testing is indicated in patients with signs and symptoms of disease and in those at increased risk.

Abbreviations: BMI, body mass index; BP, blood pressure; CAD, coronary artery disease; DHEAS, dehydroepiandrosterone; FSH, follicle-stimulating hormone; HDL, high-density lipoprotein; LDL, low-density lipoprotein; LH, luteinizing hormone; MRI, magnetic resonance imaging; PRL, prolactin; PTH, parathyroid hormone; TSH, thyroid-stimulating hormone.

response in patients with suspected adrenal insufficiency. Other stimulation tests use hypothalamic-releasing factors such as corticotropin-releasing hormone (CRH) and growth hormone–releasing hormone (GHRH) to evaluate pituitary hormone reserve **(Chap. 5)**. Insulin-induced hypoglycemia also evokes pituitary ACTH and GH responses. Stimulation tests based on reduction or inhibition of endogenous hormones are now used infrequently. Examples include metyrapone inhibition of cortisol synthesis and clomiphene inhibition of estrogen feedback.

SCREENING AND ASSESSMENT OF COMMON ENDOCRINE DISORDERS

Many endocrine disorders are prevalent in the adult population (Table 1-2) and can be diagnosed and managed by general internists, family practitioners, or other primary health care providers. The high prevalence and clinical impact of certain endocrine diseases justifies vigilance for features of these disorders during routine physical examinations; laboratory screening is indicated in selected high-risk populations.

CHAPTER 2

MECHANISMS OF HORMONE ACTION

J. Larry Jameson

CLASSES OF HORMONES

Hormones can be divided into five major types: (1) *amino acid derivatives* such as dopamine, catecholamine, and thyroid hormone; (2) *small neuropeptides* such as gonadotropin-releasing hormone (GnRH), thyrotropin-releasing hormone (TRH), somatostatin, and vasopressin; (3) *large proteins* such as insulin, luteinizing hormone (LH), and parathyroid hormone (PTH); (4) *steroid hormones* such as cortisol and estrogen that are synthesized from cholesterol-based precursors; and (5) *vitamin derivatives* such as retinoids (vitamin A) and vitamin D. A variety of *peptide growth factors*, most of which act locally, share actions with hormones. As a rule, amino acid derivatives and peptide hormones interact with cell-surface membrane receptors. Steroids, thyroid hormones, vitamin D, and retinoids are lipid-soluble and interact with intracellular nuclear receptors, although many also interact with membrane receptors or intracellular signaling proteins as well.

HORMONE AND RECEPTOR FAMILIES

Hormones and receptors can be grouped into families, reflecting structural similarities and evolutionary origins (Table 2-1). The evolution of these families generates diverse but highly selective pathways of hormone action. Recognition of these relationships has proven useful for extrapolating information gleaned from one hormone or receptor to other family members.

The glycoprotein hormone family, consisting of thyroid-stimulating hormone (TSH), follicle-stimulating hormone (FSH), LH, and human chorionic gonadotropin (hCG), illustrates many features of related hormones. The glycoprotein hormones are heterodimers that share the α subunit in common; the β subunits are distinct and confer specific biologic actions. The overall three-dimensional architecture of the β subunits is similar, reflecting the locations of conserved disulfide bonds that restrain protein conformation. The cloning of the β-subunit genes from multiple species suggests that this family arose from a common ancestral gene, probably by gene duplication and subsequent divergence to evolve new biologic functions.

As hormone families enlarge and diverge, their receptors must co-evolve to derive new biologic functions. Related G protein–coupled receptors (GPCRs), for example, have evolved for each of the glycoprotein hormones. These receptors are structurally similar, and each is coupled predominantly to the $G_s\alpha$ signaling pathway. However, there is minimal overlap of hormone binding. For example, TSH binds with high specificity to the TSH receptor but interacts minimally with the LH or FSH receptors. Nonetheless, there can be subtle physiologic consequences of hormone cross-reactivity with other receptors. Very high levels of hCG during pregnancy stimulate the TSH receptor and increase thyroid hormone levels, resulting in a compensatory decrease in TSH.

Insulin and insulin-like growth factor I (IGF-I) and IGF-II have structural similarities that are most apparent when precursor forms of the proteins are compared. In contrast to the high degree of specificity seen with the glycoprotein hormones, there is moderate cross-talk among the members of the insulin/IGF family. High concentrations of an IGF-II precursor produced by certain tumors (e.g., sarcomas) can cause hypoglycemia, partly because of binding to insulin and IGF-I receptors **(Chap. 34)**. High concentrations of insulin also bind to the IGF-I receptor, perhaps accounting for some of the clinical manifestations seen in conditions with chronic hyperinsulinemia.

Another important example of receptor cross-talk is seen with PTH and parathyroid hormone–related peptide (PTHrP) **(Chap. 34)**. PTH is produced by the parathyroid glands, whereas PTHrP is expressed at high levels during development and by a variety of tumors **(Chap. 31)**. These hormones have amino acid sequence

TABLE 2-1

EXAMPLES OF MEMBRANE RECEPTOR FAMILIES AND SIGNALING PATHWAYS

RECEPTORS	EFFECTORS	SIGNALING PATHWAYS
G Protein–Coupled Seven-Transmembrane Receptor (GPCR)		
β-Adrenergic, LH, FSH, TSH	$G_S\alpha$, adenylate cyclase	Stimulation of cyclic AMP production, protein kinase A
Glucagon, PTH, PTHrP, ACTH, MSH, GHRH, CRH	Ca^{2+} channels	Calmodulin, Ca^{2+}-dependent kinases
α-Adrenergic, somatostatin	$G_i\alpha$	Inhibition of cyclic AMP production Activation of K^+, Ca^{2+} channels
TRH, GnRH	G_q, G_{11}	Phospholipase C, diacyl-glycerol, IP_3, protein kinase C, voltage-dependent Ca^{2+} channels
Receptor Tyrosine Kinase		
Insulin, IGF-I	Tyrosine kinases, IRS	MAP kinases, PI 3-kinase; AKT
EGF, NGF	Tyrosine kinases, ras	Raf, MAP kinases, RSK
Cytokine Receptor–Linked Kinase		
GH, PRL	JAK, tyrosine kinases	STAT, MAP kinase, PI 3-kinase, IRS-1
Serine Kinase		
Activin, TGF-β, MIS	Serine kinase	Smads

Abbreviations: IP_3, inositol triphosphate; IRS, insulin receptor substrates; MAP, mitogen-activated protein; MSH, melanocyte-stimulating hormone; NGF, nerve growth factor; PI, phosphatidylinositol; RSK, ribosomal S6 kinase; TGF-β, transforming growth factor β. For all other abbreviations, see text. Note that most receptors interact with multiple effectors and activate networks of signaling pathways.

similarity, particularly in their amino-terminal regions. Both hormones bind to a single PTH receptor that is expressed in bone and kidney. Hypercalcemia and hypophosphatemia therefore may result from excessive production of either hormone, making it difficult to distinguish hyperparathyroidism from hypercalcemia of malignancy solely on the basis of serum chemistries. However, sensitive and specific assays for PTH and PTHrP now allow these disorders to be distinguished more readily.

Based on their specificities for DNA binding sites, the nuclear receptor family can be subdivided into type 1 receptors (glucocorticoid receptor, mineralocorticoid receptor, androgen receptor, estrogen receptor, progesterone receptor) that bind steroids and type 2 receptors (thyroid hormone receptor, vitamin D receptor, retinoic acid receptor, peroxisome proliferator activated receptor) that bind thyroid hormone, vitamin D, retinoic acid, or lipid derivatives. Certain functional domains in nuclear receptors, such as the zinc finger DNA-binding domains, are highly conserved. However, selective amino acid differences within this domain confer DNA sequence specificity. The hormone-binding domains are more variable, providing great diversity in the array of small molecules that bind to different nuclear receptors. With few exceptions, hormone binding is highly specific for a single type of nuclear receptor. One exception involves the glucocorticoid and mineralocorticoid receptors. Because the mineralocorticoid receptor also binds glucocorticoids with high affinity, an enzyme (11β-hydroxysteroid dehydrogenase) in renal tubular cells inactivates glucocorticoids, allowing selective responses to mineralocorticoids such as aldosterone. However, when very high glucocorticoid concentrations occur, as in Cushing's syndrome, the glucocorticoid degradation pathway becomes saturated, allowing excessive cortisol levels to exert mineralocorticoid effects (sodium retention, potassium wasting). This phenomenon is particularly pronounced in ectopic adrenocorticotropic hormone (ACTH) syndromes **(Chap. 8)**. Another example of relaxed nuclear receptor specificity involves the estrogen receptor, which can bind an array of compounds, some of which have little apparent structural similarity to the high-affinity ligand estradiol. This feature of the estrogen receptor makes it susceptible to activation by "environmental estrogens" such as resveratrol, octylphenol, and many other aromatic hydrocarbons. However, this lack of specificity provides an opportunity to synthesize a remarkable series of clinically useful antagonists (e.g., tamoxifen) and selective estrogen response modulators (SERMs) such as raloxifene. These compounds generate distinct conformations that alter receptor interactions with components of the transcription machinery (see below), thereby conferring their unique actions.

HORMONE SYNTHESIS AND PROCESSING

The synthesis of peptide hormones and their receptors occurs through a classic pathway of gene expression: transcription → mRNA → protein → posttranslational protein processing → intracellular sorting, followed by membrane integration or secretion.

Many hormones are embedded within larger precursor polypeptides that are proteolytically processed to yield the biologically active hormone. Examples include proopiomelanocortin (POMC) → ACTH; proglucagon → glucagon; proinsulin → insulin; and pro-PTH → PTH, among others. In many cases, such as POMC and proglucagon, these precursors generate multiple biologically active peptides. It is provocative that hormone precursors are typically inactive, presumably adding an additional level of regulatory control. Prohormone conversion occurs not only for peptide hormones but also for certain steroids (testosterone → dihydrotestosterone) and thyroid hormone ($T_4 \rightarrow T_3$).

Peptide precursor processing is intimately linked to intracellular sorting pathways that transport proteins to appropriate vesicles and enzymes, resulting in specific cleavage steps, followed by protein folding and translocation to secretory vesicles. Hormones destined for secretion are translocated across the endoplasmic reticulum under the guidance of an amino-terminal signal sequence that subsequently is cleaved. Cell-surface receptors are inserted into the membrane via short segments of hydrophobic amino acids that remain embedded within the lipid bilayer. During translocation through the Golgi and endoplasmic reticulum, hormones and receptors are subject to a variety of post-translational modifications, such as glycosylation and phosphorylation, which can alter protein conformation, modify circulating half-life, and alter biologic activity.

Synthesis of most steroid hormones is based on modifications of the precursor, cholesterol. Multiple regulated enzymatic steps are required for the synthesis of testosterone **(Chap. 11)**, estradiol **(Chap. 13)**, cortisol **(Chap. 8)**, and vitamin D **(Chap. 32)**. This large number of synthetic steps predisposes to multiple genetic and acquired disorders of steroidogenesis.

Endocrine genes contain regulatory DNA elements similar to those found in many other genes, but their exquisite control by hormones reflects the presence of specific hormone response elements. For example, the TSH genes are repressed directly by thyroid hormones acting through the thyroid hormone receptor (TR), a member of the nuclear receptor family. Steroidogenic enzyme gene expression requires specific transcription factors, such as steroidogenic factor-1 (SF-1), acting in conjunction with signals transmitted by trophic hormones (e.g., ACTH or LH). For some hormones, substantial regulation occurs at the level of translational efficiency. Insulin biosynthesis, although it requires ongoing gene transcription, is regulated primarily at the translational and secretory levels in response to elevated levels of glucose or amino acids.

HORMONE SECRETION, TRANSPORT, AND DEGRADATION

The level of a hormone is determined by its rate of secretion and its circulating half-life. After protein processing, peptide hormones (e.g., GnRH, insulin, growth hormone [GH]) are stored in secretory granules. As these granules mature, they are poised beneath the plasma membrane for imminent release into the circulation. In most instances, the stimulus for hormone secretion is a releasing factor or neural signal that induces rapid changes in intracellular calcium concentrations, leading to secretory granule fusion with the plasma membrane and release of its contents into the extracellular environment and bloodstream. Steroid hormones, in contrast, diffuse into the circulation as they are synthesized. Thus, their secretory rates are closely aligned with rates of synthesis. For example, ACTH and LH induce steroidogenesis by stimulating the activity of the *st*eroidogenic *a*cute *r*egulatory (StAR) protein (transports cholesterol into the mitochondrion) along with other rate-limiting steps (e.g., cholesterol side-chain cleavage enzyme, CYP11A1) in the steroidogenic pathway.

Hormone transport and degradation dictate the rapidity with which a hormonal signal decays. Some hormone signals are evanescent (e.g., somatostatin), whereas others are longer-lived (e.g., TSH). Because somatostatin exerts effects in virtually every tissue, a short half-life allows its concentrations and actions to be controlled locally. Structural modifications that impair somatostatin degradation have been useful for generating long-acting therapeutic analogues such as octreotide **(Chap. 5)**. In contrast, the actions of TSH are highly specific for the thyroid gland. Its prolonged half-life accounts for relatively constant serum levels even though TSH is secreted in discrete pulses.

An understanding of circulating hormone half-life is important for achieving physiologic hormone replacement, as the frequency of dosing and the time required to reach steady state are intimately linked to rates of hormone decay. T_4, for example, has a circulating half-life of 7 days. Consequently, >1 month is required to reach a new steady state, and single daily doses are sufficient to achieve constant hormone levels. T_3, in contrast, has a half-life of 1 day. Its administration is associated with more dynamic serum levels, and it must be administered two to three times per day. Similarly, synthetic glucocorticoids vary widely in their half-lives; those with longer half-lives (e.g., dexamethasone) are associated with greater suppression of the hypothalamic-pituitary-adrenal (HPA) axis. Most protein hormones (e.g., ACTH, GH, prolactin [PRL], PTH, LH) have relatively short half-lives (<20 min), leading to sharp peaks of secretion and decay. The only accurate way to profile the pulse frequency and amplitude of these hormones is to measure levels in frequently sampled blood (every 10 min or less) over long durations (8–24 h). Because this is not practical in a clinical setting, an alternative strategy is to pool three to four samples drawn at about 30-min intervals, or interpret the results in the context of a relatively wide normal range. Rapid hormone decay is useful in certain clinical settings. For example, the short half-life of PTH allows the use of intraoperative PTH determinations to confirm successful removal of an adenoma. This is particularly valuable diagnostically when there is a possibility of multicentric disease or parathyroid hyperplasia, as occurs with multiple endocrine neoplasia (MEN) or renal insufficiency.

Many hormones circulate in association with serum-binding proteins. Examples include (1) T_4 and T_3 binding to thyroxine-binding globulin (TBG), albumin, and thyroxine-binding prealbumin (TBPA); (2) cortisol binding to cortisol-binding globulin (CBG); (3) androgen and estrogen binding to sex hormone–binding globulin (SHBG); (4) IGF-I and -II binding to multiple IGF-binding proteins (IGFBPs); (5) GH interactions with GH-binding protein (GHBP), a circulating fragment of the GH receptor extracellular domain; and (6) activin binding to follistatin. These interactions provide a hormonal reservoir, prevent otherwise rapid degradation of unbound hormones, restrict hormone access to certain sites (e.g., IGFBPs), and modulate the unbound, or "free," hormone concentrations. Although a variety of binding protein abnormalities have been identified, most have little clinical consequence aside from creating diagnostic problems. For example, TBG deficiency can reduce total thyroid hormone levels greatly but the free concentrations of T_4 and T_3 remain normal. Liver disease and certain medications can also influence binding protein levels (e.g., estrogen increases TBG) or cause displacement of hormones from binding proteins (e.g., salsalate displaces T_4 from TBG). In general, only unbound hormone is available to interact with receptors and thus elicit a biologic response. Short-term perturbations in binding proteins change the free hormone concentration, which in turn induces compensatory adaptations through feedback loops. SHBG changes in women are an exception to this self-correcting mechanism. When SHBG decreases because of insulin resistance or androgen excess, the unbound testosterone concentration is increased, potentially leading to hirsutism **(Chap. 17)**. The increased unbound testosterone level does not result in an adequate compensatory feedback correction because estrogen, not testosterone, is the primary regulator of the reproductive axis.

An additional exception to the unbound hormone hypothesis involves megalin, a member of the low-density lipoprotein (LDL) receptor family that serves as an endocytotic receptor for carrier-bound vitamins A and D and SHBG-bound androgens and estrogens. After internalization, the carrier proteins are degraded in lysosomes and release their bound ligands within the cells. Membrane transporters have also been identified for thyroid hormones.

Hormone degradation can be an important mechanism for regulating concentrations locally. As noted above, 11β-hydroxysteroid dehydrogenase inactivates glucocorticoids in renal tubular cells, preventing actions through the mineralocorticoid receptor. Thyroid hormone deiodinases convert T_4 to T_3 and can inactivate T_3. During development, degradation of retinoic acid by Cyp26b1 prevents primordial germ cells in the male from entering meiosis, as occurs in the female ovary.

HORMONE ACTION THROUGH RECEPTORS

Receptors for hormones are divided into two major classes: membrane and nuclear. *Membrane receptors* primarily bind peptide hormones and catecholamines. *Nuclear receptors* bind small molecules that can diffuse across the cell membrane, such as steroids and vitamin D. Certain general principles apply to hormone-receptor interactions regardless of the class of receptor. Hormones bind to receptors with specificity and an affinity that generally coincides with the dynamic range of circulating hormone concentrations. Low concentrations of free hormone (usually 10^{-12} to 10^{-9} *M*) rapidly associate and dissociate from receptors in a bimolecular reaction such that the occupancy of the receptor at any given moment is a function of hormone concentration and the receptor's affinity for the hormone. Receptor numbers vary greatly in different target tissues, providing one of the major determinants of specific tissue responses to circulating hormones. For example, ACTH receptors are located almost exclusively in the adrenal cortex, and FSH receptors are found predominantly in the gonads. In contrast, insulin and TRs are widely distributed, reflecting the need for metabolic responses in all tissues.

MEMBRANE RECEPTORS

Membrane receptors for hormones can be divided into several major groups: (1) seven transmembrane GPCRs, (2) tyrosine kinase receptors, (3) cytokine receptors, and (4) serine kinase receptors (Fig. 2-1). The *seven transmembrane GPCR family* binds a remarkable array of hormones, including large proteins (e.g., LH, PTH), small peptides (e.g., TRH, somatostatin), catecholamines (epinephrine, dopamine), and even minerals (e.g., calcium). The extracellular domains of GPCRs vary widely in size and are the major binding site for large hormones. The transmembrane-spanning regions are composed of hydrophobic α-helical domains that traverse the lipid bilayer. Like some channels, these domains are thought to circularize and form a hydrophobic pocket into which certain small ligands fit. Hormone binding induces conformational changes in these domains, transducing structural changes to the intracellular domain, which is a docking site for G proteins.

The large family of *G proteins*, so named because they bind guanine nucleotides (guanosine triphosphate [GTP], guanosine diphosphate [GDP]), provides great

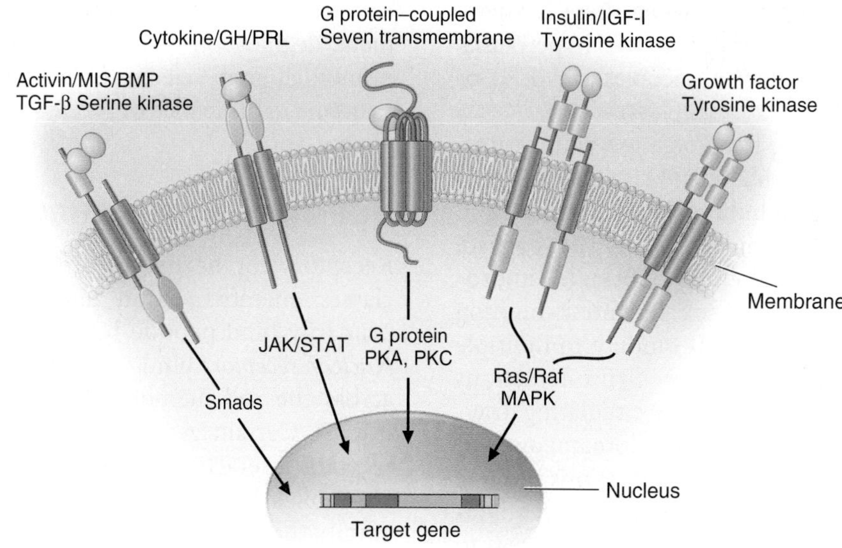

FIGURE 2-1

Membrane receptor signaling. MAPK, mitogen-activated protein kinase; PKA, C, protein kinase A, C; TGF, transforming growth factor. For other abbreviations, see text.

diversity for coupling receptors to different signaling pathways. G proteins form a heterotrimeric complex that is composed of various α and βγ subunits. The α subunit contains the guanine nucleotide–binding site and hydrolyzes GTP → GDP. The βγ subunits are tightly associated and modulate the activity of the α subunit as well as mediating their own effector signaling pathways. G protein activity is regulated by a cycle that involves GTP hydrolysis and dynamic interactions between the α and αβ subunits. Hormone binding to the receptor induces GDP dissociation, allowing Gα to bind GTP and dissociate from the αβ complex. Under these conditions, the Gα subunit is activated and mediates signal transduction through various enzymes, such as adenylate cyclase and phospholipase C. GTP hydrolysis to GDP allows reassociation with the βγ subunits and restores the inactive state. As described below, a variety of endocrinopathies result from G protein mutations or from mutations in receptors that modify their interactions with G proteins. G proteins interact with other cellular proteins, including kinases, channels, G protein–coupled receptor kinases (GRKs), and arrestins, that mediate signaling as well as receptor desensitization and recycling.

The *tyrosine kinase receptors* transduce signals for insulin and a variety of growth factors, such as IGF-I, epidermal growth factor (EGF), nerve growth factor, platelet-derived growth factor, and fibroblast growth factor. The cysteine-rich extracellular ligand-binding domains contain growth factor binding sites. After ligand binding, this class of receptors undergoes autophosphorylation, inducing interactions with intracellular adaptor proteins such as Shc and insulin receptor substrates (IRS). In the case of the insulin receptor, multiple kinases are activated, including the Raf-Ras-MAPK and the Akt/protein kinase B pathways. The tyrosine kinase receptors play a prominent role in cell growth and differentiation as well as in intermediary metabolism.

The GH and PRL receptors belong to the *cytokine receptor* family. Analogous to the tyrosine kinase receptors, ligand binding induces receptor interaction with intracellular kinases—the Janus kinases (JAKs), which phosphorylate members of the signal transduction and activators of transcription (STAT) family—as well as with other signaling pathways (Ras, PI3-K, MAPK). The activated STAT proteins translocate to the nucleus and stimulate expression of target genes.

The *serine kinase receptors* mediate the actions of activins, transforming growth factor β, müllerian-inhibiting substance (MIS, also known as anti-müllerian hormone, AMH), and bone morphogenic proteins (BMPs). This family of receptors (consisting of type I and II subunits) signals through proteins termed *smads* (fusion of terms for *Caenorhabditis elegans* sma + mammalian mad). Like the STAT proteins, the smads serve a dual role of transducing the receptor signal and acting as transcription factors. The pleomorphic actions of these growth factors dictate that they act primarily in a local (paracrine or autocrine) manner. Binding proteins such as follistatin (which binds activin and other members of this family) function to inactivate the growth factors and restrict their distribution.

NUCLEAR RECEPTORS

The family of nuclear receptors has grown to nearly 100 members, many of which are still classified as

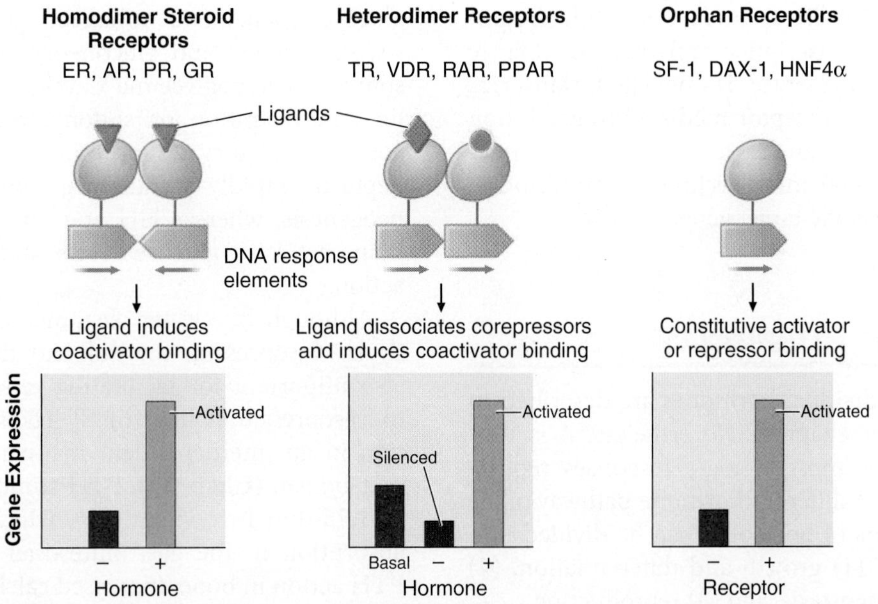

FIGURE 2-2

Nuclear receptor signaling. AR, androgen receptor; DAX, *d*osage-sensitive sex-reversal, *a*drenal hypoplasia congenita, *X*-chromosome; ER, estrogen receptor; GR, glucocorticoid receptor; HNF4α, hepatic nuclear factor 4α; PPAR, peroxisome proliferator activated receptor; PR, progesterone receptor; RAR, retinoic acid receptor; SF-1, steroidogenic factor-1; TR, thyroid hormone receptor; VDR, vitamin D receptor.

orphan receptors because their ligands, if they exist, have not been identified (Fig. 2-2). Otherwise, most nuclear receptors are classified on the basis of their ligands. Although all nuclear receptors ultimately act to increase or decrease gene transcription, some (e.g., glucocorticoid receptor) reside primarily in the cytoplasm, whereas others (e.g., TR) are located in the nucleus. After ligand binding, the cytoplasmically localized receptors translocate to the nucleus. There is growing evidence that certain nuclear receptors (e.g., glucocorticoid, estrogen) can also act at the membrane or in the cytoplasm to activate or repress signal transduction pathways, providing a mechanism for cross-talk between membrane and nuclear receptors.

The structures of nuclear receptors have been studied extensively, including by x-ray crystallography. The DNA binding domain, consisting of two zinc fingers, contacts specific DNA recognition sequences in target genes. Most nuclear receptors bind to DNA as dimers. Consequently, each monomer recognizes an individual DNA motif, referred to as a "half-site." The steroid receptors, including the glucocorticoid, estrogen, progesterone, and androgen receptors, bind to DNA as homodimers. Consistent with this twofold symmetry, their DNA recognition half-sites are palindromic. The thyroid, retinoid, peroxisome proliferator activated, and vitamin D receptors bind to DNA preferentially as heterodimers in combination with retinoid X receptors (RXRs). Their DNA half-sites are typically arranged as direct repeats.

The carboxy-terminal hormone-binding domain mediates transcriptional control. For type II receptors such as TR and retinoic acid receptor (RAR), co-repressor proteins bind to the receptor in the absence of ligand and silence gene transcription. Hormone binding induces conformational changes, triggering the release of co-repressors and inducing the recruitment of coactivators that stimulate transcription. Thus, these receptors are capable of mediating dramatic changes in the level of gene activity. Certain disease states are associated with defective regulation of these events. For example, mutations in the TR prevent co-repressor dissociation, resulting in an autosomal dominant form of hormone resistance **(Chap. 7)**. In promyelocytic leukemia, fusion of RARα to other nuclear proteins causes aberrant gene silencing that prevents normal cellular differentiation. Treatment with retinoic acid reverses this repression and allows cellular differentiation and apoptosis to occur. Most type 1 steroid receptors interact weakly with co-repressors, but ligand binding still induces interactions with an array of coactivators. X-ray crystallography shows that various SERMs induce distinct estrogen receptor conformations. The tissue-specific responses caused by these agents in breast, bone, and uterus appear to reflect distinct interactions with coactivators. The receptor-coactivator complex stimulates gene transcription by several pathways, including (1) recruitment of enzymes (histone acetyl transferases) that modify chromatin structure, (2) interactions with additional transcription factors on the target gene, and (3) direct interactions with components of the general transcription apparatus to enhance the rate of RNA polymerase II–mediated transcription. Studies of nuclear receptor-mediated transcription show that these are dynamic events that involve relatively rapid (e.g., 30–60 min) cycling of transcription complexes on any specific target gene.

FUNCTIONS OF HORMONES

The functions of individual hormones are described in detail in subsequent chapters. Nevertheless, it is useful to illustrate how most biologic responses require integration of several different hormone pathways. The physiologic functions of hormones can be divided into three general areas: (1) growth and differentiation, (2) maintenance of homeostasis, and (3) reproduction.

GROWTH

Multiple hormones and nutritional factors mediate the complex phenomenon of growth **(Chap. 3)**. Short stature may be caused by GH deficiency, hypothyroidism, Cushing's syndrome, precocious puberty, malnutrition, chronic illness, or genetic abnormalities that affect the epiphyseal growth plates (e.g., *FGFR3* and *SHOX* mutations). Many factors (GH, IGF-I, thyroid hormones) stimulate growth, whereas others (sex steroids) lead to epiphyseal closure. Understanding these hormonal interactions is important in the diagnosis and management of growth disorders. For example, delaying exposure to high levels of sex steroids may enhance the efficacy of GH treatment.

MAINTENANCE OF HOMEOSTASIS

Although virtually all hormones affect homeostasis, the most important among them are the following:

1. Thyroid hormone—controls about 25% of basal metabolism in most tissues
2. Cortisol—exerts a permissive action for many hormones in addition to its own direct effects
3. PTH—regulates calcium and phosphorus levels
4. Vasopressin—regulates serum osmolality by controlling renal free-water clearance
5. Mineralocorticoids—control vascular volume and serum electrolyte (Na^+, K^+) concentrations
6. Insulin—maintains euglycemia in the fed and fasted states

The defense against hypoglycemia is an impressive example of integrated hormone action **(Chap. 26)**. In response to the fasting state and falling blood glucose, insulin secretion is suppressed, resulting in decreased glucose uptake and enhanced glycogenolysis, lipolysis, proteolysis, and gluconeogenesis to mobilize fuel sources. If hypoglycemia develops (usually from insulin administration or sulfonylureas), an orchestrated counterregulatory response occurs—glucagon and epinephrine rapidly stimulate glycogenolysis and gluconeogenesis, whereas GH and cortisol act over several hours to raise glucose levels and antagonize insulin action.

Although free-water clearance is controlled primarily by vasopressin, cortisol and thyroid hormone are also important for facilitating renal tubular responses to vasopressin **(Chap. 6)**. PTH and vitamin D function in an interdependent manner to control calcium metabolism **(Chap. 32)**. PTH stimulates renal synthesis of 1,25-dihydroxyvitamin D, which increases calcium absorption in the gastrointestinal tract and enhances PTH action in bone. Increased calcium, along with vitamin D, feeds back to suppress PTH, thus maintaining calcium balance.

Depending on the severity of a specific stress and whether it is acute or chronic, multiple endocrine and cytokine pathways are activated to mount an appropriate physiologic response. In severe acute stress such as trauma or shock, the sympathetic nervous system is activated and catecholamines are released, leading to increased cardiac output and a primed musculoskeletal system. Catecholamines also increase mean blood pressure and stimulate glucose production. Multiple stress-induced pathways converge on the hypothalamus, stimulating several hormones, including vasopressin and corticotropin-releasing hormone (CRH). These hormones, in addition to cytokines (tumor necrosis factor α, interleukin [IL] 2, IL-6) increase ACTH and GH production. ACTH stimulates the adrenal gland, increasing cortisol, which in turn helps sustain blood pressure and dampen the inflammatory response. Increased vasopressin acts to conserve free water.

REPRODUCTION

The stages of reproduction include (1) sex determination during fetal development **(Chap. 10)**; (2) sexual maturation during puberty **(Chaps. 11 and 13)**; (3) conception, pregnancy, lactation, and child rearing **(Chap. 13)**; and (4) cessation of reproductive capability at menopause **(Chap. 16)**. Each of these stages involves an orchestrated interplay of multiple hormones, a phenomenon well illustrated by the dynamic hormonal changes that occur during each 28-day menstrual cycle. In the early follicular phase, pulsatile secretion of LH and FSH stimulates the progressive maturation of the ovarian follicle. This results in gradually increasing estrogen and progesterone levels, leading to enhanced pituitary sensitivity to GnRH, which, when combined with accelerated GnRH secretion, triggers the LH surge and rupture of the mature follicle. Inhibin, a protein produced by the granulosa cells, enhances follicular growth and feeds back to the pituitary to selectively suppress FSH without affecting LH. Growth factors such as EGF and IGF-I modulate follicular responsiveness to gonadotropins. Vascular endothelial growth factor and prostaglandins play a role in follicle vascularization and rupture.

During pregnancy, the increased production of prolactin, in combination with placentally derived steroids (e.g., estrogen and progesterone), prepares the breast for lactation. Estrogens induce the production of progesterone receptors, allowing for increased responsiveness to progesterone. In addition to these and other hormones involved in lactation, the nervous system and oxytocin mediate the suckling response and milk release.

HORMONAL FEEDBACK REGULATORY SYSTEMS

Feedback control, both negative and positive, is a fundamental feature of endocrine systems. Each of the major hypothalamic-pituitary-hormone axes is governed by negative feedback, a process that maintains hormone levels within a relatively narrow range **(Chap. 3)**. Examples of hypothalamic-pituitary negative feedback include (1) thyroid hormones on the TRH-TSH axis, (2) cortisol on the CRH-ACTH axis, (3) gonadal steroids on the GnRH-LH/FSH axis, and (4) IGF-I on the growth hormone–releasing hormone (GHRH)-GH axis (Fig. 2-3). These regulatory loops include both positive (e.g., TRH, TSH) and negative (e.g., T_4, T_3) components, allowing for exquisite control of hormone levels. As an example, a small reduction of thyroid hormone triggers a rapid increase of TRH and TSH secretion, resulting in thyroid gland stimulation and increased thyroid hormone production. When thyroid hormone reaches a normal level, it feeds back to suppress TRH and TSH, and a new steady state is attained. Feedback regulation also occurs for endocrine systems that do not involve the pituitary gland, such as calcium feedback on PTH, glucose inhibition of insulin secretion, and leptin feedback on the hypothalamus. An understanding of feedback regulation provides important insights into endocrine testing paradigms (see below).

Positive feedback control also occurs but is not well understood. The primary example is estrogen-mediated stimulation of the midcycle LH surge. Although chronic low levels of estrogen are inhibitory, gradually rising estrogen levels stimulate LH secretion. This effect, which is illustrative of an endocrine rhythm (see below), involves activation of the hypothalamic GnRH pulse generator. In addition, estrogen-primed gonadotropes are extraordinarily sensitive to GnRH, leading to amplification of LH release.

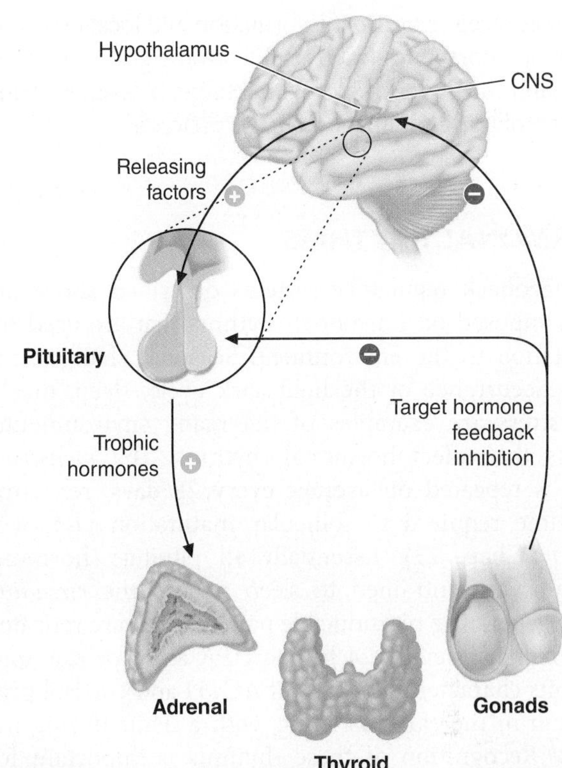

FIGURE 2-3
Feedback regulation of endocrine axes. CNS, central nervous system.

PARACRINE AND AUTOCRINE CONTROL

The previously mentioned examples of feedback control involve classic endocrine pathways in which hormones are released by one gland and act on a distant target gland. However, local regulatory systems, often involving growth factors, are increasingly recognized. *Paracrine regulation* refers to factors released by one cell that act on an adjacent cell in the same tissue. For example, somatostatin secretion by pancreatic islet δ cells inhibits insulin secretion from nearby β cells. *Autocrine regulation* describes the action of a factor on the same cell from which it is produced. IGF-I acts on many cells that produce it, including chondrocytes, breast epithelium, and gonadal cells. Unlike endocrine actions, paracrine and autocrine control are difficult to document because local growth factor concentrations cannot be measured readily.

Anatomic relationships of glandular systems also greatly influence hormonal exposure: the physical organization of islet cells enhances their intercellular communication; the portal vasculature of the hypothalamic-pituitary system exposes the pituitary to high concentrations of hypothalamic releasing factors; testicular seminiferous tubules gain exposure to high testosterone levels produced by the interdigitated Leydig cells; the pancreas receives nutrient information and local exposure to peptide hormones (incretins) from the gastrointestinal tract; and the liver is the proximal target of insulin action because of portal drainage from the pancreas.

HORMONAL RHYTHMS

The feedback regulatory systems described above are superimposed on hormonal rhythms that are used for adaptation to the environment. Seasonal changes, the daily occurrence of the light-dark cycle, sleep, meals, and stress are examples of the many environmental events that affect hormonal rhythms. The *menstrual cycle* is repeated on average every 28 days, reflecting the time required to follicular maturation and ovulation **(Chap. 13)**. Essentially all pituitary hormone rhythms are entrained to sleep and to the *circadian cycle*, generating reproducible patterns that are repeated approximately every 24 h. The HPA axis, for example, exhibits characteristic peaks of ACTH and cortisol production in the early morning, with a nadir during the night. Recognition of these rhythms is important for endocrine testing and treatment. Patients with Cushing's syndrome characteristically exhibit increased midnight cortisol levels compared with normal individuals **(Chap. 8)**. In contrast, morning cortisol levels are similar in these groups, as cortisol is normally high at this time of day in normal individuals. The HPA axis is more susceptible to suppression by glucocorticoids administered at night as they blunt the early-morning rise of ACTH. Understanding these rhythms allows glucocorticoid replacement that mimics diurnal production by administering larger doses in the morning than in the afternoon. Disrupted sleep rhythms can alter hormonal regulation. For example, sleep deprivation causes mild insulin resistance, food craving, and hypertension, which are reversible, at least in the short term. Emerging evidence indicates that circadian clock pathways not only regulate sleep-wake cycles but also play important roles in virtually every cell type. For example, tissue-specific deletion of clock genes alters rhythms and levels of gene expression, as well as metabolic responses in liver, adipose, and other tissues.

Other endocrine rhythms occur on a more rapid time scale. Many peptide hormones are secreted in discrete bursts every few hours. LH and FSH secretion are exquisitely sensitive to GnRH pulse frequency. Intermittent pulses of GnRH are required to maintain pituitary sensitivity, whereas continuous exposure to GnRH causes pituitary gonadotrope desensitization. This feature of the hypothalamic-pituitary-gonadotrope axis forms the basis for using long-acting GnRH agonists to treat central precocious puberty or to decrease testosterone levels in the management of prostate cancer. It is important to be aware of the pulsatile nature of hormone secretion and the rhythmic patterns of hormone production in relating serum hormone measurements to normal values. For some hormones, integrated markers have been developed to circumvent hormonal fluctuations. Examples include 24-h urine collections for cortisol, IGF-I as a biologic marker of GH action, and HbA1c as an index of long-term (weeks to months) blood glucose control.

Often, one must interpret endocrine data only in the context of other hormones. For example, PTH levels typically are assessed in combination with serum calcium concentrations. A high serum calcium level in association with elevated PTH is suggestive of hyperparathyroidism, whereas a suppressed PTH in this situation is more likely to be caused by hypercalcemia of malignancy or other causes of hypercalcemia. Similarly, TSH should be elevated when T_4 and T_3 concentrations are low, reflecting reduced feedback inhibition. When this is not the case, it is important to consider secondary hypothyroidism, which is caused by a defect at the level of the pituitary.

SECTION II

PITUITARY, THYROID, AND ADRENAL DISORDERS

CHAPTER 3

ANTERIOR PITUITARY: PHYSIOLOGY OF PITUITARY HORMONES

Shlomo Melmed ■ J. Larry Jameson

The anterior pituitary often is referred to as the "master gland" because, together with the hypothalamus, it orchestrates the complex regulatory functions of many other endocrine glands. The anterior pituitary gland produces six major hormones: (1) prolactin (PRL), (2) growth hormone (GH), (3) adrenocorticotropic hormone (ACTH), (4) luteinizing hormone (LH), (5) follicle-stimulating hormone (FSH), and (6) thyroid-stimulating hormone (TSH) (Table 3-1). Pituitary hormones are secreted in a pulsatile manner, reflecting stimulation by an array of specific hypothalamic releasing factors. Each of these pituitary hormones elicits specific responses in peripheral target tissues. The hormonal products of those peripheral glands, in turn, exert feedback control at the level of the hypothalamus and pituitary to modulate pituitary function (Fig. 3-1). Pituitary tumors cause characteristic hormone excess syndromes. Hormone deficiency may be inherited or acquired. Fortunately, there are efficacious treatments for many pituitary hormone excess and deficiency syndromes. Nonetheless, these diagnoses are often elusive; this emphasizes the importance of recognizing subtle clinical manifestations and performing the correct laboratory diagnostic tests. **For discussion of disorders of the posterior pituitary, or neurohypophysis, see Chap. 6.**

ANATOMY AND DEVELOPMENT

ANATOMY

The pituitary gland weighs ~600 mg and is located within the sella turcica ventral to the diaphragma sella; it consists of anatomically and functionally distinct anterior and posterior lobes. The bony sella is contiguous to vascular and neurologic structures, including the cavernous sinuses, cranial nerves, and optic chiasm. Thus, expanding intrasellar pathologic processes may have significant central mass effects in addition to their endocrinologic impact.

Hypothalamic neural cells synthesize specific releasing and inhibiting hormones that are secreted directly into the portal vessels of the pituitary stalk. Blood supply of the pituitary gland comes from the superior and inferior hypophyseal arteries (Fig. 3-2). The hypothalamic-pituitary portal plexus provides the major blood source for the anterior pituitary, allowing reliable transmission of hypothalamic peptide pulses without significant systemic dilution; consequently, pituitary cells are exposed to releasing or inhibiting factors and in turn release their hormones as discrete pulses into the systemic circulation (Fig. 3-3).

The posterior pituitary is supplied by the inferior hypophyseal arteries. In contrast to the anterior pituitary, the posterior lobe is directly innervated by hypothalamic neurons (supraopticohypophyseal and tuberohypophyseal nerve tracts) via the pituitary stalk **(Chap. 6)**. Thus, posterior pituitary production of vasopressin (antidiuretic hormone [ADH]) and oxytocin is particularly sensitive to neuronal damage by lesions that affect the pituitary stalk or hypothalamus.

PITUITARY DEVELOPMENT

The embryonic differentiation and maturation of anterior pituitary cells have been elucidated in considerable detail. Pituitary development from Rathke's pouch involves a complex interplay of lineage-specific transcription factors expressed in pluripotent precursor cells and gradients of locally produced growth factors (Table 3-1). The transcription factor Prop-1 induces pituitary development of Pit-1-specific lineages as well as gonadotropes. The transcription factor Pit-1 determines cell-specific expression of GH, PRL, and TSH in somatotropes, lactotropes, and thyrotropes.

TABLE 3-1

ANTERIOR PITUITARY HORMONE EXPRESSION AND REGULATION

CELL	CORTICOTROPE	SOMATOTROPE	LACTOTROPE	THYROTROPE	GONADOTROPE
Tissue-specific-transcription factor	T-Pit	Prop-1, Pit-1	Prop-1, Pit-1	Prop-1, Pit-1, TEF	SF-1, DAX-1
Fetal appearance	6 weeks	8 weeks	12 weeks	12 weeks	12 weeks
Hormone	POMC	GH	PRL	TSH	FSH, LH
Protein	Polypeptide	Polypeptide	Polypeptide	Glycoprotein α, βsubunits	Glycoprotein α, βsubunits
Amino acids	266 (ACTH 1–39)	191	199	211	210, 204
Stimulators	CRH, AVP, gp-130 cytokines	GHRH, ghrelin	Estrogen, TRH, VIP	TRH	GnRH, activins, estrogen
Inhibitors	Glucocorticoids	Somatostatin, IGF-I	Dopamine	T_3, T_4, dopamine, somatostatin, glucocorticoids	Sex steroids, inhibin
Target gland	Adrenal	Liver, bone, other tissues	Breast, other tissues	Thyroid	Ovary, testis
Trophic effect	Steroid production	IGF-I production, growth induction, insulin antagonism	Milk production	T_4 synthesis and secretion	Sex steroid production, follicle growth, germ cell maturation
Normal range	ACTH, 4–22 pg/L	<0.5 μg/L[a]	M <15 μg/L; F <20 μg/L	0.1–5 mU/L	M, 5–20 IU/L, F (basal), 5–20 IU/L

[a]Hormone secretion integrated over 24 h.

Abbreviations: M, male; F, female. For other abbreviations, see text.

Source: Adapted from I Shimon, S Melmed, in S Melmed, P Conn (eds): *Endocrinology: Basic and Clinical Principles*. Totowa, NJ, Humana, 2005.

Expression of high levels of estrogen receptors in cells that contain Pit-1 favors PRL expression, whereas thyrotrope embryonic factor (TEF) induces TSH expression. Pit-1 binds to GH, PRL, and TSH gene regulatory elements as well as to recognition sites on its own promoter, providing a mechanism for maintaining specific pituitary hormone phenotypic stability. Gonadotrope cell development is further defined by the cell-specific expression of the nuclear receptors steroidogenic factor (SF-1) and *d* osage-sensitive sex reversal, *a* drenal hypoplasia critical region, on chromosome *X*, gene *1* (DAX-1). Development of corticotrope cells, which express the proopiomelanocortin (POMC) gene, requires the T-Pit transcription factor. Abnormalities of pituitary development caused by mutations of Pit-1, Prop-1, SF-1, DAX-1, and T-Pit result in a rare, selective or combined pituitary hormone deficit syndromes.

ANTERIOR PITUITARY HORMONES

Each anterior pituitary hormone is under unique control, and each exhibits highly specific normal and dysregulated secretory characteristics.

PROLACTIN

Synthesis

PRL consists of 198 amino acids and has a molecular mass of 21,500 kDa; it is weakly homologous to GH and human placental lactogen (hPL), reflecting the duplication and divergence of a common GH-PRL-hPL precursor gene. PRL is synthesized in lactotropes, which constitute about 20% of anterior pituitary cells. Lactotropes and somatotropes are derived from a common precursor cell that may give rise to a tumor that secretes both PRL and GH. Marked lactotrope cell hyperplasia develops during pregnancy and the first few months of lactation. These transient functional changes in the lactotrope population are induced by estrogen.

Secretion

Normal adult serum PRL levels are about 10–25 μg/L in women and 10–20 μg/L in men. PRL secretion is pulsatile, with the highest secretory peaks occurring during rapid eye movement sleep. Peak serum PRL levels (up to 30 μg/L) occur between 4:00 and 6:00 A.M. The circulating half-life of PRL is about 50 min.

PRL is unique among the pituitary hormones in that the predominant central control mechanism is

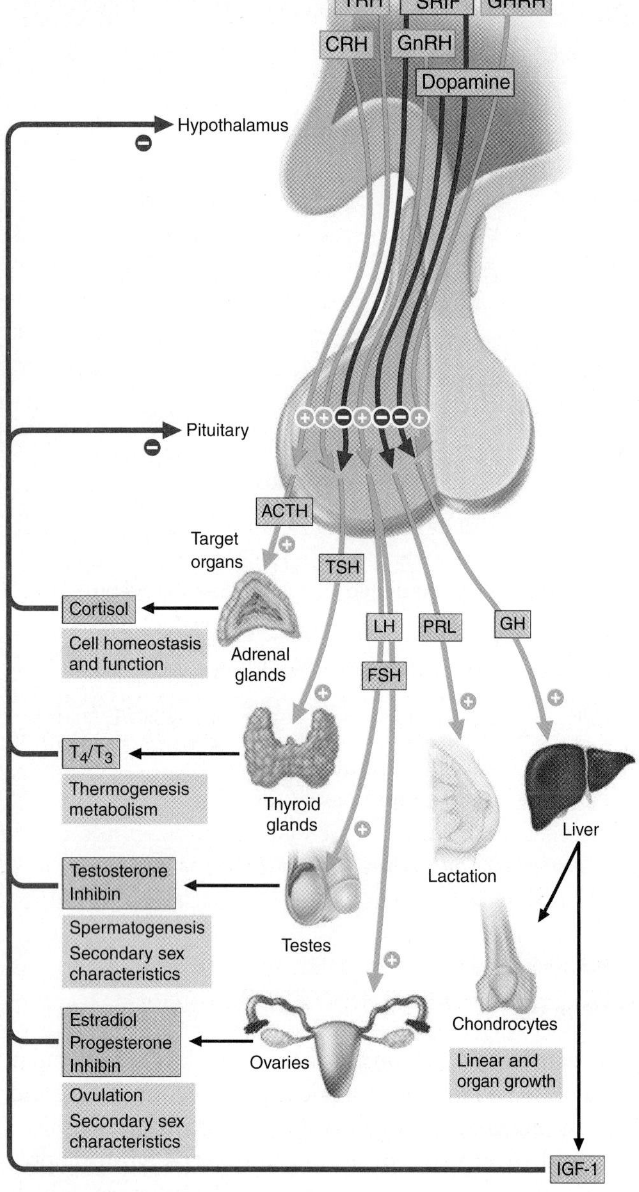

FIGURE 3-1

Diagram of pituitary axes. Hypothalamic hormones regulate anterior pituitary trophic hormones that in turn determine target gland secretion. Peripheral hormones feed back to regulate hypothalamic and pituitary hormones. For abbreviations, see text.

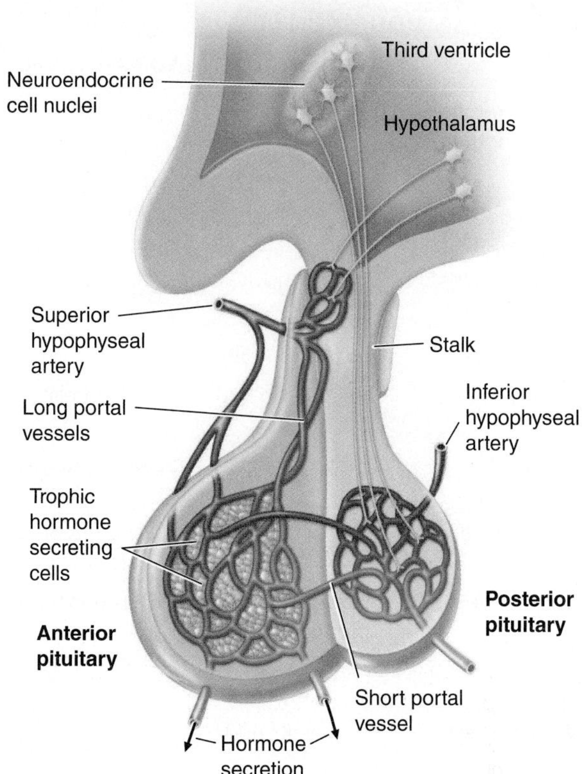

FIGURE 3-2

Diagram of hypothalamic-pituitary vasculature. The hypothalamic nuclei produce hormones that traverse the portal system and impinge on anterior pituitary cells to regulate pituitary hormone secretion. Posterior pituitary hormones are derived from direct neural extensions.

inhibitory, reflecting dopamine-mediated suppression of PRL release. This regulatory pathway accounts for the spontaneous PRL hypersecretion that occurs with pituitary stalk section, often a consequence of compressive mass lesions at the skull base. Pituitary dopamine type 2 (D_2) receptors mediate inhibition of PRL synthesis and secretion. Targeted disruption (gene knockout) of the murine D_2 receptor in mice results in hyperprolactinemia and lactotrope proliferation. As discussed below, dopamine agonists play a central role in the management of hyperprolactinemic disorders.

Thyrotropin-releasing hormone (TRH) (pyro Glu-His-Pro-NH_2) is a hypothalamic tripeptide that elicits PRL release within 15–30 min after intravenous injection. The physiologic relevance of TRH for PRL regulation is unclear, and it appears primarily to regulate TSH **(Chap. 7)**. *Vasoactive intestinal peptide* (VIP) also induces PRL release, whereas glucocorticoids and thyroid hormone weakly suppress PRL secretion.

Serum PRL levels rise transiently after exercise, meals, sexual intercourse, minor surgical procedures,

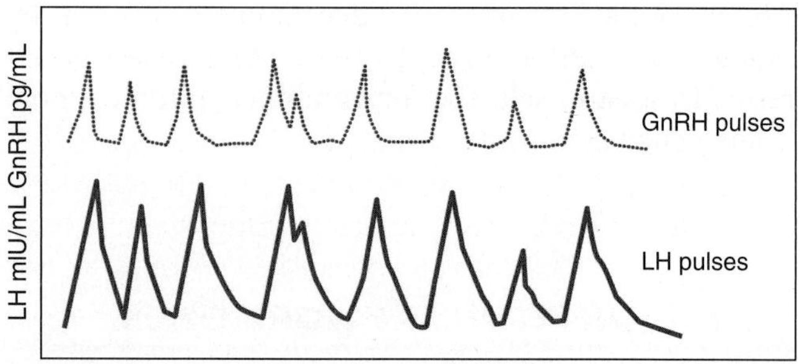

FIGURE 3-3

Hypothalamic gonadotropin-releasing hormone (GnRH) pulses induce secretory pulses of luteinizing hormone (LH).

general anesthesia, chest wall injury, acute myocardial infarction, and other forms of acute stress. PRL levels increase markedly (about tenfold) during pregnancy and decline rapidly within 2 weeks of parturition. If breast-feeding is initiated, basal PRL levels remain elevated; suckling stimulates transient reflex increases in PRL levels that last for about 30–45 min. Breast suckling activates neural afferent pathways in the hypothalamus that induce PRL release. With time, suckling-induced responses diminish and interfeeding PRL levels return to normal.

Action

The PRL receptor is a member of the type I cytokine receptor family that also includes GH and interleukin (IL) 6 receptors. Ligand binding induces receptor dimerization and intracellular signaling by Janus kinase (JAK), which stimulates translocation of the signal transduction and activators of transcription (STAT) family to activate target genes. In the breast, the lobuloalveolar epithelium proliferates in response to PRL, placental lactogens, estrogen, progesterone, and local paracrine growth factors, including insulin-like growth factor I (IGF-I).

PRL acts to induce and maintain lactation, decrease reproductive function, and suppress sexual drive. These functions are geared toward ensuring that maternal lactation is sustained and not interrupted by pregnancy. PRL inhibits reproductive function by suppressing hypothalamic gonadotropin-releasing hormone (GnRH) and pituitary gonadotropin secretion and by impairing gonadal steroidogenesis in both women and men. In the ovary, PRL blocks folliculogenesis and inhibits granulosa cell aromatase activity, leading to hypoestrogenism and anovulation. PRL also has a luteolytic effect, generating a shortened, or inadequate, luteal phase of the menstrual cycle. In men, attenuated LH secretion leads to low testosterone levels and decreased spermatogenesis. These hormonal changes decrease libido and reduce fertility in patients with hyperprolactinemia.

GROWTH HORMONE

Synthesis

GH is the most abundant anterior pituitary hormone, and GH-secreting somatotrope cells constitute up to 50% of the total anterior pituitary cell population. Mammosomatotrope cells, which coexpress PRL with GH, can be identified by using double immunostaining techniques. Somatotrope development and GH transcription are determined by expression of the cell-specific Pit-1 nuclear transcription factor. Five distinct genes encode GH and related proteins. The pituitary GH gene (*hGH-N*) produces two alternatively spliced products that give rise to 22-kDa GH (191 amino acids) and a less abundant 20-kDa GH molecule with similar biologic activity. Placental syncytiotrophoblast cells express a GH variant (*hGH-V*) gene; the related hormone human chorionic somatotropin (HCS) is expressed by distinct members of the gene cluster.

Secretion

GH secretion is controlled by complex hypothalamic and peripheral factors. *GH-releasing hormone* (GHRH) is a 44-amino-acid hypothalamic peptide that stimulates GH synthesis and release. Ghrelin, an octanoylated gastric-derived peptide, and synthetic agonists of the *GHS-R* induce GHRH and also directly stimulate GH release. *Somatostatin* (somatotropin-release inhibiting factor [SRIF]) is synthesized in the medial preoptic area of the hypothalamus and inhibits GH secretion. GHRH is secreted in discrete spikes that elicit GH pulses, whereas SRIF sets basal GH secretory tone. SRIF also is expressed in many extrahypothalamic tissues, including the central nervous system (CNS), gastrointestinal tract, and pancreas, where it also acts to inhibit islet hormone secretion. *IGF-I*, the peripheral target hormone for GH, feeds back to inhibit GH; estrogen induces GH, whereas chronic glucocorticoid excess suppresses GH release.

Surface receptors on the somatotrope regulate GH synthesis and secretion. The GHRH receptor is a G protein–coupled receptor (GPCR) that signals through the intracellular cyclic AMP pathway to stimulate somatotrope cell proliferation as well as GH production. Inactivating mutations of the GHRH receptor cause profound dwarfism. A distinct surface receptor for ghrelin, the gastric-derived GH secretagogue, is expressed in both the hypothalamus and pituitary. Somatostatin binds to five distinct receptor subtypes (SSTR1 to SSTR5); SSTR2 and SSTR5 subtypes preferentially suppress GH (and TSH) secretion.

GH secretion is pulsatile, with highest peak levels occurring at night, generally correlating with sleep onset. GH secretory rates decline markedly with age so that hormone levels in middle age are about 15% of pubertal levels. These changes are paralleled by an age-related decline in lean muscle mass. GH secretion is also reduced in obese individuals, although IGF-I levels may not be suppressed, suggesting a change in the setpoint for feedback control. Elevated GH levels occur within an hour of deep sleep onset as well as after exercise, physical stress, and trauma and during sepsis. Integrated 24-h GH secretion is higher in women and is also enhanced by estrogen replacement likely reflective of increased peripheral GH-resistance. Using standard assays, random GH measurements are undetectable in ~50% of daytime samples obtained from healthy subjects and are also undetectable in most obese and elderly subjects. Thus, single random GH measurements do not distinguish patients with adult GH deficiency from normal persons.

GH secretion is profoundly influenced by nutritional factors. Using newer ultrasensitive GH assays with a sensitivity of 0.002 μg/L, a glucose load suppresses GH to <0.7 μg/L in women and to <0.07 μg/L in men. Increased GH pulse frequency and peak amplitudes occur with chronic malnutrition or prolonged fasting. GH is stimulated by intravenous L-arginine, dopamine, and apomorphine (a dopamine receptor agonist), as well as by α-adrenergic pathways. β-Adrenergic blockade induces basal GH and enhances GHRH- and insulin-evoked GH release.

Action

The pattern of GH secretion may affect tissue responses. The higher GH pulsatility observed in men compared with the relatively continuous basal GH secretion in women may be an important biologic determinant of linear growth patterns and liver enzyme induction.

The 70-kDa peripheral GH receptor protein has structural homology with the cytokine/hematopoietic superfamily. A fragment of the receptor extracellular domain generates a soluble GH binding protein (GHBP) that interacts with GH in the circulation. The liver and cartilage contain the greatest number of GH receptors. GH binding to preformed receptor dimers is followed by internal rotation and subsequent signaling through the JAK/STAT pathway. Activated STAT proteins translocate to the nucleus, where they modulate expression of GH-regulated target genes. GH analogues that bind to the receptor but are incapable of mediating receptor signaling are potent antagonists of GH action. A GH receptor antagonist (pegvisomant) is approved for treatment of acromegaly.

GH induces protein synthesis and nitrogen retention and impairs glucose tolerance by antagonizing insulin action. GH also stimulates lipolysis, leading to increased circulating fatty acid levels, reduced omental fat mass, and enhanced lean body mass. GH promotes sodium, potassium, and water retention and elevates serum levels of inorganic phosphate. Linear bone growth occurs as a result of complex hormonal and growth factor actions, including those of IGF-I. GH stimulates epiphyseal prechondrocyte differentiation. These precursor cells produce IGF-I locally, and their proliferation is also responsive to the growth factor.

Insulin-like growth factors

Although GH exerts direct effects in target tissues, many of its physiologic effects are mediated indirectly through IGF-I, a potent growth and differentiation factor. The liver is the major source of circulating IGF-I. In peripheral tissues, IGF-I also exerts local paracrine actions that appear to be both dependent on and independent of GH. Thus, GH administration induces circulating IGF-I as well as stimulating local IGF-I production in multiple tissues.

Both IGF-I and IGF-II are bound to high-affinity circulating IGF-binding proteins (IGFBPs) that regulate IGF bioactivity. Levels of IGFBP3 are GH-dependent, and it serves as the major carrier protein for circulating IGF-I. GH deficiency and malnutrition usually are associated with low IGFBP3 levels. IGFBP1 and IGFBP2 regulate local tissue IGF action but do not bind appreciable amounts of circulating IGF-I.

Serum IGF-I concentrations are profoundly affected by physiologic factors. Levels increase during puberty, peak at 16 years, and subsequently decline by >80% during the aging process. IGF-I concentrations are higher in women than in men. Because GH is the major determinant of hepatic IGF-I synthesis, abnormalities of GH synthesis or action (e.g., pituitary failure, GHRH receptor defect, GH receptor defect or pharmacologic GH receptor blockade) reduce IGF-I levels. Hypocaloric states are associated with GH resistance; IGF-I levels are therefore low with cachexia, malnutrition, and sepsis. In acromegaly, IGF-I levels are invariably high and reflect a log-linear relationship with circulating GH concentrations.

IGF-I physiology

Injected IGF-I (100 μg/kg) induces hypoglycemia, and lower doses improve insulin sensitivity in patients with severe insulin resistance and diabetes. In cachectic subjects, IGF-I infusion (12 μg/kg per hour) enhances nitrogen retention and lowers cholesterol levels. Longer-term subcutaneous IGF-I injections enhance protein synthesis and are anabolic. Although bone formation markers are induced, bone turnover also may be stimulated by IGF-I. IGF-I has only been approved for use in patients with GH-resistance syndromes.

IGF-I side effects are dose-dependent, and overdose may result in hypoglycemia, hypotension, fluid retention, temporomandibular jaw pain, and increased intracranial pressure, all of which are reversible. Avascular femoral head necrosis has been reported. Chronic excess IGF-I administration presumably would result in features of acromegaly.

ADRENOCORTICOTROPIC HORMONE

(See also Chap. 8)

Synthesis

ACTH-secreting corticotrope cells constitute about 20% of the pituitary cell population. ACTH (39 amino acids) is derived from the POMC precursor protein (266 amino acids) that also generates several other peptides, including β-lipotropin, β-endorphin, met-enkephalin, α-melanocyte-stimulating hormone (α-MSH), and corticotropin-like intermediate lobe protein (CLIP). The POMC gene is potently suppressed by glucocorticoids and induced by corticotropin-releasing hormone (CRH), arginine vasopressin (AVP), and proinflammatory cytokines, including IL-6, as well as leukemia inhibitory factor.

CRH, a 41-amino-acid hypothalamic peptide synthesized in the paraventricular nucleus as well as in higher brain centers, is the predominant stimulator of ACTH synthesis and release. The CRH receptor is a GPCR that is expressed on the corticotrope and signals to induce POMC transcription.

Secretion

ACTH secretion is pulsatile and exhibits a characteristic circadian rhythm, peaking at about 6 A.M. and reaching a nadir about midnight. Adrenal glucocorticoid secretion, which is driven by ACTH, follows a parallel diurnal pattern. ACTH circadian rhythmicity is determined by variations in secretory pulse amplitude rather than changes in pulse frequency. Superimposed on this endogenous rhythm, ACTH levels are increased by physical and psychological stress, exercise, acute illness, and insulin-induced hypoglycemia.

Glucocorticoid-mediated negative regulation of the hypothalamic-pituitary-adrenal (HPA) axis occurs as a consequence of both hypothalamic CRH suppression and direct attenuation of pituitary POMC gene expression and ACTH release. In contrast, loss of cortisol feedback inhibition, as occurs in primary adrenal failure, results in extremely high ACTH levels.

Acute inflammatory or septic insults activate the HPA axis through the integrated actions of proinflammatory cytokines, bacterial toxins, and neural signals. The overlapping cascade of ACTH-inducing cytokines (tumor necrosis factor [TNF]; IL-1, -2, and -6; and leukemia inhibitory factor) activates hypothalamic CRH and AVP secretion, pituitary POMC gene expression, and local pituitary paracrine cytokine networks. The resulting cortisol elevation restrains the inflammatory response and enables host protection. Concomitantly, cytokine-mediated central glucocorticoid receptor resistance impairs glucocorticoid suppression of the HPA. Thus, the neuroendocrine stress response reflects the net result of highly integrated hypothalamic, intrapituitary, and peripheral hormone and cytokine signals acting to regulate cortisol secretion.

Action

The major function of the HPA axis is to maintain metabolic homeostasis and mediate the neuroendocrine stress response. ACTH induces adrenocortical steroidogenesis by sustaining adrenal cell proliferation and function. The receptor for ACTH, designated *melanocortin-2 receptor*, is a GPCR that induces steroidogenesis by stimulating a cascade of steroidogenic enzymes **(Chap. 8)**.

GONADOTROPINS: FSH AND LH

Synthesis and secretion

Gonadotrope cells constitute about 10% of anterior pituitary cells and produce two gonadotropin hormones—LH and FSH. Like TSH and hCG, LH and FSH are glycoprotein hormones that comprise α and β subunits. The α subunit is common to these glycoprotein hormones; specificity of hormone function is conferred by the β subunits, which are expressed by separate genes.

Gonadotropin synthesis and release are dynamically regulated. This is particularly true in women, in whom rapidly fluctuating gonadal steroid levels vary throughout the menstrual cycle. Hypothalamic GnRH, a 10-amino-acid peptide, regulates the synthesis and secretion of both LH and FSH. Brain kisspeptin, a product of the *KISSI* gene regulates hypothalamic GnRH release. GnRH is secreted in discrete pulses every 60–120 min, and the pulses in turn elicit LH and FSH pulses (Fig. 3-3). The pulsatile mode of GnRH input is essential to its action; pulses prime gonadotrope responsiveness, whereas continuous GnRH exposure induces desensitization. Based on this phenomenon, long-acting GnRH agonists are used to suppress gonadotropin levels in children with precocious puberty and in men with prostate cancer and are used in some ovulation-induction protocols to reduce levels of endogenous gonadotropins **(Chap. 13)**. Estrogens act at both the hypothalamus and the pituitary to modulate gonadotropin secretion. Chronic estrogen exposure is inhibitory, whereas rising estrogen levels, as occur during the preovulatory surge, exert positive feedback to increase gonadotropin pulse frequency and amplitude. Progesterone slows GnRH pulse frequency but enhances gonadotropin responses to GnRH. Testosterone feedback in men also occurs at the hypothalamic and pituitary levels and is mediated in part by its conversion to estrogens.

Although GnRH is the main regulator of LH and FSH secretion, FSH synthesis is also under separate control by the gonadal peptides inhibin and activin, which are members of the transforming growth factor β (TGF-β) family. Inhibin selectively suppresses FSH, whereas activin stimulates FSH synthesis **(Chap. 13)**.

Action

The gonadotropin hormones interact with their respective GPCRs expressed in the ovary and testis, evoking germ cell development and maturation and steroid hormone biosynthesis. In women, FSH regulates ovarian follicle development and stimulates ovarian estrogen production. LH mediates ovulation and maintenance of the corpus luteum. In men, LH induces Leydig cell testosterone synthesis and secretion, and FSH stimulates seminiferous tubule development and regulates spermatogenesis.

THYROID-STIMULATING HORMONE

Synthesis and secretion

TSH-secreting thyrotrope cells constitute 5% of the anterior pituitary cell population. TSH shares a common α subunit with LH and FSH but contains a specific TSH β subunit. TRH is a hypothalamic tripeptide (pyroglutamyl histidylprolinamide) that acts through a pituitary GPCR to stimulate TSH synthesis and secretion; it also stimulates the lactotrope cell to secrete PRL. TSH secretion is stimulated by TRH, whereas thyroid hormones, dopamine, somatostatin, and glucocorticoids suppress TSH by overriding TRH induction.

Thyrotrope cell proliferation and TSH secretion are both induced when negative feedback inhibition by thyroid hormones is removed. Thus, thyroid damage (including surgical thyroidectomy), radiation-induced hypothyroidism, chronic thyroiditis, and prolonged goitrogen exposure are associated with increased TSH levels. Long-standing untreated hypothyroidism can lead to elevated TSH levels as well as thyrotrope hyperplasia and pituitary enlargement, which may be evident on magnetic resonance imaging.

Action

TSH is secreted in pulses, although the excursions are modest in comparison to other pituitary hormones because of the low amplitude of the pulses and the relatively long half-life of TSH. Consequently, single determinations of TSH suffice to precisely assess its circulating levels. TSH binds to a GPCR on thyroid follicular cells to stimulate thyroid hormone synthesis and release **(Chap. 7)**.

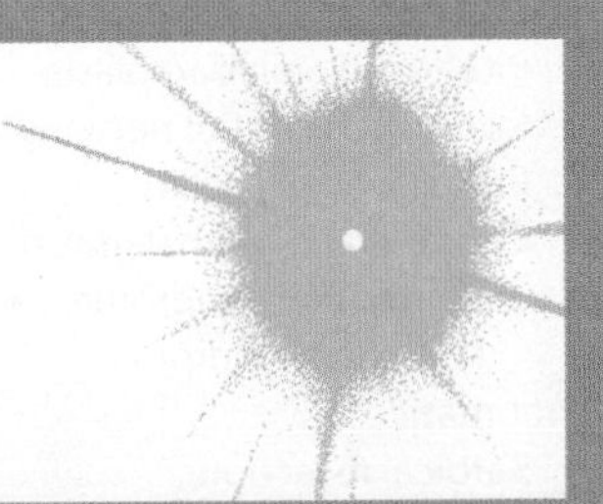

CHAPTER 4
HYPOPITUITARISM

Shlomo Melmed ■ J. Larry Jameson

Inadequate production of anterior pituitary hormones leads to features of hypopituitarism. Impaired production of one or more of the anterior pituitary trophic hormones can result from inherited disorders; more commonly, adult hypopituitarism is acquired and reflects the compressive mass effects of tumors or the consequences of local pituitary or hypothalamic traumatic, inflammatory, or vascular damage. These processes also may impair synthesis or secretion of hypothalamic hormones, with resultant pituitary failure (Table 4-1).

DEVELOPMENTAL AND GENETIC CAUSES OF HYPOPITUITARISM

Pituitary dysplasia

Pituitary dysplasia may result in aplastic, hypoplastic, or ectopic pituitary gland development. Because pituitary development follows midline cell migration from the nasopharyngeal Rathke's pouch, midline craniofacial disorders may be associated with pituitary dysplasia. Acquired pituitary failure in the newborn also can be caused by birth trauma, including cranial hemorrhage, asphyxia, and breech delivery.

SEPTO-optic dysplasia

Hypothalamic dysfunction and hypopituitarism may result from dysgenesis of the septum pellucidum or corpus callosum. Affected children have mutations in the *HESX1* gene, which is involved in early development of the ventral prosencephalon. These children exhibit variable combinations of cleft palate, syndactyly, ear deformities, hypertelorism, optic nerve hypoplasia, micropenis, and anosmia. Pituitary dysfunction leads to diabetes insipidus, growth hormone (GH) deficiency and short stature, and, occasionally, thyroid-stimulating hormone (TSH) deficiency.

Tissue-specific factor mutations

Several pituitary cell–specific transcription factors, such as Pit-1 and Prop-1, are critical for determining the development and committed function of differentiated anterior pituitary cell lineages. Autosomal dominant or recessive Pit-1 mutations cause combined GH, prolactin (PRL), and TSH deficiencies. These patients usually present with growth failure and varying degrees of hypothyroidism. The pituitary may appear hypoplastic on magnetic resonance imaging (MRI).

Prop-1 is expressed early in pituitary development and appears to be required for Pit-1 function. Familial and sporadic *PROP1* mutations result in combined GH, PRL, TSH, and gonadotropin deficiency. Over 80% of these patients have growth retardation; by adulthood, all are deficient in TSH and gonadotropins, and a small minority later develop adrenocorticotropic hormone (ACTH) deficiency. Because of gonadotropin deficiency, these individuals do not enter puberty spontaneously. In some cases, the pituitary gland appears enlarged on MRI. *TPIT* mutations result in ACTH deficiency associated with hypocortisolism.

Developmental hypothalamic dysfunction

Kallmann syndrome

Kallmann syndrome results from defective hypothalamic gonadotropin-releasing hormone (GnRH) synthesis and is associated with anosmia or hyposmia due to olfactory bulb agenesis or hypoplasia **(Chap. 11)**. Classically, the syndrome may also be associated with color blindness, optic atrophy, nerve deafness, cleft palate, renal abnormalities, cryptorchidism, and neurologic abnormalities such as mirror movements. The initial genetic cause was identified in the X-linked *KAL* gene, mutations of which impair embryonic migration of GnRH neurons from the hypothalamic olfactory placode to the hypothalamus. Based on further

TABLE 4-1

ETIOLOGY OF HYPOPITUITARISM[a]

Development/structural
- Transcription factor defect
- Pituitary dysplasia/aplasia
- Congenital central nervous system mass, encephalocele
- Primary empty sella
- Congenital hypothalamic disorders (septo-optic dysplasia, Prader-Willi syndrome, Laurence-Moon-Biedl syndrome, Kallmann syndrome)

Traumatic
- Surgical resection
- Radiation damage
- Head injuries

Neoplastic
- Pituitary adenoma
- Parasellar mass (germinoma, ependymoma, glioma)
- Rathke's cyst
- Craniopharyngioma
- Hypothalamic hamartoma, gangliocytoma
- Pituitary metastases (breast, lung, colon carcinoma)
- Lymphoma and leukemia
- Meningioma

Infiltrative/inflammatory
- Lymphocytic hypophysitis
- Hemochromatosis
- Sarcoidosis
- Histiocytosis X
- Granulomatous hypophysitis
- Transcription factor antibodies

Vascular
- Pituitary apoplexy
- Pregnancy-related (infarction with diabetes; postpartum necrosis)
- Sickle cell disease
- Arteritis

Infections
- Fungal (histoplasmosis)
- Parasitic (toxoplasmosis)
- Tuberculosis
- *Pneumocystis carinii*

[a]Trophic hormone failure associated with pituitary compression or destruction usually occurs sequentially: growth hormone > follicle-stimulating hormone > luteinizing hormone > thyroid-stimulating hormone > adrenocorticotropic hormone. During childhood, growth retardation is often the presenting feature, and in adults, hypogonadism is the earliest symptom.

studies, at least a dozen other genetic abnormalities, in addition to KAL mutations, have been found to cause isolated GnRH deficiency. Autosomal recessive (i.e., *GPR54, KISS1*) and dominant (i.e., *FGFR1*) modes of transmission have been described, and there is a growing list of genes associated with GnRH deficiency (*GNRH1, PROK2, PROKR2, CH7, PCSK1, FGF8, NELF, WDR11, TAC3, TACR3*). A fraction of patients have digenic mutations. Associated clinical features, in addition to GnRH deficiency, vary depending on the genetic cause. GnRH deficiency prevents progression through puberty. Males present with delayed puberty and pronounced hypogonadal features, including micropenis, probably the result of low testosterone levels during infancy. Females present with primary amenorrhea and failure of secondary sexual development.

Kallmann syndrome and other causes of congenital GnRH deficiency are characterized by low luteinizing hormone (LH) and follicle-stimulating hormone (FSH) levels and low concentrations of sex steroids (testosterone or estradiol). In sporadic cases of isolated gonadotropin deficiency, the diagnosis is often one of exclusion after other known causes of hypothalamic-pituitary dysfunction have been eliminated. Repetitive GnRH administration restores normal pituitary gonadotropin responses, pointing to a hypothalamic defect in these patients.

Long-term treatment of males with human chorionic gonadotropin (hCG) or testosterone restores pubertal development and secondary sex characteristics; women can be treated with cyclic estrogen and progestin. Fertility also may be restored by the administration of gonadotropins or by using a portable infusion pump to deliver subcutaneous, pulsatile GnRH.

Bardet-Biedl syndrome

This very rare genetically heterogeneous disorder is characterized by mental retardation, renal abnormalities, obesity, and hexadactyly, brachydactyly, or syndactyly. Central diabetes insipidus may or may not be associated. GnRH deficiency occurs in 75% of males and half of affected females. Retinal degeneration begins in early childhood, and most patients are blind by age 30. Numerous subtypes of Bardet-Biedl syndrome (BBS) have been identified, with genetic linkage to at least nine different loci. Several of the loci encode genes involved in basal body cilia function, and this may account for the diverse clinical manifestations.

Leptin and leptin receptor mutations

Deficiencies of leptin or its receptor cause a broad spectrum of hypothalamic abnormalities, including hyperphagia, obesity, and central hypogonadism **(Chap. 20)**. Decreased GnRH production in these patients results in attenuated pituitary FSH and LH synthesis and release.

Prader-Willi syndrome

This is a contiguous gene syndrome that results from deletion of the paternal copies of the imprinted *SNRPN* gene, the *NECDIN* gene, and possibly other genes on chromosome 15q. Prader-Willi syndrome is associated with hypogonadotropic hypogonadism, hyperphagia-obesity, chronic muscle hypotonia, mental retardation, and adult-onset diabetes mellitus. Multiple somatic defects also involve the skull, eyes, ears, hands, and feet. Diminished hypothalamic oxytocin- and vasopressin-producing nuclei have been reported. Deficient GnRH synthesis is suggested by the observation that chronic GnRH treatment restores pituitary LH and FSH release.

ACQUIRED HYPOPITUITARISM

Hypopituitarism may be caused by accidental or neurosurgical trauma; vascular events such as apoplexy; pituitary or hypothalamic neoplasms, craniopharyngioma, lymphoma, or metastatic tumors; inflammatory disease such as lymphocytic hypophysitis; infiltrative disorders such as sarcoidosis, hemochromatosis, and tuberculosis; or irradiation.

Increasing evidence suggests that patients with brain injury, including contact sports trauma, subarachnoid hemorrhage, and irradiation, have transient hypopituitarism and require intermittent long-term endocrine follow-up, because permanent hypothalamic or pituitary dysfunction will develop in 25–40% of these patients.

Hypothalamic infiltration disorders

These disorders—including sarcoidosis, histiocytosis X, amyloidosis, and hemochromatosis—frequently involve both hypothalamic and pituitary neuronal and neurochemical tracts. Consequently, diabetes insipidus occurs in half of patients with these disorders. Growth retardation is seen if attenuated GH secretion occurs before puberty. Hypogonadotropic hypogonadism and hyperprolactinemia are also common.

Inflammatory lesions

Pituitary damage and subsequent secretory dysfunction can be seen with chronic site infections such as tuberculosis, with opportunistic fungal infections associated with AIDS, and in tertiary syphilis. Other inflammatory processes, such as granulomas and sarcoidosis, may mimic the features of a pituitary adenoma. These lesions may cause extensive hypothalamic and pituitary damage, leading to trophic hormone deficiencies.

Cranial irradiation

Cranial irradiation may result in long-term hypothalamic and pituitary dysfunction, especially in children and adolescents, as they are more susceptible to damage after whole-brain or head and neck therapeutic irradiation. The development of hormonal abnormalities correlates strongly with irradiation dosage and the time interval after completion of radiotherapy. Up to two-thirds of patients ultimately develop hormone insufficiency after a median dose of 50 Gy (5000 rad) directed at the skull base. The development of hypopituitarism occurs over 5–15 years and usually reflects hypothalamic damage rather than primary destruction of pituitary cells. Although the pattern of hormone loss is variable, GH deficiency is most common, followed by gonadotropin and ACTH deficiency. When deficiency of one or more hormones is documented, the possibility of diminished reserve of other hormones is likely. Accordingly, anterior pituitary function should be continually evaluated over the long term in previously irradiated patients, and replacement therapy instituted when appropriate (see below).

Lymphocytic hypophysitis

This occurs most often in postpartum women; it usually presents with hyperprolactinemia and MRI evidence of a prominent pituitary mass that often resembles an adenoma, with mildly elevated PRL levels. Pituitary failure caused by diffuse lymphocytic infiltration may be transient or permanent but requires immediate evaluation and treatment. Rarely, isolated pituitary hormone deficiencies have been described, suggesting a selective autoimmune process targeted to specific cell types. Most patients manifest symptoms of progressive mass effects with headache and visual disturbance. The erythrocyte sedimentation rate often is elevated. Because the MRI image may be indistinguishable from that of a pituitary adenoma, hypophysitis should be considered in a postpartum woman with a newly diagnosed pituitary mass before an unnecessary surgical intervention is undertaken. The inflammatory process often resolves after several months of glucocorticoid treatment, and pituitary function may be restored, depending on the extent of damage.

Pituitary apoplexy

Acute intrapituitary hemorrhagic vascular events can cause substantial damage to the pituitary and surrounding sellar structures. Pituitary apoplexy may occur spontaneously in a preexisting adenoma; postpartum (Sheehan's syndrome); or in association with diabetes, hypertension, sickle cell anemia, or acute shock. The hyperplastic enlargement of the pituitary, which occurs normally during pregnancy, increases the risk for hemorrhage and infarction. Apoplexy is an endocrine emergency that may result in severe hypoglycemia, hypotension and shock, central nervous system (CNS) hemorrhage, and death. Acute symptoms may include severe headache with signs of meningeal irritation, bilateral visual changes, ophthalmoplegia, and, in severe cases, cardiovascular collapse and loss of consciousness. Pituitary computed tomography (CT) or MRI may reveal signs of intratumoral or sellar hemorrhage, with pituitary stalk deviation and compression of pituitary tissue.

Patients with no evident visual loss or impaired consciousness can be observed and managed conservatively with high-dose glucocorticoids. Those with significant or progressive visual loss, cranial nerve palsy, or loss of consciousness require urgent surgical decompression. Visual recovery after sellar surgery is inversely correlated with the length of time after the acute event. Therefore, severe ophthalmoplegia or visual deficits are indications for early surgery. Hypopituitarism is common after apoplexy.

Empty sella

A partial or apparently totally empty sella is often an incidental MRI finding, and may be associated with intracranial hypertension. These patients usually have normal pituitary function, implying that the surrounding rim of pituitary tissue is fully functional. Hypopituitarism, however, may develop insidiously. Pituitary masses also may undergo clinically silent infarction and involution with development of a partial or totally empty sella by cerebrospinal fluid (CSF) filling the dural herniation. Rarely, small but functional pituitary adenomas may arise within the rim of normal pituitary tissue, and they are not always visible on MRI.

PRESENTATION AND DIAGNOSIS

The clinical manifestations of hypopituitarism depend on which hormones are lost and the extent of the hormone deficiency. GH deficiency causes growth disorders in children and leads to abnormal body composition in adults (see below). Gonadotropin deficiency causes menstrual disorders and infertility in women and decreased sexual function, infertility, and loss of secondary sexual characteristics in men. TSH and ACTH deficiency usually develop later in the course of pituitary failure. TSH deficiency causes growth retardation in children and features of hypothyroidism in children and adults. The secondary form of adrenal insufficiency caused by ACTH deficiency leads to hypocortisolism with relative preservation of mineralocorticoid production. PRL deficiency causes failure of lactation. When lesions involve the posterior pituitary, polyuria and polydipsia reflect loss of vasopressin secretion. In patients with long-standing pituitary damage, epidemiologic studies document an increased mortality rate, primarily from increased cardiovascular and cerebrovascular disease. Previous head or neck irradiation is also a determinant of increased mortality rates in patients with hypopituitarism, especially from cerebrovascular disease.

LABORATORY INVESTIGATION

Biochemical diagnosis of pituitary insufficiency is made by demonstrating low levels of respective pituitary trophic hormones in the setting of low levels of target hormones. For example, low free thyroxine in the setting of a low or inappropriately normal TSH level suggests secondary hypothyroidism. Similarly, a low testosterone level without elevation of gonadotropins suggests hypogonadotropic hypogonadism. Provocative tests may be required to assess pituitary reserve (Table 4-2). GH responses to insulin-induced hypoglycemia, arginine, L-dopa, growth hormone–releasing hormone (GHRH), or growth hormone–releasing peptides (GHRPs) can be used to assess GH reserve. Corticotropin-releasing hormone (CRH) administration induces ACTH release, and administration of synthetic ACTH (cosyntropin) evokes adrenal cortisol release as an indirect indicator of pituitary ACTH reserve **(Chap. 8)**. ACTH reserve is most reliably assessed by measuring ACTH and cortisol levels during insulin-induced hypoglycemia. However, this test should be performed cautiously in patients with suspected adrenal insufficiency because of enhanced susceptibility to hypoglycemia and hypotension. Administering insulin to induce hypoglycemia is contraindicated in patients with active coronary artery disease or known seizure disorders.

TREATMENT Hypopituitarism

Hormone replacement therapy, including glucocorticoids, thyroid hormone, sex steroids, growth hormone, and vasopressin, is usually safe and free of complications. Treatment regimens that mimic physiologic hormone production allow for maintenance of satisfactory clinical homeostasis. Effective dosage schedules are outlined in Table 4-3. Patients in need of glucocorticoid replacement require careful dose adjustments during stressful events such as acute illness, dental procedures, trauma, and acute hospitalization.

DISORDERS OF GROWTH AND DEVELOPMENT

Skeletal maturation and somatic growth

The growth plate is dependent on a variety of hormonal stimuli, including GH, insulin-like growth factor (IGF) I, sex steroids, thyroid hormones, paracrine growth factors, and cytokines. The growth-promoting process also requires caloric energy, amino acids, vitamins, and trace metals and consumes about 10% of normal energy production. Malnutrition impairs chondrocyte activity, increases GH resistance, and reduces circulating IGF-I and IGFBP3 levels.

Linear bone growth rates are very high in infancy and are pituitary-dependent. Mean growth velocity is ~6 cm/year in later childhood and usually is maintained within a given range on a standardized percentile chart. Peak growth rates occur during midpuberty when bone age is

TABLE 4-2
TESTS OF PITUITARY SUFFICIENCY

HORMONE	TEST	BLOOD SAMPLES	INTERPRETATION
Growth hormone (GH)	Insulin tolerance test: Regular insulin (0.05–0.15 U/kg IV)	−30, 0, 30, 60, 120 min for glucose and GH	Glucose <40 mg/dL; GH should be >3 μg/L
	GHRH test: 1 μg/kg IV	0, 15, 30, 45, 60, 120 min for GH	Normal response is GH >3 μg/L
	L-Arginine test: 30 g IV over 30 min	0, 30, 60, 120 min for GH	Normal response is GH >3 μg/L
	L-Dopa test: 500 mg PO	0, 30, 60, 120 min for GH	Normal response is GH >3 μg/L
Prolactin	TRH test: 200–500 μg IV	0, 20, and 60 min for TSH and PRL	Normal prolactin is >2 μg/L and increase >200% of baseline
ACTH	Insulin tolerance test: regular insulin (0.05–0.15 U/kg IV)	−30, 0, 30, 60, 90 min for glucose and cortisol	Glucose <40 mg/dL Cortisol should increase by >7 μg/dL or to >20 μg/dL
	CRH test: 1 μg/kg ovine CRH IV at 8 A.M.	0, 15, 30, 60, 90, 120 min for ACTH and cortisol	Basal ACTH increases 2- to 4-fold and peaks at 20–100 pg/mL Cortisol levels >20–25 μg/dL
	Metyrapone test: Metyrapone (30 mg/kg) at midnight	Plasma 11-deoxycortisol and cortisol at 8 A.M.; ACTH can also be measured	Plasma cortisol should be <4 g/dL to assure an adequate response Normal response is 11-deoxycortisol >7.5 μg/dL or ACTH >75 pg/mL
	Standard ACTH stimulation test: ACTH 1-24 (cosyntropin), 0.25 mg IM or IV	0, 30, 60 min for cortisol and aldosterone	Normal response is cortisol >21 g/dL and aldosterone response of >4 ng/dL above baseline
	Low-dose ACTH test: ACTH 1-24 (cosyntropin), 1 μg IV	0, 30, 60 min for cortisol	Cortisol should be >21 g/dL
	3-day ACTH stimulation test consists of 0.25 mg ACTH 1-24 given IV over 8 h each day		Cortisol >21 g/dL
TSH	Basal thyroid function tests: T_4, T_3, TSH	Basal measurements	Low free thyroid hormone levels in the setting of TSH levels that are not appropriately increased indicate pituitary insufficiency
	TRH test: 200–500 μg IV	0, 20, 60 min for TSH and PRL[a]	TSH should increase by >5 mU/L unless thyroid hormone levels are increased
LH, FSH	LH, FSH, testosterone, estrogen	Basal measurements	Basal LH and FSH should be increased in postmenopausal women Low testosterone levels in the setting of low LH and FSH indicate pituitary insufficiency
	GnRH test: GnRH (100 μg) IV	0, 30, 60 min for LH and FSH	In most adults, LH should increase by 10 IU/L and FSH by 2 IU/L Normal responses are variable
Multiple hormones	Combined anterior pituitary test: GHRH (1 g/kg), CRH (1 μg/kg), GnRH (100 g), TRH (200 μg) are given IV	−30, 0, 15, 30, 60, 90, 120 min for GH, ACTH, cortisol, LH, FSH, and TSH	Combined or individual releasing hormone responses must be elevated in the context of basal target gland hormone values and may not be uniformly diagnostic (see text)

[a]Evoked PRL response indicates lactotrope integrity.
Abbreviations: T_3, triiodothyronine; T_4, thyroxine; TRH, thyrotropin-releasing hormone. For other abbreviations, see text.

TABLE 4-3

HORMONE REPLACEMENT THERAPY FOR ADULT HYPOPITUITARISM[a]

TROPHIC HORMONE DEFICIT	HORMONE REPLACEMENT
ACTH	Hydrocortisone (10–20 mg A.M.; 5–10 mg P.M.) Cortisone acetate (25 mg A.M.; 12.5 mg P.M.) Prednisone (5 mg A.M.)
TSH	L-Thyroxine (0.075–0.15 mg daily)
FSH/LH	Males Testosterone gel (5–10 g/d) Testosterone skin patch (5 mg/d) Testosterone enanthate (200 mg IM every 2 weeks) Females Conjugated estrogen (0.65–1.25 mg qd for 25 days) Progesterone (5–10 mg qd) on days 16–25 Estradiol skin patch (0.025–0.1 mg every week), adding progesterone on days 16–25 if uterus intact For fertility: menopausal gonadotropins, human chorionic gonadotropins
GH	Adults: Somatotropin (0.1–1.25 mg SC qd) Children: Somatotropin (0.02–0.05 mg/kg per day)
Vasopressin	Intranasal desmopressin (5–20 g twice daily) Oral 300–600 μg qd

[a]All doses shown should be individualized for specific patients and should be reassessed during stress, surgery, or pregnancy. Male and female fertility requirements should be managed as discussed in **Chaps. 11 and 13**.
Note: For abbreviations, see text.

12 (girls) or 13 (boys). Secondary sexual development is associated with elevated sex steroids that cause progressive epiphyseal growth plate closure. *Bone age* is delayed in patients with all forms of true GH deficiency or GH receptor defects that result in attenuated GH action.

Short stature may occur as a result of constitutive intrinsic growth defects or because of acquired extrinsic factors that impair growth. In general, delayed bone age in a child with short stature is suggestive of a hormonal or systemic disorder, whereas normal bone age in a short child is more likely to be caused by a genetic cartilage dysplasia or growth plate disorder.

GH deficiency in children

GH deficiency

Isolated GH deficiency is characterized by short stature, micropenis, increased fat, high-pitched voice, and a propensity to hypoglycemia due to relatively unopposed insulin action. Familial modes of inheritance are seen in at least one-third of these individuals and may be autosomal dominant, recessive, or X-linked. About 10% of children with GH deficiency have mutations in the *GH-N* gene, including gene deletions and a wide range of point mutations. Mutations in transcription factors Pit-1 and Prop-1, which control somatotrope development, result in GH deficiency in combination with other pituitary hormone deficiencies, which may become manifest only in adulthood. The diagnosis of *idiopathic GH deficiency* (IGHD) should be made only after known molecular defects have been rigorously excluded.

GHRH receptor mutations

Recessive mutations of the GHRH receptor gene in subjects with severe proportionate dwarfism are associated with low basal GH levels that cannot be stimulated by exogenous GHRH, GHRP, or insulin-induced hypoglycemia, as well as anterior pituitary hypoplasia The syndrome exemplifies the importance of the GHRH receptor for somatotrope cell proliferation and hormonal responsiveness.

GH insensitivity

This is caused by defects of GH receptor structure or signaling. Homozygous or heterozygous mutations of the GH receptor are associated with partial or complete GH insensitivity and growth failure (*Laron's syndrome*). The diagnosis is based on normal or high GH levels, with decreased circulating GH-binding protein (GHBP), and low IGF-I levels. Very rarely, defective IGF-I, IGF-I receptor, or IGF-I signaling defects are also encountered. *STAT5B* mutations result in both immunodeficiency as well as abrogated GH signaling, leading to short stature with normal or elevated GH levels and low IGF-I levels. Circulating GH receptor antibodies may rarely cause peripheral GH insensitivity.

Nutritional short stature

Caloric deprivation and malnutrition, uncontrolled diabetes, and chronic renal failure represent secondary causes of abrogated GH receptor function. These conditions also stimulate production of proinflammatory cytokines, which act to exacerbate the block of GH-mediated signal transduction. Children with these conditions typically exhibit features of acquired short stature with normal or elevated GH and low IGF-I levels.

Psychosocial short stature

Emotional and social deprivation lead to growth retardation accompanied by delayed speech, discordant hyperphagia, and an attenuated response to administered GH. A nurturing environment restores growth rates.

PRESENTATION AND DIAGNOSIS

Short stature is commonly encountered in clinical practice, and the decision to evaluate these children requires clinical judgment in association with auxologic data and family history. Short stature should be evaluated comprehensively if a patient's height is >3 standard deviations (SD) below the mean for age or if the growth rate has decelerated. Skeletal maturation is best evaluated by measuring a radiologic bone age, which is based mainly on the degree of wrist bone growth plate fusion. Final height can be predicted using standardized scales (Bayley-Pinneau or Tanner-Whitehouse) or estimated by adding 6.5 cm (boys) or subtracting 6.5 cm (girls) from the midparental height.

LABORATORY INVESTIGATION

Because GH secretion is pulsatile, GH deficiency is best assessed by examining the response to provocative stimuli, including exercise, insulin-induced hypoglycemia, and other pharmacologic tests that normally increase GH to >7 μg/L in children. Random GH measurements do not distinguish normal children from those with true GH deficiency. Adequate adrenal and thyroid hormone replacement should be assured before testing. Age- and sex-matched IGF-I levels are not sufficiently sensitive or specific to make the diagnosis but can be useful to confirm GH deficiency. Pituitary MRI may reveal pituitary mass lesions or structural defects. Molecular analyses for known mutations should be undertaken when the cause of short stature remains cryptic, or when additional clinical features suggest a genetic cause.

TREATMENT Disorders of Growth and Development

Replacement therapy with recombinant GH (0.02–0.05 mg/kg per day SC) restores growth velocity in GH-deficient children to ~10 cm/year. If pituitary insufficiency is documented, other associated hormone deficits should be corrected, especially adrenal steroids. GH treatment is also moderately effective for accelerating growth rates in children with Turner's syndrome and chronic renal failure.

In patients with GH insensitivity and growth retardation due to mutations of the GH receptor, treatment with IGF-I bypasses the dysfunctional GH receptor.

ADULT GH DEFICIENCY (AGHD)

This disorder usually is caused by acquired hypothalamic or pituitary somatotrope damage. Acquired pituitary hormone deficiency follows a typical pattern in which loss of adequate GH reserve foreshadows subsequent hormone deficits. The sequential order of hormone loss is usually GH → FSH/LH → TSH → ACTH. Patients previously diagnosed with childhood-onset GH deficiency should be retested as adults to affirm the diagnosis.

PRESENTATION AND DIAGNOSIS

The clinical features of AGHD include changes in body composition, lipid metabolism, and quality of life and cardiovascular dysfunction (Table 4-4). Body

TABLE 4-4

FEATURES OF ADULT GROWTH HORMONE DEFICIENCY

Clinical
- Impaired quality of life
  - Decreased energy and drive
  - Poor concentration
  - Low self-esteem
  - Social isolation
- Body composition changes
  - Increased body fat mass
  - Central fat deposition
  - Increased waist-to-hip ratio
  - Decreased lean body mass
- Reduced exercise capacity
  - Reduced maximum O_2uptake
  - Impaired cardiac function
  - Reduced muscle mass
- Cardiovascular risk factors
  - Impaired cardiac structure and function
  - Abnormal lipid profile
  - Decreased fibrinolytic activity
  - Atherosclerosis
  - Omental obesity

Imaging
- Pituitary: mass or structural damage
- Bone: reduced bone mineral density
- Abdomen: excess omental adiposity

Laboratory
- Evoked GH <3 ng/mL
- IGF-I and IGFBP3 low or normal
- Increased LDL cholesterol
- Concomitant gonadotropin, TSH, and/or ACTH reserve deficits may be present

Abbreviation: LDL, low-density lipoprotein. For other abbreviations, see text.

composition changes are common and include reduced lean body mass, increased fat mass with selective deposition of intraabdominal visceral fat, and increased waist-to-hip ratio. Hyperlipidemia, left ventricular dysfunction, hypertension, and increased plasma fibrinogen levels also may be present. Bone mineral content is reduced, with resultant increased fracture rates. Patients may experience social isolation, depression, and difficulty maintaining gainful employment. Adult hypopituitarism is associated with a threefold increase in cardiovascular mortality rates in comparison to age- and sex-matched controls, and this may be due to GH deficiency, as patients in these studies were replaced with other deficient pituitary hormones.

LABORATORY INVESTIGATION

AGHD is rare, and in light of the nonspecific nature of associated clinical symptoms, patients appropriate for testing should be selected carefully on the basis of well-defined criteria. With few exceptions, testing should be restricted to patients with the following predisposing factors: (1) pituitary surgery, (2) pituitary or hypothalamic tumor or granulomas, (3) history of cranial irradiation, (4) radiologic evidence of a pituitary lesion, (5) childhood requirement for GH replacement therapy, and rarely (6) unexplained low age- and sex-matched IGF-I levels. The transition of a GH-deficient adolescent to adulthood requires retesting to document subsequent adult GH deficiency. Up to 20% of patients previously treated for childhood-onset GH deficiency are found to be GH-sufficient on repeat testing as adults.

A significant proportion (~25%) of truly GH-deficient adults have low-normal IGF-I levels. Thus, as in the evaluation of GH deficiency in children, valid age- and sex-matched IGF-I measurements provide a useful index of therapeutic responses but are not sufficiently sensitive for diagnostic purposes. The most validated test to distinguish pituitary-sufficient patients from those with AGHD is insulin-induced (0.05–0.1 U/kg) hypoglycemia. After glucose reduction to ~40 mg/dL, most individuals experience neuroglycopenic symptoms **(Chap. 26)**, and peak GH release occurs at 60 min and remains elevated for up to 2 h. About 90% of healthy adults exhibit GH responses >5 μg/L; AGHD is defined by a peak GH response to hypoglycemia of <3 μg/L. Although insulin-induced hypoglycemia is safe when performed under appropriate supervision, it is contraindicated in patients with diabetes, ischemic heart disease, cerebrovascular disease, or epilepsy and in elderly patients. Alternative stimulatory tests include intravenous arginine (30 g), GHRH (1 μg/kg), GHRP-6 (90 μg), and glucagon (1 mg). Combinations of these tests may evoke GH secretion in subjects who are not responsive to a single test.

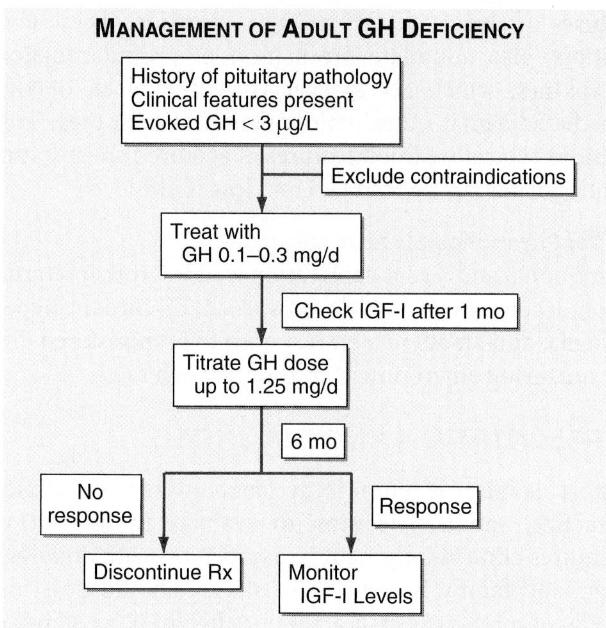

FIGURE 4-1
Management of adult growth hormone (GH) deficiency. IGF, insulin-like growth factor; Rx, Treatment.

TREATMENT Adult GH Deficiency

Once the diagnosis of AGHD is unequivocally established, replacement of GH may be indicated. Contraindications to therapy include the presence of an active neoplasm, intracranial hypertension, and uncontrolled diabetes and retinopathy. The starting dose of 0.1–0.2 mg/d should be titrated (up to a maximum of 1.25 mg/d) to maintain IGF-I levels in the mid-normal range for age- and sex-matched controls (Fig. 4-1). Women require higher doses than men, and elderly patients require less GH. Long-term GH maintenance sustains normal IGF-I levels and is associated with persistent body composition changes (e.g., enhanced lean body mass and lower body fat). High-density lipoprotein cholesterol increases, but total cholesterol and insulin levels may not change significantly. Lumbar spine bone mineral density increases, but this response is gradual (>1 year). Many patients note significant improvement in quality of life when evaluated by standardized questionnaires. The effect of GH replacement on mortality rates in GH-deficient patients is currently the subject of long-term prospective investigation.

About 30% of patients exhibit reversible dose-related fluid retention, joint pain, and carpal tunnel syndrome, and up to 40% exhibit myalgias and paresthesia. Patients receiving insulin require careful monitoring for dosing adjustments, as GH is a potent counterregulatory hormone for insulin action. Patients with type 2 diabetes mellitus initially develop further insulin resistance. However, glycemic control usually improves with the sustained loss of abdominal fat associated with long-term GH replacement. Headache, increased intracranial pressure, hypertension, and tinnitus occur rarely. Pituitary tumor regrowth and progression of skin lesions or other tumors are being assessed in long-term surveillance programs. To date, development of these potential side effects does not appear significant.

ACTH DEFICIENCY

PRESENTATION AND DIAGNOSIS

Secondary adrenal insufficiency occurs as a result of pituitary ACTH deficiency. It is characterized by fatigue, weakness, anorexia, nausea, vomiting, and, occasionally, hypoglycemia. In contrast to primary adrenal failure, hypocortisolism associated with pituitary failure usually is not accompanied by hyperpigmentation or mineralocorticoid deficiency.

ACTH deficiency is commonly due to glucocorticoid withdrawal after treatment-associated suppression of the hypothalamic-pituitary-adrenal (HPA) axis. Isolated ACTH deficiency may occur after surgical resection of an ACTH-secreting pituitary adenoma that has suppressed the HPA axis; this phenomenon is in fact suggestive of a surgical cure. The mass effects of other pituitary adenomas or sellar lesions may lead to ACTH deficiency, but usually in combination with other pituitary hormone deficiencies. Partial ACTH deficiency may be unmasked in the presence of an acute medical or surgical illness, when clinically significant hypocortisolism reflects diminished ACTH reserve. Rarely, *TPIT* or *POMC* mutations result in primary ACTH deficiency.

LABORATORY DIAGNOSIS

Inappropriately low ACTH levels in the setting of low cortisol levels are characteristic of diminished ACTH reserve. Low basal serum cortisol levels are associated with blunted cortisol responses to ACTH stimulation and impaired cortisol response to insulin-induced hypoglycemia, or testing with metyrapone or CRH. **For a description of provocative ACTH tests, see Chap. 8.**

TREATMENT ACTH Deficiency

Glucocorticoid replacement therapy improves most features of ACTH deficiency. The total daily dose of hydrocortisone replacement preferably should not exceed 25 mg daily, divided into two or three doses. Prednisone (5 mg each morning) is longer acting and has fewer mineralocorticoid effects than hydrocortisone. Some authorities advocate lower maintenance doses in an effort to avoid cushingoid side effects. Doses should be increased severalfold during periods of acute illness or stress.

GONADOTROPIN DEFICIENCY

Hypogonadism is the most common presenting feature of adult hypopituitarism even when other pituitary hormones are also deficient. It is often a harbinger of hypothalamic or pituitary lesions that impair GnRH production or delivery through the pituitary stalk. As noted below, hypogonadotropic hypogonadism is a common presenting feature of hyperprolactinemia.

A variety of inherited and acquired disorders are associated with *isolated hypogonadotropic hypogonadism* (IHH) **(Chap. 11)**. Hypothalamic defects associated with GnRH deficiency include Kallmann syndrome and mutations in more than a dozen genes that regulate GnRH neuron migration, development, and function (see above). Mutations in GPR54, DAX1, kisspeptin, the GnRH receptor, and the LHβ or FSHβ subunit genes also cause pituitary gonadotropin deficiency. Acquired forms of GnRH deficiency leading to hypogonadotropism are seen in association with anorexia nervosa, stress, starvation, and extreme exercise but also may be idiopathic. Hypogonadotropic hypogonadism in these disorders is reversed by removal of the stressful stimulus or by caloric replenishment.

PRESENTATION AND DIAGNOSIS

In premenopausal women, hypogonadotropic hypogonadism presents as diminished ovarian function leading to oligomenorrhea or amenorrhea, infertility, decreased vaginal secretions, decreased libido, and breast atrophy. In hypogonadal adult men, secondary testicular failure is associated with decreased libido and potency, infertility, decreased muscle mass with weakness, reduced beard and body hair growth, soft testes, and characteristic fine facial wrinkles. Osteoporosis occurs in both untreated hypogonadal women and men.

LABORATORY INVESTIGATION

Central hypogonadism is associated with low or inappropriately normal serum gonadotropin levels in the setting of low sex hormone concentrations (testosterone in men, estradiol in women). Because gonadotropin secretion is pulsatile, valid assessments may require repeated measurements or the use of pooled serum samples. Men have reduced sperm counts.

Intravenous GnRH (100 μg) stimulates gonadotropes to secrete LH (which peaks within 30 min) and FSH (which plateaus during the ensuing 60 min). Normal responses vary according to menstrual cycle stage, age, and sex of the patient. Generally, LH levels increase about threefold, whereas FSH responses are less pronounced. In the setting of gonadotropin deficiency, a normal gonadotropin response to GnRH indicates intact pituitary gonadotrope function and suggests a hypothalamic abnormality. An absent response, however, does not reliably distinguish pituitary from hypothalamic causes of hypogonadism. For this reason, GnRH testing usually adds little to the information gained from baseline evaluation of the hypothalamic-pituitary-gonadotrope axis except in cases of isolated GnRH deficiency (e.g., Kallmann syndrome).

TREATMENT Gonadotropin Deficiency

In males, testosterone replacement is necessary to achieve and maintain normal growth and development of the external genitalia, secondary sex characteristics, male sexual behavior, and androgenic anabolic effects, including maintenance of muscle function and bone mass. Testosterone may be administered by intramuscular injections every 1–4 weeks or by using skin patches that are replaced daily **(Chap. 11)**. Testosterone gels are also available. Gonadotropin injections (hCG or human menopausal gonadotropin [hMG]) over 12–18 months are used to restore fertility. Pulsatile GnRH therapy (25–150 ng/kg every 2 h), administered by a subcutaneous infusion pump, is also effective for treatment of hypothalamic hypogonadism when fertility is desired.

In premenopausal women, cyclical replacement of estrogen and progesterone maintains secondary sexual characteristics and integrity of genitourinary tract mucosa and prevents premature osteoporosis **(Chap. 13)**. Gonadotropin therapy is used for ovulation induction. Follicular growth and maturation are initiated using hMG or recombinant FSH; hCG or human luteinizing hormone (hLH) is subsequently injected to induce ovulation. As in men, pulsatile GnRH therapy can be used to treat hypothalamic causes of gonadotropin deficiency.

MRI examination of the sellar region and assessment of other pituitary functions usually are indicated in patients with documented central hypogonadism.

DIABETES INSIPIDUS

See Chap. 6 for diagnosis and treatment of diabetes insipidus.

CHAPTER 5

ANTERIOR PITUITARY TUMOR SYNDROMES

Shlomo Melmed ■ J. Larry Jameson

HYPOTHALAMIC, PITUITARY, AND OTHER SELLAR MASSES

EVALUATION OF SELLAR MASSES

Local mass effects

Clinical manifestations of sellar lesions vary, depending on the anatomic location of the mass and the direction of its extension (Table 5-1). The dorsal sellar diaphragm presents the least resistance to soft tissue expansion from the sella; consequently, pituitary adenomas frequently extend in a suprasellar direction. Bony invasion may occur as well.

Headaches are common features of small intrasellar tumors, even with no demonstrable suprasellar extension. Because of the confined nature of the pituitary, small changes in intrasellar pressure stretch the dural plate; however, headache severity correlates poorly with adenoma size or extension.

Suprasellar extension can lead to visual loss by several mechanisms, the most common being compression of the optic chiasm, but rarely, direct invasion of the optic nerves or obstruction of cerebrospinal fluid (CSF) flow leading to secondary visual disturbances can occur. Pituitary stalk compression by a hormonally active or inactive intrasellar mass may compress the portal vessels, disrupting pituitary access to hypothalamic hormones and dopamine; this results in early hyperprolactinemia and later concurrent loss of other pituitary hormones. This "stalk section" phenomenon may also be caused by trauma, whiplash injury with posterior clinoid stalk compression, or skull base fractures. Lateral mass invasion may impinge on the cavernous sinus and compress its neural contents, leading to cranial nerve III, IV, and VI palsies as well as effects on the ophthalmic and maxillary branches of the fifth cranial nerve. Patients may present with diplopia, ptosis, ophthalmoplegia, and decreased facial sensation, depending on the extent of neural damage. Extension into the sphenoid sinus indicates that the pituitary mass has eroded through the sellar floor. Aggressive tumors rarely invade the palate roof and cause nasopharyngeal obstruction, infection, and CSF leakage. Temporal and frontal lobe involvement may rarely lead to uncinate seizures, personality disorders, and anosmia. Direct hypothalamic encroachment by an invasive pituitary mass may cause important metabolic sequelae, including precocious puberty or hypogonadism, diabetes insipidus, sleep disturbances, dysthermia, and appetite disorders.

Magnetic resonance imaging

Sagittal and coronal T1-weighted magnetic resonance imaging (MRI) before and after administration of gadolinium allows precise visualization of the pituitary gland with clear delineation of the hypothalamus, pituitary stalk, pituitary tissue and surrounding suprasellar cisterns, cavernous sinuses, sphenoid sinus, and optic chiasm. Pituitary gland height ranges from 6 mm in children to 8 mm in adults; during pregnancy and puberty, the height may reach 10–12 mm. The upper aspect of the adult pituitary is flat or slightly concave, but in adolescent and pregnant individuals, this surface may be convex, reflecting physiologic pituitary enlargement. The stalk should be midline and vertical. Computed tomography (CT) scan is reserved to define the extent of bony erosion or the presence of calcification.

Anterior pituitary gland soft tissue consistency is slightly heterogeneous on MRI, and signal intensity resembles that of brain matter on T1-weighted imaging (Fig. 5-1). Adenoma density is usually lower than that of surrounding normal tissue on T1-weighted imaging, and the signal intensity increases with T2-weighted images. The high phospholipid content of the posterior pituitary results in a "pituitary bright spot."

Sellar masses are encountered commonly as incidental findings on MRI, and most of them are pituitary

TABLE 5-1

FEATURES OF SELLAR MASS LESIONS[a]

IMPACTED STRUCTURE	CLINICAL IMPACT
Pituitary	Hypogonadism Hypothyroidism Growth failure and adult hyposomatotropism Hypoadrenalism
Optic chiasm	Loss of red perception Bitemporal hemianopia Superior or bitemporal field defect Scotoma Blindness
Hypothalamus	Temperature dysregulation Appetite and thirst disorders Obesity Diabetes insipidus Sleep disorders Behavioral dysfunction Autonomic dysfunction
Cavernous sinus	Ophthalmoplegia with or without ptosis or diplopia Facial numbness
Frontal lobe	Personality disorder Anosmia
Brain	Headache Hydrocephalus Psychosis Dementia Laughing seizures

[a]As the intrasellar mass expands, it first compresses intrasellar pituitary tissue, then usually invades dorsally through the dura to lift the optic chiasm or laterally to the cavernous sinuses. Bony erosion is rare, as is direct brain compression. Microadenomas may present with headache.

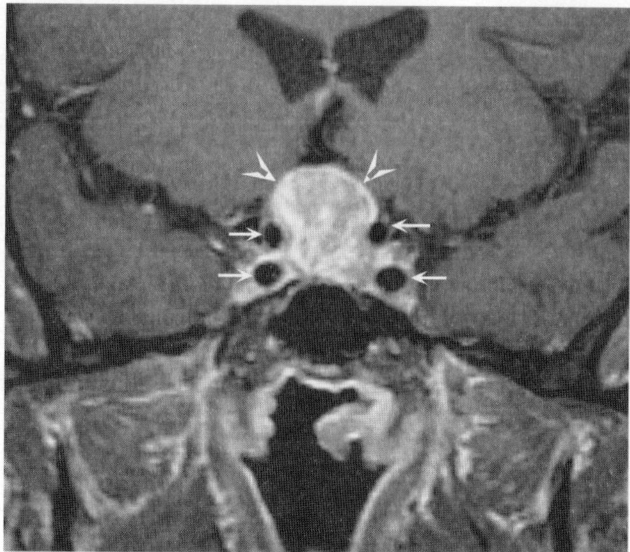

FIGURE 5-1

Pituitary adenoma. Coronal T1-weighted postcontrast magnetic resonance image shows a homogeneously enhancing mass (*arrowheads*) in the sella turcica and suprasellar region compatible with a pituitary adenoma; the *small arrows* outline the carotid arteries.

adenomas (incidentalomas). In the absence of hormone hypersecretion, these small intrasellar lesions can be monitored safely with MRI, which is performed annually and then less often if there is no evidence of further growth. Resection should be considered for incidentally discovered larger macroadenomas, because about one-third become invasive or cause local pressure effects. If hormone hypersecretion is evident, specific therapies are indicated as described below. When larger masses (>1 cm) are encountered, they should also be distinguished from nonadenomatous lesions. Meningiomas often are associated with bony hyperostosis; craniopharyngiomas may be calcified and are usually hypodense, whereas gliomas are hyperdense on T2-weighted images.

Ophthalmologic evaluation

Because optic tracts may be contiguous to an expanding pituitary mass, reproducible visual field assessment using perimetry techniques should be performed on all patients with sellar mass lesions that impinge the optic chiasm. Bitemporal hemianopia, often more pronounced superiorly, is observed classically. It occurs because nasal ganglion cell fibers, which cross in the optic chiasm, are especially vulnerable to compression of the ventral optic chiasm. Occasionally, homonymous hemianopia occurs from postchiasmal compression or monocular temporal field loss from prechiasmal compression. Invasion of the cavernous sinus can produce diplopia from ocular motor nerve palsy. Early diagnosis reduces the risk of optic atrophy, vision loss, or eye misalignment.

Laboratory investigation

The presenting clinical features of functional pituitary adenomas (e.g., acromegaly, prolactinomas, or Cushing's syndrome) should guide the laboratory studies (Table 5-2). However, for a sellar mass with no obvious clinical features of hormone excess, laboratory studies are geared toward determining the nature of the tumor and assessing the possible presence of hypopituitarism. When a pituitary adenoma is suspected based on MRI, initial hormonal evaluation usually includes (1) basal prolactin (PRL); (2) insulin-like growth factor (IGF) I; (3) 24-h urinary free cortisol (UFC) and/or overnight oral dexamethasone (1 mg) suppression test; (4) α subunit, follicle-stimulating hormone (FSH), and luteinizing hormone (LH); and (5) thyroid function tests. Additional hormonal evaluation may be indicated based on the results of these tests. Pending more detailed assessment of hypopituitarism, a menstrual history, measurement of testosterone and 8 A.M. cortisol levels, and thyroid function

TABLE 5-2

SCREENING TESTS FOR FUNCTIONAL PITUITARY ADENOMAS

	TEST	COMMENTS
Acromegaly	Serum IGF-I	Interpret IGF-I relative to age- and sex-matched controls
	Oral glucose tolerance test with GH obtained at 0, 30, and 60 min	Normal subjects should suppress growth hormone to <1 g/L
Prolactinoma	Serum PRL	Exclude medications MRI of the sella should be ordered if PRL is elevated
Cushing's disease	24-h urinary free cortisol	Ensure urine collection is total and accurate
	Dexamethasone (1 mg) at 11 P.M. and fasting plasma cortisol measured at 8 A.M.	Normal subjects suppress to <5 g/dL
	ACTH assay	Distinguishes adrenal adenoma (ACTH suppressed) from ectopic ACTH or Cushing's disease (ACTH normal or elevated)

Abbreviations: ACTH, adrenocorticotropin hormone; GH, growth hormone; IGF-I, insulin-like growth factor I; MRI, magnetic resonance imaging; PRL, prolactin.

tests usually identify patients with pituitary hormone deficiencies that require hormone replacement before further testing or surgery.

Histologic evaluation

Immunohistochemical staining of pituitary tumor specimens obtained at transsphenoidal surgery confirms clinical and laboratory studies and provides a histologic diagnosis when hormone studies are equivocal and in cases of clinically nonfunctioning tumors. Occasionally, ultrastructural assessment by electron microscopy is required for diagnosis.

TREATMENT Hypothalamic, Pituitary, and Other Sellar Masses

OVERVIEW Successful management of sellar masses requires accurate diagnosis as well as selection of optimal therapeutic modalities. Most pituitary tumors are benign and slow-growing. Clinical features result from local mass effects and hormonal hyper- or hyposecretion syndromes caused directly by the adenoma or occurring as a consequence of treatment. Thus, lifelong management and follow-up are necessary for these patients.

MRI with gadolinium enhancement for pituitary visualization, new advances in transsphenoidal surgery and in stereotactic radiotherapy (including gamma-knife radiotherapy), and novel therapeutic agents have improved pituitary tumor management. The goals of pituitary tumor treatment include normalization of excess pituitary secretion, amelioration of symptoms and signs of hormonal hypersecretion syndromes, and shrinkage or ablation of large tumor masses with relief of adjacent structure compression. Residual anterior pituitary function should be preserved during treatment and sometimes can be restored by removing the tumor mass. Ideally, adenoma recurrence should be prevented.

TRANSSPHENOIDAL SURGERY Transsphenoidal rather than transfrontal resection is the desired surgical approach for pituitary tumors, except for the rare invasive suprasellar mass surrounding the frontal or middle fossa or the optic nerves or invading posteriorly behind the clivus. Intraoperative microscopy facilitates visual distinction between adenomatous and normal pituitary tissue as well as microdissection of small tumors that may not be visible by MRI (Fig. 5-2). Transsphenoidal surgery also avoids the cranial invasion and manipulation of brain tissue required by subfrontal surgical approaches. Endoscopic techniques with three-dimensional intraoperative localization have also improved visualization and access to tumor tissue. Individual surgical experience is a major determinant of outcome efficacy with these techniques.

In addition to correction of hormonal hypersecretion, pituitary surgery is indicated for mass lesions that impinge on surrounding structures. Surgical decompression and resection are required for an expanding pituitary mass accompanied by persistent headache, progressive visual field defects, cranial nerve palsies, hydrocephalus, and, occasionally, intrapituitary hemorrhage and apoplexy. Transsphenoidal surgery sometimes is used for pituitary tissue biopsy to establish a histologic diagnosis. Whenever possible, the pituitary mass lesion should be selectively excised; normal pituitary tissue should be manipulated or resected only when critical for effective mass dissection. Nonselective hemihypophysectomy or total hypophysectomy may be indicated if no hypersecreting mass lesion is clearly discernible, multifocal lesions are present, or the remaining nontumorous pituitary tissue is obviously necrotic. This strategy, however, increases the likelihood of hypopituitarism and the need for lifelong hormone replacement.

Preoperative mass effects, including visual field defects and compromised pituitary function, may be reversed by surgery, particularly when the deficits are not long-standing. For large and invasive tumors, it is necessary to determine the optimal balance between maximal tumor resection and preservation of anterior pituitary function, especially for

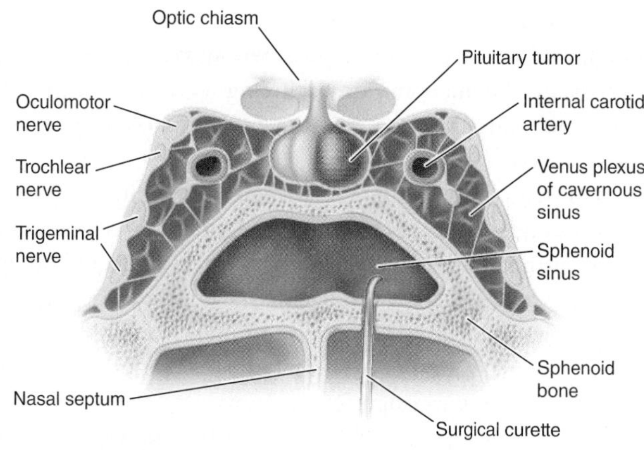

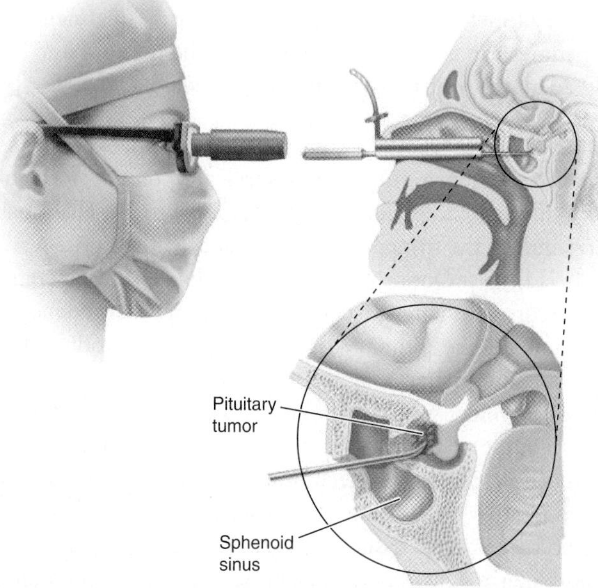

FIGURE 5-2

Transsphenoidal resection of pituitary mass via the endonasal approach. *(Adapted from R Fahlbusch: Endocrinol Metab Clin 21:669, 1992.)*

preserving growth and reproductive function in younger patients. Similarly, tumor invasion outside the sella is rarely amenable to surgical cure; the surgeon must judge the risk-versus-benefit ratio of extensive tumor resection.

Side Effects Tumor size, the degree of invasiveness, and experience of the surgeon largely determine the incidence of surgical complications. Operative mortality rate is about 1%. Transient diabetes insipidus and hypopituitarism occur in up to 20% of patients. Permanent diabetes insipidus, cranial nerve damage, nasal septal perforation, or visual disturbances may be encountered in up to 10% of patients. CSF leaks occur in 4% of patients. Less common complications include carotid artery injury, loss of vision, hypothalamic damage, and meningitis. Permanent side effects are rare after surgery for microadenomas.

RADIATION Radiation is used either as a primary therapy for pituitary or parasellar masses or, more commonly, as an adjunct to surgery or medical therapy. Focused megavoltage irradiation is achieved by precise MRI localization, using a high-voltage linear accelerator and accurate isocentric rotational arcing. A major determinant of accurate irradiation is reproduction of the patient's head position during multiple visits and maintenance of absolute head immobility. A total of <50 Gy (5000 rad) is given as 180-cGy (180-rad) fractions divided over about 6 weeks. Stereotactic radiosurgery delivers a large single high-energy dose from a cobalt-60 source (gamma knife), linear accelerator, or cyclotron. Long-term effects of gamma-knife surgery are unclear but appear to be similar to those encountered with conventional radiation. Proton beam therapy is available in some centers and provides concentrated radiation doses within a localized region.

The role of radiation therapy in pituitary tumor management depends on multiple factors, including the nature of the tumor, the age of the patient, and the availability of surgical and radiation expertise. Because of its relatively slow onset of action, radiation therapy is usually reserved for postsurgical management. As an adjuvant to surgery, radiation is used to treat residual tumor and in an attempt to prevent regrowth. Irradiation offers the only means for potentially ablating significant postoperative residual nonfunctioning tumor tissue. In contrast, PRL- and growth hormone (GH)-secreting tumor tissues are amenable to medical therapy.

Side Effects In the short term, radiation may cause transient nausea and weakness. Alopecia and loss of taste and smell may be more long-lasting. Failure of pituitary hormone synthesis is common in patients who have undergone head and neck or pituitary-directed irradiation. More than 50% of patients develop loss of GH, adrenocorticotropin hormone (ACTH), thyroid-stimulating hormone (TSH), and/or gonadotropin secretion within 10 years, usually due to hypothalamic damage. Lifelong follow-up with testing of anterior pituitary hormone reserve is therefore required after radiation treatment. Optic nerve damage with impaired vision due to optic neuritis is reported in about 2% of patients who undergo pituitary irradiation. Cranial nerve damage is uncommon now that radiation doses are ≤2 Gy (200 rad) at any one treatment session and the maximum dose is <50 Gy (5000 rad). The use of stereotactic radiotherapy may reduce damage to adjacent structures. Radiotherapy for pituitary tumors has been associated with adverse mortality rates, mainly from cerebrovascular disease. The cumulative risk of developing a secondary tumor after conventional radiation is 1.3% after 10 years and 1.9% after 20 years.

MEDICAL Medical therapy for pituitary tumors is highly specific and depends on tumor type. For prolactinomas, dopamine agonists are the treatment of choice. For acromegaly, somatostatin analogues and GH receptor antagonists are indicated. For TSH-secreting tumors, somatostatin analogues and occasionally dopamine agonists are indicated. ACTH-secreting tumors and nonfunctioning tumors are generally not responsive to medications and require surgery and/or irradiation.

SELLAR MASSES

Sellar masses other than pituitary adenomas may arise from brain, hypothalamic, or pituitary tissues. Each exhibit features related to the lesion location but also unique to the specific etiology.

Hypothalamic lesions

Lesions involving the anterior and preoptic hypothalamic regions cause paradoxical vasoconstriction, tachycardia, and hyperthermia. Acute hyperthermia usually is due to a hemorrhagic insult, but poikilothermia may also occur. Central disorders of thermoregulation result from posterior hypothalamic damage. The *periodic hypothermia syndrome* is characterized by episodic attacks of rectal temperatures <30°C (86°F), sweating, vasodilation, vomiting, and bradycardia. Damage to the ventromedial hypothalamic nuclei by craniopharyngiomas, hypothalamic trauma, or inflammatory disorders may be associated with *hyperphagia* and *obesity*. This region appears to contain an energy-satiety center where melanocortin receptors are influenced by leptin, insulin, pro-opiomelanocortin (POMC) products, and gastrointestinal peptides **(Chap. 20)**. Polydipsia and hypodipsia are associated with damage to central osmoreceptors located in preoptic nuclei **(Chap. 6)**. Slow-growing hypothalamic lesions can cause increased somnolence and disturbed sleep cycles as well as obesity, hypothermia, and emotional outbursts. Lesions of the central hypothalamus may stimulate sympathetic neurons, leading to elevated serum catecholamine and cortisol levels. These patients are predisposed to cardiac arrhythmias, hypertension, and gastric erosions.

Craniopharyngiomas are benign, suprasellar cystic masses that present with headaches, visual field deficits, and variable degrees of hypopituitarism. They are derived from Rathke's pouch and arise near the pituitary stalk, commonly extending into the suprasellar cistern. Craniopharyngiomas are often large, cystic, and locally invasive. Many are partially calcified, exhibiting a characteristic appearance on skull x-ray and CT images. More than half of all patients present before age 20, usually with signs of increased intracranial pressure, including headache, vomiting, papilledema, and hydrocephalus. Associated symptoms include visual field abnormalities, personality changes and cognitive deterioration, cranial nerve damage, sleep difficulties, and weight gain. Hypopituitarism can be documented in about 90%, and diabetes insipidus occurs in about 10% of patients. About half of affected children present with growth retardation. MRI is generally superior to CT for evaluating cystic structure and tissue components of craniopharyngiomas. CT is useful to define calcifications and evaluate invasion into surrounding bony structures and sinuses.

Treatment usually involves transcranial or transsphenoidal surgical resection followed by postoperative radiation of residual tumor. Surgery alone is curative in less than half of patients because of recurrences due to adherence to vital structures or because of small tumor deposits in the hypothalamus or brain parenchyma. The goal of surgery is to remove as much tumor as possible without risking complications associated with efforts to remove firmly adherent or inaccessible tissue. In the absence of radiotherapy, about 75% of craniopharyngiomas recur, and 10-year survival is less than 50%. In patients with incomplete resection, radiotherapy improves 10-year survival to 70–90% but is associated with increased risk of secondary malignancies. Most patients require lifelong pituitary hormone replacement.

Developmental failure of Rathke's pouch obliteration may lead to *Rathke's cysts*, which are small (<5 mm) cysts entrapped by squamous epithelium and are found in about 20% of individuals at autopsy. Although Rathke's cleft cysts do not usually grow and are often diagnosed incidentally, about a third present in adulthood with compressive symptoms, diabetes insipidus, and hyperprolactinemia due to stalk compression. Rarely, hydrocephalus develops. The diagnosis is suggested preoperatively by visualizing the cyst wall on MRI, which distinguishes these lesions from craniopharyngiomas. Cyst contents range from CSF-like fluid to mucoid material. *Arachnoid cysts* are rare and generate an MRI image that is isointense with CSF.

Sella chordomas usually present with bony clival erosion, local invasiveness, and, on occasion, calcification. Normal pituitary tissue may be visible on MRI, distinguishing chordomas from aggressive pituitary adenomas. Mucinous material may be obtained by fine-needle aspiration.

Meningiomas arising in the sellar region may be difficult to distinguish from nonfunctioning pituitary adenomas. Meningiomas typically enhance on MRI and may show evidence of calcification or bony erosion. Meningiomas may cause compressive symptoms.

Histiocytosis X includes a variety of syndromes associated with foci of eosinophilic granulomas. Diabetes insipidus, exophthalmos, and punched-out lytic bone lesions (*Hand-Schüller-Christian disease*) are associated with granulomatous lesions visible on MRI, as well as a characteristic axillary skin rash. Rarely, the pituitary stalk may be involved.

Pituitary metastases occur in ~3% of cancer patients. Bloodborne metastatic deposits are found almost exclusively in the posterior pituitary. Accordingly, diabetes insipidus can be a presenting feature of lung, gastrointestinal, breast, and other pituitary metastases. About half of pituitary metastases originate from breast cancer; about 25% of patients with metastatic breast cancer have such deposits. Rarely, pituitary stalk involvement results in anterior pituitary insufficiency. The MRI diagnosis of a metastatic lesion may be difficult to distinguish from an aggressive pituitary adenoma; the diagnosis may require histologic examination of excised tumor tissue. Primary or metastatic lymphoma, leukemias, and plasmacytomas also occur within the sella.

Hypothalamic hamartomas and *gangliocytomas* may arise from astrocytes, oligodendrocytes, and neurons with varying degrees of differentiation. These tumors may overexpress hypothalamic neuropeptides, including gonadotropin-releasing hormone (GnRH), growth hormone–releasing hormone (GHRH), and corticotropin-releasing hormone (CRH). With GnRH-producing tumors, children present with precocious puberty, psychomotor delay, and laughing-associated seizures. Medical treatment of GnRH-producing hamartomas with long-acting GnRH analogues effectively suppresses gonadotropin secretion and controls premature pubertal development. Rarely, hamartomas also are associated with craniofacial abnormalities; imperforate anus; cardiac, renal, and lung disorders; and pituitary failure as features of *Pallister-Hall syndrome*, which is caused by mutations in the carboxy terminus of the *GLI3* gene. Hypothalamic hamartomas are often contiguous with the pituitary, and preoperative MRI diagnosis may not be possible. Histologic evidence of hypothalamic neurons in tissue resected at transsphenoidal surgery may be the first indication of a primary hypothalamic lesion.

Hypothalamic gliomas and *optic gliomas* occur mainly in childhood and usually present with visual loss. Adults have more aggressive tumors; about a third are associated with neurofibromatosis.

Brain germ cell tumors may arise within the sellar region. They include *dysgerminomas*, which frequently are associated with diabetes insipidus and visual loss. They rarely metastasize. *Germinomas, embryonal carcinomas, teratomas*, and *choriocarcinomas* may arise in the parasellar region and produce hCG. These germ cell tumors present with precocious puberty, diabetes insipidus, visual field defects, and thirst disorders. Many patients are GH-deficient with short stature.

PITUITARY ADENOMAS AND HYPERSECRETION SYNDROMES

Pituitary adenomas are the most common cause of pituitary hormone hypersecretion and hyposecretion syndromes in adults. They account for ~15% of all intracranial neoplasms and have been identified with a population prevalence of ~80/100,000. At autopsy, up to one-quarter of all pituitary glands harbor an unsuspected microadenoma (<10 mm diameter). Similarly, pituitary imaging detects small clinically inapparent pituitary lesions in at least 10% of individuals.

Pathogenesis

Pituitary adenomas are benign neoplasms that arise from one of the five anterior pituitary cell types. The clinical and biochemical phenotypes of pituitary adenomas depend on the cell type from which they are derived. Thus, tumors arising from lactotrope (PRL), somatotrope (GH), corticotrope (ACTH), thyrotrope (TSH), or gonadotrope (LH, FSH) cells hypersecrete their respective hormones (Table 5-3). Plurihormonal tumors express various combinations of GH, PRL, TSH, ACTH, or the glycoprotein hormone α or β subunits. They may be diagnosed by careful immunocytochemistry or may manifest as clinical syndromes that combine features of these hormonal hypersecretory syndromes. Morphologically, these tumors may arise from a single polysecreting cell type or include cells with mixed function within the same tumor.

Hormonally active tumors are characterized by autonomous hormone secretion with diminished feedback responsiveness to physiologic inhibitory pathways. Hormone production does not always correlate with

TABLE 5-3

CLASSIFICATION OF PITUITARY ADENOMAS[a]

ADENOMA CELL ORIGIN	HORMONE PRODUCT	CLINICAL SYNDROME
Lactotrope	PRL	Hypogonadism, galactorrhea
Gonadotrope	FSH, LH, subunits	Silent or hypogonadism
Somatotrope	GH	Acromegaly/ gigantism
Corticotrope	ACTH	Cushing's disease
Mixed growth hormone and prolactin cell	GH, PRL	Acromegaly, hypogonadism, galactorrhea
Other plurihormonal cell	Any	Mixed
Acidophil stem cell	PRL, GH	Hypogonadism, galactorrhea, acromegaly
Mammosomatotrope	PRL, GH	Hypogonadism, galactorrhea, acromegaly
Thyrotrope	TSH	Thyrotoxicosis
Null cell	None	Pituitary failure
Oncocytoma	None	Pituitary failure

[a]Hormone-secreting tumors are listed in decreasing order of frequency. All tumors may cause local pressure effects, including visual disturbances, cranial nerve palsy, and headache.

Note: For abbreviations, see text.

Source: Adapted from S Melmed, in JL Jameson (ed): *Principles of Molecular Medicine*. Totowa, NJ, Humana Press, 1998.

tumor size. Small hormone-secreting adenomas may cause significant clinical perturbations, whereas larger adenomas that produce less hormone may be clinically silent and remain undiagnosed (if no central compressive effects occur). About one-third of all adenomas are clinically nonfunctioning and produce no distinct clinical hypersecretory syndrome. Most of them arise from gonadotrope cells and may secrete small amounts of α- and β-glycoprotein hormone subunits or, very rarely, intact circulating gonadotropins. True pituitary carcinomas with documented extracranial metastases are exceedingly rare.

Almost all pituitary adenomas are monoclonal in origin, implying the acquisition of one or more somatic mutations that confer a selective growth advantage. Consistent with their clonal origin, complete surgical resection of small pituitary adenomas usually cures hormone hypersecretion. Nevertheless, hypothalamic hormones such as GHRH and CRH also enhance mitotic activity of their respective pituitary target cells in addition to their role in pituitary hormone regulation. Thus, patients who harbor rare abdominal or chest tumors that elaborate ectopic GHRH or CRH may present with somatotrope or corticotrope hyperplasia with GH or ACTH hypersecretion.

Several etiologic genetic events have been implicated in the development of pituitary tumors. The pathogenesis of sporadic forms of acromegaly has been particularly informative as a model of tumorigenesis. GHRH, after binding to its G protein–coupled somatotrope receptor, uses cyclic adenosine monophosphate (AMP) as a second messenger to stimulate GH secretion and somatotrope proliferation. A subset (~35%) of GH-secreting pituitary tumors contains sporadic mutations in Gsα (Arg 201 → Cys or His; Gln 227 → Arg). These mutations attenuate intrinsic GTPase activity, resulting in constitutive elevation of cyclic AMP, Pit-1 induction, and activation of cyclic AMP response element binding protein (CREB), thereby promoting somatotrope cell proliferation and GH secretion.

Characteristic loss of heterozygosity (LOH) in various chromosomes has been documented in large or invasive macroadenomas, suggesting the presence of putative tumor suppressor genes at these loci in up to 20% of sporadic pituitary tumors, including GH-, PRL-, and ACTH-producing adenomas and some nonfunctioning tumors. Lineage-specific cell cycle disruptions with elevated levels of CDK inhibitors are present in most of these adenomas.

Compelling evidence also favors growth factor promotion of pituitary tumor proliferation. Basic fibroblast growth factor (bFGF) is abundant in the pituitary and stimulates pituitary cell mitogenesis, whereas epithelial growth factor (EGF) receptor signaling induces both hormone synthesis and cell proliferation. Other factors involved in initiation and promotion of pituitary tumors include loss of negative-feedback inhibition (as seen with primary hypothyroidism or hypogonadism) and estrogen-mediated or paracrine angiogenesis. Growth characteristics and neoplastic behavior also may be influenced by several activated oncogenes, including *RAS* and pituitary tumor transforming gene (*PTTG*), or inactivation of growth suppressor genes, including *MEG3*.

Genetic syndromes associated with pituitary tumors

Several familial syndromes are associated with pituitary tumors, and the genetic mechanisms for some of them have been unraveled (Table 5-4).

Multiple endocrine neoplasia (MEN) 1 is an autosomal dominant syndrome characterized primarily by a genetic predisposition to parathyroid, pancreatic islet, and pituitary adenomas (**Chap. 29**). MEN1 is caused by inactivating germline mutations in *MENIN*, a constitutively expressed tumor-suppressor gene located on chromosome 11q13. Loss of heterozygosity or a somatic mutation of the remaining normal *MENIN* allele leads to tumorigenesis. About half of affected patients

TABLE 5-4

FAMILIAL PITUITARY TUMOR SYNDROMES

	GENE MUTATED	CLINICAL FEATURES
Multiple endocrine neoplasia 1 (MEN 1)	*MEN1* (11q13)	Hyperparathyroidism Pancreatic neuroendocrine tumors Foregut carcinoids Adrenal adenomas Skin lesions Pituitary adenomas (40%)
Multiple endocrine neoplasia 4 (MEN 4)	*CDKNIB* (12p13)	Hyperparathyroidism Pituitary adenomas Other tumors
Carney complex	*PRKAR1A* (17q23–24)	Pituitary hyperplasia andadenomas (10%) Atrial myxomas Schwannomas Adrenal hyperplasia Lentigines
Familial pituitary adenomas	*AIP* (11q13.3)	Acromegaly/gigantism (~15% of afflicted families)

develop prolactinomas; acromegaly and Cushing's syndrome are less commonly encountered.

Carney's syndrome is characterized by spotty skin pigmentation, myxomas, and endocrine tumors, including testicular, adrenal, and pituitary adenomas. Acromegaly occurs in about 20% of these patients. A subset of patients have mutations in the R1α regulatory subunit of protein kinase A (*PRKAR1A*).

McCune-Albright syndrome consists of polyostotic fibrous dysplasia, pigmented skin patches, and a variety of endocrine disorders, including acromegaly, adrenal adenomas, and autonomous ovarian function (**Chap. 36**). Hormonal hypersecretion results from constitutive cyclic AMP production caused by inactivation of the GTPase activity of Gsα. The Gsα mutations occur postzygotically, leading to a mosaic pattern of mutant expression.

Familial acromegaly is a rare disorder in which family members may manifest either acromegaly or gigantism. A subset of families with a predisposition for familial pituitary tumors, especially acromegaly, have been found to harbor germline mutations in the *AIP* gene, which encodes the aryl hydrocarbon receptor interacting protein.

HYPERPROLACTINEMIA

Etiology

Hyperprolactinemia is the most common pituitary hormone hypersecretion syndrome in both men and women. PRL-secreting pituitary adenomas (prolactinomas) are the most common cause of PRL levels >200 μg/L (see below). Less pronounced PRL elevation can also be seen with microprolactinomas but is more commonly caused by drugs, pituitary stalk compression, hypothyroidism, or renal failure (Table 5-5).

Pregnancy and lactation are the important physiologic causes of hyperprolactinemia. Sleep-associated hyperprolactinemia reverts to normal within an hour of awakening. Nipple stimulation and sexual orgasm also may increase PRL. Chest wall stimulation or trauma (including chest surgery and herpes zoster) invoke the reflex suckling arc with resultant hyperprolactinemia. Chronic renal failure elevates PRL by decreasing peripheral clearance. Primary hypothyroidism is associated with mild hyperprolactinemia, probably because of compensatory TRH secretion.

Lesions of the hypothalamic-pituitary region that disrupt hypothalamic dopamine synthesis, portal vessel delivery, or lactotrope responses are associated with hyperprolactinemia. Thus, hypothalamic tumors, cysts, infiltrative disorders, and radiation-induced damage cause elevated PRL levels, usually in the range of 30–100 μg/L. Plurihormonal adenomas (including GH and ACTH tumors) may hypersecrete PRL directly.

TABLE 5-5

ETIOLOGY OF HYPERPROLACTINEMIA

I. Physiologic hypersecretion
- Pregnancy
- Lactation
- Chest wall stimulation
- Sleep
- Stress

II. Hypothalamic–pituitary stalk damage
- Tumors
  - Craniopharyngioma
  - Suprasellar pituitary mass
  - Meningioma
  - Dysgerminoma
  - Metastases
- Empty sella
- Lymphocytic hypophysitis
- Adenoma with stalk
- Compression
- Granulomas
- Rathke's cyst
- Irradiation
- Trauma
  - Pituitary stalk section
  - Suprasellar surgery

III. Pituitary hypersecretion
- Prolactinoma
- Acromegaly

IV. Systemic disorders
- Chronic renal failure
- Hypothyroidism
- Cirrhosis
- Pseudocyesis
- Epileptic seizures

V. Drug-induced hypersecretion
- Dopamine receptor blockers
  - Atypical antipsychotics: risperidone
  - Phenothiazines: chlorpromazine, perphenazine
  - Butyrophenones: haloperidol
  - Thioxanthenes
  - Metoclopramide
- Dopamine synthesis inhibitors
  - α-Methyldopa
- Catecholamine depletors
  - Reserpine
- Opiates
- H_2 antagonists
  - Cimetidine, ranitidine
- Imipramines
  - Amitriptyline, amoxapine
- Serotonin reuptake inhibitors
  - Fluoxetine
- Calcium channel blockers
  - Verapamil
  - Estrogens
  - Thyrotropin-releasing hormone

Note: Hyperprolactinemia >200 μg/L almost invariably is indicative of a prolactin-secreting pituitary adenoma. Physiologic causes, hypothyroidism, and drug-induced hyperprolactinemia should be excluded before extensive evaluation.

Pituitary masses, including clinically nonfunctioning pituitary tumors, may compress the pituitary stalk to cause hyperprolactinemia.

Drug-induced inhibition or disruption of dopaminergic receptor function is a common cause of hyperprolactinemia (Table 5-5). Thus, antipsychotics and antidepressants are a relatively common cause of mild hyperprolactinemia. Most patients receiving risperidone have elevated prolactin levels, sometimes exceeding 200 μg/L. Methyldopa inhibits dopamine synthesis, and verapamil blocks dopamine release, also leading to hyperprolactinemia. Hormonal agents that induce PRL include estrogens and thyrotropin-releasing hormone (TRH).

Presentation and diagnosis

Amenorrhea, galactorrhea, and infertility are the hallmarks of hyperprolactinemia in women. If hyperprolactinemia develops before menarche, primary amenorrhea results. More commonly, hyperprolactinemia develops later in life and leads to oligomenorrhea and ultimately to amenorrhea. If hyperprolactinemia is sustained, vertebral bone mineral density can be reduced compared with age-matched controls, particularly when it is associated with pronounced hypoestrogenemia. Galactorrhea is present in up to 80% of hyperprolactinemic women. Although usually bilateral and spontaneous, it may be unilateral or expressed only manually. Patients also may complain of decreased libido, weight gain, and mild hirsutism.

In men with hyperprolactinemia, diminished libido, infertility, and visual loss (from optic nerve compression) are the usual presenting symptoms. Gonadotropin suppression leads to reduced testosterone, impotence, and oligospermia. True galactorrhea is uncommon in men with hyperprolactinemia. If the disorder is long-standing, secondary effects of hypogonadism are evident, including osteopenia, reduced muscle mass, and decreased beard growth.

The diagnosis of idiopathic hyperprolactinemia is made by exclusion of known causes of hyperprolactinemia in the setting of a normal pituitary MRI. Some of these patients may harbor small microadenomas below visible MRI sensitivity (~2 mm).

GALACTORRHEA

Galactorrhea, the inappropriate discharge of milk-containing fluid from the breast, is considered abnormal if it persists longer than 6 months after childbirth or discontinuation of breast-feeding. Postpartum galactorrhea associated with amenorrhea is a self-limiting disorder usually associated with moderately elevated PRL levels. Galactorrhea may occur spontaneously, or it may be elicited by nipple pressure. In both men and women, galactorrhea may vary in color and consistency (transparent, milky, or bloody) and arise either unilaterally or bilaterally. Mammography or ultrasound is indicated for bloody discharges (particularly from a single nipple), which may be caused by breast cancer. Galactorrhea is commonly associated with hyperprolactinemia caused by any of the conditions listed in Table 5-5. Acromegaly is associated with galactorrhea in about one-third of patients. Treatment of galactorrhea usually involves managing the underlying disorder (e.g., replacing T_4 for hypothyroidism, discontinuing a medication, treating prolactinoma).

Laboratory investigation

Basal, fasting morning PRL levels (normally <20 μg/L) should be measured to assess hypersecretion. Both false-positive and false-negative results may be encountered. In patients with markedly elevated PRL levels (>1000 μg/L), reported results may be falsely lowered because of assay artifacts; sample dilution is required to measure these high values accurately. Falsely elevated values may be caused by aggregated forms of circulating PRL, which are usually biologically inactive (macroprolactinemia). Hypothyroidism should be excluded by measuring TSH and T_4 levels.

TREATMENT Hyperprolactinemia

Treatment of hyperprolactinemia depends on the cause of elevated PRL levels. Regardless of the etiology, however, treatment should be aimed at normalizing PRL levels to alleviate suppressive effects on gonadal function, halt galactorrhea, and preserve bone mineral density. Dopamine agonists are effective for most causes of hyperprolactinemia (see the treatment section for prolactinoma, below) regardless of the underlying cause.

If the patient is taking a medication known to cause hyperprolactinemia, the drug should be withdrawn, if possible. For psychiatric patients who require neuroleptic agents, supervised dose titration or the addition of a dopamine agonist can help restore normoprolactinemia and alleviate reproductive symptoms. However, dopamine agonists may worsen the underlying psychiatric condition, especially at high doses. Hyperprolactinemia usually resolves after adequate thyroid hormone replacement in hypothyroid patients or after renal transplantation in patients undergoing dialysis. Resection of hypothalamic or sellar mass lesions can reverse hyperprolactinemia caused by stalk compression and reduced dopamine tone. Granulomatous infiltrates occasionally respond to glucocorticoid administration. In patients with irreversible hypothalamic damage, no treatment may be warranted. In up to 30% of patients with hyperprolactinemia—usually without a visible pituitary microadenoma—the condition may resolve spontaneously.

PROLACTINOMA

Etiology and prevalence

Tumors arising from lactotrope cells account for about half of all functioning pituitary tumors, with a population prevalence of ~10/100,000 in men and ~30/100,000 in women. Mixed tumors that secrete combinations of GH and PRL, ACTH and PRL, and rarely TSH and PRL are also seen. These plurihormonal tumors are usually recognized by immunohistochemistry, sometimes without apparent clinical manifestations from the production of additional hormones. Microadenomas are classified as <1 cm in diameter and usually do not invade the parasellar region. Macroadenomas are >1 cm in diameter and may be locally invasive and impinge on adjacent structures. The female-to-male ratio for microprolactinomas is 20:1, whereas the sex ratio is near 1:1 for macroadenomas. Tumor size generally correlates directly with PRL concentrations; values >250 μg/L usually are associated with macroadenomas. Men tend to present with larger tumors than women, possibly because the features of male hypogonadism are less readily evident. PRL levels remain stable in most patients, reflecting the slow growth of these tumors. About 5% of microadenomas progress in the long term to macroadenomas.

Presentation and diagnosis

Women usually present with amenorrhea, infertility, and galactorrhea. If the tumor extends outside the sella, visual field defects or other mass effects may be seen. Men often present with impotence, loss of libido, infertility, or signs of central nervous system (CNS) compression, including headaches and visual defects. Assuming that physiologic and medication-induced causes of hyperprolactinemia are excluded (Table 5-5), the diagnosis of prolactinoma is likely with a PRL level >200 μg/L. PRL levels <100 μg/L may be caused by microadenomas, other sellar lesions that decrease dopamine inhibition, or nonneoplastic causes of hyperprolactinemia. For this reason, an MRI should be performed in all patients with hyperprolactinemia. It is important to remember that hyperprolactinemia caused secondarily by the mass effects of nonlactotrope lesions is also corrected by treatment with dopamine agonists despite failure to shrink the underlying mass. Consequently, PRL suppression by dopamine agonists does not necessarily indicate that the underlying lesion is a prolactinoma.

TREATMENT Prolactinoma

Because microadenomas rarely progress to become macroadenomas, no treatment may be needed if patients are asymptomatic and fertility is not desired; these patients should be monitored by regular serial PRL measurements and MRI scans. For symptomatic microadenomas, therapeutic goals include control of hyperprolactinemia, reduction of tumor size, restoration of menses and fertility, and resolution of galactorrhea. Dopamine agonist doses should be titrated to achieve maximal PRL suppression and restoration of reproductive function (Fig. 5-3). A normalized PRL level does not ensure reduced tumor size. However, tumor shrinkage usually is not seen in those who do not respond with lowered PRL levels. For macroadenomas, formal visual field testing should be performed before initiating dopamine agonists. MRI and visual fields should be assessed at 6- to 12-month intervals until the mass shrinks and annually thereafter until maximum size reduction has occurred.

MEDICAL Oral dopamine agonists (cabergoline and bromocriptine) are the mainstay of therapy for patients with micro- or macroprolactinomas. Dopamine agonists suppress PRL secretion and synthesis as well as lactotrope cell proliferation. In patients with microadenomas who have achieved normoprolactinemia and significant reduction of tumor mass, the dopamine agonist may be withdrawn after 2 years. These patients should be monitored carefully for evidence of prolactinoma recurrence. About 20% of patients (especially males) are resistant to dopaminergic treatment; these adenomas may exhibit decreased D_2 dopamine receptor numbers or a postreceptor defect. D_2 receptor gene mutations in the pituitary have not been reported.

Cabergoline An ergoline derivative, cabergoline is a long-acting dopamine agonist with high D_2 receptor affinity. The drug effectively suppresses PRL for >14 days after a single oral dose and induces prolactinoma shrinkage in most patients. Cabergoline (0.5–1.0 mg twice weekly) achieves normoprolactinemia and resumption of normal gonadal function in ~80% of patients with microadenomas; galactorrhea improves or resolves in 90% of patients. Cabergoline normalizes PRL and shrinks ~70% of macroprolactinomas. Mass effect symptoms, including headaches and visual disorders, usually improve dramatically within days after cabergoline initiation; improvement of sexual function requires several weeks of treatment but may occur before complete normalization of prolactin levels. After initial control of PRL levels has been achieved, cabergoline should be reduced to the lowest effective maintenance dose. In ~5% of treated patients harboring a microadenoma, hyperprolactinemia may resolve and not recur when dopamine agonists are discontinued after long-term treatment. Cabergoline also may be effective in patients resistant to bromocriptine. Adverse effects and drug intolerance are encountered less commonly than with bromocriptine.

BROMOCRIPTINE The ergot alkaloid bromocriptine mesylate is a dopamine receptor agonist that suppresses prolactin secretion. Because it is short-acting, the drug is preferred when pregnancy is desired. In microadenomas, bromocriptine rapidly lowers serum prolactin levels to normal in up to 70% of

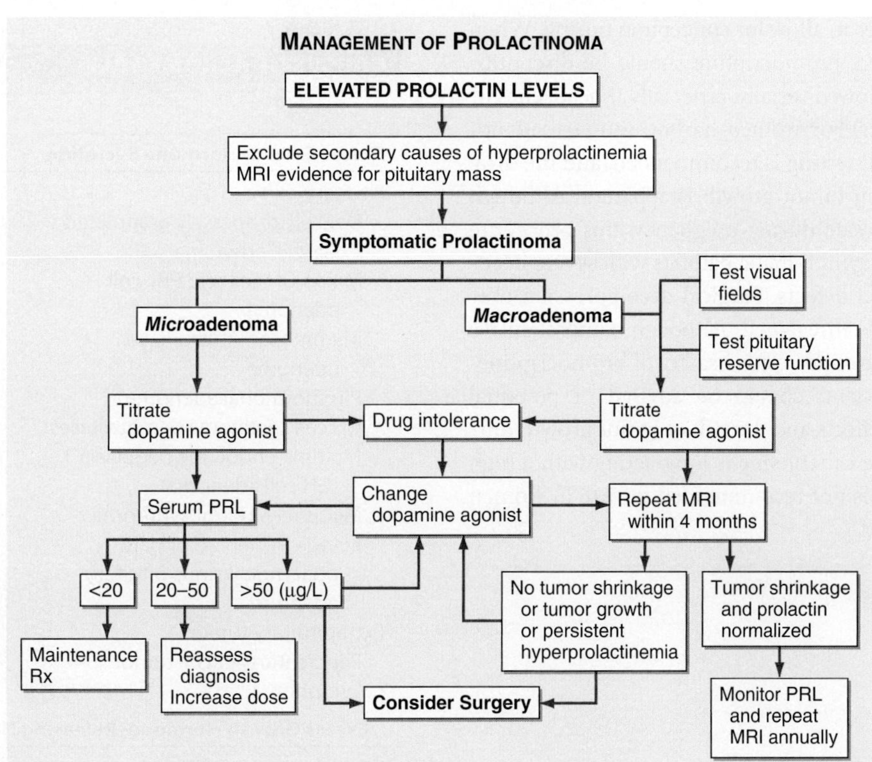

FIGURE 5-3
Management of prolactinoma. MRI, magnetic resonance imaging; PRL, prolactin.

patients, decreases tumor size, and restores gonadal function. In patients with macroadenomas, prolactin levels are also normalized in 70% of patients, and tumor mass shrinkage (≥50%) is achieved in most patients.

Therapy is initiated by administering a low bromocriptine dose (0.625–1.25 mg) at bedtime with a snack, followed by gradually increasing the dose. Most patients are controlled with a daily dose of ≤7.5 mg (2.5 mg tid).

Side Effects Side effects of dopamine agonists include constipation, nasal stuffiness, dry mouth, nightmares, insomnia, and vertigo; decreasing the dose usually alleviates these problems. Nausea, vomiting, and postural hypotension with faintness may occur in ~25% of patients after the initial dose. These symptoms may persist in some patients. In general, fewer side effects are reported with cabergoline. For the approximately 15% of patients who are intolerant of oral bromocriptine, cabergoline may be better tolerated. Intravaginal administration of bromocriptine is often efficacious in patients with intractable gastrointestinal side effects. Auditory hallucinations, delusions, and mood swings have been reported in up to 5% of patients and may be due to the dopamine agonist properties or to the lysergic acid derivative of the compounds. Rare reports of leukopenia, thrombocytopenia, pleural fibrosis, cardiac arrhythmias, and hepatitis have been described. Patients with Parkinson's disease who receive at least 3 mg of cabergoline daily have been reported to be at risk for development of cardiac valve regurgitation. Studies analyzing over 500 prolactinoma patients receiving recommended doses of cabergoline (up to 2 mg weekly) have shown no evidence for an increased incidence of valvular disorders. Nevertheless, because no controlled prospective studies in pituitary tumor patients are available, it is prudent to perform echocardiograms before initiating standard-dose cabergoline therapy.

Surgery Indications for surgical adenoma debulking include dopamine resistance or intolerance and the presence of an invasive macroadenoma with compromised vision that fails to improve after drug treatment. Initial PRL normalization is achieved in about 70% of microprolactinomas after surgical resection, but only 30% of macroadenomas can be resected successfully. Follow-up studies have shown that hyperprolactinemia recurs in up to 20% of patients within the first year after surgery; long-term recurrence rates exceed 50% for macroadenomas. Radiotherapy for prolactinomas is reserved for patients with aggressive tumors that do not respond to maximally tolerated dopamine agonists and/or surgery.

PREGNANCY The pituitary increases in size during pregnancy, reflecting the stimulatory effects of estrogen and perhaps other growth factors on pituitary vascularity and lactotrope cell hyperplasia. About 5% of microadenomas significantly increase in size, but 15–30% of macroadenomas grow during pregnancy. Bromocriptine has been used for more than 30 years to restore fertility in women with hyperprolactinemia, without evidence of teratogenic effects. Nonetheless, most authorities recommend strategies to minimize fetal exposure to the drug. For women taking bromocriptine who desire pregnancy, mechanical contraception should be used through three regular menstrual cycles to allow for conception timing. When pregnancy is confirmed, bromocriptine should be discontinued and PRL levels followed serially, especially if headaches or visual symptoms occur. For women harboring macroadenomas, regular visual field testing is recommended, and the drug should be reinstituted if tumor growth is apparent. Although pituitary MRI may be safe during pregnancy, this procedure should be reserved for symptomatic patients with severe headache and/or visual field defects. Surgical decompression may be indicated if vision is threatened. Although comprehensive data support the efficacy and relative safety of bromocriptine-facilitated fertility, patients should be advised of potential unknown deleterious effects and the risk of tumor growth during pregnancy. Because cabergoline is long-acting with a high D_2-receptor affinity, it is not recommended for use in women when fertility is desired.

ACROMEGALY

Etiology

GH hypersecretion is usually the result of a somatotrope adenoma but may rarely be caused by extrapituitary lesions (Table 5-6). In addition to the more common GH-secreting somatotrope adenomas, mixed mammosomatotrope tumors and acidophilic stem-cell adenomas secrete both GH and PRL. In patients with acidophilic stem-cell adenomas, features of hyperprolactinemia (hypogonadism and galactorrhea) predominate over the less clinically evident signs of acromegaly. Occasionally, mixed plurihormonal tumors are encountered that also secrete ACTH, the glycoprotein hormone α subunit, or TSH in addition to GH. Patients with partially empty sellas may present with GH hypersecretion due to a small GH-secreting adenoma within the compressed rim of pituitary tissue; some of these may reflect the spontaneous necrosis of tumors that were previously larger. GH-secreting tumors rarely arise from ectopic pituitary tissue remnants in the nasopharynx or midline sinuses.

There are case reports of ectopic GH secretion by tumors of pancreatic, ovarian, lung, or hematopoietic origin. Rarely, excess GHRH production may cause acromegaly because of chronic stimulation of somatotropes. These patients present with classic features of acromegaly, elevated GH levels, pituitary enlargement on MRI, and pathologic characteristics of pituitary hyperplasia. The most common cause of GHRH-mediated acromegaly is a chest or abdominal carcinoid tumor. Although these tumors usually express positive GHRH immunoreactivity, clinical features of acromegaly are evident in only a minority of patients with carcinoid disease. Excessive GHRH also may be elaborated by hypothalamic tumors, usually choristomas or neuromas.

TABLE 5-6
CAUSES OF ACROMEGALY

	PREVALENCE, %
Excess Growth Hormone Secretion	
Pituitary	98
Densely or sparsely granulated GH cell adenoma	60
Mixed GH cell and PRL cell adenoma	25
Mammosomatotrope cell adenoma	10
Plurihormonal adenoma	
GH cell carcinoma or metastases	
Multiple endocrine neoplasia 1 (GH cell adenoma)	
McCune-Albright syndrome	
Ectopic sphenoid or parapharyngeal sinus pituitary adenoma	
Extrapituitary tumor	
Pancreatic islet cell tumor	<1
Lymphoma	
Excess Growth Hormone–Releasing Hormone Secretion	
Central	<1
Hypothalamic hamartoma, choristoma, ganglioneuroma	<1
Peripheral	<1
Bronchial carcinoid, pancreatic islet cell tumor, small cell lung cancer, adrenal adenoma, medullary thyroid carcinoma, pheochromocytoma	

Abbreviations: GH, growth hormone; PRL, prolactin.
Source: Adapted from S Melmed: N Engl J Med 355:2558–2573, 2006.

Presentation and diagnosis

Protean manifestations of GH and IGF-I hypersecretion are indolent and often are not clinically diagnosed for 10 years or more. Acral bony overgrowth results in frontal bossing, increased hand and foot size, mandibular enlargement with prognathism, and widened space between the lower incisor teeth. In children and adolescents, initiation of GH hypersecretion before epiphyseal long bone closure is associated with development of pituitary gigantism (Fig. 5-4). Soft tissue swelling results in increased heel pad thickness, increased shoe or glove size, ring tightening, characteristic coarse facial features, and a large fleshy nose. Other commonly encountered clinical features include hyperhidrosis, a deep and hollow-sounding voice, oily skin, arthropathy, kyphosis, carpal tunnel syndrome, proximal muscle weakness and fatigue, acanthosis nigricans, and skin tags. Generalized visceromegaly occurs, including cardiomegaly, macroglossia, and thyroid gland enlargement.

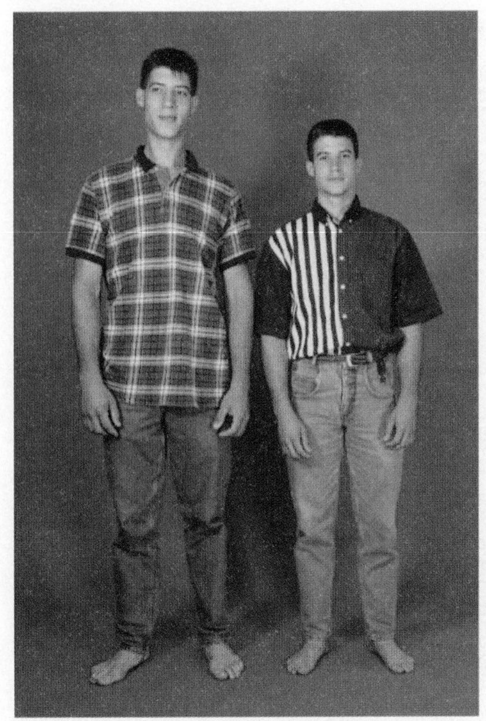

A

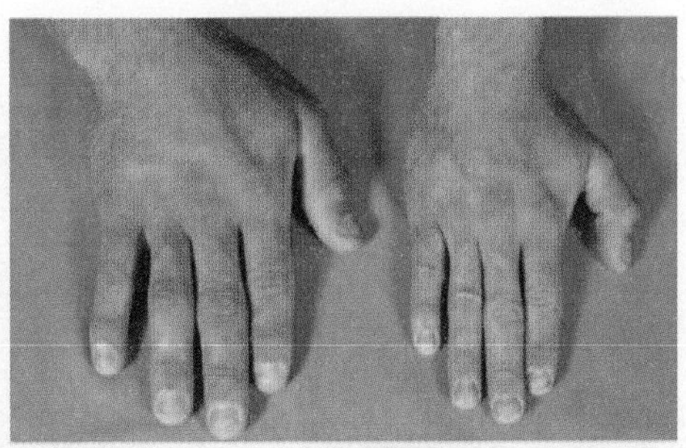

B

C

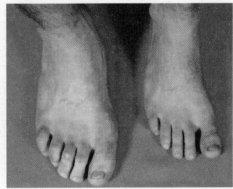

FIGURE 5-4
Features of acromegaly/gigantism. A 22-year-old man with gigantism due to excess growth hormone is shown to the left of his identical twin. The increased height and prognathism ***A.*** and enlarged hand ***B.*** and foot ***C.*** of the affected twin are apparent. Their clinical features began to diverge at the age of approximately 13 years. *(Reproduced from R Gagel, IE McCutcheon: N Engl J Med 324:524, 1999; with permission.)*

The most significant clinical impact of GH excess occurs with respect to the cardiovascular system. Coronary heart disease, cardiomyopathy with arrhythmias, left ventricular hypertrophy, decreased diastolic function, and hypertension ultimately occur in most patients if untreated. Upper airway obstruction with sleep apnea occurs in more than 60% of patients and is associated with both soft tissue laryngeal airway obstruction and central sleep dysfunction. Diabetes mellitus develops in 25% of patients with acromegaly, and most patients are intolerant of a glucose load (as GH counteracts the action of insulin). Acromegaly is associated with an increased risk of colon polyps and mortality from colonic malignancy; polyps are diagnosed in up to one-third of patients. Overall mortality is increased about threefold and is due primarily to cardiovascular and cerebrovascular disorders and respiratory disease. Unless GH levels are controlled, survival is reduced by an average of 10 years compared with an age-matched control population.

Laboratory investigation

Age-matched serum IGF-I levels are elevated in acromegaly. Consequently, an IGF-I level provides a useful laboratory screening measure when clinical features raise the possibility of acromegaly. Due to the pulsatility of GH secretion, measurement of a single random GH level is not useful for the diagnosis or exclusion of acromegaly and does not correlate with disease severity. The diagnosis of acromegaly is confirmed by demonstrating the failure of GH suppression to <0.4 μg/L within 1–2 h of an oral glucose load (75 g). When newer ultrasensitive GH assays are used, normal nadir GH levels are even lower (<0.05 μg/L). About 20% of patients exhibit a paradoxical GH rise after glucose. PRL should be measured, as it is elevated in ~25% of patients with acromegaly. Thyroid function, gonadotropins, and sex steroids may be attenuated because of tumor mass effects. Because most patients will undergo surgery with glucocorticoid coverage, tests of ACTH reserve in asymptomatic patients are more efficiently deferred until after surgery.

TREATMENT Acromegaly

The goal of treatment is to control GH and IGF-I hypersecretion, ablate or arrest tumor growth, ameliorate comorbidities, restore mortality rates to normal, and preserve pituitary function.

Surgical resection of GH-secreting adenomas is the initial treatment for most patients (Fig. 5-5). Somatostatin analogues are used as adjuvant treatment for preoperative

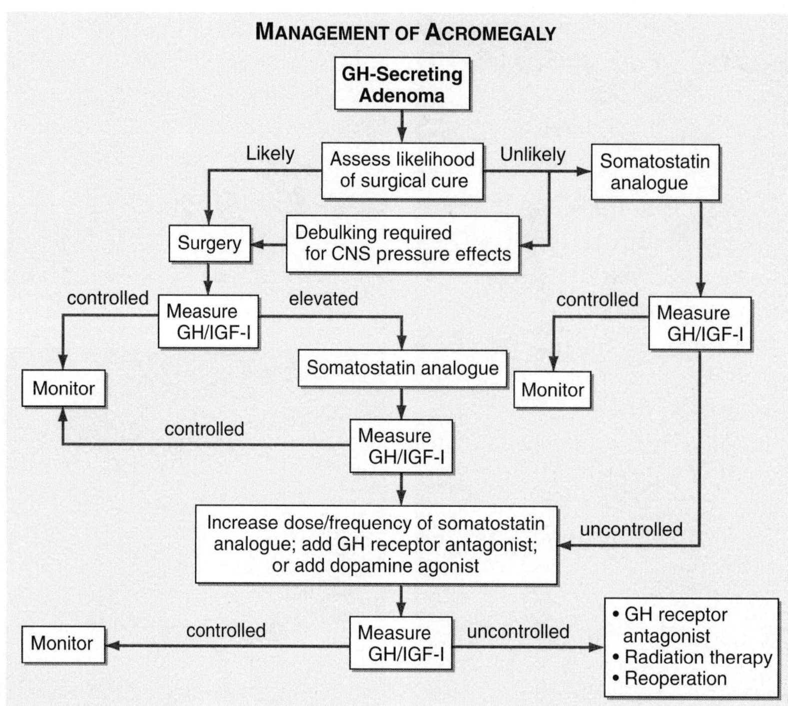

FIGURE 5-5

Management of acromegaly. GH, growth hormone; CNS, central nervous system; IGF, insulin-like growth factor. *(Adapted from S Melmed et al: J Clin Endocrinol Metab 94:1509–1517, 2009; © The Endocrine Society.)*

shrinkage of large invasive macroadenomas, immediate relief of debilitating symptoms, and reduction of GH hypersecretion; in frail patients experiencing morbidity; and in patients who decline surgery or, when surgery fails, to achieve biochemical control. Irradiation or repeat surgery may be required for patients who cannot tolerate or do not respond to adjunctive medical therapy. The high rate of late hypopituitarism and the slow rate (5–15 years) of biochemical response are the main disadvantages of radiotherapy. Irradiation is also relatively ineffective in normalizing IGF-I levels. Stereotactic ablation of GH-secreting adenomas by gamma-knife radiotherapy is promising, but initial reports suggest that long-term results and side effects are similar to those observed with conventional radiation. Somatostatin analogues may be required while awaiting the full benefits of radiotherapy. Systemic co-morbid sequelae of acromegaly, including cardiovascular disease, diabetes, and arthritis, should be managed aggressively. Mandibular surgical repair may be indicated.

SURGERY Transsphenoidal surgical resection by an experienced surgeon is the preferred primary treatment for both microadenomas (remission rate ~70%) and macroadenomas (<50% in remission). Soft tissue swelling improves immediately after tumor resection. GH levels return to normal within an hour, and IGF-I levels are normalized within 3–4 days. In ~10% of patients, acromegaly may recur several years after apparently successful surgery; hypopituitarism develops in up to 15% of patients after surgery.

SOMATOSTATIN ANALOGUES Somatostatin analogues exert their therapeutic effects through SSTR2 and SSTR5 receptors, both of which are expressed by GH-secreting tumors. Octreotide acetate is an eight-amino-acid synthetic somatostatin analogue. In contrast to native somatostatin, the analogue is relatively resistant to plasma degradation. It has a 2-h serum half-life and possesses fortyfold greater potency than native somatostatin to suppress GH. Octreotide is administered by subcutaneous injection, beginning with 50 μg tid; the dose can be increased gradually up to 1500 μg/d. Fewer than 10% of patients do not respond to the analogue. Octreotide suppresses integrated GH levels and normalizes IGF-I levels in ~60% of treated patients.

The long-acting somatostatin depot formulations, octreotide and lanreotide, are the preferred medical treatment for patients with acromegaly. *Sandostatin-LAR* is a sustained-release, long-acting formulation of octreotide incorporated into microspheres that sustain drug levels for several weeks after intramuscular injection. GH suppression occurs for as long as 6 weeks after a 30-mg intramuscular injection; long-term monthly treatment sustains GH and IGF-I suppression and also reduces pituitary tumor size in ~50% of patients. *Lanreotide* autogel, a slow-release depot somatostatin preparation, is a cyclic somatostatin octapeptide analogue that suppresses GH and IGF-I hypersecretion after a 60-mg subcutaneous injection. Long-term (4–6 weeks) administration controls GH hypersecretion in about two-thirds of treated patients and improves patient compliance because of the long interval required between drug injections. Rapid relief of headache and soft tissue swelling occurs in ~75% of patients within days to weeks of somatostatin analogue initiation. Most patients report symptomatic improvement, including amelioration of headache, perspiration, obstructive apnea, and cardiac failure.

Side Effects Somatostatin analogues are well tolerated in most patients. Adverse effects are short-lived and mostly relate to drug-induced suppression of gastrointestinal motility and secretion. Transient nausea, abdominal discomfort, fat malabsorption, diarrhea, and flatulence occur in one-third of patients, and these symptoms usually remit within 2 weeks. Octreotide suppresses postprandial gallbladder contractility and delays gallbladder emptying; up to 30% of patients develop long-term echogenic sludge or asymptomatic cholesterol gallstones. Other side effects include mild glucose intolerance due to transient insulin suppression, asymptomatic bradycardia, hypothyroxinemia, and local injection site discomfort.

GH RECEPTOR ANTAGONIST Pegvisomant antagonizes endogenous GH action by blocking peripheral GH binding to its receptor. Consequently, serum IGF-I levels are suppressed, reducing the deleterious effects of excess endogenous GH. Pegvisomant is administered by daily subcutaneous injection (10–20 mg) and normalizes IGF-I in ~70% of patients. GH levels, however, remain elevated as the drug does not target the pituitary adenoma. Side effects include reversible liver enzyme elevation, lipodystrophy, and injection site pain. Tumor size should be monitored by MRI.

Combined treatment with monthly somatostatin analogues and weekly or biweekly pegvisomant injections has been used effectively in resistant patients.

DOPAMINE AGONISTS Bromocriptine and cabergoline may modestly suppress GH secretion in some patients. Very high doses of bromocriptine (≥20 mg/d) or cabergoline (0.5 mg/d) are usually required to achieve modest GH therapeutic efficacy. Combined treatment with octreotide and cabergoline may induce additive biochemical control compared with either drug alone.

RADIATION External radiation therapy or high-energy stereotactic techniques are used as adjuvant therapy for acromegaly. An advantage of radiation is that patient compliance with long-term treatment is not required. Tumor mass is reduced, and GH levels are attenuated over time. However, 50% of patients require at least 8 years for GH levels to be suppressed to <5 μg/L; this level of GH reduction is achieved in about 90% of patients after 18 years but represents suboptimal GH suppression. Patients may require interim medical therapy for several years before attaining maximal radiation benefits. Most patients also experience hypothalamic-pituitary damage, leading to gonadotropin, ACTH, and/or TSH deficiency within 10 years of therapy.

In summary, surgery is the preferred primary treatment for GH-secreting microadenomas (Fig. 5-5). The high frequency of GH hypersecretion after macroadenoma resection usually necessitates adjuvant or primary medical therapy for these larger tumors. Patients unable to receive or respond to unimodal medical treatment may benefit from combined treatments, or can be offered radiation.

CUSHING'S SYNDROME (ACTH-PRODUCING ADENOMA)

(See also Chap. 8)

Etiology and prevalence

Pituitary corticotrope adenomas account for 70% of patients with endogenous causes of Cushing's syndrome. However, it should be emphasized that iatrogenic hypercortisolism is the most common cause of cushingoid features. Ectopic tumor ACTH production, cortisol-producing adrenal adenomas, adrenal carcinoma, and adrenal hyperplasia account for the other causes; rarely, ectopic tumor CRH production is encountered.

ACTH-producing adenomas account for about 10–15% of all pituitary tumors. Because the clinical features of Cushing's syndrome often lead to early diagnosis, most ACTH-producing pituitary tumors are relatively small microadenomas. However, macroadenomas also are seen and some ACTH-expressing adenomas are clinically silent. Cushing's disease is 5–10 times more common in women than in men. These pituitary adenomas exhibit unrestrained ACTH secretion, with resultant hypercortisolemia. However, they retain partial suppressibility in the presence of high doses of administered glucocorticoids, providing the basis for dynamic testing to distinguish pituitary from nonpituitary causes of Cushing's syndrome.

Presentation and diagnosis

The diagnosis of Cushing's syndrome presents two great challenges: (1) to distinguish patients with pathologic cortisol excess from those with physiologic or other disturbances of cortisol production and (2) to determine the etiology of pathologic cortisol excess.

Typical features of chronic cortisol excess include thin skin, central obesity, hypertension, plethoric moon facies, purple striae and easy bruisability, glucose intolerance or diabetes mellitus, gonadal dysfunction, osteoporosis, proximal muscle weakness, signs of hyperandrogenism (acne, hirsutism), and psychological disturbances (depression, mania, and psychoses) (Table 5-7). Hematopoietic features of hypercortisolism include leukocytosis, lymphopenia, and eosinopenia. Immune suppression includes delayed hypersensitivity and infection propensity. These protean yet commonly encountered manifestations of hypercortisolism make it challenging to decide which patients mandate formal laboratory evaluation. Certain features make pathologic

TABLE 5-7

CLINICAL FEATURES OF CUSHING'S SYNDROME (ALL AGES)

SYMPTOMS/SIGNS	FREQUENCY, %
Obesity or weight gain (>115% ideal body weight)	80
Thin skin	80
Moon facies	75
Hypertension	75
Purple skin striae	65
Hirsutism	65
Menstrual disorders (usually amenorrhea)	60
Plethora	60
Abnormal glucose tolerance	55
Impotence	55
Proximal muscle weakness	50
Truncal obesity	50
Acne	45
Bruising	45
Mental changes	45
Osteoporosis	40
Edema of lower extremities	30
Hyperpigmentation	20
Hypokalemic alkalosis	15
Diabetes mellitus	15

Source: Adapted from MA Magiokou et al, in ME Wierman (ed): *Diseases of the Pituitary*. Totowa, NJ, Humana, 1997.

causes of hypercortisolism more likely; they include characteristic central redistribution of fat, thin skin with striae and bruising, and proximal muscle weakness. In children and young females, early osteoporosis may be particularly prominent. The primary cause of death is cardiovascular disease, but life-threatening infections and risk of suicide are also increased.

Rapid development of features of hypercortisolism associated with skin hyperpigmentation and severe myopathy suggests an ectopic tumor source of ACTH. Hypertension, hypokalemic alkalosis, glucose intolerance, and edema are also more pronounced in these patients. Serum potassium levels <3.3 mmol/L are evident in ~70% of patients with ectopic ACTH secretion but are seen in <10% of patients with pituitary-dependent Cushing's syndrome.

Laboratory investigation

The diagnosis of Cushing's syndrome is based on laboratory documentation of endogenous hypercortisolism. Measurement of 24-h urine free cortisol (UFC) is a precise and cost-effective screening test. Alternatively, the failure to suppress plasma cortisol after an overnight 1-mg dexamethasone suppression test can be used to identify patients with hypercortisolism. As nadir levels of cortisol occur at night, elevated midnight serum or salivary samples of cortisol are suggestive of Cushing's syndrome. Basal plasma ACTH levels often distinguish patients with ACTH-independent (adrenal or exogenous glucocorticoid) from those with ACTH-dependent (pituitary, ectopic ACTH) Cushing's syndrome. Mean basal ACTH levels are about eightfold higher in patients with ectopic ACTH secretion than in those with pituitary ACTH-secreting adenomas. However, extensive overlap of ACTH levels in these two disorders precludes using ACTH measurements to make the distinction. Preferably, dynamic testing based on differential sensitivity to glucocorticoid feedback or ACTH stimulation in response to CRH or cortisol reduction is used to distinguish ectopic from pituitary sources of excess ACTH (Table 5-8). Very rarely, circulating CRH levels are elevated, reflecting ectopic tumor-derived secretion of CRH and often ACTH. **For further discussion of dynamic testing for Cushing's syndrome, see Chap. 8.**

Most ACTH-secreting pituitary tumors are <5 mm in diameter, and about half are undetectable by sensitive MRI. The high prevalence of incidental pituitary microadenomas diminishes the ability to distinguish ACTH-secreting pituitary tumors accurately from nonsecreting incidentalomas.

Inferior petrosal venous sampling

Because pituitary MRI with gadolinium enhancement is insufficiently sensitive to detect small (<2 mm) pituitary ACTH-secreting adenomas, bilateral inferior petrosal sinus ACTH sampling before and after CRH administration may be required to distinguish these lesions from ectopic ACTH-secreting tumors that may have similar clinical and biochemical characteristics. Simultaneous assessment of ACTH in each inferior petrosal vein and in the diagnosis of peripheral circulation provides a strategy for confirming and localizing pituitary ACTH production. Sampling is performed at baseline and 2, 5, and 10 min after intravenous bovine CRH (1 μg/kg) injection. An increased ratio (>2) of inferior petrosal:peripheral vein ACTH confirms pituitary Cushing's syndrome. After CRH injection, peak petrosal:peripheral ACTH ratios ≥3 confirm the presence of a pituitary ACTH-secreting tumor. The sensitivity of this test is >95%, with very rare false-positive results. False-negative results may be encountered in patients with aberrant venous drainage. Petrosal sinus catheterizations are technically difficult, and about 0.05% of patients develop neurovascular complications. The procedure should not be performed in patients

TABLE 5-8

DIFFERENTIAL DIAGNOSIS OF ACTH-DEPENDENT CUSHING'S SYNDROME[a]

	ACTH-SECRETING PITUITARY TUMOR	ECTOPIC ACTH SECRETION
Etiology	Pituitary corticotrope adenoma Plurihormonal adenoma	Bronchial, abdominal carcinoid Small cell lung cancer Thymoma
Sex	F > M	M > F
Clinical features	Slow onset	Rapid onset Pigmentation Severe myopathy
Serum potassium <3.3 μg/L	<10%	75%
24-h urinary free cortisol (UFC)	High	High
Basal ACTH level	Inappropriately high	Very high
Dexamethasone suppression		
1 mg overnight		
Low-dose (0.5 mg q6h)	Cortisol >5 μg/dL	Cortisol >5 μg/dL
High-dose (2 mg q6h)	Cortisol <5 μg/dL	Cortisol >5 μg/dL
UFC >80% suppressed	Microadenomas: 90% Macroadenomas: 50%	10%
Inferior petrosal sinus sampling (IPSS)		
Basal IPSS: peripheral	>2	<2
CRH-induced IPSS: peripheral	>3	<3

[a]ACTH-independent causes of Cushing's syndrome are diagnosed by suppressed ACTH levels and an adrenal mass in the setting of hypercortisolism. Iatrogenic Cushing's syndrome is excluded by history.

Abbreviations: ACTH, adrenocorticotropic hormone; CRH, corticotropin-releasing hormone; F, female; M, male.

with hypertension, in patients with known cerebrovascular disease, or in the presence of a well-visualized pituitary adenoma on MRI.

TREATMENT Cushing's Syndrome

Selective transsphenoidal resection is the treatment of choice for Cushing's disease (Fig. 5-6). The remission rate for this procedure is ~80% for microadenomas but <50% for macroadenomas. However, surgery is rarely successful when the adenoma is not visible on MRI. After successful tumor resection, most patients experience a postoperative period of symptomatic ACTH deficiency that may last up to 12 months. This usually requires low-dose cortisol replacement, as patients experience both steroid withdrawal symptoms and have a suppressed hypothalamic-pituitary-adrenal axis. Biochemical recurrence occurs in approximately 5% of patients in whom surgery was initially successful.

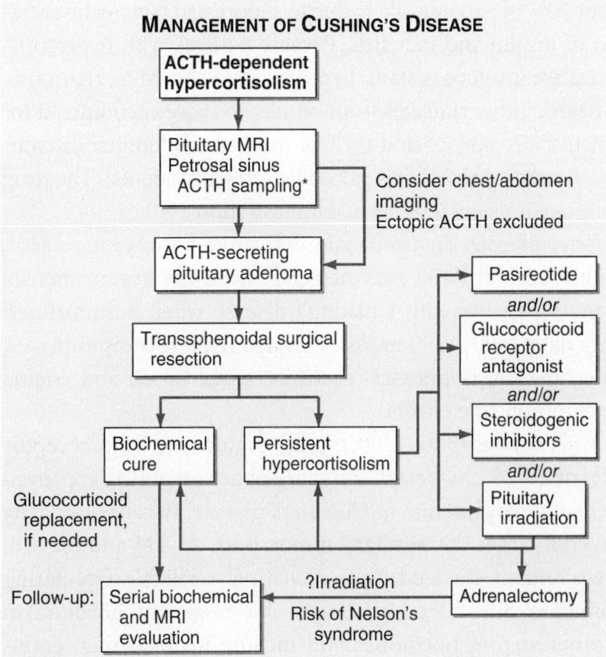

FIGURE 5-6

Management of Cushing's syndrome. ACTH, adrenocorticotropin hormone; MRI, magnetic resonance imaging. *, Not usually required.

When initial surgery is unsuccessful, repeat surgery is sometimes indicated, particularly when a pituitary source for ACTH is well documented. In older patients, in whom issues of growth and fertility are less important, hemi- or total hypophysectomy may be necessary if a discrete pituitary adenoma is not recognized. Pituitary irradiation may be used after unsuccessful surgery, but it cures only about 15% of patients. Because the effects of radiation are slow and only partially effective in adults, steroidogenic inhibitors are used in combination with pituitary irradiation to block adrenal effects of persistently high ACTH levels.

Pasireotide (600 or 900 ug/day subcutaneously), a somatostatin analog with high affinity for SST5 > SST2 receptors, has been approved for treating patients with ACTH-secreting pituitary tumors when surgery is not an option or has been unsuccessful. In clinical trials, the drug lowered plasma ACTH levels, normalized 24-h urinary free cortisol levels in about 25% of patients, and resulted in up to 40% mean pituitary tumor shrinkage. Side effects include development of hyperglycemia and diabetes in about 70% of patients, likely due to suppressed pancreatic secretion of insulin and incretins. Because patients with hypercortisolism are insulin-resistant, hyperglycemia should be rigorously managed. Other side effects are similar to those encountered for somatostatin analogs and include transient abdominal discomfort, diarrhea, nausea, and gallstones (20% of patients). The drug requires consistent long-term administration.

Ketoconazole, an imidazole derivative antimycotic agent, inhibits several P450 enzymes and effectively lowers cortisol in most patients with Cushing's disease when administered twice daily (600–1200 mg/d). Elevated hepatic transaminases, gynecomastia, impotence, gastrointestinal upset, and edema are common side effects.

Mifepristone (300–1200 mg/d), a glucocorticoid receptor antagonist, blocks peripheral cortisol action and is approved to treat hyperglycemia in Cushing's disease. Because the drug does not target the pituitary tumor, both ACTH and cortisol levels remain elevated, thus obviating a reliable circulating biomarker. Side effects are largely due to general antagonism of other steroid hormones and include hypokalemia, endometrial hyperplasia, hypoadrenalism, and hypertension.

Metyrapone (2–4 g/d) inhibits 11β-hydroxylase activity and normalizes plasma cortisol in up to 75% of patients. Side effects include nausea and vomiting, rash, and exacerbation of acne or hirsutism. *Mitotane* (*o,p* '-DDD; 3–6 g/d orally in four divided doses) suppresses cortisol hypersecretion by inhibiting 11β-hydroxylase and cholesterol side-chain cleavage enzymes and by destroying adrenocortical cells. Side effects of mitotane include gastrointestinal symptoms, dizziness, gynecomastia, hyperlipidemia, skin rash, and hepatic enzyme elevation. It also may lead to hypoaldosteronism. Other agents include *aminoglutethimide* (250 mg tid), *trilostane* (200–1000 mg/d), *cyproheptadine* (24 mg/d), and IV *etomidate* (0.3 mg/kg per hour). Glucocorticoid insufficiency is a potential side effect of agents used to block steroidogenesis.

The use of steroidogenic inhibitors has decreased the need for bilateral adrenalectomy. Surgical removal of both adrenal glands corrects hypercortisolism but may be associated with significant morbidity rates and necessitates permanent glucocorticoid and mineralocorticoid replacement. Adrenalectomy in the setting of residual corticotrope adenoma tissue predisposes to the development of *Nelson's syndrome*, a disorder characterized by rapid pituitary tumor enlargement and increased pigmentation secondary to high ACTH levels. Prophylactic radiation therapy may be indicated to prevent the development of Nelson's syndrome after adrenalectomy.

NONFUNCTIONING AND GONADOTROPIN-PRODUCING PITUITARY ADENOMAS

Etiology and prevalence

Nonfunctioning pituitary adenomas include those that secrete little or no pituitary hormones as well as tumors that produce too little hormone to result in recognizable clinical features. They are the most common type of pituitary adenoma and are usually macroadenomas at the time of diagnosis because clinical features are not apparent until tumor mass effects occur. Based on immunohistochemistry, most clinically nonfunctioning adenomas can be shown to originate from gonadotrope cells. These tumors typically produce small amounts of intact gonadotropins (usually FSH) as well as uncombined α, LH β, and FSH β subunits. Tumor secretion may lead to elevated α and FSH β subunits and, rarely, to increased LH β subunit levels. Some adenomas express α subunits without FSH or LH. TRH administration often induces an atypical increase of tumor-derived gonadotropins or subunits.

Presentation and diagnosis

Clinically nonfunctioning tumors often present with optic chiasm pressure and other symptoms of local expansion or may be incidentally discovered on an MRI performed for another indication (incidentaloma). Rarely, menstrual disturbances or ovarian hyperstimulation occur in women with large tumors that produce FSH and LH. More commonly, adenoma compression of the pituitary stalk or surrounding pituitary tissue leads to attenuated LH and features of hypogonadism. PRL levels are usually slightly increased, also because of stalk compression. It is important to distinguish this circumstance from true prolactinomas, as nonfunctioning tumors do not shrink in response to treatment with dopamine agonists.

Laboratory investigation

The goal of laboratory testing in clinically nonfunctioning tumors is to classify the type of the tumor, identify hormonal markers of tumor activity, and detect possible hypopituitarism. Free α subunit levels may be elevated in 10–15% of patients with nonfunctioning tumors. In female patients, peri- or postmenopausal basal FSH concentrations are difficult to distinguish from tumor-derived FSH elevation. Premenopausal women have cycling FSH levels, also preventing clear-cut diagnostic distinction from tumor-derived FSH. In men, gonadotropin-secreting tumors may be diagnosed because of slightly increased gonadotropins (FSH > LH) in the setting of a pituitary mass. Testosterone levels are usually low despite the normal or increased LH level, perhaps reflecting reduced LH bioactivity or the loss of normal LH pulsatility. Because this pattern of hormone test results is also seen in primary gonadal failure and, to some extent, with aging **(Chap. 11)**, the finding of increased gonadotropins alone is insufficient for the diagnosis of a gonadotropin-secreting tumor. In the majority of patients with gonadotrope adenomas,

TRH administration stimulates LH β subunit secretion; this response is not seen in normal individuals. GnRH testing, however, is not helpful for making the diagnosis. For nonfunctioning and gonadotropin-secreting tumors, the diagnosis usually rests on immunohistochemical analyses of surgically resected tumor tissue, as the mass effects of these tumors usually necessitate resection.

Although acromegaly or Cushing's syndrome usually presents with unique clinical features, clinically inapparent (silent) somatotrope or corticotrope adenomas may only be diagnosed by immunostaining of resected tumor tissue. If PRL levels are <100 μg/L in a patient harboring a pituitary mass, a nonfunctioning adenoma causing pituitary stalk compression should be considered.

TREATMENT Nonfunctioning and Gonadotropin-Producing Pituitary Adenomas

Asymptomatic small nonfunctioning microadenomas adenomas with no threat to vision may be followed with regular MRI and visual field testing without immediate intervention. However, for macroadenomas, transsphenoidal surgery is indicated to reduce tumor size and relieve mass effects (Fig. 5-7). Although it is not usually possible to remove all adenoma tissue surgically, vision improves in 70% of patients with preoperative visual field defects. Preexisting hypopituitarism that results from tumor mass effects may improve or resolve completely. Beginning about 6 months postoperatively, MRI scans should be performed yearly to detect tumor regrowth. Within 5–6 years after successful surgical resection, ~15% of nonfunctioning tumors recur. When substantial tumor remains after transsphenoidal surgery, adjuvant radiotherapy may be indicated to prevent tumor regrowth. Radiotherapy may be deferred if no postoperative residual mass is evident. Nonfunctioning pituitary tumors respond poorly to dopamine agonist treatment and somatostatin analogues are largely ineffective for shrinking these tumors. The selective GnRH antagonist Nal-Glu GnRH suppresses FSH hypersecretion but has no effect on adenoma size.

TSH-SECRETING ADENOMAS

TSH-producing macroadenomas are very rare but are often large and locally invasive when they occur. Patients usually present with thyroid goiter and hyperthyroidism, reflecting overproduction of TSH. Diagnosis is based on demonstrating elevated serum free T_4 levels, inappropriately normal or high TSH secretion, and MRI evidence of a pituitary adenoma. Elevated uncombined α subunits are seen in many patients.

It is important to exclude other causes of inappropriate TSH secretion, such as resistance to thyroid hormone, an autosomal dominant disorder caused by mutations in the thyroid hormone β receptor (**Chap. 7**). The presence of a pituitary mass and elevated β subunit levels are suggestive of a TSH-secreting tumor. Dysalbuminemic hyperthyroxinemia syndromes, caused by mutations in serum thyroid hormone binding proteins,

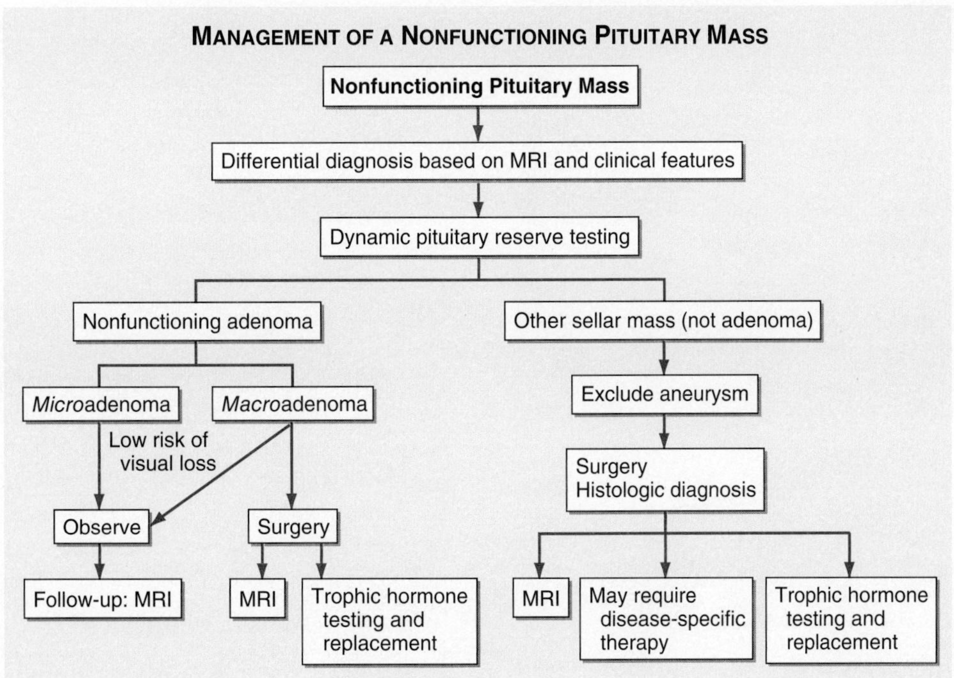

FIGURE 5-7
Management of a nonfunctioning pituitary mass. MRI, magnetic resonance imaging.

are also characterized by elevated thyroid hormone levels, but with normal rather than suppressed TSH levels. Moreover, free thyroid hormone levels are normal in these disorders, most of which are familial.

TREATMENT TSH-Secreting Adenomas

The initial therapeutic approach is to remove or debulk the tumor mass surgically, usually using a transsphenoidal approach. Total resection is not often achieved as most of these adenomas are large and locally invasive. Normal circulating thyroid hormone levels are achieved in about two-thirds of patients after surgery. Thyroid ablation or antithyroid drugs (methimazole and propylthiouracil) can be used to reduce thyroid hormone levels. Somatostatin analogue treatment effectively normalizes TSH and α subunit hypersecretion, shrinks the tumor mass in 50% of patients, and improves visual fields in 75% of patients; euthyroidism is restored in most patients. Because somatostatin analogues markedly suppress TSH, biochemical hypothyroidism often requires concomitant thyroid hormone replacement, which may also further control tumor growth.

CHAPTER 6

DISORDERS OF THE NEUROHYPOPHYSIS

Gary L. Robertson

The neurohypophysis, or posterior pituitary, is formed by axons that originate in large cell bodies in the supraoptic and paraventricular nuclei of the hypothalamus. It produces two hormones: (1) arginine vasopressin (AVP), also known as antidiuretic hormone, and (2) oxytocin. AVP acts on the renal tubules to reduce water loss by concentrating the urine. Oxytocin stimulates postpartum milk letdown in response to suckling. A deficiency of AVP secretion or action causes diabetes insipidus (DI), a syndrome characterized by the production of large amounts of dilute urine. Excessive or inappropriate AVP production impairs urinary water excretion and predisposes to hyponatremia if water intake is not reduced in parallel with urine output.

VASOPRESSIN

SYNTHESIS AND SECRETION

AVP is a nonapeptide composed of a six-member disulfide ring and a tripeptide tail (Fig. 6-1). It is synthesized via a polypeptide precursor that includes AVP, neurophysin, and copeptin, all encoded by a single gene on chromosome 20. After preliminary processing and folding, the precursor is packaged in neurosecretory vesicles, where it is transported down the axon; further processed to AVP, neurophysin, and copeptin; and stored in neurosecretory vesicles until released by exocytosis into peripheral blood.

AVP secretion is regulated primarily by the "effective" osmotic pressure of body fluids. This control is mediated by specialized hypothalamic cells known as *osmoreceptors*, which are extremely sensitive to small changes in the plasma concentration of sodium and its anions but normally are insensitive to other solutes such as urea and glucose. The osmoreceptors appear to include inhibitory as well as stimulatory components that function in concert to form a threshold, or set point, control system. Below this threshold, plasma AVP is suppressed to levels that permit the development of a maximum water diuresis. Above it, plasma AVP rises steeply in direct proportion to plasma osmolarity, quickly reaching levels sufficient to effect a maximum antidiuresis. The absolute levels of plasma osmolarity/sodium at which minimally and maximally effective levels of plasma AVP occur, vary appreciably from person to person, apparently due to genetic influences on the set and sensitivity of the system. However, the average threshold, or set point, for AVP release corresponds to a plasma osmolarity or sodium of about 280 mosmol/L or 135 meq/L, respectively; levels only 2–4% higher normally result in maximum antidiuresis.

Although it is relatively stable in a healthy adult, the set point of the osmoregulatory system can be lowered by pregnancy, the menstrual cycle, estrogen, and relatively large, acute reductions in blood pressure or volume. Those reductions are mediated largely by neuronal afferents that originate in transmural pressure receptors of the heart and large arteries and project via the vagus and glossopharyngeal nerves to the brainstem, from which postsynaptic projections ascend to the hypothalamus. These pathways maintain a tonic inhibitory tone that decreases when blood volume or pressure falls by >10–20%. This baroregulatory system is probably of minor importance in the physiology of AVP secretion because the hemodynamic changes required to affect it usually do not occur during normal activities. However, the baroregulatory system undoubtedly plays an important role in AVP secretion in patients with disorders that produce large, acute disturbances of hemodynamic function. However, the baroregulatory system undoubtedly plays an important role in AVP secretion in patients with disorders that produce large, acute disturbances of hemodynamic function.

AVP secretion also can be stimulated by nausea, acute hypoglycemia, glucocorticoid deficiency, smoking, and, possibly, hyperangiotensinemia. The emetic stimuli are

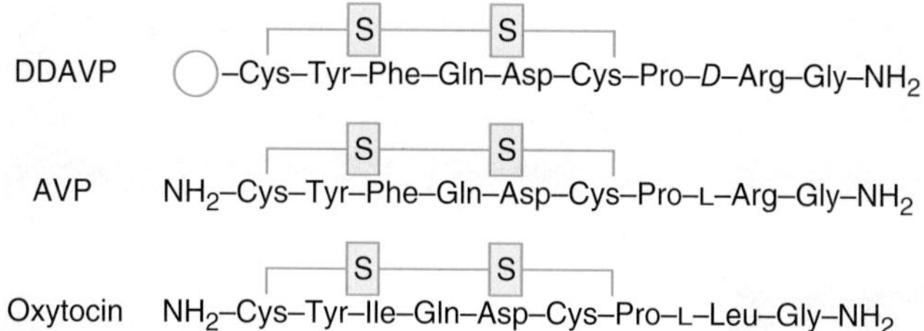

FIGURE 6-1
Primary structures of arginine vasopressin (AVP), oxytocin, and desmopressin (DDAVP).

extremely potent since they typically elicit immediate, 50- to 100-fold increases in plasma AVP even when the nausea is transient and is not associated with vomiting or other symptoms. They appear to act via the emetic center in the medulla and can be blocked completely by treatment with antiemetics such as fluphenazine. There is no evidence that pain or other noxious stresses have any effect on AVP unless they elicit a vasovagal reaction with its associated nausea and hypotension.

ACTION

The most important, if not the only, physiologic action of AVP is to reduce water excretion by promoting concentration of urine. This antidiuretic effect is achieved by increasing the hydroosmotic permeability of cells that line the distal tubule and medullary collecting ducts of the kidney (Fig. 6-2). In the absence of AVP, these cells are impermeable to water and reabsorb little, if any, of the relatively large volume of dilute filtrate that enters from the proximal nephron. The lack of reabsorption results in the excretion of very large volumes (as much as 0.2 mL/kg per min) of maximally dilute urine (specific gravity and osmolarity ~1.000 and 50 mosmol/L, respectively), a condition known as *water diuresis*. In the presence of AVP, these cells become selectively permeable to water, allowing the water to diffuse back down the osmotic gradient created by the hypertonic renal medulla. As a result, the dilute fluid passing through the tubules is concentrated and the rate of urine flow decreases. The magnitude of this effect varies in direct proportion to the plasma AVP concentration and the

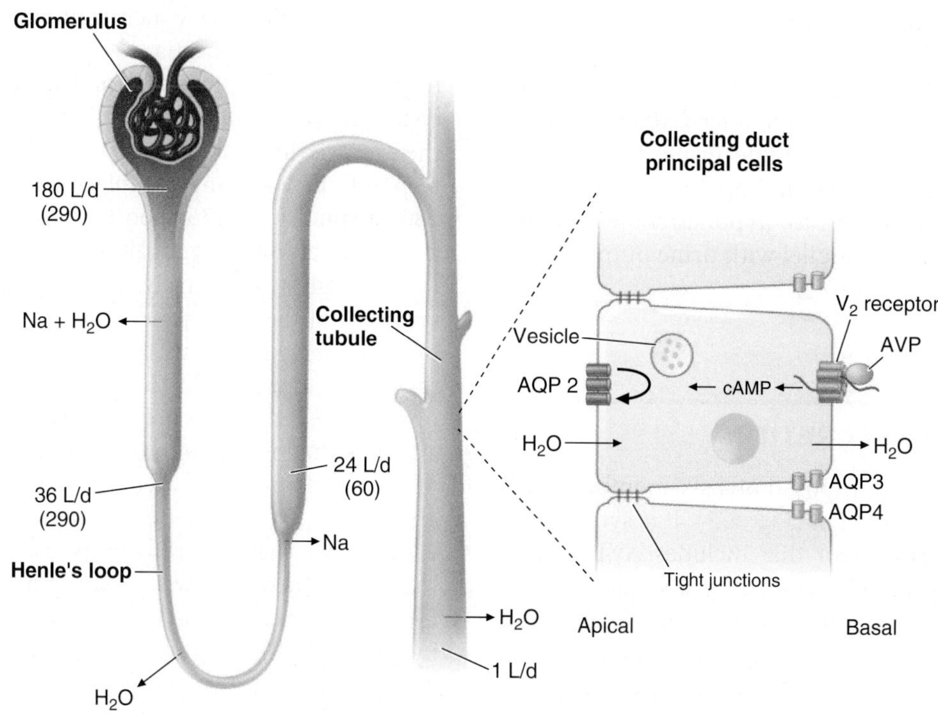

FIGURE 6-2
Antidiuretic effect of arginine vasopressin (AVP) in the regulation of urine volume. In a typical 70-kg adult, the kidney filters ~180 L/d of plasma. Of this, ~144 L (80%) is reabsorbed isosmotically in the proximal tubule and another 8 L (4–5%) is reabsorbed without solute in the descending limb of Henle's loop. The remainder is diluted to an osmolarity of ~60 mmol/kg by selective reabsorption of sodium and chloride in the ascending limb. In the absence of AVP, the urine issuing from the loop passes largely unmodified through the distal tubules and collecting ducts, resulting in a maximum water diuresis. In the presence of AVP, solute-free water is reabsorbed osmotically through the principal cells of the collecting ducts, resulting in the excretion of a much smaller volume of concentrated urine. This antidiuretic effect is mediated via a G protein–coupled V_2 receptor that increases intracellular cyclic AMP, thereby inducing translocation of aquaporin 2 (AQP 2) water channels into the apical membrane. The resultant increase in permeability permits an influx of water that diffuses out of the cell through AQP 3 and AQP 4 water channels on the basal-lateral surface. The net rate of flux across the cell is determined by the number of AQP 2 water channels in the apical membrane and the strength of the osmotic gradient between tubular fluid and the renal medulla. Tight junctions on the lateral surface of the cells serve to prevent unregulated water flow.

rate of solute excretion. At maximum levels of AVP and normal rates of solute excretion, it approximates a urine flow rate as low as 0.35 mL/min and a urine osmolarity as high as 1200 mosmol/L. This effect is reduced by a solute diuresis such as glucosuria in diabetes mellitus. Antidiuresis is mediated via binding to G protein–coupled V_2 receptors on the serosal surface of the cell, activation of adenyl cyclase, and insertion into the luminal surface of water channels composed of a protein known as *aquaporin 2* (AQP2). The V_2 receptors and aquaporin 2 are encoded by genes on chromosomes Xq28 and 12q13, respectively.

At high concentrations, AVP also causes contraction of smooth muscle in blood vessels in the skin and gastrointestinal tract, induces glycogenolysis in the liver, and potentiates adrenocorticotropic hormone (ACTH) release by corticotropin-releasing factor. These effects are mediated by V_{1a} or V_{1b} receptors that are coupled to phospholipase C. Their role, if any, in human physiology/pathophysiology is uncertain.

METABOLISM

AVP distributes rapidly into a space roughly equal to the extracellular fluid volume. It is cleared irreversibly with a half-life ($t_{1/2}$) of 10–30 min. Most AVP clearance is due to degradation in the liver and kidneys. During pregnancy, the metabolic clearance of AVP is increased three- to fourfold due to placental production of an N-terminal peptidase.

THIRST

Because AVP cannot reduce water loss below a certain minimum level obligated by urinary solute load and evaporation from skin and lungs, a mechanism for ensuring adequate intake is essential for preventing dehydration. This vital function is performed by the thirst mechanism. Like AVP, thirst is regulated primarily by an osmostat that is situated in the anteromedial hypothalamus and is able to detect very small changes in the plasma concentration of sodium and its anions. The thirst osmostat appears to be "set" about 3% higher than the AVP osmostat. This arrangement ensures that thirst, polydipsia, and dilution of body fluids do not occur until plasma osmolarity/sodium starts to exceed the defensive capacity of the antidiuretic mechanism.

OXYTOCIN

Oxytocin is also a nonapeptide that differs from AVP only at positions 3 and 8 (Fig. 6-1). However, it has relatively little antidiuretic effect and seems to act mainly on mammary ducts to facilitate milk letdown during nursing. It also may help initiate or facilitate labor by stimulating contraction of uterine smooth muscle, but it is not clear if this action is physiologic or necessary for normal delivery.

DEFICIENCIES OF AVP SECRETION AND ACTION

DIABETES INSIPIDUS

Clinical characteristics

A decrease of 75% or more in the secretion or action of AVP usually results in DI, a syndrome characterized by the production of abnormally large volumes of dilute urine. The 24-h urine volume exceeds 50 mL/kg body weight, and the osmolarity is less than 300 mosmol/L. The polyuria produces symptoms of urinary frequency, enuresis, and/or nocturia, which may disturb sleep and cause mild daytime fatigue or somnolence. It also results in a slight rise in plasma osmolarity that stimulates thirst and a commensurate increase in fluid intake (polydipsia). Overt clinical signs of dehydration are uncommon unless thirst and/or the compensatory increase of fluid intake are also impaired.

Etiology

A primary deficiency of AVP secretion usually results from agenesis or irreversible destruction of the neurohypophysis. It is referred to variously as *neurohypophyseal DI, neurogenic DI, pituitary DI, cranial DI*, or *central DI*. It can be caused by a variety of congenital, acquired, or genetic disorders, but in about one-half of all adult patients, it is idiopathic (Table 6-1). Pituitary DI caused by surgery in or around the neurohypophysis usually appears within 24 h. After a few days, it may transition to a 2- to 3-week period of inappropriate antidiuresis, after which the DI may or may not recur permanently. Five genetic forms of pituitary DI are now known. By far, the most common is transmitted in an autosomal dominant mode and is caused by diverse mutations in the coding region of one allele of the AVP–neurophysin II (or *AVP-NPII*) gene. All the mutations alter one or more amino acids known to be critical for correct processing and/or folding of the prohormone, thus interfering with its trafficking through the endoplasmic reticulum. The misfolded mutant precursor accumulates and interferes with production of AVP by the normal allele, eventually destroying the magnocellular neurons in which it is produced. The AVP deficiency and DI are usually not present at birth but develop gradually over a period of several months to years, progressing from partial to

TABLE 6-1

CAUSES OF DIABETES INSIPIDUS

PITUITARY DIABETES INSIPIDUS

- Acquired
  - Head trauma (closed and penetrating) including pituitary surgery
  - Neoplasms
    - Primary
      - Craniopharyngioma
      - Pituitary adenoma (suprasellar)
      - Dysgerminoma
      - Meningioma
    - Metastatic (lung, breast)
    - Hematologic (lymphoma, leukemia)
  - Granulomas
    - Sarcoidosis
    - Histiocytosis
    - Xanthoma disseminatum
  - Infectious
    - Chronic meningitis
    - Viral encephalitis
    - Toxoplasmosis
  - Inflammatory
    - Lymphocytic infundibuloneurohypophysitis
    - Granulomatosis with polyangiitis (Wegener's)
    - Lupus erythematosus
    - Scleroderma
  - Chemical toxins
    - Tetrodotoxin
    - Snake venom
  - Vascular
    - Sheehan's syndrome
    - Aneurysm (internal carotid)
    - Aortocoronary bypass
    - Hypoxic encephalopathy
  - Idiopathic
- Congenital malformations
  - Septo-optic dysplasia
  - Midline craniofacial defects
  - Holoprosencephaly
  - Hypogenesis, ectopia of pituitary
- Genetic
  - Autosomal dominant *(AVP-neurophysin gene)*
  - Autosomal recessive
  - Type A *(AVP-neurophysin gene)*
  - Type B *(AVP-neurophysin gene)*
  - Type C *(Wolfram's [4p-WFS 1] gene)*
  - X-linked recessive (Xq28)

GESTATIONAL DIABETES INSIPIDUS

- Pregnancy (second and third trimesters)

Nephrogenic diabetes insipidus

- Acquired
  - Drugs
    - Lithium
    - Demeclocycline
    - Methoxyflurane
    - Amphotericin B
    - Aminoglycosides
    - Cisplatin
    - Rifampin
    - Foscarnet
  - Metabolic
    - Hypercalcemia, hypercalciuria
    - Hypokalemia
  - Obstruction (ureter or urethra)
  - Vascular
    - Sickle cell disease and trait
    - Ischemia (acute tubular necrosis)
  - Granulomas
    - Sarcoidosis
  - Neoplasms
    - Sarcoma
  - Infiltration
    - Amyloidosis
  - Idiopathic
- Genetic
  - X-linked recessive *(AVP receptor-2 gene)*
  - Autosomal recessive *(AQP2 gene)*
  - Autosomal dominant *(AQP2 gene)*

Primary polydipsia

- Acquired
  - Psychogenic
    - Schizophrenia
    - Obsessive compulsive disorder
  - Dipsogenic (abnormal thirst)
    - Granulomas (sarcoidosis)
    - Infectious (tuberculous meningitis)
    - Head trauma (closed and penetrating)
    - Demyelination (multiple sclerosis)
    - Drugs
    - Idiopathic
    - Iatrogenic

severe at different rates depending on the mutation. Once established, the deficiency of AVP is permanent, but for unknown reasons, the DI occasionally improves or remits spontaneously in late middle age. The parvocellular neurons that make AVP and the magnocellular neurons that make oxytocin appear to be unaffected. There are also rare autosomal recessive forms of pituitary DI. One is due to an inactivating mutation in the AVP portion of the gene; another is due to a large deletion involving the majority of the AVP gene and regulatory sequences in the intergenic region. A third form is caused by mutations of the *WFS 1* gene responsible for Wolfram's syndrome (DI, diabetes mellitus, optic atrophy, and neural deafness [DIDMOAD]). An X-linked recessive form linked to a region on Xq28 has also been described.

A primary deficiency of plasma AVP also can result from increased metabolism by an N-terminal aminopeptidase produced by the placenta. It is referred to as *gestational DI* because the signs and symptoms manifest during pregnancy and usually remit several weeks after delivery.

Secondary deficiencies of AVP secretion result from inhibition by excessive intake of fluids. They are referred to as *primary polydipsia* and can be divided into three subcategories. One of them, *dipsogenic DI*, is characterized by inappropriate thirst caused by a reduction in the set of the osmoregulatory mechanism. It sometimes occurs in association with multifocal diseases of the brain such as neurosarcoid, tuberculous meningitis, and multiple sclerosis but is often idiopathic. The second subtype, *psychogenic polydipsia*, is not associated with thirst, and the polydipsia seems to be a feature of psychosis or obsessive compulsive disorder. The third subtype, *iatrogenic polydipsia*, results from recommendations to increase fluid intake for its presumed health benefits.

Primary deficiencies in the antidiuretic action of AVP result in *nephrogenic DI*. The causes can be genetic, acquired, or drug induced (Table 6-1). The most common genetic form is transmitted in a semirecessive X-linked manner. It is caused by mutations in the coding region of the V_2 receptor gene that impair trafficking and/or ligand binding of the mutant receptor. There are also autosomal recessive or dominant forms of nephrogenic DI. They are caused by *AQP2* gene mutations that result in complete or partial defects in trafficking and function of the water channels that mediate antidiuresis in the distal and collecting tubules of the kidney.

Secondary deficiencies in the antidiuretic response to AVP result from polyuria per se. They are caused by washout of the medullary concentration gradient and/or suppression of aquaporin function. They usually resolve 24–48 h after the polyuria is corrected but can

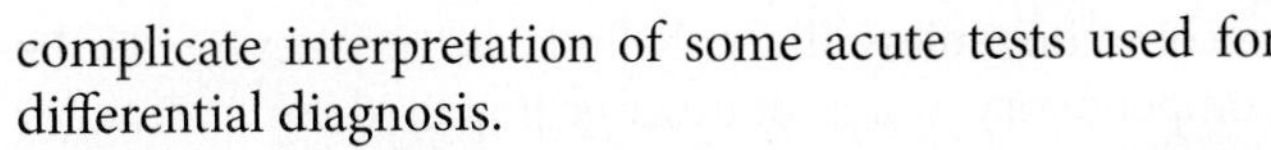

complicate interpretation of some acute tests used for differential diagnosis.

Pathophysiology

In pituitary, gestational, or nephrogenic DI, the polyuria results in a small (1–2%) decrease in body water and a commensurate increase in plasma osmolarity and sodium that stimulates thirst and a compensatory increase in water intake. As a result, *hypernatremia and other overt physical or laboratory signs of dehydration do not develop unless the patient also has a defect in thirst or fails to increase fluid intake for some other reason.*

In pituitary and nephrogenic DI, the severity of the defect in AVP secretion or action varies significantly from patient to patient. In some, the defect is so severe that it cannot be overcome by even an intense stimulus such as nausea or severe dehydration. In others, the defect in AVP secretion or action is incomplete, and a modest stimulus such as a few hours of fluid deprivation, smoking, or a vasovagal reaction can raise urine osmolarity as high as 800 mosmol/L. However, even when the defects are partial, the relation of urine osmolarity to plasma AVP in patients with nephrogenic DI (Fig. 6-3A) or of plasma AVP to plasma osmolarity and sodium in patients with pituitary DI (Fig. 6-3B) is subnormal.

In primary polydipsia, the pathogenesis of the polydipsia and polyuria is the reverse of that in pituitary, nephrogenic, and gestational DI. In primary polydipsia, an abnormality in cognition or thirst causes excessive intake of fluids and an increase in body water that reduces plasma osmolarity/sodium, AVP secretion, and urinary concentration. Dilution of the urine, in turn, results in a compensatory increase in urinary free-water excretion that usually offsets the increase in intake and stabilizes plasma osmolarity/sodium at a level only 1–2% below basal. Thus, hyponatremia or clinically appreciable overhydration is

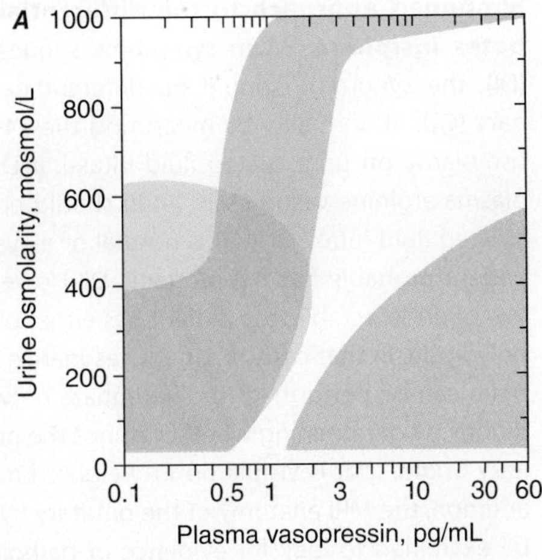

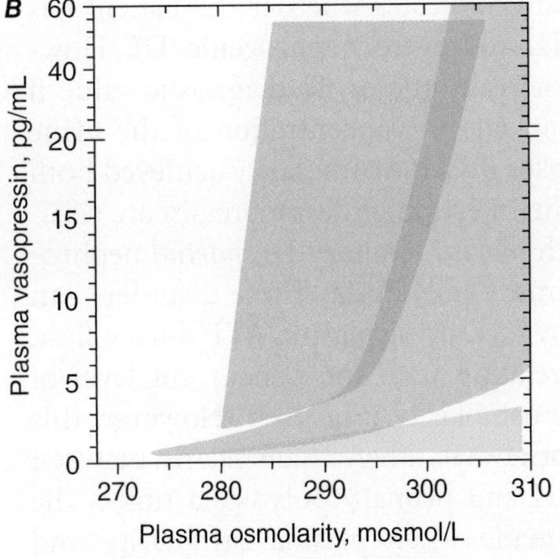

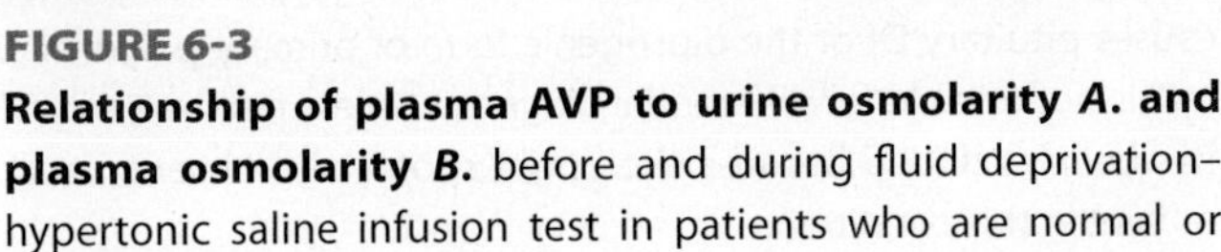

FIGURE 6-3
Relationship of plasma AVP to urine osmolarity *A.* and plasma osmolarity *B.* before and during fluid deprivation–hypertonic saline infusion test in patients who are normal or have primary polydipsia (blue zones), pituitary diabetes insipidus (green zones), or nephrogenic diabetes insipidus (pink zones).

uncommon unless the polydipsia is very severe or the compensatory water diuresis is impaired by a drug or disease that stimulates or mimics the antidiuretic effect of endogenous AVP. A rise in plasma osmolarity and sodium produced by fluid deprivation or hypertonic saline infusion increases plasma AVP normally. However, the resultant increase in urine concentration is often subnormal because polyuria per se temporarily reduces the capacity of the kidney to concentrate the urine. Thus, the maximum level of urine osmolarity achieved during fluid deprivation is often indistinguishable from that in patients with partial pituitary or partial nephrogenic DI.

Differential diagnosis

When symptoms of urinary frequency, enuresis, nocturia, and/or persistent thirst are present in the absence of glucosuria, the possibility of DI should be evaluated by collecting a 24-h urine on ad libitum fluid intake. If the volume exceeds 50 mL/kg per day (3500 mL in a 70-kg male) and the osmolarity is below 300 mosmol/L, DI is confirmed and the patient should be evaluated further to determine the type in order to select the appropriate therapy.

The type of DI can sometimes be inferred from the clinical setting or medical history. Often, however, such information is lacking, ambiguous, or misleading, and other approaches to differential diagnosis are needed. If basal plasma osmolarity and sodium are within normal limits, the traditional approach is to determine the effect of fluid deprivation and injection of antidiuretic hormone on urine osmolarity. This approach suffices for differential diagnosis *if* fluid deprivation raises plasma osmolarity and sodium above the normal range *without* inducing concentration of the urine. In that event, primary polydipsia and partial defects in AVP secretion and action are excluded, and the effect on urine osmolarity of injecting 2 μg of the AVP analogue, desmopressin, indicates whether the patient has severe pituitary DI or severe nephrogenic DI. However, this approach is of little or no diagnostic value if fluid deprivation results in concentration of the urine because the increases in urine osmolarity achieved both before and after the injection of desmopressin are similar in patients with *partial* pituitary DI, *partial* nephrogenic DI, and primary polydipsia. These disorders can be differentiated by measuring plasma AVP during fluid deprivation and relating it to the concurrent level of plasma and urine osmolarity (Fig. 6-3). However, this approach does not always differentiate clearly between partial pituitary DI and primary polydipsia unless the measurement is made when plasma osmolarity and sodium are at or above the normal range. This level is difficult to achieve by fluid deprivation alone once urinary concentration occurs. Therefore it is usually necessary to give a short infusion of 3% saline condition (0.1 mL/kg body weight per minute for 60 to 90 minutes) and repeat the measurement of plasma AVP.

A simpler but equally reliable way to differentiate between pituitary DI, nephrogenic DI, and primary polydipsia is to measure basal plasma AVP to determine if a brain magnetic resonance imaging (MRI) is needed and sufficient for diagnosis (Fig. 6-4). If plasma AVP *on ad libitum fluid intake* is normal or elevated (>1 pg/mL) when measured by a sensitive and specific assay, both primary polydipsia and pituitary DI are excluded and the diagnosis of nephrogenic DI can be confirmed, if desired, by a 1- to 2-day outpatient trial of desmopressin therapy. If, however, basal plasma AVP is low or undetectable (<1 pg/mL), nephrogenic DI is very unlikely and MRI of the brain can be used to differentiate pituitary DI from primary polydipsia. In

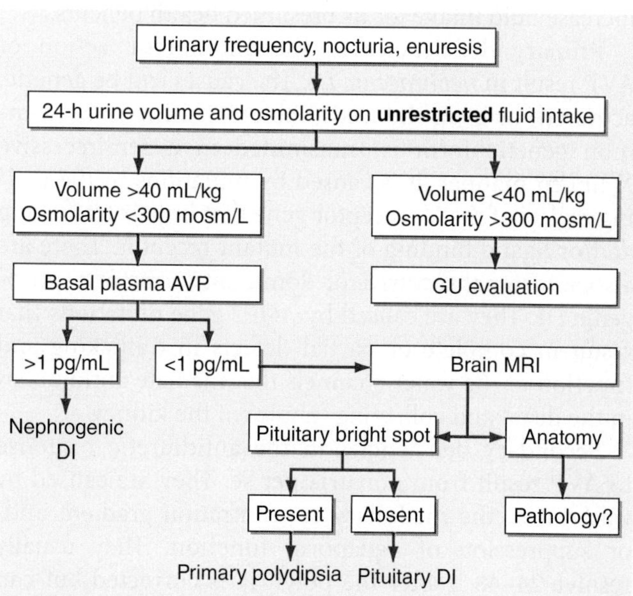

FIGURE 6-4
Simplified approach to the differential diagnosis of diabetes insipidus. When symptoms suggest diabetes insipidus (DI), the syndrome should be differentiated from a genitourinary (GU) abnormality by measuring the 24-h urine volume and osmolarity on unrestricted fluid intake. If DI is confirmed, basal plasma arginine vasopressin (AVP) should be measured on unrestricted fluid intake. If AVP is normal or elevated (>1 pg/mL), the patient probably has nephrogenic DI. However, if plasma AVP is low or undetectable, the patient has either pituitary DI or primary polydipsia. In that case, magnetic resonance imaging (MRI) of the brain can be performed to differentiate between these two conditions by determining whether or not the normal posterior pituitary bright spot is visible on T1-weighted midsagittal images. In addition, the MRI anatomy of the pituitary hypothalamic area can be examined to look for evidence of pathology that sometimes causes pituitary DI or the dipsogenic form of primary polydipsia. MRI is not reliable for differential diagnosis unless nephrogenic DI has been excluded because the bright spot is also absent, small, or faint in this condition.

most healthy adults and children, the posterior pituitary emits a hyperintense signal visible in T1-weighted midsagittal images. This "bright spot" is almost always present in patients with primary polydipsia but is always absent or abnormally small in patients with pituitary DI, even if their AVP deficiency is partial. The MRI is also useful in searching for pathology responsible for pituitary DI or the dipsogenic form of primary polydipsia (Fig. 6-2). The principal caveat is that MRI is not reliable for differential diagnosis of DI in patients with empty sella because they typically lack a bright spot even when their AVP secretion and action are normal. MRI also cannot be used to differentiate pituitary from nephrogenic DI because many patients with nephrogenic DI also lack a posterior pituitary bright spot, probably because they have an abnormally high rate of AVP secretion and turnover.

TREATMENT Diabetes Insipidus

The signs and symptoms of uncomplicated pituitary DI can be eliminated by treatment with desmopressin (DDAVP), a synthetic analogue of AVP (Fig. 6-1). DDAVP acts selectively at V_2 receptors to increase urine concentration and decrease urine flow in a dose-dependent manner. It is also more resistant to degradation than is AVP and has a three- to fourfold longer duration of action. DDAVP can be given by IV or SC injection, nasal inhalation, or orally by means of a tablet of melt. The doses required to control pituitary DI completely vary widely, depending on the patient and the route of administration. However, among adults, they usually range from 1–2 μg qd or bid by injection, 10–20 μg bid or tid by nasal spray, or 100–400 μg bid or tid orally. The onset of antidiuresis is rapid, ranging from as little as 15 min after injection to 60 min after oral administration. When given in a dose that normalizes 24-h urinary osmolarity (400–800 mosmol/L) and volume (15–30 mL/kg body weight), DDAVP produces a slight (1–3%) increase in total body water and a decrease in plasma osmolarity/sodium that rapidly eliminates thirst and polydipsia (Fig. 6-5). Consequently, water balance is maintained within the normal range. Hyponatremia does not develop unless urine volume is reduced too far (to less than 10 mL/kg per day) or fluid intake is excessive due to an associated abnormality in thirst or cognition. Fortunately, thirst abnormalities are rare, and if the patient is taught to drink only when truly thirsty, DDAVP can be given safely in doses sufficient to normalize urine output (~15–30 mL/kg per day) without the need for allowing intermittent escape to prevent water intoxication.

Primary polydipsia cannot be treated safely with DDAVP or any other antidiuretic drug because eliminating the polyuria does not eliminate the urge to drink. Therefore, it invariably produces hyponatremia and/or other signs of water intoxication, usually within 8–24 h if urine output is normalized completely. There is no consistently effective way to correct dipsogenic or psychogenic polydipsia, but the iatrogenic form may respond to patient education. To minimize the risk of water intoxication, all patients should be warned about the use of other drugs such as thiazide diuretics or carbamazepine (Tegretol) that can impair urinary free-water excretion directly or indirectly.

The polyuria and polydipsia of nephrogenic DI are not affected by treatment with standard doses of DDAVP. If resistance is partial, it may be overcome by tenfold higher doses, but this treatment is too expensive and inconvenient for long-term use. However, treatment with conventional doses of a thiazide diuretic and/or amiloride in conjunction with a low-sodium diet and a prostaglandin synthesis inhibitor (e.g., indomethacin) usually reduces the polyuria and polydipsia by 30–70% and may eliminate them completely in some patients. Side effects such as hypokalemia and gastric irritation can be minimized by the use of amiloride or potassium supplements and by taking medications with meals.

If MRI and/or AVP assays with the requisite sensitivity and specificity are unavailable and a fluid deprivation test is impractical or undesirable, a third way to differentiate between pituitary DI, nephrogenic DI, and primary polydipsia is a trial of desmopressin therapy. Such a trial should be conducted with very close monitoring of serum sodium as well as urine output, preferably in hospital, because desmopressin will produce hyponatremia in 8–24 h if the patient has primary polydipsia.

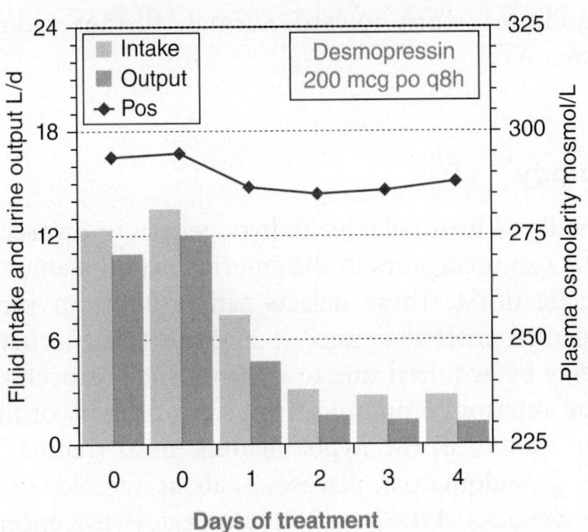

FIGURE 6-5

Effect of desmopressin therapy on fluid intake (*blue bars*), urine output (*orange bars*), and plasma osmolarity (*red line*) in a patient with uncomplicated pituitary diabetes insipidus. Note that treatment rapidly reduces fluid intake and urine output tonormal, with only a slight increase in body water as evidenced by the slight decrease in plasma osmolarity.

HYPODIPSIC HYPERNATREMIA

An increase in plasma osmolarity/sodium above the normal range (hypertonic hypernatremia) can be caused by either a decrease in total body water or an increase in total body sodium. The former results from a failure to drink enough to replace normal or increased urinary and insensible water loss. The deficient intake can be due either to water deprivation or a lack of thirst (hypodipsia). The most common cause of an increase in total body sodium is primary hyperaldosteronism **(Chap. 8)**. Rarely, it can also result from ingestion of hypertonic saline in the form of sea water or incorrectly prepared infant formula. However, even in these forms of hypernatremia, inadequate intake of water also contributes. This chapter focuses on hypodipsic hypernatremia, the form of hypernatremia due to a primary defect in the thirst mechanism.

Clinical characteristics

Hypodipsic hypernatremia is a syndrome characterized by chronic or recurrent hypertonic dehydration. The hypernatremia varies widely in severity and usually is associated with signs of hypovolemia such as tachycardia, postural hypotension, azotemia, hyperuricemia, and hypokalemia due to secondary hyperaldosteronism. Muscle weakness, pain, rhabdomyolysis, hyperglycemia, hyperlipidemia, and acute renal failure may also occur. Obtundation or coma may be present but are often absent. Despite inappropriately low levels of plasma AVP, DI usually is not evident at presentation but may develop during rehydration as blood volume, blood pressure, and plasma osmolarity/sodium return toward normal, further reducing plasma AVP.

Etiology

Hypodipsia is usually due to hypogenesis or destruction of the osmoreceptors in the anterior hypothalamus that regulate thirst. These defects can result from various congenital malformations of midline brain structures or may be acquired due to diseases such as occlusions of the anterior communicating artery, primary or metastatic tumors in the hypothalamus, head trauma, surgery, granulomatous diseases such as sarcoidosis and histiocytosis, AIDS, and cytomegalovirus encephalitis. Because of their proximity, the osmoreceptors that regulate AVP secretion also are usually impaired. Thus, AVP secretion responds poorly or not at all to hyperosmotic stimulation (Fig. 6-6) but, in most cases, increases normally to nonosmotic stimuli such as nausea or large reductions in blood volume or blood pressure, indicating that the neurohypophysis is intact.

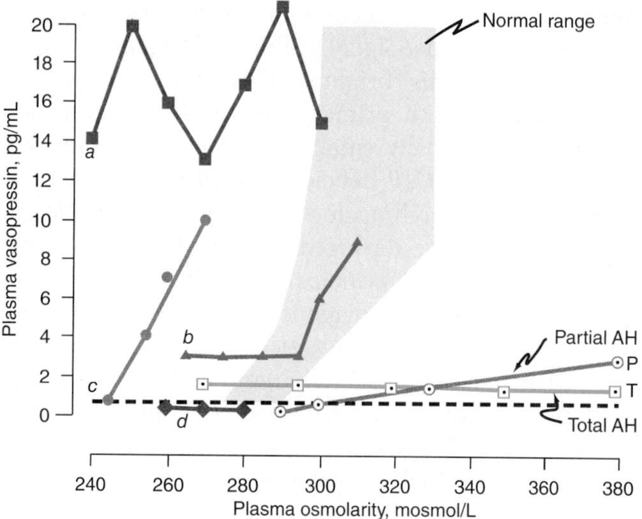

FIGURE 6-6

Heterogeneity of osmoregulatory dysfunction in adipsic hypernatremia (AH) and the syndrome of inappropriate antidiuresis (SIAD). Each line depicts schematically the relationship of plasma arginine vasopressin (AVP) to plasma osmolarity during water loading and/or infusion of 3% saline in a patient with either AH (*open symbols*) or SIAD (*closed symbols*). The shaded area indicates the normal range of the relationship. The horizontal broken line indicates the plasma AVP level below which the hormone is undetectable and urinary concentration usually does not occur. Lines P and T represent patients with a selective deficiency in the osmoregulation of thirst and AVP that is either partial (○) or total (□). In the latter, plasma AVP does not change in response to increases or decreases in plasma osmolarity but remains within a range sufficient to concentrate the urine even if overhydration produces hypotonic hyponatremia. In contrast, if the osmoregulatory deficiency is partial (○), rehydration of the patient suppresses plasma AVP to levels that result in urinary dilution and polyuria before plasma osmolarity and sodium are reduced to normal. Lines *a* –*d* represent different defects in the osmoregulation of plasma AVP observed in patients with SIADH or SIAD. In *a* (■), plasma AVP is markedly elevated and fluctuates widely without relation to changes in plasma osmolarity, indicating complete loss of osmoregulation. In *b* (▲), plasma AVP remains fixed at a slightly elevated level until plasma osmolarity reaches the normal range, at which point it begins to rise appropriately, indicating a selective defect in the inhibitory component of the osmoregulatory mechanism. In *c* (●), plasma AVP rises in close correlation with plasma osmolarity before the latter reaches the normal range, indicating downward resetting of the osmostat. In *d* (◆), plasma AVP appears to be osmoregulated normally, suggesting that the inappropriate antidiuresis is caused by some other abnormality.

Pathophysiology

Hypodipsia results in a failure to drink enough water to replenish obligatory renal and extrarenal losses. Consequently, plasma osmolarity and sodium rise often to extremely high levels before the disorder is recognized. In most cases, urinary loss of water contributes little, if any, to the dehydration because AVP continues to be secreted in the small amounts necessary to concentrate the urine. In some patients this appears to be due to hypovolemic stimulation and/or incomplete destruction of AVP osmoreceptors because plasma AVP declines and DI develops during rehydration (Fig. 6-6). In others, however, plasma AVP does not decline during rehydration even if they are overhydrated. Consequently, they develop a hyponatremic syndrome indistinguishable from inappropriate antidiuresis. This suggests that the AVP osmoreceptors normally provide inhibitory and stimulatory input to the neurohypophysis and the patients can no longer osmotically stimulate or suppress tonic secretion of the hormone because both inputs have been totally eliminated by the same pathology that destroyed the osmoregulation of thirst. In a few patients, the neurohypophysis is also destroyed, resulting in a combination of chronic pituitary DI and hypodipsia that is particularly difficult to manage.

Differential diagnosis

Hypodipsic hypernatremia usually can be distinguished from other causes of inadequate fluid intake (e.g., coma, paralysis, restraints, absence of fresh water) by the clinical history and setting. Previous episodes and/or denial of thirst and failure to drink spontaneously when the patient is conscious, unrestrained, and hypernatremic are virtually diagnostic. The hypernatremia caused by excessive retention or intake of sodium can be distinguished by the presence of thirst as well as the physical and laboratory signs of hypervolemia rather than hypovolemia.

TREATMENT Hypodipsic Hypernatremia

Hypodipsic hypernatremia should be treated by administering water orally if the patient is alert and cooperative or by infusing hypotonic fluids (0.45% saline or 5% dextrose and water) if the patient is not. The amount of free water in liters required to correct the deficit (ΔFW) can be estimated from body weight in kg (BW) and the serum sodium concentration in mmol/L (S_{Na}) by the formula $\Delta FW = 0.5BW \times ([S_{Na} - 140]/140)$. If serum glucose ($S_{Glu}$) is elevated, the measured S_{Na} should be corrected (S_{Na}^*) by the formula $S_{Na}^* = S_{Na} + ([S_{Glu} - 90]/36)$. This amount plus an allowance for continuing insensible and urinary losses should be given over a 24- to 48-h period. Close monitoring of serum sodium as well as fluid intake and urinary output is essential because, depending on the extent of osmoreceptor deficiency, some patients will develop AVP-deficient DI, requiring DDAVP therapy to complete rehydration; others will develop hyponatremia and a syndrome of inappropriate antidiuresis (SIAD)-like picture if overhydrated. If hyperglycemia and/or hypokalemia are present, insulin and/or potassium supplements should be given with the expectation that both can be discontinued soon after rehydration is complete. Plasma urea/creatinine should be monitored closely for signs of acute renal failure caused by rhabdomyolysis, hypovolemia, and hypotension.

Once the patient has been rehydrated, an MRI of the brain and tests of anterior pituitary function should be performed to look for the cause and collateral defects in other hypothalamic functions. A long-term management plan to prevent or minimize recurrence of the fluid and electrolyte imbalance also should be developed. This should include a practical method to regulate fluid intake in accordance with variations in water balance as indicated by changes in body weight or serum sodium determined by home monitoring analyzers. Prescribing a constant fluid intake is ineffective and potentially dangerous because it does not take into account the large, uncontrolled variations in insensible loss that inevitably result from changes in ambient temperature and physical activity.

HYPONATREMIA DUE TO INAPPROPRIATE ANTIDIURESIS

A decrease in plasma osmolarity/sodium below the normal range (hypotonic hyponatremia) can be due to any of three different types of salt and water imbalance: (1) an increase in total body water that exceeds the increase in total body sodium (hypervolemic hyponatremia); (2) a decrease in body sodium greater than the decrease in body water (hypovolemic hyponatremia); or (3) an increase in body water with little or no change in body sodium (euvolemic hyponatremia). All three forms are associated with a failure to fully dilute the urine and mount a water diuresis in the face of hypotonic hyponatremia. The hypervolemic form typically occurs in disorders like severe congestive heart failure or cirrhosis. The hypovolemic form typically occurs in disorders such as severe diarrhea, diuretic abuse, or mineralocorticoid deficiency. Euvolemic hyponatremia, however, is due mainly to expansion of total body water caused by excessive intake in the face of a defect in urinary dilution. The impaired dilution is usually caused by a defect in the osmotic suppression of AVP that can have either of two causes. One is a nonhemodynamic stimulus such as nausea or a cortisol deficiency, which can be corrected quickly by treatment with antiemetics or cortisol. The other is a primary defect in osmoregulation caused by another disorder such as malignancy, stroke, or pneumonia that cannot be easily or quickly corrected. The latter is commonly known as the syndrome of inappropriate antidiuretic hormone (SIADH). Much less often, euvolemic hyponatremia can also result from AVP-independent activation of renal V_2 receptors, a variant known as nephrogenic inappropriate antidiuresis or NSIAD. Both of the latter will be discussed in this chapter.

Clinical characteristics

Antidiuresis of any cause decreases the volume and increases the concentration of urine. If not accompanied by a commensurate reduction in fluid intake or an increase in insensible loss, the reduction in urine output results in excess water retention which expands and dilutes body fluids. If the hyponatremia develops gradually or has been present for more than a few days, it may be largely asymptomatic. However, if it develops acutely, it is usually accompanied by symptoms and signs of water intoxication that may include mild headache, confusion, anorexia, nausea, vomiting, coma, and convulsions. Severe acute hyponatremia may be lethal. Other clinical signs and symptoms vary greatly, depending on the type of hyponatremia. The hypervolemic form is characterized by generalized edema and other signs of marked volume expansion. The opposite is evident in the hypovolemic form. However, overt signs of volume expansion or contraction are absent in SIADH, SIAD, and other forms of euvolemic hyponatremia.

Etiology

In SIADH, the inappropriate secretion of AVP can have many different causes. They include ectopic production of AVP by lung cancer or other neoplasms; eutopic release induced by various diseases or drugs; and exogenous administration of AVP, DDAVP, or large doses of oxytocin (Table 6-2). The ectopic forms result from abnormal expression of the *AVP-NPII* gene by primary or metastatic malignancies. The eutopic forms occur most often in patients with acute infections or strokes but have also been associated with many other neurologic diseases and injuries. The mechanisms by which these diseases interfere with osmotic suppression of AVP are not known. The defect in osmoregulation can take any of four distinct forms (Fig. 6-6). In one of the most common (reset osmostat), AVP secretion remains fully responsive to changes in plasma osmolarity/sodium, but the threshold, or set point, of the osmoregulatory system is abnormally low. These patients differ from those with the other types of SIADH in that they are able to maximally suppress plasma AVP and dilute their urine if their fluid intake is high enough to reduce their plasma osmolarity and/or sodium to the new set point. In most patients, SIADH is self-limited and remits spontaneously within 2–3 weeks, but about 10% of cases are chronic. Another, smaller subgroup (~10% of the total) has inappropriate antidiuresis without a demonstrable defect in the osmoregulation of plasma AVP (Fig. 6-6). In some of them, all young boys, the inappropriate antidiuresis has been traced to a constitutively activating mutation of the V_2 receptor gene. This unusual variant may be referred to as familial nephrogenic SIAD (NSIAD) to distinguish it from other possible causes of the syndrome. The inappropriate antidiuresis in these patients appears to be permanent, although the hyponatremia is variable owing presumably to individual differences in fluid intake.

TABLE 6-2

CAUSES OF SYNDROME OF INAPPROPRIATE ANTIDIURETIC HORMONE (SIADH)

Neoplasms	Neurologic
Carcinomas	Guillain-Barré syndrome
Lung	Multiple sclerosis
Duodenum	Delirium tremens
Pancreas	Amyotrophic lateral sclerosis
Ovary	Hydrocephalus
Bladder, ureter	Psychosis
Other neoplasms	Peripheral neuropathy
Thymoma	Congenital malformations
Mesothelioma	Agenesis corpus callosum
Bronchial adenoma	Cleft lip/palate
Carcinoid	Other midline defects
Gangliocytoma	Metabolic
Ewing's sarcoma	Acute intermittent porphyria
Head trauma (closed and penetrating)	Pulmonary
Infections	Asthma
Pneumonia, bacterial or viral	Pneumothorax
Abscess, lung or brain	Positive-pressure respiration
Cavitation (aspergillosis)	Drugs
Tuberculosis, lung or brain	Vasopressin or desmopressin
Meningitis, bacterial or viral	Serotonin reuptake inhibitors
Encephalitis	Oxytocin, high dose
AIDS	Vincristine
Vascular	Carbamazepine
Cerebrovascular occlusions, hemorrhage	Nicotine
Cavernous sinus thrombosis	Phenothiazines
	Cyclophosphamide
	Tricyclic antidepressants
	Monoamine oxidase inhibitors

Pathophysiology

Impaired osmotic suppression of antidiuresis results in excessive retention of water and dilution of body fluids only if water intake exceeds insensible and urinary losses. The excess intake is sometimes due to an associated defect in the osmoregulation of thirst (dipsogenic) but can also be psychogenic or iatrogenic, including excessive IV administration of hypotonic fluids. In SIADH and other forms of euvolemic hyponatremia, the decrease in plasma osmolarity/sodium and the increase in extracellular and intracellular volume are proportional to the amount of water retained. Thus, an increase in body water of 10% (~4 L in a 70-kg adult) reduces plasma osmolarity and sodium by approximately 10% (~28 mosmol/L or 14 meq/L). An increase in body water of this magnitude is rarely detectable on physical examination but will be reflected in a weight gain of about 4 kg. It also increases glomerular filtration and atrial natriuretic hormone and suppresses plasma renin activity, thereby increasing urinary sodium excretion. The resultant reduction in total body sodium decreases the expansion of extracellular volume but aggravates the hyponatremia and further expands intracellular volume. The latter further increases brain swelling and intracranial pressure, which probably produces most of the symptoms of acute water intoxication. Within a few days, this swelling may be counteracted by inactivation or elimination of intracellular solutes, resulting in the remission of symptoms even though the hyponatremia persists.

In type I (hypervolemic) or type II (hypovolemic) hyponatremia, osmotic suppression of AVP secretion appears to be counteracted by a hemodynamic stimulus resulting from a large reduction in cardiac output and/or effective blood volume. The resultant antidiuresis is enhanced by decreased distal delivery of glomerular filtrate that results from increased reabsorption of sodium in proximal nephron. If the reduction in urine output is not associated with a commensurate reduction in water intake or an increase in insensible loss, body fluids are expanded and diluted, resulting in hyponatremia despite an increase in body sodium. Unlike SIADH and other forms of euvolemic hyponatremia, however, glomerular filtration is reduced and plasma renin activity and aldosterone are elevated. Thus, the rate of urinary sodium excretion is low (unless sodium reabsorption is impaired by a diuretic), and the hyponatremia is usually accompanied by edema, hypokalemia, azotemia, and hyperuricemia. In type II (hypovolemic) hyponatremia, sodium and water are also retained as an appropriate compensatory response to the severe depletion.

Differential diagnosis

SIADH is a diagnosis of exclusion that usually can be made from the history, physical examination, and basic laboratory data. If hyperglycemia is present, its contribution to the reduction in plasma sodium can be estimated either by measuring plasma osmolarity for a more accurate estimate of the true "effective" tonicity of body fluids or by correcting the measured plasma sodium for the reduction caused by the hyperglycemia using the simplified formula

$$\text{corrected } P_{na} = \text{measured } P_{na} + (P_{glu} - 90)/36$$

If the plasma osmolarity and/or corrected plasma sodium are below normal limits, hypotonic hyponatremia is present and further evaluation to determine the type should be undertaken in order to administer safe and effective treatment. This differentiation is usually possible by evaluating standard clinical indicators of the extracellular fluid volume (Table 6-3). If these findings are ambiguous or contradictory, measuring plasma renin activity or the *rate* of urinary sodium excretion may be helpful *provided* that the hyponatremia is not in the recovery phase or is due to a primary defect in renal conservation of sodium, diuretic abuse, or hyporeninemic hypoaldosteronism. The latter may be suspected if serum potassium is elevated instead of low, as it usually is in types I and II hyponatremia. Measurements of plasma AVP are currently of no value in differentiating SIADH from the other types of hyponatremia since the plasma levels are elevated similarly in all. In patients who fulfill the clinical criteria for type III (euvolemic) hyponatremia, morning plasma cortisol should also be measured to exclude secondary adrenal insufficiency. If it is normal and there is no history of nausea/vomiting, the diagnosis of SIADH is confirmed, and a careful search for occult lung cancer or other common causes of the syndrome (Table 6-2) should be undertaken.

SIAD due to an activating mutation of the V_2 receptor gene should be suspected if the hyponatremia occurs in a child or several members of the family or is refractory to treatment with a vaptan (see below). In that case, plasma AVP should be measured to confirm that it is appropriately suppressed while the hyponatremia and antidiuresis are present, and the V_2 receptor gene should be sequenced, if possible.

TREATMENT Hyponatremia

The management of hyponatremia differs depending on the type and the severity and duration of symptoms. In acute symptomatic SIADH, the aim should be to raise plasma osmolarity and/or plasma sodium at a rate approximating 1% an hour until they reach levels of about 270 mosmol/L or 130 meq/L, respectively. This can be accomplished in either of two ways. One is to infuse hypertonic (3%) saline at a rate of about 0.05 mL/kg body weight per minute. This treatment also has the advantage of correcting the sodium deficiency that is partly responsible for the hyponatremia and often produces a solute diuresis that serves to remove some of the excess water. The other treatment is to reduce body water by giving an AVP receptor-2 antagonist (vaptan) to block the antidiuretic effect of AVP and increase urine output (Fig. 6-7). One of the vaptans, a combined V_2/V_{1a} antagonist (Conivaptan), has been approved for short-term, in-hospital IV treatment of SIADH, and others are in various stages of development. With either approach, fluid intake should be restricted to less than urine output, and serum sodium should be checked at least once every 2h to ensure it is not raised too fast or too far. Doing so may result in central pontine myelinolysis, an acute, potentially fatal neurologic syndrome characterized by quadriparesis, ataxia, and abnormal extraocular movements.

In chronic and/or minimally symptomatic SIADH, the hyponatremia can and should be corrected more gradually.

TABLE 6-3

DIFFERENTIAL DIAGNOSIS OF HYPONATREMIA BASED ON CLINICAL ASSESSMENT OF EXTRACELLULAR FLUID VOLUME (ECFV)

CLINICAL FINDINGS	TYPE I, HYPERVOLEMIC	TYPE II, HYPOVOLEMIC	TYPE III, EUVOLEMIC	SIADH AND SIAD EUVOLEMIC
History				
CHF, cirrhosis, or nephrosis	Yes	No	No	No
Salt and water loss	No	Yes	No	No
ACTH–cortisol deficiency and/or nausea and vomiting	No	No	Yes	No
Physical examination				
Generalized edema, ascites	Yes	No	No	No
Postural hypotension	Maybe	Maybe	Maybe[a]	No
Laboratory				
BUN, creatinine	High-normal	High-normal	Low-normal	Low-normal
Uric acid	High-normal	High-normal	Low-normal	Low-normal
Serum potassium	Low-normal	Low-normal[b]	Normal[c]	Normal
Serum urate	High	High	Low	Low
Serum albumin	Low-normal	High-normal	Normal	Normal
Serum cortisol	Normal-high	Normal-high[d]	Low[e]	Normal
Plasma renin activity	High	High	Low[f]	Low
Urinary sodium (meq per unit of time)[g]	Low	Low[h]	High[i]	High[i]

[a]Postural hypotension may occur in secondary (ACTH-dependent) adrenal insufficiency even though extracellular fluid volume and aldosterone are usually normal.
[b]Serum potassium may be high if hypovolemia is due to aldosterone deficiency.
[c]Serum potassium may be low if vomiting causes alkalosis.
[d]Serum cortisol is low if hypovolemia is due to primary adrenal insufficiency (Addison's disease).
[e]Serum cortisol will be normal or high if the cause is nausea and vomiting rather than secondary (ACTH-dependent) adrenal insufficiency.
[f]Plasma renin activity may be high if the cause is secondary (ACTH) adrenal insufficiency.
[g]Urinary sodium should be expressed as the *rate of excretion* rather than the concentration. In a hyponatremic adult, an excretion rate >25 meq/d (or 25 µeq/mg of creatinine) could be considered high.
[h]The rate of urinary sodium excretion may be high if the hypovolemia is due to diuretic abuse, primary adrenal insufficiency, or other causes of renal sodium wasting.
[i]The rate of urinary sodium excretion may be low if intake is curtailed by symptoms or treatment.
Abbreviations: ACTH, adrenocorticotropic hormone; BUN, blood urea nitrogen; CHF, congestive heart failure; SIAD, syndrome of inappropriate antidiuresis.

This can be achieved by restricting total fluid intake to less than the sum of urinary and insensible losses. Because the water derived from food (300–700 mL/d) usually approximates basal insensible losses in adults, the aim should be to reduce total discretionary intake (all liquids) to approximately 500 mL less than urinary output. Adherence to this regimen is often problematic and, even if achieved, usually reduces body water and increases serum sodium by only about 1–2% per day. Hence, additional approaches are usually desirable if not necessary. The best approach for treatment of chronic SIADH is the administration of an oral vaptan, tolvaptan, a selective V_2 antagonist that also increases urinary water excretion by blocking the antidiuretic effect of AVP. Some restriction of fluid intake may also be necessary to achieve satisfactory control of the hyponatremia. It is approved for treatment of nonemergent SIADH with initial in-hospital dosing. Other approaches include demeclocycline, 150–300 mg PO tid or qid, or fludrocortisone, 0.05–0.2 mg PO bid. The effect of the demeclocycline manifests in 7–14 days and is due to induction of a reversible form of nephrogenic DI. Potential side effects include phototoxicity and azotemia. The effect of fludrocortisone also requires 1–2 weeks and is partly due to increased retention of sodium and possibly inhibition of thirst. It also increases urinary potassium excretion, which may require replacement through dietary adjustments or supplements and may induce hypertension, occasionally necessitating discontinuation of the treatment.

In euvolemic hyponatremia caused by protracted nausea and vomiting or isolated glucocorticoid deficiency (type III), all abnormalities can be corrected quickly and completely by giving an antiemetic or stress doses of hydrocortisone (for glucocorticoid deficiency). As with other treatments, care must be taken to ensure that serum sodium does not rise too quickly or too far.

In SIAD due to an activating mutation of the V_2 receptor, the V_2 antagonists usually do not block the antidiuresis or raise plasma osmolarity/sodium. In that condition, use of an osmotic diuretic such as urea is reported to be effective in preventing or correcting hyponatremia. However, some vaptans may be effective in patients with a different type of activating mutation so the response to this therapy may be neither predictable nor diagnostic.

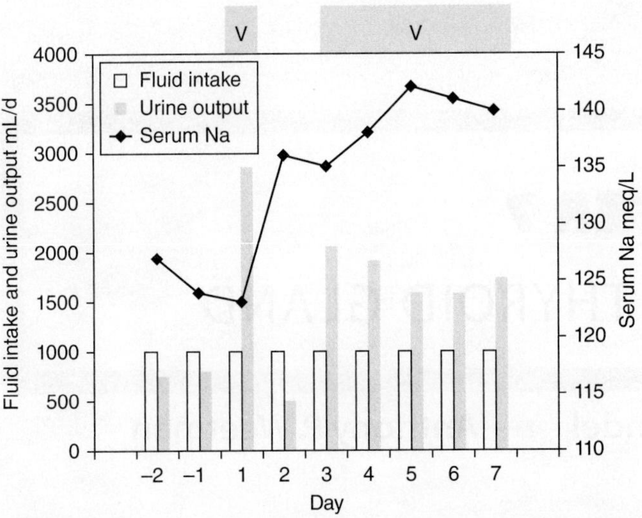

FIGURE 6-7
The effect of vaptan therapy on water balance in a patient with chronic syndrome of inappropriate antidiuretic hormone (SIADH). The periods of vaptan (V) therapy are indicated by the green shaded boxes at the top. Urine output is indicated by orange bars. Fluid intake is shown by the open bars. Intake was restricted to 1 L/d throughout. Serum sodium is indicated by the black line. Note that sodium increased progressively when vaptan increased urine output to levels that clearly exceeded fluid intake.

In hypervolemic hyponatremia, fluid restriction is also appropriate and somewhat effective if it can be maintained. However, infusion of hypertonic saline is contraindicated because it further increases total body sodium and edema and may precipitate cardiovascular decompensation. However, as in SIADH, the V_2 receptor antagonists are also safe and effective in the treatment of hypervolemic hyponatremia caused by congestive heart failure. Tolvaptan is approved by the Food and Drug Administration for this indication with the caveat that treatment should be initiated or reinitiated in hospital. Its use should also be limited to 30 days at a time because of reports that longer periods may be associated with abnormal liver chemistries.

In hypovolemic hyponatremia, the defect in AVP secretion and water balance usually can be corrected easily and quickly by stopping the loss of sodium and water and/or replacing the deficits by mouth or IV infusion of normal or hypertonic saline. As with the treatment of other forms of hyponatremia, care must be taken to ensure that plasma sodium does not increase too rapidly or too far. Fluid restriction and administration of AVP antagonists are contraindicated in type II hyponatremia because they would only aggravate the underlying volume depletion and could result in hemodynamic collapse.

GLOBAL PERSPECTIVES

The incidence, clinical characteristics, etiology, pathophysiology, differential diagnosis, and treatments of fluid and electrolyte disorders in tropical and nonindustrialized countries differ in some respects from those in the United States and other industrialized parts of the world. Hyponatremia, for example, appears to be more common and is more likely to be due to infectious diseases such as cholera, shigellosis, and other diarrheal disorders. In these circumstances, hyponatremia is probably due to gastrointestinal losses of salt and water (hypovolemia type II), but other abnormalities, including undefined infectious toxins, also may contribute. The causes of DI are similar worldwide except that malaria and venoms from snake or insect bites are much more common.

CHAPTER 7

DISORDERS OF THE THYROID GLAND

J. Larry Jameson ■ Susan J. Mandel ■ Anthony P. Weetman

The thyroid gland produces two related hormones, thyroxine (T_4) and triiodothyronine (T_3) (Fig. 7-1). Acting through thyroid hormone receptors α and β, these hormones play a critical role in cell differentiation during development and help maintain thermogenic and metabolic homeostasis in the adult. Autoimmune disorders of the thyroid gland can stimulate overproduction of thyroid hormones (*thyrotoxicosis*) or cause glandular destruction and hormone deficiency (*hypothyroidism*). In addition, benign nodules and various forms of thyroid cancer are relatively common and amenable to detection by physical examination.

ANATOMY AND DEVELOPMENT

The thyroid (Greek *thyreos*, shield, plus *eidos*, form) consists of two lobes connected by an isthmus. It is located anterior to the trachea between the cricoid cartilage and the suprasternal notch. The normal thyroid is 12–20 g in size, highly vascular, and soft in consistency. Four parathyroid glands, which produce parathyroid hormone **(Chap. 34)**, are located posterior to each pole of the thyroid. The recurrent laryngeal nerves traverse the lateral borders of the thyroid gland and must be identified during thyroid surgery to avoid injury and vocal cord paralysis.

The thyroid gland develops from the floor of the primitive pharynx during the third week of gestation. The developing gland migrates along the thyroglossal duct to reach its final location in the neck. This feature accounts for the rare ectopic location of thyroid tissue at the base of the tongue (lingual thyroid) as well as the occurrence of thyroglossal duct cysts along this developmental tract. Thyroid hormone synthesis normally begins at about 11 weeks' gestation.

Neural crest derivatives from the ultimobranchial body give rise to thyroid medullary C cells that produce calcitonin, a calcium-lowering hormone. The C cells are interspersed throughout the thyroid gland, although their density is greatest in the juncture of the upper one-third and lower two-thirds of the gland. Calcitonin plays a minimal role in calcium homeostasis in humans but the C-cells are important because of their involvement in medullary thyroid cancer.

Thyroid gland development is orchestrated by the coordinated expression of several developmental transcription factors. Thyroid transcription factor (TTF)-1, TTF-2, and paired homeobox-8 (PAX-8) are expressed selectively, but not exclusively, in the thyroid gland. In combination, they dictate thyroid cell development and the induction of thyroid-specific genes such as thyroglobulin (Tg), thyroid peroxidase (TPO), the sodium iodide symporter (Na^+/I^-, NIS), and the thyroid-stimulating hormone receptor (TSH-R). Mutations in these developmental transcription factors or their downstream target genes are rare causes of thyroid agenesis or dyshormonogenesis, although the causes of most forms of congenital hypothyroidism remain unknown (Table 7-1). Because congenital hypothyroidism occurs in approximately 1 in 4000 newborns, neonatal screening is now performed in most industrialized countries (see below). Transplacental passage of maternal thyroid hormone occurs before the fetal thyroid gland begins to function and provides partial hormone support to a fetus with congenital hypothyroidism. Early thyroid hormone replacement in newborns with congenital hypothyroidism prevents potentially severe developmental abnormalities.

The thyroid gland consists of numerous spherical follicles composed of thyroid follicular cells that surround secreted colloid, a proteinaceous fluid containing large amounts of thyroglobulin, the protein precursor of thyroid hormones (Fig. 7-2). The thyroid follicular cells are polarized—the basolateral surface is apposed to the bloodstream and an apical surface faces the follicular lumen. Increased demand for thyroid hormone is regulated by thyroid-stimulating hormone (TSH), which binds to its receptor on the basolateral surface of

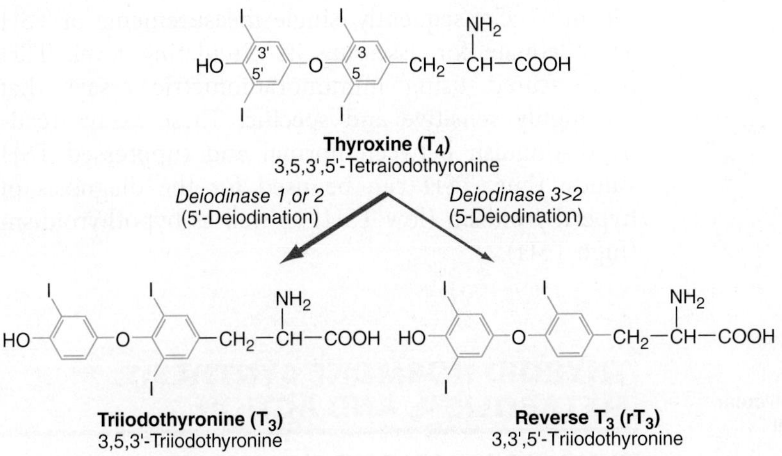

FIGURE 7-1
Structures of thyroid hormones. Thyroxine (T_4) contains four iodine atoms. Deiodination leads to production of the potent hormone triiodothyronine (T_3) or the inactive hormone reverse T_3.

the follicular cells. This binding leads to Tg reabsorption from the follicular lumen and proteolysis within the cytoplasm, yielding thyroid hormones for secretion into the bloodstream.

REGULATION OF THE THYROID AXIS

TSH, secreted by the thyrotrope cells of the anterior pituitary, plays a pivotal role in control of the thyroid axis and serves as the most useful physiologic marker of thyroid hormone action. TSH is a 31-kDa hormone composed of α and β subunits; the α subunit is common to the other glycoprotein hormones (luteinizing hormone, follicle-stimulating hormone, human chorionic gonadotropin [hCG]), whereas the TSH β subunit is unique to TSH. The extent and nature of carbohydrate modification are modulated by thyrotropin-releasing hormone (TRH) stimulation and influence the biologic activity of the hormone.

The thyroid axis is a classic example of an endocrine feedback loop. Hypothalamic TRH stimulates pituitary production of TSH, which, in turn, stimulates thyroid hormone synthesis and secretion. Thyroid hormones act via negative feedback predominantly through thyroid hormone receptor β2 (TRβ2) to inhibit TRH and TSH production (Fig. 7-2). The "set-point" in this axis is established by TSH. TRH is the major positive

TABLE 7-1
GENETIC CAUSES OF CONGENITAL HYPOTHYROIDISM

DEFECTIVE GENE PROTEIN	INHERITANCE	CONSEQUENCES
PROP-1	Autosomal recessive	Combined pituitary hormone deficiencies with preservation of adrenocorticotropic hormone
PIT-1	Autosomal recessive Autosomal dominant	Combined deficiencies of growth hormone, prolactin, thyroid-stimulating hormone (TSH)
TSHβ	Autosomal recessive	TSH deficiency
TTF-1 (TITF-1)	Autosomal dominant	Variable thyroid hypoplasia, choreoathetosis, pulmonary problems
TTF-2 (FOXE-1)	Autosomal recessive	Thyroid agenesis, choanal atresia, spiky hair
PAX-8	Autosomal dominant	Thyroid dysgenesis
TSH-receptor	Autosomal recessive	Resistance to TSH
$G_{S\alpha}$ (Albright hereditary osteodystrophy)	Autosomal dominant	Resistance to TSH
Na^+/I^- symporter	Autosomal recessive	Inability to transport iodide
DUOX2 (THOX2)	Autosomal dominant	Organification defect
DUOXA2	Autosomal recessive	Organification defect
Thyroid peroxidase	Autosomal recessive	Defective organification of iodide
Thyroglobulin	Autosomal recessive	Defective synthesis of thyroid hormone
Pendrin	Autosomal recessive	Pendred syndrome: sensorineural deafness and partial organification defect in thyroid
Dehalogenase 1	Autosomal recessive	Loss of iodide reutilization

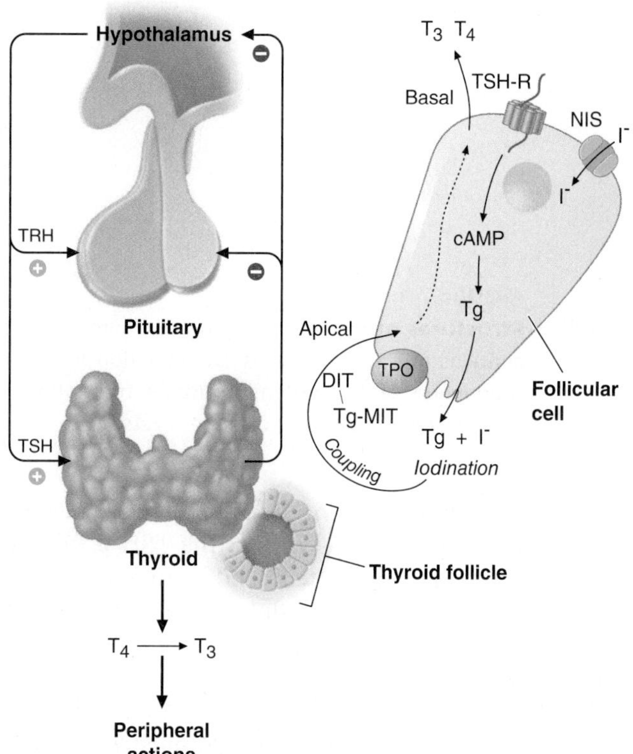

FIGURE 7-2

Regulation of thyroid hormone synthesis. *Left.* Thyroid hormones T_4 and T_3 feed back to inhibit hypothalamic production of thyrotropin-releasing hormone (TRH) and pituitary production of thyroid-stimulating hormone (TSH). TSH stimulates thyroid gland production of T_4 and T_3. ***Right.*** Thyroid follicles are formed by thyroid epithelial cells surrounding proteinaceous colloid, which contains thyroglobulin. Follicular cells, which are polarized, synthesize thyroglobulin and carry out thyroid hormone biosynthesis (see text for details). DIT, diiodotyrosine; MIT, monoiodotyrosine; NIS, sodium iodide symporter; Tg, thyroglobulin; TPO, thyroid peroxidase; TSH-R, thyroid-stimulating hormone receptor.

regulator of TSH synthesis and secretion. Peak TSH secretion occurs ~15 min after administration of exogenous TRH. Dopamine, glucocorticoids, and somatostatin suppress TSH but are not of major physiologic importance except when these agents are administered in pharmacologic doses. Reduced levels of thyroid hormone increase basal TSH production and enhance TRH-mediated stimulation of TSH. High thyroid hormone levels rapidly and directly suppress TSH gene expression secretion and inhibit TRH stimulation of TSH, indicating that thyroid hormones are the dominant regulator of TSH production. Like other pituitary hormones, TSH is released in a pulsatile manner and exhibits a diurnal rhythm; its highest levels occur at night. However, these TSH excursions are modest in comparison to those of other pituitary hormones, in part, because TSH has a relatively long plasma half-life (50 min). Consequently, single measurements of TSH are adequate for assessing its circulating level. TSH is measured using immunoradiometric assays that are highly sensitive and specific. These assays readily distinguish between normal and suppressed TSH values; thus, TSH can be used for the diagnosis of hyperthyroidism (low TSH) as well as hypothyroidism (high TSH).

THYROID HORMONE SYNTHESIS, METABOLISM, AND ACTION

THYROID HORMONE SYNTHESIS

Thyroid hormones are derived from Tg, a large iodinated glycoprotein. After secretion into the thyroid follicle, Tg is iodinated on tyrosine residues that are subsequently coupled via an ether linkage. Reuptake of Tg into the thyroid follicular cell allows proteolysis and the release of newly synthesized T_4 and T_3.

Iodine metabolism and transport

Iodide uptake is a critical first step in thyroid hormone synthesis. Ingested iodine is bound to serum proteins, particularly albumin. Unbound iodine is excreted in the urine. The thyroid gland extracts iodine from the circulation in a highly efficient manner. For example, 10–25% of radioactive tracer (e.g., ^{123}I) is taken up by the normal thyroid gland over 24 h; this value can rise to 70–90% in Graves' disease. Iodide uptake is mediated by NIS, which is expressed at the basolateral membrane of thyroid follicular cells. NIS is most highly expressed in the thyroid gland, but low levels are present in the salivary glands, lactating breast, and placenta. The iodide transport mechanism is highly regulated, allowing adaptation to variations in dietary supply. Low iodine levels increase the amount of NIS and stimulate uptake, whereas high iodine levels suppress NIS expression and uptake. The selective expression of NIS in the thyroid allows isotopic scanning, treatment of hyperthyroidism, and ablation of thyroid cancer with radioisotopes of iodine, without significant effects on other organs. Mutation of the *NIS* gene is a rare cause of congenital hypothyroidism, underscoring its importance in thyroid hormone synthesis. Another iodine transporter, pendrin, is located on the apical surface of thyroid cells and mediates iodine efflux into the lumen. Mutation of the *pendrin* gene causes *Pendred syndrome*, a disorder characterized by defective organification of iodine, goiter, and sensorineural deafness.

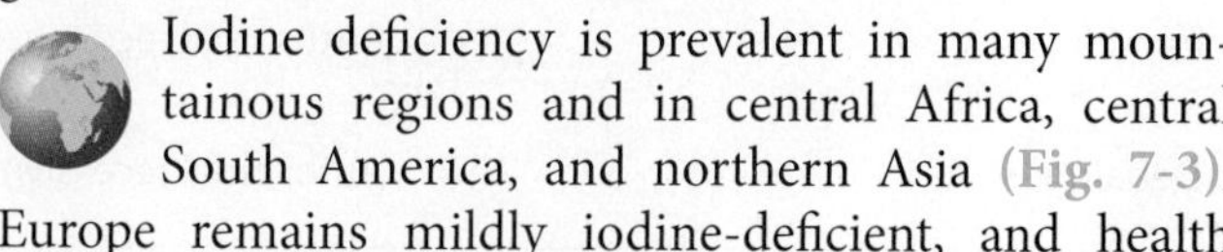

Iodine deficiency is prevalent in many mountainous regions and in central Africa, central South America, and northern Asia (Fig. 7-3). Europe remains mildly iodine-deficient, and health

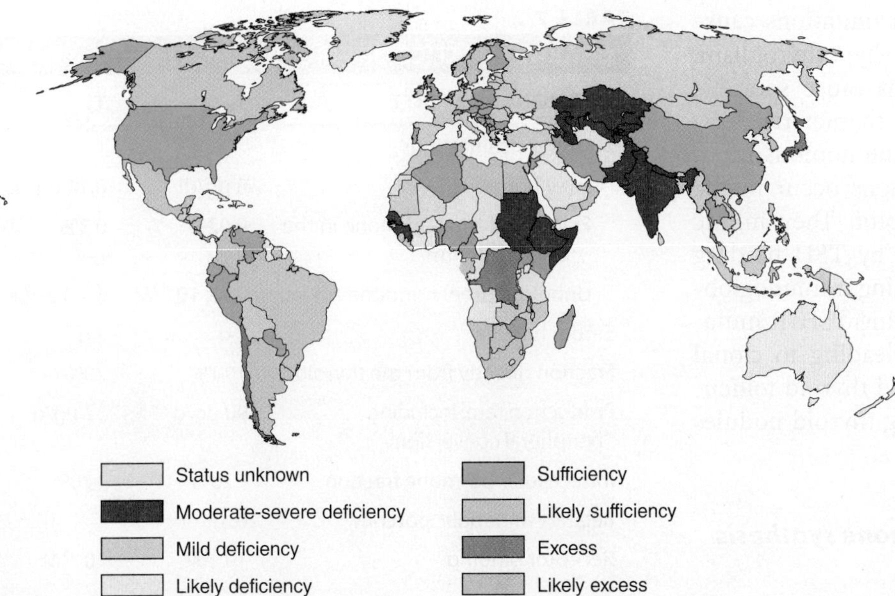

FIGURE 7-3 **Worldwide iodine nutrition.** Data are from the World Health Organization and the International Council for the Control of Iodine Deficiency Disorders (http://indorgs.virginia.edu/iccidd/mi/cidds.html).

surveys indicate that iodine intake has been falling in the United States and Australia. The World Health Organization (WHO) estimates that about 2 billion people are iodine-deficient, based on urinary excretion data. In areas of relative iodine deficiency, there is an increased prevalence of goiter and, when deficiency is severe, hypothyroidism and cretinism. *Cretinism* is characterized by mental and growth retardation and occurs when children who live in iodine-deficient regions are not treated with iodine or thyroid hormone to restore normal thyroid hormone levels during early life. These children are often born to mothers with iodine deficiency, and it is likely that maternal thyroid hormone deficiency worsens the condition. Concomitant selenium deficiency may also contribute to the neurologic manifestations of cretinism. Iodine supplementation of salt, bread, and other food substances has markedly reduced the prevalence of cretinism. Unfortunately, however, iodine deficiency remains the most common cause of preventable mental deficiency, often because of societal resistance to food additives or the cost of supplementation. In addition to overt cretinism, mild iodine deficiency can lead to subtle reduction of IQ. Oversupply of iodine, through supplements or foods enriched in iodine (e.g., shellfish, kelp), is associated with an increased incidence of autoimmune thyroid disease. The recommended average daily intake of iodine is 150–250 μg/d for adults, 90–120 μg/d for children, and 250 μg/d for pregnant and lactating women. Urinary iodine is >10 μg/dL in iodine-sufficient populations.

Organification, coupling, storage, and release

After iodide enters the thyroid, it is trapped and transported to the apical membrane of thyroid follicular cells, where it is oxidized in an organification reaction that involves TPO and hydrogen peroxide produced by dual oxidase (DUOX) and DUOX maturation factor (DUOXA). The reactive iodine atom is added to selected tyrosyl residues within Tg, a large (660 kDa) dimeric protein that consists of 2769 amino acids. The iodotyrosines in Tg are then coupled via an ether linkage in a reaction that is also catalyzed by TPO. Either T_4 or T_3 can be produced by this reaction, depending on the number of iodine atoms present in the iodotyrosines. After coupling, Tg is taken back into the thyroid cell, where it is processed in lysosomes to release T_4 and T_3. Uncoupled mono- and diiodotyrosines (MIT, DIT) are deiodinated by the enzyme dehalogenase, thereby recycling any iodide that is not converted into thyroid hormones.

Disorders of thyroid hormone synthesis are rare causes of congenital hypothyroidism. The vast majority of these disorders are due to recessive mutations in TPO or Tg, but defects have also been identified in the TSH-R, NIS, pendrin, hydrogen peroxide generation, and dehalogenase. Because of the biosynthetic defect, the gland is incapable of synthesizing adequate amounts of hormone, leading to increased TSH and a large goiter.

TSH action

TSH regulates thyroid gland function through the TSH-R, a seven-transmembrane G protein–coupled receptor (GPCR). The TSH-R is coupled to the α subunit of stimulatory G protein ($G_{S\alpha}$), which activates adenylyl cyclase, leading to increased production of cyclic adenosine monophosphate (AMP). TSH also stimulates phosphatidylinositol turnover by activating phospholipase C. The functional role of the TSH-R is exemplified by the consequences of naturally occurring mutations. Recessive loss-of-function mutations cause thyroid hypoplasia and congenital hypothyroidism. Dominant gain-of-function mutations cause sporadic or familial hyperthyroidism that is characterized by goiter, thyroid cell hyperplasia, and autonomous function. Most of these activating mutations occur in the transmembrane domain of the receptor. They mimic the conformational changes induced by TSH binding or the interactions of thyroid-stimulating immunoglobulins (TSI) in Graves' disease. Activating TSH-R mutations also occur as somatic events, leading to clonal selection and expansion of the affected thyroid follicular cell and autonomously functioning thyroid nodules (see below).

Other factors that influence hormone synthesis and release

Although TSH is the dominant hormonal regulator of thyroid gland growth and function, a variety of growth factors, most produced locally in the thyroid gland, also influence thyroid hormone synthesis. These include insulin-like growth factor I (IGF-I), epidermal growth factor, transforming growth factor β (TGF-β), endothelins, and various cytokines. The quantitative roles of these factors are not well understood, but they are important in selected disease states. In acromegaly, for example, increased levels of growth hormone and IGF-I are associated with goiter and predisposition to multinodular goiter (MNG). Certain cytokines and interleukins (ILs) produced in association with autoimmune thyroid disease induce thyroid growth, whereas others lead to apoptosis. Iodine deficiency increases thyroid blood flow and upregulates the NIS, stimulating more efficient iodine uptake. Excess iodide transiently inhibits thyroid iodide organification, a phenomenon known as the *Wolff-Chaikoff effect*. In individuals with a normal thyroid, the gland escapes from this inhibitory effect and iodide organification resumes; the suppressive action of high iodide may persist, however, in patients with underlying autoimmune thyroid disease.

THYROID HORMONE TRANSPORT AND METABOLISM

Serum binding proteins

T_4 is secreted from the thyroid gland in about twentyfold excess over T_3 (Table 7-2). Both hormones are bound to plasma proteins, including thyroxine-binding globulin (TBG), transthyretin (TTR, formerly known as thyroxine-binding prealbumin, or TBPA), and albumin. The plasma-binding proteins increase the pool of circulating hormone, delay hormone clearance, and may modulate hormone delivery to selected tissue sites. The concentration of TBG is relatively low (1–2 mg/dL), but because of its high affinity for thyroid hormones ($T_4 > T_3$), it carries about 80% of the bound hormones. Albumin has relatively low affinity for thyroid hormones but has a high plasma concentration (~3.5 g/dL), and it binds up to 10% of T_4 and 30% of T_3. TTR carries about 10% of T_4 but little T_3.

TABLE 7-2

CHARACTERISTICS OF CIRCULATING T_4 AND T_3

HORMONE PROPERTY	T_4	T_3
Serum concentrations		
Total hormone	8 μg/dL	0.14 μg/dL
Fraction of total hormone in the unbound form	0.02%	0.3%
Unbound (free) hormone	$21 \times 10^{-12} M$	$6 \times 10^{-12} M$
Serum half-life	7 d	2 d
Fraction directly from the thyroid	100%	20%
Production rate, including peripheral conversion	90 μg/d	32 μg/d
Intracellular hormone fraction	~20%	~70%
Relative metabolic potency	0.3	1
Receptor binding	$10^{-10} M$	$10^{-11} M$

When the effects of the various binding proteins are combined, approximately 99.98% of T_4 and 99.7% of T_3 are protein-bound. Because T_3 is less tightly bound than T_4, the fraction of unbound T_3 is greater than unbound T_4, but there is less unbound T_3 in the circulation because it is produced in smaller amounts and cleared more rapidly than T_4. The unbound or "free" concentrations of the hormones are $\sim 2 \times 10^{-11}$ *M* for T_4 and $\sim 6 \times 10^{-12}$ *M* for T_3, which roughly correspond to the thyroid hormone receptor binding constants for these hormones (see below). The unbound hormone is thought to be biologically available to tissues. Nonetheless, the homeostatic mechanisms that regulate the thyroid axis are directed toward maintenance of normal concentrations of unbound hormones.

Abnormalities of thyroid hormone binding proteins

A number of inherited and acquired abnormalities affect thyroid hormone binding proteins. X-linked TBG deficiency is associated with very low levels of total T_4 and T_3. However, because unbound hormone levels are normal, patients are euthyroid and TSH levels are normal. It is important to recognize this disorder to avoid efforts to normalize total T_4 levels, because this leads to thyrotoxicosis and is futile because of rapid hormone clearance in the absence of TBG. TBG levels are elevated by estrogen, which increases sialylation and delays TBG clearance. Consequently, in women who are pregnant or taking estrogen-containing contraceptives, elevated TBG increases total T_4 and T_3 levels; however, unbound T_4 and T_3 levels are normal. These features are part of the explanation for why women with hypothyroidism require increased amounts of L-thyroxine replacement as TBG levels are increased by pregnancy or estrogen treatment. Mutations in TBG, TTR, and albumin may increase the binding affinity for T_4 and/or T_3 and cause disorders known as *euthyroid hyperthyroxinemia* or *familial dysalbuminemic hyperthyroxinemia* (FDH) (Table 7-3). These disorders result in increased total T_4 and/or T_3, but unbound hormone levels are normal. The familial nature of the disorders, and the fact that TSH levels are normal rather than suppressed, should suggest this diagnosis. Unbound hormone levels (ideally measured by dialysis) are normal in FDH. The diagnosis can be confirmed by using tests that measure the affinities of radiolabeled hormone binding to specific transport proteins or by performing DNA sequence analyses of the abnormal transport protein genes.

Certain medications, such as salicylates and salsalate, can displace thyroid hormones from circulating binding proteins. Although these drugs transiently perturb the thyroid axis by increasing free thyroid hormone levels, TSH is suppressed until a new steady state is reached, thereby restoring euthyroidism. Circulating factors associated with acute illness may also displace thyroid hormone from binding proteins (see "Sick Euthyroid Syndrome," below).

Deiodinases

T_4 may be thought of as a precursor for the more potent T_3. T_4 is converted to T_3 by the deiodinase enzymes (Fig. 7-1). Type I deiodinase, which is located primarily in thyroid, liver, and kidneys, has a relatively low affinity for T_4. Type II deiodinase has a higher affinity for T_4 and is found primarily in the pituitary gland, brain, brown fat, and thyroid gland. Expression of type II deiodinase allows it to regulate T_3 concentrations locally, a property that may be important in the context of levothyroxine (T_4) replacement. Type II deiodinase is also regulated by thyroid hormone; hypothyroidism induces the enzyme, resulting in enhanced $T_4 \rightarrow T_3$ conversion in tissues such as brain and pituitary. $T_4 \rightarrow T_3$ conversion is impaired by fasting, systemic illness or acute trauma, oral contrast agents, and a variety of medications (e.g., propylthiouracil, propranolol, amiodarone, glucocorticoids). Type III deiodinase inactivates T_4 and T_3 and is the most important source of reverse T_3 (rT_3), including in the sick euthyroid syndrome. This enzyme is expressed in the human placenta but is not active in healthy individuals. In the sick euthyroid syndrome, especially with hypoperfusion, the type III

TABLE 7-3

CONDITIONS ASSOCIATED WITH EUTHYROID HYPERTHYROXINEMIA

DISORDER	CAUSE	TRANSMISSION	CHARACTERISTICS
Familial dysalbuminemic hyperthyroxinemia (FDH)	Albumin mutations, usually R218H	AD	Increased T_4 Normal unbound T_4 Rarely increased T_3
TBG			
Familial excess	Increased TBG production	XL	Increased total T_4, T_3 Normal unbound T_4, T_3
Acquired excess	Medications (estrogen), pregnancy, cirrhosis, hepatitis	Acquired	Increased total T_4, T_3 Normal unbound T_4, T_3
Transthyretin[a]			
Excess	Islet tumors	Acquired	Usually normal T_4, T_3
Mutations	Increased affinity for T_4 or T_3	AD	Increased total T_4, T_3 Normal unbound T_4, T_3
Medications: propranolol, ipodate, iopanoic acid, amiodarone	Decreased $T_4 \rightarrow T_3$ conversion	Acquired	Increased T_4 Decreased T_3 Normal or increased TSH
Resistance to thyroid hormone (RTH)	Thyroid hormone receptor β mutations	AD	Increased unbound T_4, T_3 Normal or increased TSH Some patients clinically thyrotoxic

[a]Also known as thyroxine-binding prealbumin (TBPA).

Abbreviations: AD, autosomal dominant; TBG, thyroxine-binding globulin; TSH, thyroid-stimulating hormone; XL, X-linked.

deiodinase is activated in muscle and liver. Massive hemangiomas that express type III deiodinase are a rare cause of hypothyroidism in infants.

THYROID HORMONE ACTION

Thyroid hormone transport

Circulating thyroid hormones enter cells by passive diffusion and via specific transporters such as the monocarboxylate 8 transporter (MCT8), MCT10, and organic anion-transporting polypeptide 1C1. Mutations in the *MCT8* gene have been identified in patients with X-linked psychomotor retardation and thyroid function abnormalities (low T_4, high T_3, and high TSH). After entering cells, thyroid hormones act primarily through nuclear receptors, although they also have nongenomic actions through stimulating mitochondrial enzymatic responses and may act directly on blood vessels and the heart through integrin receptors.

Nuclear thyroid hormone receptors

Thyroid hormones bind with high affinity to nuclear *thyroid hormone receptors* (TRs) α and β. Both TRα and TRβ are expressed in most tissues, but their relative expression levels vary among organs; TRα is particularly abundant in brain, kidneys, gonads, muscle, and heart, whereas TRβ expression is relatively high in the pituitary and liver. Both receptors are variably spliced to form unique isoforms. The TRβ2 isoform, which has a unique amino terminus, is selectively expressed in the hypothalamus and pituitary, where it plays a role in feedback control of the thyroid axis (see above). The TRα2 isoform contains a unique carboxy terminus that precludes thyroid hormone binding; it may function to block the action of other TR isoforms.

The TRs contain a central DNA-binding domain and a C-terminal ligand-binding domain. They bind to specific DNA sequences, termed *thyroid response elements* (TREs), in the promoter regions of target genes (Fig. 7-4). The receptors bind as homodimers or, more commonly, as heterodimers with retinoic acid X receptors (RXRs) **(Chap. 2)**. The activated receptor can either stimulate gene transcription (e.g., myosin heavy chain α) or inhibit transcription (e.g., TSH β-subunit gene), depending on the nature of the regulatory elements in the target gene.

Thyroid hormones (T_3 and T_4) bind with similar affinities to TRα and TRβ. However, structural differences in the ligand binding domains provide the potential for developing receptor-selective agonists or antagonists, and these are under investigation. T_3 is bound with 10–15 times greater affinity than T_4, which explains its increased hormonal potency. Although T_4 is produced in excess of T_3, receptors are occupied

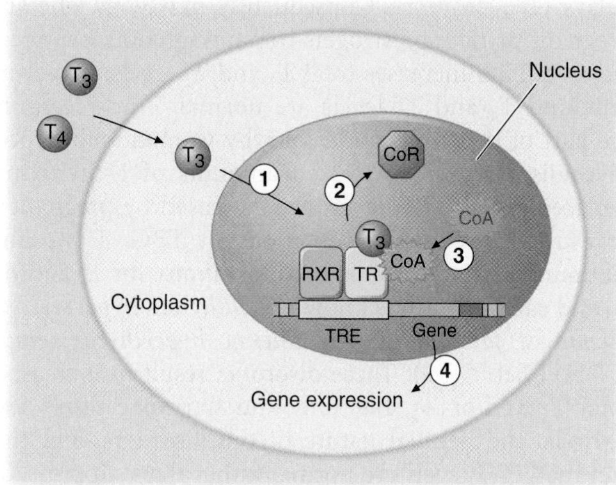

FIGURE 7-4

Mechanism of thyroid hormone receptor action. The thyroid hormone receptor (TR) and retinoid X receptor (RXR) form heterodimers that bind specifically to thyroid hormone response elements (TRE) in the promoter regions of target genes. In the absence of hormone, TR binds co-repressor (CoR) proteins that silence gene expression. The numbers refer to a series of ordered reactions that occur in response to thyroid hormone: (1) T_4 or T_3 enters the nucleus; (2) T_3 binding dissociates CoR from TR; (3) coactivators (CoA) are recruited to the T_3-bound receptor; and (4) gene expression is altered.

mainly by T_3, reflecting $T_4 \rightarrow T_3$ conversion by peripheral tissues, greater T_3 bioavailability in the plasma, and the greater affinity of receptors for T_3. After binding to TRs, thyroid hormone induces conformational changes in the receptors that modify its interactions with accessory transcription factors. Importantly, in the absence of thyroid hormone binding, the aporeceptors bind to co-repressor proteins that inhibit gene transcription. Hormone binding dissociates the co-repressors and allows the recruitment of co-activators that enhance transcription. The discovery of TR interactions with co-repressors explains the fact that TR silences gene expression in the absence of hormone binding. Consequently, hormone deficiency has a profound effect on gene expression because it causes gene repression as well as loss of hormone-induced stimulation. This concept has been corroborated by the finding that targeted deletion of the TR genes in mice has a less pronounced phenotypic effect than hormone deficiency.

Thyroid hormone resistance

Resistance to thyroid hormone (RTH) is an autosomal dominant disorder characterized by elevated thyroid hormone levels and inappropriately normal or elevated TSH. Individuals with RTH do not, in general, exhibit signs and symptoms that are typical of hypothyroidism because hormone resistance is partial and is compensated by increased levels of thyroid hormone. The clinical features of RTH can include goiter, attention deficit disorder, mild reduction in IQ, delayed skeletal maturation, tachycardia, and impaired metabolic responses to thyroid hormone.

Classical forms of RTH are caused by mutations in the TRβ gene. These mutations, located in restricted regions of the ligand-binding domain, cause loss of receptor function. However, because the mutant receptors retain the capacity to dimerize with RXRs, bind to DNA, and recruit co-repressor proteins, they function as antagonists of the remaining normal TRβ and TRα receptors. This property, referred to as "dominant negative" activity, explains the autosomal dominant mode of transmission. The diagnosis is suspected when unbound thyroid hormone levels are increased without suppression of TSH. Similar hormonal abnormalities are found in other affected family members, although the TRβ mutation arises de novo in about 20% of patients. DNA sequence analysis of the TRβ gene provides a definitive diagnosis. RTH must be distinguished from other causes of euthyroid hyperthyroxinemia (e.g., FDH) and inappropriate secretion of TSH by TSH-secreting pituitary adenomas **(Chap. 5)**. In most patients, no treatment is indicated; the importance of making the diagnosis is to avoid inappropriate treatment of mistaken hyperthyroidism and to provide genetic counseling.

A distinct form of RTH is caused by mutations in the TRα gene. Affected patients have many clinical features of congenital hypothyroidism including growth retardation, skeletal dysplasia, and severe constipation. In contrast to RTH caused by mutations in TRβ, thyroid function tests include normal TSH, low or normal T_4, and normal or elevated T_3 levels. These distinct clinical and laboratory features underscore the different tissue distribution and functional roles of TRβ and TRα. Optimal treatment of patients with RTH caused by TRα mutations has not been established.

PHYSICAL EXAMINATION

In addition to the examination of the thyroid itself, the physical examination should include a search for signs of abnormal thyroid function and the extrathyroidal features of ophthalmopathy and dermopathy (see below). Examination of the neck begins by inspecting the seated patient from the front and side and noting any surgical scars, obvious masses, or distended veins. The thyroid can be palpated with both hands from behind or while facing the patient, using the thumbs to palpate each lobe. It is best to use a combination of these methods, especially when nodules are small. The patient's neck should be slightly flexed to relax the neck muscles. After locating the cricoid cartilage, the isthmus, which is attached to the lower one-third of the thyroid lobes, can be identified and then followed laterally to locate either lobe (normally, the right lobe is slightly larger than the left). By asking the patient to swallow sips of water, thyroid consistency can be better appreciated as the gland moves beneath the examiner's fingers.

Features to be noted include thyroid size, consistency, nodularity, and any tenderness or fixation. An estimate of thyroid size (normally 12–20 g) should be made, and a drawing is often the best way to record findings. However, ultrasound is the method of choice when it is important to determine thyroid size accurately. The size, location, and consistency of any nodules should also be defined. A bruit or thrill over the gland, located over the insertion of the superior and inferior thyroid arteries (supero- or inferolaterally), indicates increased vascularity, as occurs in hyperthyroidism. If the lower borders of the thyroid lobes are not clearly felt, a goiter may be retrosternal. Large retrosternal goiters can cause venous distention over the neck and difficulty breathing, especially when the arms are raised (Pemberton's sign). With any central mass above the thyroid, the tongue should be extended, as thyroglossal cysts then move upward. The thyroid examination is not complete without assessment for lymphadenopathy in the supraclavicular and cervical regions of the neck.

LABORATORY EVALUATION

Measurement of thyroid hormones

The enhanced sensitivity and specificity of *TSH assays* have greatly improved laboratory assessment of thyroid function. Because TSH levels change dynamically in response to alterations of T_4 and T_3, a logical approach to thyroid testing is to first determine whether TSH is suppressed, normal, or elevated. With rare exceptions (see below), a normal TSH level excludes a primary abnormality of thyroid function. This strategy depends on the use of immunochemiluminometric assays (ICMAs) for TSH that are sensitive enough to discriminate between the lower limit of the reference range and the suppressed values that occur with thyrotoxicosis. Extremely sensitive (fourth-generation) assays can detect TSH levels ≤0.004 mIU/L, but, for practical purposes, assays sensitive to ≤0.1 mIU/L are sufficient. The widespread availability of the TSH ICMA has rendered the TRH stimulation test obsolete, because the failure of TSH to rise after an intravenous bolus of 200–400 μg TRH has the same implications as a suppressed basal TSH measured by ICMA.

The finding of an abnormal TSH level must be followed by measurements of circulating thyroid hormone levels to confirm the diagnosis of hyperthyroidism (suppressed TSH) or hypothyroidism (elevated TSH). Radioimmunoassays are widely available for serum *total* T_4 and *total* T_3. T_4 and T_3 are highly protein-bound, and numerous factors (illness, medications, genetic factors) can influence protein binding. It is useful, therefore, to measure the free, or unbound, hormone levels, which correspond to the biologically available hormone pool. Two direct methods are used to measure *unbound thyroid hormones*: (1) unbound thyroid hormone competition with radiolabeled T_4 (or an analogue) for binding to a solid-phase antibody, and (2) physical separation of the unbound hormone fraction by ultracentrifugation or equilibrium dialysis. Although early unbound hormone immunoassays suffered from artifacts, newer assays correlate well with the results of the more technically demanding and expensive physical separation methods. An indirect method that is now less commonly used to estimate unbound thyroid hormone levels is to calculate the free T_3 or free T_4 index from the total T_4 or T_3 concentration and the *thyroid hormone binding ratio* (THBR). The latter is derived from the *T_3-resin uptake test*, which determines the distribution of radiolabeled T_3 between an absorbent resin and the unoccupied thyroid hormone binding proteins in the sample. The binding of the labeled T_3 to the resin is increased when there is reduced unoccupied protein binding sites (e.g., TBG deficiency) or increased total thyroid hormone in the sample; it is decreased under the opposite circumstances. The product of THBR and total T_3 or T_4 provides the *free T_3 or T_4 index*. In effect, the index corrects for anomalous total hormone values caused by abnormalities in hormone-protein binding.

Total thyroid hormone levels are *elevated* when TBG is increased due to estrogens (pregnancy, oral contraceptives, hormone therapy, tamoxifen, selective estrogen receptor modulators, inflammatory liver disease) and *decreased* when TBG binding is reduced (androgens, nephrotic syndrome). Genetic disorders and acute illness can also cause abnormalities in thyroid hormone binding proteins, and various drugs (phenytoin, carbamazepine, salicylates, and nonsteroidal anti-inflammatory drugs [NSAIDs]) can interfere with thyroid hormone binding. Because unbound thyroid hormone levels are normal and the patient is euthyroid in all of these circumstances, assays that measure unbound hormone are preferable to those for total thyroid hormones.

For most purposes, the unbound T_4 level is sufficient to confirm thyrotoxicosis, but 2–5% of patients have only an elevated T_3 level (T_3 toxicosis). Thus, unbound T_3 levels should be measured in patients with a suppressed TSH but normal unbound T_4 levels.

There are several clinical conditions in which the use of TSH as a screening test may be misleading, particularly without simultaneous unbound T_4 determinations. Any severe nonthyroidal illness can cause abnormal TSH levels (see below). Although hypothyroidism is the most common cause of an elevated TSH level, rare causes include a TSH-secreting pituitary tumor **(Chap. 5)**, thyroid hormone resistance, and assay artifact. Conversely, a suppressed TSH level, particularly <0.01 mIU/L, usually indicates thyrotoxicosis. However, subnormal TSH levels between 0.01 and 0.1 mIU/L may be seen during the first trimester of pregnancy (due to hCG secretion), after treatment of hyperthyroidism (because TSH can remain suppressed for several months), and in response to certain medications (e.g., high doses of glucocorticoids or dopamine). Importantly, secondary hypothyroidism, caused by hypothalamic-pituitary disease, is associated with a variable (low to high-normal) TSH level, which is inappropriate for the low T_4 level. Thus, *TSH should not be used as an isolated laboratory test to assess thyroid function in patients with suspected or known pituitary disease.*

Tests for the end-organ effects of thyroid hormone excess or depletion, such as estimation of basal metabolic rate, tendon reflex relaxation rates, or serum cholesterol, are not useful as clinical determinants of thyroid function.

Tests to determine the etiology of thyroid dysfunction

Autoimmune thyroid disease is detected most easily by measuring circulating antibodies against TPO and Tg. Because antibodies to Tg alone are uncommon, it is reasonable to measure only TPO antibodies. About 5–15% of euthyroid women and up to 2% of euthyroid men have thyroid antibodies; such individuals are at increased risk of developing thyroid dysfunction. Almost all patients with autoimmune hypothyroidism, and up to 80% of those with Graves' disease, have TPO antibodies, usually at high levels.

TSIs are antibodies that stimulate the TSH-R in Graves' disease. They are most commonly measured by commercially available tracer displacement assays called TRAb (TSH receptor antibody) with the assumption that elevated levels in the setting of clinical hyperthyroidism reflect stimulatory effects on the TSH receptor. A bioassay is less commonly used. The main use of these assays is to predict neonatal thyrotoxicosis caused by high maternal levels of TRAb or TSI (>3× upper limit of normal) in the last trimester of pregnancy.

Serum Tg levels are increased in all types of thyrotoxicosis except *thyrotoxicosis factitia* caused by self-administration of thyroid hormone. Tg levels are particularly increased in thyroiditis, reflecting thyroid tissue destruction and release of Tg. The main role for Tg measurement, however, is in the follow-up of thyroid cancer patients. After total thyroidectomy and radioablation, Tg levels should be undetectable; in the absence of anti-Tg antibodies, measurable levels indicate incomplete ablation or recurrent cancer.

Radioiodine uptake and thyroid scanning

The thyroid gland selectively transports radioisotopes of iodine (^{123}I, ^{125}I, ^{131}I) and ^{99m}Tc pertechnetate, allowing thyroid imaging and quantitation of radioactive tracer fractional uptake.

Nuclear imaging of Graves' disease is characterized by an enlarged gland and increased tracer uptake that is distributed homogeneously. Toxic adenomas appear as focal areas of increased uptake, with suppressed tracer uptake in the remainder of the gland. In toxic MNG, the gland is enlarged—often with distorted architecture—and there are multiple areas of relatively increased (functioning nodules) or decreased tracer uptake (suppressed thyroid parenchyma or nonfunctioning nodules). Subacute, viral, and postpartum thyroiditis are associated with very low uptake because of follicular cell damage and TSH suppression. Thyrotoxicosis factitia is also associated with low uptake. In addition, if there is excessive circulating exogenous iodine (e.g., from dietary sources of iodinated contrast dye), the radionuclide uptake is low even in the presence of increased thyroid hormone production.

Thyroid scintigraphy is not used in the routine evaluation of patients with thyroid nodules, but should be performed if the serum TSH level is subnormal to determine if functioning thyroid nodules are present. Functioning or "hot" nodules are almost never malignant, and fine-needle aspiration (FNA) biopsy is not indicated. The vast majority of thyroid nodules do not produce thyroid hormone ("cold" nodules), and these are more likely to be malignant (~5–10%). Whole-body and thyroid scanning is also used in the treatment and surveillance of thyroid cancer. After thyroidectomy for thyroid cancer, the TSH level is raised by either using a thyroid hormone withdrawal protocol or recombinant human TSH injection (see below). Administration of ^{131}I allows whole-body scanning (WBS) to confirm remnant ablation and to detect any functioning metastases. In addition, WBS may be helpful in surveillance of patients at risk for recurrence.

Thyroid ultrasound

Ultrasonography is valuable for the diagnosis and evaluation of patients with nodular thyroid disease (Table 7-4). Evidence-based guidelines recommend thyroid ultrasonography for all patients suspected of having thyroid nodules by either physical examination or another imaging study. Using 10- to 12-MHz linear transducers, resolution and image quality are excellent, allowing the characterization of nodules and cysts >3 mm. Certain sonographic patterns are highly suggestive of malignancy (e.g., hypoechoic solid nodules with infiltrative borders and microcalcifications), whereas other features correlate with benignity (e.g., spongiform nodules defined as those with multiple small internal cystic areas) (Fig. 7-5). In addition to evaluating thyroid nodules, ultrasound is useful for monitoring nodule size and for the aspiration of nodules or cystic lesions. Ultrasound-guided FNA biopsy of thyroid lesions lowers the rate of inadequate sampling and decreases sample error, thereby reducing the false-negative rate of FNA cytology. Ultrasonography of the central and lateral cervical lymph node compartments is indispensable in the evaluation thyroid cancer patients, preoperatively and during follow-up.

TABLE 7-4

GRAYSCALE SONOGRAPHIC FEATURES ASSOCIATED WITH THYROID CANCER

	MEDIAN SENSITIVITY [RANGE]	MEDIAN SPECIFICITY [RANGE]
Hypoechoic compared with surrounding thyroid	81% [48–90%]	53% [36–92%]
Marked hypoechogenicity	41% [27–59%]	94% [92–94%]
Microcalcifications	44% [26–73%]	89% [69–98%]
Irregular, microlobulated margins	55% [17–84%]	79% [62–85%]
Solid consistency	86% [78–91%]	48% [30–58%]
Taller than wide shape on transverse view	48% [33–84%]	92% [82–93%]

HYPOTHYROIDISM

Iodine deficiency remains a common cause of hypothyroidism worldwide. In areas of iodine sufficiency, autoimmune disease (Hashimoto's thyroiditis) and iatrogenic causes (treatment of hyperthyroidism) are most common (Table 7-5).

CONGENITAL HYPOTHYROIDISM

Prevalence

Hypothyroidism occurs in about 1 in 4000 newborns. It may be transient, especially if the mother has TSH-R blocking antibodies or has received antithyroid drugs, but permanent hypothyroidism occurs in the majority. Neonatal hypothyroidism is due to thyroid gland

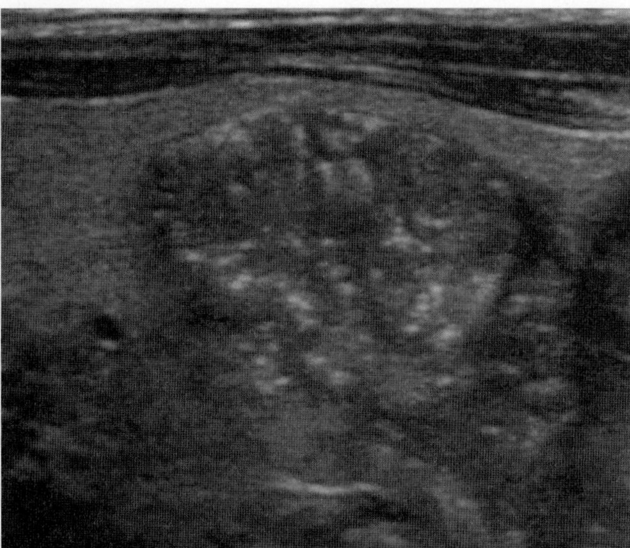

A

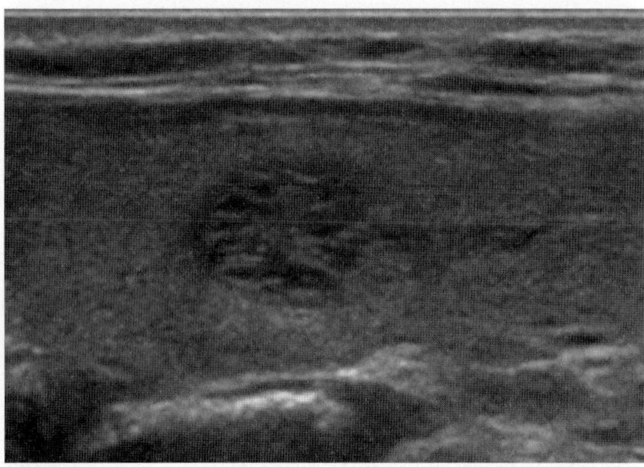

B

FIGURE 7-5

Sonographic patterns of thyroid nodules. *A.* High suspicion ultrasound pattern for thyroid malignancy (hypoechoic solid nodule with irregular borders and microcalcifications). ***B.*** Very low suspicion ultrasound pattern for thyroid malignancy (spongiform nodule with microcystic areas comprises over >50% of nodule volume).

TABLE 7-5

CAUSES OF HYPOTHYROIDISM

Primary
Autoimmune hypothyroidism: Hashimoto's thyroiditis, atrophic thyroiditis
Iatrogenic: ^{131}I treatment, subtotal or total thyroidectomy, external irradiation of neck for lymphoma or cancer
Drugs: iodine excess (including iodine-containing contrast media and amiodarone), lithium, antithyroid drugs, *p*-aminosalicylic acid, interferon α and other cytokines, aminoglutethimide, tyrosine kinase inhibitors (e.g., sunitinib)
Congenital hypothyroidism: absent or ectopic thyroid gland, dyshormonogenesis, TSH-R mutation
Iodine deficiency
Infiltrative disorders: amyloidosis, sarcoidosis, hemochromatosis, scleroderma, cystinosis, Riedel's thyroiditis
Overexpression of type 3 deiodinase in infantile hemangioma and other tumors
Transient
Silent thyroiditis, including postpartum thyroiditis
Subacute thyroiditis
Withdrawal of supraphysiologic thyroxine treatment in individuals with an intact thyroid
After ^{131}I treatment or subtotal thyroidectomy for Graves' disease
Secondary
Hypopituitarism: tumors, pituitary surgery or irradiation, infiltrative disorders, Sheehan's syndrome, trauma, genetic forms of combined pituitary hormone deficiencies
Isolated TSH deficiency or inactivity
Bexarotene treatment
Hypothalamic disease: tumors, trauma, infiltrative disorders, idiopathic

Abbreviations: TSH, thyroid-stimulating hormone; TSH-R, TSH receptor.

dysgenesis in 80–85%, to inborn errors of thyroid hormone synthesis in 10–15%, and is TSH-R antibody-mediated in 5% of affected newborns. The developmental abnormalities are twice as common in girls. Mutations that cause congenital hypothyroidism are being increasingly identified, but most remain idiopathic (Table 7-1).

Clinical manifestations

The majority of infants appear normal at birth, and <10% are diagnosed based on clinical features, which include prolonged jaundice, feeding problems, hypotonia, enlarged tongue, delayed bone maturation, and umbilical hernia. Importantly, permanent neurologic damage results if treatment is delayed. Typical features of adult hypothyroidism may also be present (Table 7-6). Other congenital malformations, especially cardiac, are four times more common in congenital hypothyroidism.

Diagnosis and treatment

Because of the severe neurologic consequences of untreated congenital hypothyroidism, neonatal screening programs have been established. These are generally based on measurement of TSH or T_4 levels in heel-prick blood specimens. When the diagnosis is confirmed, T_4 is instituted at a dose of 10–15 μg/kg per day, and the dose is adjusted by close monitoring of TSH levels. T_4

TABLE 7-6

SIGNS AND SYMPTOMS OF HYPOTHYROIDISM (DESCENDING ORDER OF FREQUENCY)

SYMPTOMS	SIGNS
Tiredness, weakness	Dry coarse skin; cool peripheral extremities
Dry skin	Puffy face, hands, and feet (myxedema)
Feeling cold	Diffuse alopecia
Hair loss	Bradycardia
Difficulty concentrating and poor memory	Peripheral edema
Constipation	Delayed tendon reflex relaxation
Weight gain with poor appetite	Carpal tunnel syndrome
Dyspnea	Serous cavity effusions
Hoarse voice	
Menorrhagia (later oligomenorrhea or amenorrhea)	
Paresthesia	
Impaired hearing	

requirements are relatively great during the first year of life, and a high circulating T_4 level is usually needed to normalize TSH. Early treatment with T_4 results in normal IQ levels, but subtle neurodevelopmental abnormalities may occur in those with the most severe hypothyroidism at diagnosis or when treatment is delayed or suboptimal.

AUTOIMMUNE HYPOTHYROIDISM

Classification

Autoimmune hypothyroidism may be associated with a goiter (Hashimoto's, or *goitrous thyroiditis*) or, at the later stages of the disease, minimal residual thyroid tissue (*atrophic thyroiditis*). Because the autoimmune process gradually reduces thyroid function, there is a phase of compensation when normal thyroid hormone levels are maintained by a rise in TSH. Although some patients may have minor symptoms, this state is called *subclinical hypothyroidism*. Later, unbound T_4 levels fall and TSH levels rise further; symptoms become more readily apparent at this stage (usually TSH >10 mIU/L), which is referred to as *clinical hypothyroidism* or *overt hypothyroidism*.

Prevalence

The mean annual incidence rate of autoimmune hypothyroidism is up to 4 per 1000 women and 1 per 1000 men. It is more common in certain populations, such as the Japanese, probably because of genetic factors and chronic exposure to a high-iodine diet. The mean age at diagnosis is 60 years, and the prevalence of overt hypothyroidism increases with age. Subclinical hypothyroidism is found in 6–8% of women (10% over the age of 60) and 3% of men. The annual risk of developing clinical hypothyroidism is about 4% when subclinical hypothyroidism is associated with positive TPO antibodies.

Pathogenesis

In Hashimoto's thyroiditis, there is a marked lymphocytic infiltration of the thyroid with germinal center formation, atrophy of the thyroid follicles accompanied by oxyphil metaplasia, absence of colloid, and mild to moderate fibrosis. In atrophic thyroiditis, the fibrosis is much more extensive, lymphocyte infiltration is less pronounced, and thyroid follicles are almost completely absent. Atrophic thyroiditis likely represents the end stage of Hashimoto's thyroiditis rather than a distinct disorder.

As with most autoimmune disorders, susceptibility to autoimmune hypothyroidism is determined by a combination of genetic and environmental factors, and the risk of either autoimmune hypothyroidism or Graves' disease is increased among siblings. HLA-DR polymorphisms are the best documented genetic risk factors for autoimmune hypothyroidism, especially HLA-DR3, -DR4, and -DR5 in Caucasians. A weak association also exists between polymorphisms in *CTLA-4*, a T cell–regulatory gene, and autoimmune hypothyroidism. Both of these genetic associations are shared by other autoimmune diseases, which may explain the relationship between autoimmune hypothyroidism and other autoimmune diseases, especially type 1 diabetes mellitus, Addison's disease, pernicious anemia, and vitiligo. HLA-DR and *CTLA-4* polymorphisms account for approximately half of the genetic susceptibility to autoimmune hypothyroidism. Other contributory loci remain to be identified. A gene on chromosome 21 may be responsible for the association between autoimmune hypothyroidism and Down's syndrome. The female preponderance of thyroid autoimmunity is most likely due to sex steroid effects on the immune response, but an X chromosome–related genetic factor is also possible and may account for the high frequency of autoimmune hypothyroidism in Turner's syndrome. Environmental susceptibility factors are poorly defined at present. A high iodine intake and decreased exposure to microorganisms in childhood increase the risk of autoimmune hypothyroidism. These factors may account for the increase in prevalence over the last two to three decades.

The thyroid lymphocytic infiltrate in autoimmune hypothyroidism is composed of activated CD4+ and CD8+ T cells as well as B cells. Thyroid cell destruction is primarily mediated by the CD8+ cytotoxic T cells, which destroy their targets by either perforin-induced cell necrosis or granzyme B–induced apoptosis. In addition, local T cell production of cytokines, such as tumor necrosis factor (TNF), IL-1, and interferon γ (IFN-γ), may render thyroid cells more susceptible to apoptosis mediated by death receptors, such as Fas, which are activated by their respective ligands on T cells. These cytokines also impair thyroid cell function directly and induce the expression of other proinflammatory molecules by the thyroid cells themselves, such as cytokines, HLA class I and class II molecules, adhesion molecules, CD40, and nitric oxide. Administration of high concentrations of cytokines for therapeutic purposes (especially IFN-α) is associated with increased autoimmune thyroid disease, possibly through mechanisms similar to those in sporadic disease.

Antibodies to TPO and Tg are clinically useful markers of thyroid autoimmunity, but any pathogenic effect is restricted to a secondary role in amplifying an ongoing autoimmune response. TPO antibodies fix complement, and complement membrane-attack complexes are present in the thyroid in autoimmune hypothyroidism. However, transplacental passage of Tg or TPO antibodies has no effect on the fetal thyroid, which suggests that T cell–mediated injury is required to initiate autoimmune damage to the thyroid.

Up to 20% of patients with autoimmune hypothyroidism have antibodies against the TSH-R, which, in contrast to TSI, do not stimulate the receptor but prevent the binding of TSH. These TSH-R-blocking antibodies, therefore, cause hypothyroidism and, especially in Asian patients, thyroid atrophy. Their transplacental passage may induce transient neonatal hypothyroidism. Rarely, patients have a mixture of TSI and TSH-R-blocking antibodies, and thyroid function can oscillate between hyperthyroidism and hypothyroidism as one or the other antibody becomes dominant. Predicting the course of disease in such individuals is difficult, and they require close monitoring of thyroid function. Bioassays can be used to document that TSH-R-blocking antibodies reduce the cyclic AMP–inducing effect of TSH on cultured TSH-R-expressing cells, but these assays are difficult to perform. Thyrotropin-binding inhibitory immunoglobulin (TBII) assays that measure the binding of antibodies to the receptor by competition with radiolabeled TSH do not distinguish between TSI- and TSH-R-blocking antibodies, but a positive result in a patient with spontaneous hypothyroidism is strong evidence for the presence of blocking antibodies. The use of these assays does not generally alter clinical management, although it may be useful to confirm the cause of transient neonatal hypothyroidism.

Clinical manifestations

The main clinical features of hypothyroidism are summarized in Table 7-6. The onset is usually insidious, and the patient may become aware of symptoms only when euthyroidism is restored. Patients with Hashimoto's thyroiditis may present because of goiter rather than symptoms of hypothyroidism. The goiter may not be large, but it is usually irregular and firm in consistency. It is often possible to palpate a pyramidal lobe, normally a vestigial remnant of the thyroglossal duct. Rarely is uncomplicated Hashimoto's thyroiditis associated with pain.

Patients with atrophic thyroiditis or the late stage of Hashimoto's thyroiditis present with symptoms and signs of hypothyroidism. The skin is dry, and there is decreased sweating, thinning of the epidermis, and hyperkeratosis of the stratum corneum. Increased dermal glycosaminoglycan content traps water, giving rise to skin thickening without pitting (*myxedema*). Typical features include a puffy face with edematous eyelids and nonpitting pretibial edema (Fig. 7-6). There is pallor, often with a yellow tinge to the skin due to carotene accumulation. Nail growth is retarded, and hair is dry, brittle, difficult to manage, and falls out easily. In addition to diffuse alopecia, there is thinning of the outer third of the eyebrows, although this is not a specific sign of hypothyroidism.

Other common features include constipation and weight gain (despite a poor appetite). In contrast to popular perception, the weight gain is usually modest and due mainly to fluid retention in the myxedematous tissues. Libido is decreased in both sexes, and there may be oligomenorrhea or amenorrhea in long-standing disease, but menorrhagia is also common. Fertility is

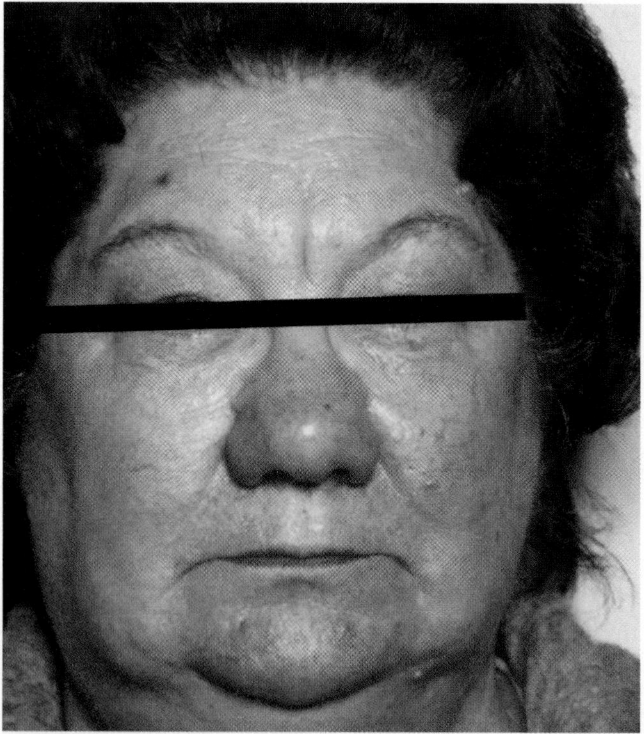

FIGURE 7-6
Facial appearance in hypothyroidism. Note puffy eyes and thickened skin.

reduced, and the incidence of miscarriage is increased. Prolactin levels are often modestly increased **(Chap. 5)** and may contribute to alterations in libido and fertility and cause galactorrhea.

Myocardial contractility and pulse rate are reduced, leading to a reduced stroke volume and bradycardia. Increased peripheral resistance may be accompanied by hypertension, particularly diastolic. Blood flow is diverted from the skin, producing cool extremities. Pericardial effusions occur in up to 30% of patients but rarely compromise cardiac function. Although alterations in myosin heavy chain isoform expression have been documented, cardiomyopathy is unusual. Fluid may also accumulate in other serous cavities and in the middle ear, giving rise to conductive deafness. Pulmonary function is generally normal, but dyspnea may be caused by pleural effusion, impaired respiratory muscle function, diminished ventilatory drive, or sleep apnea.

Carpal tunnel and other entrapment syndromes are common, as is impairment of muscle function with stiffness, cramps, and pain. On examination, there may be slow relaxation of tendon reflexes and pseudomyotonia. Memory and concentration are impaired. Experimentally, positron emission tomography (PET) scans examining glucose metabolism in hypothyroid subjects show lower regional activity in the amygdala, hippocampus, and perigenual anterior cingulated cortex, among other regions, and this activity corrects after thyroxine replacement. Rare neurologic problems include reversible cerebellar ataxia, dementia, psychosis, and myxedema coma. *Hashimoto's encephalopathy* has been defined as a steroid-responsive syndrome associated with TPO antibodies, myoclonus, and slow-wave activity on electroencephalography, but the relationship with thyroid autoimmunity or hypothyroidism is not established. The hoarse voice and occasionally clumsy speech of hypothyroidism reflect fluid accumulation in the vocal cords and tongue.

The features described above are the consequence of thyroid hormone deficiency. However, autoimmune hypothyroidism may be associated with signs or symptoms of other autoimmune diseases, particularly vitiligo, pernicious anemia, Addison's disease, alopecia areata, and type 1 diabetes mellitus. Less common associations include celiac disease, dermatitis herpetiformis, chronic active hepatitis, rheumatoid arthritis, systemic lupus erythematosus (SLE), myasthenia gravis, and Sjögren's syndrome. Thyroid-associated ophthalmopathy, which usually occurs in Graves' disease (see below), occurs in about 5% of patients with autoimmune hypothyroidism.

Autoimmune hypothyroidism is uncommon in children and usually presents with slow growth and delayed facial maturation. The appearance of permanent teeth is also delayed. Myopathy, with muscle swelling, is more common in children than in adults. In most cases, puberty is delayed, but precocious puberty sometimes occurs. There may be intellectual impairment if the onset is before 3 years and the hormone deficiency is severe.

Laboratory evaluation

A summary of the investigations used to determine the existence and cause of hypothyroidism is provided in Fig. 7-7. A normal TSH level excludes primary (but not secondary) hypothyroidism. If the TSH is elevated, an unbound T_4 level is needed to confirm the presence of clinical hypothyroidism, but T_4 is inferior to TSH when used as a screening test, because it will not detect

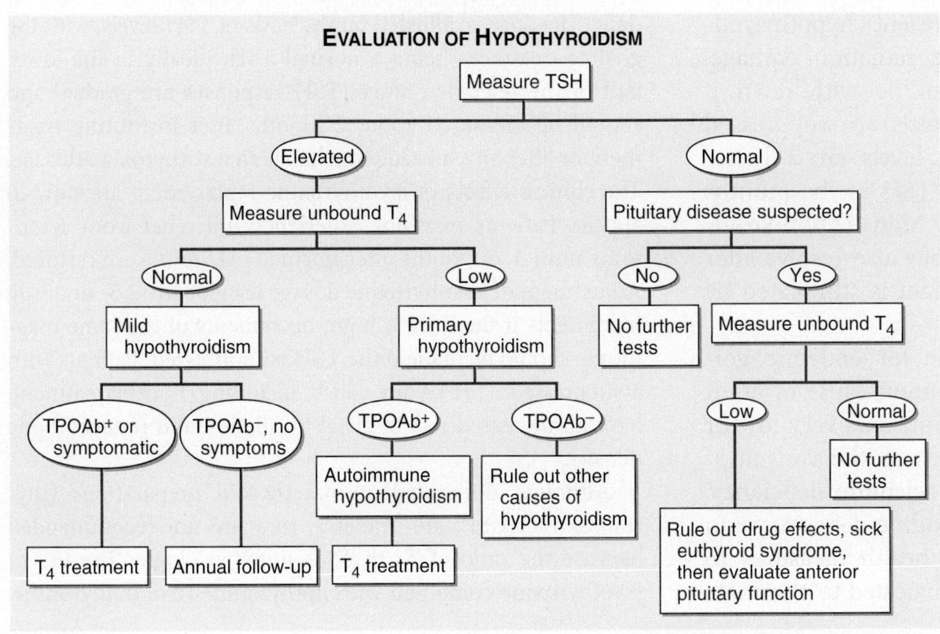

FIGURE 7-7
Evaluation of hypothyroidism. $TPOAb^+$, thyroid peroxidase antibodies present; $TPOAb^-$, thyroid peroxidase antibodies not present; TSH, thyroid-stimulating hormone.

subclinical hypothyroidism. Circulating unbound T_3 levels are normal in about 25% of patients, reflecting adaptive deiodinase responses to hypothyroidism. T_3 measurements are, therefore, not indicated.

Once clinical or subclinical hypothyroidism is confirmed, the etiology is usually easily established by demonstrating the presence of TPO antibodies, which are present in >90% of patients with autoimmune hypothyroidism. TBII can be found in 10–20% of patients, but measurement is not needed routinely. If there is any doubt about the cause of a goiter associated with hypothyroidism, FNA biopsy can be used to confirm the presence of autoimmune thyroiditis. Other abnormal laboratory findings in hypothyroidism may include increased creatine phosphokinase, elevated cholesterol and triglycerides, and anemia (usually normocytic or macrocytic). Except when accompanied by iron deficiency, the anemia and other abnormalities gradually resolve with thyroxine replacement.

Differential diagnosis

An asymmetric goiter in Hashimoto's thyroiditis may be confused with a MNG or thyroid carcinoma, in which thyroid antibodies may also be present. Ultrasound can be used to show the presence of a solitary lesion or an MNG rather than the heterogeneous thyroid enlargement typical of Hashimoto's thyroiditis. FNA biopsy is useful in the investigation of focal nodules. Other causes of hypothyroidism are discussed below and in Table 7-5 but rarely cause diagnostic confusion.

OTHER CAUSES OF HYPOTHYROIDISM

Iatrogenic hypothyroidism is a common cause of hypothyroidism and can often be detected by screening before symptoms develop. In the first 3–4 months after radioiodine treatment, transient hypothyroidism may occur due to reversible radiation damage. Low-dose thyroxine treatment can be withdrawn if recovery occurs. Because TSH levels are suppressed by hyperthyroidism, unbound T_4 levels are a better measure of thyroid function than TSH in the months following radioiodine treatment. Mild hypothyroidism after subtotal thyroidectomy may also resolve after several months, as the gland remnant is stimulated by increased TSH levels.

Iodine deficiency is responsible for endemic goiter and cretinism but is an uncommon cause of adult hypothyroidism unless the iodine intake is very low or there are complicating factors, such as the consumption of thiocyanates in cassava or selenium deficiency. Although hypothyroidism due to iodine deficiency can be treated with thyroxine, public health measures to improve iodine intake should be advocated to eliminate this problem. Iodized salt or bread or a single bolus of oral or intramuscular iodized oil have all been used successfully.

Paradoxically, chronic iodine excess can also induce goiter and hypothyroidism. The intracellular events that account for this effect are unclear, but individuals with autoimmune thyroiditis are especially susceptible. Iodine excess is responsible for the hypothyroidism that occurs in up to 13% of patients treated with amiodarone (see below). Other drugs, particularly lithium, may also cause hypothyroidism. Transient hypothyroidism caused by thyroiditis is discussed below.

Secondary hypothyroidism is usually diagnosed in the context of other anterior pituitary hormone deficiencies; isolated TSH deficiency is very rare **(Chap. 4)**. TSH levels may be low, normal, or even slightly increased in secondary hypothyroidism; the latter is due to secretion of immunoactive but bioinactive forms of TSH. The diagnosis is confirmed by detecting a low unbound T_4 level. The goal of treatment is to maintain T_4 levels in the upper half of the reference range, because TSH levels cannot be used to monitor therapy.

TREATMENT Hypothyroidism

CLINICAL HYPOTHYROIDISM If there is no residual thyroid function, the daily replacement dose of levothyroxine is usually 1.6 μg/kg body weight (typically 100–150 μg), ideally taken at least 30 min before breakfast. In many patients, however, lower doses suffice until residual thyroid tissue is destroyed. In patients who develop hypothyroidism after the treatment of Graves' disease, there is often underlying autonomous function, necessitating lower replacement doses (typically 75–125 μg/d).

Adult patients under 60 years old without evidence of heart disease may be started on 50–100 μg levothyroxine (T_4) daily. The dose is adjusted on the basis of TSH levels, with the goal of treatment being a normal TSH, ideally in the lower half of the reference range. TSH responses are gradual and should be measured about 2 months after instituting treatment or after any subsequent change in levothyroxine dosage. The clinical effects of levothyroxine replacement are slow to appear. Patients may not experience full relief from symptoms until 3–6 months after normal TSH levels are restored. Adjustment of levothyroxine dosage is made in 12.5- or 25-μg increments if the TSH is high; decrements of the same magnitude should be made if the TSH is suppressed. Patients with a suppressed TSH of any cause, including T_4 overtreatment, have an increased risk of atrial fibrillation and reduced bone density.

Although desiccated animal thyroid preparations (thyroid extract USP) are available, they are not recommended because the ratio of T_3 to T_4 is nonphysiologic. The use of levothyroxine combined with liothyronine (triiodothyronine,

T_3) has been investigated, but benefit has not been confirmed in prospective studies. There is no place for liothyronine alone as long-term replacement, because the short half-life necessitates three or four daily doses and is associated with fluctuating T_3 levels.

Once full replacement is achieved and TSH levels are stable, follow-up measurement of TSH is recommended at annual intervals and may be extended to every 2–3 years if a normal TSH is maintained over several years. It is important to ensure ongoing adherence, however, as patients do not feel any symptomatic difference after missing a few doses of levothyroxine, and this sometimes leads to self-discontinuation.

In patients of normal body weight who are taking ≥200 μg of levothyroxine per day, an elevated TSH level is often a sign of poor adherence to treatment. This is also the likely explanation for fluctuating TSH levels, despite a constant levothyroxine dosage. Such patients often have normal or high unbound T_4 levels, despite an elevated TSH, because they remember to take medication for a few days before testing; this is sufficient to normalize T_4, but not TSH levels. It is important to consider variable adherence, because this pattern of thyroid function tests is otherwise suggestive of disorders associated with inappropriate TSH secretion (Table 7-3). Because T_4 has a long half-life (7 days), patients who miss a dose can be advised to take two doses of the skipped tablets at once. Other causes of increased levothyroxine requirements must be excluded, particularly malabsorption (e.g., celiac disease, small-bowel surgery), estrogen or selective estrogen receptor modulator therapy, ingestion with a meal, and drugs that interfere with T_4 absorption or metabolism such as cholestyramine, ferrous sulfate, calcium supplements, proton pump inhibitors, lovastatin, aluminum hydroxide, rifampicin, amiodarone, carbamazepine, phenytoin, and tyrosine kinase inhibitors.

SUBCLINICAL HYPOTHYROIDISM By definition, subclinical hypothyroidism refers to biochemical evidence of thyroid hormone deficiency in patients who have few or no apparent clinical features of hypothyroidism. There are no universally accepted recommendations for the management of subclinical hypothyroidism, but levothyroxine is recommended if the patient is a woman who wishes to conceive or is pregnant, or when TSH levels are above 10 mIU/L. When TSH levels are below 10 mIU/L, treatment should be considered when patients have suggestive symptoms of hypothyroidism, positive TPO antibodies, or any evidence of heart disease. It is important to confirm that any elevation of TSH is sustained over a 3-month period before treatment is given. As long as excessive treatment is avoided, there is no risk in correcting a slightly increased TSH. Treatment is administered by starting with a low dose of levothyroxine (25–50 μg/d) with the goal of normalizing TSH. If levothyroxine is not given, thyroid function should be evaluated annually.

SPECIAL TREATMENT CONSIDERATIONS Rarely, levothyroxine replacement is associated with pseudotumor cerebri in children. Presentation appears to be idiosyncratic and occurs months after treatment has begun.

Women with a history or high risk of hypothyroidism should ensure that they are euthyroid prior to conception and during early pregnancy because maternal hypothyroidism may adversely affect fetal neural development and cause preterm delivery. The presence of thyroid autoantibodies alone, in a euthyroid patient, is also associated with miscarriage and preterm delivery; it is unclear if levothyroxine therapy improves outcomes. Thyroid function should be evaluated immediately after pregnancy is confirmed and every 4 weeks during the first half of the pregnancy, with less frequent testing after 20 weeks' gestation (every 6–8 weeks depending on whether levothyroxine dose adjustment is ongoing). The levothyroxine dose may need to be increased by up to 50% during pregnancy, with a goal TSH of less than 2.5 mIU/L during the first trimester and less than 3.0 mIU/L during the second and third trimesters. After delivery, thyroxine doses typically return to prepregnancy levels. Pregnant women should be counseled to separate ingestion of prenatal vitamins and iron supplements from levothyroxine by at least 4 h.

Elderly patients may require 20% less thyroxine than younger patients. In the elderly, especially patients with known coronary artery disease, the starting dose of levothyroxine is 12.5–25 μg/d with similar increments every 2–3 months until TSH is normalized. In some patients, it may be impossible to achieve full replacement despite optimal antianginal treatment. *Emergency surgery* is generally safe in patients with untreated hypothyroidism, although routine surgery in a hypothyroid patient should be deferred until euthyroidism is achieved.

Myxedema coma still has a 20–40% mortality rate, despite intensive treatment, and outcomes are independent of the T_4 and TSH levels. Clinical manifestations include reduced level of consciousness, sometimes associated with seizures, as well as the other features of hypothyroidism (Table 7-6). Hypothermia can reach 23°C (74°F). There may be a history of treated hypothyroidism with poor compliance, or the patient may be previously undiagnosed. Myxedema coma almost always occurs in the elderly and is usually precipitated by factors that impair respiration, such as drugs (especially sedatives, anesthetics, and antidepressants), pneumonia, congestive heart failure, myocardial infarction, gastrointestinal bleeding, or cerebrovascular accidents. Sepsis should also be suspected. Exposure to cold may also be a risk factor. Hypoventilation, leading to hypoxia and hypercapnia, plays a major role in pathogenesis; hypoglycemia and dilutional hyponatremia also contribute to the development of myxedema coma.

Levothyroxine can initially be administered as a single IV bolus of 500 μg, which serves as a loading dose. Although further levothyroxine is not strictly necessary for several days, it is usually continued at a dose of 50–100 μg/d. If suitable IV preparation is not available, the same initial dose of levothyroxine can be given by nasogastric tube (although absorption may be impaired in myxedema). An alternative is to give liothyronine (T_3) intravenously or via nasogastric tube, in doses ranging from 10 to 25 μg every 8–12 h. This treatment has been advocated because $T_4 \rightarrow T_3$ conversion is impaired in myxedema coma. However, excess liothyronine has the potential to provoke arrhythmias. Another option is to combine levothyroxine (200 μg) and liothyronine (25 μg) as a single, initial IV bolus followed by daily treatment with levothyroxine (50–100 μg/d) and liothyronine (10 μg every 8 h).

Supportive therapy should be provided to correct any associated metabolic disturbances. External warming is indicated only if the temperature is <30°C, as it can result in cardiovascular collapse. Space blankets should be used to prevent further heat loss. Parenteral hydrocortisone (50 mg every 6 h) should be administered, because there is impaired adrenal reserve in profound hypothyroidism. Any precipitating factors should be treated, including the early use of broad-spectrum antibiotics, pending the exclusion of infection. Ventilatory support with regular blood gas analysis is usually needed during the first 48 h. Hypertonic saline or IV glucose may be needed if there is severe hyponatremia or hypoglycemia; hypotonic IV fluids should be avoided because they may exacerbate water retention secondary to reduced renal perfusion and inappropriate vasopressin secretion. The metabolism of most medications is impaired, and sedatives should be avoided if possible or used in reduced doses. Medication blood levels should be monitored, when available, to guide dosage.

TABLE 7-7

CAUSES OF THYROTOXICOSIS

Primary Hyperthyroidism
Graves' disease
Toxic multinodular goiter
Toxic adenoma
Functioning thyroid carcinoma metastases
Activating mutation of the TSH receptor
Activating mutation of $G_{S\alpha}$ (McCune-Albright syndrome)
Struma ovarii
Drugs: iodine excess (Jod-Basedow phenomenon)
Thyrotoxicosis Without Hyperthyroidism
Subacute thyroiditis
Silent thyroiditis
Other causes of thyroid destruction: amiodarone, radiation, infarction of adenoma
Ingestion of excess thyroid hormone (thyrotoxicosis factitia) or thyroid tissue
Secondary Hyperthyroidism
TSH-secreting pituitary adenoma
Thyroid hormone resistance syndrome: occasional patients may have features of thyrotoxicosis
Chorionic gonadotropin-secreting tumors[a]
Gestational thyrotoxicosis[a]

[a]Circulating TSH levels are low in these forms of secondary hyperthyroidism.
Abbreviations: TSH, thyroid-stimulating hormone.

THYROTOXICOSIS

Thyrotoxicosis is defined as the state of thyroid hormone excess and is not synonymous with *hyperthyroidism*, which is the result of excessive thyroid function. However, the major etiologies of thyrotoxicosis are hyperthyroidism caused by Graves' disease, toxic MNG, and toxic adenomas. Other causes are listed in Table 7-7.

GRAVES' DISEASE

Epidemiology

Graves' disease accounts for 60–80% of thyrotoxicosis. The prevalence varies among populations, reflecting genetic factors and iodine intake (high iodine intake is associated with an increased prevalence of Graves' disease). Graves' disease occurs in up to 2% of women but is one-tenth as frequent in men. The disorder rarely begins before adolescence and typically occurs between 20 and 50 years of age; it also occurs in the elderly.

Pathogenesis

As in autoimmune hypothyroidism, a combination of environmental and genetic factors, including polymorphisms in HLA-DR, the immunoregulatory genes *CTLA-4*, *CD25*, *PTPN22*, *FCRL3*, and *CD226*, as well as the TSH-R, contribute to Graves' disease susceptibility. The concordance for Graves' disease in monozygotic twins is 20–30%, compared to <5% in dizygotic twins. Indirect evidence suggests that stress is an important environmental factor, presumably operating through neuroendocrine effects on the immune system. Smoking is a minor risk factor for Graves' disease and a major risk factor for the development of ophthalmopathy. Sudden increases in iodine intake may precipitate Graves' disease, and there is a threefold increase in the occurrence of Graves' disease in the postpartum period. Graves' disease may occur during the immune reconstitution phase after highly active antiretroviral therapy (HAART) or alemtuzumab treatment.

The hyperthyroidism of Graves' disease is caused by TSI that are synthesized in the thyroid gland as well as in bone marrow and lymph nodes. Such antibodies can be detected by bioassays or by using the more widely available TBII assays. The presence of TBII in a patient with thyrotoxicosis implies the existence of TSI, and these assays are useful in monitoring pregnant Graves' patients in whom high levels of TSI can cross the placenta and cause neonatal thyrotoxicosis. Other thyroid autoimmune responses, similar to those in autoimmune hypothyroidism (see above), occur concurrently in patients with Graves' disease. In particular, TPO antibodies occur in up to 80% of cases and serve as a readily measurable marker of autoimmunity. Because the coexisting thyroiditis can also affect thyroid function, there is no direct correlation between the level of TSI and thyroid hormone levels in Graves' disease. In the long term, spontaneous autoimmune hypothyroidism may develop in up to 15% of patients with Graves' disease.

Cytokines appear to play a major role in thyroid-associated ophthalmopathy. There is infiltration of the extraocular muscles by activated T cells; the release of cytokines such as IFN-γ, TNF, and IL-1 results in fibroblast activation and increased synthesis of glycosaminoglycans that trap water, thereby leading to characteristic muscle swelling. Late in the disease, there is irreversible fibrosis of the muscles. Orbital fibroblasts may be particularly sensitive to cytokines, perhaps explaining the anatomic localization of the immune response. Though the pathogenesis of thyroid-associated ophthalmopathy remains unclear, there is mounting evidence that the TSH-R may be a shared autoantigen that is expressed in the orbit; this would explain the close association with autoimmune thyroid disease. Increased fat is an additional cause of retrobulbar tissue expansion. The increase in intraorbital pressure can lead to proptosis, diplopia, and optic neuropathy.

Clinical manifestations

Signs and symptoms include features that are common to any cause of thyrotoxicosis (Table 7-8) as well as those specific for Graves' disease. The clinical presentation depends on the severity of thyrotoxicosis, the duration of disease, individual susceptibility to excess thyroid hormone, and the patient's age. In the elderly, features of thyrotoxicosis may be subtle or masked, and patients may present mainly with fatigue and weight loss, a condition known as *apathetic thyrotoxicosis*.

TABLE 7-8

SIGNS AND SYMPTOMS OF THYROTOXICOSIS (DESCENDING ORDER OF FREQUENCY)

SYMPTOMS	SIGNS[a]
Hyperactivity, irritability, dysphoria	Tachycardia; atrial fibrillation in the elderly
Heat intolerance and sweating	Tremor
Palpitations	Goiter
Fatigue and weakness	Warm, moist skin
Weight loss with increased appetite	Muscle weakness, proximal myopathy
Diarrhea	Lid retraction or lag
Polyuria	Gynecomastia
Oligomenorrhea, loss of libido	

[a]Excludes the signs of ophthalmopathy and dermopathy specific for Graves' disease.

Thyrotoxicosis may cause unexplained weight loss, despite an enhanced appetite, due to the increased metabolic rate. Weight gain occurs in 5% of patients, however, because of increased food intake. Other prominent features include hyperactivity, nervousness, and irritability, ultimately leading to a sense of easy fatigability in some patients. Insomnia and impaired concentration are common; apathetic thyrotoxicosis may be mistaken for depression in the elderly. Fine tremor is a frequent finding, best elicited by having patients stretch out their fingers while feeling the fingertips with the palm. Common neurologic manifestations include hyperreflexia, muscle wasting, and proximal myopathy without fasciculation. Chorea is rare. Thyrotoxicosis is sometimes associated with a form of hypokalemic periodic paralysis; this disorder is particularly common in Asian males with thyrotoxicosis, but it occurs in other ethnic groups as well.

The most common cardiovascular manifestation is sinus tachycardia, often associated with palpitations, occasionally caused by supraventricular tachycardia. The high cardiac output produces a bounding pulse, widened pulse pressure, and an aortic systolic murmur and can lead to worsening of angina or heart failure in the elderly or those with preexisting heart disease. Atrial fibrillation is more common in patients >50 years of age. Treatment of the thyrotoxic state alone converts atrial fibrillation to normal sinus rhythm in about half of patients, suggesting the existence of an underlying cardiac problem in the remainder.

The skin is usually warm and moist, and the patient may complain of sweating and heat intolerance, particularly during warm weather. Palmar erythema, onycholysis, and, less commonly, pruritus, urticaria, and diffuse hyperpigmentation may be evident. Hair texture may become fine, and a diffuse alopecia occurs in up to 40% of patients, persisting for months after restoration of euthyroidism. Gastrointestinal transit time is decreased, leading to increased stool frequency, often with diarrhea and occasionally mild steatorrhea. Women frequently experience oligomenorrhea or amenorrhea; in men, there may be impaired sexual function and, rarely, gynecomastia. The direct effect of thyroid hormones on bone resorption leads to osteopenia in long-standing thyrotoxicosis; mild hypercalcemia occurs in up to 20% of patients, but hypercalciuria is more common. There is a small increase in fracture rate in patients with a previous history of thyrotoxicosis.

In Graves' disease, the thyroid is usually diffusely enlarged to two to three times its normal size. The consistency is firm, but not nodular. There may be a thrill or bruit, best detected at the inferolateral margins of the thyroid lobes, due to the increased vascularity of the gland and the hyperdynamic circulation.

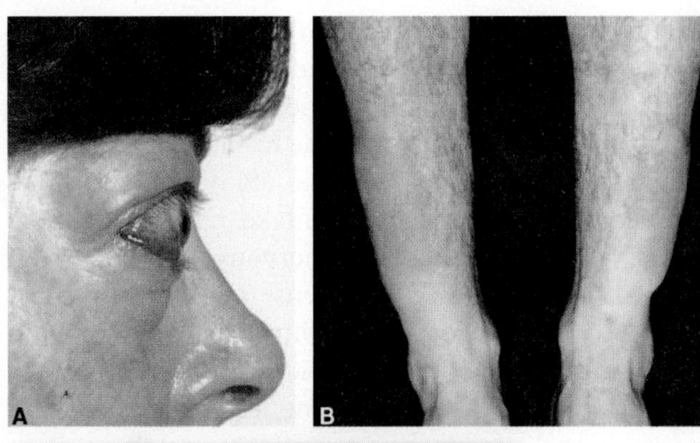

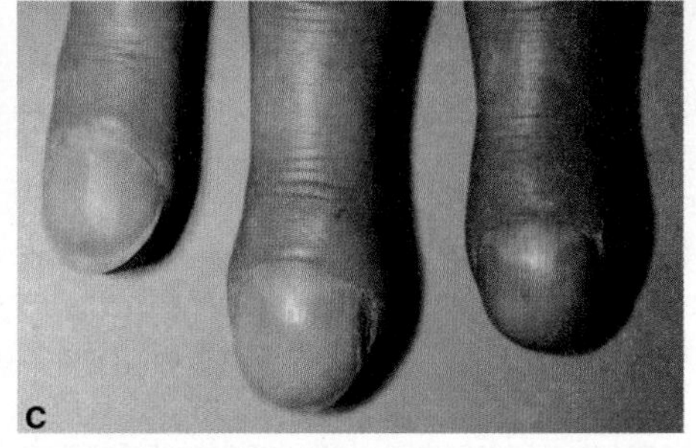

FIGURE 7-8

Features of Graves' disease. *A.* Ophthalmopathy in Graves' disease; lid retraction, periorbital edema, conjunctival injection, and proptosis are marked. ***B.*** Thyroid dermopathy over the lateral aspects of the shins. ***C.*** Thyroid acropachy.

Lid retraction, causing a staring appearance, can occur in any form of thyrotoxicosis and is the result of sympathetic overactivity. However, Graves' disease is associated with specific eye signs that comprise *Graves' ophthalmopathy* (Fig. 7-8A). This condition is also called *thyroid-associated ophthalmopathy*, because it occurs in the absence of hyperthyroidism in 10% of patients. Most of these individuals have autoimmune hypothyroidism or thyroid antibodies. The onset of Graves' ophthalmopathy occurs within the year before or after the diagnosis of thyrotoxicosis in 75% of patients but can sometimes precede or follow thyrotoxicosis by several years, accounting for some cases of euthyroid ophthalmopathy.

Some patients with Graves' disease have little clinical evidence of ophthalmopathy. However, the enlarged extraocular muscles typical of the disease, and other subtle features, can be detected in almost all patients when investigated by ultrasound or computed tomography (CT) imaging of the orbits. Unilateral signs are found in up to 10% of patients. The earliest manifestations of ophthalmopathy are usually a sensation of grittiness, eye discomfort, and excess tearing. About one-third of patients have proptosis, best detected by visualization of the sclera between the lower border of the iris and the lower eyelid, with the eyes in the primary position. Proptosis can be measured using an exophthalmometer. In severe cases, proptosis may cause corneal exposure and damage, especially if the lids fail to close during sleep. Periorbital edema, scleral injection, and chemosis are also frequent. In 5–10% of patients, the muscle swelling is so severe that diplopia results, typically, but not exclusively, when the patient looks up and laterally. The most serious manifestation is compression of the optic nerve at the apex of the orbit, leading to papilledema; peripheral field defects; and, if left untreated, permanent loss of vision.

The "NO SPECS" scoring system to evaluate ophthalmopathy is an acronym derived from the following changes:

0 = **N**o signs or symptoms
1 = **O**nly signs (lid retraction or lag), no symptoms
2 = **S**oft tissue involvement (periorbital edema)
3 = **P**roptosis (>22 mm)
4 = **E**xtraocular muscle involvement (diplopia)
5 = **C**orneal involvement
6 = **S**ight loss

Although useful as a mnemonic, the NO SPECS scheme is inadequate to describe the eye disease fully, and patients do not necessarily progress from one class to another; alternative scoring systems that assess disease activity are preferable for monitoring purposes. When Graves' eye disease is active and severe, referral to an ophthalmologist is indicated and objective measurements are needed, such as lid-fissure width; corneal staining with fluorescein; and evaluation of extraocular muscle function (e.g., Hess chart), intraocular pressure and visual fields, acuity, and color vision.

Thyroid dermopathy occurs in <5% of patients with Graves' disease (Fig. 7-8B), almost always in the presence of moderate or severe ophthalmopathy. Although most frequent over the anterior and lateral aspects of the lower leg (hence the term *pretibial myxedema*), skin changes can occur at other sites, particularly after trauma. The typical lesion is a noninflamed, indurated plaque with a deep pink or purple color and an "orange skin" appearance. Nodular involvement can occur, and the condition can rarely extend over the whole lower leg and foot, mimicking elephantiasis. *Thyroid acropachy* refers to a form of clubbing found in <1% of patients with Graves' disease (Fig. 7-8C). It is so strongly associated with thyroid dermopathy that an alternative cause of clubbing should be sought in a Graves' patient without coincident skin and orbital involvement.

Laboratory evaluation

Investigations used to determine the existence and cause of thyrotoxicosis are summarized in Fig. 7-9. In Graves' disease, the TSH level is suppressed, and total and unbound thyroid hormone levels are increased. In 2–5% of patients (and more in areas of borderline iodine intake), only T_3 is increased (T_3 toxicosis). The

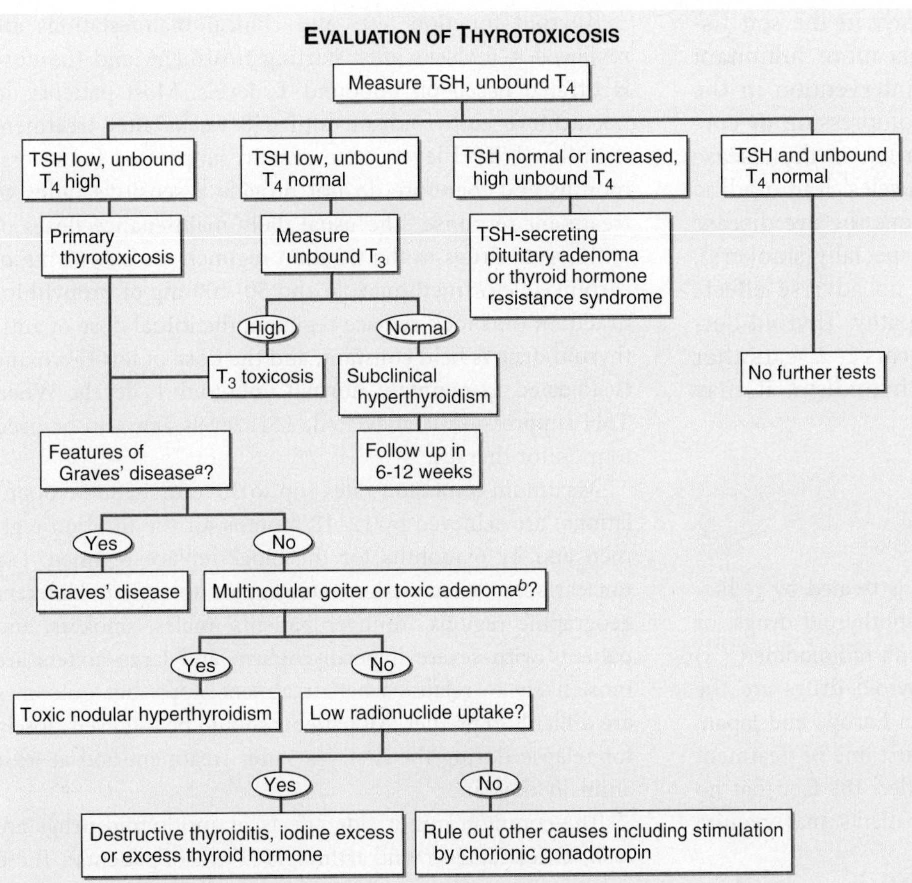

FIGURE 7-9

Evaluation of thyrotoxicosis. [a]Diffuse goiter, positive TPO antibodies or TRAb, ophthalmopathy, dermopathy. [b]Can be confirmed by radionuclide scan. TSH, thyroid-stimulating hormone.

converse state of T_4 toxicosis, with elevated total and unbound T_4 and normal T_3 levels, is occasionally seen when hyperthyroidism is induced by excess iodine, providing surplus substrate for thyroid hormone synthesis. Measurement of TPO antibodies or TRAb may be useful if the diagnosis is unclear clinically but is not needed routinely. Associated abnormalities that may cause diagnostic confusion in thyrotoxicosis include elevation of bilirubin, liver enzymes, and ferritin. Microcytic anemia and thrombocytopenia may occur.

Differential diagnosis

Diagnosis of Graves' disease is straightforward in a patient with biochemically confirmed thyrotoxicosis, diffuse goiter on palpation, ophthalmopathy, and often a personal or family history of autoimmune disorders. For patients with thyrotoxicosis who lack these features, the diagnosis is generally established by a radionuclide (^{99m}Tc, ^{123}I, or ^{131}I) scan and uptake of the thyroid, which will distinguish the diffuse, high uptake of Graves' disease from destructive thyroiditis, ectopic thyroid tissue, and factitious thyrotoxicosis. Scintigraphy is the preferred diagnostic test; however, TRAb measurement can be used to assess autoimmune activity. In secondary hyperthyroidism due to a TSH-secreting pituitary tumor, there is also a diffuse goiter. The presence of a nonsuppressed TSH level and the finding of a pituitary tumor on CT or magnetic resonance scan (MRI) scan suggest this diagnosis.

Clinical features of thyrotoxicosis can mimic certain aspects of other disorders, including panic attacks, mania, pheochromocytoma, and weight loss associated with malignancy. The diagnosis of thyrotoxicosis can be easily excluded if the TSH and unbound T_4 and T_3 levels are normal. A normal TSH also excludes Graves' disease as a cause of diffuse goiter.

Clinical course

Clinical features generally worsen without treatment; mortality was 10–30% before the introduction of satisfactory therapy. Some patients with mild Graves' disease experience spontaneous relapses and remissions. Rarely, there may be fluctuation between hypo- and hyperthyroidism due to changes in the functional activity of TSH-R antibodies. About 15% of patients who enter remission after treatment develop hypothyroidism 10–15 years later as a result of the destructive autoimmune process.

The clinical course of ophthalmopathy does not follow that of the thyroid disease. Ophthalmopathy typically worsens over the initial 3–6 months, followed by a plateau phase over the next 12–18 months, with spontaneous improvement, particularly in the soft tissue changes. However, the course is more fulminant in up to 5% of patients, requiring intervention in the acute phase if there is optic nerve compression or corneal ulceration. Diplopia may appear late in the disease due to fibrosis of the extraocular muscles. Radioiodine treatment for hyperthyroidism worsens the eye disease in a small proportion of patients (especially smokers). Antithyroid drugs or surgery have no adverse effects on the clinical course of ophthalmopathy. Thyroid dermopathy, when it occurs, usually appears 1–2 years after the development of Graves' hyperthyroidism; it may improve spontaneously.

TREATMENT Graves' Disease

The *hyperthyroidism* of Graves' disease is treated by reducing thyroid hormone synthesis, using antithyroid drugs, or reducing the amount of thyroid tissue with radioiodine (^{131}I) treatment or by thyroidectomy. Antithyroid drugs are the predominant therapy in many centers in Europe and Japan, whereas radioiodine is more often the first line of treatment in North America. These differences reflect the fact that no single approach is optimal and that patients may require multiple treatments to achieve remission.

The main *antithyroid drugs* are the thionamides, such as propylthiouracil, carbimazole (not available in the United States), and the active metabolite of the latter, methimazole. All inhibit the function of TPO, reducing oxidation and organification of iodide. These drugs also reduce thyroid antibody levels by mechanisms that remain unclear, and they appear to enhance rates of remission. Propylthiouracil inhibits deiodination of $T_4 \rightarrow T_3$. However, this effect is of minor benefit, except in the most severe thyrotoxicosis, and is offset by the much shorter half-life of this drug (90 min) compared to methimazole (6 h). Due to the hepatotoxicity of propylthiouracil, the U.S. Food and Drug Administration (FDA) has limited indications for its use to the first trimester of pregnancy, the treatment of thyroid storm, and patients with minor adverse reactions to methimazole. If propylthiouracil is used, monitoring of liver function tests is recommended.

There are many variations of antithyroid drug regimens. The initial dose of carbimazole or methimazole is usually 10–20 mg every 8 or 12 h, but once-daily dosing is possible after euthyroidism is restored. Propylthiouracil is given at a dose of 100–200 mg every 6–8 h, and divided doses are usually given throughout the course. Lower doses of each drug may suffice in areas of low iodine intake. The starting dose of antithyroid drugs can be gradually reduced (titration regimen) as thyrotoxicosis improves. Alternatively, high doses may be given combined with levothyroxine supplementation (block-replace regimen) to avoid drug-induced hypothyroidism. The titration regimen is preferred to minimize the dose of antithyroid drug and provide an index of treatment response.

Thyroid function tests and clinical manifestations are reviewed 4–6 weeks after starting treatment, and the dose is titrated based on unbound T_4 levels. Most patients do not achieve euthyroidism until 6–8 weeks after treatment is initiated. TSH levels often remain suppressed for several months and therefore do not provide a sensitive index of treatment response. The usual daily maintenance doses of antithyroid drugs in the titration regimen are 2.5–10 mg of carbimazole or methimazole and 50–100 mg of propylthiouracil. In the block-replace regimen, the initial dose of antithyroid drug is held constant, and the dose of levothyroxine is adjusted to maintain normal unbound T_4 levels. When TSH suppression is alleviated, TSH levels can also be used to monitor therapy.

Maximum remission rates (up to 30–60% in some populations) are achieved by 12–18 months for the titration regimen and by 6 months for the block-replace regimen. For unclear reasons, remission rates appear to vary in different geographic regions. Younger patients, males, smokers, and patients with severe hyperthyroidism and large goiters are most likely to relapse when treatment stops, but outcomes are difficult to predict. All patients should be followed closely for relapse during the first year after treatment and at least annually thereafter.

The common minor side effects of antithyroid drugs are rash, urticaria, fever, and arthralgia (1–5% of patients). These may resolve spontaneously or after substituting an alternative antithyroid drug. Rare but major side effects include hepatitis (propylthiouracil; avoid use in children) and cholestasis (methimazole and carbimazole); an SLE-like syndrome; and, most important, agranulocytosis (<1%). It is essential that antithyroid drugs are stopped and not restarted if a patient develops major side effects. Written instructions should be provided regarding the symptoms of possible agranulocytosis (e.g., sore throat, fever, mouth ulcers) and the need to stop treatment pending an urgent complete blood count to confirm that agranulocytosis is not present. It is not useful to monitor blood counts prospectively, because the onset of agranulocytosis is idiosyncratic and abrupt.

Propranolol (20–40 mg every 6 h) or longer-acting selective β_1 receptor blockers such as atenolol may be helpful to control adrenergic symptoms, especially in the early stages before antithyroid drugs take effect. Beta blockers are also useful in patients with thyrotoxic periodic paralysis, pending correction of thyrotoxicosis. In consultation with a cardiologist, anticoagulation with warfarin should be considered in all patients with atrial fibrillation who often spontaneously revert to sinus rhythm with control of hyperthyroidism. Decreased warfarin doses are required when patients are thyrotoxic. If digoxin is used, increased doses are often needed in the thyrotoxic state.

Radioiodine causes progressive destruction of thyroid cells and can be used as initial treatment or for relapses after a trial of antithyroid drugs. There is a small risk of thyrotoxic crisis (see below) after radioiodine, which can be minimized by pretreatment with antithyroid drugs for at least a month before treatment. Antecedent treatment with antithyroid drugs should be considered for all elderly patients or for those with cardiac problems to deplete thyroid hormone stores before administration of radioiodine. Carbimazole or methimazole must be stopped 3–5 days before radioiodine administration to achieve optimum iodine uptake. Propylthiouracil appears to have a prolonged radioprotective effect and should be stopped for a longer period before radioiodine is given, or a larger dose of radioiodine will be necessary.

Efforts to calculate an optimal dose of radioiodine that achieves euthyroidism without a high incidence of relapse or progression to hypothyroidism have not been successful. Some patients inevitably relapse after a single dose because the biologic effects of radiation vary between individuals, and hypothyroidism cannot be uniformly avoided even using accurate dosimetry. A practical strategy is to give a fixed dose based on clinical features, such as the severity of thyrotoxicosis, the size of the goiter (increases the dose needed), and the level of radioiodine uptake (decreases the dose needed). ^{131}I dosage generally ranges between 370 MBq (10 mCi) and 555 MBq (15 mCi). Most authorities favor an approach aimed at thyroid ablation (as opposed to euthyroidism), given that levothyroxine replacement is straightforward and most patients ultimately progress to hypothyroidism over 5–10 years, frequently with some delay in the diagnosis of hypothyroidism.

Certain radiation safety precautions are necessary in the first few days after radioiodine treatment, but the exact guidelines vary depending on local protocols. In general, patients need to avoid close, prolonged contact with children and pregnant women for 5–7 days because of possible transmission of residual isotope and exposure to radiation emanating from the gland. Rarely, there may be mild pain due to radiation thyroiditis 1–2 weeks after treatment. Hyperthyroidism can persist for 2–3 months before radioiodine takes full effect. For this reason, β-adrenergic blockers or antithyroid drugs can be used to control symptoms during this interval. Persistent hyperthyroidism can be treated with a second dose of radioiodine, usually 6 months after the first dose. The risk of hypothyroidism after radioiodine depends on the dosage but is at least 10–20% in the first year and 5% per year thereafter. Patients should be informed of this possibility before treatment and require close follow-up during the first year followed by annual thyroid function testing.

Pregnancy and breast-feeding are absolute contraindications to radioiodine treatment, but patients can conceive safely 6 months after treatment. The presence of severe ophthalmopathy requires caution, and some authorities advocate the use of prednisone, 40 mg/d, at the time of radioiodine treatment, tapered over 6–12 weeks to prevent exacerbation of ophthalmopathy. The overall risk of cancer after radioiodine treatment in adults is not increased. Although many physicians avoid radioiodine in children and adolescents because of the theoretical risks of malignancy, emerging evidence suggests that radioiodine can be used safely in older children.

Subtotal or near-total thyroidectomy is an option for patients who relapse after antithyroid drugs and prefer this treatment to radioiodine. Some experts recommend surgery in young individuals, particularly when the goiter is very large. Careful control of thyrotoxicosis with antithyroid drugs, followed by potassium iodide (3 drops SSKI orally tid), is needed prior to surgery to avoid thyrotoxic crisis and to reduce the vascularity of the gland. The major complications of surgery—bleeding, laryngeal edema, hypoparathyroidism, and damage to the recurrent laryngeal nerves—are unusual when the procedure is performed by highly experienced surgeons. Recurrence rates in the best series are <2%, but the rate of hypothyroidism is only slightly less than that following radioiodine treatment.

The titration regimen of antithyroid drugs should be used to manage Graves' disease in *pregnancy* because transplacental passage of these drugs may produce fetal hypothyroidism and goiter if the maternal dose is excessive. If available, propylthiouracil should be used in early gestation because of the association of rare cases of fetal *aplasia cutis* and other defects, such as choanal atresia with carbimazole and methimazole. As noted above, because of its rare association with hepatotoxicity, propylthiouracil should be limited to the first trimester and then maternal therapy should be converted to methimazole (or carbimazole) at a ratio of 15–20 mg of propylthiouracil to 1 mg of methimazole The lowest effective antithyroid drug dose should be used throughout gestation to maintain the maternal serum free T_4 level at the upper limit of the nonpregnant normal reference range. It is often possible to stop treatment in the last trimester because TSIs tend to decline in pregnancy. Nonetheless, the transplacental transfer of these antibodies rarely causes *fetal* or *neonatal thyrotoxicosis*. Poor intrauterine growth, a fetal heart rate of >160 beats/min, and high levels of maternal TSI in the last trimester may herald this complication. Antithyroid drugs given to the mother can be used to treat the fetus and may be needed for 1–3 months after delivery, until the maternal antibodies disappear from the baby's circulation. The postpartum period is a time of major risk for relapse of Graves' disease. Breast-feeding is safe with low doses of antithyroid drugs. Graves' disease in *children* is usually managed with methimazole or carbimazole (avoid propylthiouracil), often given as a prolonged course of the titration regimen. Surgery or radioiodine may be indicated for severe disease.

Thyrotoxic crisis, or *thyroid storm*, is rare and presents as a life-threatening exacerbation of hyperthyroidism, accompanied by fever, delirium, seizures, coma, vomiting, diarrhea, and jaundice. The mortality rate due to cardiac failure, arrhythmia, or hyperthermia is as high as 30%, even with treatment. Thyrotoxic crisis is usually precipitated by acute illness (e.g., stroke, infection, trauma, diabetic ketoacidosis), surgery (especially on the thyroid), or radioiodine treatment of a patient with partially treated or untreated hyperthyroidism. Management requires intensive monitoring and supportive care, identification and treatment of the precipitating cause, and measures that reduce thyroid hormone synthesis.

Large doses of propylthiouracil (500–1000 mg loading dose and 250 mg every 4 h) should be given orally or by nasogastric tube or per rectum; the drug's inhibitory action on $T_4 \rightarrow T_3$ conversion makes it the antithyroid drug of choice. If not available, methimazole can be used in doses up to 30 mg every 12 h. One hour after the first dose of propylthiouracil, stable iodide is given to block thyroid hormone synthesis via the Wolff-Chaikoff effect (the delay allows the antithyroid drug to prevent the excess iodine from being incorporated into new hormone). A saturated solution of potassium iodide (5 drops SSKI every 6 h) or, where available, ipodate or iopanoic acid (500 mg per 12 h) may be given orally. Sodium iodide, 0.25 g IV every 6 h, is an alternative but is not generally available. Propranolol should also be given to reduce tachycardia and other adrenergic manifestations (60–80 mg PO every 4 h; or 2 mg IV every 4 h). Although other β-adrenergic blockers can be used, high doses of propranolol decrease $T_4 \rightarrow T_3$ conversion, and the doses can be easily adjusted. Caution is needed to avoid acute negative inotropic effects, but controlling the heart rate is important, as some patients develop a form of high-output heart failure. Short-acting IV esmolol can be used to decrease heart rate while monitoring for signs of heart failure. Additional therapeutic measures include glucocorticoids (e.g., hydrocortisone 300 mg IV bolus, then 100 mg every 8 h), antibiotics if infection is present, cooling, oxygen, and IV fluids.

Ophthalmopathy requires no active treatment when it is mild or moderate, because there is usually spontaneous improvement. General measures include meticulous control of thyroid hormone levels, cessation of smoking, and an explanation of the natural history of ophthalmopathy. Discomfort can be relieved with artificial tears (e.g., 1% methylcellulose), eye ointment, and the use of dark glasses with side frames. Periorbital edema may respond to a more upright sleeping position or a diuretic. Corneal exposure during sleep can be avoided by using patches or taping the eyelids shut. Minor degrees of diplopia improve with prisms fitted to spectacles. Severe ophthalmopathy, with optic nerve involvement or chemosis resulting in corneal damage, is an emergency requiring joint management with an ophthalmologist. Pulse therapy with IV methylprednisolone (e.g., 500 mg of methylprednisolone once weekly for 6 weeks, then 250 mg once weekly for 6 weeks) is preferable to oral glucocorticoids, which are used for moderately active disease. When glucocorticoids are ineffective, orbital decompression can be achieved by removing bone from any wall of the orbit, thereby allowing displacement of fat and swollen extraocular muscles. The transantral route is used most often because it requires no external incision. Proptosis recedes an average of 5 mm, but there may be residual or even worsened diplopia. Once the eye disease has stabilized, surgery may be indicated for relief of diplopia and correction of the appearance. External beam radiotherapy of the orbits has been used for many years, but the efficacy of this therapy remains unclear, and it is best reserved for those with moderately active disease who have failed or are not candidates for glucocorticoid therapy. Other immunosuppressive agents such as rituximab have shown some benefit, but their role is yet to be established.

Thyroid dermopathy does not usually require treatment, but it can cause cosmetic problems or interfere with the fit of shoes. Surgical removal is not indicated. If necessary, treatment consists of topical, high-potency glucocorticoid ointment under an occlusive dressing. Octreotide may be beneficial in some cases.

OTHER CAUSES OF THYROTOXICOSIS

Destructive thyroiditis (subacute or silent thyroiditis) typically presents with a short thyrotoxic phase due to the release of preformed thyroid hormones and catabolism of Tg (see "Subacute Thyroiditis," below). True hyperthyroidism is absent, as demonstrated by a low radionuclide uptake. Circulating Tg levels are usually increased. Other causes of thyrotoxicosis with low or absent thyroid radionuclide uptake include *thyrotoxicosis factitia*, iodine excess, and, rarely, ectopic thyroid tissue, particularly teratomas of the ovary (*struma ovarii*) and functional metastatic follicular carcinoma. Whole-body radionuclide studies can demonstrate ectopic thyroid tissue, and thyrotoxicosis factitia can be distinguished from destructive thyroiditis by the clinical features and low levels of Tg. Amiodarone treatment is associated with thyrotoxicosis in up to 10% of patients, particularly in areas of low iodine intake (see below).

TSH-secreting pituitary adenoma is a rare cause of thyrotoxicosis. It is characterized by the presence of an inappropriately normal or increased TSH level in a patient with hyperthyroidism, diffuse goiter, and elevated T_4 and T_3 levels **(Chap. 5)**. Elevated levels of the α-subunit of TSH, released by the TSH-secreting adenoma, support this diagnosis, which can be confirmed by demonstrating the pituitary tumor on MRI or CT scan. A combination of transsphenoidal surgery, sella irradiation, and octreotide may be required to normalize TSH, because many of these tumors are large and locally invasive at the time of diagnosis. Radioiodine or antithyroid drugs can be used to control thyrotoxicosis.

Thyrotoxicosis caused by *toxic MNG* and *hyperfunctioning solitary nodules* is discussed below.

THYROIDITIS

A clinically useful classification of thyroiditis is based on the onset and duration of disease (Table 7-9).

ACUTE THYROIDITIS

Acute thyroiditis is rare and due to suppurative infection of the thyroid. In children and young adults, the most common cause is the presence of a piriform

TABLE 7-9

CAUSES OF THYROIDITIS
Acute
Bacterial infection: especially *Staphylococcus, Streptococcus,* and *Enterobacter*
Fungal infection: *Aspergillus, Candida, Coccidioides, Histoplasma,* and *Pneumocystis*
Radiation thyroiditis after ^{131}I treatment
Amiodarone (may also be subacute or chronic)
Subacute
Viral (or granulomatous) thyroiditis
Silent thyroiditis (including postpartum thyroiditis)
Mycobacterial infection
Drug induced (interferon, amiodarone)
Chronic
Autoimmunity: focal thyroiditis, Hashimoto's thyroiditis, atrophic thyroiditis
Riedel's thyroiditis
Parasitic thyroiditis: echinococcosis, strongyloidiasis, cysticercosis
Traumatic: after palpation

sinus, a remnant of the fourth branchial pouch that connects the oropharynx with the thyroid. Such sinuses are predominantly left-sided. A long-standing goiter and degeneration in a thyroid malignancy are risk factors in the elderly. The patient presents with thyroid pain, often referred to the throat or ears, and a small, tender goiter that may be asymmetric. Fever, dysphagia, and erythema over the thyroid are common, as are systemic symptoms of a febrile illness and lymphadenopathy.

The differential diagnosis of *thyroid pain* includes subacute or, rarely, chronic thyroiditis; hemorrhage into a cyst; malignancy including lymphoma; and, rarely, amiodarone-induced thyroiditis or amyloidosis. However, the abrupt presentation and clinical features of acute thyroiditis rarely cause confusion. The erythrocyte sedimentation rate (ESR) and white cell count are usually increased, but thyroid function is normal. FNA biopsy shows infiltration by polymorphonuclear leukocytes; culture of the sample can identify the organism. Caution is needed in immunocompromised patients as fungal, mycobacterial, or *Pneumocystis* thyroiditis can occur in this setting. Antibiotic treatment is guided initially by Gram stain and, subsequently, by cultures of the FNA biopsy. Surgery may be needed to drain an abscess, which can be localized by CT scan or ultrasound. Tracheal obstruction, septicemia, retropharyngeal abscess, mediastinitis, and jugular venous thrombosis may complicate acute thyroiditis but are uncommon with prompt use of antibiotics.

SUBACUTE THYROIDITIS

This is also termed *de Quervain's thyroiditis, granulomatous thyroiditis,* or *viral thyroiditis.* Many viruses have been implicated, including mumps, coxsackie, influenza, adenoviruses, and echoviruses, but attempts to identify the virus in an individual patient are often unsuccessful and do not influence management. The diagnosis of subacute thyroiditis is often overlooked because the symptoms can mimic pharyngitis. The peak incidence occurs at 30–50 years, and women are affected three times more frequently than men.

Pathophysiology

The thyroid shows a characteristic patchy inflammatory infiltrate with disruption of the thyroid follicles and multinucleated giant cells within some follicles. The follicular changes progress to granulomas accompanied by fibrosis. Finally, the thyroid returns to normal, usually several months after onset. During the initial phase of follicular destruction, there is release of Tg and thyroid hormones, leading to increased circulating T_4 and T_3 and suppression of TSH (Fig. 7-10). During this destructive phase, radioactive iodine uptake is low or undetectable. After several weeks, the thyroid is depleted of stored thyroid hormone and a phase of hypothyroidism typically occurs, with low unbound T_4 (and sometimes T_3) and moderately increased TSH levels. Radioactive iodine uptake returns to normal or is even increased as a result of the rise in TSH. Finally,

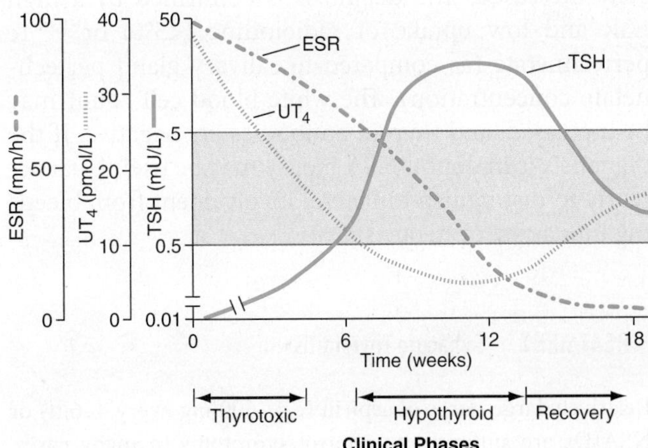

FIGURE 7-10

Clinical course of subacute thyroiditis. The release of thyroid hormones is initially associated with a thyrotoxic phase and suppressed thyroid-stimulating hormone (TSH). A hypothyroid phase then ensues, with low T_4 and TSH levels that are initially low but gradually increase. During the recovery phase, increased TSH levels combined with resolution of thyroid follicular injury lead to normalization of thyroid function, often several months after the beginning of the illness. ESR, erythrocyte sedimentation rate; UT_4, free or unbound T_4.

thyroid hormone and TSH levels return to normal as the disease subsides.

Clinical manifestations

The patient usually presents with a painful and enlarged thyroid, sometimes accompanied by fever. There may be features of thyrotoxicosis or hypothyroidism, depending on the phase of the illness. Malaise and symptoms of an upper respiratory tract infection may precede the thyroid-related features by several weeks. In other patients, the onset is acute, severe, and without obvious antecedent. The patient typically complains of a sore throat, and examination reveals a small goiter that is exquisitely tender. Pain is often referred to the jaw or ear. Complete resolution is the usual outcome, but late-onset permanent hypothyroidism occurs in 15% of cases, particularly in those with coincidental thyroid autoimmunity. A prolonged course over many months, with one or more relapses, occurs in a small percentage of patients.

Laboratory evaluation

As depicted in Fig. 7-10, thyroid function tests characteristically evolve through three distinct phases over about 6 months: (1) thyrotoxic phase, (2) hypothyroid phase, and (3) recovery phase. In the thyrotoxic phase, T_4 and T_3 levels are increased, reflecting their discharge from the damaged thyroid cells, and TSH is suppressed. The T_4/T_3 ratio is greater than in Graves' disease or thyroid autonomy, in which T_3 is often disproportionately increased. The diagnosis is confirmed by a high ESR and low uptake of radioiodine (<5%) or ^{99m}Tc pertechnetate (as compared to salivary gland pertechnetate concentration). The white blood cell count may be increased, and thyroid antibodies are negative. If the diagnosis is in doubt, FNA biopsy may be useful, particularly to distinguish unilateral involvement from bleeding into a cyst or neoplasm.

TREATMENT Subacute Thyroiditis

Relatively large doses of aspirin (e.g., 600 mg every 4–6 h) or NSAIDs are sufficient to control symptoms in many cases. If this treatment is inadequate, or if the patient has marked local or systemic symptoms, glucocorticoids should be given. The usual starting dose is 40–60 mg of prednisone, depending on severity. The dose is gradually tapered over 6–8 weeks, in response to improvement in symptoms and the ESR. If a relapse occurs during glucocorticoid withdrawal, treatment should be started again and withdrawn more gradually. In these patients, it is useful to wait until the radioactive iodine uptake normalizes before stopping treatment. Thyroid function should be monitored every 2–4 weeks using TSH and unbound T_4 levels. Symptoms of thyrotoxicosis improve spontaneously but may be ameliorated by β-adrenergic blockers; antithyroid drugs play no role in treatment of the thyrotoxic phase. Levothyroxine replacement may be needed if the hypothyroid phase is prolonged, but doses should be low enough (50–100 μg daily) to allow TSH-mediated recovery.

SILENT THYROIDITIS

Painless thyroiditis, or *"silent" thyroiditis*, occurs in patients with underlying autoimmune thyroid disease and has a clinical course similar to that of subacute thyroiditis. The condition occurs in up to 5% of women 3–6 months after pregnancy and is then termed *postpartum thyroiditis*. Typically, patients have a brief phase of thyrotoxicosis lasting 2–4 weeks, followed by hypothyroidism for 4–12 weeks, and then resolution; often, however, only one phase is apparent. The condition is associated with the presence of TPO antibodies antepartum, and it is three times more common in women with type 1 diabetes mellitus. As in subacute thyroiditis, the uptake of ^{99m}Tc pertechnetate or radioactive iodine is initially suppressed. In addition to the painless goiter, silent thyroiditis can be distinguished from subacute thyroiditis by a normal ESR and the presence of TPO antibodies. Glucocorticoid treatment is not indicated for silent thyroiditis. Severe thyrotoxic symptoms can be managed with a brief course of propranolol, 20–40 mg three or four times daily. Thyroxine replacement may be needed for the hypothyroid phase but should be withdrawn after 6–9 months, as recovery is the rule. Annual follow-up thereafter is recommended, because a proportion of these individuals develop permanent hypothyroidism. The condition may recur in subsequent pregnancies.

DRUG-INDUCED THYROIDITIS

Patients receiving cytokines such as IFN-α or IL-2 may develop painless thyroiditis. IFN-α, which is used to treat chronic hepatitis B or C and hematologic and skin malignancies, causes thyroid dysfunction in up to 5% of treated patients. It has been associated with painless thyroiditis, hypothyroidism, and Graves' disease, and is most common in women with TPO antibodies prior to treatment. For discussion of amiodarone, see "Amiodarone Effects on Thyroid Function," below.

CHRONIC THYROIDITIS

Focal thyroiditis is present in 20–40% of euthyroid autopsy cases and is associated with serologic evidence of autoimmunity, particularly the presence of TPO antibodies. The most common clinically apparent cause of chronic thyroiditis is *Hashimoto's thyroiditis*, an autoimmune disorder that often presents as a firm or hard goiter of variable size (see above). *Riedel's thyroiditis* is a rare disorder that typically occurs in middle-aged women. It presents with an insidious, painless goiter with local symptoms due to compression of the esophagus, trachea, neck veins, or recurrent laryngeal nerves. Dense fibrosis disrupts normal gland architecture and can extend outside the thyroid capsule. Despite these extensive histologic changes, thyroid dysfunction is uncommon. The goiter is hard, nontender, often asymmetric, and fixed, leading to suspicion of a malignancy. Diagnosis requires open biopsy as FNA biopsy is usually inadequate. Treatment is directed to surgical relief of compressive symptoms. Tamoxifen may also be beneficial. There is an association between Riedel's thyroiditis and IgG4-related systemic disease causing idiopathic fibrosis at other sites (retroperitoneum, mediastinum, biliary tree, lung, and orbit).

SICK EUTHYROID SYNDROME (NONTHYROIDAL ILLNESS)

Any acute, severe illness can cause abnormalities of circulating TSH or thyroid hormone levels in the absence of underlying thyroid disease, making these measurements potentially misleading. The major cause of these hormonal changes is the release of cytokines such as IL-6. Unless a thyroid disorder is strongly suspected, the routine testing of thyroid function should be avoided in acutely ill patients.

The most common hormone pattern in sick euthyroid syndrome (SES) is a decrease in total and unbound T_3 levels (low T_3 syndrome) with normal levels of T_4 and TSH. The magnitude of the fall in T_3 correlates with the severity of the illness. T_4 conversion to T_3 via peripheral 5′ (outer ring) deiodination is impaired, leading to increased reverse T_3 (rT_3). Since rT_3 is metabolized by 5′ deiodination, its clearance is also reduced. Thus, decreased clearance rather than increased production is the major basis for increased rT_3. Also, T_4 is alternately metabolized to the hormonally inactive T_3 sulfate. It is generally assumed that this low T_3 state is adaptive, because it can be induced in normal individuals by fasting. Teleologically, the fall in T_3 may limit catabolism in starved or ill patients.

Very sick patients may exhibit a dramatic fall in total T_4 and T_3 levels (low T_4 syndrome). With decreased tissue perfusion, muscle and liver expression of the type 3 deiodinase leads to accelerated T_4 and T_3 metabolism. This state has a poor prognosis. Another key factor in the fall in T_4 levels is altered binding to TBG. The commonly used free T_4 assays are subject to artifact when serum binding proteins are low and underestimate the true free T_4 level. Fluctuation in TSH levels also creates challenges in the interpretation of thyroid function in sick patients. TSH levels may range from <0.1 mIU/L in very ill patients, especially with dopamine or glucocorticoid therapy, to >20 mIU/L during the recovery phase of SES. The exact mechanisms underlying the subnormal TSH seen in 10% of sick patients and the increased TSH seen in 5% remain unclear but may be mediated by cytokines including IL-12 and IL-18.

Any severe illness can induce changes in thyroid hormone levels, but certain disorders exhibit a distinctive pattern of abnormalities. Acute liver disease is associated with an initial rise in total (but not unbound) T_3 and T_4 levels due to TBG release; these levels become subnormal with progression to liver failure. A transient increase in total and unbound T_4 levels, usually with a normal T_3 level, is seen in 5–30% of acutely ill psychiatric patients. TSH values may be transiently low, normal, or high in these patients. In the early stage of HIV infection, T_3 and T_4 levels rise, even if there is weight loss. T_3 levels fall with progression to AIDS, but TSH usually remains normal. Renal disease is often accompanied by low T_3 concentrations, but with normal rather than increased rT_3 levels, due to an unknown factor that increases uptake of rT_3 into the liver.

The diagnosis of SES is challenging. Historic information may be limited, and patients often have multiple metabolic derangements. Useful features to consider include previous history of thyroid disease and thyroid function tests, evaluation of the severity and time course of the patient's acute illness, documentation of medications that may affect thyroid function or thyroid hormone levels, and measurements of rT_3 together with unbound thyroid hormones and TSH. The diagnosis of SES is frequently presumptive, given the clinical context and pattern of laboratory values; only resolution of the test results with clinical recovery can clearly establish this disorder. Treatment of SES with thyroid hormone (T_4 and/or T_3) is controversial, but most authorities recommend monitoring the patient's thyroid function tests during recovery, without administering thyroid hormone, unless there is historic or clinical evidence suggestive of hypothyroidism. Sufficiently large randomized controlled trials using thyroid hormone are unlikely to resolve this therapeutic controversy in the near future, because clinical presentations and outcomes are highly variable.

AMIODARONE EFFECTS ON THYROID FUNCTION

Amiodarone is a commonly used type III antiarrhythmic agent. It is structurally related to thyroid hormone and contains 39% iodine by weight. Thus, typical doses of amiodarone (200 mg/d) are associated with very high iodine intake, leading to greater than fortyfold increases in plasma and urinary iodine levels. Moreover, because amiodarone is stored in adipose tissue, high iodine levels persist for >6 months after discontinuation of the drug. Amiodarone inhibits deiodinase activity, and its metabolites function as weak antagonists of thyroid hormone action. Amiodarone has the following effects on thyroid function: (1) acute, transient suppression of thyroid function; (2) hypothyroidism in patients susceptible to the inhibitory effects of a high iodine load; and (3) thyrotoxicosis that may be caused by either a Jod-Basedow effect from the iodine load, in the setting of MNG or incipient Graves' disease, or a thyroiditis-like condition.

The initiation of amiodarone treatment is associated with a transient decrease of T_4 levels, reflecting the inhibitory effect of iodine on T_4 release. Soon thereafter, most individuals escape from iodide-dependent suppression of the thyroid (Wolff-Chaikoff effect), and the inhibitory effects on deiodinase activity and thyroid hormone receptor action become predominant. These events lead to the following pattern of thyroid function tests: increased T_4, decreased T_3, increased rT_3, and a transient TSH increase (up to 20 mIU/L). TSH levels normalize or are slightly suppressed within 1–3 months.

The incidence of hypothyroidism from amiodarone varies geographically, apparently correlating with iodine intake. Hypothyroidism occurs in up to 13% of amiodarone-treated patients in iodine-replete countries, such as the United States, but is less common (<6% incidence) in areas of lower iodine intake, such as Italy or Spain. The pathogenesis appears to involve an inability of the thyroid gland to escape from the Wolff-Chaikoff effect in autoimmune thyroiditis. Consequently, amiodarone-associated hypothyroidism is more common in women and individuals with positive TPO antibodies. It is usually unnecessary to discontinue amiodarone for this side effect, because levothyroxine can be used to normalize thyroid function. TSH levels should be monitored, because T_4 levels are often increased for the reasons described above.

The management of amiodarone-induced thyrotoxicosis (AIT) is complicated by the fact that there are different causes of thyrotoxicosis and because the increased thyroid hormone levels exacerbate underlying arrhythmias and coronary artery disease. Amiodarone treatment causes thyrotoxicosis in 10% of patients living in areas of low iodine intake and in 2% of patients in regions of high iodine intake. There are two major forms of AIT, although some patients have features of both. Type 1 AIT is associated with an underlying thyroid abnormality (preclinical Graves' disease or nodular goiter). Thyroid hormone synthesis becomes excessive as a result of increased iodine exposure (Jod-Basedow phenomenon). Type 2 AIT occurs in individuals with no intrinsic thyroid abnormalities and is the result of drug-induced lysosomal activation leading to destructive thyroiditis with histiocyte accumulation in the thyroid; the incidence rises as cumulative amiodarone dosage increases. Mild forms of type 2 AIT can resolve spontaneously or can occasionally lead to hypothyroidism. Color-flow Doppler thyroid scanning shows increased vascularity in type 1 AIT but decreased vascularity in type 2 AIT. Thyroid scintiscans are difficult to interpret in this setting because the high endogenous iodine levels diminish tracer uptake. However, the presence of normal or rarely increased uptake favors type 1 AIT.

In AIT, the drug should be stopped, if possible, although this is often impractical because of the underlying cardiac disorder. Discontinuation of amiodarone will not have an acute effect because of its storage and prolonged half-life. High doses of antithyroid drugs can be used in type 1 AIT but are often ineffective. In type 2 AIT, oral contrast agents, such as sodium ipodate (500 mg/d) or sodium tyropanoate (500 mg, 1–2 doses/d), rapidly reduce T_4 and T_3 levels, decrease $T_4 \rightarrow T_3$ conversion, and may block tissue uptake of thyroid hormones. Potassium perchlorate, 200 mg every 6 h, has been used to reduce thyroidal iodide content. Perchlorate treatment has been associated with agranulocytosis, although the risk appears relatively low with short-term use. Glucocorticoids, as administered for subacute thyroiditis, have modest benefit in type 2 AIT. Lithium blocks thyroid hormone release and can also provide some benefit. Near-total thyroidectomy rapidly decreases thyroid hormone levels and may be the most effective long-term solution if the patient can undergo the procedure safely.

THYROID FUNCTION IN PREGNANCY

Five factors alter thyroid function in pregnancy: (1) the transient increase in hCG during the first trimester, which stimulates the TSH-R; (2) the estrogen-induced rise in TBG during the first trimester, which is sustained during pregnancy; (3) alterations in the immune system, leading to the onset, exacerbation, or amelioration of an underlying autoimmune thyroid disease (see above); (4) increased thyroid hormone metabolism by the placenta; and (5) increased urinary iodide excretion, which can cause impaired thyroid hormone production in areas of marginal iodine sufficiency. Women with a precarious iodine intake (<50 μg/d) are most at risk of developing a goiter during pregnancy or giving birth to an infant with a goiter and hypothyroidism. The World Health Organization recommends a daily iodine intake of 250 μg during pregnancy and prenatal vitamins should contain 150 μg per tablet.

The rise in circulating hCG levels during the first trimester is accompanied by a reciprocal fall in TSH that persists into the middle of pregnancy. This reflects the weak binding of hCG, which is present at very high levels, to the TSH-R. Rare individuals have been described with variant TSH-R sequences that enhance hCG binding and TSH-R activation. hCG-induced changes in thyroid function can result in transient gestational hyperthyroidism that may be associated with *hyperemesis gravidarum*, a condition characterized by severe nausea and vomiting and risk of volume depletion. However, since the hyperthyroidism is not causal, antithyroid drugs are not indicated unless concomitant Graves' disease is suspected. Parenteral fluid replacement usually suffices until the condition resolves.

During pregnancy, subclinical hypothyroidism occurs in 2% of women, but overt hypothyroidism is present in only 1 in 500. Prospective randomized controlled trials have not shown a benefit for universal thyroid disease screening in pregnancy. Targeted TSH testing for hypothyroidism is recommended for women planning a pregnancy if they have a strong family history of autoimmune thyroid disease, other autoimmune disorders (e.g., type 1 diabetes), prior preterm delivery or recurrent miscarriage, or signs or symptoms of thyroid disease. Thyroid hormone requirements are increased by up to 50% during pregnancy in levothyroxine-treated hypothyroid women (see above section on treatment of hypothyroidism).

GOITER AND NODULAR THYROID DISEASE

Goiter refers to an enlarged thyroid gland. Biosynthetic defects, iodine deficiency, autoimmune disease, and nodular diseases can each lead to goiter, although by different mechanisms. Biosynthetic defects and iodine deficiency are associated with reduced efficiency of thyroid hormone synthesis, leading to increased TSH, which stimulates thyroid growth as a compensatory mechanism to overcome the block in hormone synthesis. Graves' disease and Hashimoto's thyroiditis are also associated with goiter. In Graves' disease, the goiter results mainly from the TSH-R–mediated effects of TSI. The goitrous form of Hashimoto's thyroiditis occurs because of acquired defects in hormone synthesis, leading to elevated levels of TSH and its consequent growth effects. Lymphocytic infiltration and immune system–induced growth factors also contribute to thyroid enlargement in Hashimoto's thyroiditis. Nodular disease is characterized by the disordered growth of thyroid cells, often combined with the gradual development of fibrosis. Because the management of goiter depends on the etiology, the detection of thyroid enlargement on physical examination should prompt further evaluation to identify its cause.

Nodular thyroid disease is common, occurring in about 3–7% of adults when assessed by physical examination. Using ultrasound, nodules are present in up to 50% of adults, with the majority being <1 cm in diameter. Thyroid nodules may be solitary or multiple, and they may be functional or nonfunctional.

DIFFUSE NONTOXIC (SIMPLE) GOITER

Etiology and pathogenesis

When diffuse enlargement of the thyroid occurs in the absence of nodules and hyperthyroidism, it is referred to as a *diffuse nontoxic goiter*. This is sometimes called *simple goiter*, because of the absence of nodules, or *colloid goiter*, because of the presence of uniform follicles that are filled with colloid. Worldwide, diffuse goiter is most commonly caused by iodine deficiency and is termed *endemic goiter* when it affects >5% of the population. In nonendemic regions, *sporadic goiter* occurs, and the cause is usually unknown. Thyroid enlargement in teenagers is sometimes referred to as *juvenile goiter*. In general, goiter is more common in women than men, probably because of the greater prevalence of underlying autoimmune disease and the increased iodine demands associated with pregnancy.

In *iodine-deficient areas*, thyroid enlargement reflects a compensatory effort to trap iodide and produce sufficient hormone under conditions in which hormone synthesis is relatively inefficient. Somewhat surprisingly, TSH levels are usually normal or only slightly increased, suggesting increased sensitivity to TSH or activation of other pathways that lead to thyroid growth. Iodide appears to have direct actions on thyroid vasculature and may indirectly affect growth through vasoactive substances such as endothelins and nitric oxide. Endemic goiter is also caused by exposure to environmental *goitrogens* such as cassava root, which contains a thiocyanate; vegetables of the Cruciferae family (known as cruciferous vegetables) (e.g., Brussels sprouts, cabbage, and cauliflower); and milk from regions where goitrogens are present in grass. Although relatively rare, inherited defects in thyroid hormone synthesis lead to a diffuse nontoxic goiter. Abnormalities at each step in hormone synthesis, including iodide transport (NIS), Tg synthesis, organification and coupling (TPO), and the regeneration of iodide (dehalogenase), have been described.

CLINICAL MANIFESTATIONS AND DIAGNOSIS

If thyroid function is preserved, most goiters are asymptomatic. Examination of a diffuse goiter reveals a symmetrically enlarged, nontender, generally soft gland without palpable nodules. Goiter is defined, somewhat arbitrarily, as a lateral lobe with a volume greater than the thumb of the individual being examined. If the thyroid is markedly enlarged, it can cause tracheal or esophageal compression. These features are unusual, however, in the absence of nodular disease and fibrosis. *Substernal goiter* may obstruct the thoracic inlet. *Pemberton's sign* refers to symptoms of faintness with evidence of facial congestion and external jugular venous obstruction when the arms are raised above the head, a maneuver that draws the thyroid into the thoracic inlet. Respiratory flow measurements and CT or MRI should be used to evaluate substernal goiter in patients with obstructive signs or symptoms.

Thyroid function tests should be performed in all patients with goiter to exclude thyrotoxicosis or hypothyroidism. It is not unusual, particularly in iodine deficiency, to find a low total T_4, with normal T_3 and TSH, reflecting enhanced $T_4 \rightarrow T_3$ conversion. A low TSH with a normal free T_3 and free T_4, particularly in older patients, suggests the possibility of thyroid autonomy or undiagnosed Graves' disease, and is termed *subclinical thyrotoxicosis*. The benefit of treatment (typically with radioiodine) in subclinical thyrotoxicosis, versus follow-up and implementing treatment if free T_3 or free T_4 levels become abnormal, is unclear, but treatment is increasingly recommended in the elderly to reduce the risk of atrial fibrillation and bone loss. TPO antibodies may be useful to identify patients at increased risk of autoimmune thyroid disease. Low urinary iodine levels (<50 μg/L) support a diagnosis of iodine deficiency. Thyroid scanning is not generally necessary but will reveal increased uptake in iodine deficiency and most cases of dyshormonogenesis. Ultrasound is not generally indicated in the evaluation of diffuse goiter unless a nodule is palpable on physical examination.

TREATMENT **Diffuse Nontoxic (Simple) Goiter**

Iodine replacement induces variable regression of goiter in iodine deficiency, depending on how long it has been present and the degree of fibrosis that has developed. Surgery is rarely indicated for diffuse goiter. Exceptions include documented evidence of tracheal compression or obstruction of the thoracic inlet, which are more likely to be associated with substernal MNGs (see below). Subtotal or near-total thyroidectomy for these or cosmetic reasons should be performed by an experienced surgeon to minimize complication rates. Surgery should be followed by replacement with levothyroxine, with the aim of keeping the TSH level at the lower end of the reference range to prevent regrowth of the goiter.

NONTOXIC MULTINODULAR GOITER

Etiology and pathogenesis

Depending on the population studied, MNG or nodular enlargement of the thyroid occurs in up to 12% of adults. MNG is more common in women than men and increases in prevalence with age. It is more common in iodine-deficient regions but also occurs in regions of iodine sufficiency, reflecting multiple genetic, autoimmune, and environmental influences on the pathogenesis.

There is typically wide variation in nodule size. Histology reveals a spectrum of morphologies ranging from hypercellular regions to cystic areas filled with colloid. Fibrosis is often extensive, and areas of hemorrhage or lymphocytic infiltration may be seen. Using molecular techniques, most nodules within an MNG are polyclonal in origin, suggesting a hyperplastic response to locally produced growth factors and cytokines. TSH, which is usually not elevated, may play a permissive or contributory role. Monoclonal lesions also occur within an MNG, reflecting mutations in genes that confer a selective growth advantage to the progenitor cell.

Clinical manifestations

Most patients with nontoxic MNG are asymptomatic and euthyroid. MNG typically develops over many years and is detected on routine physical examination, when an individual notices an enlargement in the neck, or as an incidental finding on imaging. If the goiter is large enough, it can ultimately lead to compressive symptoms including difficulty swallowing, respiratory distress (tracheal compression), or plethora (venous congestion), but these symptoms are uncommon. Symptomatic MNGs are usually extraordinarily large and/or develop fibrotic areas that cause compression. Sudden pain in an MNG is usually caused by hemorrhage into a nodule but should raise the possibility of invasive malignancy. Hoarseness, reflecting laryngeal nerve involvement, also suggests malignancy.

Diagnosis

On examination, thyroid architecture is distorted, and multiple nodules of varying size can be appreciated. Because many nodules are deeply embedded in thyroid tissue or reside in posterior or substernal locations, it is not possible to palpate all nodules. Pemberton's sign, characterized by facial suffusion when the patient's arms are elevated above the head, suggests that the goiter has increased pressure in the thoracic inlet. A TSH level should be measured to exclude subclinical hyper- or hypothyroidism, but thyroid function is usually normal. Tracheal deviation is common, but compression must usually exceed 70% of the tracheal diameter before there is significant airway compromise. Pulmonary function testing can be used to assess the functional effects of compression, which characteristically causes inspiratory stridor. CT or MRI can be used to evaluate the anatomy of the goiter and the extent of substernal extension or tracheal narrowing. A barium swallow may reveal the extent of esophageal compression. The risk of malignancy in MNG is similar to that in solitary nodules. Ultrasonography can be used to identify which nodules should be biopsied based on sonographic features (see section above on ultrasound) and size. For nodules with more suspicious imaging characteristics (e.g., hypoechogenicity, microcalcifications, irregular margins), biopsy is recommended when ≥1 cm.

TREATMENT Nontoxic Multinodular Goiter

Most nontoxic MNGs can be managed conservatively. T_4 suppression is rarely effective for reducing goiter size and introduces the risk of subclinical or overt thyrotoxicosis, particularly if there is underlying autonomy or if it develops during treatment. If levothyroxine is used, it should be started at low doses (50 μg daily) and advanced gradually while monitoring the TSH level to avoid excessive suppression. Contrast agents and other iodine-containing substances should be avoided because of the risk of inducing the *Jod-Basedow effect*, characterized by enhanced thyroid hormone production by autonomous nodules. Radioiodine is used with increasing frequency in areas where large goiters are more prevalent because it can decrease goiter size and may selectively ablate regions of autonomy. Dosage of ^{131}I depends on the size of the goiter and radioiodine uptake but is usually about 3.7 MBq (0.1 mCi) per gram of tissue, corrected for uptake (typical dose 370–1070 MBq [10 to 29 mCi]). Repeat treatment may be needed and effectiveness may be increased by concurrent administration of low-dose recombinant TSH (0.1 mg IM). It is possible to achieve a 40–50% reduction in goiter size in most patients. Earlier concerns about radiation-induced thyroid swelling and tracheal compression have diminished, as studies have shown this complication to be rare. When acute compression occurs, glucocorticoid treatment or surgery may be needed. Radiation-induced hypothyroidism is less common than after treatment for Graves' disease. However, post-treatment autoimmune thyrotoxicosis may occur in up to 5% of patients treated for nontoxic MNG. Surgery remains highly effective but is not without risk, particularly in older patients with underlying cardiopulmonary disease.

TOXIC MULTINODULAR GOITER

The pathogenesis of toxic MNG appears to be similar to that of nontoxic MNG; the major difference is the presence of functional autonomy in toxic MNG. The molecular basis for autonomy in toxic MNG remains unknown. As in nontoxic goiters, many nodules are polyclonal, whereas others are monoclonal and vary in their clonal origins. Genetic abnormalities known to confer functional autonomy, such as activating TSH-R or $G_s\alpha$ mutations (see below), are not usually found in the autonomous regions of toxic MNG goiter.

In addition to features of goiter, the clinical presentation of toxic MNG includes subclinical hyperthyroidism or mild thyrotoxicosis. The patient is usually elderly and may present with atrial fibrillation or palpitations, tachycardia, nervousness, tremor, or weight loss. Recent exposure to iodine, from contrast dyes or other sources, may precipitate or exacerbate thyrotoxicosis. The TSH level is low. The uncombined T_4 level may be normal or minimally increased; T_3 is often elevated to a greater degree than T_4. Thyroid scan shows heterogeneous uptake with multiple regions of increased and decreased uptake; 24-h uptake of radioiodine may not be increased but is usually in the upper normal range.

Prior to definitive treatment of the hyperthyroidism, ultrasound imaging should be performed to assess the presence of discrete nodules corresponding to areas of decreased uptake ("cold" nodules). If present, FNA may be indicated based on sonographic features and size cutoffs. The cytology results, if indeterminate or suspicious, may direct the therapy to surgery.

TREATMENT Toxic Multinodular Goiter

Antithyroid drugs normalize thyroid function and are particularly useful in the elderly or ill patients with limited lifespan. In contrast to Graves' disease, spontaneous remission does not occur and so treatment is long-term. Radioiodine is generally the treatment of choice; it treats areas of autonomy as well as decreasing the mass of the goiter. Sometimes, however, a degree of autonomy remains, presumably because multiple autonomous regions emerge as soon as others are treated, and further radioiodine treatment may be necessary. Surgery provides definitive treatment of underlying thyrotoxicosis as well as goiter. Patients should be rendered euthyroid using an antithyroid drug before operation.

HYPERFUNCTIONING SOLITARY NODULE

A solitary, autonomously functioning thyroid nodule is referred to as *toxic adenoma*. The pathogenesis of this disorder has been unraveled by demonstrating the functional effects of mutations that stimulate the TSH-R signaling pathway. Most patients with solitary hyperfunctioning nodules have acquired somatic, activating mutations in

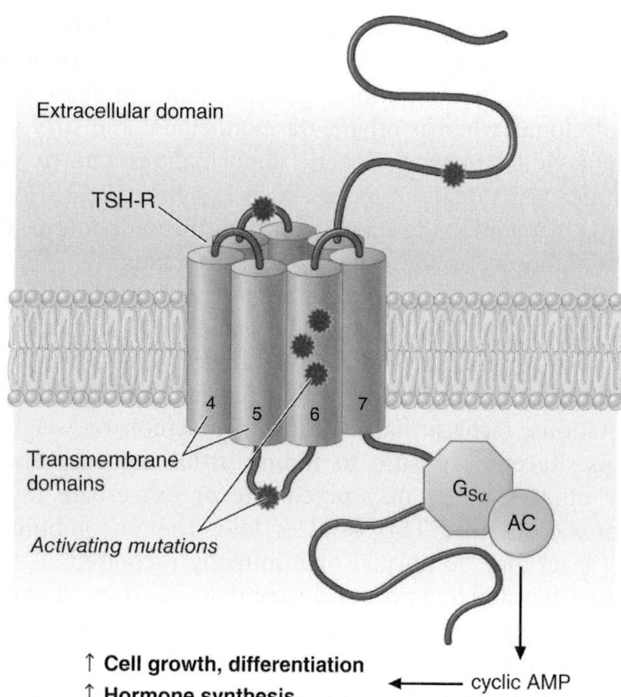

FIGURE 7-11

Activating mutations of the thyroid-stimulating hormone receptor (TSH-R). Mutations (*) that activate TSH-R reside mainly in transmembrane 5 and intracellular loop 3, although mutations have occurred in a variety of different locations. The effect of these mutations is to induce conformational changes that mimic TSH binding, thereby leading to coupling to stimulatory G protein ($G_{S\alpha}$) and activation of adenylate cyclase (AC), an enzyme that generates cyclic AMP.

the TSH-R (Fig. 7-11). These mutations, located primarily in the receptor transmembrane domain, induce constitutive receptor coupling to $G_{S\alpha}$, increasing cyclic AMP levels and leading to enhanced thyroid follicular cell proliferation and function. Less commonly, somatic mutations are identified in $G_{S\alpha}$. These mutations, which are similar to those seen in McCune-Albright syndrome **(Chap. 13)** or in a subset of somatotrope adenomas **(Chap. 5)**, impair guanosine triphosphate (GTP) hydrolysis, causing constitutive activation of the cyclic AMP signaling pathway. In most series, activating mutations in either the TSH-R or the $G_{S\alpha}$ subunit genes are identified in >90% of patients with solitary hyperfunctioning nodules.

Thyrotoxicosis is usually mild. The disorder is suggested by a subnormal TSH level; the presence of the thyroid nodule, which is generally large enough to be palpable; and the absence of clinical features suggestive of Graves' disease or other causes of thyrotoxicosis. A thyroid scan provides a definitive diagnostic test, demonstrating focal uptake in the hyperfunctioning nodule and diminished uptake in the remainder of the gland, as activity of the normal thyroid is suppressed.

TREATMENT Hyperfunctioning Solitary Nodule

Radioiodine ablation is usually the treatment of choice. Because normal thyroid function is suppressed, ^{131}I is concentrated in the hyperfunctioning nodule with minimal uptake and damage to normal thyroid tissue. Relatively large radioiodine doses (e.g., 370–1110 MBq [10–29.9 mCi] ^{131}I) have been shown to correct thyrotoxicosis in about 75% of patients within 3 months. Hypothyroidism occurs in <10% of those patients over the next 5 years. Surgical resection is also effective and is usually limited to enucleation of the adenoma or lobectomy, thereby preserving thyroid function and minimizing risk of hypoparathyroidism or damage to the recurrent laryngeal nerves. Medical therapy using antithyroid drugs and beta blockers can normalize thyroid function but is not an optimal long-term treatment. Using ultrasound guidance, repeated ethanol injections and percutaneous radiofrequency thermal ablation have been used successfully in some centers to ablate hyperfunctioning nodules, and these techniques have also been used to reduce the size of nonfunctioning thyroid nodules.

BENIGN NEOPLASMS

The various types of benign thyroid nodules are listed in Table 7-10. These lesions are common (5–10% adults), particularly when assessed by sensitive techniques such as ultrasound. The risk of malignancy is very low for *macrofollicular adenomas* and *normofollicular adenomas. Microfollicular, trabecular, and Hürthle cell variants* raise greater concern, and the histology is more difficult to interpret. Many are mixed cystic/solid lesions on ultrasound and may appear spongiform reflecting the pathology of macrofollicular structure. However, the majority of solid nodules (whether hypo-, iso-, or hyperechoic) are also benign. FNA, usually performed with ultrasound guidance, is the diagnostic procedure of choice to evaluate thyroid nodules (see the "Approach to the Patient" section on thyroid nodules). Pure thyroid cysts, <2% of all thyroid growths, consist of colloid and are benign as well. Cysts frequently recur, even after repeated aspiration, and may require surgical excision if they are large. Ethanol ablation to sclerose the cyst has been used successfully for patients who are symptomatic.

TSH suppression with levothyroxine therapy does not decrease thyroid nodule size in iodine-sufficient populations. However, if there is relative iodine deficiency, both iodine and levothyroxine therapy may decrease nodule volume. If levothyroxine is administered in this situation and the nodule has not decreased in size after 6–12 months of suppressive therapy, treatment should be discontinued because little benefit is likely to accrue from long-term

TABLE 7-10

CLASSIFICATION OF THYROID NEOPLASMS

Benign	
Follicular epithelial cell adenomas	
Macrofollicular (colloid)	
Normofollicular (simple)	
Microfollicular (fetal)	
Trabecular (embryonal)	
Hürthle cell variant (oncocytic)	
Malignant	**Approximate Prevalence, %**
Follicular epithelial cell	
Well-differentiated carcinomas	
Papillary carcinomas	80–90
Pure papillary	
Follicular variant	
Diffuse sclerosing variant	
Tall cell, columnar cell variants	
Follicular carcinomas	5–10
Minimally invasive	
Widely invasive	
Hürthle cell carcinoma (oncocytic)	
Insular carcinoma	
Undifferentiated (anaplastic) carcinomas	
C cell (calcitonin-producing)	
Medullary thyroid cancer	<10
Sporadic	
Familial	
MEN 2	
Other malignancies	
Lymphomas	1–2
Sarcomas	
Metastases	
Others	

Abbreviation: MEN, multiple endocrine neoplasia.

treatment; the risk of iatrogenic subclinical thyrotoxicosis should also be considered.

THYROID CANCER

Thyroid carcinoma is the most common malignancy of the endocrine system. Malignant tumors derived from the follicular epithelium are classified according to histologic features. Differentiated tumors, such as papillary thyroid cancer (PTC) or follicular thyroid cancer (FTC), are often curable, and the prognosis is good for patients identified with early-stage disease. In contrast, anaplastic thyroid cancer (ATC) is aggressive, responds poorly to treatment, and is associated with a bleak prognosis.

The incidence of thyroid cancer is ~12/100,000 per year in the United States and increases with age.

TABLE 7-11

RISK FACTORS FOR THYROID CARCINOMA IN PATIENTS WITH THYROID NODULE

History of head and neck irradiation, including total-body irradiation for bone marrow transplant and brain radiation for childhood leukemia	Family history of thyroid cancer, MEN 2, or other genetic syndromes associated with thyroid malignancy (e.g., Cowden's syndrome, familial polyposis, Carney complex)
Exposure to ionizing radiation from fallout in childhood or adolescence	Vocal cord paralysis, hoarse voice
Age <20 or >65 years	Nodule fixed to adjacent structures
Increased nodule size (>4 cm)	Extrathyroidal extension
New or enlarging neck mass	Lateral cervical lymphadenopathy
Male gender	

Abbreviation: MEN, multiple endocrine neoplasia.

Prognosis is worse in older persons (>65 years). Thyroid cancer is twice as common in women as men, but male gender is associated with a worse prognosis. Additional important risk factors include a history of childhood head or neck irradiation, large nodule size (≥4 cm), evidence for local tumor fixation or invasion into lymph nodes, and the presence of metastases (Table 7-11). Several unique features of thyroid cancer facilitate its management: (1) thyroid nodules are amenable to biopsy by FNA; (2) iodine radioisotopes can be used to diagnose (^{123}I) and treat (^{131}I) differentiated thyroid cancer, reflecting the unique uptake of this anion by the thyroid gland; and (3) serum markers allow the detection of residual or recurrent disease, including the use of Tg levels for PTC and FTC, and calcitonin for medullary thyroid cancer (MTC).

CLASSIFICATION

Thyroid neoplasms can arise in each of the cell types that populate the gland, including thyroid follicular cells, calcitonin-producing C cells, lymphocytes, and stromal and vascular elements, as well as metastases from other sites (Table 7-10). The American Joint Committee on Cancer (AJCC) has designated a staging system using the tumor, node, metastasis (TNM) classification (Table 7-12). Several other classification and staging systems are also widely used, some of which place greater emphasis on histologic features or risk factors such as age or gender.

PATHOGENESIS AND GENETIC BASIS

Radiation

Early studies of the pathogenesis of thyroid cancer focused on the role of external radiation, which predisposes to chromosomal breaks, leading to genetic rearrangements and loss of tumor-suppressor genes.

TABLE 7-12

THYROID CANCER CLASSIFICATION[a]

Papillary or Follicular Thyroid Cancers		
	<45 years	>45 years
Stage I	Any T, any N, M0	T1, N0, M0
Stage II	Any T, any N, M1	T2, N0, M0
Stage III	—	T3, N0, M0
		T1–T3, N1a, M0
Stage IVA	—	T4a, any N, M0
		T1–T3, N1b, M0
Stage IVB		T4b, any N, M0
Stage IVC		Any T, any N, M1
Anaplastic Thyroid Cancer		
Stage IV	All cases are stage IV	
Medullary Thyroid Cancer		
Stage I	T1, N0, M0	
Stage II	T2 or T3, N0, M0	
Stage III	T1–T3, N1a, M0	
Stage IVA	T4a, any N, M0	
	T1–T3, N1b, M0	
Stage IVB	T4b, any N, M0	
Stage IVC	Any T, any N, M1	

[a]Criteria include: T, the size and extent of the primary tumor (T1a ≤1 cm; T1b >1 cm but ≤2 cm; T2 >2 cm but ≤4 cm; T3 >4 cm or any tumor with extension into perithyroidal soft tissue or sternothyroid muscle; T4a invasion into subcutaneous soft tissues, larynx, trachea, esophagus, or recurrent laryngeal nerve; T4b invasion into prevertebral fascia or encasement of carotid artery or mediastinal vessels); N, the absence (N0) or presence (N1a level IV central compartment; N1b levels II–V lateral compartment, upper mediastinal or retro/parapharyngeal) of regional node involvement; M, the absence (M0) or presence (M1) of distant metastases.
Source: American Joint Committee on Cancer staging system for thyroid cancers using the TNM classification, 7th edition.

External radiation of the mediastinum, face, head, and neck region was administered in the past to treat an array of conditions, including acne and enlargement of the thymus, tonsils, and adenoids. Radiation exposure increases the risk of benign and malignant thyroid nodules, is associated with multicentric cancers, and shifts the incidence of thyroid cancer to an earlier age group. Radiation from nuclear fallout also increases the risk of thyroid cancer. Children seem more predisposed to the effects of radiation than adults. Of note, radiation derived from ^{131}I therapy appears to contribute minimal increased risk of thyroid cancer.

TSH and growth factors

Many differentiated thyroid cancers express TSH receptors and, therefore, remain responsive to TSH. Higher serum TSH levels, even within normal range, are associated with increased thyroid cancer risk in patients with thyroid nodules. These observations provide the rationale for T_4 suppression of TSH in patients with thyroid cancer. Residual expression of TSH receptors also allows TSH-stimulated uptake of ^{131}I therapy (see below).

Oncogenes and tumor-suppressor genes

Thyroid cancers are monoclonal in origin, consistent with the idea that they originate as a consequence of mutations that confer a growth advantage to a single cell. In addition to increased rates of proliferation, some thyroid cancers exhibit impaired apoptosis and features that enhance invasion, angiogenesis, and metastasis. Thyroid neoplasms have been analyzed for a variety of genetic alterations, but without clear evidence of an ordered acquisition of somatic mutations as they progress from the benign to the malignant state. On the other hand, certain mutations are relatively specific for thyroid neoplasia, some of which correlate with histologic classification (Table 7-13).

As described above, activating mutations of the TSH-R and the $G_{S\alpha}$ subunit are associated with autonomously functioning nodules. Although these mutations induce thyroid cell growth, this type of nodule is almost always benign.

Activation of the RET-RAS-BRAF signaling pathway is seen in up to 70% of PTCs, although the types of mutations are heterogeneous. A variety of rearrangements involving the *RET* gene on chromosome 10 bring this receptor tyrosine kinase under the control of other promoters, leading to receptor overexpression. *RET* rearrangements occur in 20–40% of PTCs in different series and were observed with increased frequency in tumors developing after the Chernobyl radiation accident. Rearrangements in PTC have also been observed for another tyrosine kinase gene, *TRK1*, which is located on chromosome 1. To date, the identification of PTC with *RET* or *TRK1* rearrangements has not proven useful for predicting prognosis or treatment responses. *BRAF V600E* mutations appear to be the most common genetic alteration in PTC. These mutations activate the kinase, which stimulates the mitogen-activated protein MAP kinase (MAPK) cascade. *RAS* mutations, which also stimulate the MAPK cascade, are found in about 20–30% of thyroid neoplasms (*NRAS* > *HRAS* > *KRAS*), including both PTC and FTC. Of note, simultaneous *RET*, *BRAF*, and *RAS* mutations rarely occur in the same tumor, suggesting that activation of the MAPK cascade is critical for tumor development, independent of the step that initiates the cascade.

RAS mutations also occur in FTCs. In addition, a rearrangement of the thyroid developmental transcription factor PAX8 with the nuclear receptor PPARγ is identified in a significant fraction of FTCs. Overall,

TABLE 7-13

GENETIC ALTERATIONS IN THYROID NEOPLASIA

GENE/PROTEIN	TYPE OF GENE	CHROMOSOMAL LOCATION	GENETIC ABNORMALITY	TUMOR
TSH receptor	GPCR receptor	14q31	Point mutations	Toxic adenoma, differentiated carcinomas
$G_{S\alpha}$	G protein	20q13.2	Point mutations	Toxic adenoma, differentiated carcinomas
RET/PTC	Receptor tyrosine kinase	10q11.2	Rearrangements PTC1: inv(10)(q11.2q21) PTC2: t(10;17)(q11.2;q23) PTC3: ELE1/TK	PTC (more common in radiation-induced tumors)
RET	Receptor tyrosine kinase	10q11.2	Point mutations	MEN 2, medullary thyroid cancer
BRAF	MEK kinase	7q24	Point mutations, rearrangements	PTC, ATC
TRK	Receptor tyrosine kinase	1q23-24	Rearrangements	Multinodular goiter, papillary thyroid cancer
RAS	Signal transducing p21	NRAS 1p13.2 (most common); HRAS 11p15.5; KRAS 12p12.1	Point mutations	Follicular thyroid cancer, PTC follicular variant, adenomas
p53	Tumor suppressor, cell cycle control, apoptosis	17p13	Point mutations Deletion, insertion	Anaplastic cancer
APC	Tumor suppressor, adenomatous polyposis coli gene	5q21-q22	Point mutations	Anaplastic cancer, also associated with familial polyposis coli
p16 (MTS1, CDKN2A)	Tumor suppressor, cell cycle control	9p21	Deletions	Differentiated carcinomas
p21/WAF	Tumor suppressor, cell cycle control	6p21.2	Overexpression	Anaplastic cancer
MET	Receptor tyrosine kinase	7q31	Overexpression	Follicular thyroid cancer
c-MYC	Receptor tyrosine kinase	8q24.12-13	Overexpression	Differentiated carcinoma
PTEN	Phosphatase	10q23	Point mutations	PTC in Cowden's syndrome (multiple hamartomas, breast tumors, gastrointestinal polyps, thyroid tumors)
CTNNB1	β-Catenin	3p22	Point mutations	Anaplastic cancer
Loss of heterozygosity (LOH)	? Tumor suppressors	3p; 11q13, other loci	Deletions	Differentiated thyroid carcinomas, anaplastic cancer
PAX8-PPARγ1	Transcription factor-nuclear receptor fusion	t(2;3)(q13;p25)	Translocation	Follicular adenoma or carcinoma, rare PTC follicular variant

Abbreviations: APC, adenomatous polyposis coli; ATC, anaplastic thyroid cancer; BRAF, v-raf homologue, B1; CDKN2A, cyclin-dependent kinase inhibitor 2A; c-MYC, cellular homologue of myelocytomatosis virus protooncogene; ELE1/TK, RET-activating gene ele1/tyrosine kinase; GPCR, G protein–coupled receptor; $G_{S\alpha}$, G-protein stimulating α-subunit; MEK, mitogen extracellular signal-regulated kinase; MEN 2, multiple endocrine neoplasia-2; MET, met protooncogene (hepatocyte growth factor receptor); MTS, multiple tumor suppressor; p53, p53 tumor suppressor gene; PTC, papillary thyroid cancer; PTEN, phosphatase and tensin homologue; RAS, rat sarcoma protooncogene; RET, rearranged during transfection protooncogene; p21, p21 tumor suppressor; PAX8, paired domain transcription factor; PPARγ1, peroxisome-proliferator activated receptor γ1; TRK, tyrosine kinase receptor; TSH, thyroid-stimulating hormone; WAF, wild-type p53 activated fragment.

Source: Adapted with permission from P Kopp, JL Jameson, in JL Jameson (ed): *Principles of Molecular Medicine*. Totowa, NJ, Humana Press, 1998.

about 70% of follicular cancers have mutations or genetic rearrangements. Loss of heterozygosity of 3p or 11q, consistent with deletions of tumor-suppressor genes, is also common in FTCs.

Most of the mutations seen in differentiated thyroid cancers have also been detected in ATCs. *BRAF* mutations are seen in up to 50% of ATCs. Mutations in *CTNNB1,* which encodes β-catenin, occur in about two-thirds of ATCs, but not in PTC or FTC. Mutations of the tumor-suppressor *P53* also play an important role in the development of ATC. Because *P53* plays a role in cell cycle surveillance, DNA repair, and apoptosis, its loss may contribute to the rapid acquisition of genetic instability as well as poor treatment responses (Table 7-13).

The role of molecular diagnostics in the clinical management of thyroid cancer is under investigation. In principle, analyses of specific mutations might aid in classification, prognosis, or choice of treatment. Although *BRAF V600E* mutations are associated with loss of iodine uptake by tumor cells, there is no clear evidence to date that this information alters clinical decision making. Higher recurrence rates have been variably reported in patients with *BRAF*-positive PTC, but the impact on survival rates is unclear. Sequencing of thyroid cancers as part of the Cancer Genome Atlas (TCGA) is likely to lead to new classification schemes based on molecular abnormalities in tumors.

MTC, when associated with multiple endocrine neoplasia (MEN) type 2, harbors an inherited mutation of the *RET* gene. Unlike the rearrangements of *RET* seen in PTC, the mutations in MEN 2 are point mutations that induce constitutive activity of the tyrosine kinase **(Chap. 29)**. MTC is preceded by hyperplasia of the C cells, raising the likelihood that as-yet-unidentified "second hits" lead to cellular transformation. A subset of sporadic MTC contains somatic mutations that activate *RET*.

WELL-DIFFERENTIATED THYROID CANCER

Papillary

PTC is the most common type of thyroid cancer, accounting for 70–90% of well-differentiated thyroid malignancies. Microscopic PTC is present in up to 25% of thyroid glands at autopsy, but most of these lesions are very small (several millimeters) and are not clinically significant. Characteristic cytologic features of PTC help make the diagnosis by FNA or after surgical resection; these include psammoma bodies, cleaved nuclei with an "orphan-Annie" appearance caused by large nucleoli, and the formation of papillary structures.

PTC tends to be multifocal and to invade locally within the thyroid gland as well as through the thyroid capsule and into adjacent structures in the neck. It has a propensity to spread via the lymphatic system but can metastasize hematogenously as well, particularly to bone and lung. Because of the relatively slow growth of the tumor, a significant burden of pulmonary metastases may accumulate, sometimes with remarkably few symptoms. The prognostic implication of lymph node spread is debated. Lymph node involvement by thyroid cancer can be well tolerated but appears to increase the risk of recurrence and mortality, particularly in older patients. The staging of PTC by the TNM system is outlined in Table 7-12. Most papillary cancers are identified in the early stages (>80% stages I or II) and have an excellent prognosis, with survival curves similar to expected survival (Fig. 7-12). Mortality is markedly increased in stage IV disease, especially in the presence of distant metastases (stage IVC), but this group comprises only about 1% of patients. The treatment of PTC is described below.

Follicular

The incidence of FTC varies widely in different parts of the world; it is more common in iodine-deficient regions. Currently, FTC accounts for only about 5% of all thyroid cancers diagnosed in the United States. FTC is difficult to diagnose by FNA because the distinction between benign and malignant follicular neoplasms rests largely on evidence of invasion into vessels, nerves, or adjacent structures. FTC tends to spread by hematogenous routes leading to bone, lung, and central nervous system metastases. Mortality rates associated with FTC are less favorable than for PTC, in part because a larger proportion of patients present with stage IV disease. Poor prognostic features include distant metastases, age >50 years, primary tumor size >4 cm, Hürthle cell histology, and the presence of marked vascular invasion.

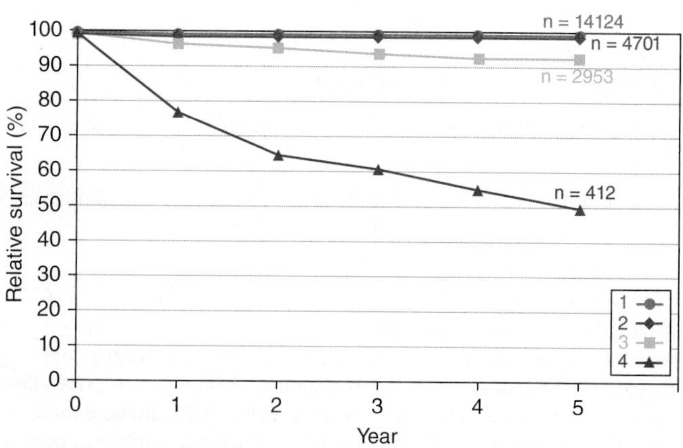

FIGURE 7-12

Survival rates of patients with different stages of papillary cancer. *(Adapted with permission from Edge SB, Byrd DR: Thyroid, in Compton CC, Fritz AB, Greene FL, Trotti A [eds]: AJCC Cancer Staging Manual, 7th ed. New York, Springer, 2010, pp 87–92.)*

TREATMENT Well-Differentiated Thyroid Cancer

SURGERY All well-differentiated thyroid cancers should be surgically excised. In addition to removing the primary lesion, surgery allows accurate histologic diagnosis and staging, and multicentric disease is commonly found in the contralateral thyroid lobe. Preoperative sonography should be performed in all patients to assess the central and lateral cervical lymph node compartments for suspicious adenopathy, which if present, can undergo FNA and then be removed at surgery. Bilateral, near-total thyroidectomy has been shown to reduce recurrence rates in all patients except those with T1a tumors (≤1 cm). If cytology is diagnostic for thyroid cancer, bilateral surgery should be done. If malignancy is identified pathologically after lobectomy, completion surgery is recommended unless the tumor is T1a or is a minimally invasive follicular cancer. Bilateral surgery for patients at higher risk allows monitoring of serum Tg levels and administration of radioiodine for remnant ablation and potential treatment of iodine-avid metastases, if indicated. Therefore, near-total thyroidectomy is preferable in almost all patients; complication rates are acceptably low if the surgeon is highly experienced in the procedure.

TSH SUPPRESSION THERAPY Because most tumors are still TSH-responsive, levothyroxine suppression of TSH is a mainstay of thyroid cancer treatment. Although TSH suppression clearly provides therapeutic benefit, there are no prospective studies that define the optimal level of TSH suppression. The degree of TSH suppression should be individualized based on a patient's risk of recurrence. It should be adjusted over time as surveillance blood tests and imaging confirm absence of disease or, alternatively, indicate possible residual/recurrent cancer. For patients at low risk of recurrence, TSH should be suppressed into the low but detectable range (0.1–0.5 mIU/L). If subsequent surveillance testing indicates no evidence of disease, the TSH target may rise to the lower half of the normal range. For patients at high risk of recurrence or with known metastatic disease, TSH levels should be kept to <0.1 mIU/L if there are no strong contraindications to mild thyrotoxicosis. In this instance, unbound T_4 must also be monitored to avoid excessive treatment.

RADIOIODINE TREATMENT After near-total thyroidectomy, substantial thyroid tissue often remains, particularly in the thyroid bed and surrounding the parathyroid glands. Postsurgical radioablation of the remnant thyroid eliminates residual normal thyroid, facilitating the use of Tg determinations and radioiodine scanning for long-term follow-up. In addition, well-differentiated thyroid cancer often incorporates radioiodine, although less efficiently than normal thyroid follicular cells. Radioiodine uptake is determined primarily by expression of the NIS and is stimulated by TSH, requiring expression of the TSH-R. The retention time for radioactivity is influenced by the extent to which the tumor retains differentiated functions such as iodide trapping and organification. Consequently, for patients at risk of recurrence and for those with known distant metastatic disease, ^{131}I ablation may also potentially treat residual tumor cells.

Indications Not all patients benefit from radioiodine therapy. Neither recurrence nor survival rates are improved in stage I patients with T1 tumors (≤2 cm) confined to the thyroid. However, in higher risk patients (larger tumors, more aggressive variants of papillary cancer, tumor vascular invasion, presence of large-volume lymph node metastases), radioiodine reduces recurrence and may increase survival.

^{131}I Thyroid Ablation and Treatment As noted above, the decision to use ^{131}I for thyroid ablation should be coordinated with the surgical approach, because radioablation is much more effective when there is minimal remaining normal thyroid tissue. Radioiodine is administered after iodine depletion (patient follows a low-iodine diet for 1≤2 weeks) and in the presence of elevated serum TSH levels to stimulate uptake of the isotope into both the remnant and potentially any residual tumor. To achieve high serum TSH levels, there are two approaches. A patient may be withdrawn from thyroid hormone so that endogenous TSH is secreted and, ideally, the serum TSH level is >25 mIU/L at the time of ^{131}I therapy. A typical strategy is to treat the patient for several weeks postoperatively with liothyronine (25 μg qd or bid), followed by thyroid hormone withdrawal for 2 weeks. Alternatively, recombinant human TSH (rhTSH) is administered as two daily consecutive injections (0.9 mg) with administration of ^{131}I 24 h after the second injection. The patient can continue to take levothyroxine and remains euthyroid. Both approaches have equal success in achieving remnant ablation.

A pretreatment scanning dose of ^{131}I (usually 111–185 MBq [3–5 mCi]) or ^{123}I (74 MBq [2 mCi]) can reveal the amount of residual tissue and provides guidance about the dose needed to accomplish ablation. However, because of concerns about radioactive "stunning" that impairs subsequent treatment, there is a trend to avoid pretreatment scanning with ^{131}I and use either ^{123}I or proceed directly to ablation, unless there is suspicion that the amount of residual tissue will alter therapy or that there is distant metastatic disease. In the United States, outpatient doses of up to 6475 MBq (175 mCi) can be given at most centers. The administered dose depends on the indication for therapy with lower doses of 1850–2775 MBq (50–75 mCi) given for remnant ablation but higher doses of 3700–5500 MBq (100–150 mCi) used as adjuvant therapy when residual disease may be present. A WBS following radioiodine treatment is used to confirm the ^{131}I uptake in the remnant and to identify possible metastatic disease.

Follow-Up Whole-Body Thyroid Scanning and Thyroglobulin Determinations Serum thyroglobulin is a sensitive marker of residual/recurrent thyroid cancer after ablation of the residual postsurgical thyroid tissue. However, newer Tg assays have functional sensitivities as low as 0.1 ng/mL, as opposed to older assays with functional sensitivities of 1 ng/mL, reducing the number of patients with truly undetectable serum Tg levels. Because the vast majority of papillary thyroid cancer recurrences are in cervical lymph nodes, a neck ultrasound should be performed about 6 months after thyroid ablation; ultrasound has been shown to be more sensitive than WBS in this scenario.

In low-risk patients who have no clinical evidence of residual disease after ablation and a basal Tg <1 ng/mL on levothyroxine, an rhTSH-stimulated Tg level should be obtained 6–12 months after ablation, without WBS. If stimulated Tg levels are low (<1 ng/mL) and, ideally, undetectable, the risk of recurrence is <5% at 5 years. Newer data indicate that rhTSH stimulation may not be required for patients with undetectable basal Tg levels in sensitive assays, if there is documented absence of Tg antibodies. These patients can be followed with unstimulated Tg every 6–12 months and neck ultrasound as indicated. Levothyroxine dosing may then be titrated to a higher TSH level of 0.5–1.5 mIU/L.

The use of WBS is reserved for patients with known iodine-avid metastases or those with elevated serum thyroglobulin levels and negative imaging with ultrasound, chest CT, and neck cross-sectional imaging who may require additional ^{131}I therapy.

In addition, most authorities advocate radioiodine treatment for scan-negative, Tg-positive (Tg >5–10 ng/mL) patients, as many derive therapeutic benefit from a large dose of ^{131}I. For such patients, rhTSH preparation is not FDA approved for the treatment of metastatic disease, and the traditional approach of thyroid hormone withdrawal should be followed. This involves switching patients from levothyroxine (T_4) to the more rapidly cleared hormone liothyronine (T_3), thereby allowing TSH to increase more quickly. Whenever ^{131}I is administered, posttherapy WBS is the gold standard to assess iodine-avid metastases.

In addition to radioiodine, external beam radiotherapy is also used to treat specific metastatic lesions, particularly when they cause bone pain or threaten neurologic injury (e.g., vertebral metastases).

New Potential Therapies Kinase inhibitors are being explored as a means to target pathways known to be active in thyroid cancer, including the RAS, BRAF, EGFR, VEGFR, and angiogenesis pathways. A multicenter randomized controlled trial of the multikinase inhibitor sorafenib in 417 patients with progressive metastatic thyroid cancer reported a doubling of progression-free survival to 10.8 months in the treatment group compared with the placebo group. Ongoing trials are exploring whether differentiation protocols with kinase inhibitors or other approaches might enhance radioiodine uptake and efficacy.

ANAPLASTIC AND OTHER FORMS OF THYROID CANCER

Anaplastic thyroid cancer

As noted above, ATC is a poorly differentiated and aggressive cancer. The prognosis is poor, and most patients die within 6 months of diagnosis. Because of the undifferentiated state of these tumors, the uptake of radioiodine is usually negligible, but it can be used therapeutically if there is residual uptake. Chemotherapy has been attempted with multiple agents, including anthracyclines and paclitaxel, but it is usually ineffective. External beam radiation therapy can be attempted and continued if tumors are responsive.

Thyroid lymphoma

Lymphoma in the thyroid gland often arises in the background of Hashimoto's thyroiditis. A rapidly expanding thyroid mass suggests the possibility of this diagnosis. Diffuse large-cell lymphoma is the most common type in the thyroid. Biopsies reveal sheets of lymphoid cells that can be difficult to distinguish from small-cell lung cancer or ATC. These tumors are often highly sensitive to external radiation. Surgical resection should be avoided as initial therapy because it may spread disease that is otherwise localized to the thyroid. If staging indicates disease outside of the thyroid, treatment should follow guidelines used for other forms of lymphoma.

MEDULLARY THYROID CARCINOMA

MTC can be sporadic or familial and accounts for about 5% of thyroid cancers. There are three familial forms of MTC: MEN 2A, MEN 2B, and familial MTC without other features of MEN **(Chap. 29)**. In general, MTC is more aggressive in MEN 2B than in MEN 2A, and familial MTC is more aggressive than sporadic MTC. Elevated serum calcitonin provides a marker of residual or recurrent disease. All patients with MTC should be tested for *RET* mutations, because genetic counseling and testing of family members can be offered to those individuals who test positive for mutations.

The management of MTC is primarily surgical. Unlike tumors derived from thyroid follicular cells, these tumors do not take up radioiodine. External radiation treatment and chemotherapy may provide palliation in patients with advanced disease **(Chap. 29)**.

APPROACH TO THE PATIENT: Thyroid Nodules

Palpable thyroid nodules are found in about 5% of adults, but the prevalence varies considerably worldwide. Given this high prevalence rate, practitioners commonly identify thyroid nodules either on physical examination or as incidental findings on imaging performed for another indication (e.g., carotid ultrasound, cervical spine MRI). The main goal of this evaluation is to identify, in a cost-effective manner, the small subgroup of individuals with malignant lesions.

Nodules are more common in iodine-deficient areas, in women, and with aging. Most palpable nodules are >1 cm in diameter, but the ability to feel a nodule is influenced by its location within the gland (superficial versus deeply embedded), the anatomy of the patient's neck, and the experience of the examiner. More sensitive methods of detection, such as CT, thyroid ultrasound, and pathologic studies, reveal thyroid nodules in up to 50% of glands in individuals over the age of 50. The presence of these thyroid incidentalomas has led to much debate about how to detect nodules and which nodules to investigate further.

An approach to the evaluation of a solitary nodule is outlined in Fig. 7-13. Most patients with thyroid nodules have normal thyroid function tests. Nonetheless, thyroid function should be assessed by measuring a TSH level, which may be suppressed by one or more autonomously functioning nodules. If the TSH is suppressed, a radionuclide scan is indicated to determine if the identified nodule is "hot," as lesions with increased uptake are almost never malignant and FNA is unnecessary. Otherwise, the next step in evaluation is performance of a thyroid ultrasound for three reasons: (1) Ultrasound will confirm if the palpable nodule is indeed a nodule. About 15% of "palpable" nodules are not confirmed on imaging, and therefore, no further evaluation is required. (2) Ultrasound will assess if there are additional nonpalpable nodules for which FNA may be recommended based on imaging features and size. (3) Ultrasound will characterize the imaging features of the nodule, which, combined with the nodule's size, facilitate decision making about FNA.

Evidence-based guidelines from both the American Thyroid Association and the American Association of Clinical Endocrinologists provide recommendations for nodule FNA based on sonographic imaging features and size cut offs, with lower size cut offs for nodules with more suspicious ultrasound characteristics. FNA biopsy, ideally

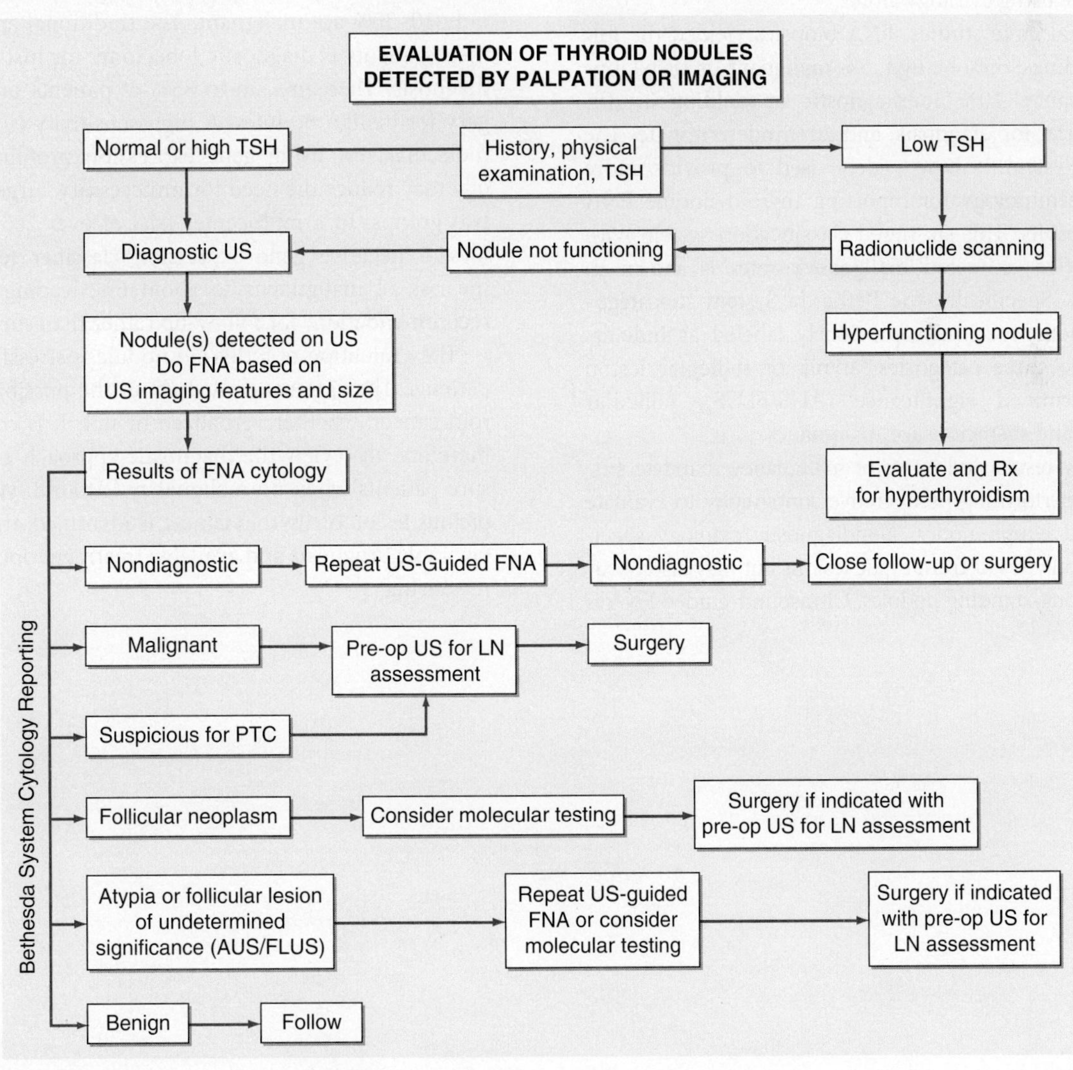

FIGURE 7-13

Approach to the patient with a thyroid nodule. See text and references for details. FNA, fine-needle aspiration; LN, lymph node; PTC, papillary thyroid cancer; TSH, thyroid-stimulating hormone; US, ultrasound.

TABLE 7-14

BETHESDA CLASSIFICATION FOR THYROID CYTOLOGY

DIAGNOSTIC CATEGORY	RISK OF MALIGNANCY
Nondiagnostic or unsatisfactory	1–5%
Benign	2–4%
Atypia or follicular lesion of unknown significance (AUS/FLUS)	15–20%
Follicular neoplasm	20–30%
Suspicious for malignancy	60–75%
Malignant	97–100%

performed with ultrasound guidance, has good sensitivity and specificity when performed by physicians familiar with the procedure and when the results are interpreted by experienced cytopathologists. The technique is particularly useful for detecting PTC. However, the distinction between benign and malignant follicular lesions is often not possible using cytology alone.

In several large studies, FNA biopsies yielded the following findings: 65% benign, 5% malignant or suspicious for malignancy, 10% nondiagnostic or yielding insufficient material for diagnosis, and 20% indeterminate. The Bethesda System is now widely used to provide more uniform terminology for reporting thyroid nodule FNA cytology results. This six-tiered classification system with the respective estimated malignancy rates is shown in Table 7-14. Specifically, the Bethesda System subcategorized cytology specimens previously labeled as indeterminate into three categories: atypia or follicular lesion of undetermined significance (AUS/FLUS), follicular neoplasm, and suspicious for malignancy.

Cytology results indicative of malignancy mandate surgery, after performing preoperative sonography to evaluate the cervical lymph nodes. Nondiagnostic cytology specimens generally result from cystic lesions but may also occur in fibrous long-standing nodules. Ultrasound-guided FNA is indicated when a repeat FNA is necessary. Repeat FNA will yield a diagnostic cytology in about 50% of cases. Benign nodules should be monitored by ultrasound for growth, and repeat FNA should be considered if the nodule enlarges. The use of levothyroxine to suppress serum TSH is not effective in shrinking nodules in iodine-replete populations, and therefore, levothyroxine should not be used.

The three new cytology classifications introduced by the Bethesda System are associated with different risks of malignancy (Table 7-14).

For nodules with suspicious for malignancy cytology, surgery is recommended after ultrasound assessment of cervical lymph nodes. Options to be discussed with the patient include: (1) lobectomy with intraoperative frozen section; (2) near-total thyroidectomy; and (3) mutational analysis mainly for *BRAF V600E*, which is virtually diagnostic of PTC, and bilateral rather than unilateral thyroid surgery is required.

On the other hand, the majority of nodules with AUS/FLUS and follicular neoplasm cytology results are benign; only 10–30% are malignant. The traditional approach for these patients is diagnostic lobectomy for histopathologic diagnosis. Therefore, up to 85% of patients undergo surgery for benign nodules. A high-sensitivity (~90%) novel molecular test using gene expression profiling technology may reduce the need for unnecessary surgery in these two groups. In a multicenter trial of over 265 such nodules, a negative gene expression classifier test reduced the risk of malignancy to about 6%, leading to clinical recommendations for follow-up rather than surgery.

The evaluation of a thyroid nodule is stressful for most patients. They are concerned about the possibility of thyroid cancer, whether verbalized or not. It is constructive, therefore, to review the diagnostic approach and to reassure patients when no malignancy is found. When a suspicious lesion or thyroid cancer is identified, the generally favorable prognosis and available treatment options can be reassuring.

CHAPTER 8

DISORDERS OF THE ADRENAL CORTEX

Wiebke Arlt

The adrenal cortex produces three classes of corticosteroid hormones: glucocorticoids (e.g., cortisol), mineralocorticoids (e.g., aldosterone), and adrenal androgen precursors (e.g., dehydroepiandrosterone [DHEA]) (Fig. 8-1). Glucocorticoids and mineralocorticoids act through specific nuclear receptors, regulating aspects of the physiologic stress response as well as blood pressure and electrolyte homeostasis. Adrenal androgen precursors are converted in the gonads and peripheral target cells to sex steroids that act via nuclear androgen and estrogen receptors.

Disorders of the adrenal cortex are characterized by deficiency or excess of one or several of the three major corticosteroid classes. Hormone deficiency can be caused by inherited glandular or enzymatic disorders or by destruction of the pituitary or adrenal gland by autoimmune disorders, infection, infarction, or iatrogenic events such as surgery or hormonal suppression. Hormone excess is usually the result of neoplasia, leading to increased production of adrenocorticotropic hormone (ACTH) by the pituitary or neuroendocrine cells (ectopic ACTH) or increased production of glucocorticoids, mineralocorticoids, or adrenal androgen precursors by adrenal nodules. Adrenal nodules are increasingly identified incidentally during abdominal imaging performed for other reasons.

ADRENAL ANATOMY AND DEVELOPMENT

The normal adrenal glands weigh 6–11 g each. They are located above the kidneys and have their own blood supply. Arterial blood flows initially to the subcapsular region and then meanders from the outer cortical zona glomerulosa through the intermediate zona fasciculata to the inner zona reticularis and eventually to the adrenal medulla. The right suprarenal vein drains directly into the vena cava, while the left suprarenal vein drains into the left renal vein.

During early embryonic development, the adrenals originate from the urogenital ridge and then separate from gonads and kidneys at about the sixth week of gestation. Concordant with the time of sexual differentiation (seventh to ninth week of gestation, **Chap. 10**), the adrenal cortex starts to produce cortisol and the adrenal sex steroid precursor DHEA. The orphan nuclear receptors SF1 (steroidogenic factor 1; encoded by the gene *NR5A1*) and DAX1 (dosage-sensitive sex reversal gene 1; encoded by the gene *NR0B1*), among others, play a crucial role during this period of development, as they regulate a multitude of adrenal genes involved in steroidogenesis.

REGULATORY CONTROL OF STEROIDOGENESIS

Production of glucocorticoids and adrenal androgens is under the control of the hypothalamic-pituitary-adrenal (HPA) axis, whereas mineralocorticoids are regulated by the renin-angiotensin-aldosterone (RAA) system.

Glucocorticoid synthesis is under inhibitory feedback control by the hypothalamus and the pituitary (Fig. 8-2). Hypothalamic release of corticotropin-releasing hormone (CRH) occurs in response to endogenous or exogenous stress. CRH stimulates the cleavage of the 241–amino acid polypeptide proopiomelanocortin (POMC) by pituitary-specific prohormone convertase 1 (PC1), yielding the 39–amino acid peptide ACTH. ACTH is released by the corticotrope cells of the anterior pituitary and acts as the pivotal regulator of adrenal cortisol synthesis, with additional short-term effects on mineralocorticoid and adrenal androgen synthesis. The release of CRH, and subsequently ACTH, occurs in a pulsatile fashion that follows a circadian rhythm under the control of the hypothalamus, specifically its suprachiasmatic nucleus (SCN), with additional

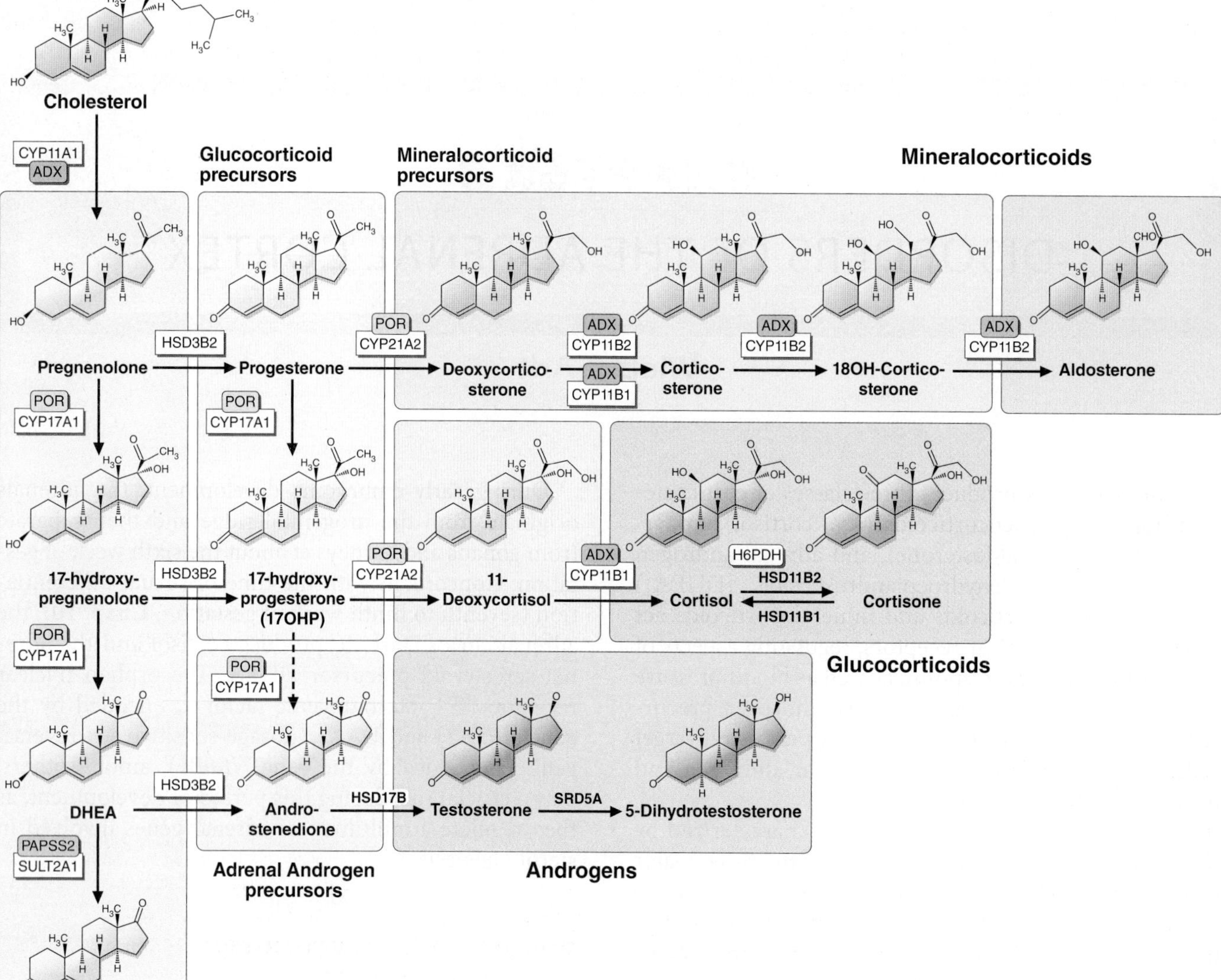

FIGURE 8-1

Adrenal steroidogenesis. ADX, adrenodoxin; CYP11A1, side chain cleavage enzyme; CYP11B1, 11β-hydroxylase; CYP11B2, aldosterone synthase; CYP17A1, 17α-hydroxylase/17,20 lyase; CYP21A2, 21-hydroxylase; DHEA, dehydroepiandrosterone; DHEAS, dehydroepiandrosterone sulfate; H6PDH, hexose-6-phosphate dehydrogenase; HSD11B1, 11β-hydroxysteroid dehydrogenase type 1; HSD11B2, 11β-hydroxysteroid dehydrogenase type 2; HSD17B, 17β-hydroxysteroid dehydrogenase; HSD3B2, 3β-hydroxysteroid dehydrogenase type 2; PAPSS2, PAPS synthase type 2; POR, P450 oxidoreductase; SRD5A, 5α-reductase; SULT2A1, DHEA sulfotransferase.

regulation by a complex network of cell-specific clock genes. Reflecting the pattern of ACTH secretion, adrenal cortisol secretion exhibits a distinct circadian rhythm, starting to rise in the early morning hours prior to awakening, with peak levels in the morning and low levels in the evening (Fig. 8-3).

Diagnostic tests assessing the HPA axis make use of the fact that it is regulated by negative feedback. Glucocorticoid excess is diagnosed by employing a dexamethasone suppression test. Dexamethasone, a potent synthetic glucocorticoid, suppresses CRH/ACTH by binding hypothalamic-pituitary glucocorticoid receptors and, therefore, results in downregulation of endogenous cortisol synthesis. Various versions of the dexamethasone suppression test are described in detail in **Chap. 5**. If cortisol production is autonomous (e.g., adrenal nodule), ACTH is already suppressed and dexamethasone has little additional effect. If cortisol production is driven by an ACTH-producing pituitary adenoma, dexamethasone suppression is ineffective at low doses but usually induces suppression at high doses. If cortisol production is driven by an ectopic

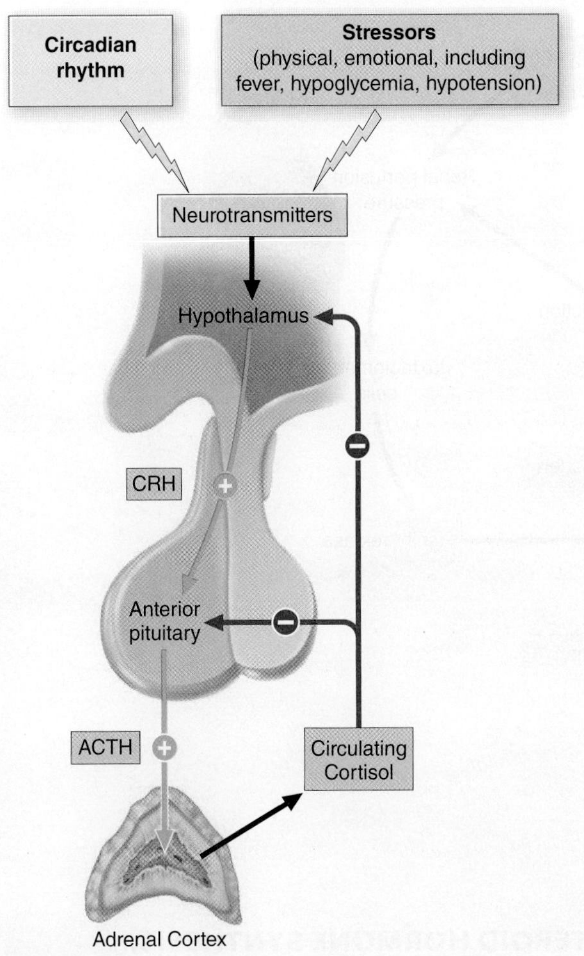

FIGURE 8-2

Regulation of the hypothalamic-pituitary-adrenal (HPA) axis. ACTH, adrenocorticotropic hormone; CRH, corticotropin-releasing hormone.

source of ACTH, the tumors are usually resistant to dexamethasone suppression. Thus, the dexamethasone suppression test is useful to establish the diagnosis of Cushing's syndrome and to assist with the differential diagnosis of cortisol excess.

Conversely, to assess glucocorticoid deficiency, ACTH stimulation of cortisol production is used. The ACTH peptide contains 39 amino acids but the first 24 are sufficient to elicit a physiologic response. The standard ACTH stimulation test involves administration of cosyntropin (ACTH 1-24), 0.25 mg IM or IV, and collection of blood samples at 0, 30, and 60 min for cortisol. A normal response is defined as a cortisol level >20 μg/dL (>550 nmol/L) 30–60 min after cosyntropin stimulation. A low-dose (1 μg cosyntropin IV) version of this test has been advocated; however, it has no superior diagnostic value and is more cumbersome to carry out. Alternatively, an insulin tolerance test (ITT) can be used to assess adrenal function. It involves injection of insulin to induce hypoglycemia, which represents a strong stress signal that triggers hypothalamic CRH release and activation of the entire HPA axis. The ITT involves administration of regular insulin 0.1 U/kg IV (dose should be lower if hypopituitarism is likely) and collection of blood samples at 0, 30, 60, and 120 min for glucose, cortisol, and growth hormone (GH), if also assessing the GH axis. Oral or IV glucose is administered after the patient has achieved symptomatic hypoglycemia (usually glucose <40 mg/dL). A normal response is defined as a cortisol >20 μg/dL and GH >5.1 μg/L. The ITT requires careful clinical monitoring and sequential measurements of glucose. It is contraindicated in patients with coronary disease,

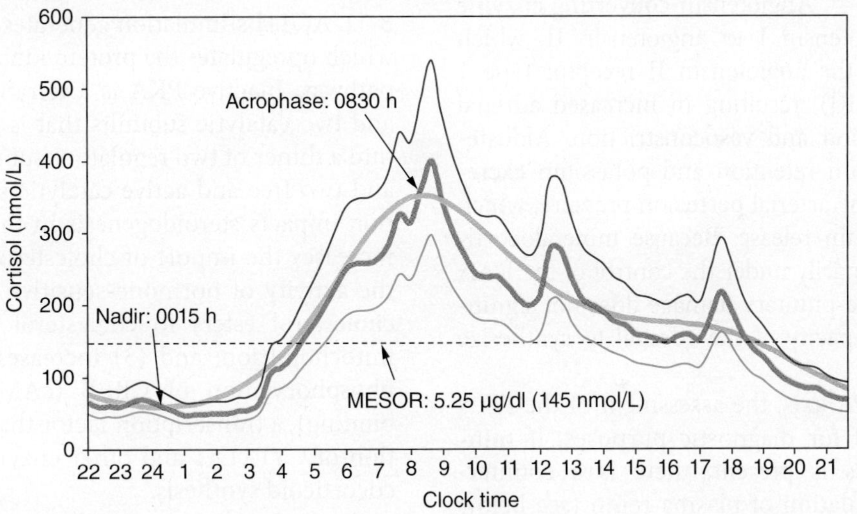

FIGURE 8-3

Physiologic cortisol circadian rhythm. Circulating cortisol concentrations (geometrical mean ± standard deviation values and fitted cosinor) drop under the rhythm-adjusted mean (MESOR) in the early evening hours, with nadir levels around midnight and a rise in the early morning hours; peak levels are observed ~8:30 AM (acrophase). *(Modified after M Debono et al: Modified-release hydrocortisone to provide circadian cortisol profiles. J Clin Endocrinol Metab 94:1548, 2009.)*

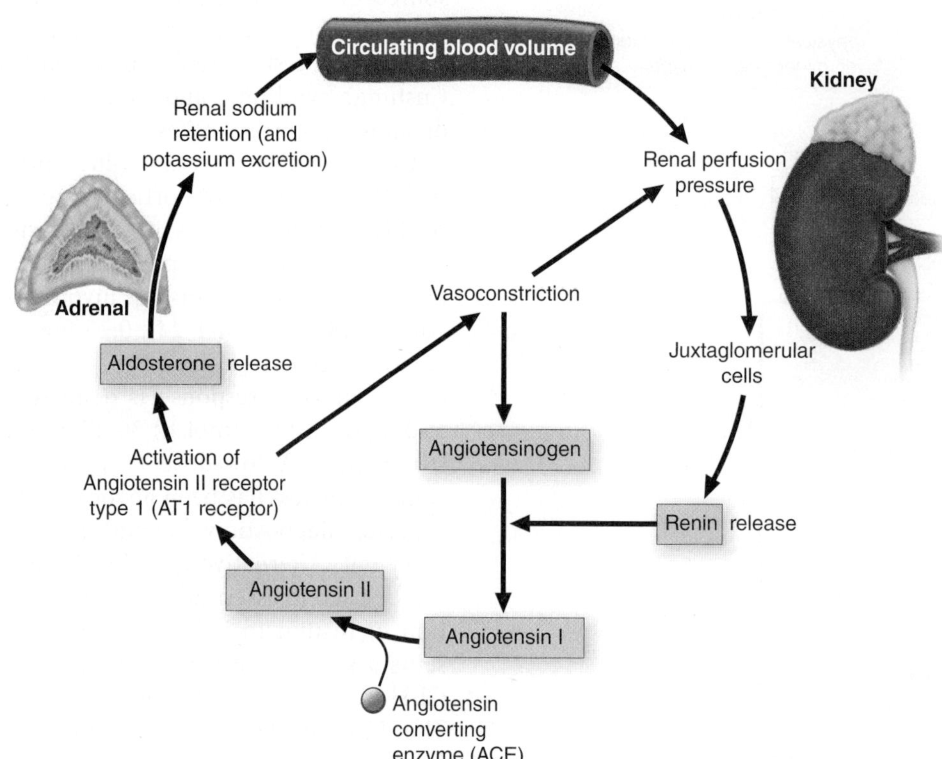

FIGURE 8-4
Regulation of the renin-angiotensin-aldosterone (RAA) system.

cerebrovascular disease, or seizure disorders, which has made the short cosyntropin test the commonly accepted first-line test.

Mineralocorticoid production is controlled by the RAA regulatory cycle, which is initiated by the release of renin from the juxtaglomerular cells in the kidney, resulting in cleavage of angiotensinogen to angiotensin I in the liver (Fig. 8-4). Angiotensin-converting enzyme (ACE) cleaves angiotensin I to angiotensin II, which binds and activates the angiotensin II receptor type 1 (AT1 receptor [AT1R]), resulting in increased adrenal aldosterone production and vasoconstriction. Aldosterone enhances sodium retention and potassium excretion, and increases the arterial perfusion pressure, which in turn regulates renin release. Because mineralocorticoid synthesis is primarily under the control of the RAA system, hypothalamic-pituitary damage does not significantly impact the capacity of the adrenal to synthesize aldosterone.

Similar to the HPA axis, the assessment of the RAA system can be used for diagnostic purposes. If mineralocorticoid excess is present, there is a counter-regulatory downregulation of plasma renin (see below for testing). Conversely, in mineralocorticoid deficiency, plasma renin is markedly increased. Physiologically, oral or IV sodium loading results in suppression of aldosterone, a response that is attenuated or absent in patients with autonomous mineralocorticoid excess.

STEROID HORMONE SYNTHESIS, METABOLISM, AND ACTION

ACTH stimulation is required for the initiation of steroidogenesis. The ACTH receptor MC2R (melanocortin 2 receptor) interacts with the MC2R-accessory protein MRAP, and the complex is transported to the adrenocortical cell membrane, where it binds to ACTH (Fig. 8-5). ACTH stimulation generates cyclic AMP (cAMP), which upregulates the protein kinase A (PKA) signaling pathway. Inactive PKA is a tetramer of two regulatory and two catalytic subunits that is dissociated by cAMP into a dimer of two regulatory subunits bound to cAMP and two free and active catalytic subunits. PKA activation impacts steroidogenesis in three distinct ways: (1) increases the import of cholesterol esters; (2) increases the activity of hormone-sensitive lipase, which cleaves cholesterol esters to cholesterol for import into the mitochondrion; and (3) increases the availability and phosphorylation of CREB (cAMP response element binding), a transcription factor that enhances transcription of CYP11A1 and other enzymes required for glucocorticoid synthesis.

Adrenal steroidogenesis occurs in a zone-specific fashion, with mineralocorticoid synthesis occurring in the outer zona glomerulosa, glucocorticoid synthesis in the zona fasciculata, and adrenal androgen synthesis in the inner zona reticularis (Fig. 8-1). All steroidogenic

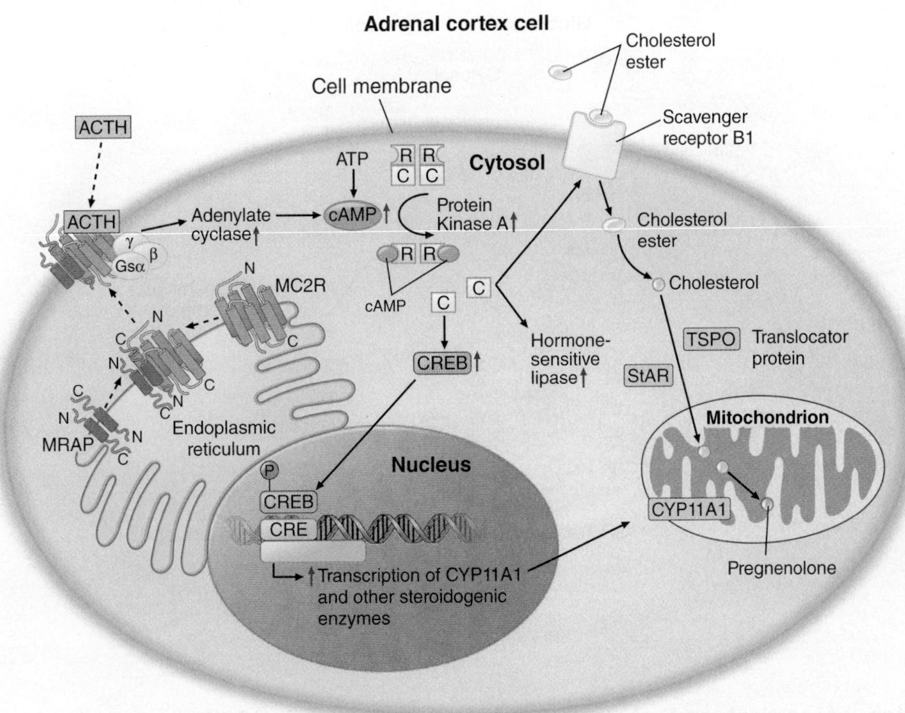

FIGURE 8-5
ACTH effects on adrenal steroidogenesis. ACTH, adrenocorticotropic hormone; binding protein; MRAP, MC2R-accessory protein; protein kinase A catalytic subunit (C; *PRKACA*), PKA regulatory subunit (R; *PRKAR1A*); StAR, steroidogenic acute regulatory (protein); TSPO, translocator protein.

pathways require cholesterol import into the mitochondrion, a process initiated by the action of the steroidogenic acute regulatory (StAR) protein, which shuttles cholesterol from the outer to the inner mitochondrial membrane. The majority of steroidogenic enzymes are cytochrome P450 (CYP) enzymes, which are either located in the mitochondrion (side chain cleavage enzyme, CYP11A1; 11β-hydroxylase, CYP11B1; aldosterone synthase, CYP11B2) or in the endoplasmic reticulum membrane (17α-hydroxylase, CYP17A1; 21-hydroxylase, CYP21A2; aromatase, CYP19A1). These enzymes require electron donation via specific redox cofactor enzymes, P450 oxidoreductase (POR), and adrenodoxin/adrenodoxin reductase (ADX/ADR) for the microsomal and mitochondrial CYP enzymes, respectively. In addition, the short-chain dehydrogenase 3β-hydroxysteroid dehydrogenase type 2 (3β-HSD2), also termed Δ4,Δ5 isomerase, plays a major role in adrenal steroidogenesis.

The cholesterol side chain cleavage enzyme CYP11A1 generates pregnenolone. Glucocorticoid synthesis requires conversion of pregnenolone to progesterone by 3β-HSD2, followed by conversion to 17-hydroxyprogesterone by CYP17A1, further hydroxylation at carbon 21 by CYP21A2, and eventually, 11β-hydroxylation by CYP11B1 to generate active cortisol (Fig. 8-1). Mineralocorticoid synthesis also requires progesterone, which is first converted to deoxycorticosterone by CYP21A2 and then converted via corticosterone and 18-hydroxycorticosterone to aldosterone in three steps catalyzed by CYP11B2. For adrenal androgen synthesis, pregnenolone undergoes conversion by CYP17A1, which uniquely catalyzes two enzymatic reactions. Via its 17α-hydroxylase activity, CYP17A1 converts pregnenolone to 17-hydroxypregnenolone, followed by generation of the universal sex steroid precursor DHEA via CYP17A1 17, 20 lyase activity. The majority of DHEA is secreted by the adrenal in the form of its sulfate ester, DHEAS, generated by DHEA sulfotransferase (SULT2A1).

Following its release from the adrenal, cortisol circulates in the bloodstream mainly bound to cortisol-binding globulin (CBG) and to a lesser extent to albumin, with only a minor fraction circulating as free, unbound hormone. Free cortisol is thought to enter cells directly, not requiring active transport. In addition, in a multitude of peripheral target tissues of glucocorticoid action, including adipose, liver, muscle, and brain, cortisol is generated from inactive cortisone within the cell by the enzyme 11β-hydroxysteroid dehydrogenase type 1 (11β-HSD1) (Fig. 8-6). Thereby, 11β-HSD1 functions as a tissue-specific prereceptor regulator of glucocorticoid action. For the conversion of inactive cortisone to active cortisol, 11β-HSD1 requires nicotinamide adenine dinucleotide phosphate (NADPH [reduced form]), which is provided by the enzyme hexose-6-phosphate dehydrogenase (H6PDH).

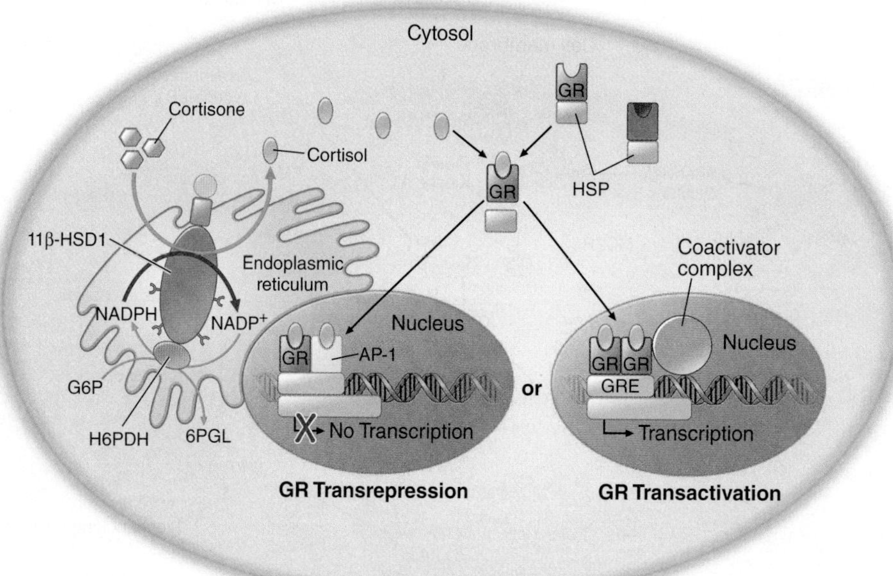

FIGURE 8-6

Prereceptor activation of cortisol and glucocorticoid receptor (GR) action. AP-1 activator protein-1; G6P, glucose-6-phosphate; GRE, glucocorticoid response elements; HSP, heat shock proteins; NADPH, nicotinamide adenine dinucleotide phosphate (reduced form); 6PGL, 6-phosphogluconate.

Like the catalytic domain of 11β-HSD1, H6PDH is located in the lumen of the endoplasmic reticulum, and converts glucose-6-phosphate (G6P) to 6-phosphogluconate (6PGL), thereby regenerating NADP+ to NADPH, which drives the activation of cortisol from cortisone by 11β-HSD1.

In the cytosol of target cells, cortisol binds and activates the glucocorticoid receptor (GR), which results in dissociation of heat shock proteins (HSP) from the receptor and subsequent dimerization (Fig. 8-6). Cortisol-bound GR dimers translocate to the nucleus and activate glucocorticoid response elements (GRE) in the DNA sequence, thereby enhancing transcription of glucocorticoid-regulated genes (GR transactivation). However, cortisol-bound GR can also form heterodimers with transcription factors such as AP-1 or NF-κB, resulting in transrepression of proinflammatory genes, a mechanism of major importance for the anti-inflammatory action of glucocorticoids. It is important to note that corticosterone also exerts glucocorticoid activity, albeit much weaker than cortisol itself. However, in rodents, corticosterone is the major glucocorticoid, and in patients with 17-hydroxylase deficiency, lack of cortisol can be compensated for by higher concentrations of corticosterone that accumulates as a consequence of the enzymatic block.

Cortisol is inactivated to cortisone by the microsomal enzyme 11β-hydroxysteroid dehydrogenase type 2 (11β-HSD2) (Fig. 8-7), mainly in the kidney, but also in the colon, salivary glands, and other target tissues. Cortisol and aldosterone bind the mineralocorticoid receptor (MR) with equal affinity; however, cortisol circulates in the bloodstream at about a thousandfold higher concentration. Thus, only rapid inactivation of cortisol to cortisone by 11β-HSD2 prevents MR activation by excess cortisol, thereby acting as a tissue-specific modulator of the MR pathway. In addition to cortisol and aldosterone, deoxycorticosterone (DOC) (Fig. 8-1) also exerts mineralocorticoid activity. DOC accumulation due to 11β-hydroxylase deficiency or due to tumor-related excess production can result in mineralocorticoid excess.

Aldosterone synthesis in the adrenal zona glomerulosa cells is driven by the enzyme aldosterone synthase (CYP11B2). The binding of angiotensin II to the AT1 receptor causes glomerulosa cell membrane depolarization by increasing intracellular sodium through inhibition of sodium potassium (Na^+/K^+) ATPase enzymes as well as potassium channels. This drives an increase in intracellular calcium by opening of voltage-dependent calcium channels or inhibition of calcium (Ca^{2+}) ATPase enzymes. Consequently, the calcium signaling pathway is triggered, resulting in upregulation of CYP11B2 transcription (Fig. 8-8).

Analogous to cortisol action via the GR, aldosterone (or cortisol) binding to the MR in the kidney tubule cell dissociates the HSP–receptor complex, allowing homodimerization of the MR, and translocation of the hormone-bound MR dimer to the nucleus (Fig. 8-7). The activated MR enhances transcription of the epithelial sodium channel (ENaC) and serum glucocorticoid-inducible kinase 1 (SGK-1). In the cytosol, interaction

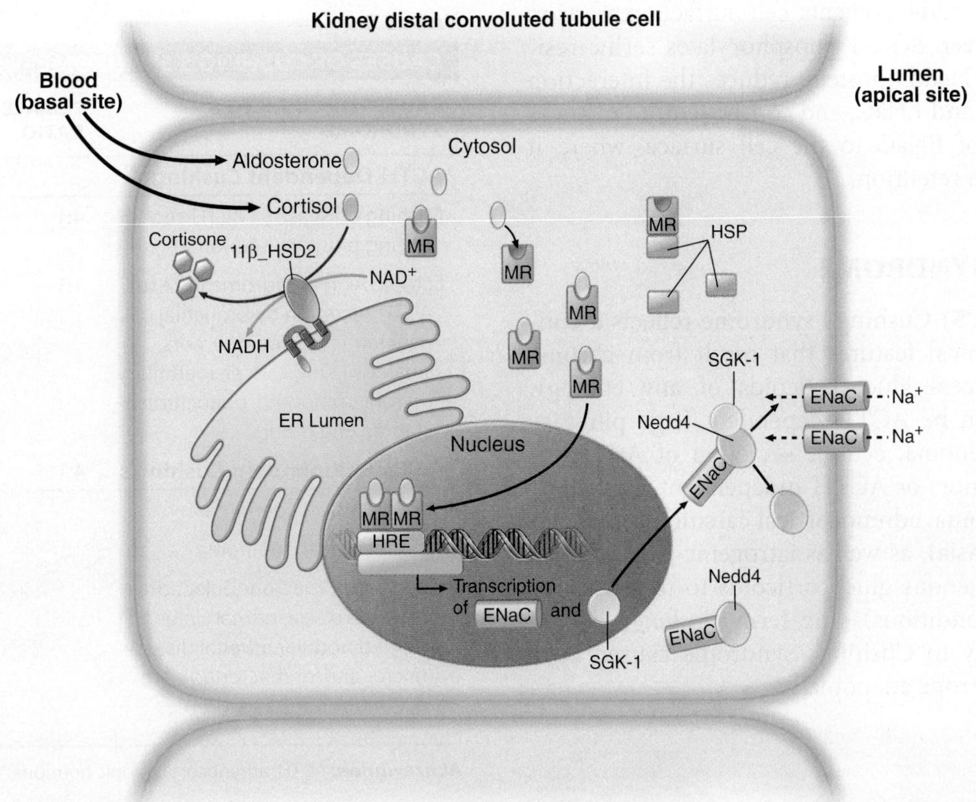

FIGURE 8-7

Prereceptor inactivation of cortisol and mineralocorticoid receptor action. ENaC, epithelial sodium channel; HRE, hormone response element; NADH, nicotinamide adenine dinucleotide; SGK-1, serum glucocorticoid-inducible kinase-1.

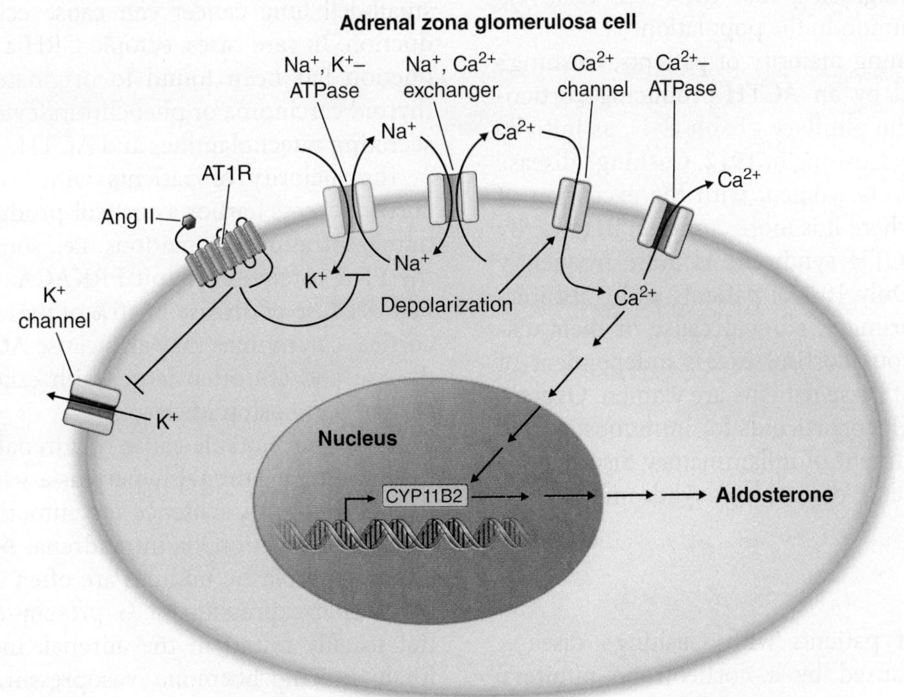

FIGURE 8-8

Regulation of adrenal aldosterone synthesis. AngII, angiotensin II; AT1R, angiotensin II receptor type 1; CYP11B2, aldosterone synthase. *(Modified after F Beuschlein: Regulation of aldosterone secretion: from physiology to disease. Eur J Endocrinol 168:R85, 2013.)*

of ENaC with Nedd4 prevents cell surface expression of ENaC. However, SGK-1 phosphorylates serine residues within the Nedd4 protein, reduces the interaction between Nedd4 and ENaC, and consequently, enhances the trafficking of ENaC to the cell surface, where it mediates sodium retention.

CUSHING'S SYNDROME

(See also Chap. 5) Cushing's syndrome reflects a constellation of clinical features that result from chronic exposure to excess glucocorticoids of any etiology. The disorder can be ACTH-dependent (e.g., pituitary corticotrope adenoma, ectopic secretion of ACTH by nonpituitary tumor) or ACTH-independent (e.g., adrenocortical adenoma, adrenocortical carcinoma, nodular adrenal hyperplasia), as well as iatrogenic (e.g., administration of exogenous glucocorticoids to treat various inflammatory conditions). The term *Cushing's disease* refers specifically to Cushing's syndrome caused by a pituitary corticotrope adenoma.

Epidemiology

Cushing's syndrome is generally considered a rare disease. It occurs with an incidence of 1–2 per 100,000 population per year. However, it is debated whether mild cortisol excess may be more prevalent among patients with several features of Cushing's such as centripetal obesity, type 2 diabetes, and osteoporotic vertebral fractures, recognizing that these are relatively nonspecific and common in the population.

In the overwhelming majority of patients, Cushing's syndrome is caused by an ACTH-producing corticotrope adenoma of the pituitary (Table 8-1), as initially described by Harvey Cushing in 1912. Cushing's disease more frequently affects women, with the exception of prepubertal cases, where it is more common in boys. By contrast, ectopic ACTH syndrome is more frequently identified in men. Only 10% of patients with Cushing's syndrome have a primary, adrenal cause of their disease (e.g., autonomous cortisol excess independent of ACTH), and most of these patients are women. Overall, the medical use of glucocorticoids for immunosuppression, or for the treatment of inflammatory disorders, is the most common cause of Cushing's syndrome.

TABLE 8-1

CAUSES OF CUSHING'S SYNDROME

CAUSES OF CUSHING'S SYNDROME	FEMALE: MALE RATIO	%
ACTH-Dependent Cushing's		90
Cushing's disease (= ACTH-producing pituitary adenoma)	4:1	75
Ectopic ACTH syndrome (due to ACTH secretion by bronchial or pancreatic carcinoid tumors, small-cell lung cancer, medullary thyroid carcinoma, pheochromocytoma and others)	1:1	15
ACTH-Independent Cushing's	4:1	10
Adrenocortical adenoma		5–10
Adrenocortical carcinoma		1
Rare causes: macronodular adrenal hyperplasia; primary pigmented nodular adrenal disease (micro- and/or macronodular); McCune-Albright syndrome		<1

Abbreviation: ACTH, adrenocorticotropic hormone.

Etiology

In at least 90% of patients with Cushing's disease, ACTH excess is caused by a corticotrope pituitary microadenoma, often only a few millimeters in diameter. Pituitary macroadenomas (i.e., tumors >1 cm in size) are found in only 5–10% of patients. Pituitary corticotrope adenomas usually occur sporadically but very rarely can be found in the context of multiple endocrine neoplasia type 1 (MEN 1) **(Chap. 29)**.

Ectopic ACTH production is predominantly caused by occult carcinoid tumors, most frequently in the lung, but also in thymus or pancreas. Because of their small size, these tumors are often difficult to locate. Advanced small-cell lung cancer can cause ectopic ACTH production. In rare cases, ectopic CRH and/or ACTH production has been found to originate from medullary thyroid carcinoma or pheochromocytoma, the latter cosecreting catecholamines and ACTH.

The majority of patients with ACTH-independent cortisol excess harbor a cortisol-producing adrenal adenoma; intratumor mutations, i.e., somatic mutations in the PKA catalytic subunit PRKACA, have been identified as cause of disease in 40% of these tumors. Adrenocortical carcinomas may also cause ACTH-independent disease and are often large, with excess production of several corticosteroid classes.

A rare but notable cause of adrenal cortisol excess is macronodular adrenal hyperplasia with low circulating ACTH, but with evidence for autocrine stimulation of cortisol production via intraadrenal ACTH production. These hyperplastic nodules are often also characterized by ectopic expression of G protein–coupled receptors not usually found in the adrenal, including receptors for luteinizing hormone, vasopressin, serotonin, interleukin 1, catecholamines, or gastric inhibitory peptide (GIP), the cause of food-dependent Cushing's. Activation of these receptors results in upregulation of PKA signaling, as physiologically occurs with ACTH, with a subsequent increase in cortisol production. A combination of germline and somatic mutations in the tumor-suppressor gene *ARMC5* have been identified as a prevalent cause of Cushing's due to macronodular adrenal hyperplasia. Germline mutations in the PKA catalytic subunit PRKACA can represent a rare cause of macronodular adrenal hyperplasia associated with cortisol excess.

Mutations in one of the regulatory subunits of PKA, PRKAR1A, are found in patients with primary pigmented nodular adrenal disease (PPNAD) as part of *Carney's complex*, an autosomal dominant multiple neoplasia condition associated with cardiac myxomas, hyperlentiginosis, Sertoli cell tumors, and PPNAD. PPNAD can present as micronodular or macronodular hyperplasia, or both. Phosphodiesterases can influence intracellular cAMP and can thereby impact PKA activation. Mutations in PDE11A and PDE8B have been identified in patients with bilateral adrenal hyperplasia and Cushing's, with and without evidence of PPNAD.

Another rare cause of ACTH-independent Cushing's is *McCune-Albright syndrome*, also associated with polyostotic fibrous dysplasia, unilateral café-au-lait spots, and precocious puberty. McCune-Albright syndrome is caused by activating mutations in the stimulatory G protein alpha subunit 1, GNAS-1 (guanine nucleotide binding protein alpha stimulating activity polypeptide 1), and such mutations have also been found in bilateral macronodular hyperplasia without other McCune-Albright features and, in rare instances, also in isolated cortisol-producing adrenal adenomas (Table 8-1; **Chap. 36**).

Clinical manifestations

Glucocorticoids affect almost all cells of the body, and thus signs of cortisol excess impact multiple physiologic systems (Table 8-2), with upregulation of gluconeogenesis, lipolysis, and protein catabolism causing the most prominent features. In addition, excess glucocorticoid secretion overcomes the ability of 11β-HSD2 to rapidly inactivate cortisol to cortisone in the kidney, thereby exerting mineralocorticoid actions, manifest as diastolic hypertension, hypokalemia, and edema. Excess glucocorticoids also interfere with central regulatory systems, leading to suppression of gonadotropins with subsequent hypogonadism and amenorrhea, and suppression of the hypothalamic-pituitary-thyroid axis, resulting in decreased thyroid-stimulating hormone (TSH) secretion.

The majority of clinical signs and symptoms observed in Cushing's syndrome are relatively nonspecific and include features such as obesity, diabetes, diastolic hypertension, hirsutism, and depression that are commonly found in patients who do not have Cushing's. Therefore, careful clinical assessment is an important aspect of evaluating suspected cases. A diagnosis of Cushing's should be considered when several clinical features are found in the same patient, in particular when more specific features are found. These include fragility of the skin, with easy bruising and broad (>1 cm), purplish striae (Fig. 8-9), and signs of proximal myopathy, which becomes most obvious when trying to stand up from a chair without the use of hands or when climbing stairs. Clinical manifestations of Cushing's do not differ substantially among the different causes of Cushing's. In ectopic ACTH syndrome, hyperpigmentation of the knuckles, scars, or skin areas exposed to increased friction can be observed (Fig. 8-9)

TABLE 8-2

SIGNS AND SYMPTOMS OF CUSHING'S SYNDROME

BODY COMPARTMENT/ SYSTEM	SIGNS AND SYMPTOMS
Body fat	Weight gain, central obesity, rounded face, fat pad on back of neck ("buffalo hump")
Skin	Facial plethora, thin and brittle skin, easy bruising, broad and purple stretch marks, acne, hirsutism
Bone	Osteopenia, osteoporosis (vertebral fractures), decreased linear growth in children
Muscle	Weakness, proximal myopathy (prominent atrophy of gluteal and upper leg muscles with difficulty climbing stairs or getting up from a chair)
Cardiovascular system	Hypertension, hypokalemia, edema, atherosclerosis
Metabolism	Glucose intolerance/diabetes, dyslipidemia
Reproductive system	Decreased libido, in women amenorrhea (due to cortisol-mediated inhibition of gonadotropin release)
Central nervous system	Irritability, emotional lability, depression, sometimes cognitive defects; in severe cases, paranoid psychosis
Blood and immune system	Increased susceptibility to infections, increased white blood cell count, eosinopenia, hypercoagulation with increased risk of deep vein thrombosis and pulmonary embolism

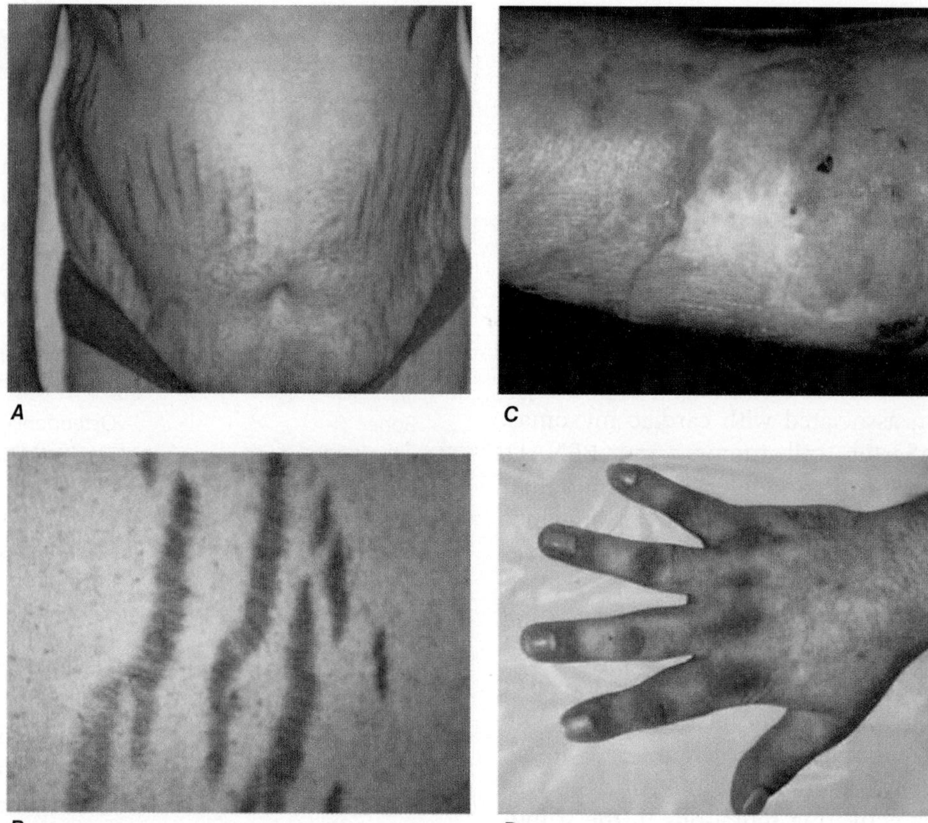

FIGURE 8-9

Clinical features of Cushing's syndrome. ***A.*** Note central obesity and broad, purple stretch marks (***B.*** close-up). ***C.*** Note thin and brittle skin in an elderly patient with Cushing's syndrome. ***D.*** Hyperpigmentation of the knuckles in a patient with ectopic adrenocorticotropic hormone (ACTH) excess.

and is caused by stimulatory effects of excess ACTH and other POMC cleavage products on melanocyte pigment production. Furthermore, patients with ectopic ACTH syndrome, and some with adrenocortical carcinoma as the cause of Cushing's, may have a more brisk onset and rapid progression of clinical signs and symptoms.

Patients with Cushing's syndrome can be acutely endangered by deep vein thrombosis, with subsequent pulmonary embolism due to a hypercoagulable state associated with Cushing's. The majority of patients also experience psychiatric symptoms, mostly in the form of anxiety or depression, but acute paranoid or depressive psychosis may also occur. Even after cure, long-term health may be affected by persistently impaired health-related quality of life and increased risk of cardiovascular disease and osteoporosis with vertebral fractures, depending on the duration and degree of exposure to significant cortisol excess.

Diagnosis

The most important first step in the management of patients with suspected Cushing's syndrome is to establish the correct diagnosis. Most mistakes in clinical management, leading to unnecessary imaging or surgery, are made because the diagnostic protocol is not followed (Fig. 8-10). This protocol requires establishing the diagnosis of Cushing's beyond doubt prior to employing any tests used for the differential diagnosis of the condition. In principle, after excluding exogenous glucocorticoid use as the cause of clinical signs and symptoms, suspected cases should be tested if there are multiple and progressive features of Cushing's, particularly features with a potentially higher discriminatory value. Exclusion of Cushing's is also indicated in patients with incidentally discovered adrenal masses.

A diagnosis of Cushing's can be considered as established if the results of several tests are consistently suggestive of Cushing's. These tests may include increased 24-h urinary free cortisol excretion in three separate collections, failure to appropriately suppress morning cortisol after overnight exposure to dexamethasone, and evidence of loss of diurnal cortisol secretion with high levels at midnight, the time of the physiologically lowest secretion (Fig. 8-10). Factors potentially affecting the outcome of these diagnostic tests have to be excluded such as incomplete 24-h urine collection or

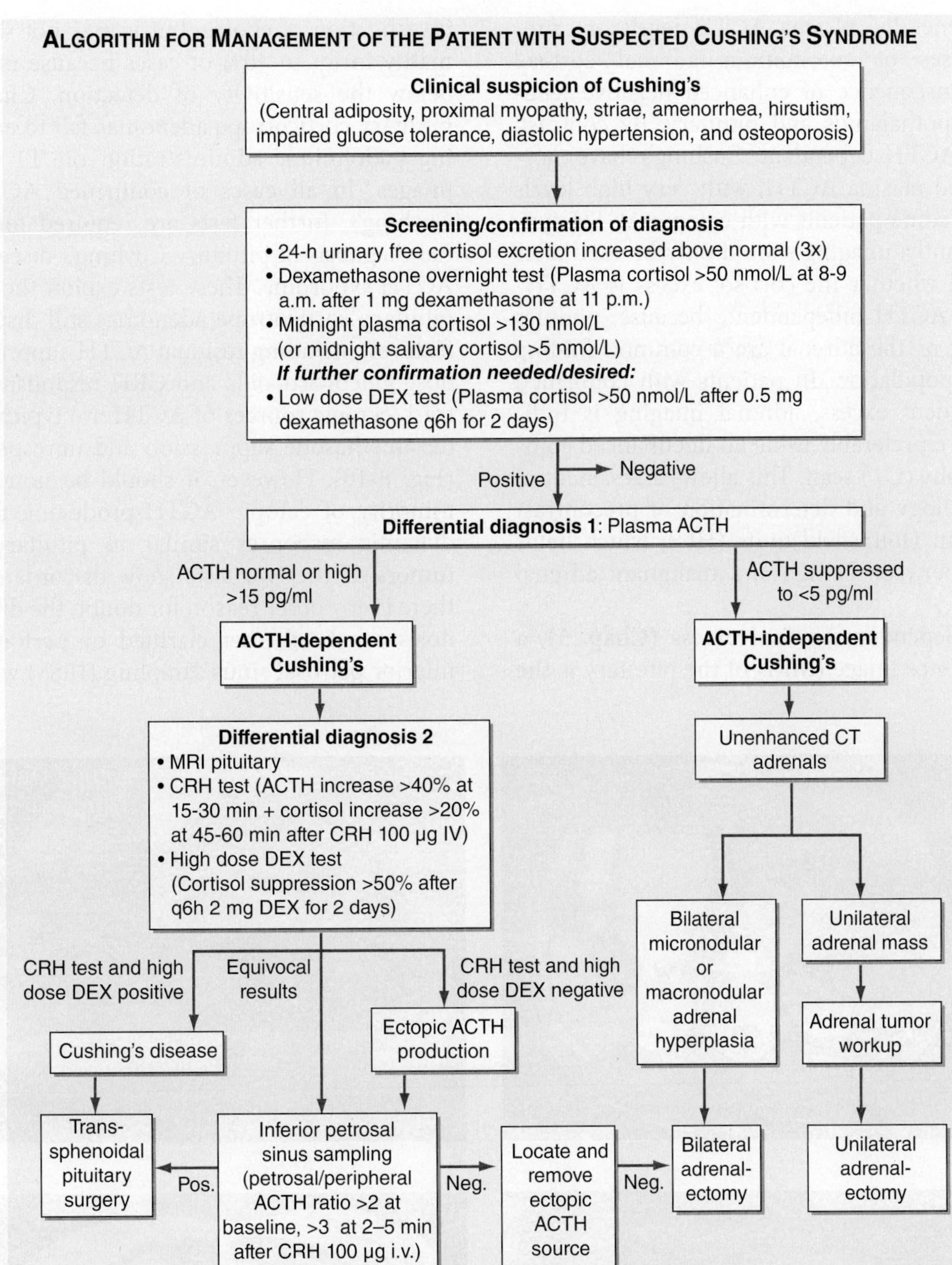

FIGURE 8-10

Management of the patient with suspected Cushing's syndrome. ACTH, adrenocorticotropic hormone; CRH, corticotropin-releasing hormone; CT, computed tomography; DEX, dexamethasone; MRI, magnetic resonance imaging.

rapid inactivation of dexamethasone due to concurrent intake of CYP3A4-inducing drugs (e.g., antiepileptics, rifampicin). Concurrent intake of oral contraceptives that raise CBG and thus total cortisol can cause failure to suppress after dexamethasone. If in doubt, testing should be repeated after 4–6 weeks off estrogens. Patients with pseudo-Cushing states, i.e., alcohol-related, and those with cyclic Cushing's may require further testing to safely confirm or exclude the diagnosis of Cushing's. In addition, the biochemical assays employed can affect the test results, with specificity representing a common problem with antibody-based assays for the measurement of urinary free cortisol. These assays have been greatly improved by the introduction of highly specific tandem mass spectrometry.

Differential diagnosis

The evaluation of patients with confirmed Cushing's should be carried out by an endocrinologist and begins with the differential diagnosis of ACTH-dependent and ACTH-independent cortisol excess

(Fig. 8-10). Generally, plasma ACTH levels are suppressed in cases of autonomous adrenal cortisol excess, as a consequence of enhanced negative feedback to the hypothalamus and pituitary. By contrast, patients with ACTH-dependent Cushing's have normal or increased plasma ACTH, with very high levels being found in some patients with ectopic ACTH syndrome. Importantly, imaging should only be used after it is established whether the cortisol excess is ACTH-dependent or ACTH-independent, because nodules in the pituitary or the adrenal are a common finding in the general population. In patients with confirmed ACTH-independent excess, adrenal imaging is indicated (Fig. 8-11), preferably using an unenhanced computed tomography (CT) scan. This allows assessment of adrenal morphology and determination of precontrast tumor density in Hounsfield units (HU), which helps to distinguish between benign and malignant adrenal lesions.

For ACTH-dependent cortisol excess **(Chap. 5)**, a magnetic resonance image (MRI) of the pituitary is the investigation of choice, but it may not show an abnormality in up to 40% of cases because of small tumors below the sensitivity of detection. Characteristically, pituitary corticotrope adenomas fail to enhance following gadolinium administration on T1-weighted MRI images. In all cases of confirmed ACTH-dependent Cushing's, further tests are required for the differential diagnosis of pituitary Cushing's disease and ectopic ACTH syndrome. These tests exploit the fact that most pituitary corticotrope adenomas still display regulatory features, including residual ACTH suppression by high-dose glucocorticoids and CRH responsiveness. In contrast, ectopic sources of ACTH are typically resistant to dexamethasone suppression and unresponsive to CRH (Fig. 8-10). However, it should be noted that a small minority of ectopic ACTH-producing tumors exhibit dynamic responses similar to pituitary corticotrope tumors. If the two tests show discordant results, or if there is any other reason for doubt, the differential diagnosis can be further clarified by performing bilateral inferior petrosal sinus sampling (IPSS) with concurrent

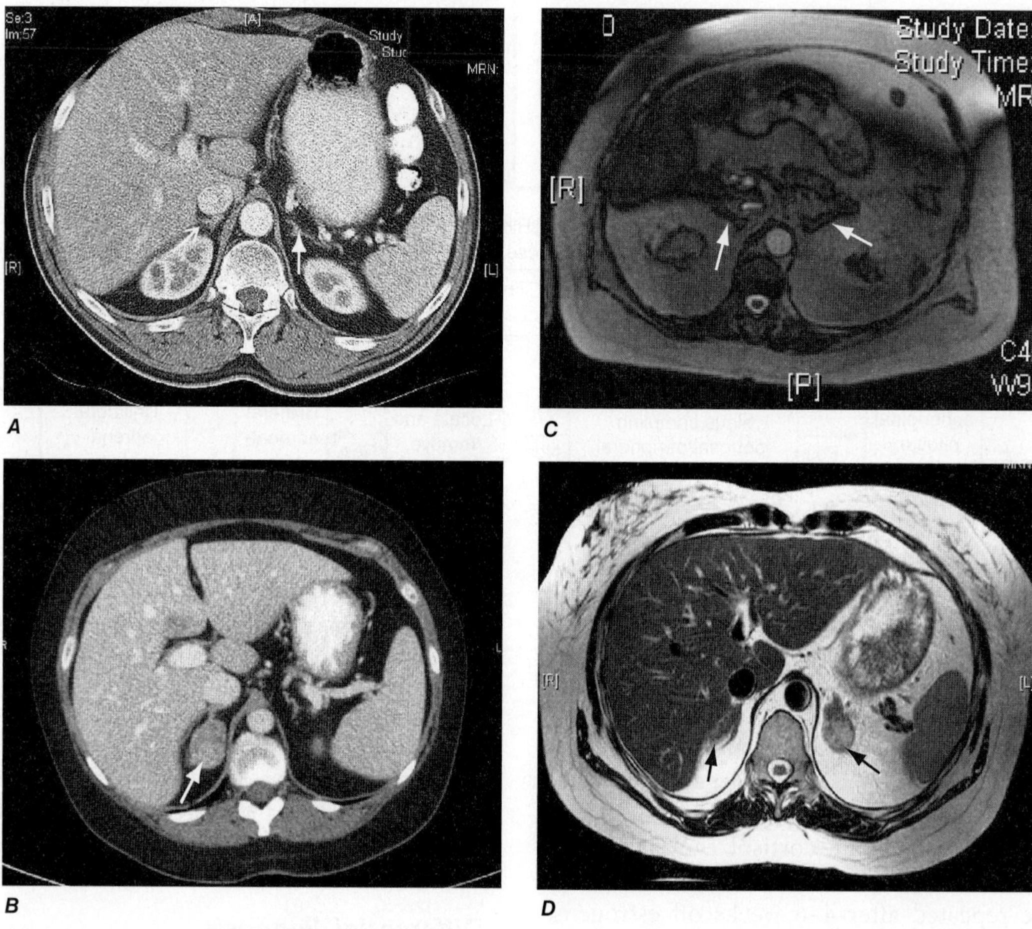

FIGURE 8-11

Adrenal imaging in Cushing's syndrome. *A.* Adrenal computed tomography (CT) showing normal bilateral adrenal morphology (*arrows*). ***B.*** CT scan depicting a right adrenocortical adenoma (*arrow*) causing Cushing's syndrome. ***C.*** Magnetic resonance imaging (MRI) showing bilateral adrenal hyperplasia due to excess adrenocorticotropic hormone stimulation in Cushing's disease. ***D.*** MRI showing bilateral macronodular hyperplasia causing Cushing's syndrome.

blood sampling for ACTH in the right and left inferior petrosal sinus and a peripheral vein. An increased central/peripheral plasma ACTH ratio >2 at baseline and >3 at 2–5 min after CRH injection is indicative of Cushing's disease (Fig. 8-10), with very high sensitivity and specificity. Of note, the results of the IPSS cannot be reliably used for lateralization (i.e., prediction of the location of the tumor within the pituitary), because there is broad interindividual variability in the venous drainage of the pituitary region. Importantly, no cortisol-lowering agents should be used prior to IPSS.

If the differential diagnostic testing indicates ectopic ACTH syndrome, then further imaging should include high-resolution, fine-cut CT scanning of the chest and abdomen for scrutiny of the lung, thymus, and pancreas. If no lesions are identified, an MRI of the chest can be considered because carcinoid tumors usually show high signal intensity on T2-weighted images. Furthermore, octreotide scintigraphy can be helpful in some cases because ectopic ACTH-producing tumors often express somatostatin receptors. Depending on the suspected cause, patients with ectopic ACTH syndrome should also undergo blood sampling for fasting gut hormones, chromogranin A, calcitonin, and biochemical exclusion of pheochromocytoma.

TREATMENT Cushing's Syndrome

Overt Cushing's is associated with a poor prognosis if left untreated. In ACTH-independent disease, treatment consists of surgical removal of the adrenal tumor. For smaller tumors, a minimally invasive approach can be used, whereas for larger tumors and those suspected of malignancy, an open approach is preferred.

In Cushing's disease, the treatment of choice is selective removal of the pituitary corticotrope tumor, usually via an endoscopic transsphenoidal approach. This results in an initial cure rate of 70–80% when performed by a highly experienced surgeon. However, even after initial remission following surgery, long-term follow-up is important because late relapse occurs in a significant number of patients. If pituitary disease recurs, there are several options, including second surgery, radiotherapy, stereotactic radiosurgery, and bilateral adrenalectomy. These options need to be applied in a highly individualized fashion.

In some patients with very severe, overt Cushing's (e.g., difficult to control hypokalemic hypertension or acute psychosis), it may be necessary to introduce medical therapy to rapidly control the cortisol excess during the period leading up to surgery. Similarly, patients with metastasized, glucocorticoid-producing carcinomas may require long-term antiglucocorticoid drug treatment. In case of ectopic ACTH syndrome, in which the tumor cannot be located, one must carefully weigh whether drug treatment or bilateral adrenalectomy is the most appropriate choice, with the latter facilitating immediate cure but requiring life-long corticosteroid replacement. In this instance, it is paramount to ensure regular imaging follow-up for identification of the ectopic ACTH source.

Oral agents with established efficacy in Cushing's syndrome are metyrapone and ketoconazole. Metyrapone inhibits cortisol synthesis at the level of 11β-hydroxylase (Fig. 8-1), whereas the antimycotic drug ketoconazole inhibits the early steps of steroidogenesis. Typical starting doses are 500 mg tid for metyrapone (maximum dose, 6 g) and 200 mg tid for ketoconazole (maximum dose, 1200 mg). Mitotane, a derivative of the insecticide o,p'DDD, is an adrenolytic agent that is also effective for reducing cortisol. Because of its side effect profile, it is most commonly used in the context of adrenocortical carcinoma, but low-dose treatment (500–1000 mg/d) has also been used in benign Cushing's. In severe cases of cortisol excess, etomidate can be used to lower cortisol. It is administered by continuous IV infusion in low, nonanesthetic doses.

After the successful removal of an ACTH- or cortisol-producing tumor, the HPA axis will remain suppressed. Thus, hydrocortisone replacement needs to be initiated at the time of surgery and slowly tapered following recovery, to allow physiologic adaptation to normal cortisol levels. Depending on degree and duration of cortisol excess, the HPA axis may require many months or even years to resume normal function.

MINERALOCORTICOID EXCESS

Epidemiology

Following the first description of a patient with an aldosterone-producing adrenal adenoma (*Conn's syndrome*), mineralocorticoid excess was thought to represent a rare cause of hypertension. However, in studies systematically screening all patients with hypertension, a much higher prevalence is now recognized, ranging from 5 to 12%. The prevalence is higher when patients are preselected for hypokalemic hypertension.

Etiology

The most common cause of mineralocorticoid excess is primary aldosteronism, reflecting excess production of aldosterone by the adrenal zona glomerulosa. Bilateral micronodular hyperplasia is somewhat more common than unilateral adrenal adenomas (Table 8-3). Somatic mutations in channels and enzymes responsible for increasing sodium and calcium influx in adrenal zona glomerulosa cells have been identified as prevalent causes of aldosterone-producing adrenal adenomas (Table 8-3) and, in the case of germline mutations, also of primary aldosteronism due to bilateral macronodular adrenal hyperplasia. However, bilateral adrenal hyperplasia as a

TABLE 8-3

CAUSES OF MINERALOCORTICOID EXCESS

CAUSES OF MINERALOCORTICOID EXCESS	MECHANISM	%
Primary Aldosteronism		
Adrenal (Conn's) adenoma	Autonomous aldosterone excess can be caused by somatic (intratumor) mutations in the potassium channel GIRK4 (encoded by *KCNJ5*; identified as cause of disease in 40% of aldosterone-producing adenomas; rare germline mutations can cause bilateral macronodular adrenal hyperplasia). Further causes include somatic mutations affecting the α-subunit of the Na^+/K^+-ATPase (encoded by *ATP1A1*), the plasma membrane calcium-transporting ATPase 3 (encoded by *ATP2B3*), and somatic or germline mutations in *CACNA1D* encoding the voltage-gated calcium channel Cav1.3. All mutations result in upregulation of CYP11B2 and hence aldosterone synthesis.	60
Bilateral (micronodular) adrenal hyperplasia	Autonomous aldosterone excess	60
Glucocorticoid-remediable hyperaldosteronism (dexamethasone-suppressible hyperaldosteronism)	Crossover between the *CYP11B1* and *CYP11B2* genes results in ACTH-driven aldosterone production	<1
Other Causes (Rare)		<1
Syndrome of apparent mineralocorticoid excess (SAME)	Mutations in *HSD11B2* result in lack of renal inactivation of cortisol to cortisone, leading to excess activation of the MR by cortisol	
Cushing's syndrome	Cortisol excess overcomes the capacity of HSD11B2 to inactivate cortisol to cortisone, consequently flooding the MR	
Glucocorticoid resistance	Upregulation of cortisol production due to GR mutations results in flooding of the MR by cortisol	
Adrenocortical carcinoma	Autonomous aldosterone and/or DOC excess	
Congenital adrenal hyperplasia	Accumulation of DOC due to mutations in *CYP11B1* or *CYP17A1*	
Progesterone-induced hypertension	Progestero ne acts as an abnormal ligand due to mutations in the MR gene	
Liddle's syndrome	Mutant ENaC β or γ subunits resulting in reduced degradation of ENaC keeping the membrane channel in open conformation for longer, enhancing mineralocorticoid action	

Abbreviations: ACTH, adrenocorticotropic hormone; DOC, deoxycorticosterone; ENaC, epithelial sodium channel; GR, glucocorticoid receptor; HSD11B2, 11β-hydroxysteroid dehydrogenase type 2; MR, mineralocorticoid receptor.

cause of mineralocorticoid excess is usually micronodular but can also contain larger nodules that might be mistaken for a unilateral adenoma. In rare instances, primary aldosteronism is caused by an adrenocortical carcinoma. Carcinomas should be considered in younger patients and in those with larger tumors, because benign aldosterone-producing adenomas usually measure <2 cm in diameter.

A rare cause of aldosterone excess is glucocorticoid-remediable aldosteronism (GRA), which is caused by a chimeric gene resulting from cross-over of promoter sequences between the *CYP11B1* and *CYP11B2* genes that are involved in glucocorticoid and mineralocorticoid synthesis, respectively (Fig. 8-1). This rearrangement brings *CYP11B2* transcription under the control of ACTH receptor signaling; consequently, aldosterone production is regulated by ACTH rather than by renin. The family history can be helpful because there may be evidence for dominant transmission of hypertension. Recognition of the disorder is important because it can be associated with early-onset hypertension and strokes. In addition, glucocorticoid suppression can reduce aldosterone production.

Other rare causes of mineralocorticoid excess are listed in Table 8-3. An important cause is excess binding and activation of the mineralocorticoid receptor by a steroid other than aldosterone. Cortisol acts as a potent mineralocorticoid if it escapes efficient inactivation to cortisone by 11β-HSD2 in the kidney (Fig. 8-7). This can be caused by inactivating mutations in the *HSD11B2* gene resulting in the syndrome of apparent mineralocorticoid excess (SAME) that characteristically manifests with severe hypokalemic hypertension in childhood. However, milder mutations may cause normokalemic hypertension manifesting in adulthood (type II SAME). Inhibition of 11β-HSD2 by excess licorice ingestion also results in hypokalemic hypertension, as does overwhelming of

11β-HSD2 conversion capacity by cortisol excess in Cushing's syndrome. Deoxycorticosterone (DOC) also binds and activates the mineralocorticoid receptor and can cause hypertension if its circulating concentrations are increased. This can arise through autonomous DOC secretion by an adrenocortical carcinoma, but also when DOC accumulates as a consequence of an adrenal enzymatic block, as seen in congenital adrenal hyperplasia due to CYP11B1 (11β-hydroxylase) or CYP17A1 (17α-hydroxylase) deficiency (Fig. 8-1). Progesterone can cause hypokalemic hypertension in rare individuals who harbor a mineralocorticoid receptor mutation that enhances binding and activation by progesterone; physiologically, progesterone normally exerts antimineralocorticoid activity. Finally, excess mineralocorticoid activity can be caused by mutations in the β or γ subunits of the ENaC, disrupting its interaction with Nedd4 (Fig. 8-7), and thereby decreasing receptor internalization and degradation. The constitutively active ENAC drives hypokalemic hypertension, resulting in an autosomal dominant disorder termed *Liddle's syndrome*.

Clinical manifestations

Excess activation of the mineralocorticoid receptor leads to potassium depletion and increased sodium retention, with the latter causing an expansion of extracellular and plasma volume. Increased ENaC activity also results in hydrogen depletion that can cause metabolic alkalosis. Aldosterone also has direct effects on the vascular system, where it increases cardiac remodeling and decreases compliance. Aldosterone excess may cause direct damage to the myocardium and the kidney glomeruli, in addition to secondary damage due to systemic hypertension.

The clinical hallmark of mineralocorticoid excess is hypokalemic hypertension; serum sodium tends to be normal due to the concurrent fluid retention, which in some cases can lead to peripheral edema. Hypokalemia can be exacerbated by thiazide drug treatment, which leads to increased delivery of sodium to the distal renal tubule, thereby driving potassium excretion. Severe hypokalemia can be associated with muscle weakness, overt proximal myopathy, or even hypokalemic paralysis. Severe alkalosis contributes to muscle cramps and, in severe cases, can cause tetany.

Diagnosis

Diagnostic screening for mineralocorticoid excess is not currently recommended for all patients with hypertension, but should be restricted to those who exhibit hypertension associated with drug resistance, hypokalemia, an adrenal mass, or onset of disease before the age of 40 years (Fig. 8-12). The accepted screening test is concurrent measurement of plasma renin and aldosterone with subsequent calculation of the aldosterone-renin ratio (ARR) (Fig. 8-12); serum potassium needs to be normalized prior to testing. Stopping antihypertensive medication can be cumbersome, particularly in patients with severe hypertension. Thus, for practical purposes, in the first instance the patient can remain on the usual antihypertensive medications, with the exception that mineralocorticoid receptor antagonists need to be ceased at least 4 weeks prior to ARR measurement. The remaining antihypertensive drugs usually do not affect the outcome of ARR testing, except that beta blocker treatment can cause false-positive results and ACE/AT1R inhibitors can cause false-negative results in milder cases (Table 8-4).

ARR screening is positive if the ratio is >750 pmol/L per ng/mL per hour, with a concurrently high normal or increased aldosterone (Fig. 8-12). If one relies on the ARR only, the likelihood of a false-positive ARR becomes greater when renin levels are very low. The characteristics of the biochemical assays are also important. Some labs measure plasma renin activity, whereas others measure plasma renin concentrations. Antibody-based assays for the measurement of serum aldosterone lack the reliability of tandem mass spectrometry assays, but these are not yet ubiquitously available.

Diagnostic confirmation of mineralocorticoid excess in a patient with positive ARR screening result should be undertaken by an endocrinologist as the tests lack optimized validation. The most straightforward is the saline infusion test, which involves the IV administration of 2 L of physiologic saline over a 4-h period. Failure of aldosterone to suppress below 140 pmol/L (5 ng/dL) is indicative of autonomous mineralocorticoid excess. Alternative tests are the oral sodium loading test (300 mmol NaCl/d for 3 days) or the fludrocortisone suppression test (0.1 mg q6h with 30 mmol NaCl q8h for 4 days); the latter can be difficult because of the risk of profound hypokalemia and increased hypertension. In patients with overt hypokalemic hypertension, strongly positive ARR, and concurrently increased aldosterone levels, confirmatory testing is usually not necessary.

Differential diagnosis and treatment

After the diagnosis of hyperaldosteronism is established, the next step is to use adrenal imaging to further assess the cause. Fine-cut CT scanning of the adrenal region is the method of choice because it provides excellent visualization of adrenal morphology. CT will readily identify larger tumors suspicious of malignancy but may miss lesions smaller than 5 mm. The differentiation between bilateral micronodular hyperplasia and a unilateral adenoma is only required if a surgical approach is feasible and desired. Consequently, selective adrenal vein sampling (AVS) should only be carried out

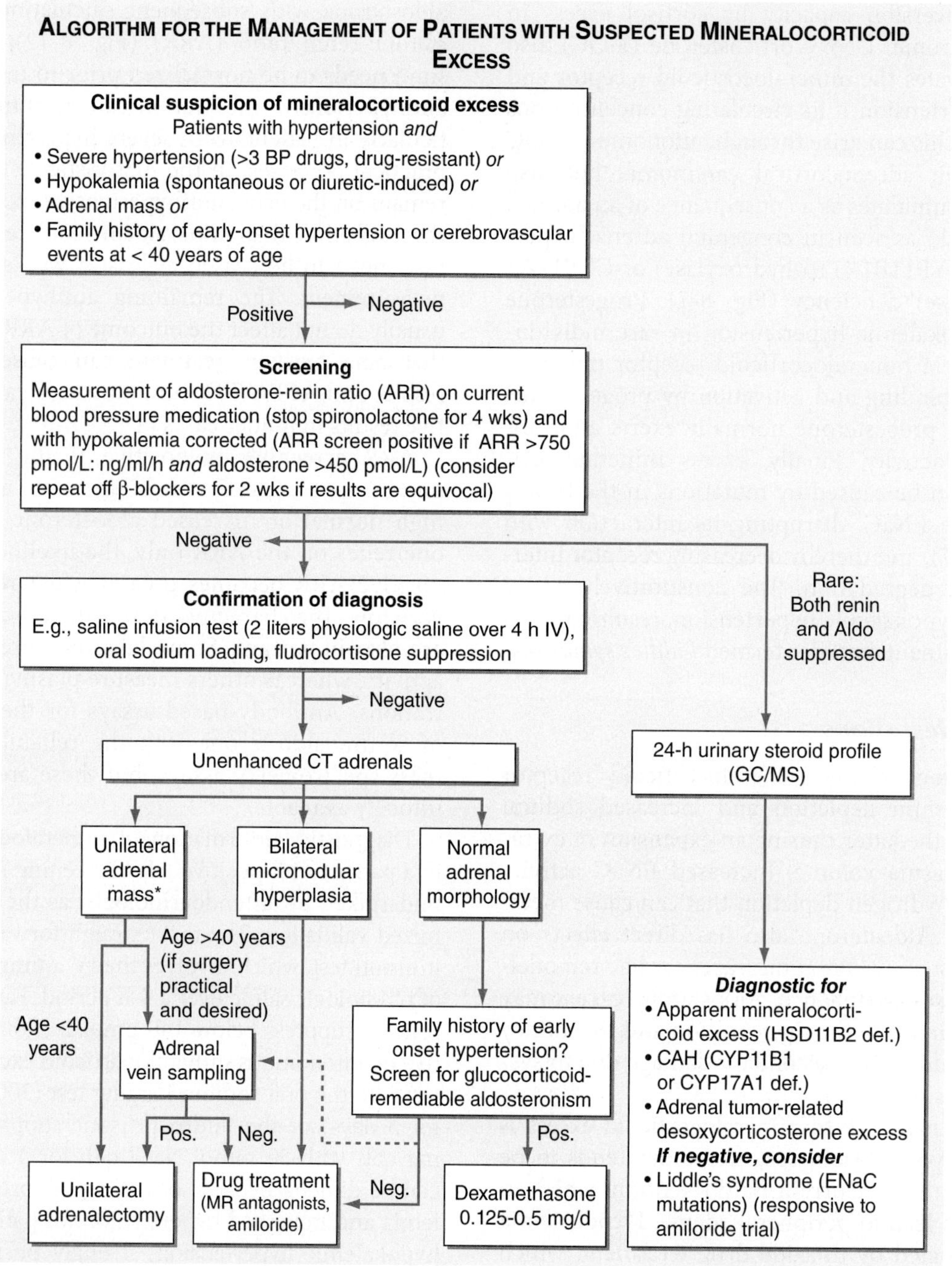

ALGORITHM FOR THE MANAGEMENT OF PATIENTS WITH SUSPECTED MINERALOCORTICOID EXCESS

Clinical suspicion of mineralocorticoid excess
Patients with hypertension *and*
- Severe hypertension (>3 BP drugs, drug-resistant) *or*
- Hypokalemia (spontaneous or diuretic-induced) *or*
- Adrenal mass *or*
- Family history of early-onset hypertension or cerebrovascular events at < 40 years of age

Positive → Negative

Screening
Measurement of aldosterone-renin ratio (ARR) on current blood pressure medication (stop spironolactone for 4 wks) and with hypokalemia corrected (ARR screen positive if ARR >750 pmol/L: ng/ml/h *and* aldosterone >450 pmol/L) (consider repeat off β-blockers for 2 wks if results are equivocal)

Negative

Rare: Both renin and Aldo suppressed

Confirmation of diagnosis
E.g., saline infusion test (2 liters physiologic saline over 4 h IV), oral sodium loading, fludrocortisone suppression

Negative

Unenhanced CT adrenals

24-h urinary steroid profile (GC/MS)

Unilateral adrenal mass*

Bilateral micronodular hyperplasia

Normal adrenal morphology

Age >40 years (if surgery practical and desired)

Age <40 years

Adrenal vein sampling

Family history of early onset hypertension? Screen for glucocorticoid-remediable aldosteronism

Diagnostic for
- Apparent mineralocorticoid excess (HSD11B2 def.)
- CAH (CYP11B1 or CYP17A1 def.)
- Adrenal tumor-related desoxycorticosterone excess

If negative, consider
- Liddle's syndrome (ENaC mutations) (responsive to amiloride trial)

Pos. Neg. Pos. Neg.

Unilateral adrenalectomy

Drug treatment (MR antagonists, amiloride)

Dexamethasone 0.125-0.5 mg/d

FIGURE 8-12

Management of patients with suspected mineralocorticoid excess. *Perform adrenal tumor workup (see Fig. 8-13). BP, blood pressure; CAH, congenital adrenal hyperplasia; CT, computed tomography; GC/MS, gas chromatography/mass spectrometry; PRA, plasma renin activity.

in surgical candidates with either no obvious lesion on CT or evidence of a unilateral lesion in patients older than 40 years, because the latter patients have a high likelihood of harboring a coincidental, endocrine-inactive adrenal adenoma (Fig. 8-12). AVS is used to compare aldosterone levels in the inferior vena cava and between the right and left adrenal veins. AVS requires concurrent measurement of cortisol to document correct placement of the catheter in the adrenal veins and should demonstrate a cortisol gradient >3 between the vena cava and each adrenal vein. Lateralization is confirmed by an aldosterone/cortisol ratio that is at least twofold higher on one side than the other. AVS is a complex procedure that requires a highly skilled interventional radiologist. Even then, the right adrenal vein can be difficult to cannulate correctly, which, if not achieved, invalidates the procedure. There is also no agreement as to whether the two adrenal veins should

TABLE 8-4

EFFECTS OF ANTIHYPERTENSIVE DRUGS ON THE ALDOSTERONE-RENIN-RATIO (ARR)

DRUG	EFFECT ON RENIN	EFFECT ON ALDOSTERONE	NET EFFECT ON ARR
β Blockers	↓	↑	↑
$α_1$ Blockers	→	→	→
$α_2$ Sympathomimetics	→	→	→
ACE inhibitors	↑	↓	↓
AT1R blockers	↑	↓	↓
Calcium antagonists	→	→	→
Diuretics	(↑)	(↑)	→/(↓)

Abbreviations: ACE, angiotensin-converting enzyme; AT1R, angiotensin II receptor type 1.

be cannulated simultaneously or successively and whether ACTH stimulation enhances the diagnostic value of AVS.

Patients younger than 40 years with confirmed mineralocorticoid excess and a unilateral lesion on CT can go straight to surgery, which is also indicated in patients with confirmed lateralization documented by a valid AVS procedure. Laparoscopic adrenalectomy is the preferred approach. Patients who are not surgical candidates, or with evidence of bilateral hyperplasia based on CT or AVS, should be treated medically (Fig. 8-12). Medical treatment, which can also be considered prior to surgery to avoid postsurgical hypoaldosteronism, consists primarily of the mineralocorticoid receptor antagonist spironolactone. It can be started at 12.5–50 mg bid and titrated up to a maximum of 400 mg/d to control blood pressure and normalize potassium. Side effects include menstrual irregularity, decreased libido, and gynecomastia. The more selective MR antagonist eplerenone can also be used. Doses start at 25 mg bid, and it can be titrated up to 200 mg/d. Another useful drug is the sodium channel blocker amiloride (5–10 mg bid).

In patients with normal adrenal morphology and family history of early-onset, severe hypertension, a diagnosis of GRA should be considered and can be evaluated using genetic testing. Treatment of GRA consists of administering dexamethasone, using the lowest dose possible to control blood pressure. Some patients also require additional MR antagonist treatment.

The diagnosis of nonaldosterone-related mineralocorticoid excess is based on documentation of suppressed renin and suppressed aldosterone in the presence of hypokalemic hypertension. This testing is best carried out by employing urinary steroid metabolite profiling by gas chromatography/mass spectrometry (GC/MS). An increased free cortisol over free cortisone ratio is suggestive of SAME and can be treated with dexamethasone. Steroid profiling by GC/MS also detects the steroids associated with CYP11B1 and CYP17A1 deficiency or the irregular steroid secretion pattern in a DOC-producing adrenocortical carcinoma (Fig. 8-12). If the GC/MS profile is normal, then Liddle's syndrome should be considered. It is very sensitive to amiloride treatment but will not respond to MR antagonist treatment, because the defect is due to a constitutively active ENaC.

APPROACH TO THE PATIENT: INCIDENTALLY DISCOVERED ADRENAL MASS

Epidemiology

Incidentally discovered adrenal masses, commonly termed adrenal "incidentalomas," are common, with a prevalence of at least 2% in the general population as documented in CT and autopsy series. The prevalence increases with age, with 1% of 40-year-olds and 7% of 70-year-olds harboring an adrenal mass.

Etiology

Most solitary adrenal tumors are monoclonal neoplasms. Several genetic syndromes, including MEN 1 (*MEN1*), MEN 2 (*RET*), Carney's complex (*PRKAR1A*), and McCune-Albright (*GNAS1*), can have adrenal tumors as one of their features. Somatic mutations in *MEN1*, *GNAS1*, and *PRKAR1A* have been identified in a small proportion of sporadic adrenocortical adenomas. Aberrant expression of membrane receptors (gastric inhibitory peptide, α- and β-adrenergic, luteinizing hormone, vasopressin V1, and interleukin 1 receptors) have been identified in some sporadic cases of macronodular adrenocortical hyperplasia.

The majority of adrenal nodules are endocrine-inactive adrenocortical adenomas. However, larger series suggest that up to 25% of adrenal nodules are hormonally active, due to a cortisol- or aldosterone-producing adrenocortical adenoma or a pheochromocytoma associated with catecholamine excess (Table 8-5). Adrenocortical carcinoma is rare but is the cause of an adrenal mass in 5% of patients. However, the most common cause of a malignant adrenal mass is metastasis originating from another solid tissue tumor (Table 8-5).

Differential diagnosis and treatment

Patients with an adrenal mass >1 cm require a diagnostic evaluation. Two key questions need to be addressed: (1) Does the tumor autonomously secrete hormones that could have a detrimental effect on health? (2) Is the adrenal mass benign or malignant?

Hormone secretion by an adrenal mass occurs along a continuum, with a gradual increase in clinical manifestations in parallel with hormone levels. Exclusion of

TABLE 8-5

CLASSIFICATION OF UNILATERAL ADRENAL MASSES

MASS	APPROXIMATE PREVALENCE (%)
Benign	
Adrenocortical adenoma	
Endocrine-inactive	60–85
Cortisol-producing	5–10
Aldosterone-producing	2–5
Pheochromocytoma	5–10
Adrenal myelolipoma	<1
Adrenal ganglioneuroma	<0.1
Adrenal hemangioma	<0.1
Adrenal cyst	<1
Adrenal hematoma/hemorrhagic infarction	<1
Indeterminate	
Adrenocortical oncocytoma	<1
Malignant	
Adrenocortical carcinoma	2–5
Malignant pheochromocytoma	<1
Adrenal neuroblastoma	<0.1
Lymphomas (including primary adrenal lymphoma)	<1
Metastases (most frequent: breast, lung)	15

Note: Bilateral adrenal enlargement/masses may be caused by congenital adrenal hyperplasia, bilateral macronodular hyperplasia, bilateral hemorrhage (due to antiphospholipid syndrome or sepsis-associated Waterhouse-Friderichsen syndrome), granuloma, amyloidosis, or infiltrative disease including tuberculosis.

catecholamine excess from a pheochromocytoma arising from the adrenal medulla is a mandatory part of the diagnostic workup (Fig. 8-13). Furthermore, autonomous cortisol and aldosterone secretion resulting in Cushing's syndrome or primary aldosteronism, respectively, require exclusion. Adrenal incidentalomas can be associated with lower levels of autonomous cortisol secretion, and patients may lack overt clinical features of Cushing's syndrome. Nonetheless, they may exhibit one or more components of the metabolic syndrome (e.g., obesity, type 2 diabetes, or hypertension). There is ongoing debate about the optimal treatment for these patients with mild or subclinical Cushing's syndrome. Overproduction of adrenal androgen precursors, DHEA and its sulfate, is rare and most frequently seen in the context of adrenocortical carcinoma, as are increased levels of steroid precursors such as 17-hydroxyprogesterone.

For the differentiation of benign from malignant adrenal masses, imaging is relatively sensitive, although specificity is suboptimal. CT is the procedure of choice for imaging the adrenal glands (Fig. 8-11). The risk of adrenocortical carcinoma, pheochromocytoma, and benign adrenal myelolipoma increases with the diameter of the adrenal mass. However, size alone is of poor predictive value, with only 80% sensitivity and 60% specificity for the differentiation of benign from malignant masses when using a 4-cm cut-off. Metastases are found with similar frequency in adrenal masses of all sizes. Tumor density on unenhanced CT is of additional diagnostic value, with most adrenocortical adenomas being lipid rich and thus presenting with low attenuation values (i.e., densities of <10 HU). By contrast, adrenocortical carcinomas, but also pheochromocytomas, usually have high attenuation values (i.e., densities >20 HU on precontrast scans). Generally, benign lesions are rounded and homogenous, whereas most malignant lesions appear lobulated and inhomogeneous. Pheochromocytoma and adrenomyelolipoma may also exhibit lobulated and inhomogeneous features. Additional information can be obtained from CT by assessment of contrast wash-out after 15 min, which is >50% in benign lesions but <40% in malignant lesions, which usually have a more extensive vascularization. MRI also allows for the visualization of the adrenal glands with somewhat lower resolution than CT. However, because it does not involve exposure to ionizing radiation, it is preferred in children, young adults, and during pregnancy. MRI has a valuable role in the characterization of indeterminate adrenal lesions using chemical shift analysis, with malignant tumors rarely showing loss of signal on opposed-phase MRI.

Fine-needle aspiration (FNA) or CT-guided biopsy of an adrenal mass is almost never indicated. FNA of a pheochromocytoma can cause a life-threatening hypertensive crisis. FNA of an adrenocortical carcinoma violates the tumor capsule and can cause needle track metastasis. FNA should only be considered in a patient with a history of nonadrenal malignancy and a newly detected adrenal mass, after careful exclusion of pheochromocytoma, and if the outcome will influence therapeutic management. It is important to recognize that in 25% of patients with a previous history of nonadrenal malignancy, a newly detected mass on CT is not a metastasis.

Adrenal masses associated with confirmed hormone excess or suspected malignancy are usually treated surgically (Fig. 8-13) or, if adrenalectomy is not feasible or desired, with medication. Preoperative exclusion of glucocorticoid excess is particularly important for the prediction of postoperative suppression of the contralateral adrenal gland, which requires glucocorticoid replacement peri- and postoperatively. If the initial

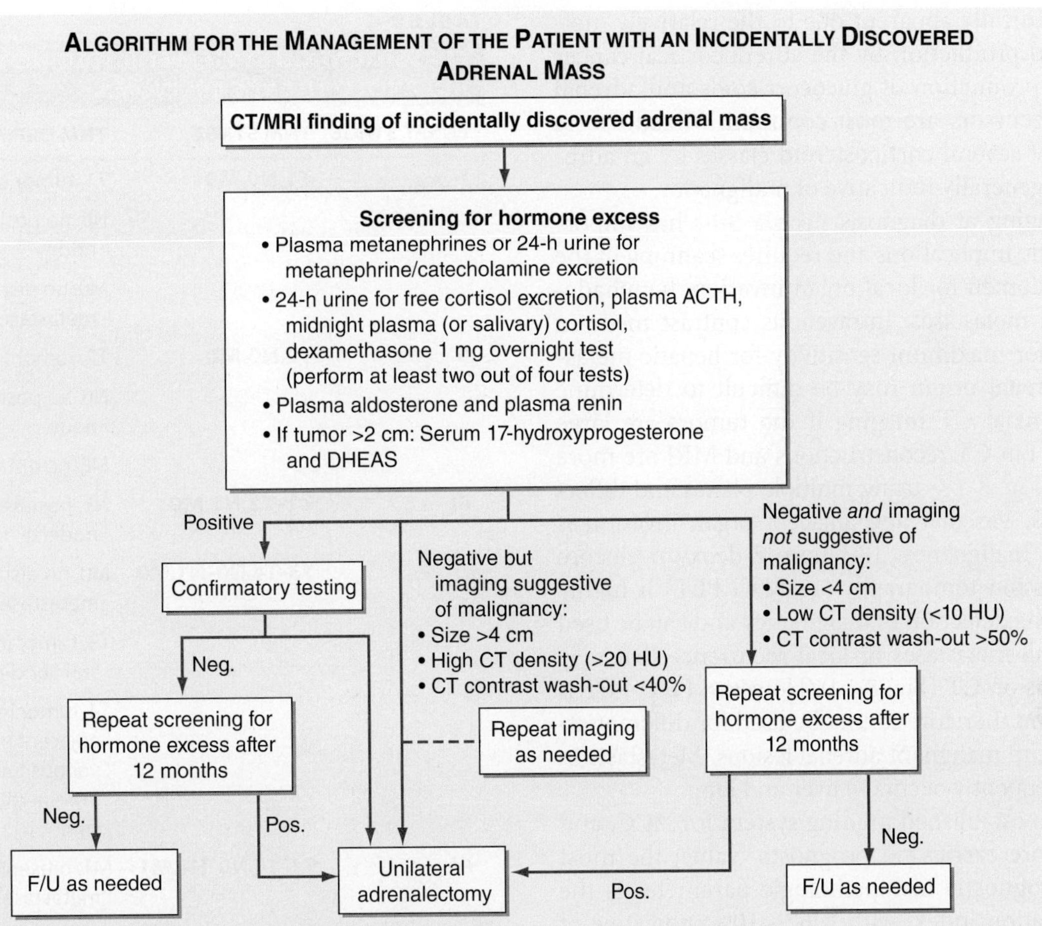

FIGURE 8-13

Management of the patient with an incidentally discovered adrenal mass. CT, computed tomography; F/U, follow-up; MRI, magnetic resonance imaging.

decision is for observation, imaging and biochemical testing should be repeated about a year after the first assessment. However, this may be performed earlier in patients with borderline imaging or hormonal findings. There is no agreement with regard to the required long-term follow-up beyond 1 year in patients with normal biochemistry and no evidence of increased tumor size at follow-up.

ADRENOCORTICAL CARCINOMA

Adrenocortical carcinoma (ACC) is a rare malignancy with an annual incidence of 1–2 per million population. ACC is generally considered a highly malignant tumor; however, it presents with broad interindividual variability with regard to biologic characteristics and clinical behavior. Somatic mutations in the tumor-suppressor gene *TP53* are found in 25% of apparently sporadic ACC. Germline *TP53* mutations are the cause of the Li-Fraumeni syndrome associated with multiple solid organ cancers including ACC and are found in 25% of pediatric ACC cases; the *TP53* mutation R337H is found in almost all pediatric ACC in Brazil. Other genetic changes identified in ACC include alterations in the Wnt/β-catenin pathway and in the insulin-like growth factor 2 (IGF2) cluster; IGF2 overexpression is found in 90% of ACC.

Patients with large adrenal tumors suspicious of malignancy should be managed by a multidisciplinary specialist team, including an endocrinologist, an oncologist, a surgeon, a radiologist, and a histopathologist. FNA is not indicated in suspected ACC: first, cytology and also histopathology of a core biopsy cannot differentiate between benign and malignant primary adrenal masses; second, FNA violates the tumor capsule and may even cause needle canal metastasis. Even when the entire tumor specimen is available, the histopathologic differentiation between benign and malignant lesions is a diagnostic challenge. The most common histopathologic classification is the Weiss score, taking into account high nuclear grade; mitotic rate (>5/HPF); atypical mitosis; <25% clear cells; diffuse architecture; and presence of necrosis, venous invasion, and invasion of sinusoidal structures and tumor capsule. The presence of three or more elements suggests ACC.

Although 60–70% of ACCs show biochemical evidence of steroid overproduction, in many patients, this is not clinically apparent due to the relatively inefficient steroid production by the adrenocortical cancer cells. Excess production of glucocorticoids and adrenal androgen precursors are most common. Mixed excess production of several corticosteroid classes by an adrenal tumor is generally indicative of malignancy.

Tumor staging at diagnosis (Table 8-6) has important prognostic implications and requires scanning of the chest and abdomen for local organ invasion, lymphadenopathy, and metastases. Intravenous contrast medium is necessary for maximum sensitivity for hepatic metastases. An adrenal origin may be difficult to determine on standard axial CT imaging if the tumors are large and invasive, but CT reconstructions and MRI are more informative (Fig. 8-14) using multiple planes and different sequences. Vascular and adjacent organ invasion is diagnostic of malignancy. 18-Fluoro-2-deoxy-D-glucose positron emission tomography (18-FDG PET) is highly sensitive for the detection of malignancy and can be used to detect small metastases or local recurrence that may not be obvious on CT (Fig. 8-14). However, FDG PET is not specific and therefore cannot be used for differentiating benign from malignant adrenal lesions. Metastasis in ACC most frequently occurs to liver and lung.

There is no established grading system for ACC, and the Weiss score carries no prognostic value; the most important prognostic histopathologic parameter is the Ki67 proliferation index, with Ki67 <10% indicative of slow to moderate growth velocity, whereas a Ki67 ≥10% is associated with poor prognosis including high risk of recurrence and rapid progression.

TABLE 8-6

CLASSIFICATION SYSTEM FOR STAGING OF ADRENOCORTICAL CARCINOMA

ENSAT STAGE	TNM STAGE	TNM DEFINITIONS
I	T1,N0,M0	T1, tumor ≤5 cm N0, no positive lymph node M0, no distant metastases
II	T2,N0,M0	T2, tumor >5 cm N0, no positive lymph node M0, no distant metastases
III	T1–T2,N1,M0	N1, positive lymph node(s)
	T3–T4,N0–N1,M0	M0, no distant metastases T3, tumor infiltration into surrounding tissue T4, tumor invasion into adjacent organs *or* venous tumor thrombus in vena cava or renal vein
IV	T1–T4,N0–N1,M1	M1, presence of distant metastases

Abbreviations: ENSAT, European Network for the Study of Adrenal Tumors; TNM, tumor, node, metastasis.

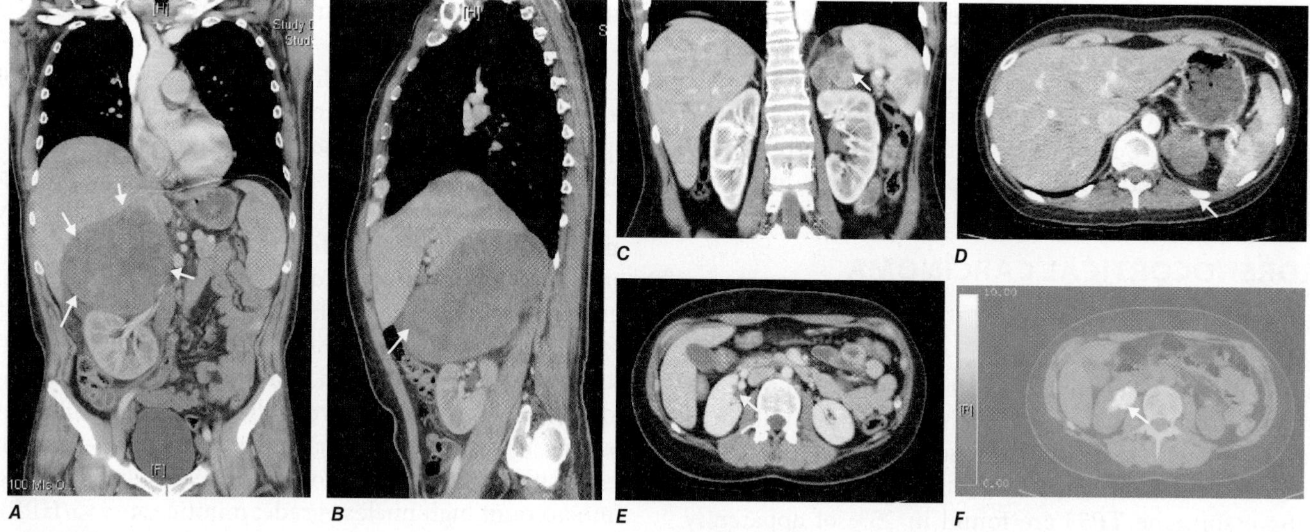

FIGURE 8-14

Imaging in adrenocortical carcinoma. Magnetic resonance imaging scan with ***A.*** frontal and ***B.*** lateral views of a right adrenocortical carcinoma that was detected incidentally. Computed tomography (CT) scan with ***C.*** coronal and ***D.*** transverse views depicting a right-sided adrenocortical carcinoma. Note the irregular border and inhomogeneous structure. CT scan ***E.*** and positron emission tomography/CT ***F.*** visualizing a peritoneal metastasis of an adrenocortical carcinoma in close proximity to the right kidney (*arrow*).

Cure of ACC can only be achieved by early detection and complete surgical removal. Capsule violation during primary surgery, metastasis at diagnosis, and primary treatment in a nonspecialist center are major determinants of poor survival. If the primary tumor invades adjacent organs, en bloc removal of kidney and spleen should be considered to reduce the risk of recurrence. Surgery can also be considered in a patient with metastases if there is severe tumor-related hormone excess. This indication needs to be carefully weighed against surgical risk, including thromboembolic complications, and the resulting delay in the introduction of other therapeutic options. Patients with confirmed ACC and successful removal of the primary tumor should receive adjuvant treatment with mitotane (o,p'DDD), particularly in patients with a high risk of recurrence as determined by tumor size >8 cm, histopathologic signs of vascular invasion, capsule invasion or violation, and a Ki67 proliferation index ≥10%. Adjuvant mitotane should be continued for at least 2 years, if the patient can tolerate side effects. Regular monitoring of plasma mitotane levels is mandatory (therapeutic range 14–20 mg/L; neurotoxic complications more frequent at >20 mg/L). Mitotane is usually started at 500 mg tid, with stepwise increases to a maximum dose of 2000 mg tid in days (high-dose saturation) or weeks (low-dose saturation) as tolerated. Once therapeutic range plasma mitotane levels are achieved, the dose can be tapered to maintenance doses mostly ranging from 1000 to 1500 mg tid. Mitotane treatment results in disruption of cortisol synthesis and thus requires glucocorticoid replacement; glucocorticoid replacement dose should be at least double of that usually used in adrenal insufficiency (i.e., 20 mg tid) because mitotane induces hepatic CYP3A4 activity resulting in rapid inactivation of glucocorticoids. Mitotane also increases circulating CBG, thereby decreasing the available free cortisol fraction. Single metastases can be addressed surgically or with radiofrequency ablation as appropriate. If the tumor recurs or progresses during mitotane treatment, chemotherapy should be considered; the established first-line chemotherapy regimen is the combination of cisplatin, etoposide, and doxorubicin plus continuing mitotane. Painful bone metastasis responds to irradiation. Overall survival in ACC is still poor, with 5-year survival rates of 30–40% and a median survival of 15 months in metastatic ACC.

ADRENAL INSUFFICIENCY

Epidemiology

The prevalence of well-documented, permanent adrenal insufficiency is 5 in 10,000 in the general population. Hypothalamic-pituitary origin of disease is most frequent, with a prevalence of 3 in 10,000, whereas primary adrenal insufficiency has a prevalence of 2 in 10,000. Approximately one-half of the latter cases are acquired, mostly caused by autoimmune destruction of the adrenal glands; the other one-half are genetic, most commonly caused by distinct enzymatic blocks in adrenal steroidogenesis affecting glucocorticoid synthesis (i.e., congenital adrenal hyperplasia.)

Adrenal insufficiency arising from suppression of the HPA axis as a consequence of exogenous glucocorticoid treatment is much more common, occurring in 0.5–2% of the population in developed countries.

Etiology

Primary adrenal insufficiency is most commonly caused by autoimmune adrenalitis. Isolated autoimmune adrenalitis accounts for 30–40%, whereas 60–70% develop adrenal insufficiency as part of autoimmune polyglandular syndromes (APS) **(Chap. 29)** (Table 8-7). APS1, also termed APECED (autoimmune polyendocrinopathy-candidiasis-ectodermal dystrophy), is the underlying cause in 10% of patients affected by APS. APS1 is transmitted in an autosomal recessive manner and is caused by mutations in the autoimmune regulator gene *AIRE*. Associated autoimmune conditions overlap with those seen in APS2, but may also include total alopecia, primary hypoparathyroidism, and, in rare cases, lymphoma. APS1 patients invariably develop chronic mucocutaneous candidiasis, usually manifest in childhood, and preceding adrenal insufficiency by years or decades. The much more prevalent APS2 is of polygenic inheritance, with confirmed associations with the *HLA-DR3* gene region in the major histocompatibility complex and distinct gene regions involved in immune regulation (*CTLA-4, PTPN22, CLEC16A*). Coincident autoimmune disease most frequently includes thyroid autoimmune disease, vitiligo, and premature ovarian failure. Less commonly, additional features may include type 1 diabetes and pernicious anemia caused by vitamin B_{12} deficiency.

X-linked adrenoleukodystrophy has an incidence of 1:20,000 males and is caused by mutations in the *X-ALD* gene encoding the peroxisomal membrane transporter protein ABCD1; its disruption results in accumulation of very long chain (>24 carbon atoms) fatty acids. Approximately 50% of cases manifest in early childhood with rapidly progressive white matter disease (cerebral ALD); 35% present during adolescence or in early adulthood with neurologic features indicative of myelin and peripheral nervous system involvement (adrenomyeloneuropathy [AMN]). In the remaining 15%, adrenal insufficiency is the sole manifestation of disease. Of note, distinct mutations manifest with variable penetrance and phenotypes within affected families.

Rarer causes of adrenal insufficiency involve destruction of the adrenal glands as a consequence of infection, hemorrhage, or infiltration (Table 8-7); tuberculous adrenalitis is still a frequent cause of disease in developing countries.

TABLE 8-7

CAUSES OF PRIMARY ADRENAL INSUFFICIENCY

DIAGNOSIS	GENE	ASSOCIATED FEATURES
Autoimmune polyglandular syndrome 1 (APS1)	*AIRE*	Hypoparathyroidism, chronic mucocutaneous candidiasis, other autoimmune disorders, rarely lymphomas
Autoimmune polyglandular syndrome 2 (APS2)	Associations with HLA-DR3, CTLA-4	Hypothyroidism, hyperthyroidism, premature ovarian failure, vitiligo, type 1 diabetes mellitus, pernicious anemia
Isolated autoimmune adrenalitis	Associations with HLA-DR3, CTLA-4	
Congenital adrenal hyperplasia (CAH)	*CYP21A2, CYP11B1, CYP17A1, HSD3B2, POR*	See Table 8-10 (see also **Chap. 10**)
Congenital lipoid adrenal hyperplasia (CLAH)	*STAR, CYP11A1*	46,XY DSD, gonadal failure (see also **Chap. 10**)
Adrenal hypoplasia congenita (AHC)	*NR0B1 (DAX-1), NR5A1 (SF-1)*	46,XY DSD, gonadal failure (see also **Chap. 10**)
Adrenoleukodystrophy (ALD), adrenomyeloneuropathy (AMN)	*X-ALD*	Demyelination of central nervous system (ALD) or spinal cord and peripheral nerves (AMN)
Familial glucocorticoid deficiency	*MC2R*	Tall stature
	MRAP	None
	STAR	None
	NNT	None
	MCM4	Growth retardation, natural killer cell deficiency
Triple A syndrome	*AAAS*	Alacrima, achalasia, neurologic impairment
Smith-Lemli-Opitz syndrome	*SLOS*	Cholesterol synthesis disorder associated with mental retardation, craniofacial malformations, growth failure
Kearns-Sayre syndrome	Mitochondrial DNA deletions	Progressive external ophthalmoplegia, pigmentary retinal degeneration, cardiac conduction defects, gonadal failure, hypoparathyroidism, type 1 diabetes,
IMAGe syndrome	*CDKN1C*	Intrauterine growth retardation, metaphyseal dysplasia, genital anomalies
Adrenal infections		Tuberculosis, HIV, CMV, cryptococcosis, histoplasmosis, coccidioidomycosis
Adrenal infiltration		Metastases, lymphomas, sarcoidosis, amyloidosis, hemochromatosis
Adrenal hemorrhage		Meningococcal sepsis (Waterhouse-Friderichsen syndrome), primary antiphospholipid syndrome
Drug-induced		Mitotane, aminoglutethimide, abiraterone, trilostane, etomidate, ketoconazole, suramin, RU486
Bilateral adrenalectomy		E.g., in the management of Cushing's or after bilateral nephrectomy

Abbreviations: AIRE, autoimmune regulator; CMV, cytomegalovirus; DSD, disordered sex development; MC2R, ACTH receptor; MCM4, mini chromosome maintenance-deficient 4 homologue; MRAP, MC2R-accessory protein; NNT, nicotinamide nucleotide transhydrogenase.

TABLE 8-8

CAUSES OF SECONDARY ADRENAL INSUFFICIENCY

DIAGNOSIS	GENE	ASSOCIATED FEATURES
Pituitary tumors (endocrine active and inactive adenomas, very rare: carcinoma)		Depending on tumor size and location: visual field impairment (bilateral hemianopia), hyperprolactinemia, secondary hypothyroidism, hypogonadism, growth hormone deficiency
Other mass lesions affecting the hypothalamic-pituitary region		Craniopharyngioma, meningioma, ependymoma, metastases
Pituitary irradiation		Radiotherapy administered for pituitary tumors, brain tumors, or craniospinal irradiation in leukemia
Autoimmune hypophysitis		Often associated with pregnancy; may present with panhypopituitarism or isolated ACTH deficiency; can be associated with autoimmune thyroid disease, more rarely with vitiligo, premature ovarian failure, type 1 diabetes, pernicious anemia
Pituitary apoplexy/hemorrhage		Hemorrhagic infarction of large pituitary adenomas or pituitary infarction consequent to traumatic major blood loss (e.g., surgery or pregnancy: Sheehan's syndrome)
Pituitary infiltration		Tuberculosis, actinomycosis, sarcoidosis, histiocytosis X, granulomatosis with polyangiitis (Wegener's), metastases
Drug-induced		Chronic glucocorticoid excess (endogenous or exogenous)
Congenital isolated ACTH deficiency	*TBX19* (Tpit)	
Combined pituitary hormone deficiency (CPHD)	*PROP-1*	Progressive development of CPHD in the order GH, PRL, TSH, LH/FSH, ACTH
	HESX1	CPHD and septo-optic dysplasia
	LHX3	CPHD and limited neck rotation, sensorineural deafness
	LHX4	CPHD and cerebellar abnormalities
	SOX3	CPHD and variable mental retardation
Proopiomelanocortin (POMC) deficiency	*POMC*	Early-onset obesity, red hair pigmentation

Abbreviations: ACTH, adrenocorticotropic hormone; GH, growth hormone; LH/FSH, luteinizing hormone/follicle-stimulating hormone; PRL, prolactin; TSH, thyroid-stimulating hormone.

Adrenal metastases rarely cause adrenal insufficiency, and this occurs only with bilateral, bulky metastases.

Inborn causes of primary adrenal insufficiency other than congenital adrenal hyperplasia are rare, causing less than 1% of cases. However, their elucidation provides important insights into adrenal gland development and physiology. Mutations causing primary adrenal insufficiency (Table 8-7) include factors regulating adrenal development and steroidogenesis (DAX-1, SF-1), cholesterol synthesis, import and cleavage (DHCR7, StAR, CYP11A1), and elements of the adrenal ACTH response pathway (MC2R, MRAP) (Fig. 8-5), and factors involved in redox regulation (NNT) and DNA repair (MCM4, CDKN1C).

Secondary adrenal insufficiency is the consequence of dysfunction of the hypothalamic-pituitary component of the HPA axis (Table 8-8). Excluding iatrogenic suppression, the overwhelming majority of cases are caused by pituitary or hypothalamic tumors or their treatment by surgery or irradiation **(Chap. 5)**. Rarer causes include pituitary apoplexy, either as a consequence of an infarcted pituitary adenoma or transient reduction in the blood supply of the pituitary during surgery or after rapid blood loss associated with parturition, also termed Sheehan's syndrome. Isolated ACTH deficiency is rarely caused by autoimmune disease or pituitary infiltration (Table 8-8). Mutations in the ACTH precursor POMC or in factors regulating pituitary development are genetic causes of ACTH deficiency (Table 8-8).

Clinical manifestations

In principle, the clinical features of primary adrenal insufficiency (Addison's disease) are characterized by the loss of both glucocorticoid and mineralocorticoid secretion (Table 8-9). In secondary adrenal insufficiency, only glucocorticoid deficiency is present, as the adrenal itself is intact and thus still amenable to regulation by the RAA system. Adrenal androgen secretion is disrupted in both primary and secondary adrenal insufficiency (Table 8-9). Hypothalamic-pituitary disease can lead to additional clinical manifestations due to involvement of other endocrine

TABLE 8-9

SIGNS AND SYMPTOMS OF ADRENAL INSUFFICIENCY
Signs and Symptoms Caused by Glucocorticoid Deficiency
TB>Fatigue, lack of energy
Weight loss, anorexia
Myalgia, joint pain
Fever
Normochromic anemia, lymphocytosis, eosinophilia
Slightly increased TSH (due to loss of feedback inhibition of TSH release)
Hypoglycemia (more frequent in children)
Low blood pressure, postural hypotension
Hyponatremia (due to loss of feedback inhibition of AVP release)
Signs and Symptoms Caused by Mineralocorticoid Deficiency (Primary Adrenal Insufficiency Only)
Abdominal pain, nausea, vomiting
Dizziness, postural hypotension
Salt craving
Low blood pressure, postural hypotension
Increased serum creatinine (due to volume depletion)
Hyponatremia
Hyperkalemia
Signs and Symptoms Caused by Adrenal Androgen Deficiency
Lack of energy
Dry and itchy skin (in women)
Loss of libido (in women)
Loss of axillary and pubic hair (in women)
Other Signs and Symptoms
Hyperpigmentation (primary adrenal insufficiency only) (due to excess of proopiomelanocortin [POMC]-derived peptides)
Alabaster-colored pale skin (secondary adrenal insufficiency only) (due to deficiency of POMC-derived peptides)

Abbreviations: AVP, arginine vasopressin; TSH, thyroid-stimulating hormone.

axes (thyroid, gonads, growth hormone, prolactin) or visual impairment with bitemporal hemianopia caused by chiasmal compression. It is important to recognize that iatrogenic adrenal insufficiency caused by exogenous glucocorticoid suppression of the HPA axis may result in all symptoms associated with glucocorticoid deficiency (Table 8-9), if exogenous glucocorticoids are stopped abruptly. However, patients will appear clinically cushingoid as a result of the preceding overexposure to glucocorticoids.

Chronic adrenal insufficiency manifests with relatively nonspecific signs and symptoms such as fatigue and loss of energy, often resulting in delayed or missed diagnoses (e.g., as depression or anorexia). A distinguishing feature of primary adrenal insufficiency is hyperpigmentation, which is caused by excess ACTH stimulation of melanocytes. Hyperpigmentation is most pronounced in skin areas exposed to increased friction or shear stress and is increased by sunlight (Fig. 8-15). Conversely, in secondary adrenal insufficiency, the skin has an alabaster-like paleness due to lack of ACTH secretion.

Hyponatremia is a characteristic biochemical feature in primary adrenal insufficiency and is found in 80% of patients at presentation. Hyperkalemia is present in 40% of patients at initial diagnosis. Hyponatremia is primarily caused by mineralocorticoid deficiency but can also occur in secondary adrenal insufficiency due to diminished inhibition of antidiuretic hormone (ADH) release by cortisol, resulting in mild syndrome of inappropriate secretion of antidiuretic hormone (SIADH). Glucocorticoid deficiency also results in slightly increased TSH concentrations that normalize within days to weeks after initiation of glucocorticoid replacement.

Acute adrenal insufficiency usually occurs after a prolonged period of nonspecific complaints and is more frequently observed in patients with primary adrenal insufficiency, due to the loss of both glucocorticoid and mineralocorticoid secretion. Postural hypotension may progress to hypovolemic shock. Adrenal insufficiency may mimic features of acute abdomen with abdominal tenderness, nausea, vomiting, and fever. In some cases, the primary presentation may resemble neurologic disease, with decreased responsiveness, progressing to stupor and coma. An adrenal crisis can be triggered by an intercurrent illness, surgical or other stress, or increased glucocorticoid inactivation (e.g., hyperthyroidism).

Diagnosis

The diagnosis of adrenal insufficiency is established by the short cosyntropin test, a safe and reliable tool with excellent predictive diagnostic value (Fig. 8-16). The cut-off for failure is usually defined at cortisol levels of <500–550 nmol/L (18–20 μg/dL) sampled 30–60 min after ACTH stimulation; the exact cut-off is dependent on the locally available assay. During the early phase of HPA disruption (e.g., within 4 weeks of pituitary insufficiency), patients may still respond to exogenous ACTH stimulation. In this circumstance, the ITT is an alternative choice but is more invasive and should be carried out only under a specialist's supervision (see above). Induction of hypoglycemia is contraindicated in individuals with diabetes mellitus, cardiovascular disease, or history of seizures. Random serum cortisol measurements are of limited diagnostic value, because baseline cortisol levels may be coincidentally low due to the physiologic diurnal rhythm of cortisol secretion (Fig. 8-3). Similarly, many patients with secondary adrenal insufficiency have relatively normal baseline cortisol levels but fail to mount an appropriate cortisol response to ACTH, which can only

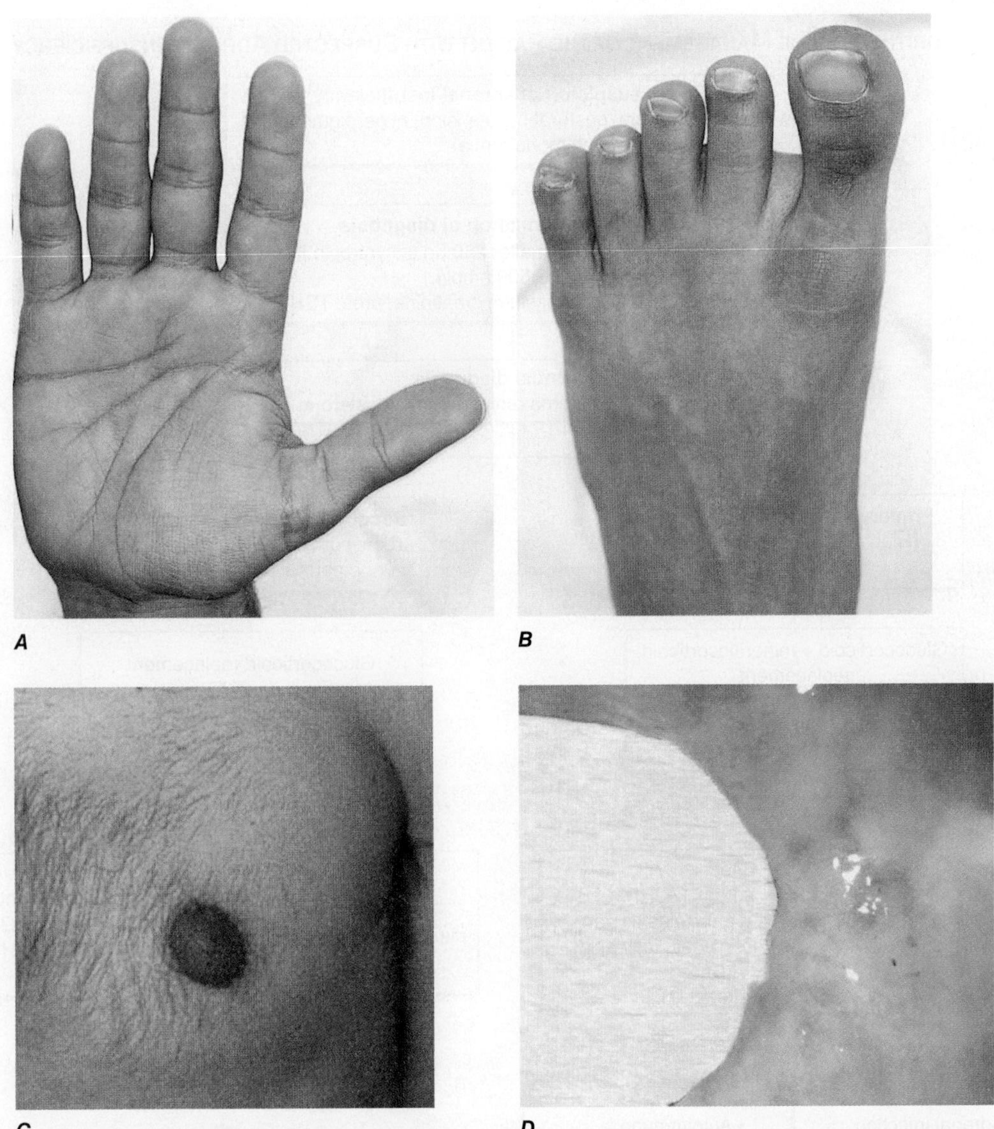

FIGURE 8-15
Clinical features of Addison's disease. Note the hyperpigmentation in areas of increased friction including ***A.*** palmar creases, ***B.*** dorsal foot, ***C.*** nipples and axillary region, and ***D.*** patchy hyperpigmentation of the oral mucosa.

be revealed by stimulation testing. Importantly, tests to establish the diagnosis of adrenal insufficiency should never delay treatment. Thus, in a patient with suspected adrenal crisis, it is reasonable to draw baseline cortisol levels, provide replacement therapy, and defer formal stimulation testing until a later time.

Once adrenal insufficiency is confirmed, measurement of plasma ACTH is the next step, with increased or inappropriately low levels defining primary and secondary origin of disease, respectively (Fig. 8-16). In primary adrenal insufficiency, increased plasma renin will confirm the presence of mineralocorticoid deficiency. At initial presentation, patients with primary adrenal insufficiency should undergo screening for steroid autoantibodies as a marker of autoimmune adrenalitis. If these tests are negative, adrenal imaging by CT is indicated to investigate possible hemorrhage, infiltration, or masses. In male patients with negative autoantibodies in the plasma, very-long-chain fatty acids should be measured to exclude X-ALD. Patients with inappropriately low ACTH, in the presence of confirmed cortisol deficiency, should undergo hypothalamic-pituitary imaging by MRI. Features suggestive of preceding pituitary apoplexy, such as sudden-onset severe headache or history of previous head trauma, should be carefully explored, particularly in patients with no obvious MRI lesion.

TREATMENT Acute Adrenal Insufficiency

Acute adrenal insufficiency requires immediate initiation of rehydration, usually carried out by saline infusion at initial rates of 1 L/h with continuous cardiac monitoring. Glucocorticoid replacement should be initiated by bolus injection of 100 mg hydrocortisone, followed by the administration of 100–200 mg hydrocortisone over 24 h, either by continuous

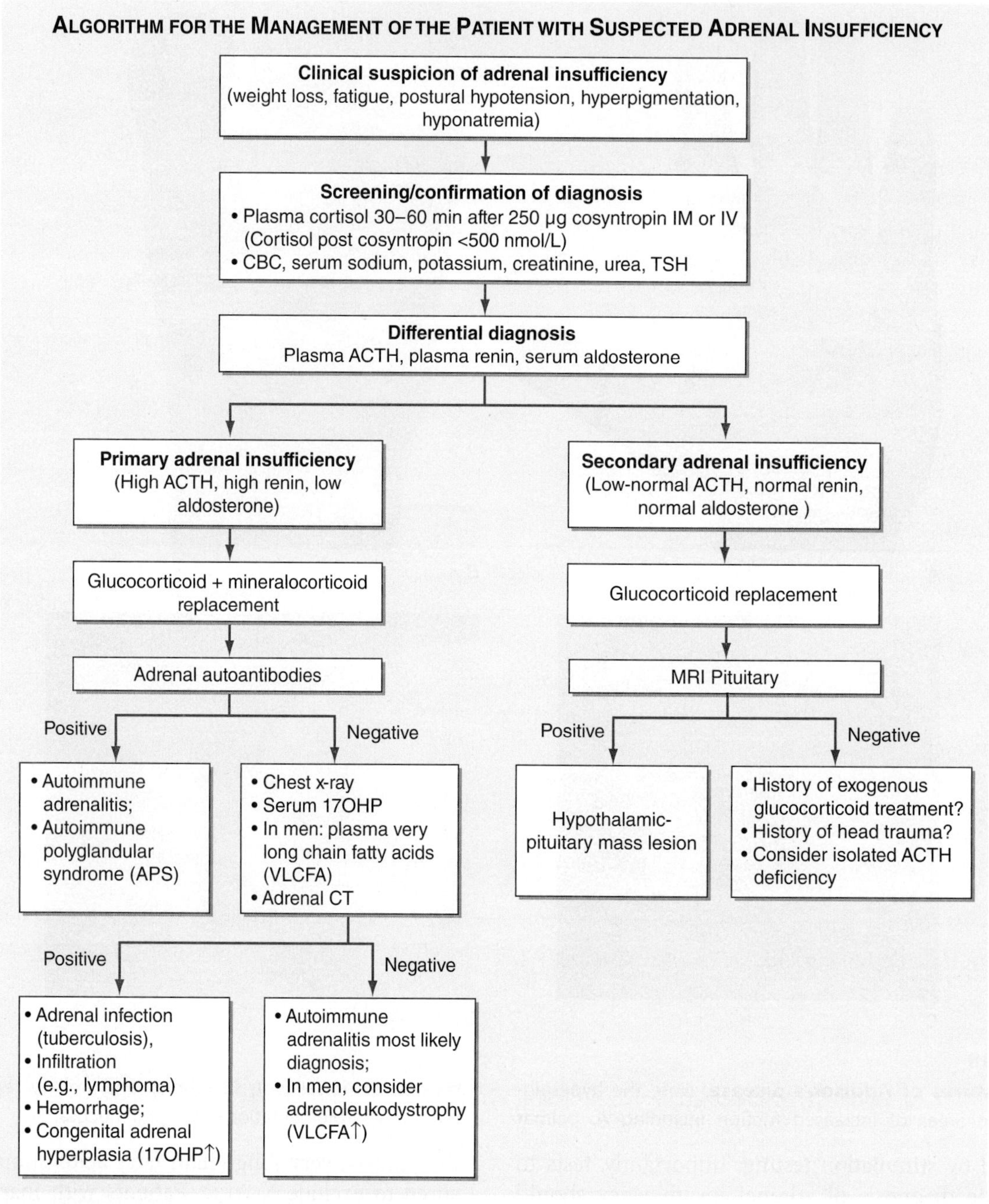

ALGORITHM FOR THE MANAGEMENT OF THE PATIENT WITH SUSPECTED ADRENAL INSUFFICIENCY

Clinical suspicion of adrenal insufficiency
(weight loss, fatigue, postural hypotension, hyperpigmentation, hyponatremia)

↓

Screening/confirmation of diagnosis
- Plasma cortisol 30–60 min after 250 µg cosyntropin IM or IV (Cortisol post cosyntropin <500 nmol/L)
- CBC, serum sodium, potassium, creatinine, urea, TSH

↓

Differential diagnosis
Plasma ACTH, plasma renin, serum aldosterone

↓

Primary adrenal insufficiency
(High ACTH, high renin, low aldosterone)

↓ Glucocorticoid + mineralocorticoid replacement

↓ Adrenal autoantibodies

- Positive:
  - Autoimmune adrenalitis;
  - Autoimmune polyglandular syndrome (APS)
- Negative:
  - Chest x-ray
  - Serum 17OHP
  - In men: plasma very long chain fatty acids (VLCFA)
  - Adrenal CT
  - Positive:
    - Adrenal infection (tuberculosis),
    - Infiltration (e.g., lymphoma)
    - Hemorrhage;
    - Congenital adrenal hyperplasia (17OHP↑)
  - Negative:
    - Autoimmune adrenalitis most likely diagnosis;
    - In men, consider adrenoleukodystrophy (VLCFA↑)

Secondary adrenal insufficiency
(Low-normal ACTH, normal renin, normal aldosterone)

↓ Glucocorticoid replacement

↓ MRI Pituitary

- Positive:
  - Hypothalamic-pituitary mass lesion
- Negative:
  - History of exogenous glucocorticoid treatment?
  - History of head trauma?
  - Consider isolated ACTH deficiency

FIGURE 8-16

Management of the patient with suspected adrenal insufficiency. ACTH, adrenocorticotropic hormone; CBC, complete blood count; MRI, magnetic resonance imaging; PRA, plasma renin activity; TSH, thyroid-stimulating hormone.

infusion or by bolus IV or IM injections. Mineralocorticoid replacement can be initiated once the daily hydrocortisone dose has been reduced to <50 mg because at higher doses hydrocortisone provides sufficient stimulation of mineralocorticoid receptors.

Glucocorticoid replacement for the treatment of chronic adrenal insufficiency should be administered at a dose that replaces the physiologic daily cortisol production, which is usually achieved by the oral administration of 15–25 mg hydrocortisone in two to three divided doses. Pregnancy may require an increase in hydrocortisone dose by 50% during the last trimester. In all patients, at least one-half of the daily dose should be administered in the morning. Currently available glucocorticoid preparations fail to mimic the physiologic cortisol secretion rhythm (Fig. 8-3). Long-acting glucocorticoids such as prednisolone or dexamethasone are not preferred because they result in increased glucocorticoid exposure due to extended glucocorticoid receptor activation at times of physiologically low cortisol secretion. There are no well-established dose equivalencies, but as a guide, equipotency can be assumed for 1 mg hydrocortisone, 1.6 mg cortisone acetate, 0.2 mg prednisolone, 0.25 mg prednisone, and 0.025 mg dexamethasone.

Monitoring of glucocorticoid replacement is mainly based on the history and examination for signs and symptoms suggestive of glucocorticoid over- or underreplacement, including assessment of body weight and blood pressure. Plasma ACTH, 24-h urinary free cortisol, or serum cortisol day curves reflect whether hydrocortisone has been taken or not, but do not convey reliable information about replacement quality. In patients with isolated primary adrenal insufficiency, monitoring should include screening for autoimmune thyroid disease, and female patients should be made aware of the possibility of premature ovarian failure. Supraphysiologic glucocorticoid treatment with doses equivalent to 30 mg hydrocortisone or more will affect bone metabolism, and these patients should undergo regular bone mineral density evaluation. All patients with adrenal insufficiency need to be instructed about the requirement for stress-related glucocorticoid dose adjustments. These generally consist of doubling the routine oral glucocorticoid dose in the case of intercurrent illness with fever and bed rest and the need for IV hydrocortisone injection at a daily dose of 100 mg in cases of prolonged vomiting, surgery, or trauma. Patients living or traveling in regions with delayed access to acute health care should carry a hydrocortisone self-injection emergency kit, in addition to their usual steroid emergency cards and bracelets.

Mineralocorticoid replacement in primary adrenal insufficiency should be initiated at a dose of 100–150 μg fludrocortisone. The adequacy of treatment can be evaluated by measuring blood pressure, sitting and standing, to detect a postural drop indicative of hypovolemia. In addition, serum sodium, potassium, and plasma renin should be measured regularly. Renin levels should be kept in the upper normal reference range. Changes in glucocorticoid dose may also impact on mineralocorticoid replacement as cortisol also binds the mineralocorticoid receptor; 40 mg hydrocortisone is equivalent to 100 μg fludrocortisone. In patients living or traveling in areas with hot or tropical weather conditions, the fludrocortisone dose should be increased by 50–100 μg during the summer. Mineralocorticoid dose may also need to be adjusted during pregnancy, due to the antimineralocorticoid activity of progesterone, but this is less often required than hydrocortisone dose adjustment. Plasma renin cannot serve as a monitoring tool during pregnancy, because renin rises physiologically during gestation.

Adrenal androgen replacement is an option in patients with lack of energy, despite optimized glucocorticoid and mineralocorticoid replacement. It may also be indicated in women with features of androgen deficiency, including loss of libido. Adrenal androgen replacement can be achieved by once-daily administration of 25–50 mg DHEA. Treatment is monitored by measurement of DHEAS, androstenedione, testosterone, and sex hormone–binding globulin (SHBG) 24 h after the last DHEA dose.

CONGENITAL ADRENAL HYPERPLASIA

(See also Chap. 10) Congenital adrenal hyperplasia (CAH) is caused by mutations in genes encoding steroidogenic enzymes involved in glucocorticoid synthesis (*CYP21A2, CYP17A1, HSD3B2, CYP11B1*) or in the cofactor enzyme P450 oxidoreductase that serves as an electron donor to CYP21A2 and CYP17A1 (Fig. 8-1). Invariably, patients affected by CAH exhibit glucocorticoid deficiency. Depending on the exact step of enzymatic block, they may also have excess production of mineralocorticoids or deficient production of sex steroids (Table 8-10). The diagnosis of CAH is readily established by measurement of the steroids accumulating before the distinct enzymatic block, either in serum or in urine, preferably by the use of mass spectrometry–based assays (Table 8-10).

TABLE 8-10

VARIANTS OF CONGENITAL ADRENAL HYPERPLASIA

VARIANT	GENE	IMPACT ON STEROID SYNTHESIS	DIAGNOSTIC MARKER STEROIDS IN SERUM (AND URINE)
21-Hydroxylase deficiency (21OHD)	*CYP21A2*	Glucocorticoid deficiency, mineralocorticoid deficiency, adrenal androgen excess	17-Hydroxyprogesterone, 21-deoxycortisol (pregnanetriol, 17-hydroxypregnanolone, pregnanetriolone)
11β-Hydroxylase deficiency (11OHD)	*CYP11B1*	Glucocorticoid deficiency, mineralocorticoid excess, adrenal androgen excess	11-Deoxycortisol, 11-deoxycorticosterone (tetrahydro-11-deoxycortisol, tetrahydro-11-deoxycorticosterone)
17α-Hydroxylase deficiency (17OHD)	*CYP17A1*	(Glucocorticoid deficiency), mineralocorticoid excess, androgen deficiency	11-Deoxycorticosterone, corticosterone, pregnenolone, progesterone (tetrahydro-11-deoxycorticosterone, tetrahydrocorticosterone, pregnenediol, pregnanediol)
3β-Hydroxysteroid dehydrogenase deficiency (3bHSDD)	*HSD3B2*	Glucocorticoid deficiency, (mineralocorticoid deficiency), adrenal androgen excess (females and males), gonadal androgen deficiency (males)	17-Hydroxypregnanolone (pregnanetriol)
P450 oxidoreductase deficiency (ORD)	*POR*	Glucocorticoid deficiency, (mineralocorticoid excess), androgen deficiency, skeletal malformations	Pregnenolone, progesterone, 17-hydroxyprogesterone (pregnanediol, pregnanetriol)

Mutations in *CYP21A2* are the most prevalent cause of CAH, responsible for 90–95% of cases. 21-Hydroxylase deficiency disrupts glucocorticoid and mineralocorticoid synthesis (Fig. 8-1), resulting in diminished negative feedback via the HPA axis. This leads to increased pituitary ACTH release, which drives increased synthesis of adrenal androgen precursors and subsequent androgen excess. The degree of impairment of glucocorticoid and mineralocorticoid secretion depends on the severity of mutations. Major loss-of-function mutations result in combined glucocorticoid and mineralocorticoid deficiency (classic CAH, neonatal presentation), whereas less severe mutations affect glucocorticoid synthesis only (simple virilizing CAH, neonatal or early childhood presentation). The mildest mutations result in the least severe clinical phenotype, nonclassic CAH, usually presenting during adolescence and early adulthood and with preserved glucocorticoid production.

Androgen excess is present in all patients and manifests with broad phenotypic variability, ranging from severe virilization of the external genitalia in neonatal girls (e.g., 46,XX disordered sex development [DSD]) to hirsutism and oligomenorrhea resembling a polycystic ovary syndrome phenotype in young women with nonclassic CAH. In countries without neonatal screening for CAH, boys with classic CAH usually present with life-threatening adrenal crisis in the first few weeks of life (salt-wasting crisis); a simple-virilizing genotype manifests with precocious pseudo-puberty and advanced bone age in early childhood, whereas men with nonclassic CAH are usually detected only through family screening.

Glucocorticoid treatment is more complex than for other causes of primary adrenal insufficiency as it not only needed to replace missing glucocorticoids but also to control the increased ACTH drive and subsequent androgen excess. Current treatment is hampered by the lack of glucocorticoid preparations that mimic the diurnal cortisol secretion profile, resulting in a prolonged period of ACTH stimulation and subsequent androgen production during the early morning hours. In childhood, optimization of growth and pubertal development are important goals of glucocorticoid treatment, in addition to prevention of adrenal crisis and treatment of 46,XX DSD. In adults, the focus shifts to preserving fertility and preventing side effects of glucocorticoid overtreatment, namely, the metabolic syndrome and osteoporosis. Fertility can be compromised in women due to oligomenorrhea/amenorrhea with chronic anovulation as a consequence of androgen excess. Men may develop so-called testicular adrenal rest tumors (Fig. 8-17). These consist of hyperplastic

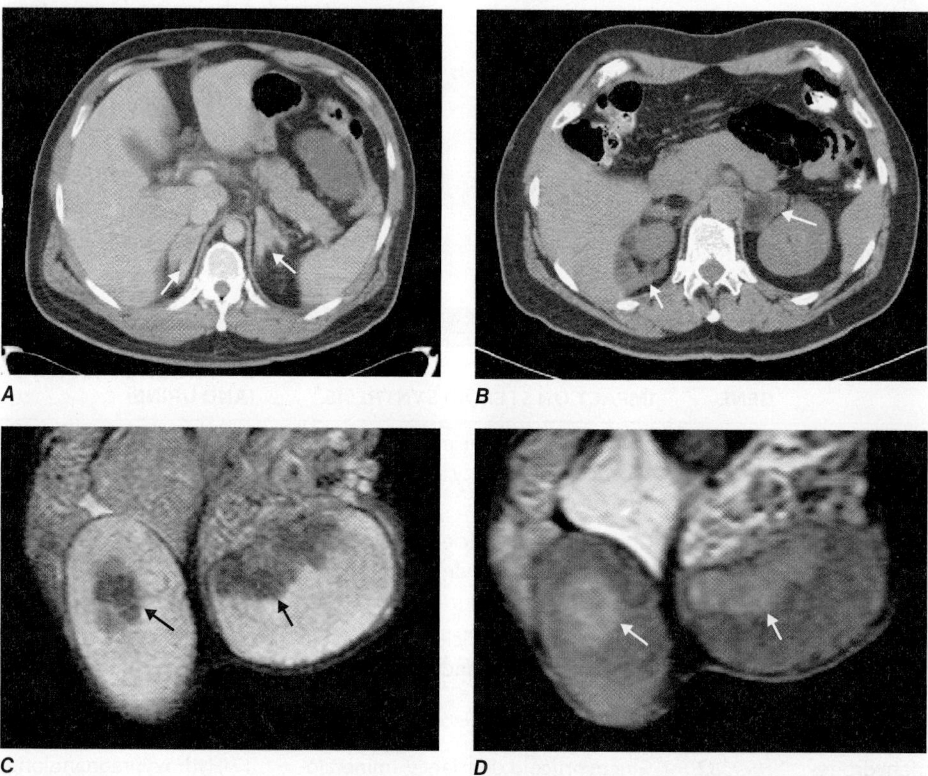

FIGURE 8-17

Imaging in congenital adrenal hyperplasia (CAH). Adrenal computed tomography scans showing homogenous bilateral hyperplasia in a young patient with classic CAH ***A.*** and macronodular bilateral hyperplasia ***B.*** in a middle-aged patient with classic CAH with longstanding poor disease control. Magnetic resonance imaging scan with T1-weighted ***C.*** and T2-weighted ***D.*** images showing bilateral testicular adrenal rest tumors (*arrows*) in a young patient with salt-wasting congenital adrenal hyperplasia. *(Courtesy of N. Reisch.)*

cells with adrenocortical characteristics located in the rete testis and should not be confused with testicular tumors. Testicular adrenal rest tissue can compromise sperm production and induce fibrosis that may be irreversible.

TREATMENT Congenital Adrenal Hyperplasia

Hydrocortisone is a good treatment option for the prevention of adrenal crisis, but longer acting prednisolone may be needed to control androgen excess. In children, hydrocortisone is given in divided doses at 1–1.5 times the normal cortisol production rate (about 10–13 mg/m^2 per day). In adults, if hydrocortisone does not suffice, intermediate-acting glucocorticoids (e.g., prednisone) may be given, using the lowest dose necessary to suppress excess androgen production. For achieving fertility, dexamethasone treatment may be required, but should be only given for the shortest possible time period to limit adverse metabolic side effects. Biochemical monitoring should include androstenedione and testosterone, aiming for the normal sex-specific reference range. 17-Hydroxyprogesterone (17OHP) is a useful marker of overtreatment, indicated by 17OHP levels within the normal range of healthy controls. Glucocorticoid overtreatment may suppress the hypothalamic-pituitary-gonadal axis. Thus, treatment needs to be carefully titrated against clinical features of disease control. Stress dose glucocorticoids should be given at double or triple the daily dose for surgery, acute illness, or severe trauma. Poorly controlled CAH can result in adrenocortical hyperplasia, which gave the disease its name, and may present as macronodular hyperplasia subsequent to long-standing ACTH excess (Fig. 8-17). The nodular areas can develop autonomous adrenal androgen production and may be unresponsive to glucocorticoid treatment.

Mineralocorticoid requirements change during life and are higher in children, explained by relative mineralocorticoid resistance that diminishes with ongoing maturation of the kidney. Children with CAH usually receive mineralocorticoid and salt replacement. However, young adults with CAH should undergo reassessment of their mineralocorticoid reserve. Plasma renin should be regularly monitored and kept within the upper half of the normal reference range.

CHAPTER 9
PHEOCHROMOCYTOMA

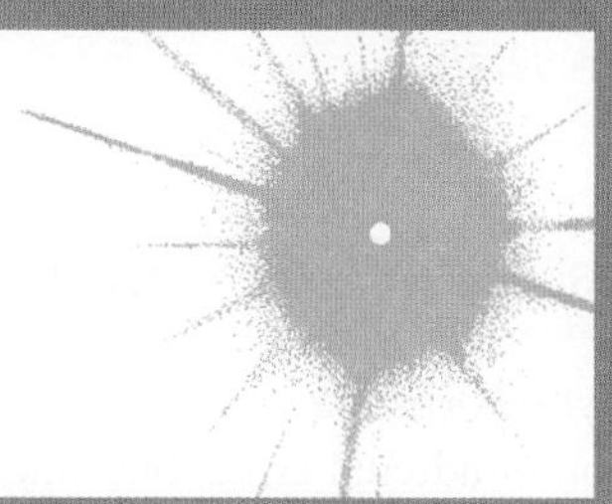

Hartmut P. H. Neumann

Pheochromocytomas and paragangliomas are catecholamine-producing tumors derived from the sympathetic or parasympathetic nervous system. These tumors may arise sporadically or be inherited as features of multiple endocrine neoplasia type 2, von Hippel–Lindau disease, or several other pheochromocytoma-associated syndromes. The diagnosis of pheochromocytomas identifies a potentially correctable cause of hypertension, and their removal can prevent hypertensive crises that can be lethal. The clinical presentation is variable, ranging from an adrenal incidentaloma to a hypertensive crisis with associated cerebrovascular or cardiac complications.

EPIDEMIOLOGY

Pheochromocytoma is estimated to occur in 2–8 of 1 million persons per year, and ~0.1% of hypertensive patients harbor a pheochromocytoma. The mean age at diagnosis is ~40 years, although the tumors can occur from early childhood until late in life. The classic "rule of tens" for pheochromocytomas states that ~10% are bilateral, 10% are extra-adrenal, and 10% are malignant.

ETIOLOGY AND PATHOGENESIS

Pheochromocytomas and paragangliomas are well-vascularized tumors that arise from cells derived from the sympathetic (e.g., adrenal medulla) or parasympathetic (e.g., carotid body, glomus vagale) paraganglia (Fig. 9-1). The name *pheochromocytoma* reflects the black-colored staining caused by chromaffin oxidation of catecholamines; although a variety of terms have been used to describe these tumors, most clinicians use this designation to describe symptomatic catecholamine-producing tumors, including those in extra-adrenal retroperitoneal, pelvic, and thoracic sites. The term *paraganglioma* is used to describe catecholamine-producing tumors in the skull base and neck; these tumors may secrete little or no catecholamine. In contrast to common clinical parlance, the World Health Organization (WHO) restricts the term *pheochromocytoma* to adrenal tumors and applies the term *paraganglioma* to tumors at all other sites.

The etiology of sporadic pheochromocytomas and paragangliomas is unknown. However, 25–33% of patients have an inherited condition, including germline mutations in the classically recognized *RET, VHL, NF1, SDHB, SDHC,* and *SDHD* genes or in the more recently recognized *SDHA, SDHAF2, TMEM127*, and *MAX* genes. Biallelic gene inactivation has been demonstrated for the *VHL, NF1*, and *SDH* genes, whereas *RET* mutations activate receptor tyrosine kinase activity. SDH is an enzyme of the Krebs cycle and the mitochondrial respiratory chain. The VHL protein is a component of a ubiquitin E3 ligase. *VHL* mutations reduce protein degradation, resulting in upregulation of components involved in cell cycle progression, glucose metabolism, and oxygen sensing.

CLINICAL FEATURES

Its clinical presentation is so variable that pheochromocytoma has been termed "the great masquerader" (Table 9-1). Among the presenting manifestations, episodes of palpitation, headache, and profuse sweating are typical, and these manifestations constitute a classic triad. The presence of all three manifestations in association with hypertension makes pheochromocytoma a likely diagnosis. However, a pheochromocytoma can be asymptomatic for years, and some tumors grow to a considerable size before patients note symptoms.

The dominant sign is hypertension. Classically, patients have episodic hypertension, but sustained hypertension is also common. Catecholamine crises can lead to heart failure, pulmonary edema, arrhythmias, and intracranial hemorrhage. During episodes of hormone release, which can occur at widely divergent

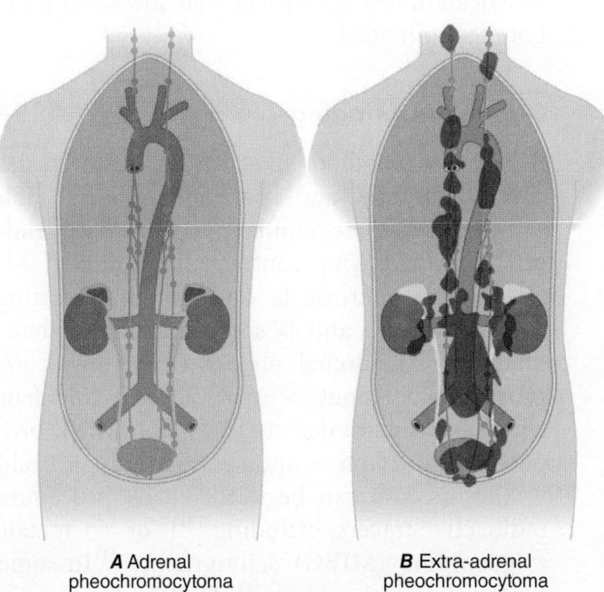

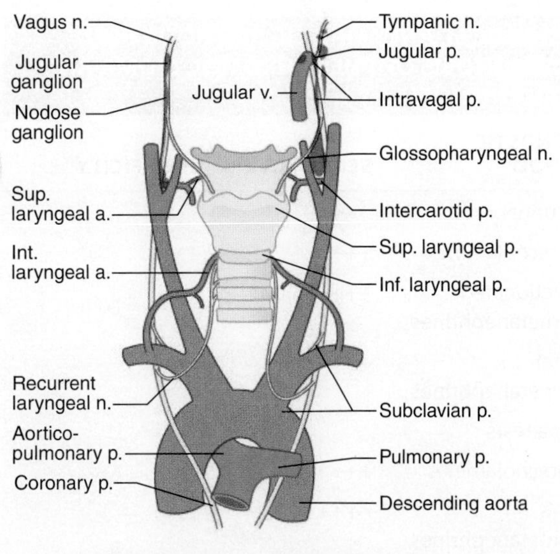

FIGURE 9-1

The paraganglial system and topographic sites (in red) of pheochromocytomas and paragangliomas. *(Parts A and B from WM Manger, RW Gifford: Clinical and experimental pheochromocytoma. Cambridge, Blackwell Science, 1996; Part C from GG Glenner, PM Grimley: Tumors of the Extra-adrenal Paraganglion System [Including Chemoreceptors], Atlas of Tumor Pathology, 2nd Series, Fascicle 9. Washington, DC, AFIP, 1974.)*

intervals, patients are anxious and pale, and they experience tachycardia and palpitations. These paroxysms generally last <1 h and may be precipitated by surgery, positional changes, exercise, pregnancy, urination (particularly with bladder pheochromocytomas), and various medications (e.g., tricyclic antidepressants, opiates, metoclopramide).

DIAGNOSIS

The diagnosis is based on documentation of catecholamine excess by biochemical testing and localization of the tumor by imaging. These two criteria are of equal importance, although measurement of catecholamines or metanephrines (their methylated metabolites) is traditionally the first step in diagnosis.

TABLE 9-1

CLINICAL FEATURES ASSOCIATED WITH PHEOCHROMOCYTOMA, LISTED BY FREQUENCY OF OCCURRENCE

1. Headaches	10. Weight loss
2. Profuse sweating	11. Paradoxical response to antihypertensive drugs
3. Palpitations and tachycardia	12. Polyuria and polydipsia
4. Hypertension, sustained or paroxysmal	13. Constipation
	14. Orthostatic hypotension
5. Anxiety and panic attacks	15. Dilated cardiomyopathy
6. Pallor	16. Erythrocytosis
7. Nausea	17. Elevated blood sugar
8. Abdominal pain	18. Hypercalcemia
9. Weakness	

Biochemical testing

Pheochromocytomas and paragangliomas synthesize and store catecholamines, which include norepinephrine (noradrenaline), epinephrine (adrenaline), and dopamine. Elevated plasma and urinary levels of catecholamines and metanephrines form the cornerstone of diagnosis. The characteristic fluctuations in the hormonal activity of tumors results in considerable variation in serial catecholamine measurements. However, most tumors continuously leak O-methylated metabolites, which are detected by measurement of metanephrines.

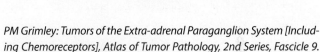

Catecholamines and metanephrines can be measured by different methods, including high-performance liquid chromatography, enzyme-linked immunosorbent assay, and liquid chromatography/mass spectrometry. When pheochromocytoma is suspected on clinical grounds (i.e., when values are three times the upper limit of normal), this diagnosis is highly likely regardless of the assay used. However, as summarized in Table 9-2, the sensitivity and specificity of available biochemical tests vary greatly, and these differences are important in assessing patients with borderline elevations of different compounds. Urinary tests for metanephrines (total or fractionated) and catecholamines are widely available and are used commonly

TABLE 9-2

BIOCHEMICAL AND IMAGING METHODS USED FOR DIAGNOSIS OF PHEOCHROMOCYTOMA AND PARAGANGLIOMA

DIAGNOSTIC METHOD	SENSITIVITY	SPECIFICITY
24-h urinary tests		
Catecholamines	+++	+++
Fractionated metanephrines	++++	++
Total metanephrines	+++	++++
Plasma tests		
Catecholamines	+++	++
Free metanephrines	++++	+++
Imaging		
CT	++++	+++
MRI	++++	+++
MIBG scintigraphy	+++	++++
Somatostatin receptor scintigraphy[a]	++	++
^{18}Fluoro-DOPA PET/CT	+++	++++

[a]Values are particularly high in head and neck paragangliomas.

Abbreviations: MIBG, metaiodobenzylguanidine; PET/CT, positron emission tomography plus CT. For the biochemical tests, the ratings correspond globally to sensitivity and specificity rates as follows: ++, <85%; +++, 85–95%; and ++++, >95%.

for initial evaluation. Among these tests, those for the fractionated metanephrines and catecholamines are the most sensitive. Plasma tests are more convenient and include measurements of catecholamines and metanephrines. Measurements of plasma metanephrine are the most sensitive and are less susceptible to false-positive elevations from stress, including venipuncture. Although the incidence of false-positive test results has been reduced by the introduction of newer assays, physiologic stress responses and medications that increase catecholamine levels still can confound testing. Because the tumors are relatively rare, borderline elevations are likely to represent false-positive results. In this circumstance, it is important to exclude dietary or drug-related factors (withdrawal of levodopa or use of sympathomimetics, diuretics, tricyclic antidepressants, alpha and beta blockers) that might cause false-positive results and then to repeat testing or perform a clonidine suppression test (i.e., the measurement of plasma normetanephrine 3 h after oral administration of 300 μg of clonidine). Other pharmacologic tests, such as the phentolamine test and the glucagon provocation test, are of relatively low sensitivity and are not recommended.

Diagnostic imaging

A variety of methods have been used to localize pheochromocytomas and paragangliomas (Table 9-2). CT and MRI are similar in sensitivity and should be performed with contrast. T2-weighted MRI with gadolinium contrast is optimal for detecting pheochromocytomas and is somewhat better than CT for imaging extraadrenal pheochromocytomas and paragangliomas. About 5% of adrenal incidentalomas, which usually are detected by CT or MRI, prove to be pheochromocytomas upon endocrinologic evaluation.

Tumors also can be localized by procedures using radioactive tracers, including ^{131}I- or ^{123}I-metaiodobenzylguanidine (MIBG) scintigraphy, ^{111}In-somatostatin analogue scintigraphy, ^{18}F-DOPA positron emission tomography (PET), or ^{18}F-fluorodeoxyglucose (FDG) PET. Because these agents exhibit selective uptake in paragangliomas, nuclear imaging is particularly useful in the hereditary syndromes.

Differential diagnosis

When the possibility of a pheochromocytoma is being entertained, other disorders to consider include essential hypertension, anxiety attacks, use of cocaine or amphetamines, mastocytosis or carcinoid syndrome (usually without hypertension), intracranial lesions, clonidine withdrawal, autonomic epilepsy, and factitious crises (usually from use of sympathomimetic amines). When an asymptomatic adrenal mass is identified, likely diagnoses other than pheochromocytoma include a nonfunctioning adrenal adenoma, an aldosteronoma, and a cortisol-producing adenoma (Cushing's syndrome).

TREATMENT Pheochromocytoma

Complete tumor removal, the ultimate therapeutic goal, can be achieved by partial or total adrenalectomy. It is important to preserve the normal adrenal cortex, particularly in hereditary disorders in which bilateral pheochromocytomas are most likely. Preoperative preparation of the patient is important. Before surgery, blood pressure should be consistently below 160/90 mmHg. Classically, blood pressure has been controlled by α-adrenergic blockers (oral phenoxybenzamine, 0.5–4 mg/kg of body weight). Because patients are volume-constricted, liberal salt intake and hydration are necessary to avoid severe orthostasis. Oral prazosin or intravenous phentolamine can be used to manage paroxysms while adequate alpha blockade is awaited. Beta blockers (e.g., 10 mg of propranolol three or four times per day) can then be added. Other antihypertensives, such as calcium channel blockers or angiotensin-converting enzyme inhibitors, have also been used effectively.

Surgery should be performed by teams of surgeons and anesthesiologists with experience in the management of pheochromocytomas. Blood pressure can be labile during surgery, particularly at the outset of intubation or when the tumor is manipulated. Nitroprusside infusion is useful for intraoperative hypertensive crises, and hypotension usually responds to volume infusion.

Minimally invasive techniques (laparoscopy or retroperitoneoscopy) have become the standard approaches in pheochromocytoma surgery. They are associated with fewer complications, a faster recovery, and optimal cosmetic results. Extra-adrenal abdominal and most thoracic pheochromocytomas also can also be removed endoscopically. Postoperatively, catecholamine normalization should be documented. An adrenocorticotropic hormone test should be used to exclude cortisol deficiency when bilateral adrenal cortex–sparing surgery has been performed.

MALIGNANT PHEOCHROMOCYTOMA

About 5–10% of pheochromocytomas and paragangliomas are malignant. The diagnosis of malignant pheochromocytoma is problematic. The typical histologic criteria of cellular atypia, presence of mitoses, and invasion of vessels or adjacent tissues are insufficient for the diagnosis of malignancy in pheochromocytoma. Thus, the term *malignant pheochromocytoma* is restricted to tumors with distant metastases, most commonly found by nuclear medicine imaging in lungs, bone, or liver—locations suggesting a vascular pathway of spread. Because hereditary syndromes are associated with multifocal tumor sites, these features should be anticipated in patients with germ-line mutations of *RET, VHL, SDHD,* or *SDHB*. However, distant metastases also occur in these syndromes, especially in carriers of *SDHB* mutations.

Treatment of malignant pheochromocytoma or paraganglioma is challenging. Options include tumor mass reduction, alpha blockers for symptoms, chemotherapy, and nuclear medicine radiotherapy. The first-line choice is nuclear medicine therapy for scintigraphically documented metastases, preferably with ^{131}I-MIBG in 200-mCi doses at monthly intervals over three to six cycles. Averbuch's chemotherapy protocol includes dacarbazine (600 mg/m^2 on days 1 and 2), cyclophosphamide (750 mg/m^2 on day 1), and vincristine (1.4 mg/m^2 on day 1), all repeated every 21 days for three to six cycles. Palliation (stable disease to shrinkage) is achieved in about one-half of patients. Other chemotherapeutic options are sunitinib and temozolomide/thalidomide. The prognosis of metastatic pheochromocytoma or paraganglioma is variable, with 5-year survival rates of 30–60%.

PHEOCHROMOCYTOMA IN PREGNANCY

Pheochromocytomas occasionally are diagnosed in pregnancy. Endoscopic removal, preferably in the fourth to sixth month of gestation, is possible and can be followed by uneventful childbirth. Regular screening in families with inherited pheochromocytomas provides an opportunity to identify and remove asymptomatic tumors in women of reproductive age.

PHEOCHROMOCYTOMA-ASSOCIATED SYNDROMES

About 25–33% of patients with a pheochromocytoma or paraganglioma have an inherited syndrome. At diagnosis, patients with inherited syndromes are a mean of ~15 years younger than patients with sporadic tumors.

Neurofibromatosis type 1 (NF1) was the first described pheochromocytoma-associated syndrome. The *NF1* gene functions as a tumor suppressor by regulating the Ras signaling cascade. Classic features of neurofibromatosis include multiple neurofibromas, café au lait spots, axillary freckling of the skin, and Lisch nodules of the iris (Fig. 9-2). Pheochromocytomas occur in only ~1% of these patients and are located predominantly in the adrenals. Malignant pheochromocytoma is not uncommon.

The best-known pheochromocytoma-associated syndrome is the autosomal dominant disorder *multiple endocrine neoplasia type 2* (MEN2) **(Chap. 29)**. Both types of MEN2 (2A and 2B) are caused by mutations in *RET* (*re*arranged during *t*ransfection), which encodes a tyrosine kinase. The locations of RET mutations correlate with the severity of disease and the type of MEN2 **(Chap. 29)**. MEN2A is characterized by medullary thyroid carcinoma (MTC), pheochromocytoma, and hyperparathyroidism; MEN2B also includes MTC and pheochromocytoma as well as multiple mucosal neuromas, marfanoid habitus, and other developmental disorders, though it typically lacks hyperparathyroidism. MTC is found in virtually all patients with MEN2, but pheochromocytoma occurs in only ~50% of these patients. Nearly all pheochromocytomas in MEN2 are benign and located in the adrenals, often bilaterally (Fig. 9-3). Pheochromocytoma may be symptomatic before MTC. Prophylactic thyroidectomy is being performed in many carriers of *RET* mutations; pheochromocytomas should be excluded before any surgery in these patients.

Von Hippel–Lindau syndrome (VHL) is an autosomal dominant disorder that predisposes to retinal and cerebellar hemangioblastomas, which also occur in the brainstem and spinal cord (Fig. 9-4). Other important

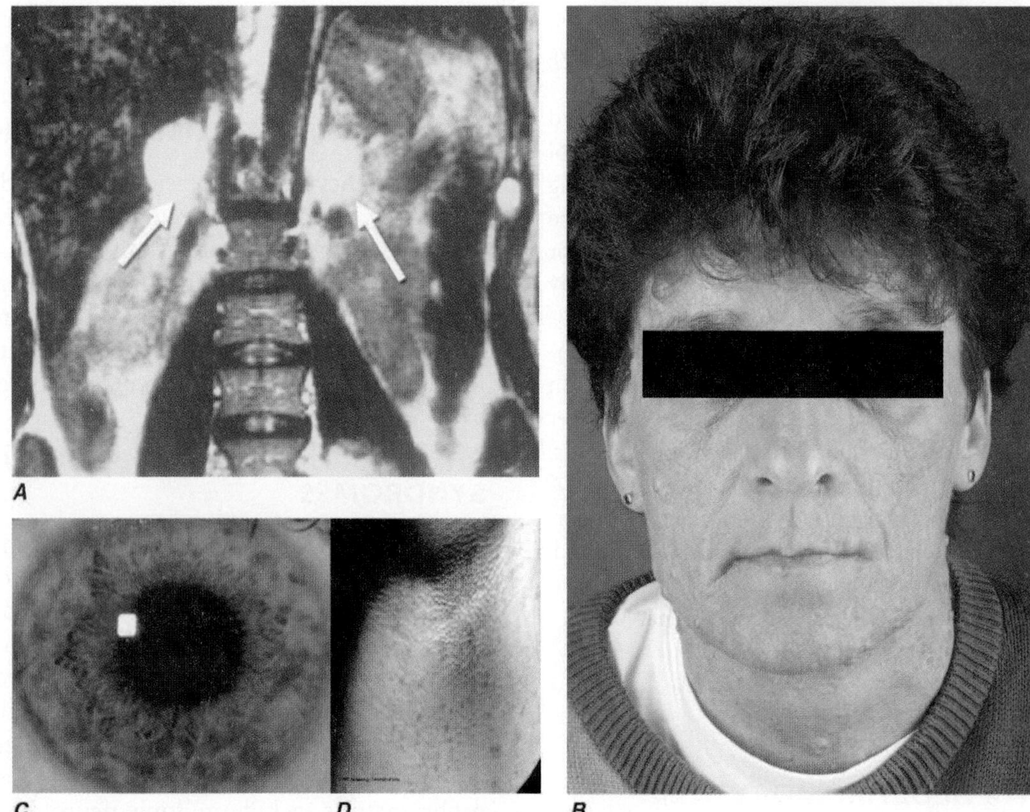

FIGURE 9-2
Neurofibromatosis. *A.* MRI of bilateral adrenal pheochromocytoma. ***B.*** Cutaneous neurofibromas. ***C.*** Lisch nodules of the iris. ***D.*** Axillary freckling. *(Part A from HPH Neumann et al: Keio J Med 54:15, 2005; with permission.)*

features of VHL are clear cell renal carcinomas, pancreatic neuroendocrine tumors, endolymphatic sac tumors of the inner ear, cystadenomas of the epididymis and broad ligament, and multiple pancreatic or renal cysts.

The *VHL* gene (among other genes) encodes an E3 ubiquitin ligase that regulates expression of hypoxia-inducible factor 1. Loss of *VHL* is associated with increased expression of vascular endothelial growth factor (VEGF), which induces angiogenesis. Although the *VHL* gene can be inactivated by all types of mutations, patients with pheochromocytoma predominantly have missense mutations. About 20–30% of patients with VHL have pheochromocytomas, but in some families the incidence can reach 90%. The recognition of pheochromocytoma as a VHL-associated feature provides an opportunity to diagnose retinal, central nervous system, renal, and pancreatic tumors at a stage when effective treatment may still be possible.

The *paraganglioma syndromes (PGLs)* have been classified by genetic analyses of families with head and neck paragangliomas. The susceptibility genes encode subunits of the enzyme succinate dehydrogenase (SDH), a component in the Krebs cycle and the mitochondrial electron transport chain. SDH is formed by four subunits (A–D). Mutations of *SDHB* (PGL4), *SDHC* (PGL3), *SDHD* (PGL1), and *SDHAF2* (PGL2) predispose to the PGLs. The transmission of the disease in carriers of *SDHB* and *SDHC* germ-line mutations is autosomal dominant. In contrast, in *SDHD* and *SDHAF2* families, only the progeny of affected fathers develop tumors if they inherit the mutation. PGL1 is most common, followed by PGL4; PGL2 and PGL3 are rare. Adrenal, extra-adrenal abdominal, and thoracic pheochromocytomas, which are components of PGL1 and PGL4, are rare in PGL3 and absent in PGL2 (Fig. 9-5). About one-third of patients with PGL4 develop metastases.

Familial pheochromocytoma (FP) has been attributed to hereditary, mainly adrenal tumors in patients with germ-line mutations in the genes *TMEM127*, *MAX*, and *SDHA*. Transmission is also autosomal dominant, and mutations of *MAX*, like those of *SDHD*, cause tumors only if inherited from the father.

GUIDELINES FOR GENETIC SCREENING OF PATIENTS WITH PHEOCHROMOCYTOMA OR PARAGANGLIOMA

In addition to family history, general features suggesting an inherited syndrome include young age, multifocal tumors, extra-adrenal tumors, and malignant

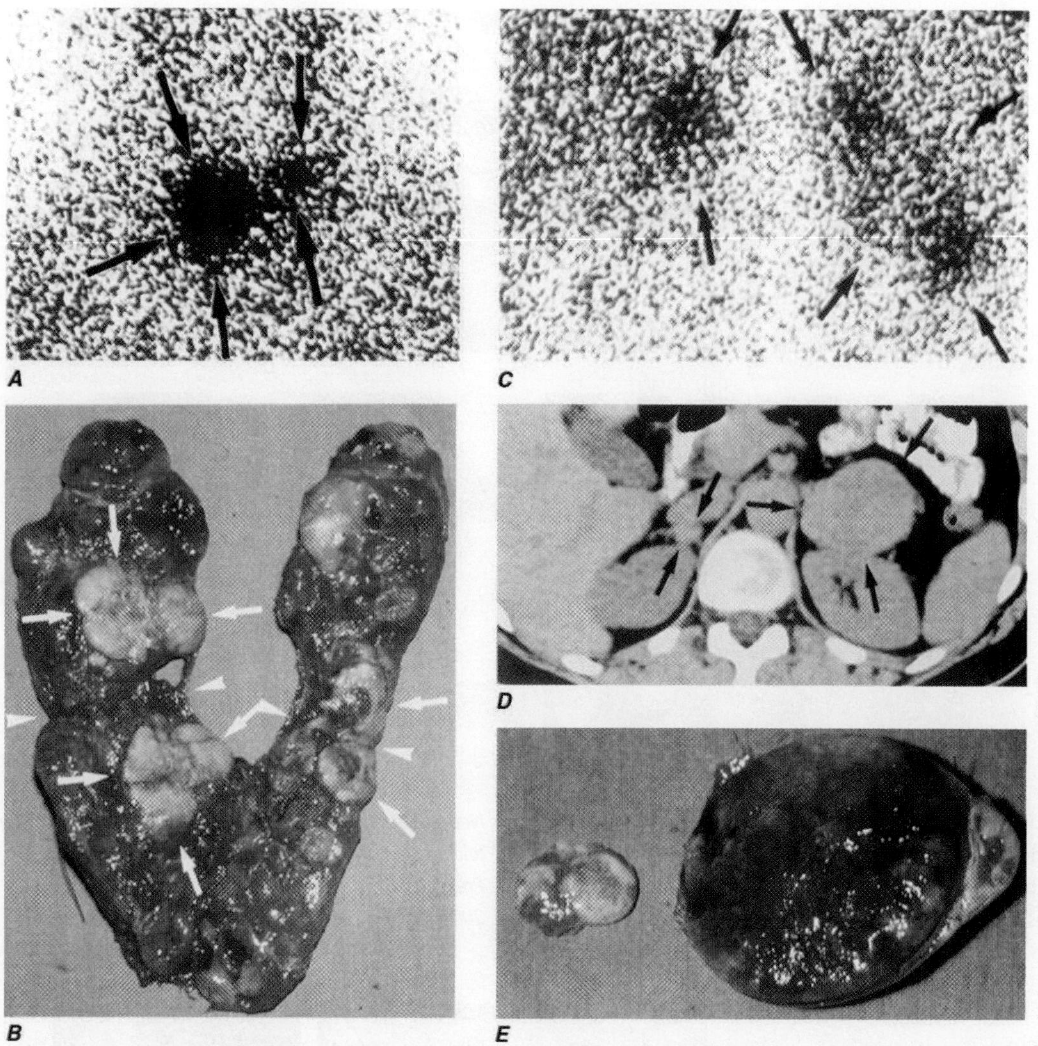

FIGURE 9-3

Multiple endocrine neoplasia type 2. *A, B.* Multifocal medullary thyroid carcinoma shown by MIBG scintigraphy (*A*) and operative specimen (*B*). Arrows demonstrate the tumors; arrowheads show the tissue bridge of the cut specimen. ***C–E.*** Bilateral adrenal pheochromocytoma shown by MIBG scintigraphy (*C*), CT imaging (*D*), and operative specimens (*E*). *(From HPH Neumann et al: Keio J Med 54:15, 2005; with permission.)*

tumors (Fig. 9-6). Because of the relatively high prevalence of familial syndromes among patients who present with pheochromocytoma or paraganglioma, it is useful to identify germ-line mutations even in patients without a known family history. A first step is to search for clinical features of inherited syndromes and to obtain an in-depth, multigenerational family history. Each of these syndromes exhibits autosomal dominant transmission with variable penetrance, but a proband with a mother affected by paraganglial tumors is not predisposed to PLG1 (*SDHD* mutation carrier). Cutaneous neurofibromas, café au lait spots, and axillary freckling suggest neurofibromatosis. Germ-line mutations in *NF1* have not been reported in patients with sporadic pheochromocytomas. Thus, *NF1* testing need not be performed in the absence of other clinical features of neurofibromatosis. A personal or family history of MTC or an elevation of serum calcitonin strongly suggests MEN 2 and should prompt testing for *RET* mutations. A history of visual impairment or tumors of the cerebellum, kidney, brainstem, or spinal cord suggests the possibility of VHL. A personal and/or family history of head and neck paraganglioma suggests PGL1 or PGL4.

A single adrenal pheochromocytoma in a patient with an otherwise unremarkable history may still be associated with mutations of *VHL, RET, SDHB*, or *SDHD* (in decreasing order of frequency). Two-thirds of extra-adrenal tumors are associated with one of these syndromes, and multifocal tumors occur with decreasing frequency in carriers of *RET, SDHD, VHL*, and *SDHB* mutations. About 30% of head and neck paragangliomas are associated with germ-line mutations of one of the SDH subunit genes (most often *SDHD*) and

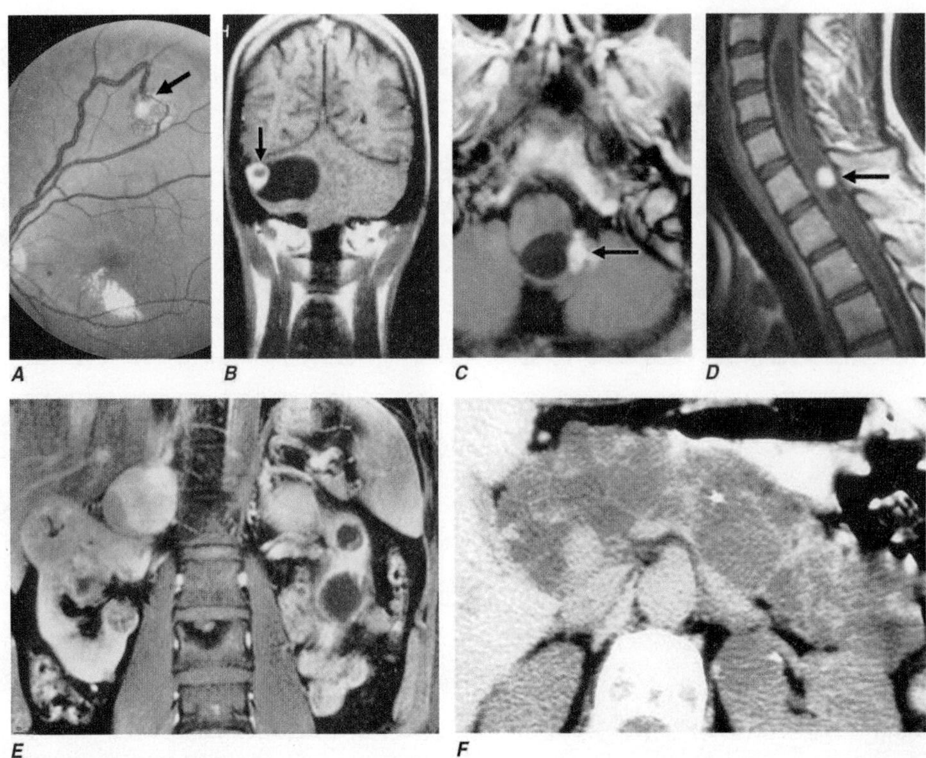

FIGURE 9-4

Von Hippel–Lindau disease. *A.* Retinal angioma. All subsequent panels show findings on MRI: ***B–D.*** Hemangioblastomas of the cerebellum (*B*) in brainstem (*C*) and spinal cord (*D*). ***E.*** Bilateral pheochromocytomas and bilateral renal clear cell carcinomas ***F.*** Multiple pancreatic cysts. *(Parts A and D from HPH Neumann et al: Adv Nephrol Necker Hosp 27:361, 1997. © Elsevier. Part B from SH Morgan, J-P Grunfeld [eds]: Inherited Disorders of the Kidney. Oxford, UK, Oxford University Press, 1998. Part F from HPH Neumann et al: Contrib Nephrol 136:193, 2001. © S. Karger AG, Basel.)*

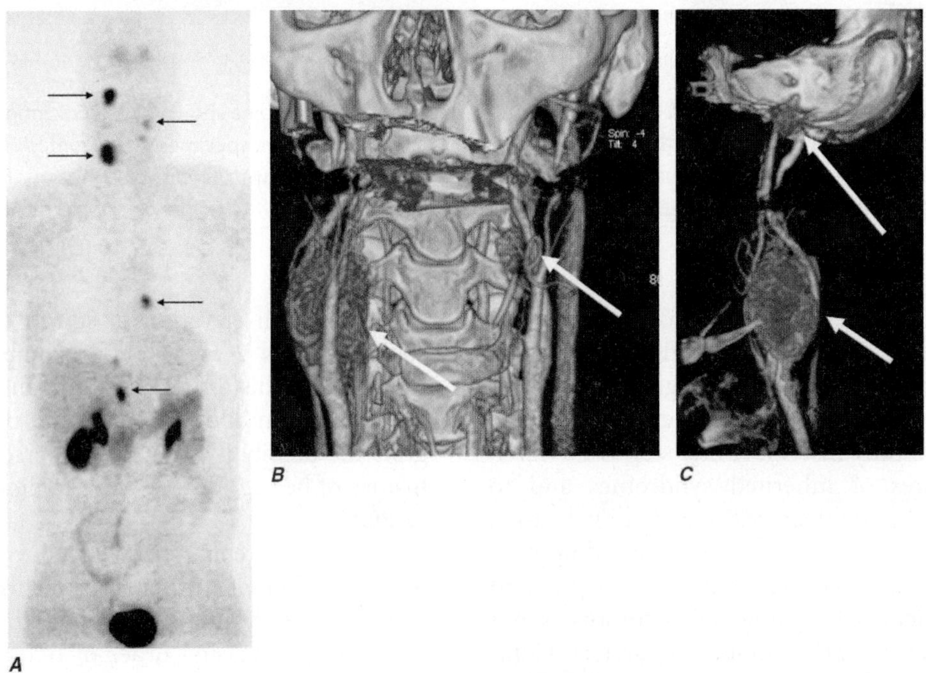

FIGURE 9-5

Paraganglioma syndrome. A patient with the SDHD W5X mutation and PGL1 underwent incomplete resection of a left carotid body tumor. ***A.*** ^{18}F-DOPA positron emission tomography demonstrating tumor uptake in the right jugular glomus, the right carotid body, the left carotid body, the left coronary glomus, and the right adrenal gland. Note the physiologic accumulation of the radiopharmaceutical agent in the kidneys, liver, gallbladder, renal pelvis, and urinary bladder. ***B*** and ***C.*** CT angiography with three-dimensional reconstruction. Arrows point to the paraganglial tumors. *(From S Hoegerle et al: Eur J Nucl Med Mol Imaging 30:689, 2003; with permission.)*

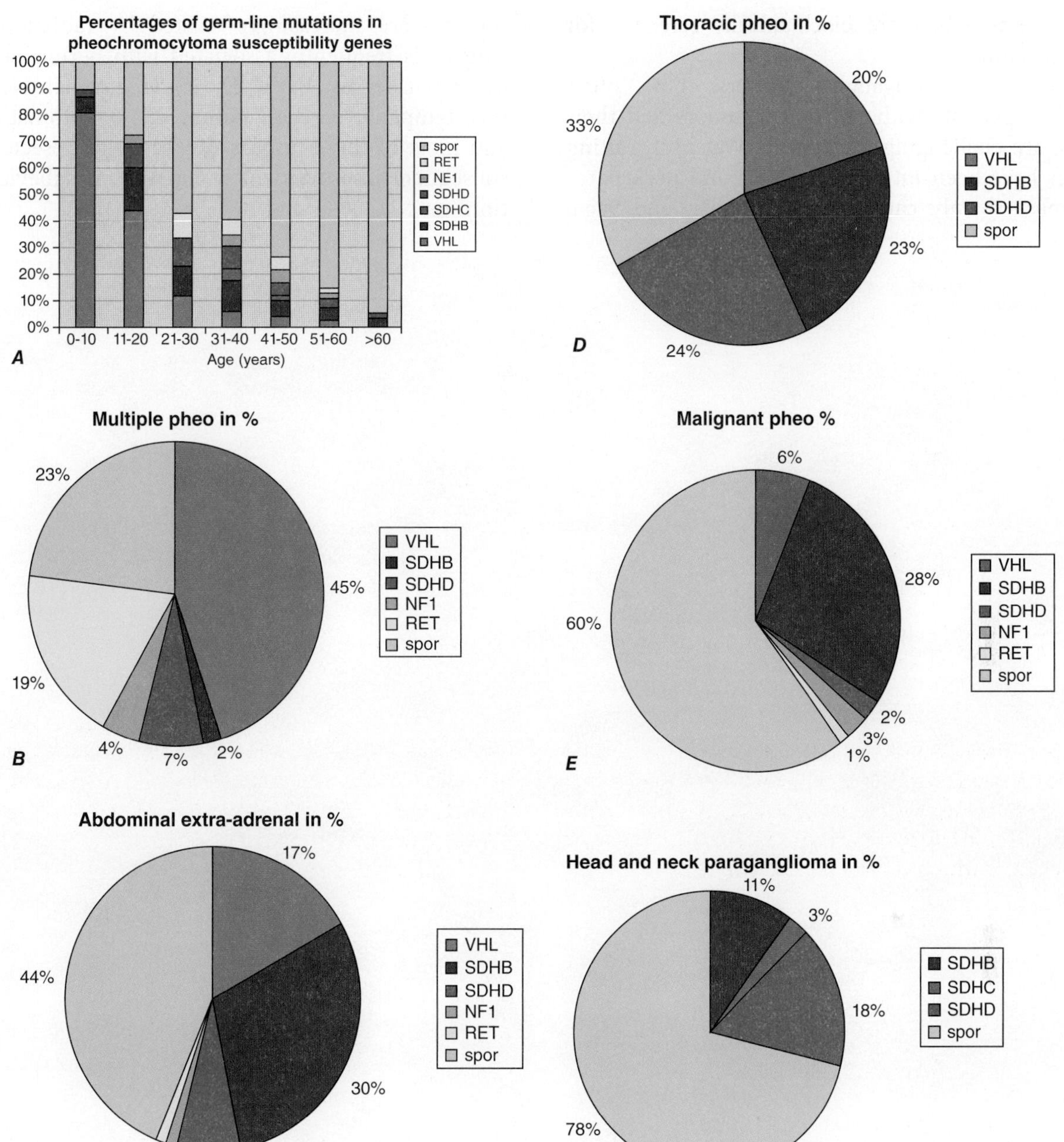

FIGURE 9-6

Mutation distribution in the *VHL, RET, SDHB, SDHC, SDHD,* and *NF1* genes in 2021 patients with pheochromocytomas and paragangliomas from the European-American Pheochromocytoma-Paraganglioma Registry based in Freiburg, Germany, as updated on March 1, 2014. ***A.*** Correlation with age. The bars depict the frequency of sporadic (spor) or various inherited forms of pheochromocytoma in different age groups. The inherited disorders are much more common among younger individuals presenting with pheochromocytoma. Patients with mutations in the *TMEM127, MAX, and SDHA genes* are not included, since they contribute <1% in decades 4–7 only. ***B–F.*** Germ-line mutations according to multiple (*B*), extra-adrenal retroperitoneal (*C*), thoracic (*D*), and malignant (*E*) pheochromocytomas and head and neck paragangliomas (*F*). *(Data from the Freiburg International Pheochromocytoma and Paraganglioma Registry, 2014.)*

are rare in carriers of *VHL, RET*, and *TMEM127* mutations (Fig. 9-6F).

Immunohistochemistry is helpful in the preselection of hereditary pheochromocytoma. Negative immunostaining with antibodies to SDHB, TMEM127, and MAX may predict mutations of the *SDH*, *TMEM127*, and *MAX* genes, respectively.

Once the underlying syndrome is diagnosed, the benefit of genetic testing can be extended to relatives. For this purpose, it is necessary to identify the germ-line mutation in the proband and, after genetic counseling, to perform DNA sequence analyses of the responsible gene in relatives to determine whether they are affected. Other family members may benefit when individuals who carry a germ-line mutation are biochemically screened for paraganglial tumors.

Asymptomatic paraganglial tumors, now often detected in patients with hereditary tumors and their relatives, are challenging to manage. Watchful waiting strategies have been introduced. Head and neck paragangliomas—mainly carotid body, jugular, and vagal tumors—are increasingly treated by radiation, since surgery is frequently associated with permanent palsy of cranial nerves II, VII, IX, X, XI, and XII. Nevertheless, tympanic paragangliomas are symptomatic early, and most of these tumors can easily be resected, with subsequent improvement of hearing and alleviation of tinnitus.

SECTION III

REPRODUCTIVE ENDOCRINOLOGY

CHAPTER 10
DISORDERS OF SEX DEVELOPMENT

John C. Achermann ■ J. Larry Jameson

Sex development begins in utero but continues into young adulthood with the achievement of sexual maturity and reproductive capability. The major determinants of sex development can be divided into three components: chromosomal sex, gonadal sex (sex determination), and phenotypic sex (sex differentiation) (Fig. 10-1). Variations at each of these stages can result in disorders (or differences) of sex development (DSDs) (Table 10-1). In the newborn period, approximately 1 in 4000 babies require investigation because of ambiguous (atypical) genitalia. Urgent assessment is required, because some causes such as congenital adrenal hyperplasia (CAH) can be associated with life-threatening adrenal crises. Support for the parents and clear communication about the diagnosis and management options are essential. The involvement of an experienced multidisciplinary team is important for counseling, planning appropriate investigations, and discussing long-term well-being. DSDs can also present at other ages and to a range of health professionals. Subtler forms of gonadal dysfunction (e.g., Klinefelter's syndrome [KS], Turner's syndrome [TS]) often are diagnosed later in life by internists. Because these conditions are associated with a variety of psychological, reproductive, and potential medical consequences, an open dialogue must be established between the patient and health care providers to ensure continuity and attention to these issues.

SEX DEVELOPMENT

Chromosomal sex, defined by a karyotype, describes the X and/or Y chromosome complement (46,XY; 46,XX) that is established at the time of fertilization. The presence of a normal Y chromosome determines that testis development will occur even in the presence of multiple X chromosomes (e.g., 47,XXY or 48,XXXY). The loss of an X chromosome impairs gonad development (45,X or 45,X/46,XY mosaicism). Fetuses with no X chromosome (45,Y) are not viable.

Gonadal sex refers to the histologic and functional characteristics of gonadal tissue as testis or ovary. The embryonic gonad is bipotential and can develop (from ~42 days after conception) into either a testis or an ovary, depending on which genes are expressed (Fig. 10-2). Testis development is initiated by expression of the Y chromosome gene *SRY* (sex-determining region on the Y chromosome) that encodes an HMG box transcription factor. *SRY* is expressed transiently in cells destined to become Sertoli cells and serves as a pivotal switch to establish the testis lineage. Mutation of *SRY* prevents testis development in 46,XY individuals, whereas translocation of *SRY* in 46,XX individuals is sufficient to induce testis development and a male phenotype. Other genes are necessary to continue testis development. *SOX9* (*SRY*-related HMG-box gene 9) is upregulated by *SRY* in the developing testis but is suppressed in the ovary. *WT1* (Wilms' tumor–related gene 1) acts early in the genetic pathway and regulates the transcription of several genes, including *SFI* (*NR5A1*), *DAX1* (*NR0B1*), and *AMH* (encoding müllerian-inhibiting substance [MIS]). *SF1* encodes steroidogenic factor 1, a nuclear receptor that functions in cooperation with other transcription factors to regulate a large array of adrenal and gonadal genes, including *SOX9* and many genes involved in steroidogenesis. *SF1* mutations causing loss of function are found in ~10% of XY patients with gonadal dysgenesis and impaired androgenization. In contrast, duplication of a related gene *DAX1* also impairs testis development, revealing the exquisite sensitivity of the testis-determining pathway to gene dosage effects. *DAX1* loss-of-function mutations cause adrenal hypoplasia, hypogonadotropic

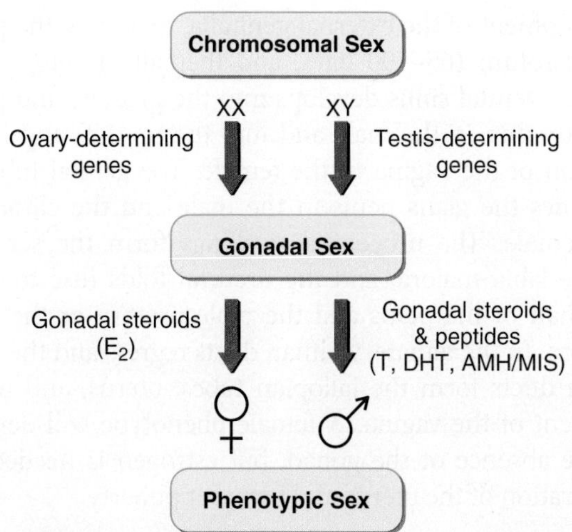

FIGURE 10-1

Sex development can be divided into three major components: chromosomal sex, gonadal sex, and phenotypic sex. DHT, dihydrotestosterone; MIS, müllerian-inhibiting substance also known as anti-müllerian hormone, AMH; T, testosterone.

hypogonadism, and testicular dysgenesis. In addition to the genes mentioned above, studies of humans and mice indicate that at least 30 other genes are also involved in gonad development (Fig. 10-2). These genes encode an array of signaling molecules and paracrine growth factors in addition to transcription factors.

Although ovarian development once was considered a "default" process, it is now clear that specific genes are expressed during the earliest stages of ovary development. Some of these factors may repress testis development (e.g., WNT4, R-spondin-1) (Fig. 10-2). Once the ovary has formed, additional factors are required for normal follicular development (e.g., follicle-stimulating hormone [FSH] receptor, *GDF9*). Steroidogenesis in the ovary requires the development of follicles that contain granulosa cells and theca cells surrounding the oocytes (**Chap. 13**). Thus, there is relatively limited ovarian steroidogenesis until puberty.

Germ cells also develop in a sex dimorphic manner. In the developing ovary, primordial germ cells (PGCs) proliferate and enter meiosis, whereas they proliferate and then undergo mitotic arrest in the developing

TABLE 10-1

CLASSIFICATION OF DISORDERS OF SEX DEVELOPMENT (DSDs)

SEX CHROMOSOME DSD	46,XY DSD (SEE TABLE 10-3)	46,XX DSD (SEE TABLE 10-4)
47,XXY (Klinefelter's syndrome and variants)	**Disorders of gonadal (testis) development**	**Disorders of gonadal (ovary) development**
45,X (Turner's syndrome and variants)	Complete or partial gonadal dysgenesis (e.g., SRY, SOX9, SF1, WT1, DHH, MAP3K1)	Gonadal dysgenesis
45,X/46,XY mosaicism (mixed gonadal dysgenesis)	Impaired fetal Leydig cell function (e.g., *SF1/NR5A1*, *CXorf6/MAMLD1*)	Ovotesticular DSD
46,XX/46,XY (chimerism/mosaicism)	Ovotesticular DSD	Testicular DSD (e.g., *SRY*+, dup *SOX9*, *RSPO1*)
	Testis regression	**Androgen excess**
	Disorders in androgen synthesis or action	Fetal
	Disorders of androgen biosynthesis	3β-Hydroxysteroid dehydrogenase II (*HSD3β2*)
	LH receptor (*LHCGR*)	21-Hydroxylase (*CYP21A2*)
	Smith-Lemli-Opitz syndrome	P450 oxidoreductase (*POR*)
	Steroidogenic acute regulatory (*StAR*) protein	11β-Hydroxylase (*CYP11B1*)
	Cholesterol side-chain cleavage (*CYP11A1*)	Glucocorticoid receptor mutations
	3β-Hydroxysteroid dehydrogenase II (*HSD3B2*)	Fetoplacental
	17α-Hydroxylase/17,20-lyase (*CYP17A1*)	Aromatase deficiency (*CYP19*)
	P450 oxidoreductase (*POR*)	Oxidoreductase deficiency (*POR*)
	Cytochrome b5 (*CYB5A*)	Maternal
	17β-Hydroxysteroid dehydrogenase III (*HSD17B3*)	Maternal virilizing tumors (e.g., luteomas)
	5α-Reductase II (*SRD5A2*)	Androgenic drugs
	Aldo-keto reductase 1C2 (*AKR1C2*)	**Other**
	Disorders of androgen action	Syndromic associations (e.g., cloacal anomalies)
	Androgen insensitivity syndrome	Müllerian agenesis/hypoplasia (e.g., MRKH)
	Drugs and environmental modulators	Uterine abnormalities (e.g., MODY5)
	Other	Vaginal atresia (e.g., McKusick-Kaufman)
	Syndromic associations of male genital development	Labial adhesions
	Persistent müllerian duct syndrome	
	Vanishing testis syndrome	
	Isolated hypospadias	
	Congenital hypogonadotropic hypogonadism	
	Cryptorchidism	
	Environmental influences	

Source: Modified from IA Hughes: Arch Dis Child 91:554, 2006.

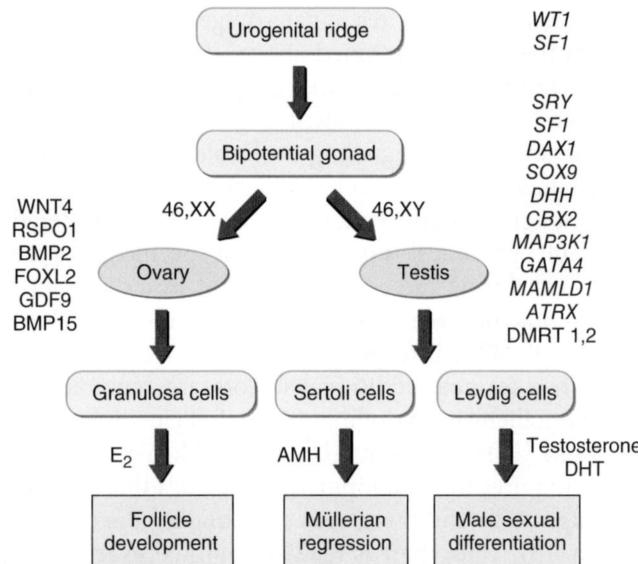

FIGURE 10-2

The genetic regulation of gonadal development. AMH, anti-müllerian hormone (müllerian-inhibiting substance); *ATRX*, α-thalassemia, mental retardation on the X; BMP2 and 15, bone morphogenic factors 2 and 15; *CBX2*, chromobox homologue 2; *DAX1*, dosage sensitive sex-reversal, adrenal hypoplasia congenita on the X chromosome, gene 1; *DHH*, desert hedgehog; DHT, dihydrotestosterone; *DMRT 1,2*, doublesex MAB3-related transcription factor 1,2; *FOXL2*, forkhead transcription factor L2; *GATA4*, GATA binding protein 4; GDF9, growth differentiation factor 9; *MAMLD1*, mastermind-like domain containing 1; *MAP3K1*, mitogen-activated protein kinase kinase kinase 1; RSPO1, R-spondin 1; *SF1*, steroidogenic factor 1 (also known as NR5A1); *SOX9*, *SRY*-related HMG-box gene 9; *SRY*, sex-determining region on the Y chromosome; *WNT4*, wingless-type MMTV integration site 4; *WT1*, Wilms' tumor–related gene 1.

testis. PGC entry into meiosis is initiated by retinoic acid that activates *STRA8* (stimulated by retinoic acid 8) and other genes involved in meiosis. The developing testis produces high levels of CYP26B1, an enzyme that degrades retinoic acid, preventing PGC entry into meiosis. Approximately 7 million germ cells are present in the fetal ovary in the second trimester, and 1 million remain at birth. Only 400 are ovulated during a woman's reproductive life span **(Chap. 13)**.

Phenotypic sex refers to the structures of the external and internal genitalia and secondary sex characteristics. The developing testis releases anti-müllerian hormone (AMH; also known as müllerian-inhibiting substance [MIS]) from Sertoli cells and testosterone from Leydig cells. AMH is a member of the transforming growth factor (TGF) β family and acts through specific receptors to cause regression of the müllerian structures from 60–80 days after conception. At ~60–140 days after conception, testosterone supports the development of wolffian structures, including the epididymides, vasa deferentia, and seminal vesicles. Testosterone is the precursor for dihydrotestosterone (DHT), a potent androgen that promotes development of the external genitalia, including the penis and scrotum (65–100 days, and thereafter) (Fig. 10-3). The urogenital sinus develops into the prostate and prostatic urethra in the male and into the urethra and lower portion of the vagina in the female. The genital tubercle becomes the glans penis in the male and the clitoris in the female. The urogenital swellings form the scrotum or the labia majora, and the urethral folds fuse to form the shaft of the penis and the male urethra or the labia minora. In the female, wolffian ducts regress and the müllerian ducts form the fallopian tubes, uterus, and upper segment of the vagina. A female phenotype will develop in the absence of the gonad, but estrogen is needed for maturation of the uterus and breast at puberty.

DISORDERS OF CHROMOSOMAL SEX

Variations in sex chromosome number and structure can present as DSDs (e.g., 45,X/46,XY). KS (47,XXY) and TS (45,X) do not usually present with genital ambiguity but are associated with gonadal dysfunction (Table 10-2).

KLINEFELTER'S SYNDROME (47,XXY)

Pathophysiology

The classic form of KS (47,XXY) occurs after meiotic nondisjunction of the sex chromosomes during gametogenesis (40% during spermatogenesis, 60% during oogenesis). Mosaic forms of KS (46,XY/47,XXY) are thought to result from chromosomal mitotic nondisjunction within the zygote and occur in at least 10% of individuals with this condition. Other chromosomal variants of KS (e.g., 48,XXYY, 48,XXXY) have been reported but are less common.

Clinical features

KS is characterized by small testes, infertility, gynecomastia, tall stature/increased leg length, and hypogonadism in phenotypic males. It has an incidence of at least 1 in 1000 men, but approximately 75% of cases are not diagnosed. Of those who are diagnosed, only 10% are identified prepubertally, usually because of small genitalia or cryptorchidism. Others are diagnosed after puberty, usually based on impaired androgenization and/or gynecomastia. Developmental delay, speech difficulties, and poor motor skills may be features but are variable, especially in adolescence. Later in life, body habitus or infertility leads to the diagnosis. Testes are small and firm (median length 2.5 cm [4 mL volume]; almost always <3.5 cm [12 mL]) and typically seem inappropriately small for the degree of androgenization. Biopsies

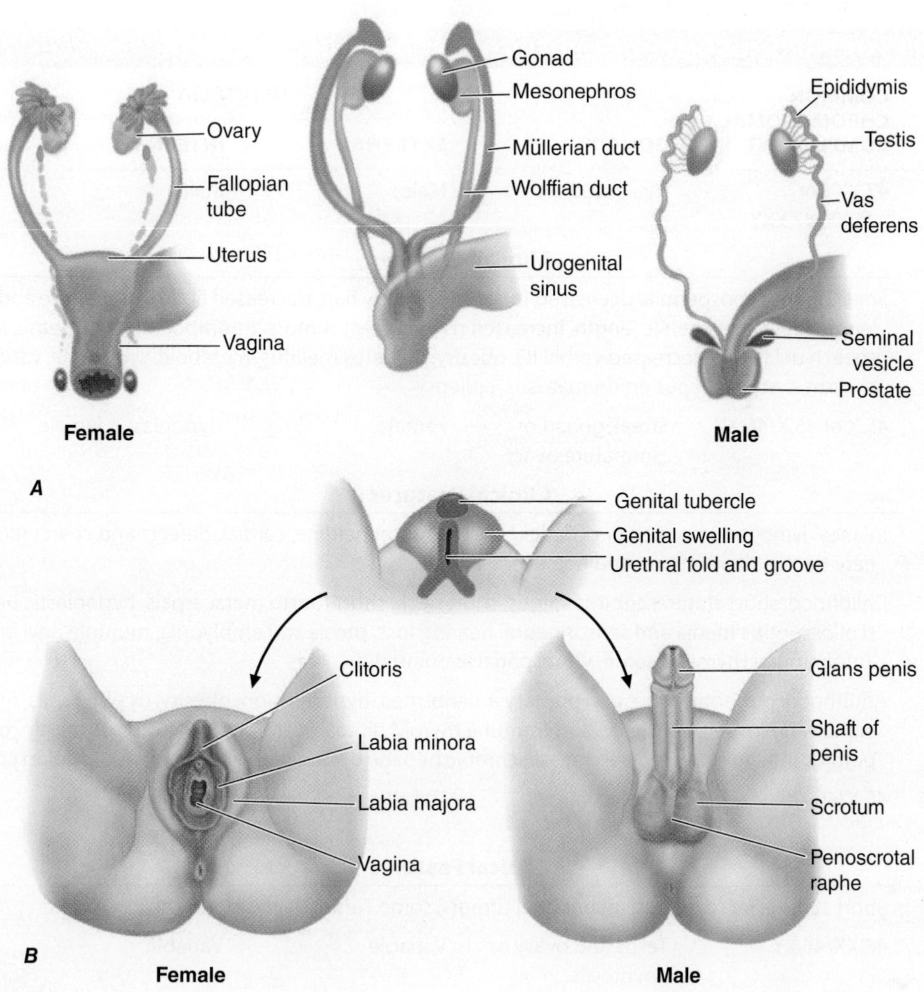

FIGURE 10-3

Sex development. *A.* Internal urogenital tract. ***B.*** External genitalia. *(After E Braunwald et al [eds]: Harrison's Principles of Internal Medicine, 15th ed. New York, McGraw-Hill, 2001.)*

are not usually necessary but typically reveal seminiferous tubule hyalinization and azoospermia. Other clinical features of KS are listed in Table 10-2. Plasma concentrations of FSH and luteinizing hormone (LH) are increased in most adults with 47,XXY, and plasma testosterone is decreased (50–75%), reflecting primary gonadal failure. Estradiol is often increased, likely because of chronic Leydig cell stimulation by LH and aromatization of androstenedione by adipose tissue; the increased ratio of estradiol-to-testosterone results in gynecomastia **(Chap. 11)**. Patients with mosaic forms of KS have less severe clinical features, have larger testes, and sometimes achieve spontaneous fertility.

TREATMENT Klinefelter's Syndrome

Growth, endocrine function, and bone mineralization should be monitored, especially from adolescence. Educational and psychological support is important for many individuals with KS. Androgen supplementation improves virilization, libido, energy, hypofibrinolysis, and bone mineralization in men with low testosterone levels but may occasionally worsen gynecomastia **(Chap. 11)**. Gynecomastia can be treated by surgical reduction if it causes concern **(Chap. 11)**. Fertility has been achieved by using in vitro fertilization in men with oligospermia or with intracytoplasmic sperm injection (ICSI) after retrieval of spermatozoa by testicular sperm extraction techniques. In specialized centers, successful spermatozoa retrieval using this technique is possible in >50% of men with nonmosaic KS. Results may be better in younger men. After ICSI and embryo transfer, successful pregnancies can be achieved in ~50% of these cases. The risk of transmission of this chromosomal abnormality needs to be considered, and preimplantation screening may be desired, although this outcome is much less common than originally predicted. Long-term monitoring of men with KS is important given the increased risk of breast cancer, cardiovascular disease, metabolic syndrome, and autoimmune disorders. Because most men with KS are never diagnosed, it is important that all internists consider this diagnosis in men with these features who might be seeking medical advice for other conditions.

TABLE 10-2

CLINICAL FEATURES OF CHROMOSOMAL DISORDERS OF SEX DEVELOPMENT (DSD)

DISORDER	COMMON CHROMOSOMAL COMPLEMENT	GONAD	GENITALIA EXTERNAL	GENITALIA INTERNAL	BREAST DEVELOPMENT
Klinefelter's syndrome	47,XXY or 46,XY/47,XXY	Hyalinized testes	Male	Male	Gynecomastia
	Clinical Features				
	Small testes, azoospermia, decreased facial and axillary hair, decreased libido, tall stature and increased leg length, decreased penile length, increased risk of breast tumors, thromboembolic disease, learning difficulties, speech delay and decreased verbal IQ, obesity, diabetes mellitus, metabolic syndrome, varicose veins, hypothyroidism, systemic lupus erythematosus, epilepsy				
Turner's syndrome	45,X or 45,X/46,XX	Streak gonad or immature ovary	Female	Hypoplastic female	Immature female
	Clinical Features				
	Infancy: lymphedema, web neck, shield chest, low-set hairline, cardiac defects and coarctation of the aorta, urinary tract malformations, and horseshoe kidney Childhood: short stature, cubitus valgus, short neck, short fourth metacarpals, hypoplastic nails, micrognathia, scoliosis, otitis media and sensorineural hearing loss, ptosis and amblyopia, multiple nevi and keloid formation, autoimmune thyroid disease, visuospatial learning difficulties Adulthood: pubertal failure and primary amenorrhea, hypertension, obesity, dyslipidemia, impaired glucose tolerance and insulin resistance, autoimmune thyroid disease, cardiovascular disease, aortic root dilation, osteoporosis, inflammatory bowel disease, chronic hepatic dysfunction, increased risk of colon cancer, hearing loss				
45,X/46,XY mosaicism	45,X/46,XY	Testis or streak gonad	Variable	Variable	Usually male
	Clinical Features				
	Short stature, increased risk of gonadal tumors, some Turner's syndrome features				
Ovotesticular DSD (true hermaphroditism)	46,XX/46,XY	Testis and ovary or ovotestis	Variable	Variable	Gynecomastia
	Clinical Features				
	Possible increased risk of gonadal tumors				

TURNER'S SYNDROME (GONADAL DYSGENESIS; 45,X)

Pathophysiology

Approximately one-half of women with TS have a 45,X karyotype, about 20% have 45,X/46,XX mosaicism, and the remainder have structural abnormalities of the X chromosome such as X fragments, isochromosomes, or rings. The clinical features of TS result from haploinsufficiency of multiple X chromosomal genes (e.g., short stature homeobox, *SHOX*). However, imprinted genes also may be affected when the inherited X has different parental origins.

Clinical features

TS is characterized by bilateral streak gonads, primary amenorrhea, short stature, and multiple congenital anomalies in phenotypic females. It affects ~1 in 2500 women and is diagnosed at different ages depending on the dominant clinical features (Table 10-2). Prenatally, a diagnosis of TS usually is made incidentally after chorionic villus sampling or amniocentesis for unrelated reasons such as advanced maternal age. Prenatal ultrasound findings include increased nuchal translucency. The postnatal diagnosis of TS should be considered in female neonates or infants with lymphedema, nuchal folds, low hairline, or left-sided cardiac defects and in girls with unexplained growth failure or pubertal delay. Although limited spontaneous pubertal development occurs in up to 30% of girls with TS (10%, 45,X; 30–40%, 45,X/46,XX) and ~2% reach menarche, the vast majority of women with TS develop complete ovarian insufficiency. Therefore, this diagnosis should be considered in all women who present with primary or secondary amenorrhea and elevated gonadotropin levels.

TREATMENT Turner's Syndrome

The management of girls and women with TS requires a multidisciplinary approach because of the number of potentially involved organ systems. Detailed cardiac and renal evaluation should be performed at the time of diagnosis. Individuals with congenital heart defects (CHDs) (30%) (bicuspid aortic valve, 30–50%; coarctation of the aorta, 30%; aortic root dilation, 5%) require long-term follow-up by an experienced cardiologist, antibiotic prophylaxis for dental or surgical procedures, and serial magnetic resonance imaging (MRI) of aortic root dimensions, because progressive aortic root dilation is associated with increased risk of aortic dissection. Individuals found to have congenital renal and urinary tract malformations (30%) are at risk for urinary tract infections, hypertension, and nephrocalcinosis. Hypertension can occur independently of cardiac and renal malformations and should be monitored and treated as in other patients with essential hypertension. Clitoral enlargement or other evidence of virilization suggests the presence of covert, translocated Y chromosomal material and is associated with increased risk of gonadoblastoma. Regular assessment of thyroid function, weight, dentition, hearing, speech, vision, and educational issues should be performed during childhood. Otitis media and middle-ear disease are prevalent in childhood (50–85%), and sensorineural hearing loss becomes progressively common with age (70–90%). Autoimmune hypothyroidism (15–30%) can occur in childhood but has a mean age of onset in the third decade. Counseling about long-term growth and fertility issues should be provided. Patient support groups are active throughout the world and can play an invaluable role.

Short stature can be an issue for some girls because untreated final height rarely exceeds 150 cm in nonmosaic 45,X TS. High-dose recombinant growth hormone stimulates growth rate in children with TS and is occasionally combined with low doses of the nonaromatizable anabolic steroid oxandrolone (up to 0.05 mg/kg per day) in an older child (>9 years). However, final height increments are often about 5–10 cm, and individualization of treatment response to regimens may be beneficial. Girls with evidence of ovarian insufficiency require estrogen replacement to induce breast and uterine development, support growth, and maintain bone mineralization. Most physicians now initiate low-dose estrogen therapy (one-tenth to one-eighth of the adult replacement dose) to induce puberty at an age-appropriate time (~12 years). Doses of estrogen are increased gradually to allow development over a 2- to 4-year period. Progestins are added later to regulate withdrawal bleeds. Some women with TS have achieved successful pregnancy after ovum donation and in vitro fertilization but are high risk, and cardiac assessment is required. Long-term follow-up of women with TS involves careful surveillance of sex hormone replacement and reproductive function, bone mineralization, cardiac function and aortic root dimensions, blood pressure, weight and glucose tolerance, hepatic and lipid profiles, thyroid function, and hearing. This service is provided by a dedicated TS clinic in some centers.

45,X/46,XY MOSAICISM (MIXED GONADAL DYSGENESIS)

The phenotype of individuals with 45,X/46,XY mosaicism (sometimes called *mixed gonadal dysgenesis*) can vary considerably. Some have a predominantly female phenotype with somatic features of TS, streak gonads, and müllerian structures, and are managed as TS with a Y chromosome. Most 45,X/46,XY individuals have a male phenotype and testes, and the diagnosis is made incidentally after amniocentesis or during investigation of infertility. In practice, most newborns referred for assessment have atypical genitalia and variable somatic features. Management is complex and needs to be individualized. A female sex-of-rearing is often assigned if uterine structures are present, gonads are intraabdominal, and phallic development is incomplete. In such situations, gonadectomy usually is considered to prevent further androgen secretion at puberty and prevent risk of gonadoblastoma (up to 25%). Individuals raised as males usually require reconstructive surgery for hypospadias and removal of dysgenetic or streak gonads if the gonads cannot be brought down into the scrotum. Scrotal testes can be preserved but require regular examination for tumor development and sonography at the time of puberty. Biopsy for carcinoma in situ is recommended in adolescence, and testosterone supplementation may be required to support androgenization in puberty or if low testosterone is detected in adulthood. Height potential is usually attenuated; some children receive recombinant growth hormone using TS protocols. Screening for cardiac, renal, and other TS features should be considered, and psychological support offered for the family and young person.

OVOTESTICULAR DSD

Ovotesticular DSD (formerly called *true hermaphroditism*) occurs when both an ovary and a testis—or when an ovotestis—are found in one individual. Most individuals with this diagnosis have a 46,XX karyotype, especially in sub-Saharan Africa, and present with ambiguous genitalia at birth or with breast development and phallic development at puberty. A 46,XX/46,XY chimeric karyotype is less common and has a variable phenotype.

DISORDERS OF GONADAL AND PHENOTYPIC SEX

Disorders of gonadal and phenotypic sex can result in underandrogenization of individuals with a 46,XY karyotype (46,XY DSD) and the excess androgenization of individuals with a 46,XX karyotype (46,XX DSD) (Table 10-1). These disorders cover a spectrum of phenotypes ranging from "46,XY phenotypic females" or "46,XX phenotypic males" to individuals with atypical genitalia.

46,XY DSD

Underandrogenization of the 46,XY fetus (formerly called *male pseudohermaphroditism*) reflects defects in androgen production or action. It can result from disorders of testis development, defects of androgen synthesis, or resistance to testosterone and DHT (Table 10-1).

Disorders of testis development

Testicular dysgenesis

Pure (or *complete*) *gonadal dysgenesis* (*Swyer's syndrome*) is associated with streak gonads, müllerian structures (due to insufficient AMH/MIS secretion), and a complete absence of androgenization. Phenotypic females with this condition often present because of absent pubertal development and are found to have a 46,XY karyotype. Serum sex steroids, AMH/MIS, and inhibin B are low, and LH and FSH are elevated. Patients with *partial gonadal dysgenesis* (*dysgenetic testes*) may produce enough MIS to regress the uterus and sufficient testosterone for partial androgenization, and therefore usually present in the newborn period with atypical genitalia. Gonadal dysgenesis can result from mutations or deletions of testis-promoting genes (*WT1*, *CBX2*, *SF1*, *SRY*, *SOX9*, *MAP3K1*, *DHH*, *GATA4*, *ATRX*, *ARX*, *DMRT*) or duplication of chromosomal loci containing "antitestis" genes (e.g., *WNT4/RSPO1*, *DAX1*) (Table 10-3). Among these, deletions or mutations of *SRY* and heterozygous mutations of *SF1* (*NR5A1*) appear to be most common but still account collectively for <25% of cases. Associated clinical features may be present, reflecting additional functional roles for these genes. For example, renal dysfunction occurs in patients with specific *WT1* mutations (Denys-Drash and Frasier's syndromes), primary adrenal failure occurs in some patients with *SF1* mutations, and severe cartilage abnormalities (campomelic dysplasia) are the predominant clinical feature of *SOX9* mutations. A family history of DSD, infertility, or early menopause is important because mutations in *SF1/NR5A1* can be inherited from a mother in a sex-limited dominant manner (which can mimic X-linked inheritance). In some cases, a woman may later develop primary ovarian insufficiency because of the effect of *SF1* on the ovary. Intraabdominal dysgenetic testes should be removed to prevent malignancy, and estrogens can be used to induce secondary sex characteristics and uterine development in 46,XY individuals raised as females, if it is felt that a female gender identity is established. *Absent (vanishing) testis syndrome* (*bilateral anorchia*) reflects regression of the testis during development. The etiology is unknown, but the absence of müllerian structures indicates adequate secretion of AMH early in utero. In most cases, androgenization of the external genitalia is either normal or slightly impaired (e.g., small penis, hypospadias). These individuals can be offered testicular prostheses and should receive androgen replacement in adolescence.

Disorders of androgen synthesis

Defects in the pathway that regulates androgen synthesis (Fig. 10-4) cause underandrogenization of the 46,XY fetus (Table 10-1). Müllerian regression is unaffected because Sertoli cell function is preserved. Most of these conditions can present with a spectrum of genital phenotypes, ranging from female-typical external genitalia or clitoromegaly in the more severe situations to penoscrotal hypospadias or a small phallus in others.

LH receptor

Mutations in the LH receptor (LHCGR) cause Leydig cell hypoplasia and androgen deficiency, due to impaired actions of human chorionic gonadotropin in utero and LH late in gestation and during the neonatal period. As a result, testosterone and DHT synthesis are insufficient for complete androgenization.

Steroidogenic enzyme pathways

Mutations in *steroidogenic acute regulatory protein* (*StAR*) and *CYP11A1* affect both adrenal and gonadal steroidogenesis (Fig. 10-4) **(Chap. 8)**. Affected individuals (46,XY) usually have severe early-onset salt-losing adrenal failure and a female phenotype, although later-onset milder variants have been reported. Defects in *3β-hydroxysteroid dehydrogenase type 2* (*HSD3β2*) also cause adrenal insufficiency in severe cases, but the accumulation of dehydroepiandrosterone (DHEA) has a mild androgenizing effect, resulting in ambiguous genitalia or hypospadias. Salt loss occurs in many but not all cases. Patients with CAH due to *17α-hydroxylase (CYP17) deficiency* have variable underandrogenization and develop hypertension and hypokalemia due to the potent salt-retaining effects of corticosterone and 11-deoxycorticosterone. Patients with complete loss of 17α-hydroxylase function often present as phenotypic females who fail to enter puberty and are found to have inguinal testes and hypertension in adolescence. Some mutations in *CYP17* selectively impair 17,20-lyase activity without altering 17α-hydroxylase activity, leading to underandrogenization without mineralocorticoid excess and hypertension. Disruption of the coenzyme, *cytochrome b5* (*CYB5A*), can present similarly, and methemoglobinemia is usually present. Mutations in *P450 oxidoreductase* (*POR*) affect multiple steroidogenic enzymes, leading to impaired androgenization and a biochemical pattern of apparent combined 21-hydroxylase and 17α-hydroxylase deficiency, sometimes with

TABLE 10-3

SELECTED GENETIC CAUSES OF 46,XY DISORDERS OF SEX DEVELOPMENT (DSDs)

GENE	INHERITANCE	GONAD	UTERUS	EXTERNAL GENITALIA	ASSOCIATED FEATURES
Disorders of Testis Development					
WT1	AD	Dysgenetic testis	+/–	Female or ambiguous	Wilms' tumor, renal abnormalities, gonadal tumors (WAGR, Denys-Drash and Frasier's syndromes)
CBX2	AD	Ovary	+	Female	
SF1	AR/AD (SL)	Dysgenetic testis/ Leydig dysfunction	+/–	Female or ambiguous	Primary adrenal failure; primary ovarian insufficiency in female (46,XX) relatives
SRY	Y	Dysgenetic testis or ovotestis	+/–	Female or ambiguous	
SOX9	AD	Dysgenetic testis or ovotestis	+/–	Female or ambiguous	Campomelic dysplasia
MAP3K1	AD (SL)	Dysgenetic testis	+/–	Female or ambiguous	
DHH	AR	Dysgenetic testis	+	Female	Minifascicular neuropathy
GATA4	AD	Dysgenetic testis	–	Ambiguous or male	Congenital heart disease
ATRX	X	Dysgenetic testis	–	Female or ambiguous	α Thalassemia, developmental delay
ARX	X	Dysgenetic testis	–	Male or ambiguous	Developmental delay; X-linked lissencephaly
MAMLD1	X	Dysgenetic testis/ Leydig dysfunction	–	Hypospadias	
DAX1	dupXp21	Dysgenetic testis	+/–	Female or ambiguous	
WNT4/RSPO1	dup1p35	Dysgenetic testis	+	Ambiguous	
Disorders of Androgen Synthesis					
LHR	AR	Testis	–	Female, ambiguous or micropenis	Leydig cell hypoplasia
DHCR7	AR	Testis	–	Variable	Smith-Lemli-Opitz syndrome: coarse facies, second-third toe syndactyly, failure to thrive, developmental delay, cardiac and visceral abnormalities
StAR	AR	Testis	–	Female or ambiguous	Congenital lipoid adrenal hyperplasia (primary adrenal failure)
CYP11A1	AR	Testis	–	Ambiguous	Primary adrenal failure
HSD3B2	AR	Testis	–	Ambiguous	CAH, primary adrenal failure ± salt loss, partial androgenization due to ↑ DHEA
CYP17	AR	Testis	–	Female or ambiguous	CAH, hypertension due to ↑ corticosterone and 11-deoxycorticosterone, except in isolated 17,20-lyase deficiency
CYB5A	AR	Testis	–	Ambiguous	Apparent isolated 17,20-lyase deficiency; methemoglobinemia
POR	AR	Testis	–	Ambiguous or male	Mixed features of 21-hydroxylase deficiency and 17α-hydroxylase/17,20-lyase deficiency, sometimes associated with Antley-Bixler craniosynostosis

(*Continued*)

TABLE 10-3

SELECTED GENETIC CAUSES OF 46,XY DISORDERS OF SEX DEVELOPMENT (DSDs) (CONTINUED)

GENE	INHERITANCE	GONAD	UTERUS	EXTERNAL GENITALIA	ASSOCIATED FEATURES
Disorders of Androgen Synthesis					
HSD17B3	AR	Testis	–	Female or ambiguous	Partial androgenization at puberty, ↑ androstenedione-to-testosterone ratio
SRD5A2	AR	Testis	–	Ambiguous or micropenis	Partial androgenization at puberty, ↑ testosterone-to-dihydrotestosterone ratio
AKR1C2 (*AKR1C4*)	AR	Testis	–	Female or ambiguous	Decreased fetal DHT production
Disorders of Androgen Action					
Androgen receptor	X	Testis	–	Female, ambiguous, micropenis or normal male	Phenotypic spectrum from complete androgen insensitivity syndrome (female external genitalia) and partial androgen insensitivity (ambiguous) to normal male genitalia and infertility

Abbreviations: AD, autosomal dominant; *AKR1C2*, aldo-keto reductase family 1 member 2; AR, autosomal recessive; *ARX*, aristaless related homeobox, X-linked; *ATRX*, α-thalassemia, mental retardation on the X; CAH, congenital adrenal hyperplasia; *CBX2*, chromobox homologue 2; *CYB5A*, cytochrome b5 POR, P450 oxidoreductase; *CYP11A1*, P450 cholesterol side-chain cleavage; *CYP17*, 17α-hydroxylase and 17,20-lyase; *DAX1*, dosage sensitive sex-reversal, adrenal hypoplasia congenita on the X chromosome, gene 1; DHEA, dehydroepiandrosterone; *DHCR7*, sterol 7 δ reductase; *DHH*, desert hedgehog; *GATA4*, GATA binding protein 4; *HSD17B3*, 17β-hydroxysteroid dehydrogenase type 3; *HSD3B2*, 3β-hydroxysteroid dehydrogenase type 2; *LHR*, LH receptor; *MAP3K1*, mitogen-activated protein kinase kinase kinase 1; *SF1*, steroidogenic factor 1; SL, sex-limited; *SOX9*, *SRY*-related HMG-box gene 9; *SRD5A2*, 5α-reductase type 2; *SRY*, sex-related gene on the Y chromosome; *StAR*, steroidogenic acute regulatory protein; WAGR, Wilms' tumor, aniridia, genitourinary anomalies, and mental retardation; *WNT4*, wingless-type mouse mammary tumor virus integration site, 4; *WT1*, Wilms' tumor–related gene 1.

skeletal abnormalities (Antley-Bixler craniosynostosis). Defects in *17β-hydroxysteroid dehydrogenase type 3* (*HSD17β3*) and *5α-reductase type 2* (*SRD5A2*) interfere with the synthesis of testosterone and DHT, respectively. These conditions are characterized by minimal or absent androgenization in utero, but some phallic development can occur during adolescence due to the action of other enzyme isoforms. Individuals with 5α-reductase type 2 deficiency have normal wolffian structures and usually do not develop breast tissue. At puberty, the increase in testosterone induces muscle mass and other virilizing features despite DHT deficiency. Some individuals change gender from female to male at puberty. Thus, the management of this disorder is challenging. DHT cream can improve prepubertal phallic growth in patients raised as male. Gonadectomy before adolescence and estrogen replacement at puberty can be considered in individuals raised as females who have a female gender identity. Disruption of alternative pathways to fetal DHT production might also present with 46,XY DSD (*AKR1C2/AKR1C4*).

Disorders of androgen action

Androgen insensitivity syndrome

Mutations in the androgen receptor cause resistance to androgen (testosterone, DHT) action or the *androgen insensitivity syndrome* (*AIS*). AIS is a spectrum of disorders that affects at least 1 in 100,000 46,XY individuals. Because the androgen receptor is X-linked, only 46,XY offspring are affected if the mother is a carrier of a mutation. XY individuals with *complete AIS* (formerly called *testicular feminization syndrome*) have a female phenotype, normal breast development (due to aromatization of testosterone), a short vagina but no uterus (because MIS production is normal), scanty pubic and axillary hair, and a female gender identity and sex role behavior. Gonadotropins and testosterone levels can be low, normal, or elevated, depending on the degree of androgen resistance and the contribution of estradiol to feedback inhibition of the hypothalamic-pituitary-gonadal axis. AMH/MIS levels in childhood are normal or high. Most patients present with inguinal hernias (containing testes) in childhood or with primary amenorrhea in late adolescence. Gonadectomy sometimes is offered for girls diagnosed in childhood, because there is a low risk of malignancy, and estrogen replacement is prescribed. Alternatively, the gonads can be left in situ until breast development is complete and removed because of tumor risk. Some adults with complete AIS decline gonadectomy, but should be counseled about the risk of malignancy, especially because early detection of premalignant changes by imaging or biomarkers is currently not possible. The use of graded dilators in adolescence is usually sufficient to dilate the vagina for sexual intercourse.

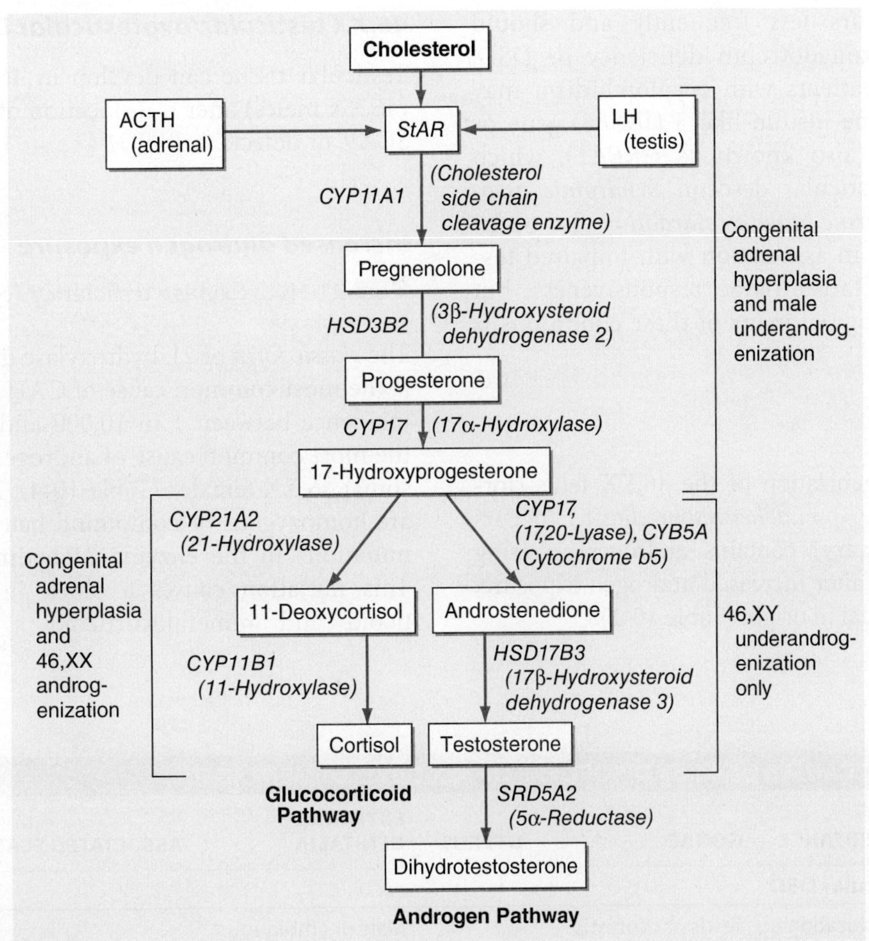

FIGURE 10-4

Simplified overview of glucocorticoid and androgen synthesis pathways. Defects in *CYP21A2* and *CYP11B1* shunt steroid precursors into the androgen pathway and cause androgenization of the 46,XX fetus. Testosterone is synthesized in the testicular Leydig cells and converted to dihydrotestosterone peripherally. Defects in enzymes involved in androgen synthesis result in underandrogenization of the 46,XY fetus. *StAR*, steroidogenic acute regulatory protein. *(After E Braunwald et al [eds]: Harrison's Principles of Internal Medicine, 15th ed. New York, McGraw-Hill, 2001.)*

Partial AIS (Reifenstein's syndrome) results from androgen receptor mutations that maintain residual function. Patients often present in infancy with penoscrotal hypospadias and small undescended testes and with gynecomastia at the time of puberty. Those individuals raised as males usually require hypospadias repair in childhood and may need breast reduction in adolescence. Some boys enter puberty spontaneously. High-dose testosterone has been given to support development if puberty does not progress, but long-term data are limited. More severely underandrogenized patients present with clitoral enlargement and labial fusion and may be raised as females. The surgical and psychosexual management of these patients is complex and requires active involvement of the parents and the patient during the appropriate stages of development. *Azoospermia* and male-factor infertility also have been described in association with mild loss-of-function mutations in the androgen receptor.

OTHER DISORDERS AFFECTING 46,XY MALES

Persistent müllerian duct syndrome is the presence of a uterus in an otherwise phenotypic male. This condition can result from mutations in AMH or its receptor (AMHR2). The uterus may be removed, but only if damage to the vasa deferentia and blood supply can be avoided. *Isolated hypospadias* occurs in ~1 in 250 males and is usually repaired surgically. Most cases are idiopathic, although evidence of penoscrotal hypospadias, poor phallic development, and/or bilateral cryptorchidism requires investigation for an underlying DSD (e.g., partial gonadal dysgenesis, mild defect in testosterone action, or even severe forms of 46,XX CAH). Unilateral undescended testes (cryptorchidism) affect more than 3% of boys at birth. Orchidopexy should be considered if the testis has not descended by 6–9 months of age. Bilateral cryptorchidism occurs less frequently and should raise suspicion of gonadotropin deficiency or DSD. A small subset of patients with cryptorchidism may have mutations in the insulin-like 3 (*INSL3*) gene or its receptor LGR8 (also known as *GREAT*), which mediates normal testicular descent. *Syndromic associations* and *intrauterine growth retardation* also occur relatively frequently in association with impaired testicular function or target tissue responsiveness, but the underlying etiology of many of these conditions is unknown.

46,XX DSD

Inappropriate androgenization of the 46,XX fetus (formerly called *female pseudohermaphroditism*) occurs when the gonad (ovary) contains androgen-secreting testicular material or after increased androgen exposure, which is usually adrenal in origin (Table 10-1).

46,XX testicular/ovotesticular DSD

Testicular tissue can develop in 46,XX testicular DSD (46,XX males) after translocation of *SRY*, duplication of *SOX9*, or defects in *RSPO1* (Table 10-4).

Increased androgen exposure

21-Hydroxylase deficiency (congenital adrenal hyperplasia)

The *classic form* of 21-hydroxylase deficiency (21-OHD) is the most common cause of CAH (**Chap. 8**). It has an incidence between 1 in 10,000 and 1 in 15,000 and is the most common cause of androgenization in chromosomal 46,XX females (Table 10-4). Affected individuals are homozygous or compound heterozygous for severe mutations in the enzyme 21-hydroxylase (*CYP21A2*). This mutation causes a block in adrenal glucocorticoid and mineralocorticoid synthesis, increasing

TABLE 10-4

SELECTED GENETIC CAUSES OF 46,XX DISORDERS OF SEX DEVELOPMENT (DSDs)

GENE	INHERITANCE	GONAD	UTERUS	EXTERNAL GENITALIA	ASSOCIATED FEATURES
Testicular/Ovotesticular DSD					
SRY	Translocation	Testis or ovotestis	–	Male or ambiguous	
SOX9	dup17q24	Unknown	–	Male or ambiguous	
RSPO1	AR	Testis or ovotestis	±	Male or ambiguous	Palmar plantar hyperkeratosis, squamous cell skin carcinoma
WNT4	AR	Testis or ovotestis	–	Male or ambiguous	SERKAL syndrome (renal dysgenesis, adrenal and lung hypoplasia)
Increased Androgen Synthesis					
HSD3B2	AR	Ovary	+	Clitoromegaly	CAH, primary adrenal failure, mild androgenization due to ↑ DHEA
CYP21A2	AR	Ovary	+	Ambiguous	CAH, phenotypic spectrum from severe salt-losing forms associated with adrenal failure to simple virilizing forms with compensated adrenal function, ↑ 17-hydroxyprogesterone
POR	AR	Ovary	+	Ambiguous or female	Mixed features of 21-hydroxylase deficiency and 17α-hydroxylase/17,20-lyase deficiency, sometimes associated with Antley-Bixler craniosynostosis
CYP11B1	AR	Ovary	+	Ambiguous	CAH, hypertension due to ↑ 11-deoxycortisol and 11-deoxycorticosterone
CYP19	AR	Ovary	+	Ambiguous	Maternal virilization during pregnancy, absent breast development at puberty
Glucocorticoid receptor	AR	Ovary	+	Ambiguous	↑ ACTH, 17-hydroxyprogesterone and cortisol; failure of dexamethasone suppression

Abbreviations: ACTH, adrenocorticotropin; AR, autosomal recessive; CAH, congenital adrenal hyperplasia; *CYP11B1*, 11β-hydroxylase; *CYP19*, aromatase; *CYP21A2*, 21-hydroxylase; DHEA, dehydroepiandrosterone; *HSD3B2*, 3β-hydroxysteroid dehydrogenase type 2; *POR*, P450 oxidoreductase; *RSPO1*, R-spondin 1; *SOX9*, *SRY*-related HMG-box gene 9; *SRY*, sex-related gene on the Y chromosome.

17-hydroxyprogesterone and shunting steroid precursors into the androgen synthesis pathway (Fig. 10-4). Glucocorticoid insufficiency causes a compensatory elevation of adrenocorticotropin (ACTH), resulting in adrenal hyperplasia and additional synthesis of steroid precursors proximal to the enzymatic block. Increased androgen synthesis in utero causes androgenization of the 46,XX fetus in the first trimester. Ambiguous genitalia are seen at birth, with varying degrees of clitoral enlargement and labial fusion. Excess androgen production causes gonadotropin-independent precocious puberty in males with 21-OHD.

The *salt-wasting* form of 21-OHD results from severe combined glucocorticoid and mineralocorticoid deficiency. A salt-wasting crisis usually manifests between 5 and 21 days of life and is a potentially life-threatening event that requires urgent fluid resuscitation and steroid treatment. Thus, a diagnosis of 21-OHD should be considered in any baby with atypical genitalia with bilateral nonpalpable gonads. Males (46,XY) with 21-OHD have no genital abnormalities at birth but are equally susceptible to adrenal insufficiency and salt-losing crises.

Females with the *classic simple virilizing* form of 21-OHD also present with genital ambiguity. They have impaired cortisol biosynthesis but do not develop salt loss. Patients with *nonclassic 21-OHD* produce normal amounts of cortisol and aldosterone but at the expense of producing excess androgens. Hirsutism (60%), oligomenorrhea (50%), and acne (30%) are the most common presenting features. This is one of the most common recessive disorders in humans, with an incidence as high as 1 in 100 to 500 in many populations and 1 in 27 in Ashkenazi Jews of Eastern European origin.

Biochemical features of acute salt-wasting 21-OHD are hyponatremia, hyperkalemia, hypoglycemia, inappropriately low cortisol and aldosterone, and elevated 17-hydroxyprogesterone, ACTH, and plasma renin activity. Presymptomatic diagnosis of classic 21-OHD is now made by neonatal screening tests for increased 17-hydroxyprogesterone in many centers. In most cases, 17-hydroxyprogesterone is markedly increased. In adults, ACTH stimulation (0.25 mg of cosyntropin IV) with assays for 17-hydroxyprogesterone at 0 and 30 min can be useful for detecting nonclassic 21-OHD and heterozygotes **(Chap. 8)**.

TREATMENT Congenital Adrenal Hyperplasia

Acute salt-wasting crises require fluid resuscitation, IV hydrocortisone, and correction of hypoglycemia. Once the patient is stabilized, glucocorticoids must be given to correct the cortisol insufficiency and suppress ACTH stimulation, thereby preventing further virilization, rapid skeletal maturation, and the development of polycystic ovaries. Typically, hydrocortisone (10–15 mg/m^2 per day in three divided doses) is used in childhood with a goal of partially suppressing 17-hydroxyprogesterone (100 to <1000 ng/dL). The aim of treatment is to use the lowest glucocorticoid dose that adequately suppresses adrenal androgen production without causing signs of glucocorticoid excess such as impaired growth and obesity. Salt-wasting conditions are treated with mineralocorticoid replacement. Infants usually need salt supplements up to the first year of life. Plasma renin activity and electrolytes are used to monitor mineralocorticoid replacement. Some patients with simple virilizing 21-OHD also benefit from mineralocorticoid supplements. Parents and patients should be educated about the need for increased doses of steroids during sickness, and patients should carry medic alert systems.

Steroid treatment for older adolescents and adults varies depending on lifestyle, age, and factors such as a desire to optimize fertility. Hydrocortisone remains a useful approach, but treatment with prednisolone at night may provide more complete ACTH suppression. Steroid doses should be adjusted to individual requirements because overtreatment can result in iatrogenic Cushing's-like features, including weight gain, insulin resistance, hypertension, and osteopenia. Because it is long acting, dexamethasone given at night is useful for ACTH suppression but is often associated with more side effects, making hydrocortisone or prednisolone preferable for most patients. Androstenedione and testosterone may be useful measurements of long-term control, with less fluctuation than 17-hydroxyprogesterone. Mineralocorticoid requirements often decrease in adulthood, and doses should be reassessed and reduced to avoid hypertension in adults. In very severe cases, adrenalectomy has been advocated but incurs the risks of surgery and total adrenal insufficiency.

Girls with significant genital androgenization due to classic 21-OHD usually undergo vaginal reconstruction and sometimes clitoral reduction (maintaining the glans and nerve supply), but the optimal timing of these procedures is debated, as is the need for the individual to be able to consent. There is a higher threshold for undertaking clitoral surgery in some centers because long-term sensation and ability to achieve orgasm can be affected, but the long-term results of newer techniques are not yet known. Full information about all options should be provided. If surgery is performed in infancy, surgical revision or regular vaginal dilatation may be needed in adolescence or adulthood, and long-term psychological support and psychosexual counseling may be appropriate. Women with 21-OHD frequently develop polycystic ovaries and have reduced fertility, especially when control is poor. Fecundity is achieved in 60–90% of women with good metabolic control, but ovulation induction (or even adrenalectomy) may be required. Dexamethasone should be avoided in pregnancy. Men with poorly controlled 21-OHD may develop testicular adrenal rests and are at risk for reduced fertility. Prenatal treatment of 21-OHD by the administration of dexamethasone to mothers is still under evaluation. However, pending methods to diagnose the disorder early in pregnancy, both affected and nonaffected fetuses will be exposed because treatment is started ideally before 6 to 7 weeks. The long-term effects of prenatal dexamethasone exposure on fetal development are still under evaluation, and current guidelines recommend full informed consent before treatment, ideally in a protocol that allows long-term follow-up of all children treated. Newer techniques such as cell-free fetal DNA testing may potentially reduce treatment of nonaffected fetuses.

The treatment of other forms of CAH includes mineralocorticoid and glucocorticoid replacement for salt-losing conditions (e.g., *StAR*, *CYP11A1*, *HSD3β2*), suppression of ACTH drive with glucocorticoids in disorders associated with hypertension (e.g., *CYP17*, *CYP11B1*), and appropriate sex hormone replacement in adolescence and adulthood, when necessary.

Other causes

Increased androgen synthesis can also occur in CAH due to defects in *POR*, *11β-hydroxylase* (*CYP11B1*), and *3β-hydroxysteroid dehydrogenase type 2* (*HSD3B2*) and with mutations in the genes encoding *aromatase* (*CYP19*) and the glucocorticoid receptor. Increased androgen exposure in utero can occur with maternal virilizing tumors and with ingestion of androgenic compounds.

OTHER DISORDERS AFFECTING 46,XX FEMALES

Congenital absence of the vagina occurs in association with *müllerian agenesis* or *hypoplasia* as part of the Mayer-Rokitansky-Kuster-Hauser (MRKH) syndrome (rarely caused by *WNT4* mutations). This diagnosis should be considered in otherwise phenotypically normal females with primary amenorrhea. Associated features include renal (agenesis) and cervical spinal abnormalities.

GLOBAL CONSIDERATIONS

The approach to a child or adolescent with ambiguous genitalia or another DSD requires cultural sensitivity, as the concepts of sex and gender vary widely. Rare genetic DSDs can occur more frequently in specific populations (e.g., *5α-reductase type 2* in the Dominican Republic). Different forms of CAH also show ethnic and geographic variability. In many countries, appropriate biochemical tests may not be readily available, and access to appropriate forms of treatment and support may be limited.

CHAPTER 11

DISORDERS OF THE TESTES AND MALE REPRODUCTIVE SYSTEM

Shalender Bhasin ■ J. Larry Jameson

The male reproductive system regulates sex differentiation, virilization, and the hormonal changes that accompany puberty, ultimately leading to spermatogenesis and fertility. Under the control of the pituitary hormones—luteinizing hormone (LH) and follicle-stimulating hormone (FSH)—the Leydig cells of the testes produce testosterone and germ cells are nurtured by Sertoli cells to divide, differentiate, and mature into sperm. During embryonic development, testosterone and dihydrotestosterone (DHT) induce the wolffian duct and virilization of the external genitalia. During puberty, testosterone promotes somatic growth and the development of secondary sex characteristics. In the adult, testosterone is necessary for spermatogenesis, stimulation of libido and normal sexual function, and maintenance of muscle and bone mass. This chapter focuses on the physiology of the testes and disorders associated with decreased androgen production, which may be caused by gonadotropin deficiency or by primary testis dysfunction. A variety of testosterone formulations now allow more physiologic androgen replacement. Infertility occurs in ~5% of men and is increasingly amenable to treatment by hormone replacement or by using sperm transfer techniques. **For further discussion of sexual dysfunction, disorders of the prostate, and testicular cancer, see Chaps. 19, and 12, respectively.**

DEVELOPMENT AND STRUCTURE OF THE TESTIS

The fetal testis develops from the undifferentiated gonad after expression of a genetic cascade that is initiated by the *SRY* (sex-related gene on the Y chromosome) **(Chap. 10)**. SRY induces differentiation of Sertoli cells, which surround germ cells and, together with peritubular myoid cells, form testis cords that will later develop into seminiferous tubules. Fetal Leydig cells and endothelial cells migrate into the gonad from the adjacent mesonephros but may also arise from interstitial cells that reside between testis cords. Leydig cells produce testosterone, which supports the growth and differentiation of wolffian duct structures that develop into the epididymis, vas deferens, and seminal vesicles. Testosterone is also converted to DHT (see below), which induces formation of the prostate and the external male genitalia, including the penis, urethra, and scrotum. Testicular descent through the inguinal canal is controlled in part by Leydig cell production of insulin-like factor 3 (INSL3), which acts via a receptor termed *Great* (*G* protein–coupled *re*ceptor *a*ffecting *t*estis descent). Sertoli cells produce müllerian-inhibiting substance (MIS), which causes regression of the müllerian structures, including the fallopian tube, uterus, and upper segment of the vagina.

NORMAL MALE PUBERTAL DEVELOPMENT

Although *puberty* commonly refers to the maturation of the reproductive axis and the development of secondary sex characteristics, it involves a coordinated response of multiple hormonal systems including the adrenal gland and the growth hormone (GH) axis (Fig. 11-1). The development of secondary sex characteristics is initiated by *adrenarche*, which usually occurs between 6 and 8 years of age when the adrenal gland begins to produce greater amounts of androgens from the zona reticularis, the principal site of dehydroepiandrosterone (DHEA) production. The sex maturation process is greatly accelerated by the activation of the hypothalamic-pituitary axis and the production

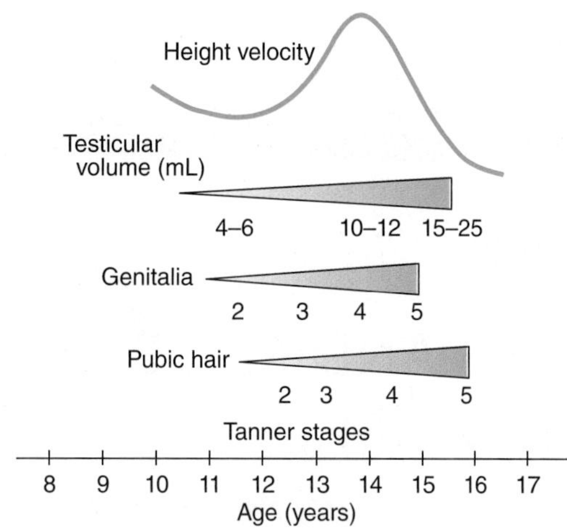

FIGURE 11-1

Pubertal events in males. Sexual maturity ratings for genitalia and pubic hair and divided into five stages. *(From WA Marshall, JM Tanner: Variations in the pattern of pubertal changes in boys. Arch Dis Child 45:13, 1970.)*

of gonadotropin-releasing hormone (GnRH). The GnRH pulse generator in the hypothalamus is active during fetal life and early infancy but is restrained until the early stages of puberty by a neuroendocrine brake imposed by the inhibitory actions of glutamate, γ-aminobutyric acid (GABA), and neuropeptide Y. Although the pathways that initiate reactivation of the GnRH pulse generator at the onset of puberty have been elusive, mounting evidence supports involvement of GPR54, a G protein–coupled receptor that binds an endogenous ligand, kisspeptin. Individuals with mutations of GPR54 fail to enter puberty, and experiments in primates demonstrate that infusion of the ligand is sufficient to induce premature puberty. Kisspeptin signaling plays an important role in mediating the feedback action of sex steroids on gonadotropin secretion and in regulating the tempo of sexual maturation at puberty. Leptin, a hormone produced by adipose cells, plays a permissive role in the resurgence of GnRH secretion at the onset of puberty, as leptin-deficient individuals also fail to enter puberty **(Chap. 20)**. The adipocyte hormone leptin, gut hormone ghrelin, neuropeptide Y, and kisspeptin integrate the signals originating in energy stores and metabolic tissues with mechanisms that control onset of puberty through regulation of GnRH secretion. Energy deficit and excess and metabolic stress are associated with disturbed reproductive maturation and timing of pubertal onset.

The early stages of puberty are characterized by nocturnal surges of LH and FSH. Growth of the testes is usually the first sign of puberty, reflecting an increase in seminiferous tubule volume. Increasing levels of testosterone deepen the voice and increase muscle growth. Conversion of testosterone to DHT leads to growth of the external genitalia and pubic hair. DHT also stimulates prostate and facial hair growth and initiates recession of the temporal hairline. The growth spurt occurs at a testicular volume of about 10–12 mL. GH increases early in puberty and is stimulated in part by the rise in gonadal steroids. GH increases the level of insulin-like growth factor I (IGF-I), which enhances linear bone growth. The prolonged pubertal exposure to gonadal steroids (mainly estradiol) ultimately causes epiphyseal closure and limits further bone growth.

REGULATION OF TESTICULAR FUNCTION

REGULATION OF THE HYPOTHALAMIC-PITUITARY-TESTIS AXIS IN ADULT MAN

Hypothalamic GnRH regulates the production of the pituitary gonadotropins LH and FSH (Fig. 11-2). GnRH is released in discrete pulses approximately every 2 h, resulting in corresponding pulses of LH and FSH. These dynamic hormone pulses account in part for the wide variations in LH and testosterone, even within the same individual. LH acts primarily on the Leydig cell to stimulate testosterone synthesis. The regulatory control of androgen synthesis is mediated by testosterone and estrogen feedback on both the hypothalamus and the pituitary. FSH acts on the Sertoli cell to regulate spermatogenesis and the production of Sertoli products such as inhibin B, which acts to selectively suppress pituitary FSH. Despite these somewhat distinct Leydig and Sertoli cell–regulated pathways, testis function is integrated at several levels: GnRH regulates both gonadotropins; spermatogenesis requires high levels of testosterone; and numerous paracrine interactions between Leydig and Sertoli cells are necessary for normal testis function.

THE LEYDIG CELL: ANDROGEN SYNTHESIS

LH binds to its seven-transmembrane, G protein–coupled receptor to activate the cyclic AMP pathway. Stimulation of the LH receptor induces *st*eroid *a*cute *r*egulatory (StAR) protein, along with several steroidogenic enzymes involved in androgen synthesis. LH receptor mutations cause Leydig cell hypoplasia or agenesis, underscoring the importance of this pathway for Leydig cell development and function. The rate-limiting process in testosterone synthesis is the delivery of cholesterol by the StAR protein to the inner mitochondrial membrane. Peripheral benzodiazepine receptor, a mitochondrial cholesterol-binding protein, is also an acute regulator of Leydig cell steroidogenesis. The five major enzymatic steps involved in testosterone synthesis are summarized in Fig. 11-3. After cholesterol transport into the mitochondrion,

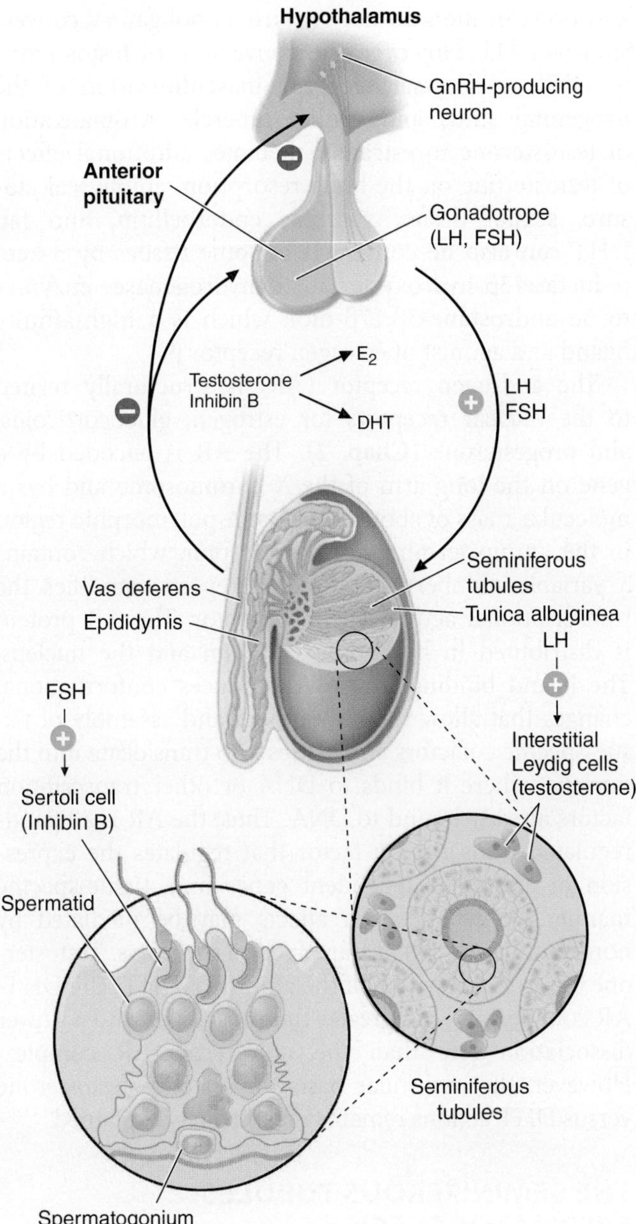

FIGURE 11-2

Human pituitary gonadotropin axis, structure of testis, and seminiferous tubule. E_2, 17β-estradiol; DHT, dihydrotestosterone; FSH, follicle-stimulating hormones; GnRH, gonadotropin-releasing; LH, luteinizing hormone.

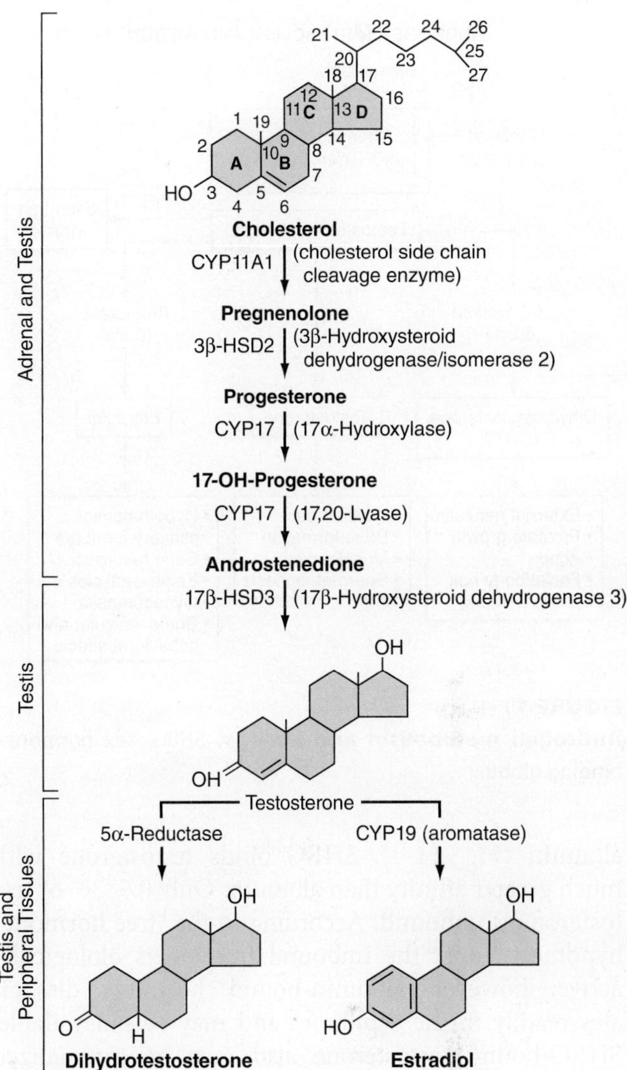

FIGURE 11-3

The biochemical pathway in the conversion of 27-carbon sterol cholesterol to androgens and estrogens.

the formation of pregnenolone by CYP11A1 (side chain cleavage enzyme) is a limiting enzymatic step. The 17α-hydroxylase and the 17,20-lyase reactions are catalyzed by a single enzyme, CYP17; posttranslational modification (phosphorylation) of this enzyme and the presence of specific enzyme cofactors confer 17,20-lyase activity selectively in the testis and zona reticularis of the adrenal gland. Testosterone can be converted to the more potent DHT by 5α-reductase, or it can be aromatized to estradiol by CYP19 (aromatase). Two isoforms of steroid 5α-reductase, SRD5A1 and SRD5A2, have been described; all known kindreds with 5α-reductase deficiency have had mutations in SRD5A2, the predominant form in the prostate and the skin.

Testosterone transport and metabolism

In males, 95% of circulating testosterone is derived from testicular production (3–10 mg/d). Direct secretion of testosterone by the adrenal and the peripheral conversion of androstenedione to testosterone collectively account for another 0.5 mg/d of testosterone. Only a small amount of DHT (70 μg/d) is secreted directly by the testis; most circulating DHT is derived from peripheral conversion of testosterone. Most of the daily production of estradiol (~45 μg/d) in men is derived from aromatase-mediated peripheral conversion of testosterone and androstenedione.

Circulating testosterone is bound to two plasma proteins: sex hormone–binding globulin (SHBG) and

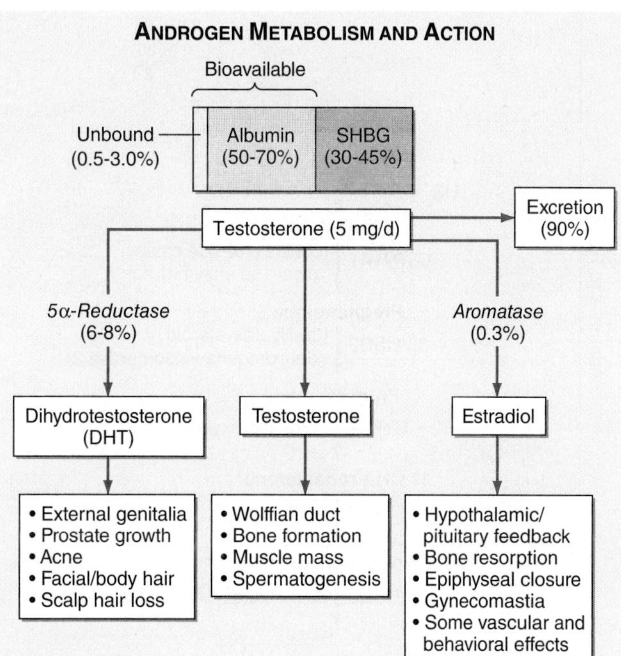

FIGURE 11-4
Androgen metabolism and actions. SHBG, sex hormone–binding globulin.

albumin (Fig. 11-4). SHBG binds testosterone with much greater affinity than albumin. Only 0.5–3% of testosterone is unbound. According to the "free hormone" hypothesis, only the unbound fraction is biologically active; however, albumin-bound hormone dissociates readily in the capillaries and may be bioavailable. SHBG-bound testosterone also may be internalized through endocytic pits by binding to a protein called megalin. SHBG concentrations are decreased by androgens, obesity, diabetes mellitus, insulin, and nephrotic syndrome. Conversely, estrogen administration, hyperthyroidism, many chronic inflammatory illnesses, infections such as HIV or hepatitis B and C, and aging are associated with high SHBG concentrations.

Testosterone is metabolized predominantly in the liver, although some degradation occurs in peripheral tissues, particularly the prostate and the skin. In the liver, testosterone is converted by a series of enzymatic steps that involve 5α- and 5β-reductases, 3α- and 3β-hydroxysteroid dehydrogenases, and 17β-hydroxysteroid dehydrogenase into androsterone, etiocholanolone, DHT, and 3-α-androstanediol. These compounds undergo glucuronidation or sulfation before being excreted by the kidneys.

Mechanism of androgen action

Testosterone exerts some of its biologic effects by binding to androgen receptor, either directly or after its conversion to DHT by the steroid 5-α reductase. Testosterone's effects on the skeletal muscle, erythropoiesis, and bone in men do not require its obligatory conversion to DHT. However, the conversion of testosterone to DHT is necessary for the masculinization of the urogenital sinus and genital tubercle. Aromatization of testosterone to estradiol mediates additional effects of testosterone on the bone resorption, epiphyseal closure, sexual desire, vascular endothelium, and fat. DHT can also be converted in some tissues by 3-keto reductase/3β-hydroxysteroid dehydrogenase enzymes to 5α-androstane-3β,17β-diol, which is a high-affinity ligand and agonist of estrogen receptor β.

The androgen receptor (AR) is structurally related to the nuclear receptors for estrogen, glucocorticoids, and progesterone **(Chap. 2)**. The AR is encoded by a gene on the long arm of the X chromosome and has a molecular mass of about 110 kDa. A polymorphic region in the amino terminus of the receptor, which contains a variable number of glutamine repeats, modifies the transcriptional activity of the receptor. The AR protein is distributed in both the cytoplasm and the nucleus. The ligand binding to the AR induces conformational changes that allow the recruitment and assembly of tissue-specific cofactors and causes it to translocate into the nucleus, where it binds to DNA or other transcription factors already bound to DNA. Thus, the AR is a ligand-regulated transcription factor that regulates the expression of androgen-dependent genes in a tissue-specific manner. Some androgen effects may be mediated by nongenomic AR signal transduction pathways. Testosterone binds to AR with half the affinity of DHT. The DHT-AR complex also has greater thermostability and a slower dissociation rate than the testosterone-AR complex. However, the molecular basis for selective testosterone versus DHT actions remains incompletely explained.

THE SEMINIFEROUS TUBULES: SPERMATOGENESIS

The seminiferous tubules are convoluted, closed loops with both ends emptying into the rete testis, a network of progressively larger efferent ducts that ultimately form the epididymis (Fig. 11-2). The seminiferous tubules total about 600 m in length and comprise about two-thirds of testis volume. The walls of the tubules are formed by polarized Sertoli cells that are apposed to peritubular myoid cells. Tight junctions between Sertoli cells create a blood-testis barrier. Germ cells compose the majority of the seminiferous epithelium (~60%) and are intimately embedded within the cytoplasmic extensions of the Sertoli cells, which function as "nurse cells." Germ cells progress through characteristic stages of mitotic and meiotic divisions. A pool of type A spermatogonia serve as stem cells capable of self-renewal. Primary spermatocytes are derived from type B spermatogonia and undergo meiosis before progressing to spermatids that undergo spermiogenesis (a differentiation process involving chromatin condensation, acquisition of an acrosome, elongation of cytoplasm, and formation of a tail) and are released from Sertoli cells as mature spermatozoa. The complete differentiation process into mature sperm requires 74 days. Peristaltic-type action by peritubular myoid cells transports sperm into the efferent ducts. The spermatozoa spend an additional 21 days in the epididymis, where they undergo further maturation and capacitation. The normal adult testes produce >100 million sperm per day.

Naturally occurring mutations in the *FSHβ* gene and in the FSH receptor confirm an important, but not essential, role for this pathway in spermatogenesis. Females with these mutations are hypogonadal and infertile because ovarian follicles do not mature; males exhibit variable degrees of reduced spermatogenesis, presumably because of impaired Sertoli cell function. Because Sertoli cells produce inhibin B, an inhibitor of FSH, seminiferous tubule damage (e.g., by radiation) causes a selective increase of FSH. Testosterone reaches very high concentrations locally in the testis and is essential for spermatogenesis. The cooperative actions of FSH and testosterone are important in the progression of meiosis and spermiation. FSH and testosterone regulate germ cell survival via the intrinsic and the extrinsic apoptotic mechanisms. FSH may also play an important role in supporting spermatogonia. Gonadotropin-regulated testicular RNA helicase (GRTH/DDX25), a testis-specific gonadotropin/androgen-regulated RNA helicase, is present in germ cells and Leydig cells and may be an important factor in the paracrine regulation of germ cell development. Several cytokines and growth factors are also involved in the regulation of spermatogenesis by paracrine and autocrine mechanisms. A number of knockout mouse models exhibit impaired germ cell development or spermatogenesis, presaging possible mutations associated with male infertility. The human Y chromosome contains a small pseudoautosomal region that can recombine with homologous regions of the X chromosome. Most of the Y chromosome does not recombine with the X chromosome and is referred to as the male-specific region of the Y (MSY). The MSY contains 156 transcription units that encode for 26 proteins, including nine families of Y-specific multicopy genes; many of these Y-specific genes are also testis-specific and necessary for spermatogenesis. Microdeletions of several Y chromosome azoospermia factor (*AZF*) genes (e.g., RNA-binding motif, *RBM*; deleted in azoospermia, *DAZ*) are associated with oligospermia or azoospermia.

TREATMENT **Male Factor Infertility**

Treatment options for male factor infertility have expanded greatly in recent years. Secondary hypogonadism is highly amenable to treatment with pulsatile GnRH or gonadotropins (see below). Assisted reproductive technologies such as the in vitro fertilization (IVF) and intracytoplasmic sperm injection (ICSI) have provided new opportunities for patients with primary testicular failure and disorders of sperm transport. Choice of initial treatment options depends on sperm concentration and motility. Expectant management should be attempted initially in men with mild male factor infertility (sperm count of 15–20 × 10^6/mL and normal motility). Moderate male factor infertility (10–15 × 10^6/mL and 20–40% motility) should begin with intrauterine insemination alone or in combination with treatment of the female partner with clomiphene or gonadotropins, but it may require IVF with or without ICSI. For men with a severe defect (sperm count of <10 × 10^6/mL, 10% motility), IVF with ICSI or donor sperm should be used.

CLINICAL AND LABORATORY EVALUATION OF MALE REPRODUCTIVE FUNCTION

HISTORY AND PHYSICAL EXAMINATION

The history should focus on developmental stages such as puberty and growth spurts, as well as androgen-dependent events such as early morning erections, frequency and intensity of sexual thoughts, and frequency of masturbation or intercourse. Although libido and the overall frequency of sexual acts are decreased in androgen-deficient men, young hypogonadal men may achieve erections in response to visual erotic stimuli. Men with acquired androgen deficiency often report decreased energy and increased irritability.

The physical examination should focus on secondary sex characteristics such as hair growth, gynecomastia, testicular volume, prostate, and height and body proportions. *Eunuchoid proportions* are defined as an arm span >2 cm greater than height and suggest that androgen deficiency occurred before epiphyseal fusion. Hair growth in the face, axilla, chest, and pubic regions is androgen-dependent; however, changes may not be noticeable unless androgen deficiency is severe and prolonged. Ethnicity also influences the intensity of hair growth **(Chap. 17)**. Testicular volume is best assessed by using a Prader orchidometer. Testes range from 3.5 to 5.5 cm in length, which corresponds to a volume of 12–25 mL. Advanced age does not influence testicular size, although the consistency becomes less firm. Asian men generally have smaller testes than Western Europeans, independent of differences in body size. Because of its possible role in infertility, the presence of varicocele should be sought by palpation while the patient is standing; it is more common on the left side. Patients with Klinefelter's syndrome have markedly reduced testicular volumes (1–2 mL). In congenital hypogonadotropic hypogonadism, testicular volumes provide a good index for the degree of gonadotropin deficiency and the likelihood of response to therapy.

GONADOTROPIN AND INHIBIN MEASUREMENTS

LH and FSH are measured using two-site immunoradiometric, immunofluorometric, or chemiluminescent assays, which have very low cross-reactivity with other pituitary glycoprotein hormones and human chorionic gonadotropin (hCG) and have sufficient sensitivity to measure the low levels present in patients with hypogonadotropic hypogonadism. In men with a low testosterone level, an LH level can distinguish primary (high LH) versus secondary (low or inappropriately normal LH) hypogonadism. An elevated LH level indicates a primary defect at the testicular level, whereas a low or inappropriately normal LH level suggests a defect at the hypothalamic-pituitary level. LH pulses occur about every 1–3 h in normal men. Thus, gonadotropin levels fluctuate, and samples should be pooled or repeated when results are equivocal. FSH is less pulsatile than LH because it has a longer half-life. Selective increase in FSH suggests damage to the seminiferous tubules. Inhibin B, a Sertoli cell product that suppresses FSH, is reduced with seminiferous tubule damage. Inhibin B is a dimer with α-β_B subunits and is measured by two-site immunoassays.

GnRH stimulation testing

The GnRH test is performed by measuring LH and FSH concentrations at baseline and at 30 and 60 min after intravenous administration of 100 μg of GnRH. A minimally acceptable response is a twofold LH increase and a 50% FSH increase. In the prepubertal period or with severe GnRH deficiency, the gonadotrope may not respond to a single bolus of GnRH because it has not been primed by endogenous hypothalamic GnRH; in these patients, GnRH responsiveness may be restored by chronic, pulsatile GnRH administration. With the availability of sensitive and specific LH assays, GnRH stimulation testing is used rarely except to evaluate gonadotrope function in patients who have undergone pituitary surgery or have a space-occupying lesion in the hypothalamic-pituitary region.

TESTOSTERONE ASSAYS

Total testosterone

Total testosterone includes both unbound and protein-bound testosterone and is measured by radioimmunoassays, immunometric assays, or liquid chromatography tandem mass spectrometry (LC-MS/MS). LC-MS/MS involves extraction of serum by organic solvents, separation of testosterone from other steroids by high-performance liquid chromatography and mass spectrometry, and quantitation of unique testosterone fragments by mass spectrometry. LC-MS/MS provides accurate and sensitive measurements of testosterone levels even in the low range and is emerging as the method of choice for testosterone measurement. Laboratories that have been certified by the Centers for Disease Control and Prevention (CDC) Hormone Standardization Program for Testosterone (HoST) can ensure that testosterone measurements are accurate and calibrated to an international standard. A single fasting morning sample provides a good approximation of the average testosterone concentration with the realization that testosterone levels fluctuate in response to pulsatile LH. Testosterone is generally lower in the late afternoon and is reduced by acute illness. The testosterone concentration in healthy young men ranges from 300 to 1000 ng/dL in most laboratories, and efforts are under way to generate harmonized population-based reference ranges that can be applied to all CDC-certified laboratories. Alterations in SHBG levels due to aging, obesity, diabetes mellitus, hyperthyroidism, some types of medications, or chronic illness or on a congenital basis can affect total testosterone levels. Heritable factors contribute substantially to the population-level variation in testosterone levels, and genome-wide association studies have revealed polymorphisms in the *SHBG* gene as important contributors to variation in testosterone levels.

Measurement of unbound testosterone levels

Most circulating testosterone is bound to SHBG and to albumin; only 0.5–3% of circulating testosterone is unbound, or "free." The unbound testosterone concentration can be measured by equilibrium dialysis or calculated from total testosterone, SHBG, and albumin concentrations. Recent research has shown that testosterone binding to SHBG is a multistep process that involves complex homoallostery within the SHBG dimer; a novel allosteric model of testosterone binding to SHBG dimers provides good estimates of free testosterone concentrations. The previous law of mass action equations based on linear models of testosterone binding to SHBG have been shown to be erroneous. Tracer analogue methods are relatively inexpensive and convenient, but they are inaccurate. *Bioavailable testosterone* refers to unbound testosterone plus testosterone that is loosely bound to albumin; it can be determined by the ammonium sulfate precipitation method.

hCG stimulation test

The hCG stimulation test is performed by administering a single injection of 1500–4000 IU of hCG intramuscularly and measuring testosterone levels at baseline and 24, 48, 72, and 120 h after hCG injection. An alternative regimen involves three injections of 1500 units of hCG on successive days and measuring testosterone levels 24 h after the last dose. An acceptable response to hCG is a doubling of the testosterone concentration in adult men. In prepubertal boys, an increase in testosterone to >150 ng/dL indicates the presence of testicular tissue. No response may indicate an absence of testicular tissue or marked impairment of Leydig cell function. Measurement of MIS, a Sertoli cell product, is also used to detect the presence of testes in prepubertal boys with cryptorchidism.

SEMEN ANALYSIS

Semen analysis is the most important step in the evaluation of male infertility. Samples are collected by masturbation following a period of abstinence for 2–3 days. Semen volumes and sperm concentrations vary considerably among fertile men, and several samples may be needed before concluding that the results are abnormal. Analysis should be performed within an hour of collection. Using semen samples from over 4500 men in 14 countries, whose partners had a time-to-pregnancy of less than 12 months, the World Health Organization (WHO) has generated the following one-sided reference limits for semen parameters: semen volume, 1.5 mL; total sperm number, 39 million per ejaculate; sperm concentration, 15 million/mL; vitality, 58% live; progressive motility, 32%; total (progressive + nonprogressive) motility, 40%; morphologically normal forms, 4.0%. Some men with low sperm counts are nevertheless fertile. A variety of tests for sperm function can be performed in specialized laboratories, but these add relatively little to the treatment options.

TESTICULAR BIOPSY

Testicular biopsy is useful in some patients with oligospermia or azoospermia as an aid in diagnosis and indication for the feasibility of treatment. Using local anesthesia, fine-needle aspiration biopsy is performed to aspirate tissue for histology. Alternatively, open biopsies can be performed under local or general anesthesia when more tissue is required. A normal biopsy in an azoospermic man with a normal FSH level suggests obstruction of the vas deferens, which may be correctable surgically. Biopsies are also used to harvest sperm for ICSI and to classify disorders such as hypospermatogenesis (all stages present but in reduced numbers), germ cell arrest (usually at primary spermatocyte stage), and Sertoli cell–only syndrome (absent germ cells) or hyalinization (sclerosis with absent cellular elements).

DISORDERS OF SEXUAL DIFFERENTIATION

See Chap. 10.

DISORDERS OF PUBERTY

The onset and tempo of puberty varies greatly in the general population and is affected by genetic and environmental factors. Although some of the variance in the timing of puberty is explained by heritable factors, the genes involved remain unknown.

PRECOCIOUS PUBERTY

Puberty in boys before age 9 is considered precocious. *Isosexual precocity* refers to premature sexual development consistent with phenotypic sex and includes features such as the development of facial hair and phallic growth. Isosexual precocity is divided into gonadotropin-dependent and gonadotropin-independent causes of androgen excess (Table 11-1). *Heterosexual precocity* refers to the premature development of estrogenic features in boys, such as breast development.

Gonadotropin-dependent precocious puberty

This disorder, called *central precocious puberty* (CPP), is less common in boys than in girls. It is caused by premature activation of the GnRH pulse generator, sometimes because of central nervous system (CNS) lesions such as hypothalamic hamartomas, but it is often idiopathic. CPP is characterized by gonadotropin levels that are inappropriately elevated for age. Because pituitary priming has occurred, GnRH elicits LH and FSH responses typical of those seen in puberty or in adults. Magnetic resonance imaging (MRI) should be performed to exclude a mass, structural defect, infection, or inflammatory process. Mutations in *MKRN3*, an imprinted gene encoding makorin ring-finger protein 3, which is expressed only from the paternally inherited allele, have been associated with CPP.

Gonadotropin-independent precocious puberty

In gonadotropin-independent precocious puberty, androgens from the testis or the adrenal are increased, but gonadotropins are low. This group of disorders includes hCG-secreting tumors; congenital adrenal hyperplasia; sex steroid–producing tumors of the testis, adrenal, and ovary; accidental or deliberate exogenous sex steroid administration; hypothyroidism; and activating mutations of the LH receptor or $G_s\alpha$ subunit.

TABLE 11-1

CAUSES OF PRECOCIOUS OR DELAYED PUBERTY IN BOYS

- I. Precocious puberty
  - A. Gonadotropin-dependent
    1. Idiopathic
    2. Hypothalamic hamartoma or other lesions
    3. CNS tumor or inflammatory state
  - B. Gonadotropin-independent
    1. Congenital adrenal hyperplasia
    2. hCG-secreting tumor
    3. McCune-Albright syndrome
    4. Activating LH receptor mutation
    5. Exogenous androgens
- II. Delayed puberty
  - A. Constitutional delay of growth and puberty
  - B. Systemic disorders
    1. Chronic disease
    2. Malnutrition
    3. Anorexia nervosa
  - C. CNS tumors and their treatment (radiotherapy and surgery)
  - D. Hypothalamic-pituitary causes of pubertal failure (low gonadotropins)
    1. Congenital disorders (see Table 11-2)
    2. Acquired disorders
       - a. Pituitary tumors
       - b. Hyperprolactinemia
  - E. Gonadal causes of pubertal failure (elevated gonadotropins)
    1. Klinefelter's syndrome
    2. Bilateral undescended testes
    3. Orchitis
    4. Chemotherapy or radiotherapy
    5. Anorchia
  - F. Androgen insensitivity

Abbreviations: CNS, central nervous system; GnRH, gonadotropin-releasing hormone; hCG, human chronic gonadotropin; LH, luteinizing hormone.

Familial male-limited precocious puberty

Also called *testotoxicosis*, familial male-limited precocious puberty is an autosomal dominant disorder caused by activating mutations in the LH receptor, leading to constitutive stimulation of the cyclic AMP pathway and testosterone production. Clinical features include premature androgenization in boys, growth acceleration in early childhood, and advanced bone age followed by premature epiphyseal fusion. Testosterone is elevated, and LH is suppressed. Treatment options include inhibitors of testosterone synthesis (e.g., ketoconazole), AR antagonists (e.g., flutamide and bicalutamide), and aromatase inhibitors (e.g., anastrazole).

McCune-Albright syndrome

This is a sporadic disorder caused by somatic (postzygotic) activating mutations in the $G_s\alpha$ subunit that links G protein–coupled receptors to intracellular signaling pathways **(Chap. 36)**. The mutations impair the guanosine triphosphatase activity of the $G_s\alpha$ protein, leading to constitutive activation of adenylyl cyclase. Like activating LH receptor mutations, this stimulates testosterone production and causes gonadotropin-independent precocious puberty. In addition to sexual precocity, affected individuals may have autonomy in the adrenals, pituitary, and thyroid glands. Café au lait spots are characteristic skin lesions that reflect the onset of the somatic mutations in melanocytes during embryonic development. Polyostotic fibrous dysplasia is caused by activation of the parathyroid hormone receptor pathway in bone. Treatment is similar to that in patients with activating LH receptor mutations. Bisphosphonates have been used to treat bone lesions.

Congenital adrenal hyperplasia

Boys with congenital adrenal hyperplasia (CAH) who are not well controlled with glucocorticoid suppression of adrenocorticotropic hormone (ACTH) can develop premature virilization because of excessive androgen production by the adrenal gland **(Chaps. 8 and 10)**. LH is low, and the testes are small. Adrenal rests may develop within the testis of poorly controlled patients with CAH because of chronic ACTH stimulation; adrenal rests do not require surgical removal and regress with effective glucocorticoid therapy. Some children with CAH may develop gonadotropin-dependent precocious puberty with early maturation of the hypothalamic-pituitary-gonadal axis, elevated gonadotropins, and testicular growth.

Heterosexual sexual precocity

Breast enlargement in prepubertal boys can result from familial aromatase excess, estrogen-producing tumors in the adrenal gland, Sertoli cell tumors in the testis, marijuana smoking, or exogenous estrogens or androgens. Occasionally, germ cell tumors that secrete hCG can be associated with breast enlargement due to excessive stimulation of estrogen production (see "Gynecomastia," below).

APPROACH TO THE PATIENT: Precocious Puberty

After verification of precocious development, serum LH and FSH levels should be measured to determine whether gonadotropins are increased in relation to chronologic age (gonadotropin-dependent) or whether sex steroid secretion is occurring independent of LH and FSH (gonadotropin-independent). In children with gonadotropin-dependent precocious puberty, CNS lesions should be excluded by history, neurologic examination, and MRI scan of the head. If organic causes are not found, one is left with the diagnosis of idiopathic central precocity. Patients with high testosterone but suppressed LH concentrations have gonadotropin-independent sexual precocity; in these patients, DHEA sulfate (DHEAS) and 17α-hydroxyprogesterone should be measured. High levels of testosterone and 17α-hydroxyprogesterone suggest the possibility of CAH due to 21α-hydroxylase or 11β-hydroxylase deficiency. If testosterone and DHEAS are elevated, adrenal tumors should be excluded by obtaining a computed tomography (CT) scan of the adrenal glands. Patients with elevated testosterone but without increased 17α-hydroxyprogesterone or DHEAS should undergo careful evaluation of the testis by palpation and ultrasound to exclude a Leydig cell neoplasm. Activating mutations of the LH receptor should be considered in children with gonadotropin-independent precocious puberty in whom CAH, androgen abuse, and adrenal and testicular neoplasms have been excluded.

TREATMENT Precocious Puberty

In patients with a known cause (e.g., a CNS lesion or a testicular tumor), therapy should be directed toward the underlying disorder. In patients with idiopathic CPP, long-acting GnRH analogues can be used to suppress gonadotropins and decrease testosterone, halt early pubertal development, delay accelerated bone maturation, prevent early epiphyseal closure, promote final height gain, and mitigate the psychosocial consequences of early pubertal development without causing osteoporosis. The treatment is most effective for increasing final adult height if it is initiated before age 6. Puberty resumes after discontinuation of the GnRH analogue. Counseling is an important aspect of the overall treatment strategy.

In children with gonadotropin-independent precocious puberty, inhibitors of steroidogenesis, such as ketoconazole, and AR antagonists have been used empirically. Long-term treatment with spironolactone (a weak androgen antagonist) and ketoconazole has been reported to normalize growth rate and bone maturation and to improve predicted height in small, nonrandomized trials in boys with familial male-limited precocious puberty. Aromatase inhibitors, such as testolactone and letrozole, have been used as an adjunct to antiandrogen and GnRH analogue therapy for children with familial male-limited precocious puberty, CAH, and McCune-Albright syndrome.

DELAYED PUBERTY

Puberty is delayed in boys if it has not ensued by age 14, an age that is 2–2.5 standard deviations above the mean for healthy children. Delayed puberty is more common in boys than in girls. There are four main categories of delayed puberty: (1) constitutional delay of growth and puberty (~60% of cases); (2) functional hypogonadotropic hypogonadism caused by systemic illness or malnutrition (~20% of cases); (3) hypogonadotropic hypogonadism caused by genetic or acquired defects in the hypothalamic-pituitary region (~10% of cases); and (4) hypergonadotropic hypogonadism secondary to primary gonadal failure (~15% of cases) (Table 11-1). Functional hypogonadotropic hypogonadism is more common in girls than in boys. Permanent causes of hypogonadotropic or hypergonadotropic hypogonadism are identified in >25% of boys with delayed puberty.

APPROACH TO THE PATIENT: Delayed Puberty

Any history of systemic illness, eating disorders, excessive exercise, social and psychological problems, and abnormal patterns of linear growth during childhood should be verified. Boys with pubertal delay may have accompanying emotional and physical immaturity relative to their peers, which can be a source of anxiety. Physical examination should focus on height; arm span; weight; visual fields; and secondary sex characteristics, including hair growth, testicular volume, phallic size, and scrotal reddening and thinning. Testicular size >2.5 cm generally indicates that the child has entered puberty.

The main diagnostic challenge is to distinguish those with constitutional delay, who will progress through puberty at a later age, from those with an underlying pathologic process. Constitutional delay should be suspected when there is a family history and when there are delayed bone age and short stature. Pituitary priming by pulsatile GnRH is required before LH and FSH are synthesized and secreted normally. Thus, blunted responses to exogenous GnRH can be seen in patients with constitutional delay, GnRH deficiency, or pituitary disorders (see "GnRH Stimulation Testing," above). On the other hand, low-normal basal gonadotropin levels or a normal response to exogenous GnRH is consistent with an early stage of puberty, which is often heralded by nocturnal GnRH secretion. Thus, constitutional delay is a diagnosis of exclusion that requires ongoing evaluation until the onset of puberty and the growth spurt.

TREATMENT Delayed Puberty

If therapy is considered appropriate, it can begin with 25–50 mg testosterone enanthate or testosterone cypionate every 2 weeks, or by using a 2.5-mg testosterone patch or 25-mg testosterone gel. Because aromatization of testosterone to estrogen is obligatory for mediating androgen effects on epiphyseal fusion, concomitant treatment with aromatase inhibitors may allow attainment of greater final adult height. Testosterone treatment should be interrupted after 6 months to determine if endogenous LH and FSH secretion have ensued. Other causes of delayed puberty should be considered when there are associated clinical features or when boys do not enter puberty spontaneously after a year of observation or treatment.

Reassurance without hormonal treatment is appropriate for many individuals with presumed constitutional delay of puberty. However, the impact of delayed growth and pubertal progression on a child's social relationships and school performance should be weighed. Also, boys with constitutional delay of puberty are less likely to achieve their full genetic height potential and have reduced total-body bone mass as adults, mainly due to narrow limb bones and vertebrae as a result of impaired periosteal expansion during puberty. Administration of androgen therapy to boys with constitutional delay does not affect final height, and when administered with an aromatase inhibitor, it may improve final height.

DISORDERS OF THE MALE REPRODUCTIVE AXIS DURING ADULTHOOD

HYPOGONADOTROPIC HYPOGONADISM

Because LH and FSH are trophic hormones for the testes, impaired secretion of these pituitary gonadotropins results in secondary hypogonadism, which is characterized by low testosterone in the setting of low LH and FSH. Those with the most severe deficiency have complete absence of pubertal development, sexual infantilism, and, in some cases, hypospadias and undescended testes. Patients with partial gonadotropin deficiency have delayed or arrested sex development. The 24-h LH secretory profiles are heterogeneous in patients with hypogonadotropic hypogonadism, reflecting variable abnormalities of LH pulse frequency or amplitude. In severe cases, basal LH is low and there are no LH pulses. A smaller subset of patients has low-amplitude LH pulses or markedly reduced pulse frequency. Occasionally, only sleep-entrained LH pulses occur, reminiscent of the pattern seen in the early stages of puberty. Hypogonadotropic hypogonadism can be classified into congenital and acquired disorders. Congenital disorders most commonly involve GnRH deficiency, which leads to gonadotropin deficiency. Acquired disorders are much more common than congenital disorders and may result from a variety of sellar mass lesions or infiltrative diseases of the hypothalamus or pituitary.

Congenital disorders associated with gonadotropin deficiency

Congenital hypogonadotropic hypogonadism is a heterogeneous group of disorders characterized by decreased gonadotropin secretion and testicular dysfunction either due to impaired function of the GnRH pulse generator or the gonadotrope. The disorders characterized by GnRH deficiency represent a family of oligogenic disorders whose phenotype spans a wide spectrum. Some individuals with GnRH deficiency may suffer from complete absence of pubertal development, while others may manifest varying degrees of gonadotropin deficiency and pubertal delay, and a subset that carries the same mutations as their affected family members may even have normal reproductive function. In approximately 10% of men with idiopathic hypogonadotropic hypogonadism, reversal of gonadotropin deficiency may occur in adult life after sex steroid therapy. Also, a small fraction of men with idiopathic hypogonadotropic hypogonadism may present with androgen deficiency and infertility in adult life after having gone through apparently normal pubertal development. Nutritional, emotional, or metabolic stress may unmask gonadotropin deficiency and reproductive dysfunction (analogous to hypothalamic amenorrhea) in some patients who harbor mutations in the candidate genes but who previously had normal reproductive function. The clinical phenotype may include isolated anosmia or hyposmia. These striking variations in phenotypic presentation of GnRH deficiency have highlighted the important role of oligogenicity and gene-gene and gene-environment interactions in shaping the clinical phenotype.

Mutations in a number of genes involved in the development and migration of GnRH neurons or in the regulation of GnRH secretion have been linked to GnRH deficiency, although the genetic defect remains elusive in nearly two-thirds of cases. Familial hypogonadotropic hypogonadism can be transmitted as an X-linked (20%), autosomal recessive (30%), or autosomal dominant (50%) trait. Some individuals with idiopathic hypogonadotropic hypogonadism (IHH) have sporadic mutations in the same genes that cause inherited forms of the disorder. The genetic defects associated with GnRH deficiency can be conveniently classified as anosmic (Kallmann's syndrome) or normosmic (Table 11-2), although the occurrence of both anosmic and normosmic forms of GnRH deficiency in the same families suggests commonality of pathophysiologic mechanisms. *Kallmann's syndrome*, the anosmic form of GnRH deficiency, can result from mutations in one or more genes associated with olfactory bulb morphogenesis and the migration of GnRH neurons from their origin in the region of the olfactory placode, along the scaffold established by the olfactory nerves, through the cribriform plate into their final location into the preoptic region of the hypothalamus. Thus, mutations in *KAL1, FGF8, FGFR1, NELF, PROK2, PROK2R,* and *CHD7* have been described in patients with Kallmann's syndrome. An X-linked form of IHH is caused by mutations in the *KAL1* gene, which encodes anosmin, a protein that mediates the migration

TABLE 11-2

CAUSES OF CONGENITAL HYPOGONADOTROPIC HYPOGONADISM

GENE	LOCUS	INHERITANCE	ASSOCIATED FEATURES
A. Hypogonadotropic Hypogonadism due to GnRH Deficiency			
A1. GnRH Deficiency Associated with Hyposmia or Anosmia			
KAL1	Xp22	X-linked	Anosmia, renal agenesis, synkinesia, cleft lip/palate, oculomotor/visuospatial defects, gut malformations
NELF	9q34.3	AR	Anosmia, hypogonadotropic hypogonadism
FGFR1	8p11-p12	AD	Anosmia, cleft lip/palate, synkinesia, syndactyly
PROK2	3p21	AR	Anosmia/sleep dysregulation
PROK2R	20p12.3	AR	Variable
CHD7	8q12.1		Anosmia, other features of CHARGE syndrome
A2. GnRH Deficiency with Normal Sense of Smell			
GNRHR	4q21	AR	None
GnRH1	8p21	AR	None
KISS1R	19p13	AR	None
TAC3	12q13	AR	Microphallus, cryptorchidism, reversal of GnRH deficiency
TAC3R	4q25	AR	Microphallus, cryptorchidism, reversal of GnRH deficiency
LEPR	1p31	AR	Obesity
LEP	7q31	AR	Obesity
FGF8	10q24	AR	Skeletal abnormalities
B. Hypogonadotropic Hypogonadism not due to GnRH Deficiency			
PC1	5q15-21	AR	Obesity, diabetes mellitus, ACTH deficiency
HESX1	3p21	AR AD	Septo-optic dysplasia, CPHD Isolated GH insufficiency
LHX3	9q34	AR	CPHD (ACTH spared), cervical spine rigidity
PROP1	5q35	AR	CPHD (ACTH usually spared)
FSHβ	11p13	AR	↑ LH
LHβ	19q13	AR	↑ FSH
SF1 (NR5A1)	9p33	AD/AR	Primary adrenal failure, XY sex reversal

Abbreviations: ACTH, adrenocorticotropic hormone; AD, autosomal dominant; AR, autosomal recessive; CHARGE, eye coloboma, choanal atresia, growth and developmental retardation, genitourinary anomalies, ear anomalies; CPHD, combined pituitary hormone deficiency; *DAX1*, dosage-sensitive sex-reversal, adrenal hypoplasia congenita, X-chromosome; *FGFR1*, fibroblast growth factor receptor 1; FSH, follicle-stimulating hormone; *FSHβ*, follicle-stimulating hormone β-subunit; GH, growth hormone; GnRH, gonadotropin-releasing hormone; *GNRHR*, gonadotropin-releasing hormone receptor; *GPR54*, G protein–coupled receptor 54; *HESX1*, homeo box gene expressed in embryonic stem cells 1; *KAL1*, interval-1 gene; *LEP*, leptin; *LEPR*, leptin receptor; LH, luteinizing hormone; *LHβ*, luteinizing hormone β-subunit; *LHX3*, LIM homeobox gene 3; *NELF*, nasal embryonic LHRH factor; *PC1*, prohormone convertase 1; *PROK2*, prokineticin 2; *PROP1*, Prophet of Pit 1; *SF1*, steroidogenic factor 1; *TAC3*, tachykinin 3; *TAC3R*, tachykinin 3 receptor.

of neural progenitors of the olfactory bulb and GnRH-producing neurons. These individuals have GnRH deficiency and variable combinations of anosmia or hyposmia, renal defects, and neurologic abnormalities including mirror movements. Mutations in the *FGFR1* gene cause an autosomal dominant form of hypogonadotropic hypogonadism that clinically resembles Kallmann's syndrome; mutations in its putative ligand, *FGF8* gene product, have also been associated with IHH. Prokineticin 2 (*PROK2*) also encodes a protein involved in migration and development of olfactory and GnRH neurons. Recessive mutations in *PROK2* or in its receptor, *PROKR2*, have been associated with both anosmic and normosmic forms of hypogonadotropic hypogonadism.

Normosmic GnRH deficiency results from defects in pulsatile GnRH secretion, its regulation, or its action on the gonadotrope and has been associated with mutations in *GnRHR*, *GNRH1*, *KISS1R*, *TAC3*, *TACR3*, and *NROB1* (*DAX1*). Some mutations, such as those in *PROK2*, *PROKR2*, and *CHD7*, have been associated with both the anosmic and normosmic forms of IHH.

GnRHR mutations, the most frequent identifiable cause of normosmic IHH, account for ~40% of autosomal recessive and 10% of sporadic cases of hypogonadotropic hypogonadism. These patients have decreased LH response to exogenous GnRH. Some receptor mutations alter GnRH binding affinity, allowing apparently normal responses to pharmacologic doses of exogenous GnRH, whereas other mutations may alter signal transduction downstream of hormone binding. Mutations of the *GnRH1* gene have also been reported in patients with hypogonadotropic hypogonadism, although they are rare. G protein–coupled receptor *KISS1R* (*GPR54*) and its cognate ligand, kisspeptin (*KISS1*), are important regulators of sexual maturation in primates. Recessive mutations in *GPR54* cause gonadotropin deficiency without anosmia. Patients retain responsiveness to exogenous GnRH, suggesting an abnormality in the neural pathways controlling GnRH release. The genes encoding neurokinin B (*TAC3*), which is involved in preferential activation of GnRH release in early development, and its receptor (*TAC3R*) have been implicated in some families with normosmic IHH. Mutations in more than one gene (digenicity or oligogenicity) may contribute to clinical heterogeneity in IHH patients. X-linked hypogonadotropic hypogonadism also occurs in *adrenal hypoplasia congenita*, a disorder caused by mutations in the *DAX1* gene, which encodes a nuclear receptor in the adrenal gland and reproductive axis. Adrenal hypoplasia congenita is characterized by absent development of the adult zone of the adrenal cortex, leading to neonatal adrenal insufficiency. Puberty usually does not occur or is arrested, reflecting variable degrees of gonadotropin deficiency. Although sexual differentiation is normal, **most** patients have testicular dysgenesis and impaired spermatogenesis despite gonadotropin replacement. Less commonly, adrenal hypoplasia congenita, sex reversal, and hypogonadotropic hypogonadism can be caused by mutations of steroidogenic factor 1 (SF1). Rarely, recessive mutations in the *LHβ* or *FSHβ* gene have been described in patients with selective deficiencies of these gonadotropins. In approximately 10% of men with IHH, reversal of gonadotropin deficiency may occur in adult life. Also, a small fraction of men with IHH may present with androgen deficiency and infertility in adult life after having gone through apparently normal pubertal development.

A number of homeodomain transcription factors are involved in the development and differentiation of the specialized hormone-producing cells within the pituitary gland (Table 11-2). Patients with mutations of *PROP1* have combined pituitary hormone deficiency that includes GH, prolactin (PRL), thyroid-stimulating hormone (TSH), LH, and FSH, but not ACTH. *LHX3* mutations cause combined pituitary hormone deficiency in association with cervical spine rigidity. *HESX1* mutations cause septo-optic dysplasia and combined pituitary hormone deficiency.

Prader-Willi syndrome is characterized by obesity, hypotonic musculature, mental retardation, hypogonadism, short stature, and small hands and feet. Prader-Willi syndrome is a genomic imprinting disorder caused by deletions of the proximal portion of the paternally derived chromosome 15q11-15q13 region, which contains a bipartite imprinting center, uniparental disomy of the maternal alleles, or mutations of the genes/loci involved in imprinting. *Laurence-Moon syndrome* is an autosomal recessive disorder characterized by obesity, hypogonadism, mental retardation, polydactyly, and retinitis pigmentosa. Recessive mutations of leptin, or its receptor, cause severe obesity and pubertal arrest, apparently because of hypothalamic GnRH deficiency **(Chap. 20)**.

Acquired hypogonadotropic disorders

Severe illness, stress, malnutrition, and exercise

These factors may cause reversible gonadotropin deficiency. Although gonadotropin deficiency and reproductive dysfunction are well documented in these conditions in women, men exhibit similar but less pronounced responses. Unlike women, most male runners and other endurance athletes have normal gonadotropin and sex steroid levels, despite low body fat and frequent intensive exercise. Testosterone levels fall at the onset of illness and recover during recuperation. The magnitude of gonadotropin suppression generally correlates with the severity of illness. Although hypogonadotropic hypogonadism is the most common cause of androgen deficiency in patients with acute illness, some have elevated levels of LH and FSH, which suggest primary gonadal dysfunction. The pathophysiology of reproductive dysfunction during acute illness is unknown but likely involves a combination of cytokine and/or glucocorticoid effects. There is a high frequency of low testosterone levels in patients with chronic illnesses such as HIV infection, end-stage renal disease, chronic obstructive lung disease, and many types of cancer and in patients receiving glucocorticoids. About 20% of HIV-infected men with low testosterone levels have elevated LH and FSH levels; these patients presumably have primary testicular dysfunction. The remaining 80% have either normal or low LH and FSH levels; these men have a central hypothalamic-pituitary defect or a dual defect involving both the testis and the hypothalamic-pituitary centers. Muscle wasting is common in chronic diseases associated with hypogonadism, which also leads to debility, poor quality of life, and adverse outcome of disease. There is great interest in exploring strategies that can reverse androgen deficiency or attenuate the sarcopenia associated with chronic illness.

Men using opioids for relief of cancer or noncancerous pain or because of addiction often have suppressed testosterone and LH levels and high prevalence of sexual dysfunction and osteoporosis; the degree of suppression is dose-related and particularly severe with long-acting opioids such as methadone. Opioids suppress GnRH secretion and alter the sensitivity to feedback inhibition by gonadal steroids. Men who are heavy users of marijuana have decreased testosterone secretion and sperm production. The mechanism of marijuana-induced hypogonadism is decreased GnRH secretion. Gynecomastia observed in marijuana users can also be caused by plant estrogens in crude preparations. Androgen deprivation therapy in men with prostate cancer has been associated with increased risk of bone fractures, diabetes mellitus, cardiovascular events, fatigue, sexual dysfunction, and poor quality of life.

Obesity

In men with mild to moderate obesity, SHBG levels decrease in proportion to the degree of obesity, resulting in lower total testosterone levels. However, free testosterone levels usually remain within the normal range. The decrease in SHBG levels is caused by increased circulating insulin, which inhibits SHBG production. Estradiol levels are higher in obese men compared to healthy, nonobese controls, because of aromatization of testosterone to estradiol in adipose tissue. Weight loss is associated with reversal of these abnormalities including an increase in total and free testosterone levels and a decrease in estradiol levels. A subset of obese men with moderate to severe obesity may have a defect in the hypothalamic-pituitary axis as suggested by low free testosterone in the absence of elevated gonadotropins. Weight gain in adult men can accelerate the rate of age-related decline in testosterone levels.

Hyperprolactinemia

(See also Chap. 5) Elevated PRL levels are associated with hypogonadotropic hypogonadism. PRL inhibits hypothalamic GnRH secretion either directly or through modulation of tuberoinfundibular dopaminergic pathways. A PRL-secreting tumor may also destroy the surrounding gonadotropes by invasion or compression of the pituitary stalk. Treatment with dopamine agonists reverses gonadotropin deficiency, although there may be a delay relative to PRL suppression.

Sellar mass lesions

Neoplastic and nonneoplastic lesions in the hypothalamus or pituitary can directly or indirectly affect gonadotrope function. In adults, pituitary adenomas constitute the largest category of space-occupying lesions affecting gonadotropin and other pituitary hormone production. Pituitary adenomas that extend into the suprasellar region can impair GnRH secretion and mildly increase PRL secretion (usually <50 μg/L) because of impaired tonic inhibition by dopaminergic pathways. These tumors should be distinguished from prolactinomas, which typically secrete higher PRL levels. The presence of diabetes insipidus suggests the possibility of a craniopharyngioma, infiltrative disorder, or other hypothalamic lesions **(Chap. 6)**.

Hemochromatosis

Both the pituitary and testis can be affected by excessive iron deposition. However, the pituitary defect is the predominant lesion in most patients with hemochromatosis and hypogonadism. The diagnosis of hemochromatosis is suggested by the association of characteristic skin discoloration, hepatic enlargement or dysfunction, diabetes mellitus, arthritis, cardiac conduction defects, and hypogonadism.

PRIMARY TESTICULAR CAUSES OF HYPOGONADISM

Common causes of primary testicular dysfunction include Klinefelter's syndrome, uncorrected cryptorchidism, cancer chemotherapy, radiation to the testes, trauma, torsion, infectious orchitis, HIV infection, anorchia syndrome, and myotonic dystrophy. Primary testicular disorders may be associated with impaired spermatogenesis, decreased androgen production, or both. **See Chap. 10 for disorders of testis development, androgen synthesis, and androgen action.**

Klinefelter's syndrome

(See also Chap. 10) Klinefelter's syndrome is the most common chromosomal disorder associated with testicular dysfunction and male infertility. It occurs in about 1 in 600 live-born males. Azoospermia is the rule in men with Klinefelter's syndrome who have the 47,XXY karyotype; however, men with mosaicism may have germ cells, especially at a younger age. The clinical phenotype of Klinefelter's syndrome can be heterogeneous possibly because of mosaicism, polymorphisms in AR gene, variable testosterone levels, or other genetic factors. Testicular histology shows hyalinization of seminiferous tubules and absence of spermatogenesis. Although their function is impaired, the number of Leydig cells appears to increase. Testosterone is decreased and estradiol is increased, leading to clinical features of undervirilization and gynecomastia. Men with Klinefelter's syndrome are at increased risk of systemic lupus erythematosus, Sjögren's syndrome, breast cancer, diabetes mellitus, osteoporosis, non-Hodgkin's lymphoma, and lung cancer, and reduced risk of prostate cancer. Periodic mammography for breast cancer surveillance is recommended for men with Klinefelter's syndrome. Fertility has been achieved by intracytoplasmic injection of sperm retrieved surgically from testicular biopsies of men with Klinefelter's syndrome, including some men with the nonmosaic form of Klinefelter's syndrome. The karyotypes 48,XXXY and 49,XXXXY are associated with a more severe phenotype, increased risk of congenital malformations, and lower intelligence than 47,XXY individuals.

Cryptorchidism

Cryptorchidism occurs when there is incomplete descent of the testis from the abdominal cavity into the scrotum. About 3% of full-term and 30% of premature male infants have at least one undescended testis at birth, but descent is usually complete by the first few weeks of life. The incidence of cryptorchidism is <1% by 9 months of age. Androgens regulate predominantly the inguinoscrotal descent of the testes through degeneration of the craniosuspensory ligament and a shortening of the gubernaculums, respectively. Mutations in *INSL3* and leucine-rich repeat family of G protein–coupled receptor 8 (*LGR8*), which regulate the transabdominal portion of testicular descent, have been found in some patients with cryptorchidism.

Cryptorchidism is associated with increased risk of malignancy, infertility, inguinal hernia, and torsion. Unilateral cryptorchidism, even when corrected before puberty, is associated with decreased sperm count, possibly reflecting unrecognized damage to the fully descended testis or other genetic factors. Epidemiologic, clinical, and molecular evidence supports the idea that cryptorchidism, hypospadias, impaired spermatogenesis, and testicular cancer may be causally related to common genetic and environment perturbations and are components of the testicular dysgenesis syndrome.

Acquired testicular defects

Viral orchitis may be caused by the mumps virus, echovirus, lymphocytic choriomeningitis virus, and group B arboviruses. Orchitis occurs in as many as one-fourth of adult men with mumps; the orchitis is unilateral in about two-thirds and bilateral in the remainder. Orchitis usually develops a few days after the onset of parotitis but may precede it. The testis may return to normal size and function or undergo atrophy. Semen analysis returns to normal for three-fourths of men with unilateral involvement but for only one-third of men with bilateral orchitis. *Trauma*, including testicular torsion, can also cause secondary atrophy of the testes. The exposed position of the testes in the scrotum renders them susceptible to both thermal and physical trauma, particularly in men with hazardous occupations.

The testes are sensitive to *radiation damage*. Doses >200 mGy (20 rad) are associated with increased FSH and LH levels and damage to the spermatogonia. After ~800 mGy (80 rad), oligospermia or azoospermia develops, and higher doses may obliterate the germinal epithelium. Permanent androgen deficiency in adult men is uncommon after therapeutic radiation; however, most boys given direct testicular radiation therapy for acute lymphoblastic leukemia have permanently low testosterone levels. Sperm banking should be considered before patients undergo radiation treatment or chemotherapy.

Drugs interfere with testicular function by several mechanisms, including inhibition of testosterone synthesis (e.g., ketoconazole), blockade of androgen action (e.g., spironolactone), increased estrogen (e.g., marijuana), or direct inhibition of spermatogenesis (e.g., chemotherapy).

Combination chemotherapy for acute leukemia, Hodgkin's disease, and testicular and other cancers may impair Leydig cell function and cause infertility. The degree of gonadal dysfunction depends on the type of chemotherapeutic agent and the dose and duration of therapy. Because of high response rates and the young age of these men, infertility and androgen deficiency have emerged as important long-term complications of cancer chemotherapy. Cyclophosphamide and combination regimens containing procarbazine are particularly toxic to germ cells. Thus, 90% of men with Hodgkin's lymphoma receiving MOPP (mechlorethamine, vincristine, procarbazine, prednisone) therapy develop azoospermia or extreme oligozoospermia; newer regimens that do not include procarbazine, such as ABVD (doxorubicin, bleomycin, vinblastine, dacarbazine), are less toxic to germ cells.

Alcohol, when consumed in excess for prolonged periods, decreases testosterone, independent of liver disease or malnutrition. Elevated estradiol and decreased testosterone levels may occur in men taking digitalis.

The occupational and recreational history should be carefully evaluated in all men with infertility because of the toxic effects of many *chemical agents* on spermatogenesis. Known environmental hazards include pesticides (e.g., vinclozolin, dicofol, atrazine), sewage contaminants (e.g., ethinyl estradiol in birth control pills, surfactants such as octylphenol, nonyphenol), plasticizers (e.g., pthalates), flame retardants (e.g., polychlorinated biphenyls, polybrominated diphenol ethers), industrial pollutants (e.g., heavy metals cadmium and lead, dioxins, polycyclic aromatic hydrocarbons), microwaves, and ultrasound. In some populations, sperm density is said to have declined by as much as 40% in the past 50 years. Environmental estrogens or antiandrogens may be partly responsible.

Testicular failure also occurs as a part of *polyglandular autoimmune insufficiency* **(Chap. 29)**. Sperm antibodies can cause isolated male infertility. In some instances, these antibodies are secondary phenomena resulting from duct obstruction or vasectomy. Granulomatous diseases can affect the testes, and testicular atrophy occurs in 10–20% of men with lepromatous leprosy because of direct tissue invasion by the mycobacteria. The tubules are involved initially, followed by endarteritis and destruction of Leydig cells.

Systemic disease can cause primary testis dysfunction in addition to suppressing gonadotropin production. In cirrhosis, a combined testicular and pituitary abnormality leads to decreased testosterone production independent of the direct toxic effects of ethanol. Impaired hepatic extraction of adrenal androstenedione leads to extraglandular conversion to estrone and estradiol, which partially suppresses LH. Testicular atrophy and gynecomastia are present in approximately one-half of men with cirrhosis. In chronic renal failure, androgen synthesis and sperm production decrease despite elevated gonadotropins. The elevated LH level is due to reduced clearance, but it does not restore normal testosterone production. About one-fourth of men with renal failure have hyperprolactinemia. Improvement in testosterone production with hemodialysis is incomplete, but successful renal transplantation may return testicular function to normal. Testicular atrophy is present in one-third of men with sickle cell anemia. The defect may be at either the testicular or the hypothalamic-pituitary level. Sperm density can decrease temporarily after acute febrile illness in the absence of a change in testosterone production. Infertility in men with celiac disease is associated with a hormonal pattern typical of androgen resistance, namely elevated testosterone and LH levels.

Neurologic diseases associated with altered testicular function include myotonic dystrophy, spinobulbar muscular atrophy, and paraplegia. In myotonic dystrophy, small testes may be associated with impairment of both spermatogenesis and Leydig cell function. Spinobulbar muscular atrophy is caused by an expansion of the glutamine repeat sequences in the amino-terminal region of the AR; this expansion impairs function of the AR, but it is unclear how the alteration is related to the neurologic manifestations. Men with spinobulbar muscular atrophy often have undervirilization and infertility as a late manifestation. Spinal cord lesions that cause paraplegia can lead to a temporary decrease in testosterone levels and may cause persistent defects in spermatogenesis; some patients retain the capacity for penile erection and ejaculation.

ANDROGEN INSENSITIVITY SYNDROMES

Mutations in the AR cause resistance to the action of testosterone and DHT. These X-linked mutations are associated with variable degrees of defective male phenotypic development and undervirilization **(Chap. 10)**. Although not technically hormone-insensitivity syndromes, two genetic disorders impair testosterone conversion to active sex steroids. Mutations in the *SRD5A2* gene, which encodes 5α-reductase type 2, prevent the conversion of testosterone to DHT, which is necessary for the normal development of the male external genitalia. Mutations in the *CYP19* gene, which encodes aromatase, prevent testosterone conversion to estradiol. Males with *CYP19* mutations have delayed epiphyseal fusion, tall stature, eunuchoid proportions, and osteoporosis, consistent with evidence from an estrogen receptor–deficient individual that these testosterone actions are mediated indirectly via estrogen.

GYNECOMASTIA

Gynecomastia refers to enlargement of the male breast. It is caused by excess estrogen action and is usually the result of an increased estrogen-to-androgen ratio. True gynecomastia is associated with glandular breast tissue that is >4 cm in diameter and often tender. Glandular tissue enlargement should be distinguished from excess adipose tissue: glandular tissue is firmer and contains fibrous-like cords. Gynecomastia occurs as a normal physiologic phenomenon in the newborn (due to transplacental transfer of maternal and placental estrogens), during puberty (high estrogen-to-androgen ratio in early stages of puberty), and with aging (increased fat tissue and increased aromatase activity), but it can also result from pathologic conditions associated with androgen deficiency or estrogen excess. The prevalence of gynecomastia increases with age and body mass index (BMI), likely because of increased aromatase activity in adipose tissue. Medications that alter androgen metabolism or action may also cause gynecomastia. The relative risk of breast cancer is increased in men with gynecomastia, although the absolute risk is relatively small.

PATHOLOGIC GYNECOMASTIA

Any cause of *androgen deficiency* can lead to gynecomastia, reflecting an increased estrogen-to-androgen ratio, because estrogen synthesis still occurs by aromatization of residual adrenal and gonadal androgens. Gynecomastia is a characteristic feature of Klinefelter's syndrome **(Chap. 10)**. *Androgen insensitivity* disorders also cause gynecomastia. *Excess estrogen production* may be caused by tumors, including Sertoli cell tumors in isolation or in association with Peutz-Jeghers syndrome or Carney complex. Tumors that produce hCG, including some testicular tumors, stimulate Leydig cell estrogen synthesis. *Increased conversion of androgens to estrogens* can be a result of increased availability of substrate (androstenedione) for extraglandular estrogen formation (CAH, hyperthyroidism, and most feminizing adrenal tumors) or of diminished catabolism of androstenedione (liver disease) so that estrogen precursors are shunted to aromatase in peripheral sites. Obesity is associated with increased aromatization of androgen precursors to estrogens. Extraglandular aromatase activity can also be increased in tumors of the liver or adrenal gland or rarely as an inherited disorder. Several families with *increased peripheral aromatase activity* inherited as an autosomal dominant or as an X-linked disorder have been described. In some families with this disorder, an inversion in chromosome 15q21.2-3 causes the CYP19 gene to be activated by the regulatory elements of contiguous genes, resulting in excessive estrogen production in the fat and other extragonadal tissues. *Drugs* can cause gynecomastia by acting directly as estrogenic substances (e.g., oral contraceptives, phytoestrogens, digitalis) or by inhibiting androgen synthesis (e.g., ketoconazole) or action (e.g., spironolactone).

Because up to two-thirds of pubertal boys and half of hospitalized men have palpable glandular tissue that is benign, detailed investigation or intervention is not indicated in all men presenting with gynecomastia (Fig. 11-5). In addition to the extent of gynecomastia, recent onset, rapid growth, tender tissue, and occurrence in a lean subject should prompt more extensive evaluation. This should include a careful drug history, measurement and examination of the testes, assessment of virilization, evaluation of liver function, and hormonal measurements including testosterone, estradiol, and androstenedione, LH, and hCG. A karyotype should be obtained in men with very small testes to exclude Klinefelter's syndrome. Despite extensive evaluation, the etiology is established in fewer than one-half of patients.

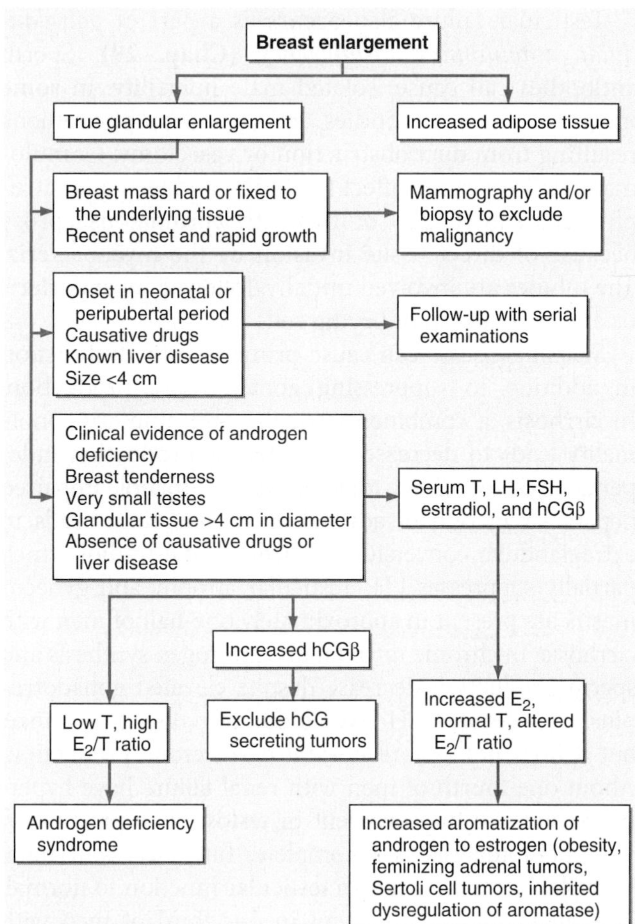

FIGURE 11-5

Evaluation of gynecomastia. E_2, 17β-estradiol; hCGβ, human chorionic gonadotropin β; T, testosterone.

TREATMENT Gynecomastia

When the primary cause can be identified and corrected, breast enlargement usually subsides over several months. However, if gynecomastia is of long duration, surgery is the most effective therapy. Indications for surgery include severe psychological and/or cosmetic problems, continued growth or tenderness, or suspected malignancy. In patients who have painful gynecomastia and in whom surgery cannot be performed, treatment with antiestrogens such as tamoxifen (20 mg/d) can reduce pain and breast tissue size in over half the patients. Estrogen receptor antagonists, tamoxifen and raloxifene, have been reported in small trials to reduce breast size in men with pubertal gynecomastia, although complete regression of breast enlargement is unusual with the use of estrogen receptor antagonists. Aromatase inhibitors can be effective in the early proliferative phase of the disorder. However, in a randomized trial in men with established gynecomastia, anastrozole proved no more effective than placebo in reducing breast size. Tamoxifen is effective in the prevention and treatment of breast enlargement and breast pain in men with prostate cancer who are receiving antiandrogen therapy.

AGING-RELATED CHANGES IN MALE REPRODUCTIVE FUNCTION

A number of cross-sectional and longitudinal studies (e.g., The Baltimore Longitudinal Study of Aging, the Framingham Heart Study, the Massachusetts Male Aging Study, and the European Male Aging Study) have established that testosterone concentrations decrease with advancing age. This age-related decline starts in the third decade of life and progresses slowly; the rate of decline in testosterone concentrations is greater in obese men, men with chronic illness, and those taking medications than in healthy older men. Because SHBG concentrations are higher in older men than in younger men, free or bioavailable testosterone concentrations decline with aging to a greater extent than total testosterone concentrations. The age-related decline in testosterone is due to defects at all levels of the hypothalamic-pituitary-testicular axis: pulsatile GnRH secretion is attenuated, LH response to GnRH is reduced, and testicular response to LH is impaired. However, the gradual rise of LH with aging suggests that testis dysfunction is the main cause of declining androgen levels. The term *andropause* has been used to denote age-related decline in testosterone concentrations; this term is a misnomer because there is no discrete time when testosterone concentrations decline abruptly. The approach to evaluating hypogonadism is summarized in Fig. 11-6.

In epidemiologic surveys, low total and bioavailable testosterone concentrations have been associated with decreased appendicular skeletal muscle mass and strength, decreased self-reported physical function, higher visceral fat mass, insulin resistance, and increased risk of coronary artery disease and mortality,

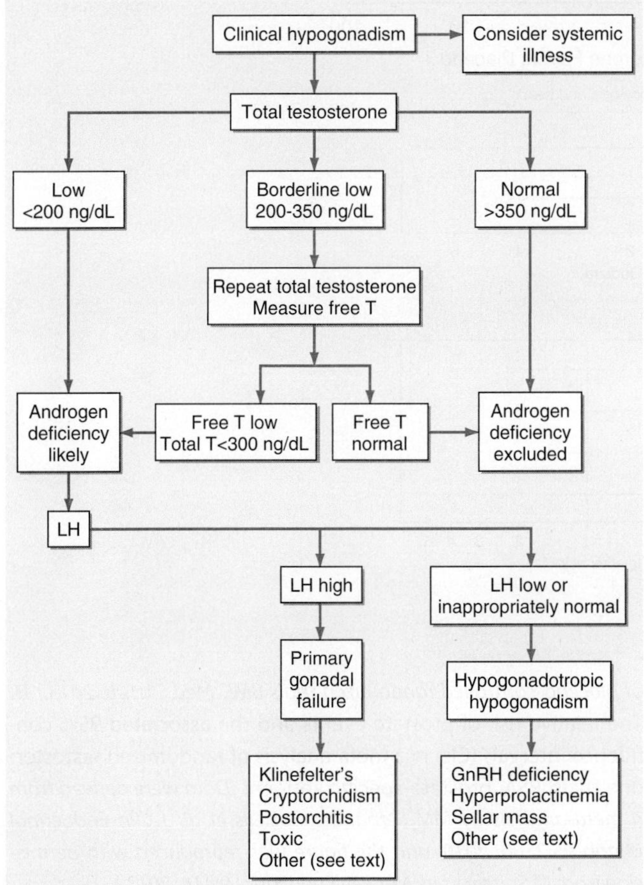

FIGURE 11-6

Evaluation of hypogonadism. GnRH, gonadotropin-releasing hormone; LH, luteinizing hormone; T, testosterone.

although the associations are weak. An analysis of signs and symptoms in older men in the European Male Aging Study revealed a syndromic association of sexual symptoms with total testosterone levels below 320 ng/dL and free testosterone levels below 64 pg/mL in community-dwelling older men. In systematic reviews of randomized controlled trials, testosterone therapy of healthy older men with low or low-normal testosterone levels was associated with greater increments in lean body mass, grip strength, and self-reported physical function compared with placebo. Testosterone therapy also induced greater improvement in vertebral but not femoral bone mineral density. Testosterone therapy of older men with sexual dysfunction and unequivocally low testosterone levels improves libido, but testosterone effects on erectile function and response to selective phosphodiesterase inhibitors have been inconsistent. Testosterone therapy has not been shown to improve depression scores, fracture risk, cognitive function, response to phosphodiesterase inhibitors, or clinical outcomes in older men. Furthermore, neither the long-term risks nor clinical benefits of testosterone therapy in older men have been demonstrated in adequately powered trials. Although there is no evidence that testosterone causes prostate cancer, there is concern that testosterone therapy might cause subclinical prostate cancers to grow. Testosterone therapy is associated with increased risk of detection of prostate events (Fig. 11-7).

One randomized testosterone trial in older men with mobility limitation and high burden of chronic conditions, such as diabetes, heart disease, hypertension, and hyperlipidemia, reported a greater number of cardiovascular events in men randomized to the testosterone arm of the study than in those randomized to the placebo arm. Since then, two large retrospective analyses of patient databases have reported higher frequency of cardiovascular events, including myocardial infarction, in older men with preexisting heart disease (Fig. 11-7).

Population screening of all older men for low testosterone levels is not recommended, and testing should be restricted to men who have symptoms or physical features attributable to androgen deficiency. Testosterone therapy is not recommended for all older men with low testosterone levels. In older men with significant symptoms of androgen deficiency who have testosterone levels below 200 ng/dL, testosterone therapy may be considered on an individualized basis and should be instituted after careful discussion of the risks and benefits (see "Testosterone Replacement," below).

Testicular morphology, semen production, and fertility are maintained up to a very old age in men. Although concern has been expressed about age-related increases in germ cell mutations and impairment of DNA repair mechanisms, there is no clear evidence that

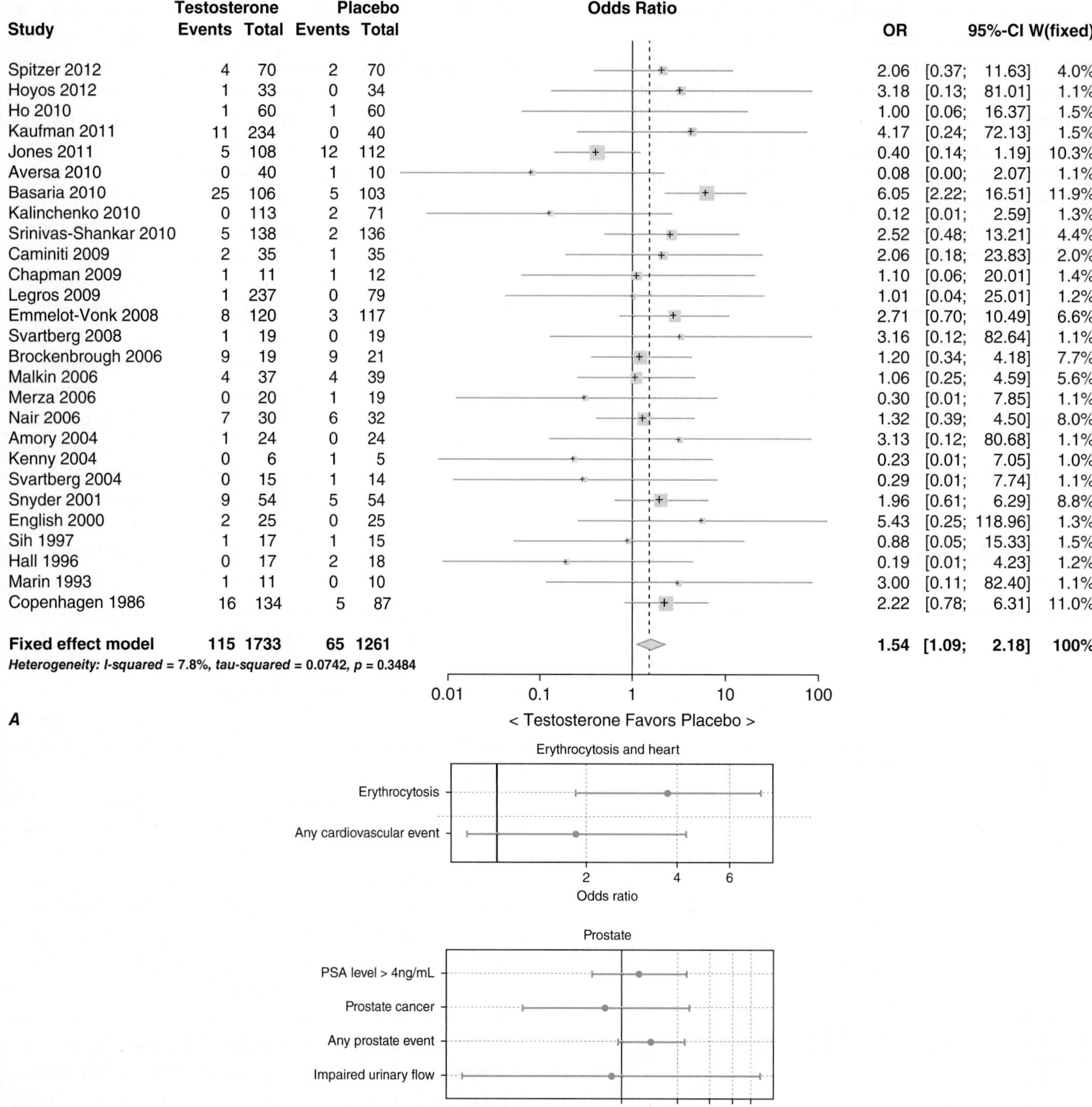

FIGURE 11-7

Meta-analyses of cardiovascular and prostate adverse events associated with testosterone therapy. *A.* A meta-analysis of cardiovascular-related events in randomized testosterone trials of 12 weeks or longer in duration. Randomization to testosterone was associated with a significantly increased risk of cardiovascular-related event (odds ratio [OR] 1.54). *(Modified with permission from L Xu et al: Testosterone therapy and cardiovascular events among men: a systematic review and meta-analysis of placebo-controlled randomized trials BMC Med 11:108, 2013.)* ***B.*** The relative risk of prostate events and the associated 95% confidence intervals (CIs) in a meta-analysis of randomized testosterone trials. PSA, prostate-specific antigen. *(Data were derived from a meta-analysis by MM Fernández-Balsells et al: J Clin Endocrinol Metab 95:2560, 2010, and the figure was reproduced with permission from M Spitzer et al: Nat Rev Endocrinol 9:414, 2013.)*

the frequency of chromosomal aneuploidy is increased in the sperm of older men. However, the incidence of autosomal dominant diseases, such as achondroplasia, polyposis coli, Marfan's syndrome, and Apert's syndrome, increases in the offspring of men who are advanced in age, consistent with transmission of sporadic missense mutations. Advanced paternal age may be associated with increased rates of de novo mutations, which may contribute to an increased risk of neurodevelopmental diseases such as schizophrenia and autism. The somatic mutations in male germ cells that enhance the proliferation of germ cells could lead to within-testis expansion of mutant clonal lines, thus favoring the propagation of germ cells carrying these pathogenic mutations and increasing the risk of mutations in the offspring of older fathers (the "selfish spermatogonial selection" hypothesis).

APPROACH TO THE PATIENT: Androgen Deficiency

Hypogonadism is often characterized by decreased sex drive, reduced frequency of sexual activity, inability to maintain erections, reduced beard growth, loss of muscle mass, decreased testicular size, and gynecomastia. Erectile dysfunction and androgen deficiency are two distinct clinical disorders that can coexist in middle-aged and older men. Less than 10% of patients with erectile dysfunction have testosterone deficiency. Thus, it is useful to evaluate men presenting with erectile dysfunction for androgen deficiency. Except when extreme, these clinical features of androgen deficiency may be difficult to distinguish from changes that occur with normal aging.

Moreover, androgen deficiency may develop gradually. Several epidemiologic studies, such as the Framingham Heart Study, the Massachusetts Male Aging Study, the Baltimore Longitudinal Study of Aging, and the Study of Osteoporotic Fractures in Men, have reported a high prevalence of low testosterone levels in middle-aged and older men. The age-related decline in testosterone should be distinguished from classical hypogonadism due to diseases of the testes, the pituitary, and the hypothalamus.

When symptoms or clinical features suggest possible androgen deficiency, the laboratory evaluation is initiated by the measurement of total testosterone, preferably in the morning using a reliable assay, such as LC-MS/MS that has been calibrated to an international testosterone standard (Fig. 11-6). A consistently low total testosterone level <300 ng/dL measured by a reliable assay, in association with symptoms, is evidence of testosterone deficiency. An early-morning testosterone level >400 ng/dL makes the diagnosis of androgen deficiency unlikely. In men with testosterone levels between 200 and 400 ng/dL, the total testosterone level should be repeated and a free testosterone level should be measured. In older men and in patients with other clinical states that are associated with alterations in SHBG levels, a direct measurement of free testosterone level by equilibrium dialysis can be useful in unmasking testosterone deficiency.

When androgen deficiency has been confirmed by the consistently low testosterone concentrations, LH should be measured to classify the patient as having primary (high LH) or secondary (low or inappropriately normal LH) hypogonadism. An elevated LH level indicates that the defect is at the testicular level. Common causes of primary testicular failure include Klinefelter's syndrome, HIV infection, uncorrected cryptorchidism, cancer chemotherapeutic agents, radiation, surgical orchiectomy, or prior infectious orchitis. Unless causes of primary testicular failure are known, a karyotype should be performed in men with low testosterone and elevated LH to exclude Klinefelter's syndrome. Men who have low testosterone levels but "inappropriately normal" or low LH levels have secondary hypogonadism; their defect resides at the hypothalamic-pituitary level. Common causes of acquired secondary hypogonadism include space-occupying lesions of the sella, hyperprolactinemia, chronic illness, hemochromatosis, excessive exercise, and the use of anabolic-androgenic steroids, opiates, marijuana, glucocorticoids, and alcohol. Measurement of PRL and MRI scan of the hypothalamic-pituitary region can help exclude the presence of a space-occupying lesion. Patients in whom known causes of hypogonadotropic hypogonadism have been excluded are classified as having IHH. It is not unusual for congenital causes of hypogonadotropic hypogonadism, such as Kallmann's syndrome, to be diagnosed in young adults.

TREATMENT Androgen Deficiency

GONADOTROPINS Gonadotropin therapy is used to establish or restore fertility in patients with gonadotropin deficiency of any cause. Several gonadotropin preparations are available. Human menopausal gonadotropin (hMG; purified from the urine of postmenopausal women) contains 75 IU FSH and 75 IU LH per vial. hCG (purified from the urine of pregnant women) has little FSH activity and resembles LH in its ability to stimulate testosterone production by Leydig cells. Recombinant LH is now available. Because of the expense of hMG, treatment is usually begun with hCG alone, and hMG is added later to promote the FSH-dependent stages of spermatid development. Recombinant human FSH (hFSH) is now available and is indistinguishable from purified urinary hFSH in its biologic activity and pharmacokinetics in vitro and in vivo, although the mature β subunit of recombinant hFSH has seven fewer amino acids. Recombinant hFSH is available in ampoules containing 75 IU (~7.5 μg FSH), which accounts for >99% of protein content. Once spermatogenesis is restored using combined FSH and LH therapy, hCG alone is often sufficient to maintain spermatogenesis.

Although a variety of treatment regimens are used, 1000–2000 IU of hCG or recombinant human LH (rhLH) administered intramuscularly three times weekly is a reasonable starting dose. Testosterone levels should be measured 6–8 weeks later and 48–72 h after the hCG or rhLH injection; the hCG/rhLH dose should be adjusted to achieve testosterone levels in the mid-normal range. Sperm counts should be monitored on a monthly basis. It may take several months for spermatogenesis to be restored; therefore, it is important to forewarn patients about the potential length and expense of the treatment and to provide conservative estimates of success rates. If testosterone levels are in the mid-normal range but the sperm concentrations are low after 6 months of therapy with hCG alone, FSH should be added. This can be done by using hMG, highly purified urinary hFSH, or recombinant hFSH. The selection of FSH dose is empirical. A common practice is to start with the addition of 75 IU FSH three times each week in conjunction with the hCG/rhLH injections. If sperm densities are still low after 3 months of combined treatment, the FSH dose should be increased to 150 IU. Occasionally, it may take ≥18–24 months for spermatogenesis to be restored.

The two best predictors of success using gonadotropin therapy in hypogonadotropic men are testicular volume at presentation and time of onset. In general, men with testicular volumes >8 mL have better response rates than those who have testicular volumes >4 mL. Patients who became hypogonadotropic after puberty experience higher success rates than those who have never undergone pubertal changes. Spermatogenesis can usually be reinitiated by hCG alone, with high rates of success for men with postpubertal onset of hypogonadotropism. The presence of a primary testicular abnormality, such as cryptorchidism, will attenuate testicular response to gonadotropin therapy. Prior androgen therapy does not preclude subsequent response to gonadotropin therapy, although some studies suggest that it may attenuate response to subsequent gonadotropin therapy.

TESTOSTERONE REPLACEMENT Androgen therapy is indicated to restore testosterone levels to normal to correct features of androgen deficiency. Testosterone replacement improves libido and overall sexual activity; increases energy, lean muscle mass, and bone density; and decreases fat mass. The benefits of testosterone replacement therapy have only been proven in men who have documented androgen deficiency, as demonstrated by testosterone levels that are well below the lower limit of normal.

Testosterone is available in a variety of formulations with distinct pharmacokinetics (Table 11-3). Testosterone serves as a prohormone and is converted to 17β-estradiol by aromatase and to 5α-dihydrotestosterone by steroid 5α-reductase. Therefore, when evaluating testosterone formulations, it is important to consider whether the formulation being used can achieve physiologic estradiol and DHT concentrations, in addition to normal testosterone concentrations. Although testosterone concentrations at the lower end of the normal male range can restore sexual function, it is not clear whether low-normal testosterone levels can maintain bone mineral density and muscle mass. The current recommendation is to restore testosterone levels to the mid-normal range.

Oral Derivatives of Testosterone Testosterone is well-absorbed after oral administration but is quickly degraded during the first pass through the liver. Therefore, it is difficult to achieve sustained blood levels of testosterone after oral administration of crystalline testosterone. 17α-Alkylated derivatives of testosterone (e.g., 17α-methyl testosterone, oxandrolone, fluoxymesterone) are relatively resistant to hepatic degradation and can be administered orally; however, because of the potential for hepatotoxicity, including cholestatic jaundice, peliosis, and hepatoma, these formulations should not be used for testosterone replacement. Hereditary angioedema due to C1 esterase deficiency is the only exception to this general recommendation; in this condition, oral 17α-alkylated androgens are useful because they stimulate hepatic synthesis of the C1 esterase inhibitor.

Injectable Forms of Testosterone The esterification of testosterone at the 17β-hydroxy position makes the molecule hydrophobic and extends its duration of action. The slow release of testosterone ester from an oily depot in the muscle accounts for its extended duration of action. The longer the side chain, the greater is the hydrophobicity of the ester and the longer is the duration of action. Thus, testosterone enanthate, cypionate, and undecanoate with longer side chains have longer duration of action than testosterone propionate. Within 24 h after intramuscular administration of 200 mg testosterone enanthate or cypionate, testosterone levels rise into the high-normal or supraphysiologic range and then gradually decline into the hypogonadal range over the next 2 weeks. A bimonthly regimen of testosterone enanthate or cypionate therefore results in peaks and troughs in testosterone levels that are accompanied by changes in a patient's mood, sexual desire, and energy level. The kinetics of testosterone enanthate and cypionate are similar. Estradiol and DHT levels are normal if testosterone replacement is physiologic.

Transdermal Testosterone Patch The nongenital testosterone patch, when applied in an appropriate dose, can normalize testosterone, DHT, and estradiol levels 4–12 h after application. Sexual function and well-being are restored in androgen-deficient men treated with the nongenital patch. One 5-mg patch may not be sufficient to increase testosterone into the mid-normal male range in all hypogonadal men; some patients may need two 5-mg patches daily to achieve the targeted testosterone concentrations. The use of testosterone

TABLE 11-3

CLINICAL PHARMACOLOGY OF SOME TESTOSTERONE FORMULATIONS

FORMULATION	REGIMEN	PHARMACOKINETIC PROFILE	DHT AND E_2	ADVANTAGES	DISADVANTAGES
Testosterone enanthate or cypionate	150–200 mg IM q2wk or 75–100 mg/wk	After a single IM injection, serum T levels rise into the supraphysiologic range, then decline gradually into the hypogonadal range by the end of the dosing interval	DHT and E_2 levels rise in proportion to the increase in T levels; T:DHT and T:E_2 ratios do not change	Corrects symptoms of androgen deficiency; relatively inexpensive, if self-administered; flexibility of dosing	Requires IM injection; peaks and valleys in serum T levels
Topical testosterone gels and axillary testosterone solution	Available in sachets, tubes, and pumps	When used in appropriate doses, these topical formulations restore serum T and E_2 levels to the physiologic male range	Serum DHT levels are higher and T:DHT ratios are lower in hypogonadal men treated with the transdermal gels than in healthy eugonadal men	Corrects symptoms of androgen deficiency, provides flexibility of dosing, ease of application, good skin tolerability	Potential of transfer to a female partner or child by direct skin-to-skin contact; skin irritation in a small proportion of treated men; moderately high DHT levels; considerable interindividual and intraindivudal variation in on-treatment T levels
Transdermal testosterone patch	1 or 2 patches, designed to nominally deliver 5–10 mg T over 24 h applied every day on nonpressure areas	Restores serum T, DHT, and E_2 levels to the physiologic male range	T:DHT and T:E_2 levels are in the physiologic male range	Ease of application, corrects symptoms of androgen deficiency	Serum T levels in some androgen-deficient men may be in the low-normal range; these men may need application of 2 patches daily; skin irritation at the application site occurs frequently in many patients
Buccal, bioadhesive, testosterone tablets	30-mg controlled-release, bioadhesive tablets bid	Absorbed from the buccal mucosa	Normalizes serum T and DHT levels in hypogonadal men	Corrects symptoms of androgen deficiency in healthy, hypogonadal men	Gum-related adverse events in 16% of treated men
Testosterone pellets	2–6 pellets implanted SC; dose and regimen vary with formulation	Serum T peaks at 1 month and then is sustained in normal range for 3–6 months, depending on formulation	T:DHT and T:E_2 ratios do not change	Corrects symptoms of androgen deficiency	Requires surgical incision for insertions; pellets may extrude spontaneously
17-α-Methyl testosterone	This 17-α-alkylated compound should *not* be used because of potential for liver toxicity	Orally active			Clinical responses are variable; potential for liver toxicity; should *not* be used for treatment of androgen deficiency

(*continued*)

TABLE 11-3

CLINICAL PHARMACOLOGY OF SOME TESTOSTERONE FORMULATIONS (CONTINUED)

FORMULATION	REGIMEN	PHARMACOKINETIC PROFILE	DHT AND E_2	ADVANTAGES	DISADVANTAGES
Oral testosterone undecanoate[a]	40–80 mg PO bid or tid with meals	When administered in oleic acid, T undecanoate is absorbed through the lymphatics, bypassing the portal system; considerable variability in the same individual on different days and among individuals	High DHT:T ratio	Convenience of oral administration	Not approved in the United States; variable clinical responses, variable serum T levels, high DHT:T ratio
Injectable long-acting testosterone undecanoate in oil[a]	European regimen 1000 mg IM, followed by 1000 mg at 6 weeks, and 1000 mg every 10–14 weeks	When administered at a dose of 750–1000 mg IM, serum T levels are maintained in the normal range in a majority of treated men	DHT and E_2 levels rise in proportion to the increase in T levels; T:DHT and T:E_2 ratios do not change	Corrects symptoms of androgen deficiency; requires infrequent administration	Requires IM injection of a large volume (4 mL); cough reported immediately after injection in a very small number of men
Testosterone-in-adhesive matrix patch[a]	2 × 60 cm^2 patches delivering approximately 4.8 mg of T/d	Restores serum T, DHT, and E_2 to the physiologic range	T:DHT and T:E_2 are in the physiologic range	Lasts 2 d	Some skin irritation

[a]These formulations are not approved for clinical use in the United States, but are available outside the United States in many countries. Physicians in those countries where these formulations are available should follow the approved drug regimens.
Abbreviations: DHT, dihydrotestosterone; E_2, estradiol; T, testosterone.

patches may be associated with skin irritation in some individuals.

Testosterone Gel Several transdermal testosterone gels (e.g., Androgel, Testim, Fortesta, and Axiron), when applied topically to the skin in appropriate doses (Table 11-3), can maintain total and free testosterone concentrations in the normal range in hypogonadal men. The current recommendations are to begin with an initial U.S. Food and Drug Administration–approved dose and adjust the dose based on testosterone levels. The advantages of the testosterone gel include the ease of application and its flexibility of dosing. A major concern is the potential for inadvertent transfer of the gel to a sexual partner or to children who may come in close contact with the patient. The ratio of DHT to testosterone concentrations is higher in men treated with the testosterone gel than in healthy men. Also, there is considerable intra- and interindividual variation in serum testosterone levels in men treated with the transdermal gel due to variations in transdermal absorption and plasma clearance of testosterone. Therefore, monitoring of serum testosterone levels and multiple dose adjustments may be required to achieve and maintain testosterone levels in the target range.

Buccal Adhesive Testosterone A buccal testosterone tablet, which adheres to the buccal mucosa and releases testosterone as it is slowly dissolved, has been approved. After twice-daily application of 30-mg tablets, serum testosterone levels are maintained within the normal male range in a majority of treated hypogonadal men. The adverse effects include buccal ulceration and gum problems in a few subjects. The effects of food and brushing on absorption have not been studied in detail.

Implants of crystalline testosterone can be inserted in the subcutaneous tissue by means of a trocar through a small skin incision. Testosterone is released by surface erosion of the implant and absorbed into the systemic circulation. Two to six 200-mg implants can maintain testosterone in the mid-to high-normal range for up to 6 months. Potential drawbacks include incising the skin for insertion and removal and spontaneous extrusions and fibrosis at the site of the implant.

Testosterone Formulations Not Available in the United States Testosterone undecanoate, when administered orally in oleic acid, is absorbed preferentially through the lymphatics into the systemic circulation and is spared the first-pass degradation in the liver. Doses of 40–80 mg orally, two or three times daily, are typically used. However, the clinical responses are variable and suboptimal. DHT-to-testosterone ratios are higher in hypogonadal men treated with oral testosterone undecanoate, as compared to eugonadal men.

After initial priming, long-acting testosterone undecanoate in oil, when administered intramuscularly every 12 weeks, maintains serum testosterone, estradiol, and DHT in the normal male range and corrects symptoms of androgen deficiency in a majority of treated men. However, large injection volume (4 mL) is its relative drawback.

Novel Androgen Formulations A number of androgen formulations with better pharmacokinetics or more selective activity profiles are under development. A long-acting ester, testosterone undecanoate, when injected intramuscularly, can maintain circulating testosterone concentrations in the male range for 7–12 weeks. Initial clinical trials have demonstrated the feasibility of administering testosterone by the sublingual or buccal routes. 7α-Methyl-19-nortestosterone is an androgen that cannot be 5α-reduced; therefore, compared to testosterone, it has relatively greater agonist activity in muscle and gonadotropin suppression but lesser activity on the prostate.

Selective AR modulators (SARMs) are a class of AR ligands that bind the AR and display tissue-selective actions. A number of nonsteroidal SARMs that act as full agonists on the muscle and bone and that spare the prostate to varying degrees have advanced to phase 3 human trials. Nonsteroidal SARMs do not serve as substrates for either the steroid 5α-reductase or the CYP19 aromatase. SARM binding to AR induces specific conformational changes in the AR protein, which then modulates protein-protein interactions between AR and its coregulators, resulting in tissue-specific regulation of gene expression.

Pharmacologic Uses of Androgens Androgens and SARMs are being evaluated as anabolic therapies for functional limitations associated with aging and chronic illness. Testosterone supplementation increases skeletal muscle mass, maximal voluntary strength, and muscle power in healthy men, hypogonadal men, older men with low testosterone levels, HIV-infected men with weight loss, and men receiving glucocorticoids. These anabolic effects of testosterone are related to testosterone dose and circulating concentrations. Systematic reviews have confirmed that testosterone therapy of HIV-infected men with weight loss promotes improvements in body weight, lean body mass, muscle strength, and depression indices, leading to the recommendation that testosterone be considered as an adjunctive therapy in HIV-infected men who are experiencing unexplained weight loss and who have low testosterone levels. Similarly, in glucocorticoid-treated men, testosterone therapy should be considered to maintain muscle mass and strength and vertebral bone mineral density. It is unknown whether testosterone therapy of older men with functional limitations is safe and effective in improving physical function, vitality, and health-related quality of life and reducing disability. Concerns about potential adverse effects of testosterone on prostate and cardiovascular event rates have encouraged the development of SARMs that are preferentially anabolic and spare the prostate.

Testosterone administration induces hypertrophy of both type 1 and 2 fibers and increases satellite cell (muscle progenitor cells) and myonuclear number. Androgens promote the differentiation of mesenchymal, multipotent progenitor cells into the myogenic lineage and inhibit their differentiation into the adipogenic lineage. Testosterone may have additional effects on satellite cell replication and muscle protein synthesis, which may contribute to an increase in skeletal muscle mass.

Other indications for androgen therapy are in selected patients with anemia due to bone marrow failure (an indication largely supplanted by erythropoietin) or for hereditary angioedema.

Male Hormonal Contraception Based on Combined Administration of Testosterone and Gonadotropin Inhibitors Supraphysiologic doses of testosterone (200 mg testosterone enanthate weekly) suppress LH and FSH secretion and induce azoospermia in 50% of Caucasian men and >95% of Chinese men. The WHO-supported multicenter efficacy trials have demonstrated that suppression of spermatogenesis to azoospermia or severe oligozoospermia (<3 million/mL) by administration of testosterone enanthate to men results in highly effective contraception. Because of concern about long-term adverse effects of supraphysiologic testosterone doses, regimens that combine other gonadotropin inhibitors, such as GnRH antagonists and progestins with replacement doses of testosterone, are being investigated. Oral etonogestrel daily in combination with intramuscular testosterone decanoate every 4–6 weeks induced azoospermia or severe oligozoospermia (sperm density <1 million/mL) in 99% of treated men over a 1-year period. This regimen was associated with weight gain, deceased testicular volume, and decreased plasma high-density lipoprotein (HDL) cholesterol, and its long-term safety has not been demonstrated. SARMs that are more potent inhibitors of gonadotropins than testosterone and spare the prostate hold promise for their contraceptive potential.

Recommended Regimens for Androgen Replacement Testosterone esters are administered typically at doses of 75–100 mg intramuscularly every week, or 150–200 mg every 2 weeks. One or two 5-mg nongenital testosterone patches can be applied daily over the skin of the back, thigh, or upper arm away from pressure areas. Testosterone gels are typically applied over a covered area of skin at initial doses that vary with the formulation; patients should wash their hands after gel application. Bioadhesive buccal testosterone tablets at a dose of 30 mg are typically applied twice daily on the buccal mucosa.

Establishing Efficacy of Testosterone Replacement Therapy Because a clinically useful marker of androgen action is not available, restoration of testosterone levels to the mid-normal range remains the goal of therapy. Measurements of LH and FSH are not useful in assessing the adequacy of testosterone replacement. Testosterone should be measured 3 months after initiating therapy to assess adequacy of therapy. There is substantial interindividual variability in serum testosterone levels, especially with transdermal gels, presumably due to genetic differences in testosterone clearance and transdermal absorption. In patients who are treated with testosterone enanthate or cypionate, testosterone levels should be 350–600 ng/dL 1 week after the injection. If testosterone levels are outside this range, adjustments should be made either in the dose or in the interval between injections. In men on transdermal patch, gel, or buccal testosterone therapy, testosterone levels should be in the mid-normal range (500–700 ng/dL) 4–12 h after application. If testosterone levels are outside this range, the dose should be adjusted. Multiple dose adjustments are often necessary to achieve testosterone levels in the desired therapeutic range.

Restoration of sexual function, secondary sex characteristics, energy, and well-being and maintenance of muscle and bone health are important objectives of testosterone replacement therapy. The patient should be asked about sexual desire and activity, the presence of early morning erections, and the ability to achieve and maintain erections adequate for sexual intercourse. Some hypogonadal men continue to complain about sexual dysfunction even after testosterone replacement has been instituted; these patients may benefit from counseling. The hair growth in response to androgen replacement is variable and depends on ethnicity. Hypogonadal men with prepubertal onset of androgen deficiency who begin testosterone therapy in their late twenties or thirties may find it difficult to adjust to their newly found sexuality and may benefit from counseling. If the patient has a sexual partner, the partner should be included in counseling because of the dramatic physical and sexual changes that occur with androgen treatment.

Contraindications for Androgen Administration Testosterone administration is contraindicated in men with a history of prostate or breast cancer (Table 11-4). Testosterone therapy should not be administered without further urologic evaluation to men with a palpable prostate nodule or induration; to men with prostate-specific antigen levels >4 ng/mL or >3 ng/mL in men at high risk for prostate cancer such as African Americans or men with first-degree relatives with prostate cancer; or to men with severe lower urinary tract symptoms (American Urological Association lower urinary tract symptom score >19). Testosterone replacement should not be administered to men with baseline hematocrit ≥50%, severe untreated obstructive sleep apnea, uncontrolled or poorly controlled congestive heart failure, or myocardial infarction, stroke, or acute coronary syndrome in the preceding 6 months.

Monitoring Potential Adverse Experiences The clinical effectiveness and safety of testosterone replacement therapy should be assessed 3 to 6 months after initiating testosterone therapy and annually thereafter (Table 11-5). Potential adverse effects include acne, oiliness of skin, erythrocytosis, breast tenderness and enlargement, leg edema, induction and exacerbation of obstructive sleep apnea, and increased risk of detection of prostate events. In addition, there may be formulation-specific adverse effects such as skin irritation with transdermal patch, risk of gel transfer to a sexual partner with testosterone gels, buccal ulceration and gum problems with buccal testosterone, and pain and mood fluctuation with injectable testosterone esters. Older men with preexisting heart disease may be at increased risk of cardiovascular events after initiation of testosterone therapy.

TABLE 11-4

CONDITIONS IN WHICH TESTOSTERONE ADMINISTRATION IS ASSOCIATED WITH A RISK OF ADVERSE OUTCOME

Conditions in which testosterone administration is associated with very high risk of serious adverse outcomes:
Metastatic prostate cancer
Breast cancer
Conditions in which testosterone administration is associated with moderate to high risk of adverse outcomes:
Undiagnosed prostate nodule or induration
PSA >4 ng/mL (>3 ng/mL in individuals at high risk for prostate cancer, such as African Americans or men with first-degree relatives who have prostate cancer)
Erythrocytosis (hematocrit >50%)
Severe lower urinary tract symptoms associated with benign prostatic hypertrophy as indicated by American Urological Association/International Prostate Symptom Score >19
Uncontrolled or poorly controlled congestive heart failure
Myocardial infarction, stroke, or acute coronary syndrome in the preceding 6 months

Abbreviation: PSA, prostate-specific antigen.
Source: Reproduced from the Endocrine Society Guideline for Testosterone Therapy of Androgen Deficiency Syndromes in Men (S Bhasin et al: J Clin Endocrinol Metab 95:2536, 2010).

HEMOGLOBIN LEVELS Administration of testosterone to androgen-deficient men is typically associated with a ~3% increase in hemoglobin levels, due to increased erythropoiesis, suppression of hepcidin, and increased iron availability for erythropoiesis. The magnitude of hemoglobin increase during testosterone therapy is greater in older men than younger men and in men who have sleep apnea, a significant smoking history, or chronic obstructive lung disease. The frequency of erythrocytosis is higher in hypogonadal men treated with injectable testosterone esters than in those treated with transdermal formulations, presumably due to the higher testosterone dose delivered by the typical regimens of testosterone esters. Erythrocytosis is the most frequent adverse event reported in testosterone trials in middle-aged and older men and is also the most frequent cause of treatment discontinuation in these trials. If hematocrit rises above 54%, testosterone therapy should be stopped until hematocrit has fallen to <50%. After evaluation of the patient for hypoxia and sleep apnea, testosterone therapy may be reinitiated at a lower dose.

PROSTATE AND SERUM PROSTATE-SPECIFIC ANTIGEN LEVELS Testosterone replacement therapy increases prostate volume to the size seen in age-matched controls but does not increase prostate volume beyond that expected for age. There

TABLE 11-5

MONITORING MEN RECEIVING TESTOSTERONE THERAPY

1. Evaluate the patient 3–6 months after treatment initiation and then annually to assess whether symptoms have responded to treatment and whether the patient is suffering from any adverse effects.
2. Monitor testosterone level 3–6 months after initiation of testosterone therapy:
   - Therapy should aim to raise serum testosterone level into the mid-normal range.
     - Injectable testosterone enanthate or cypionate: Measure serum testosterone level midway between injections. If testosterone is >700 ng/dL (24.5 nmol/L) or >400 ng/dL (14.1 nmol/L), adjust dose or frequency.
     - Transdermal patches: Assess testosterone level 3–12 h after application of the patch; adjust dose to achieve testosterone level in the mid-normal range.
     - Buccal testosterone bioadhesive tablet: Assess level immediately before or after application of fresh system.
     - Transdermal gels and solution: Assess testosterone level 2–8 h after patient has been on treatment for at least 2 weeks; adjust dose to achieve serum testosterone level in the mid-normal range.
     - Testosterone pellets: Measure testosterone levels at the end of the dosing interval. Adjust the number of pellets and/or the dosing interval to achieve serum testosterone levels in the normal range.
     - Oral testosterone undecanoate[a]: Monitor serum testosterone level 3–5 h after ingestion.
     - Injectable testosterone undecanoate: Measure serum testosterone level just prior to each subsequent injection and adjust the dosing interval to maintain serum testosterone in mid-normal range.
3. Check hematocrit at baseline, at 3–6 months, and then annually. If hematocrit is >54%, stop therapy until hematocrit decreases to a safe level; evaluate the patient for hypoxia and sleep apnea; reinitiate therapy with a reduced dose.
4. Measure bone mineral density of lumbar spine and/or femoral neck after 1–2 years of testosterone therapy in hypogonadal men with osteoporosis or low trauma fracture, consistent with regional standard of care.
5. In men 40 years of age or older with baseline PSA >0.6 ng/mL, perform digital rectal examination and check PSA level before initiating treatment, at 3–6 months, and then in accordance with guidelines for prostate cancer screening depending on the age and race of the patient.
6. Obtain urologic consultation if there is:
   - An increase in serum PSA concentration >1.4 ng/mL within any 12-month period of testosterone treatment.
   - A PSA velocity of >0.4 ng/mL per year using the PSA level after 6 months of testosterone administration as the reference (only applicable if PSA data are available for a period exceeding 2 years).
   - Detection of a prostatic abnormality on digital rectal examination.
   - An AUA/IPSS prostate symptom score of >19.
7. Evaluate formulation-specific adverse effects at each visit:
   - Buccal testosterone tablets: Inquire about alterations in taste and examine the gums and oral mucosa for irritation.
   - Injectable testosterone esters (enanthate, cypionate, and undecanoate): Ask about fluctuations in mood or libido and, rarely, cough after injections.
   - Testosterone patches: Look for skin reaction at the application site.
   - Testosterone gels: Advise patients to cover the application sites with a shirt and to wash the skin with soap and water before having skin-to-skin contact, because testosterone gels leave a testosterone residue on the skin that can be transferred to a woman or child who might come in close contact. Serum testosterone levels are maintained when the application site is washed 4–6 h after application of the testosterone gel.
   - Testosterone pellets: Look for signs of infection, fibrosis, or pellet extrusion.

[a]Not approved for clinical use in the United States.

Abbreviations: AUA/IPSS, American Urological Association/International Prostate Symptom Score; PSA, prostate-specific antigen.

Source: Reproduced with permission from the Endocrine Society Guideline for Testosterone Therapy of Androgen Deficiency Syndromes in Adult Men (S Bhasin et al: J Clin Endocrinol Metab 95:2536, 2010).

is no evidence that testosterone therapy causes prostate cancer. However, androgen administration can exacerbate preexisting metastatic prostate cancer. Many older men harbor microscopic foci of cancer in their prostates. It is not known whether long-term testosterone administration will induce these microscopic foci to grow into clinically significant cancers.

Prostate-specific antigen (PSA) levels are lower in testosterone-deficient men and are restored to normal after testosterone replacement. There is considerable test-retest variability in PSA measurements. Increments in PSA levels after testosterone supplementation in androgen-deficient men are generally <0.5 ng/mL, and increments >1.0 ng/mL over a 3- to 6-month period are unusual. The 90% confidence interval for the change in PSA values in men with benign prostatic hypertrophy, measured 3–6 months apart, is 1.4 ng/mL. Therefore, the Endocrine Society expert panel suggested that an increase in PSA >1.4 ng/mL in any 1 year after starting testosterone therapy, if confirmed, should lead to urologic evaluation. PSA velocity criterion can be used for patients who have sequential PSA measurements for >2 years; a change of >0.40 ng/mL per year merits closer urologic follow-up.

CARDIOVASCULAR RISK In epidemiologic studies, testosterone concentrations are negatively related to the risk of diabetes mellitus, heart disease, and all-cause and cardiovascular mortality. A recent testosterone trial in older men with mobility limitation was stopped early because of the higher rates of cardiovascular events in the testosterone arm than in the placebo arm of this trial. Meta-analyses of testosterone trials have found a significant increase in cardiovascular event rates in older men receiving testosterone therapy. Inferences about adverse events from previous trials included in these meta-analyses are limited by poor ascertainment, small numbers of events, heterogeneity of study populations, and small numbers of participants. Two retrospective analyses also found a higher frequency of cardiovascular events in association with testosterone therapy in older men with preexisting heart disease. Retrospective database analyses are limited by their inherent inability to verify the indication for treatment, diagnoses, or other relevant quantitative information and are susceptible to confounding by many other factors. Adequately powered prospective studies are needed to determine the effect on testosterone replacement on cardiovascular risk.

Androgen Abuse by Athletes and Recreational Bodybuilders The illicit use of androgenic-anabolic steroids (AAS) to enhance athletic performance first surfaced in the 1950s among power lifters and spread rapidly to other sports, professional as well as high school athletes, and recreational bodybuilders. In the early 1980s, the use of AAS spread beyond the athletic community into the general population, and now as many as 3 million Americans, most of them men, have likely used these compounds. Most AAS users are not athletes, but rather recreational weightlifters, who use these drugs to look lean and more muscular. The most commonly used AAS include testosterone esters, nandrolone, stanozolol, methandienone, and methenolol. AAS users generally use increasing doses of multiple steroids in a practice known as stacking.

The adverse effects of long-term AAS abuse remain poorly understood. Most of the information about the adverse effects of AAS has emerged from case reports, uncontrolled studies, or clinical trials that used replacement doses of testosterone. The adverse event data from clinical trials using physiologic replacement doses of testosterone have been extrapolated unjustifiably to AAS users who may administer 10–100 times the replacement doses of testosterone over many years and to support the claim that AAS use is safe. A substantial fraction of androgenic steroid users also use other drugs that are perceived to be muscle building or performance enhancing, such as GH; erythropoiesis-stimulating agents; insulin; and stimulants such as amphetamine, clenbuterol, cocaine, ephedrine, and thyroxine; and drugs perceived to reduce adverse effects such as hCG, aromatase inhibitors, or estrogen antagonists. The men who abuse androgenic steroids are more likely to engage in other high-risk behaviors than nonusers. The adverse events associated with AAS use may be due to AAS themselves, concomitant use of other drugs, high-risk behaviors, and host characteristics that may render these individuals more susceptible to AAS use or to other high-risk behaviors.

The high rates of mortality and morbidities observed in AAS users are alarming. One Finnish study reported 4.6 times the risk of death among elite power lifters than in age-matched men from the general population. The causes of death among power lifters included suicides, myocardial infarction, hepatic coma, and non-Hodgkin's lymphoma. A retrospective review of patient records in Sweden also reported higher standardized mortality ratios for AAS users than for nonusers. Thiblin and colleagues found that 32% of deaths among AAS users were suicidal, 26% homicidal, and 35% accidental. The median age of death among AAS users (24 years) is even lower than that for heroin or amphetamine users.

Numerous reports of cardiac death among young AAS users raise concerns about the adverse cardiovascular effects of AAS. High doses of AAS may induce proatherogenic dyslipidemia, increase thrombosis risk via effects on clotting factors and platelets, and induce vasospasm through their effects on vascular nitric oxide.

Replacement doses of testosterone, when administered parenterally, are associated with only a small decrease in HDL cholesterol and little or no effect on total cholesterol, low-density lipoprotein (LDL) cholesterol, and triglyceride levels. In contrast, supraphysiologic doses of testosterone and orally administered, 17α-alkylated, nonaromatizable AAS are associated with marked reductions in HDL cholesterol and increases in LDL cholesterol.

Recent studies of AAS users using tissue Doppler and strain imaging and MRI have reported diastolic and systolic dysfunction, including significantly lower early and late diastolic tissue velocities, reduced E/A ratio, and reduced peak systolic strain in AAS users than in nonusers. Power athletes using AAS often have short QT intervals but increased QT dispersion, which may predispose them to ventricular arrhythmias. Long-term AAS use may be associated with myocardial hypertrophy and fibrosis. Myocardial tissue of power lifters using AAS has been shown to be infiltrated with fibrous tissue and fat droplets. The finding of ARs on myocardial cells suggests that AAS might be directly toxic to myocardial cells.

Long-term AAS use suppresses LH and FSH secretion and inhibits endogenous testosterone production and spermatogenesis. Men who have used AAS for more than a few months experience marked suppression of the hypothalamic-pituitary-testicular (HPT) axis after stopping AAS that may be associated with sexual dysfunction, fatigue, infertility, and depression; in some AAS users, HPT suppression may last more than a year, and in a few individuals, complete recovery may never occur. The symptoms of androgen deficiency caused by androgen withdrawal may cause some men to revert back to using AAS, leading to continued use and AAS dependence. As many as 30% of AAS users develop a syndrome of AAS dependence, characterized by long-term AAS use despite adverse medical and psychiatric effects.

Supraphysiologic doses of testosterone may also impair insulin sensitivity. Orally administered androgens also have been associated with insulin resistance and diabetes.

Unsafe injection practices, high-risk behaviors, and increased rates of incarceration render AAS users at increased risk of HIV and hepatitis B and C. In one survey, nearly 1 in 10 gay men had injected AAS or other substances, and AAS users were more likely to report high-risk unprotected anal sex than other men.

Some AAS users develop hypomanic or manic symptoms during AAS exposure (irritability, aggressiveness, reckless behavior, and occasional psychotic symptoms, sometimes associated with violence) and major depression (sometimes associated with suicidality) during AAS withdrawal. Users may also develop other forms of illicit drug use, which may be potentiated or exacerbated by AAS.

Elevated liver enzymes, cholestatic jaundice, hepatic neoplasms, and peliosis hepatis have been reported with oral, 17α-alkylated AAS. AAS use may cause muscle hypertrophy without compensatory adaptations in tendons, ligaments, and joints, thus increasing the risk of tendon and joint injuries. AAS use is associated with acne, baldness, and increased body hair.

The suspicion of AAS use may be raised by the increased hemoglobin and hematocrit, suppressed LH and FSH and testosterone levels, low high-density lipoproteins cholesterol, and low testicular volume and sperm density in a person who looks highly muscular. Accredited laboratories use gas chromatography–mass spectrometry or liquid chromatography–mass spectrometry to detect anabolic steroid abuse. In recent years, the availability of high-resolution mass spectrometry and tandem mass spectrometry has further improved the sensitivity of detecting androgen abuse. Illicit testosterone use is detected generally by the application of the measurement of the urinary testosterone-to-epitestosterone ratio and further confirmed by the use of the $^{13}C:^{12}C$ ratio in testosterone by the use of isotope ratio combustion mass spectrometry. Exogenous testosterone administration increases urinary testosterone glucuronide excretion and consequently the testosterone-to-epitestosterone ratio. Ratios >4 suggest exogenous testosterone use but can also reflect genetic variation. Genetic variations in the uridine diphosphoglucuronyl transferase 2B17 (*UGT2B17*), the major enzyme for testosterone glucuronidation, affect the testosterone-to-epitestosterone ratio. Synthetic testosterone has a lower $^{13}C:^{12}C$ ratio than endogenously produced testosterone, and these differences in $^{13}C:^{12}C$ ratio can be detected by isotope ratio combustion mass spectrometry, which is used to confirm exogenous testosterone use in individuals with a high testosterone-to-epitestosterone ratio.

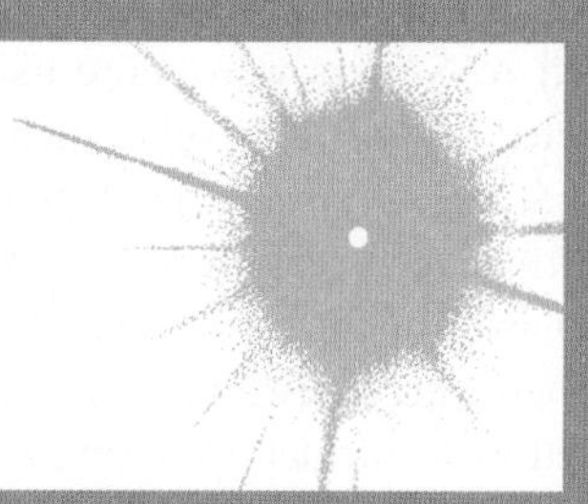

CHAPTER 12

TESTICULAR CANCER

Robert J. Motzer ■ Darren R. Feldman ■ George J. Bosl

Primary germ cell tumors (GCTs) of the testis arising by the malignant transformation of primordial germ cells constitute 95% of all testicular neoplasms. Infrequently, GCTs arise from an extragonadal site, including the mediastinum, retroperitoneum, and, very rarely, the pineal gland. This disease is notable for the young age of the afflicted patients, the totipotent capacity for differentiation of the tumor cells, and its curability; approximately 95% of newly diagnosed patients are cured. Experience in the management of GCTs leads to improved outcome.

INCIDENCE AND EPIDEMIOLOGY

The incidence of testicular GCT is now approximately 8000 cases annually in the United States, resulting in nearly 400 deaths. The tumor occurs most frequently in men between the ages of 20 and 40 years. A testicular mass in a male ≥50 years should be regarded as a lymphoma until proved otherwise. GCT is at least four to five times more common in white than in African-American males, and a higher incidence has been observed in Scandinavia and New Zealand than in the United States.

ETIOLOGY AND GENETICS

Cryptorchidism is associated with a several-fold higher risk of GCT. Abdominal cryptorchid testes are at a higher risk than inguinal cryptorchid testes. Orchiopexy should be performed before puberty, if possible. Early orchiopexy reduces the risk of GCT and improves the ability to save the testis. An abdominal cryptorchid testis that cannot be brought into the scrotum should be removed. Approximately 2% of men with GCTs of one testis will develop a primary tumor in the other testis. Testicular feminization syndromes and family history increase the risk of testicular GCT, and Klinefelter's syndrome is associated with mediastinal GCT.

An isochromosome of the short arm of chromosome 12 [i(12p)] is pathognomonic for GCT. Excess 12p copy number, either in the form of i(12p) or as increased 12p on aberrantly banded marker chromosomes, occurs in nearly all GCTs, but the gene(s) on 12p involved in the pathogenesis are not yet defined.

CLINICAL PRESENTATION

A painless testicular mass is pathognomonic for a testicular malignancy. More commonly, patients present with testicular discomfort or swelling suggestive of epididymitis and/or orchitis. In this circumstance, a trial of antibiotics is reasonable. However, if symptoms persist or a residual abnormality remains, then testicular ultrasound examination is indicated.

Ultrasound of the testis is indicated whenever a testicular malignancy is considered and for persistent or painful testicular swelling. If a testicular mass is detected, a radical inguinal orchiectomy should be performed. Because the testis develops from the gonadal ridge, its blood supply and lymphatic drainage originate in the abdomen and descend with the testis into the scrotum. An inguinal approach is taken to avoid breaching anatomic barriers and permitting additional pathways of spread.

Back pain from retroperitoneal metastases is common and must be distinguished from musculoskeletal pain. Dyspnea from pulmonary metastases occurs infrequently. Patients with increased serum levels of human chorionic gonadotropin (hCG) may present with gynecomastia. A delay in diagnosis is associated with a more advanced stage and possibly worse survival.

The staging evaluation for GCT includes a determination of serum levels of α fetoprotein (AFP), hCG, and lactate dehydrogenase (LDH). After orchiectomy, a computed tomography (CT) scan of the chest, abdomen, and pelvis is generally performed. Stage I disease is limited to the testis, epididymis, or spermatic cord.

Stage II disease is limited to retroperitoneal (regional) lymph nodes. Stage III disease is disease outside the retroperitoneum, involving supradiaphragmatic nodal sites or viscera. The staging may be "clinical"—defined solely by physical examination, blood marker evaluation, and radiographs—or "pathologic"—defined by an operative procedure.

The regional draining lymph nodes for the testis are in the retroperitoneum, and the vascular supply originates from the great vessels (for the right testis) or the renal vessels (for the left testis). As a result, the lymph nodes that are involved first by a right testicular tumor are the interaortocaval lymph nodes just below the renal vessels. For a left testicular tumor, the first involved lymph nodes are lateral to the aorta (para-aortic) and below the left renal vessels. In both cases, further retroperitoneal nodal spread is inferior, contralateral, and, less commonly, above the renal hilum. Lymphatic involvement can extend cephalad to the retrocrural, posterior mediastinal, and supraclavicular lymph nodes. Treatment is determined by tumor histology (seminoma versus nonseminoma) and clinical stage (Fig. 12–1).

PATHOLOGY

GCTs are divided into nonseminoma and seminoma subtypes. Nonseminomatous GCTs are most frequent in the third decade of life and can display the full spectrum of embryonic and adult cellular differentiation. This entity comprises four histologies: embryonal carcinoma, teratoma, choriocarcinoma, and endodermal sinus (yolk sac) tumor. Choriocarcinoma, consisting of both cytotrophoblasts and syncytiotrophoblasts, represents malignant trophoblastic differentiation and is invariably associated with secretion of hCG. Endodermal sinus tumor is the malignant counterpart of the fetal yolk sac and is associated with secretion of AFP. Pure embryonal carcinoma may secrete AFP or hCG, or both; this pattern is biochemical evidence of differentiation. Teratoma is composed of somatic cell types derived from two or more germ layers (ectoderm, mesoderm, or endoderm). Each of these histologies may be present alone or in combination with others. Nonseminomatous GCTs tend to metastasize early to sites such as the retroperitoneal lymph nodes and lung parenchyma. Sixty percent of patients present with disease limited to the testis (stage I), 20% with retroperitoneal metastases (stage II), and 20% with more extensive supradiaphragmatic nodal or visceral metastases (stage III).

Seminoma represents approximately 50% of all GCTs, has a median age in the fourth decade, and generally follows a more indolent clinical course. Eighty percent of patients present with stage I disease, approximately 10% with stage II disease, and 10% with stage III disease; lung or other visceral metastases are rare. When a tumor contains both seminoma and nonseminoma components, patient management is directed by the more aggressive nonseminoma component.

TUMOR MARKERS

Careful monitoring of the serum tumor markers AFP and hCG is essential in the management of patients with GCT, because these markers are important for diagnosis, as prognostic indicators, in monitoring treatment response, and in the early detection of relapse. Approximately 70% of patients presenting with disseminated nonseminomatous GCT have increased serum concentrations of AFP and/or hCG. Although hCG concentrations may be increased in patients with either nonseminoma or seminoma histology, the AFP concentration is increased only in patients with nonseminoma. The presence of an increased AFP level in a patient whose tumor shows only seminoma indicates that an occult nonseminomatous component exists, and the patient should be treated for nonseminomatous GCT. LDH levels are less specific than AFP or hCG but are increased in 50–60% patients with metastatic nonseminoma and in up to 80% of patients with advanced seminoma.

AFP, hCG, and LDH levels should be determined before and after orchiectomy. Increased serum AFP and hCG concentrations decay according to first-order kinetics; the half-life is 24–36 h for hCG and 5–7 days for AFP. AFP and hCG should be assayed serially during and after treatment. The reappearance of hCG and/or AFP or the failure of these markers to decline according to the predicted half-life is an indicator of persistent or recurrent tumor.

TREATMENT Testicular Cancer

STAGE I NONSEMINOMA Patients with radiographs and physical examination showing no evidence of disease and serum AFP and hCG concentrations that are either normal or declining to normal according to the known half-life have clinical stage I disease. Approximately 20–50% of such patients will have retroperitoneal lymph node metastases (pathologic stage II) but will still be cured in over 95% of cases. Depending on risk of relapse, which is determined by the pathology (see below), surveillance, a nerve-sparing retroperitoneal lymph node dissection (RPLND), or adjuvant chemotherapy (one to two cycles of bleomycin, etoposide, and cisplatin [BEP]) may be appropriate choices depending on *the availability of surgical expertise and patient and physician preference*. If the primary tumor shows no evidence for lymphatic or vascular invasion and is limited to the testis (T1, clinical stage IA), then the risk of relapse is

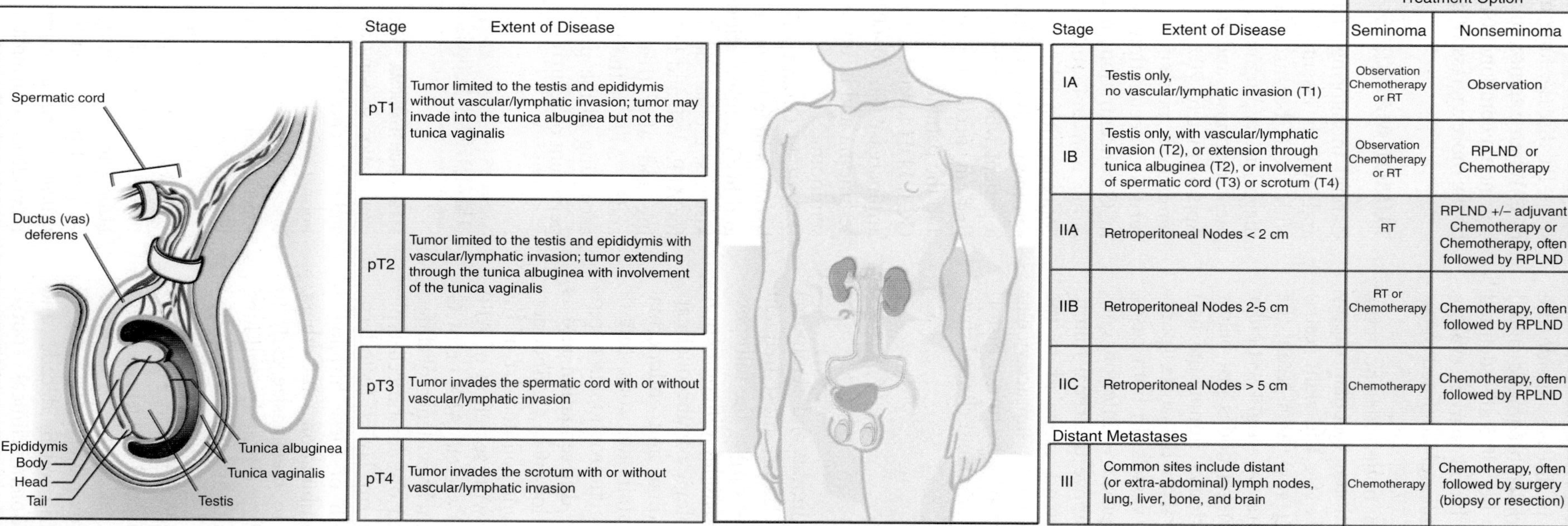

Stage	Extent of Disease
pT1	Tumor limited to the testis and epididymis without vascular/lymphatic invasion; tumor may invade into the tunica albuginea but not the tunica vaginalis
pT2	Tumor limited to the testis and epididymis with vascular/lymphatic invasion; tumor extending through the tunica albuginea with involvement of the tunica vaginalis
pT3	Tumor invades the spermatic cord with or without vascular/lymphatic invasion
pT4	Tumor invades the scrotum with or without vascular/lymphatic invasion

Stage	Extent of Disease	Treatment Option: Seminoma	Treatment Option: Nonseminoma
IA	Testis only, no vascular/lymphatic invasion (T1)	Observation Chemotherapy or RT	Observation
IB	Testis only, with vascular/lymphatic invasion (T2), or extension through tunica albuginea (T2), or involvement of spermatic cord (T3) or scrotum (T4)	Observation Chemotherapy or RT	RPLND or Chemotherapy
IIA	Retroperitoneal Nodes < 2 cm	RT	RPLND +/– adjuvant Chemotherapy or Chemotherapy, often followed by RPLND
IIB	Retroperitoneal Nodes 2-5 cm	RT or Chemotherapy	Chemotherapy, often followed by RPLND
IIC	Retroperitoneal Nodes > 5 cm	Chemotherapy	Chemotherapy, often followed by RPLND
Distant Metastases			
III	Common sites include distant (or extra-abdominal) lymph nodes, lung, liver, bone, and brain	Chemotherapy	Chemotherapy, often followed by surgery (biopsy or resection)

FIGURE 12-1
Germ cell tumor staging and treatment. RPLND, retroperitoneal lymph node dissection; RT, radiotherapy.

only 10–20%. Because over 80% of patients with clinical stage IA nonseminoma are cured with orchiectomy alone and there is no survival advantage to RPLND (or adjuvant chemotherapy), surveillance is the preferred treatment option. This avoids overtreatment with the potential for both acute and long-term toxicities (see below). Surveillance requires patients to be carefully followed with periodic chest radiography, physical examination, CT scan of the abdomen, and serum tumor marker determinations. The median time to relapse is approximately 7 months, and late relapses (>2 years) are rare. Noncompliant patients can be considered for RPLND or adjuvant BEP.

If lymphatic or vascular invasion is present or the tumor extends *through* the tunica, spermatic cord, or scrotum (T2 through T4, clinical stage IB), then the risk of relapse is approximately 50%, and RPLND and adjuvant chemotherapy can be considered. Relapse rates are reduced to 3–5% after one to two cycles of adjuvant BEP. All three approaches (surveillance, RPLND, and adjuvant BEP) should cure >95% of patients with clinical stage IB disease.

RPLND is the standard operation for removal of the regional lymph nodes of the testis (retroperitoneal nodes). The operation removes the lymph nodes draining the primary site and the nodal groups adjacent to the primary landing zone. The standard (modified bilateral) RPLND removes all node-bearing tissue down to the bifurcation of the great vessels, including the ipsilateral iliac nodes. The major long-term effect of this operation is retrograde ejaculation with resultant infertility. Nerve-sparing RPLND can preserve anterograde ejaculation in ~90% of patients. Patients with pathologic stage I disease are observed, and only the <10% who relapse require additional therapy. If nodes are found to be involved at RPLND, then a decision regarding adjuvant chemotherapy is made on the basis of the extent of retroperitoneal disease (see "Stage II Nonseminoma" below). Hence, because less than 20% of patients require chemotherapy, of the three approaches, RPLND results in the lowest number of patients at risk for the late toxicities of chemotherapy.

STAGE II NONSEMINOMA Patients with limited, ipsilateral retroperitoneal adenopathy ≤2 cm in largest diameter and normal levels of AFP and hCG can be treated with either a modified bilateral nerve-sparing RPLND or chemotherapy. The local recurrence rate after a properly performed RPLND is very low. Depending on the extent of disease, the postoperative management options include either surveillance or two cycles of adjuvant chemotherapy. Surveillance is the preferred approach for patients with resected "low-volume" metastases (tumor nodes ≤2 cm in diameter *and* <6 nodes involved) because the probability of relapse is one-third or less. For those who relapse, risk-directed chemotherapy is indicated (see section on advanced GCT below). Because relapse occurs in ≥50% of patients with "high-volume" metastases (>6 nodes involved, *or* any involved node >2 cm in largest diameter, *or* extranodal tumor extension), two cycles of adjuvant chemotherapy should be considered, as it results in a cure in ≥98% of patients. Regimens consisting of etoposide plus cisplatin (EP) with or without bleomycin every 3 weeks are effective and well tolerated.

Increased levels of either AFP or hCG imply metastatic disease outside the retroperitoneum; full-dose (not adjuvant) chemotherapy is used in this setting. Primary management with chemotherapy is also favored for patients with larger (>2 cm) or bilateral retroperitoneal nodes (see section on advanced GCT below).

STAGES I AND II SEMINOMA Inguinal orchiectomy followed by immediate retroperitoneal radiation therapy or surveillance with treatment at relapse both result in cure in nearly 100% of patients with stage I seminoma. Historically, radiation was the mainstay of treatment, but the reported association between radiation and secondary malignancies and the absence of a survival advantage of radiation over surveillance has led many to favor surveillance for compliant patients. Approximately 15% of patients relapse, which is usually treated with chemotherapy. Longterm follow-up is essential, because approximately 30% of relapses occur after 2 years and 5% occur after 5 years. A single dose of carboplatin has also been investigated as an alternative to radiation therapy; the outcome was similar, but long-term safety data are lacking, and the retroperitoneum remained the most frequent site of relapse.

Generally, nonbulky retroperitoneal disease (stage IIA and small IIB) is treated with retroperitoneal radiation therapy. Approximately 90% of patients achieve relapse-free survival with retroperitoneal masses <3 cm in diameter. Due to higher relapse rates after radiation for bulkier disease, initial chemotherapy is preferred for all stage IIC and some stage IIB patients. Chemotherapy has been studied as an alternative to radiation for stage IIA and small stage IIB seminoma with lower recurrence rates compared with historical controls. These results, combined with studies demonstrating a threefold increase in the incidence of secondary malignancies and cardiovascular disease among patients who receive both radiation and chemotherapy (patients relapsing after radiation fall into this category), have led some experts to prefer chemotherapy for all stage II seminomas.

CHEMOTHERAPY FOR ADVANCED GCT Regardless of histology, all patients with stage IIC and stage III and most with stage IIB GCT are treated with chemotherapy. Combination chemotherapy programs based on cisplatin at doses of 100 mg/m^2 plus etoposide at doses of 500 mg/m^2 per cycle cure 70–80% of such patients, with or without bleomycin, depending on risk stratification (see below). A complete response (the complete disappearance of all clinical evidence of tumor on physical examination and radiography plus normal serum levels of AFP and hCG for ≥1 month) occurs after chemotherapy alone in ~60% of patients, and another 10–20% become disease free with surgical resection of residual masses containing viable GCT. Lower doses of cisplatin result in inferior survival rates.

The toxicity of four cycles of the BEP is substantial. Nausea, vomiting, and hair loss occur in most patients, although nausea and vomiting have been markedly ameliorated by modern antiemetic regimens. Myelosuppression is frequent, and symptomatic bleomycin pulmonary toxicity occurs in ~5% of patients. Treatment-induced mortality due to neutropenia with septicemia or bleomycin-induced pulmonary failure occurs in 1–3% of patients. Dose reductions for myelosuppression are rarely indicated. Long-term permanent toxicities include nephrotoxicity (reduced glomerular filtration and persistent magnesium wasting), ototoxicity, peripheral neuropathy, and infertility. When bleomycin is administered by weekly bolus injection, Raynaud's phenomenon appears in 5–10% of patients. Other evidence of small blood vessel damage, such as transient ischemic attacks and myocardial infarction, is seen less often.

RISK-DIRECTED CHEMOTHERAPY Because not all patients are cured and treatment may cause significant toxicities, patients are stratified into "good-risk," "intermediate-risk," and "poor-risk" groups according to pretreatment clinical features established by the International Germ Cell Cancer Consensus Group (Table 12-1). For good-risk patients, the goal is to achieve maximum efficacy with minimal toxicity. For intermediate- and poor-risk patients, the goal is to identify more effective therapy with tolerable toxicity.

The marker cut offs are included in the TNM (primary tumor, regional nodes, metastasis) staging of GCT. Hence, TNM stage groupings are based on both anatomy (site and extent of disease) and biology (marker status and histology). Seminoma is either good- or intermediate-risk, based on the absence or presence of nonpulmonary visceral metastases. No poor-risk category exists for seminoma. Marker levels and primary site play no role in defining risk for seminoma. Nonseminomas have good-, intermediate-, and poor-risk categories based on the primary site of the tumor, the presence or absence of nonpulmonary visceral metastases, and marker levels.

For ~90% of patients with good-risk GCTs, four cycles of EP or three cycles of BEP produce durable complete responses, with minimal acute and chronic toxicity, and a low relapse rate. Pulmonary toxicity is absent when bleomycin is not used and is rare when therapy is limited to 9 weeks; myelosuppression with neutropenic fever is less frequent; and the treatment mortality rate is negligible. Approximately 75% of intermediate-risk patients and 50% of poor-risk patients achieve durable complete remission with four cycles of BEP, and no regimen has proved superior.

POSTCHEMOTHERAPY SURGERY Resection of residual metastases after the completion of chemotherapy is an integral part of therapy. If the initial histology is nonseminoma and the marker values have normalized, all sites of residual disease should be resected. In general, residual retroperitoneal disease requires a modified bilateral RPLND. Thoracotomy (unilateral or bilateral) and neck dissection are less frequently required to remove residual mediastinal, pulmonary parenchymal, or cervical nodal disease. Viable tumor (seminoma, embryonal carcinoma, yolk sac tumor, or choriocarcinoma) will be present in 15%, mature teratoma in 40%, and necrotic debris and fibrosis in 45% of resected specimens. The frequency of teratoma or viable disease is highest in residual mediastinal tumors. If necrotic debris or mature teratoma is present, no further chemotherapy is necessary. If viable tumor is present but is completely excised, two additional cycles of chemotherapy are given.

If the initial histology is pure seminoma, mature teratoma is rarely present, and the most frequent finding is necrotic debris. For residual retroperitoneal disease, a complete RPLND

TABLE 12-1

INTERNATIONAL GERM CELL CANCER CONSENSUS GROUP RISK CLASSIFICATION FOR ADVANCED GERM CELL TUMORS

RISK	NONSEMINOMA	SEMINOMA
Good	Gonadal or retroperitoneal primary site Absent nonpulmonary visceral metastases AFP <1000 ng/mL β-hCG <5000 mIU/mL LDH <1.5 × upper limit or normal (ULN)	Any primary site Absent nonpulmonary visceral metastases Any LDH, hCG
Intermediate	Gonadal or retroperitoneal primary site Absent nonpulmonary visceral metastases AFP 1000–10,000 ng/mL β-hCG 5000–50,000 mIU/mL LDH 1.5–10 × ULN	Any primary site Presence of nonpulmonary visceral metastases Any LDH, hCG
Poor	Mediastinal primary site Presence of nonpulmonary visceral metastases AFP >10,000 ng/mL β-hCG >50,000 mIU/mL LDH >10 × ULN	No patients classified as poor prognosis

Abbreviations: AFP, α fetoprotein; hCG, human chorionic gonadotropin; LDH, lactate dehydrogenase.
Source: From International Germ Cell Cancer Consensus Group.

is technically difficult due to extensive postchemotherapy fibrosis. Observation is recommended when no radiographic abnormality exists on CT scan. Positive findings on a positron emission tomography (PET) scan correlate with viable seminoma in residua and mandate surgical excision or biopsy.

SALVAGE CHEMOTHERAPY Of patients with advanced GCT, 20–30% fail to achieve a durable complete response to first-line chemotherapy. A combination of vinblastine, ifosfamide, and cisplatin (VeIP) will cure approximately 25% of patients as a second-line therapy. Patients are more likely to achieve a durable complete response if they had a testicular primary tumor and relapsed from a prior complete remission to first-line cisplatin-containing chemotherapy. Substitution of paclitaxel for vinblastine (TIP) in this setting was associated with durable remission in nearly two-thirds of patients. In contrast, for patients with a primary mediastinal nonseminoma or who did not achieve a complete response with first-line chemotherapy, then VeIP standard-dose salvage therapy is rarely beneficial. Such patients are usually managed with high-dose chemotherapy and/or surgical resection.

Chemotherapy consisting of dose-intensive, high-dose carboplatin plus high-dose etoposide, with peripheral blood stem cell support, induces a complete response in 25–40% of patients who have progressed after ifosfamide-containing salvage chemotherapy. Approximately one-half of the complete responses will be durable. High-dose therapy is standard of care for this patient population and has been suggested as the treatment of choice for all patients with relapsed or refractory disease. Paclitaxel is active when incorporated into high-dose combination programs. Cure is still possible in some relapsed patients.

EXTRAGONADAL GCT

The prognosis and management of patients with extragonadal GCT depends on the tumor histology and site of origin. All patients with a diagnosis of extragonadal GCT should have a testicular ultrasound examination. Nearly all patients with retroperitoneal or mediastinal seminoma achieve a durable complete response to BEP or EP. The clinical features of patients with primary retroperitoneal nonseminoma GCT are similar to those of patients with a primary tumor of testis origin, and careful evaluation will find evidence of a primary testicular GCT in about two-thirds of cases. In contrast, a primary mediastinal nonseminomatous GCT is associated with a poor prognosis; one-third of patients are cured with standard therapy (four cycles of BEP). Patients with newly diagnosed mediastinal nonseminoma are considered to have poor-risk disease and should be considered for clinical trials testing regimens of possibly greater efficacy. In addition, mediastinal nonseminoma is associated with hematologic disorders, including acute myelogenous leukemia, myelodysplastic syndrome, and essential thrombocytosis unrelated to previous chemotherapy. These hematologic disorders are very refractory to treatment. Nonseminoma of any primary site may change into other malignant histologies such as embryonal rhabdomyosarcoma or adenocarcinoma. This is called *malignant transformation*. i(12p) has been identified in the transformed cell type, indicating GCT clonal origin.

A group of patients with poorly differentiated tumors of unknown histogenesis, midline in distribution, and not associated with secretion of AFP or hCG has been described; a few (10–20%) are cured by standard cisplatin-containing chemotherapy. An i(12p) is present in ~25% of such tumors (the fraction that are cisplatin-responsive), confirming their origin from primitive germ cells. This finding is also predictive of the response to cisplatin-based chemotherapy and resulting long-term survival. These tumors are heterogeneous; neuroepithelial tumors and lymphoma may also present in this fashion.

FERTILITY

Infertility is an important consequence of the treatment of GCTs. Preexisting infertility or impaired fertility is often present. Azoospermia and/or oligospermia are present at diagnosis in at least 50% of patients with testicular GCTs. Ejaculatory dysfunction is associated with RPLND, and germ cell damage may result from cisplatin-containing chemotherapy. Nerve-sparing techniques to preserve the retroperitoneal sympathetic nerves have made retrograde ejaculation less likely in the subgroups of patients who are candidates for this operation. Spermatogenesis does recur in some patients after chemotherapy. However, because of the significant risk of impaired reproductive capacity, semen analysis and cryopreservation of sperm in a sperm bank should be recommended to all patients before treatment.

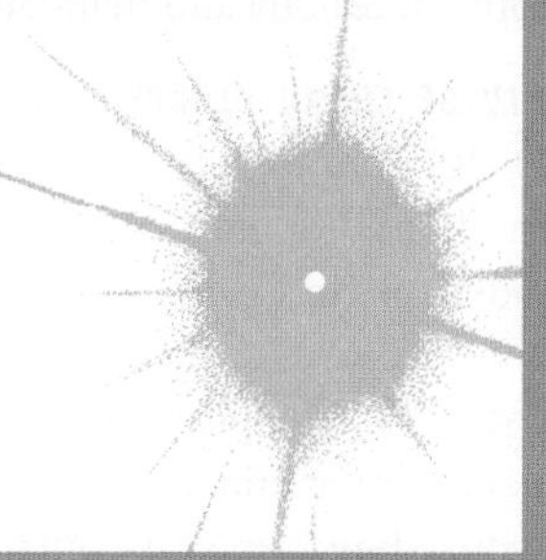

CHAPTER 13

DISORDERS OF THE FEMALE REPRODUCTIVE SYSTEM

Janet E. Hall

The female reproductive system regulates the hormonal changes responsible for puberty and adult reproductive function. Normal reproductive function in women requires the dynamic integration of hormonal signals from the hypothalamus, pituitary, and ovary, resulting in repetitive cycles of follicle development, ovulation, and preparation of the endometrial lining of the uterus for implantation should conception occur. It is critical to understand pubertal development in normal girls (and boys) as a yardstick for identifying precocious and delayed puberty.

For further discussion of related topics, see the following chapters: amenorrhea and pelvic pain (Chap. 15), infertility and contraception (Chap. 14), menopause (Chap. 16), disorders of sex development (Chap. 10), and disorders of the male reproductive system (Chap. 11).

DEVELOPMENT OF THE OVARY AND EARLY FOLLICULAR GROWTH

The ovary orchestrates the development and release of a mature oocyte and also elaborates hormones (e.g., estrogen, progesterone, inhibin, relaxin) that are critical for pubertal development and preparation of the uterus for conception, implantation, and the early stages of pregnancy. To achieve these functions in repeated monthly cycles, the ovary undergoes some of the most dynamic changes of any organ in the body. Primordial germ cells can be identified by the third week of gestation, and their migration to the genital ridge is complete by 6 weeks of gestation. Germ cells persist within the genital ridge, are then referred to as *oogonia*, and are essential for induction of ovarian development. Although one X chromosome undergoes X inactivation in somatic cells, it is reactivated in oogonia and genes on both X chromosomes are required for normal ovarian development. A streak ovary containing only stromal cells is found in patients with 45,X Turner's syndrome **(Chap. 10)**.

The germ cell population expands, and starting at ~8 weeks of gestation, oogonia begin to enter prophase of the first meiotic division and become primary oocytes. This allows the oocyte to be surrounded by a single layer of flattened granulosa cells to form a primordial follicle (Fig. 13-1). Granulosa cells are derived from mesonephric cells that invade the ovary early in its development, pushing the germ cells to the periphery. The weight of evidence supports the concept that for the most part, the ovary contains a nonrenewable pool of germ cells. Through the combined processes of mitosis, meiosis, and atresia, the population of oogonia reaches its maximum of 6–7 million by 20 weeks of gestation, after which there is a progressive loss of both oogonia and primordial follicles through the process of atresia. At birth, oogonia are no longer present in the ovary, and only 1–2 million germ cells remain in the form of primordial follicles (Fig. 13-2). The oocyte persists in prophase of the first meiotic division until just before ovulation, when meiosis resumes.

The quiescent primordial follicles are recruited to further growth and differentiation through a highly regulated process that limits the size of the developing cohort to ensure that folliculogenesis can continue throughout the reproductive life span. This initial recruitment of primordial follicles to form primary follicles (Fig. 13-1) is characterized by growth of the oocyte and the transition from squamous to cuboidal granulosa cells. The theca interna cells that surround the developing follicle begin to form as the primary follicle grows. Acquisition of a zona pellucida by the oocyte and the presence of several layers of surrounding cuboidal granulosa cells mark the development of

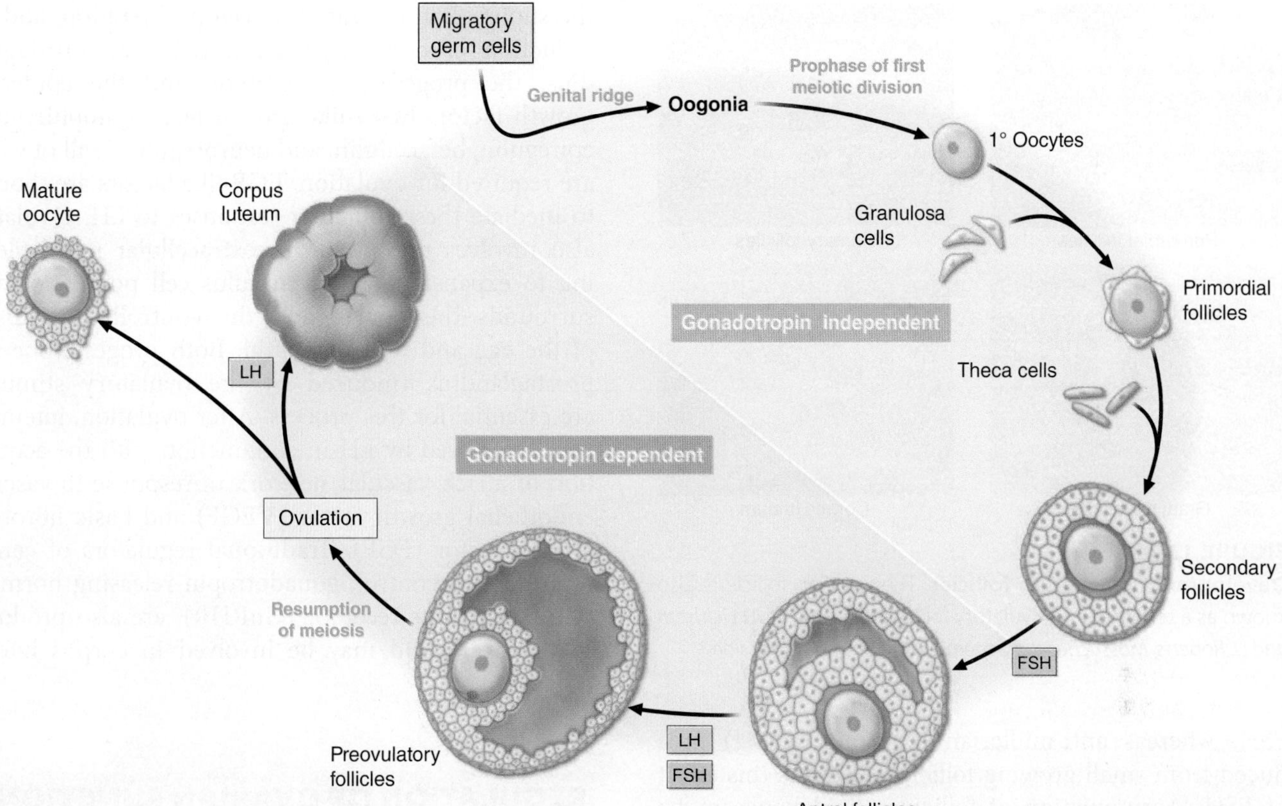

FIGURE 13-1

Stages of ovarian development from the arrival of the migratory germ cells at the genital ridge through gonadotropin-independent and gonadotropin-dependent phases that ultimately result in ovulation of a mature oocyte. FSH, follicle-stimulating hormone; LH, luteinizing hormone.

secondary follicles. It is at this stage that granulosa cells develop follicle-stimulating hormone (FSH), estradiol, and androgen receptors and communicate with one another through the development of gap junctions.

Bidirectional signaling between the germ cells and the somatic cells in the ovary is a necessary component underlying the maturation of the oocyte and the capacity for hormone secretion. For example, oocyte-derived growth differentiation factor 9 (GDF-9) and

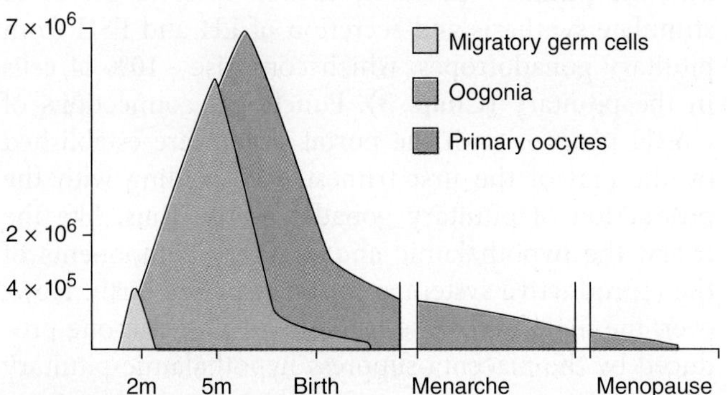

FIGURE 13-2

Ovarian germ cell number is maximal at mid-gestation and then decreases precipitously.

bone morphogenic protein-15 (BMP-15), also known as GDF-9b, are required for migration of pregranulosa and pretheca cells to the outer surface of the developing follicle and, hence, initial follicle formation. GDF-9 is also required for formation of secondary follicles, as are granulosa cell–derived KIT ligand (KITL) and the forkhead transcription factor (FOXL2). All of these genes are potential candidates for premature ovarian failure in women, and mutations in the human *FOXL2* gene have been shown to cause the syndrome of blepharophimosis/ptosis/epicanthus inversus, which is associated with ovarian failure.

DEVELOPMENT OF A MATURE FOLLICLE

The early stages of follicle growth are primarily driven by intraovarian factors and may take up to a year from development of the primary follicle to the dominant follicle stage. Further maturation to the preovulatory state, including the resumption of meiosis in the oocyte, requires the combined stimulus of FSH and luteinizing hormone (LH) (Fig. 13-1) and can be accomplished within weeks. Recruitment of secondary follicles from the resting follicle pool requires the direct action of

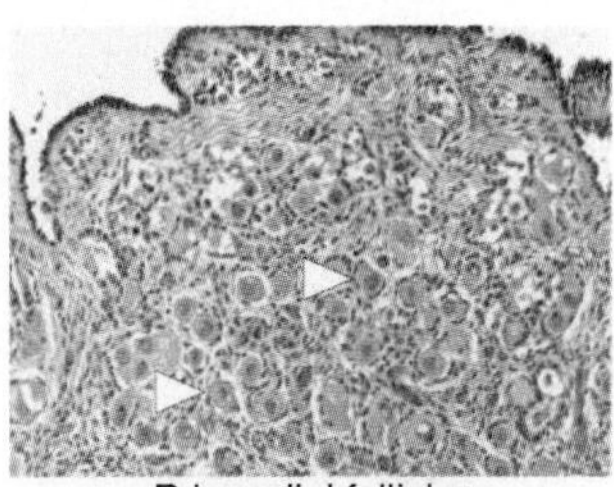

Primordial follicles

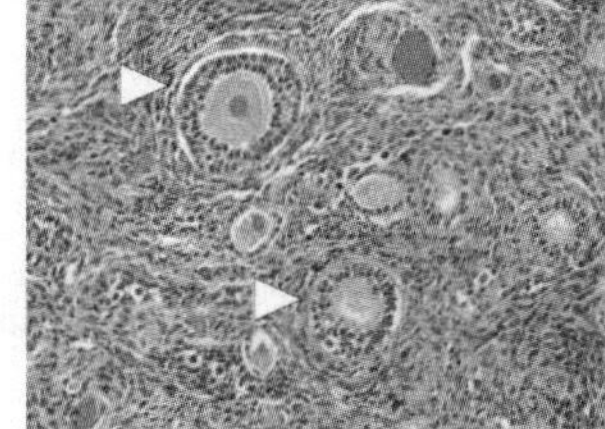

Primary follicles

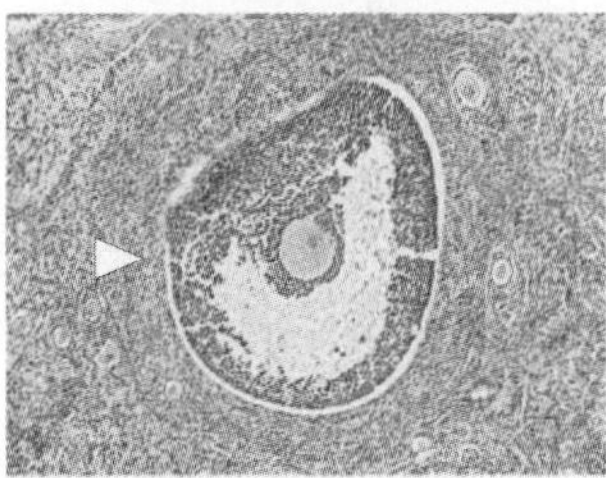

Graafian follicle

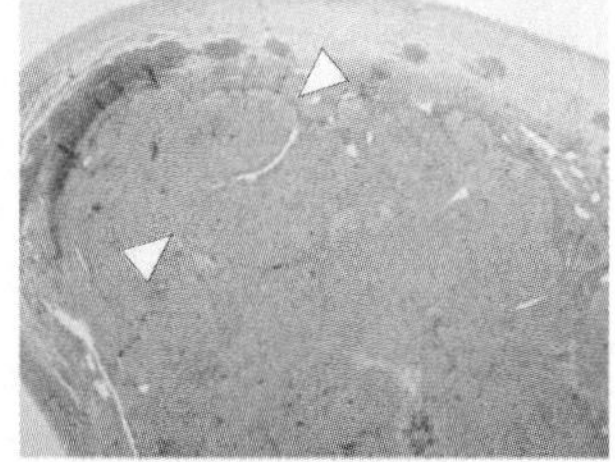

Corpus luteum

FIGURE 13-3
Development of ovarian follicles. The Graafian follicle is also known as a tertiary or preovulatory follicle. *(Courtesy of JH Eichhorn and D. Roberts, Massachusetts General Hospital; with permission.)*

FSH, whereas anti-müllerian hormone (AMH) produced from small growing follicles, restrains this effect of FSH. Accumulation of follicular fluid between the layers of granulosa cells creates an antrum that divides the granulosa cells into two functionally distinct groups: mural cells that line the follicle wall and cumulus cells that surround the oocyte (Fig. 13-3). Recent evidence suggests that, in addition to its role in normal development of the müllerian system, the WNT signaling pathway is required for normal antral follicle development and may also play a role in ovarian steroidogenesis. A single dominant follicle emerges from the growing follicle pool within the first 5–7 days after the onset of menses, and the majority of follicles fall off their growth trajectory and become atretic. Autocrine actions of activin and BMP-6, derived from the granulosa cells, and paracrine actions of GDF-9, BMP-15, BMP-6, and Gpr149, derived from the oocyte, are involved in granulosa cell proliferation and modulation of FSH responsiveness. Differential exposure to these factors may explain the mechanism whereby a given follicle is selected for continued growth to the preovulatory stage. The dominant follicle can be distinguished by its size, evidence of granulosa cell proliferation, large number of FSH receptors, high aromatase activity, and elevated concentrations of estradiol and inhibin A in follicular fluid.

The dominant follicle undergoes rapid expansion during the 5–6 days prior to ovulation, reflecting granulosa cell proliferation and accumulation of follicular fluid. FSH induces LH receptors on the granulosa cells, and the preovulatory, or Graafian, follicle moves to the outer ovarian surface in preparation for ovulation. The LH surge triggers the resumption of meiosis, the suppression of granulosa cell proliferation, and the induction of cyclooxygenase 2 (COX-2), prostaglandins, the progesterone receptor, and the epidermal growth factor (EGF)-like growth factors amphiregulin, epiregulin, betacellulin, and neuroregulin 1, all of which are required for ovulation. EGF-like factors are thought to mediate these follicular responses to LH. Ovulation also involves production of extracellular matrix leading to expansion of the cumulus cell population that surrounds the oocyte and the controlled expulsion of the egg and follicular fluid. Both progesterone and prostaglandins (induced by the ovulatory stimulus) are essential for this process. After ovulation, luteinization is induced by LH in conjunction with the acquisition of a rich vascular network in response to vascular endothelial growth factor (VEGF) and basic fibroblast growth factor (FGF). Traditional regulators of central reproductive control, gonadotropin-releasing hormone (GnRH) and its receptor (GnRHR), are also produced in the ovary and may be involved in corpus luteum function.

REGULATION OF OVARIAN FUNCTION

HYPOTHALAMIC AND PITUITARY SECRETION

GnRH neurons develop from epithelial cells outside the central nervous system and migrate, initially alongside the olfactory neurons, to the medial basal hypothalamus. Studies in GnRH-deficient patients who fail to undergo puberty have provided insights into genes that control the ontogeny and function of GnRH neurons (Fig. 13-4). *KAL1*, *FGF8/FGFR1*, *PROK2/PROKR2*, *NSMF*, and *CDH7*, among others **(Chap. 11)**, have been implicated in the migration of GnRH neurons to the hypothalamus. Approximately 7000 GnRH neurons, scattered throughout the medial basal hypothalamus, establish contacts with capillaries of the pituitary portal system in the median eminence. GnRH is secreted into the pituitary portal system in discrete pulses to stimulate synthesis and secretion of LH and FSH from pituitary gonadotropes, which comprise ~10% of cells in the pituitary **(Chap. 3)**. Functional connections of GnRH neurons with the portal system are established by the end of the first trimester, coinciding with the production of pituitary gonadotropins. Thus, like the ovary, the hypothalamic and pituitary components of the reproductive system are present before birth. However, the high levels of estradiol and progesterone produced by the placenta suppress hypothalamic-pituitary stimulation of ovarian hormonal secretion in the fetus.

After birth and the loss of placenta-derived steroids, gonadotropin levels rise. FSH levels are much higher in girls than in boys. This rise in FSH results

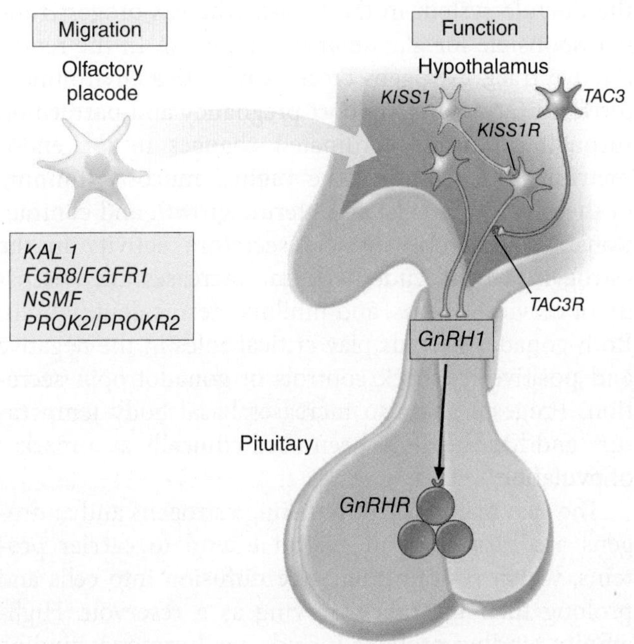

FIGURE 13-4

Establishment of a functional gonadotropin-releasing hormone (GnRH) system requires the participation of a number of genes that are essential for development and migration of GnRH neurons from the olfactory placode to the hypothalamus in addition to genes involved in the functional control of GnRH secretion and action.

in ovarian activation (evident on ultrasound) and increased inhibin B and estradiol levels. Studies that have identified mutations in *TAC3*, which encodes neurokinin B, and its receptor, *TAC3R*, in patients with GnRH deficiency indicate that both are involved in control of GnRH secretion and may be particularly important at this early stage of development. By 12–20 months of age, the reproductive axis is again suppressed, and a period of relative quiescence persists until puberty (Fig. 13-5). At the onset of puberty,

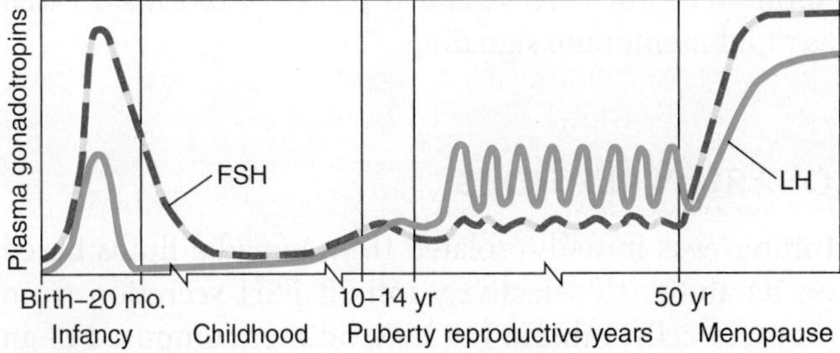

FIGURE 13-5

Follicle-stimulating hormone (FSH) and luteinizing hormone (LH) are increased during the neonatal years but go through a period of childhood quiescence before increasing again during puberty. Gonadotropin levels are cyclic during the reproductive years and increase dramatically with the loss of negative feedback that accompanies menopause.

pulsatile GnRH secretion induces pituitary gonadotropin production. In the early stages of puberty, LH and FSH secretion are apparent only during sleep, but as puberty develops, pulsatile gonadotropin secretion occurs throughout the day and night.

The mechanisms responsible for the childhood quiescence and pubertal reactivation of the reproductive axis remain incompletely understood. GnRH neurons in the hypothalamus respond to both excitatory and inhibitory factors. Increased sensitivity to the inhibitory influence of gonadal steroids has long been implicated in the inhibition of GnRH secretion during childhood but has not been definitively established in the human. Metabolic signals, such as adipocyte-derived leptin, play a permissive role in reproductive function **(Chap. 20)**. Studies of patients with isolated GnRH deficiency reveal that mutations in the G protein–coupled receptor 54 (*GPR54*) gene (now known as *KISS1R*) preclude the onset of puberty. The ligand for this receptor, metastin, is derived from the parent peptide, kisspeptin-1 (*KISS1*), and is a powerful stimulant for GnRH release. A potential role for kisspeptin in the onset of puberty has been suggested by upregulation of *KISS1* and *KISS1R* transcripts in the hypothalamus at the time of puberty. *TAC3* and dynorphin (*Dyn*), which appear to play an inhibitory rather than stimulatory role in GnRH control, are co-expressed with *KISS1* in KNDy neurons that project to GnRH neurons. This system is intimately involved with estrogen negative feedback regulation of GnRH secretion.

OVARIAN STEROIDS

Ovarian steroid-producing cells do not store hormones but produce them in response to LH and FSH during the normal menstrual cycle. The sequence of steps and the enzymes involved in the synthesis of steroid hormones are similar in the ovary, adrenal, and testis. However, the enzymes required to catalyze specific steps are compartmentalized and may not be abundant or even present in all cell types. Within the developing ovarian follicle, estrogen synthesis from cholesterol requires close integration between theca and granulosa cells—sometimes called the *two-cell model for steroidogenesis* (Fig. 13-6). FSH receptors are confined to the granulosa cells, whereas LH receptors are restricted to the theca cells until the late stages of follicular development, when they are also found on granulosa cells. The theca cells surrounding the follicle are highly vascularized and use cholesterol, derived primarily from circulating lipoproteins, as the starting point for the synthesis of androstenedione and testosterone under the control of LH. Androstenedione and testosterone are transferred across the basal lamina to the granulosa cells, which receive no direct blood supply. The mural granulosa cells

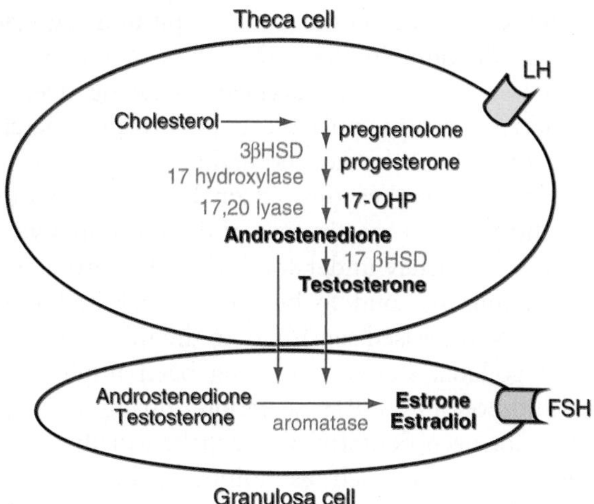

FIGURE 13-6

Estrogen production in the ovary requires the cooperative function of the theca and granulosa cells under the control of luteinizing hormone (LH) and follicle-stimulating hormone (FSH). HSD, hydroxysteroid dehydrogenase; OHP, hydroxyprogesterone.

are particularly rich in aromatase and, under the control of FSH, produce estradiol, the primary steroid secreted from the follicular phase ovary and the most potent estrogen. Theca cell–produced androstenedione and, to a lesser extent, testosterone are also secreted into peripheral blood, where they can be converted to dihydrotestosterone in skin and to estrogens in adipose tissue. The hilar interstitial cells of the ovary are functionally similar to Leydig cells and are also capable of secreting androgens. Although stromal cells proliferate in response to androgens (as in polycystic ovarian syndrome [PCOS]), they do not secrete androgens.

Development of the rich capillary network following rupture of the follicle at the time of ovulation makes it possible for large molecules such as low-density lipoprotein (LDL) to reach the luteinized granulosa and theca lutein cells. As in the follicle, both cell types are required for steroidogenesis in the corpus luteum. The large luteinized granulosa cells are the main source of progesterone production, whereas the smaller theca lutein cells produce 17-hydroxyprogesterone, a substrate for aromatization to estradiol by the luteinized granulosa cells. LH is critical for normal structure and function of the corpus luteum. Because LH and human chorionic gonadotropin (hCG) bind to a common receptor, the role of LH in support of the corpus luteum can be replaced by hCG in the first 10 weeks after conception, and hCG is commonly used for luteal phase support in the treatment of infertility.

Steroid hormone actions

Both estrogen and progesterone play critical roles in the expression of secondary sexual characteristics in women **(Chap. 2)**. Estrogen promotes development of the ductule system in the breast, whereas progesterone is responsible for glandular development. In the reproductive tract, estrogens create a receptive environment for fertilization and support pregnancy and parturition through carefully coordinated changes in the endometrium, thickening of the vaginal mucosa, thinning of the cervical mucus, and uterine growth and contractions. Progesterone induces secretory activity in the estrogen-primed endometrium, increases the viscosity of cervical mucus, and inhibits uterine contractions. Both gonadal steroids play critical roles in the negative and positive feedback controls of gonadotropin secretion. Progesterone also increases basal body temperature and has therefore been used clinically as a marker of ovulation.

The vast majority of circulating estrogens and androgens are carried in the blood bound to carrier proteins, which restrain their free diffusion into cells and prolong their clearance, serving as a reservoir. High-affinity binding proteins include sex hormone–binding globulin (SHBG), which binds androgens with somewhat greater affinity than estrogens, and corticosteroid-binding globulin (CBG), which also binds progesterone. Modulations in binding protein levels by insulin, androgens, and estrogens contribute to high bioavailable testosterone levels in PCOS and to high circulating estrogen and progesterone levels during pregnancy.

Estrogens act primarily through binding to the nuclear receptors, estrogen receptor (ER) α and β. Transcriptional coactivators and co-repressors modulate ER action **(Chap. 2)**. Both ER subtypes are present in the hypothalamus, pituitary, ovary, and reproductive tract. Although ERα and -β exhibit some functional redundancy, there is also a high degree of specificity, particularly in expression within cell types. For example, ERα functions in the ovarian theca cells, whereas ERβ is critical for granulosa cell function. There is also evidence for membrane-initiated signaling by estrogen. Similar signaling mechanisms pertain for progesterone with evidence of transcriptional regulation through progesterone receptor (PR) A and B protein isoforms, as well as rapid membrane signaling.

OVARIAN PEPTIDES

Inhibin was initially isolated from gonadal fluids based on its ability to selectively inhibit FSH secretion from pituitary cells. Inhibin is a heterodimer composed of an α subunit and a βA or βB subunit to form inhibin A or inhibin B, both of which are secreted from the ovary. Activin is a homodimer of inhibin β subunits with the capacity to stimulate the synthesis and secretion of FSH. Inhibins and activins are members of the transforming growth factor β (TGF-β) superfamily of growth and differentiation factors. During the purification of inhibin, follistatin, an unrelated monomeric protein that inhibits FSH secretion, was discovered. Within the pituitary, follistatin inhibits FSH secretion indirectly through binding and neutralizing activin.

Inhibin B is secreted from the granulosa cells of small antral follicles, whereas inhibin A is present in both granulosa and theca cells and is secreted by dominant follicles. Inhibin A is also present in luteinized granulosa cells and is a major secretory product of the corpus luteum. Inhibin B is constitutively secreted by granulosa cells and increases in serum in conjunction with recruitment of secondary follicles to the pool of actively growing follicles under the control of FSH. Inhibin B has been used clinically as a marker of ovarian reserve. Inhibin B is an important inhibitor of FSH, independent of estradiol, during the menstrual cycle. Although activin is also secreted from the ovary, the excess of follistatin in serum, combined with its nearly irreversible binding of activin, make it unlikely that ovarian activin plays an endocrine role in FSH regulation. However, there is evidence that activin plays an autocrine/paracrine role in the ovary, in addition to its intrapituitary role in modulation of FSH production.

AMH (also known as müllerian-inhibiting substance) is important in ovarian biology in addition to the function from which it derived its name (i.e., promotion of the degeneration of the müllerian system during embryogenesis in the male). AMH is produced by granulosa cells from small follicles and, like inhibin B, is a marker of ovarian reserve. AMH inhibits the recruitment of primordial follicles into the follicle pool and counters FSH stimulation of aromatase expression.

Relaxin, which is produced by the theca lutein cells of the corpus luteum, is thought to play a role in decidualization of the endometrium and suppression of myometrial contractile activity, both of which are essential for the early establishment of pregnancy.

HORMONAL INTEGRATION OF THE NORMAL MENSTRUAL CYCLE

The sequence of changes responsible for mature reproductive function is coordinated through a series of negative and positive feedback loops that alter pulsatile GnRH secretion, the pituitary response to GnRH, and the relative secretion of LH and FSH from the gonadotrope. The frequency and amplitude of pulsatile GnRH secretion differentially modulate the synthesis and secretion of LH and FSH, with slow frequencies favoring FSH synthesis and increased amplitudes favoring LH synthesis. Activin is produced in both pituitary gonadotropes and folliculostellate cells and stimulates the synthesis and secretion of FSH. Inhibins function as potent antagonists of activins through sequestration of

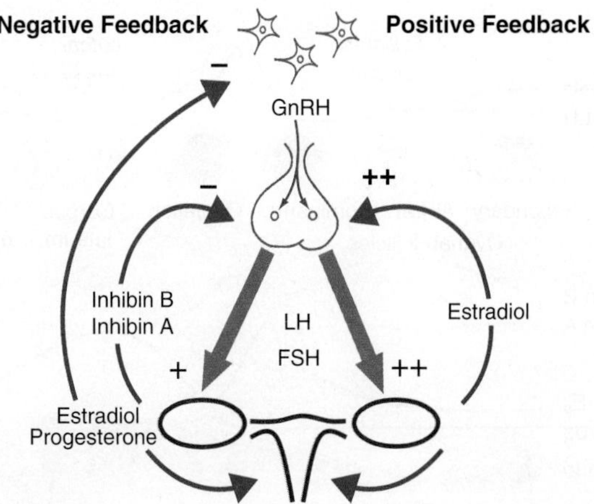

FIGURE 13-7
The reproductive system in women is critically dependent on both negative feedback of gonadal steroids and inhibin to modulate follicle-stimulating hormone (FSH) secretion and on estrogen positive feedback to generate the preovulatory luteinizing hormone (LH) surge. GnRH, gonadotropin-releasing hormone.

the activin receptors. Although inhibin is expressed in the pituitary, gonadal inhibin is the principal source of feedback inhibition of FSH.

For the majority of the cycle, the reproductive system functions in a classic endocrine negative feedback mode. Estradiol and progesterone inhibit GnRH secretion, and the inhibins act at the pituitary to selectively inhibit FSH synthesis and secretion (Fig. 13-7). This negative feedback control of FSH is critical for development of the single mature oocyte that characterizes normal reproductive function in women. In addition to these negative feedback controls, the menstrual cycle is uniquely dependent on estrogen-induced positive feedback to produce an LH surge that is essential for ovulation of a mature follicle. Estrogen negative feedback in women occurs primarily at the hypothalamus with a small pituitary contribution, whereas estrogen positive feedback occurs at the pituitary with hypothalamic GnRH secretion playing a permissive role.

THE FOLLICULAR PHASE

The follicular phase is characterized by recruitment of a cohort of secondary follicles and the ultimate selection of a dominant preovulatory follicle (Fig. 13-8). The follicular phase begins, by convention, on the first day of menses. However, follicle recruitment is initiated by the rise in FSH that begins in the late luteal phase of the previous cycle in conjunction with the loss of negative feedback of gonadal steroids and likely inhibin A. The fact that a 20–30% increase in FSH is adequate for follicular recruitment speaks to the marked sensitivity of the resting follicle pool to FSH. The resultant granulosa cell proliferation is responsible for increasing

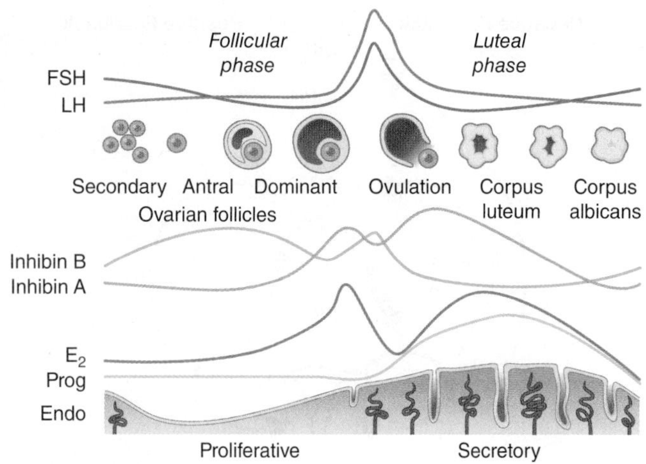

FIGURE 13-8

Relationship between gonadotropins, follicle development, gonadal secretion, and endometrial changes during the normal menstrual cycle. E_2, estradiol; Endo, endometrium; FSH, follicle-stimulating hormone; LH, luteinizing hormone; Prog, progesterone.

early follicular phase levels of inhibin B. Inhibin B in conjunction with rising levels of estradiol, and probably inhibin A, restrain FSH secretion during this critical period such that only a single follicle matures in the vast majority of cycles. The increased risk of multiple gestation associated with the increased levels of FSH characteristic of advanced maternal age, or with exogenous gonadotropin administration in the treatment of infertility, attests to the importance of negative feedback regulation of FSH. With further growth of the dominant follicle, estradiol and inhibin A increase exponentially and the follicle acquires LH receptors. Increasing levels of estradiol are responsible for proliferative changes in the endometrium. The exponential rise in estradiol results in positive feedback on the pituitary, leading to the generation of an LH surge (and a smaller FSH surge), thereby triggering ovulation and luteinization of the granulosa cells.

THE LUTEAL PHASE

The luteal phase begins with the formation of the corpus luteum from the ruptured follicle (Fig. 13-8). Progesterone and inhibin A are produced from the luteinized granulosa cells, which continue to aromatize theca-derived androgen precursors, producing estradiol. The combined actions of estrogen and progesterone are responsible for the secretory changes in the endometrium that are necessary for implantation. The corpus luteum is supported by LH but has a finite life span because of diminished sensitivity to LH. The demise of the corpus luteum results in a progressive decline in hormonal support of the endometrium. Inflammation or local hypoxia and ischemia result in vascular changes in the endometrium, leading to the release of cytokines, cell death, and shedding of the endometrium.

If conception occurs, hCG produced by the trophoblast binds to LH receptors on the corpus luteum, maintaining steroid hormone production and preventing involution of the corpus luteum. The corpus luteum is essential for the hormonal maintenance of the endometrium during the first 6–10 weeks of pregnancy until this function is taken over by the placenta.

CLINICAL ASSESSMENT OF OVARIAN FUNCTION

Menstrual bleeding should become regular within 2–4 years of menarche, although anovulatory and irregular cycles are common before that. For the remainder of adult reproductive life, the cycle length counted from the first day of menses to the first day of subsequent menses is ~28 days, with a range of 25–35 days. However, cycle-to-cycle variability for an individual woman is ±2 days. Luteal phase length is relatively constant between 12 and 14 days in normal cycles; thus, the major variability in cycle length is due to variations in the follicular phase. The duration of menstrual bleeding in ovulatory cycles varies between 4 and 6 days. There is a gradual shortening of cycle length with age such that women over the age of 35 have cycles that are shorter than during their younger reproductive years. Anovulatory cycles increase as women approach menopause, and bleeding patterns may be erratic.

Women who report regular monthly bleeding with cycles that do not vary by >4 days generally have ovulatory cycles, but several other clinical signs can be used to assess the likelihood of ovulation. Some women experience *mittelschmerz*, described as midcycle pelvic discomfort that is thought to be caused by the rapid expansion of the dominant follicle at the time of ovulation. A constellation of premenstrual moliminal symptoms such as bloating, breast tenderness, and food cravings often occur several days before menses in ovulatory cycles, but their absence cannot be used as evidence of anovulation. Methods that can be used to determine whether ovulation is likely include a serum progesterone level >5 ng/mL ~7 days before expected menses, an increase in basal body temperature of 0.24°C (>0.5°F) in the second half of the cycle due to the thermoregulatory effect of progesterone, or the detection of the urinary LH surge using ovulation predictor kits. Because ovulation occurs ~36 h after the LH surge, urinary LH can be helpful in timing intercourse to coincide with ovulation.

Ultrasound can be used to detect the growth of the fluid-filled antrum of the developing follicle and to

TABLE 13-1

MEAN AGE (YEARS) OF PUBERTAL MILESTONES IN GIRLS

	ONSET OF BREAST/ PUBIC HAIR DEVELOPMENT	AGE OF PEAK HEIGHT VELOCITY	MENARCHE	FINAL BREAST/ PUBIC HAIR DEVELOPMENT	ADULT HEIGHT
White	10.2	11.9	12.6	14.3	17.1
Black	9.6	11.5	12	13.6	16.5

Source: From FM Biro et al: J Pediatr 148:234, 2006.

assess endometrial proliferation in response to increasing estradiol levels in the follicular phase, as well as the characteristic echogenicity of the secretory endometrium of the luteal phase.

PUBERTY

NORMAL PUBERTAL DEVELOPMENT IN GIRLS

The first menstrual period (*menarche*) occurs relatively late in the series of developmental milestones that characterize normal pubertal development (Table 13-1). Menarche is preceded by the appearance of pubic and then axillary hair (*adrenarche*) as a result of maturation of the zona reticularis in the adrenal gland and increased adrenal androgen secretion, particularly dehydroepiandrosterone (DHEA). The triggers for adrenarche remain unknown but may involve increases in body mass index, as well as in utero and neonatal factors. Menarche is also preceded by breast development (*thelarche*). The breast is exquisitely sensitive to the very low levels of estrogen that result from peripheral conversion of adrenal androgens and the low levels of estrogen secreted from the ovary early in pubertal maturation. Breast development precedes the appearance of pubic and axillary hair in ~60% of girls. The interval between the onset of breast development and menarche is ~2 years. There has been a gradual decline in the age of menarche over the past century, attributed in large part to improvement in nutrition, and there is a relationship between adiposity and earlier sexual maturation in girls. In the United States, menarche occurs at an average age of 12.5 years (Table 13-1). Much of the variation in the timing of puberty is due to genetic factors, with heritability estimates of 50–80%. Both adrenarche and thelarche occur ~1 year earlier in black compared with white girls, although the timing of menarche differs by only 6 months between these ethnic groups.

Other important hormonal changes also occur in conjunction with puberty. Growth hormone (GH) levels increase early in puberty, stimulated in part by the pubertal increases in estrogen secretion. GH increases insulin-like growth factor-I (IGF-I), which enhances linear growth. The growth spurt is generally less pronounced in girls than in boys, with a peak growth velocity of ~7 cm/year. Linear growth is ultimately limited by closure of epiphyses in the long bones as a result of prolonged exposure to estrogen. Puberty is also associated with mild insulin resistance.

DISORDERS OF PUBERTY

The differential diagnosis of precocious and delayed puberty is similar in boys **(Chap. 11)** and girls. However, there are differences in the timing of normal puberty and differences in the relative frequency of specific disorders in girls compared with boys.

Precocious puberty

Traditionally, precocious puberty has been defined as the development of secondary sexual characteristics before the age of 8 in girls based on data from Marshall and Tanner in British girls studied in the 1960s. More recent studies led to recommendations that girls be evaluated for precocious puberty if breast development or pubic hair is present at <7 years of age for white girls or <6 years for black girls.

Precocious puberty in girls is most often centrally mediated (Table 13-2), resulting from early activation of the hypothalamic-pituitary-ovarian axis. It is characterized by pulsatile LH secretion (which is initially associated with deep sleep) and an enhanced LH and FSH response to exogenous GnRH (two- to threefold stimulation) (Table 13-3). True precocity is marked by advancement in bone age of >2 standard deviations, a recent history of growth acceleration, and progression of secondary sexual characteristics. In girls, centrally mediated precocious puberty is idiopathic in ~85% of cases; however, neurogenic causes must be considered. Mutations in genes associated with GnRH deficiency have been reported in small numbers of patients with idiopathic precocious puberty (*KISS, KISS1R, TAC3, TAC3R*, and *DAX-1*), but their frequency is insufficient to warrant their use in clinical testing. GnRH agonists that induce pituitary desensitization are the mainstay of

TABLE 13-2

DIFFERENTIAL DIAGNOSIS OF PRECOCIOUS PUBERTY

CENTRAL (GnRH DEPENDENT)	PERIPHERAL (GnRH INDEPENDENT)
Idiopathic	Congenital adrenal hyperplasia
CNS tumors	Estrogen-producing tumors
Hamartomas	Adrenal tumors
Astrocytomas	Ovarian tumors
Adenomyomas	Gonadotropin/hCG-producing tumors
Gliomas	
Germinomas	Exogenous exposure to estrogen or androgen
CNS infection	McCune-Albright syndrome
Head trauma	Aromatase excess syndrome
Iatrogenic	
Radiation	
Chemotherapy	
Surgical	
CNS malformation	
Arachnoid or suprasellar cysts	
Septo-optic dysplasia	
Hydrocephalus	

Abbreviations: CNS, central nervous system; GnRH, gonadotropin-releasing hormone; hCG, human chorionic gonadotropin.

treatment to prevent premature epiphyseal closure and preserve adult height, as well as to manage psychosocial repercussions of precocious puberty.

Peripherally mediated precocious puberty does not involve activation of the hypothalamic-pituitary-ovarian axis and is characterized by suppressed gonadotropins in the presence of elevated estradiol. Management of peripheral precocious puberty involves treating the underlying disorder (Table 13-2) and limiting the effects of gonadal steroids using aromatase inhibitors, inhibitors of steroidogenesis, and ER blockers. It is important to be aware that central precocious puberty can also develop in girls whose precocity was initially peripherally mediated, as in McCune-Albright syndrome and congenital adrenal hyperplasia.

Incomplete and intermittent forms of precocious puberty may also occur. For example, premature breast development may occur in girls before the age of 2 years, with no further progression and without significant advancement in bone age, estrogen production, or compromised height. Premature adrenarche can also occur in the absence of progressive pubertal development, but it must be distinguished from late-onset congenital adrenal hyperplasia and androgen-secreting

TABLE 13-3

EVALUATION OF PRECOCIOUS AND DELAYED PUBERTY

	PRECOCIOUS	DELAYED
Initial Screening Tests		
History and physical	×	×
Assessment of growth velocity	×	×
Bone age	×	×
LH, FSH	×	×
Estradiol, testosterone	×	×
DHEAS	×	×
17-Hydroxyprogesterone	×	
TSH, T_4	×	×
Complete blood count		×
Sedimentation rate, C-reactive protein		×
Electrolytes, renal function		×
Liver enzymes		×
IGF-I, IGFBP-3		×
Urinalysis		×
Secondary Tests		
Pelvic ultrasound	×	×
Cranial MRI	×	×
β-hCG	×	
GnRH/agonist stimulation test	×	×
ACTH stimulation test	×	
Inflammatory bowel disease panel	×	×
Celiac disease panel		×
Prolactin		×
Karyotype		×

Abbreviations: ACTH, adrenocorticotropic hormone; DHEAS, dehydroepiandrosterone sulfate; FSH, follicle-stimulating hormone; hCG, human chorionic gonadotropin; IGF-I, insulin-like growth factor-I; IGFBP-3, IGF-binding protein 3; LH, luteinizing hormone; MRI, magnetic resonance imaging; TSH, thyroid-stimulating hormone; T_4, thyroxine.

tumors, in which case it may be termed *heterosexual precocity*. Premature adrenarche may be associated with obesity, hyperinsulinemia, and the subsequent predisposition to PCOS.

Delayed puberty

Delayed puberty (Table 13-4) is defined as the absence of secondary sexual characteristics by age 13 in girls. The diagnostic considerations are very similar to those for primary amenorrhea **(Chap. 15)**. Between 25 and 40% of delayed puberty in girls is of ovarian origin, with Turner's syndrome accounting for the majority

TABLE 13-4

DIFFERENTIAL DIAGNOSIS OF DELAYED PUBERTY

Hypergonadotropic
Ovarian
Turner's syndrome
Gonadal dysgenesis
Chemotherapy/radiation therapy
Galactosemia
Autoimmune oophoritis
Congenital lipoid hyperplasia
Steroidogenic enzyme abnormalities
17α-Hydroxylase deficiency
Aromatase deficiency
Gonadotropin/receptor mutations
FSHβ, LHR, FSHR
Androgen resistance syndrome
Hypogonadotropic
Genetic
Hypothalamic syndromes
Leptin/leptin receptor
HESX1 (septo-optic dysplasia)
PC1 (prohormone convertase)
IHH and Kallmann's syndrome
KAL1, FGF8, FGFR1, NSMF, PROK2, PROKR2, KISS1, KISS1R, TAC3, TAC3R, GnRH1, GnRHR, SEM3A, HS6ST1, WDR11, CHD7
Abnormalities of pituitary development/function
PROP1
CNS tumors/infiltrative disorders
Craniopharyngioma
Astrocytoma, germinoma, glioma
Prolactinomas, other pituitary tumors
Histiocytosis X
Chemotherapy/radiation
Functional
Chronic diseases
Malnutrition
Excessive exercise
Eating disorders

Abbreviations: *CHD7*, chromodomain-helicase-DNA-binding protein 7; CNS, central nervous system; *FGF8*, fibroblast growth factor 8; *FGFR1*, fibroblast growth factor 1 receptor; *FSHβ*, follicle-stimulating hormone β chain; *FSHR*, FSH receptor; *GNRHR*, gonadotropin-releasing hormone receptor; *HESX1*, homeobox, embryonic stem cell expressed 1; *HS6ST1*, heparin sulfate 6-O sulfotransferase 1; IHH, idiopathic hypogonadotropic hypogonadism; KAL, Kallmann; *KISS1*, kisspeptin 1; *KISSR1*, KISS1 receptor; *LHR*, luteinizing hormone receptor; *NSMF*, NMDA receptor synaptonuclear signaling and neuronal migration factor; *PROK2*, prokineticin 2; *PROKR2* prokineticin receptor 2; *PROP1*, prophet of Pit1, paired-like homeodomain transcription factor *SEMA3A*, semaphorin-3A; *WDR11*, WD repeat-containing protein 11.

of such patients. Functional hypogonadotropic hypogonadism encompasses diverse etiologies such as systemic illnesses, including celiac disease and chronic renal disease, and endocrinopathies such as diabetes and hypothyroidism. In addition, girls appear to be particularly susceptible to the adverse effects of decreased energy balance resulting from exercise, dieting, and/or eating disorders. Together these reversible conditions account for ~25% of delayed puberty in girls. Congenital hypogonadotropic hypogonadism in girls or boys can be caused by mutations in several different genes or combinations of genes (Fig. 13-4, **Chap. 11**, Table 11-2). Approximately 50% of girls with congenital hypogonadotropic hypogonadism, with or without anosmia, have a history of some degree of breast development, and 10% report one to two episodes of vaginal bleeding. Family studies suggest that genes identified in association with absent puberty may also cause delayed puberty, and recent reports have further suggested that a genetic susceptibility to environmental stresses such as diet and exercise may account for at least some cases of functional hypothalamic amenorrhea. Although neuroanatomic causes of delayed puberty are considerably less common in girls than in boys, it is always important to rule these out in the setting of hypogonadotropic hypogonadism.

CHAPTER 14

INFERTILITY AND CONTRACEPTION

Janet E. Hall

INFERTILITY

DEFINITION AND PREVALENCE

Infertility has traditionally been defined as the inability to conceive after 12 months of unprotected sexual intercourse. In women who ultimately conceived, pregnancy occurred in ~50% within 3 months, 75–82% within 6 months, and 85–92% within 12 months. The World Health Organization (WHO) considers infertility as a disability (an impairment of function) and thus access to health care falls under the Convention on the Rights of Persons with Disability. Thirty-four million women, predominantly from developing countries, have infertility resulting from maternal sepsis and unsafe abortion. In populations <60 years old, infertility is ranked the fifth highest serious global disability. In the United States, the rate of infertility in married women age 15–44 is 6% based on the National Survey of Family Growth, although prospective studies suggest that it may be as high as 12–15%. The infertility rate has remained relatively stable over the past 30 years in most countries. However, the proportion of couples without children has risen, reflecting both higher numbers of couples in childbearing years and a trend to delay childbearing. This trend has important implications because of an age-related decrease in fecundability: the incidence of primary infertility increases from ~8% between the ages of 18 and 38 to 25% and 30% between the ages of 35 and 39 and 40 and 44, respectively. It is estimated that 14% of couples in the United States have received medical assistance for infertility; of these, two-thirds received counseling, ~12% underwent infertility testing of the female and/or male partner, and 17% received drugs to induce ovulation.

CAUSES OF INFERTILITY

The spectrum of infertility ranges from reduced conception rates or the need for medical intervention to irreversible causes of infertility. Infertility can be attributed primarily to male factors in 25% of couples and female factors in 58% of couples and is unexplained in about 17% of couples (Fig. 14-1). Not uncommonly, both male and female factors contribute to infertility. Decreases in the ability to conceive as a function of age in women has led to recommendations that women >34 years old who are not at increased risk of infertility seek attention after 6 months, rather than 12 months as suggested for younger women, and receive an expedited work-up and approach to treatment.

APPROACH TO THE PATIENT: Infertility

INITIAL EVALUATION In all couples presenting with infertility, the initial evaluation includes discussion of the appropriate timing of intercourse and discussion of modifiable risk factors such as smoking, alcohol, caffeine, and obesity. The range of required investigations should be reviewed as well as a brief description of infertility treatment options, including adoption. Initial investigations are focused on determining whether the primary cause of the infertility is male, female, or both. These investigations include a semen analysis in the male, confirmation of ovulation in the female, and, in the majority of situations, documentation of tubal patency in the female. In some cases, after an extensive workup excluding all male and female factors, a specific cause cannot be identified, and infertility may ultimately be classified as unexplained.

PSYCHOLOGICAL ASPECTS OF INFERTILITY Infertility is invariably associated with psychological stress related not only to the diagnostic and therapeutic procedures themselves but also to repeated cycles of hope and loss associated with each new procedure or cycle of treatment that does not result in the birth of a child. These

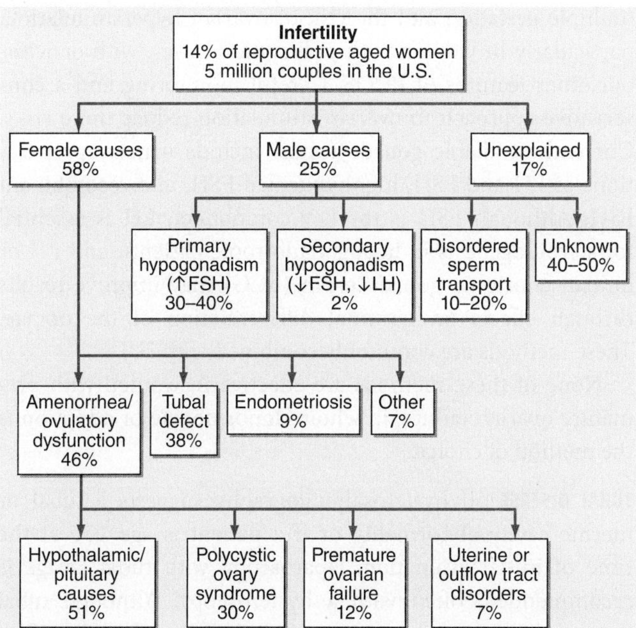

FIGURE 14-1

Causes of infertility. FSH, follicle-stimulating hormone; LH, luteinizing hormone.

feelings are often combined with a sense of isolation from friends and family. Counseling and stress-management techniques should be introduced early in the evaluation of infertility. Importantly, infertility and its treatment do not appear to be associated with long-term psychological sequelae.

FEMALE CAUSES Abnormalities in menstrual function constitute the most common cause of female infertility. These disorders, which include ovulatory dysfunction and abnormalities of the uterus or outflow tract, may present as amenorrhea or as irregular or short menstrual cycles. A careful history and physical examination and a limited number of laboratory tests will help to determine whether the abnormality is (1) hypothalamic or pituitary (low follicle-stimulating hormone [FSH], luteinizing hormone [LH], and estradiol with or without an increase in prolactin), (2) polycystic ovary syndrome (PCOS; irregular cycles and hyperandrogenism in the absence of other causes of androgen excess), (3) ovarian (low estradiol with increased FSH), or (4) a uterine or outflow tract abnormality. The frequency of these diagnoses depends on whether the amenorrhea is primary or occurs after normal puberty and menarche (see Fig. 15-2).

The approach to further evaluation of these disorders is described in detail in Chap. 15.

Ovulatory Dysfunction In women with a history of regular menstrual cycles, *evidence of ovulation* should be sought **(Chap. 13)**. Even in the presence of ovulatory cycles, evaluation of *ovarian reserve* is recommended for women age >35 years if they are interested in fertility. Measurement of FSH on day 3 of the cycle (an FSH level <10 IU/mL on cycle day 3 predicts adequate ovarian oocyte reserve) is the most cost-effective test. Other tests include measurement of FSH in response to clomiphene citrate (blocks estrogen negative feedback on FSH), antral follicle count on ultrasound, and anti-müllerian hormone (AMH; <0.5 ng/mL predicts reduced ovarian reserve although there is variability between labs).

Tubal Disease Tubal dysfunction may result from pelvic inflammatory disease (PID), appendicitis, endometriosis, pelvic adhesions, tubal surgery, previous use of an intrauterine device (IUD), and a previous ectopic pregnancy. However, a cause is not identified in up to 50% of patients with documented tubal factor infertility. Because of the high prevalence of tubal disease, evaluation of tubal patency by hysterosalpingogram (HSG) or laparoscopy should occur early in the majority of couples with infertility. Subclinical infections with *Chlamydia trachomatis* may be an underdiagnosed cause of tubal infertility and requires the treatment of both partners.

Endometriosis *Endometriosis* is defined as the presence of endometrial glands or stroma outside the endometrial cavity and uterine musculature and accounts for 40% of infertility not due to ovulatory disorders, tubal obstruction, or male factor. Its presence is suggested by a history of dyspareunia (painful intercourse), worsening dysmenorrhea that often begins before menses, or a thickened rectovaginal septum or deviation of the cervix on pelvic examination. Mild endometriosis does not appear to impair fertility; the pathogenesis of the infertility associated with moderate and severe endometriosis may be multifactorial with impairments of folliculogenesis, fertilization, and implantation, as well as adhesions. Endometriosis is often clinically silent, however, and can only be excluded definitively by laparoscopy.

MALE CAUSES Known causes of male infertility include primary testicular disease, genetic disorders (particularly Y chromosome microdeletions), disorders of sperm transport, and hypothalamic-pituitary disease resulting in secondary hypogonadism **(See also Chap. 11)**. However, the etiology is not ascertained in up to one-half of men with suspected male factor infertility. The key initial diagnostic test is a *semen analysis.* Testosterone levels should be measured if the sperm count is low on repeated examination or if there is clinical evidence of hypogonadism. Gonadotropin levels will help to determine a gonadal versus a central cause of hypogonadism.

TREATMENT Infertility

In addition to addressing the negative impact of smoking on fertility and pregnancy outcome, counseling about nutrition and weight is a fundamental component of infertility and pregnancy management. Both low and increased body mass index (BMI) are associated with infertility in women and with increased morbidity during pregnancy. Obesity has also been associated with infertility in men. The treatment of infertility should be tailored to the problems unique to each couple. In many situations, including unexplained infertility, mild-to-moderate endometriosis, and/or borderline semen parameters, a stepwise approach to infertility is optimal, beginning with low-risk interventions and moving to more invasive, higher risk interventions only if necessary. After determination of all infertility factors and their correction, if possible, this approach might include, in increasing order of complexity: (1) expectant management, (2) clomiphene citrate or an aromatase inhibitor (see below) with or without intrauterine insemination (IUI), (3) gonadotropins with or without IUI, and (4) in vitro fertilization (IVF). The time used for evaluation, correction of problems identified, and expectant management can be longer in women age <30 years, but this process should be advanced rapidly in women age >35 years. In some situations, expectant management will not be appropriate.

OVULATORY DYSFUNCTION Treatment of ovulatory dysfunction should first be directed at identification of the etiology of the disorder to allow specific management when possible. Dopamine agonists, for example, may be indicated in patients with hyperprolactinemia **(Chap. 5)**; lifestyle modification may be successful in women with obesity, low body weight, or a history of intensive exercise.

Medications used for ovulation induction include agents that increase FSH through alteration of negative feedback, gonadotropins, and pulsatile GnRH. *Clomiphene citrate* is a nonsteroidal estrogen antagonist that increases FSH and LH levels by blocking estrogen negative feedback at the hypothalamus. The efficacy of clomiphene for ovulation induction is highly dependent on patient selection. In appropriate patients, it induces ovulation in ~60% of women with PCOS and has traditionally been the initial treatment of choice. Combination with agents that modify insulin levels such as metformin does not appear to improve outcome. Clomiphene citrate is less successful in patients with hypogonadotropic hypogonadism. *Aromatase inhibitors* have also been investigated for the treatment of infertility. Studies suggest they may have advantages over clomiphene, but these medications have not been approved for this indication.

Gonadotropins are highly effective for ovulation induction in women with hypogonadotropic hypogonadism and PCOS and are used to induce the development of multiple follicles in unexplained infertility and in older reproductive-age women. Disadvantages include a significant risk of multiple gestation and the risk of ovarian hyperstimulation, particularly in women with polycystic ovaries, with or without other features of PCOS. Careful monitoring and a conservative approach to ovarian stimulation reduce these risks. Currently available gonadotropins include urinary preparations of LH and FSH, highly purified FSH, and recombinant FSH. Although FSH is the key component, LH is essential for steroidogenesis in hypogonadotropic patients, and LH or human chorionic gonadotropin (hCG) may improve results through effects on terminal differentiation of the oocyte. These methods are commonly combined with IUI.

None of these methods are effective in women with premature ovarian failure, in whom donor oocyte or adoption is the method of choice.

TUBAL DISEASE If hysterosalpingography suggests a tubal or uterine cavity abnormality or if a patient is age ≥35 at the time of initial evaluation, laparoscopy with tubal lavage is recommended, often with a hysteroscopy. Although tubal reconstruction may be attempted if tubal disease is identified, it is generally being replaced by the use of IVF. These patients are at increased risk of developing an ectopic pregnancy.

ENDOMETRIOSIS Although 60% of women with minimal or mild endometriosis may conceive within 1 year without treatment, laparoscopic resection or ablation appears to improve conception rates. Medical management of advanced stages of endometriosis is widely used for symptom control but has not been shown to enhance fertility. In moderate and severe endometriosis, conservative surgery is associated with pregnancy rates of 50 and 39%, respectively, compared with rates of 25 and 5% with expectant management alone. In some patients, IVF may be the treatment of choice.

MALE FACTOR INFERTILITY The treatment options for male factor infertility have expanded greatly in recent years **(Chap. 11)**. Secondary hypogonadism is highly amenable to treatment with gonadotropins or pulsatile gonadotropin-releasing hormone (GnRH) where available. In vitro techniques have provided new opportunities for patients with primary testicular failure and disorders of sperm transport. Choice of initial treatment options depends on sperm concentration and motility. Expectant management should be attempted initially in men with mild male factor infertility (sperm count of 15 to 20 × 10^6/mL and normal motility). Moderate male factor infertility (10 to 15 × 10^6/mL and 20–40% motility) should begin with IUI alone or in combination with treatment of the female partner with ovulation induction, but it may require IVF with or without intracytoplasmic sperm injection (ICSI). For men with a severe defect (sperm count of <10 × 10^6/mL, 10% motility), IVF with ICSI or donor sperm should be used. If ICSI is performed because of azoospermia due to congenital bilateral absence of the vas deferens, genetic testing and counseling should be provided because of the risk of cystic fibrosis.

ASSISTED REPRODUCTIVE TECHNOLOGIES The development of assisted reproductive technologies (ARTs) has dramatically altered the treatment of male and female infertility. IVF is indicated for patients with many causes of infertility that have not been successfully managed with more conservative approaches. IVF or ICSI is often the treatment of choice in couples with a significant male factor or tubal disease, whereas IVF using donor oocytes is used in patients with premature ovarian failure and in women of advanced reproductive age. Success rates are influenced by cause of infertility and age, varying between 15 and 40%. Success rates are highest in anovulatory women and lowest in women with decreased ovarian reserve. In the United States, success rates are higher in white than in black, Asian, or Hispanic women. Although often effective, IVF is expensive and requires careful monitoring of ovulation induction and invasive techniques, including the aspiration of multiple follicles. IVF is associated with a significant risk of multiple gestation, particularly in women age <35, in whom the rate can be as high as 30%, which has led to specific recommendations for numbers of embryos or blastocysts to transfer based on age and specific prognostic factors.

CONTRACEPTION

Although use of contraception worldwide has increased in the last two decades, as of 2010, 146 million women worldwide age 15–49 years who were married or in a union had an unmet need for family planning. The absolute number of married women who use contraception or have an unmet need for family planning is projected to grow from 900 million (876–922 million) in 2010 to 962 million (927–992 million) in 2015.

Only 15% of couples in the United States report having unprotected sexual intercourse in the past 3 months. However, despite the wide availability and widespread use of a variety of effective methods of contraception, approximately one-half of all births in the United States are the result of unintended pregnancy. Teenage pregnancies continue to represent a serious public health problem in the United States, with >1 million unintended pregnancies each year—a significantly greater incidence than in other industrialized nations.

Of the contraceptive methods available (Table 14-1), a reversible form of contraception is used by >50% of couples, whereas sterilization (male or female) has been

TABLE 14-1

EFFECTIVENESS OF DIFFERENT FORMS OF CONTRACEPTION

METHOD OF CONTRACEPTION	THEORETICAL[a] EFFECTIVENESS, %	ACTUAL[a] EFFECTIVENESS, %	PERCENT CONTINUING USE AT 1 YEAR[b]	CONTRACEPTIVE METHODS USED BY U.S. WOMEN[c]
Barrier methods				
Condoms	98	88	63	18
Diaphragm	94	82	58	2
Cervical cap	94	82	50	<1
Spermicides	97	79	43	1
Sterilization				
Male	99.9	99.9	100	9
Female	99.8	99.6	100	27
Intrauterine device				1
Copper T380	99	97	78	
Progestasert	98	97	81	
Mirena	99.9	99.8		
Hormonal contraceptives	99.7	92	72	31
Combination pill				
Progestin only pill				
Transdermal patch				
Vaginal ring				
Monthly injection				
Long-acting progestins				

[a]Adapted from J Trussel et al: Obstet Gynecol 76:558, 1990.
[b]Adapted from Contraceptive Technology Update. Contraceptive Technology, Feb. 1996, Vol 17, No 1, pp 13–24.
[c]Adapted from LJ Piccinino, WD Mosher: Fam Plan Perspective 30:4, 1998.

used as a permanent form of contraception by over one-third of couples. Pregnancy termination is relatively safe when directed by health care professionals but is rarely the option of choice.

No single contraceptive method is ideal, although all are safer than carrying a pregnancy to term. The effectiveness of a given method of contraception does not just depend on the efficacy of the method itself. Discrepancies between theoretical and actual effectiveness emphasize the importance of patient education and compliance when considering various forms of contraception (Table 14-1). Knowledge of the advantages and disadvantages of each contraceptive is essential for counseling an individual about the methods that are safest and most consistent with his or her lifestyle. The WHO has extensive family planning resources for the physician and patient that can be accessed online. Similar resources for determining medical eligibility are available through the Centers for Disease Control and Prevention (CDC). Considerations for contraceptive use in obese patients and after bariatric surgery are discussed below.

BARRIER METHODS

Barrier contraceptives (such as condoms, diaphragms, and cervical caps) and spermicides are easily available, reversible, and have fewer side effects than hormonal methods. However, their effectiveness is highly dependent on adherence and proper use (Table 14-1). A major advantage of barrier contraceptives is the protection provided against sexually transmitted infections (STIs). Consistent use is associated with a decreased risk of HIV, gonorrhea, nongonococcal urethritis, and genital herpes, probably due in part to the concomitant use of spermicides. Natural membrane condoms may be less effective than latex condoms, and petroleum-based lubricants can degrade condoms and decrease their efficacy for preventing HIV infection. Barrier methods used by women include the diaphragm, cervical cap, and contraceptive sponge. The cervical cap and sponge are less effective than the diaphragm, and there have been rare reports of toxic shock syndrome with the diaphragm and contraceptive sponge.

STERILIZATION

Sterilization is the method of birth control most frequently chosen by fertile men and multiparous women >30 years old (Table 14-1). Sterilization refers to a procedure that prevents fertilization by surgical interruption of the fallopian tubes in women or the vas deferens in men. Although tubal ligation and vasectomy are potentially reversible, these procedures should be considered permanent and should not be undertaken without patient counseling.

Several methods of *tubal ligation* have been developed, all of which are highly effective with a 10-year cumulative pregnancy rate of 1.85 per 100 women. However, when pregnancy does occur, the risk of ectopic pregnancy may be as high as 30%. The success rate of tubal reanastomosis depends on the method of ligation used, but even after successful reversal, the risk of ectopic pregnancy remains high. In addition to prevention of pregnancy, tubal ligation reduces the risk of ovarian cancer, possibly by limiting the upward migration of potential carcinogens.

Vasectomy is a highly effective outpatient surgical procedure that has little risk. The development of azoospermia may be delayed for 2–6 months, and other forms of contraception must be used until two sperm-free ejaculations provide proof of sterility. Reanastomosis may restore fertility in 30–50% of men, but the success rate declines with time after vasectomy and may be influenced by factors such as the development of antisperm antibodies.

INTRAUTERINE DEVICES

IUDs inhibit pregnancy through several mechanisms, primarily via a spermicidal effect caused by a sterile inflammatory reaction induced by the presence of a foreign body in the uterine cavity (copper IUDs) or by the release of progestins (Progestasert, Mirena). IUDs provide a high level of efficacy in the absence of systemic metabolic effects, and ongoing motivation is not required to ensure efficacy once the device has been placed. However, only 1% of women in the United States use this method compared to a utilization rate of 15–30% in much of Europe and Canada, despite evidence that the newer devices are not associated with increased rates of pelvic infection and infertility, as occurred with earlier devices. An IUD should not be used in women at high risk for development of STI or in women at high risk for bacterial endocarditis. The IUD may not be effective in women with uterine leiomyomas because they alter the size or shape of the uterine cavity. IUD use is associated with increased menstrual blood flow, although this is less pronounced with the progestin-releasing IUD, which is associated with a more frequent occurrence of spotting or amenorrhea.

HORMONAL METHODS

Oral contraceptive pills

Because of their ease of use and efficacy, oral contraceptive pills are the most widely used form of hormonal contraception. They act by suppressing ovulation, changing cervical mucus, and altering the endometrium. The current formulations are made from synthetic estrogens and progestins. The estrogen component of the pill consists of ethinyl estradiol or mestranol, which is metabolized to ethinyl estradiol. Multiple synthetic progestins are used. Norethindrone and its derivatives are used in many formulations. Low-dose norgestimate and the more recently developed (third-generation) progestins (desogestrel, gestodene, drospirenone) have a less androgenic profile; levonorgestrel appears to be the most androgenic of the progestins and should be avoided in patients with hyperandrogenism. The three major formulations of oral contraceptives are (1) fixed-dose estrogen-progestin combination, (2) phasic estrogen-progestin combination, and (3) progestin only. Each of these formulations is administered daily for 3 weeks followed by a week of no medication during which menstrual bleeding generally occurs. Two extended oral contraceptives are approved for use in the United States; Seasonale is a 3-month preparation with 84 days of active drug and 7 days of placebo, whereas Lybrel is a continuous preparation. Current doses of ethinyl estradiol range from 10 to 50 μg. However, indications for the 50-μg dose are rare, and the majority of formulations contain 30–35 μg of ethinyl estradiol. The reduced estrogen and progestin content in the second- and third-generation pills has decreased both side effects and risks associated with oral contraceptive use (Table 14-2). At the currently used doses, patients must be cautioned not to miss pills due to the potential for ovulation. Side effects, including breakthrough bleeding, amenorrhea, breast tenderness, and weight gain, often respond to a change in formulation. Even the lower dose oral contraceptives have been associated with an increased risk of cardiovascular disease (myocardial infarction, stroke, venous thromboembolism [VTE]), but the absolute excess risk is extremely low. VTE risk is higher with the third-generation than the second-generation progestins, and the risk of stroke and VTE is also higher with drospirenone (although not cyproterone), but the absolute excess risk is small and may be outweighed by contraceptive benefits and reduction in ovarian and endometrial cancer risk.

The microdose progestin-only minipill is less effective as a contraceptive, having a pregnancy rate of 2–7 per 100 women-years. However, it may be appropriate for women at increased risk for cardiovascular disease or for women who cannot tolerate synthetic estrogens.

TABLE 14-2

ORAL CONTRACEPTIVES: CONTRAINDICATIONS AND DISEASE RISK

Contraindications
Absolute
Previous thromboembolic event or stroke
History of an estrogen-dependent tumor
Active liver disease
Pregnancy
Undiagnosed abnormal uterine bleeding
Hypertriglyceridemia
Women age >35 years who smoke heavily
Relative
Hypertension
Women receiving anticonvulsant drug therapy
Women following bariatric surgery (malabsorptive procedure)
Disease Risks
Increased
Coronary heart disease—increased in smokers >35; no relation to progestin type
Hypertension—relative risk 1.8 (current users) and 1.2 (previous users)
Venous thrombosis—relative risk ~4; may be higher with third-generation progestin, drospirenone, and patch; compounded by obesity (tenfold increased risk compared with nonobese, no OCP); markedly increased with factor V Leiden or prothrombin gene mutations
Stroke—slight increase; unclear relation to migraine headache
Cerebral vein thrombosis—relative risk ~13–15; synergistic with prothrombin gene mutation
Cervical cancer—relative risk 2–4
Breast cancer—may increase risk in carriers of *BRCA1* and possibly *BRCA2*
Decreased
Ovarian cancer—50% reduction in risk
Endometrial cancer—40% reduction in risk

Abbreviation: OCP, oral contraceptive pill.

Alternative methods

A *weekly contraceptive patch* (Ortho Evra) is available and has similar efficacy to oral contraceptives. Approximately 2% of patches fail to adhere, and a similar percentage of women have skin reactions. Efficacy is lower in women weighing >90 kg. The amount of estrogen delivered may be comparable to that of a 40-μg ethinyl estradiol oral contraceptive, raising the possibility of increased risk of VTE, which must be balanced against potential benefits for women not able to successfully use other methods. A *monthly contraceptive estrogen/progestin injection* (Lunelle) is highly effective, with a first-year failure rate of <0.2%, but it may be less effective in obese women. Its use is associated with bleeding irregularities that diminish over time. Fertility returns rapidly after discontinuation. A *monthly vaginal ring* (NuvaRing) that is intended to be left in place during intercourse is also available for contraceptive use. It is highly effective, with a 12-month failure rate of 0.7%.

Ovulation returns within the first recovery cycle after discontinuation.

Long-term contraceptives

Long-term progestin administration acts primarily by inhibiting ovulation and causing changes in the endometrium and cervical mucus that result in decreased implantation and sperm transport. Depot medroxyprogesterone acetate (Depo-Provera, DMPA), the only injectable form available in the United States, is effective for 3 months, but return of fertility after discontinuation may be delayed for up to 12–18 months. DMPA is now available for both SC and IM injection. Irregular bleeding, amenorrhea, and weight gain are the most common side effects. This form of contraception may be particularly good for women in whom an estrogen-containing contraceptive is contraindicated (e.g., migraine exacerbation, sickle cell anemia, fibroids).

POSTCOITAL CONTRACEPTION

The probability of pregnancy without relation to time of the month is 8%, but the probability varies significantly in relation to proximity to ovulation and may be as high has 30%. In order of efficacy, methods of postcoital contraception include the following:

1. Copper IUD insertion within a maximum of 5 days has a reported efficacy of 99–100% and prevents pregnancy by its spermicidal effect; insertion is frequently available through family planning clinics.
2. Oral antiprogestins (ulipristal acetate, 30 mg single dose, available worldwide, or mifepristone, 600 mg single dose, not available for this indication in the United States) prevent pregnancy by delaying or preventing ovulation; when administered, ideally within 72 h but up to 120 h after intercourse, they have an efficacy of 98–99%; require a prescription.
3. Levonorgestrel (1.5 mg as a single dose) delays or prevents ovulation and is not effective after ovulation; should be taken within 72 h of unprotected intercourse, and has an efficacy that varies between 60 and 94%; it is available over the counter.

Combined estrogen and progestin regimens have lower efficacy and are no longer recommended. A pregnancy test is not necessary before the use of oral methods, but pregnancy should be excluded before IUD insertion. Risk factors for failure of oral regimens include close proximity to ovulation and unprotected intercourse after use. In addition, there is an increased risk of pregnancy in obese and overweight women using levonorgestrel for postcoital contraception and an increased risk in obese women using an antiprogestin.

IMPACT OF OBESITY ON CONTRACEPTIVE CHOICE

Approximately one-third of adults in the United States are obese. Although obesity is associated with some reduction in fertility, the vast majority of obese women can conceive. The risk of pregnancy-associated complications is higher in obese women. Intrauterine contraception may be more effective than oral or transdermal methods for obese women. The WHO guidelines provide no restrictions (class 1) for the use of intrauterine contraception, DMPA, and progestin-only pills for obese women (BMI ≥30) in the absence of coexistent medical problems, whereas methods that include estrogen (pill, patch, ring) are considered class 2 (advantages generally outweigh theoretical or proven risks) due to the increased risk of thromboembolic disease. There are no restrictions to the use of any contraceptive methods following restrictive bariatric surgery procedures, but both combined and progestin-only pills are relatively less effective following procedures associated with malabsorption.

CHAPTER 15

MENSTRUAL DISORDERS AND PELVIC PAIN

Janet E. Hall

Menstrual dysfunction can signal an underlying abnormality that may have long-term health consequences. Although frequent or prolonged bleeding usually prompts a woman to seek medical attention, infrequent or absent bleeding may seem less troubling and the patient may not bring it to the attention of the physician. Thus, a focused menstrual history is a critical part of every encounter with a female patient. Pelvic pain is a common complaint that may relate to an abnormality of the reproductive organs but also may be of gastrointestinal, urinary tract, or musculoskeletal origin. Depending on its cause, pelvic pain may require urgent surgical attention.

MENSTRUAL DISORDERS

DEFINITION AND PREVALENCE

Amenorrhea refers to the absence of menstrual periods. Amenorrhea is classified as *primary* if menstrual bleeding has never occurred in the absence of hormonal treatment or *secondary* if menstrual periods cease for 3–6 months. Primary amenorrhea is a rare disorder that occurs in <1% of the female population. However, between 3 and 5% of women experience at least 3 months of secondary amenorrhea in any specific year. There is no evidence that race or ethnicity influences the prevalence of amenorrhea. However, because of the importance of adequate nutrition for normal reproductive function, both the age at menarche and the prevalence of secondary amenorrhea vary significantly in different parts of the world.

Oligomenorrhea is defined as a cycle length >35 days or <10 menses per year. Both the frequency and the amount of vaginal bleeding are irregular in oligomenorrhea, and moliminal symptoms (premenstrual breast tenderness, food cravings, mood lability), suggestive of ovulation, are variably present. Anovulation can also present with intermenstrual intervals <24 days or vaginal bleeding for >7 days. Frequent or heavy irregular bleeding is termed *dysfunctional uterine bleeding* if anatomic uterine and outflow tract lesions or a bleeding diathesis has been excluded.

Primary amenorrhea

The absence of menses by age 16 has been used traditionally to define primary amenorrhea. However, other factors, such as growth, secondary sexual characteristics, the presence of cyclic pelvic pain, and the secular trend toward an earlier age of menarche, particularly in African-American girls, also influence the age at which primary amenorrhea should be investigated. Thus, an evaluation for amenorrhea should be initiated by age 15 or 16 in the presence of normal growth and secondary sexual characteristics; age 13 in the absence of secondary sexual characteristics or if height is less than the third percentile; age 12 or 13 in the presence of breast development and cyclic pelvic pain; or within 2 years of breast development if menarche, defined by the first menstrual period, has not occurred.

Secondary amenorrhea or oligomenorrhea

Anovulation and irregular cycles are relatively common for up to 2 years after menarche and for 1–2 years before the final menstrual period. In the intervening years, menstrual cycle length is ~28 days, with an intermenstrual interval normally ranging between 25 and 35 days. Cycle-to-cycle variability in an individual woman who is ovulating consistently is generally +/− 2 days. Pregnancy is the most common cause of amenorrhea and should be excluded early in any evaluation of menstrual irregularity. However, many women occasionally miss a single period. Three or more months of secondary amenorrhea should prompt an evaluation, as should a history of intermenstrual intervals >35 or <21 days or bleeding that persists for >7 days.

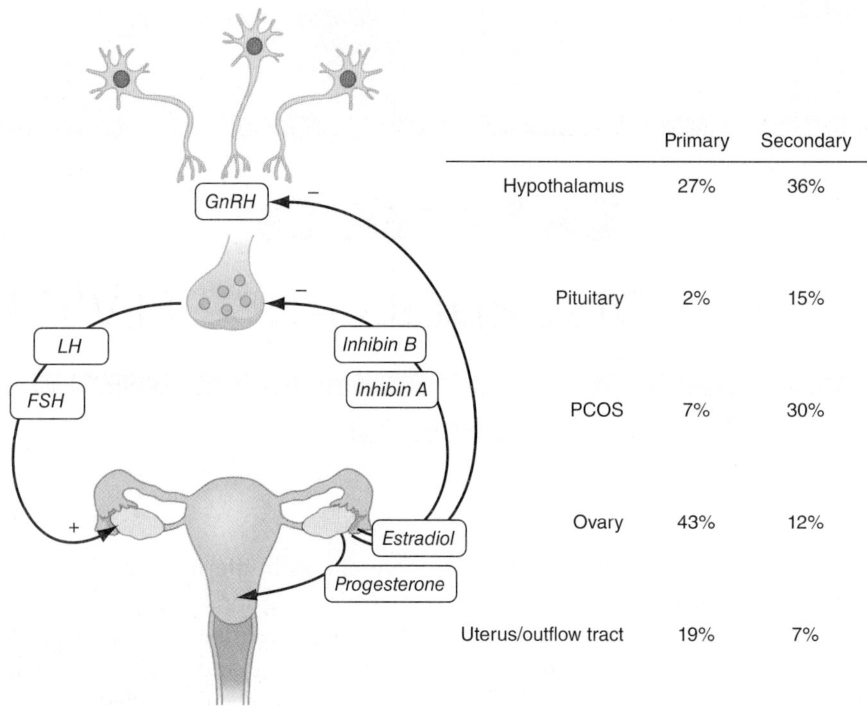

FIGURE 15-1

Role of the hypothalamic-pituitary-gonadal axis in the etiology of amenorrhea. Gonadotropin-releasing hormone (GnRH) secretion from the hypothalamus stimulates follicle-stimulating hormone (FSH) and luteinizing hormone (LH) secretion from the pituitary to induce ovarian folliculogenesis and steroidogenesis. Ovarian secretion of estradiol and progesterone controls the shedding of the endometrium, resulting in menses, and, in combination with the inhibins, provides feedback regulation of the hypothalamus and pituitary to control secretion of FSH and LH. The prevalence of amenorrhea resulting from abnormalities at each level of the reproductive system (hypothalamus, pituitary, ovary, uterus, and outflow tract) varies depending on whether amenorrhea is primary or secondary. PCOS, polycystic ovarian syndrome.

DIAGNOSIS

Evaluation of menstrual dysfunction depends on understanding the interrelationships between the four critical components of the reproductive tract: (1) the hypothalamus, (2) the pituitary, (3) the ovaries, and (4) the uterus and outflow tract (Fig. 15-1; **Chap. 13**). This system is maintained by complex negative and positive feedback loops involving the ovarian steroids (estradiol and progesterone) and peptides (inhibin B and inhibin A) and the hypothalamic (gonadotropin-releasing hormone [GnRH]) and pituitary (follicle-stimulating hormone [FSH] and luteinizing hormone [LH]) components of this system (Fig. 15-1).

Disorders of menstrual function can be thought of in two main categories: disorders of the uterus and outflow tract and disorders of ovulation. Many of the conditions that cause primary amenorrhea are congenital but go unrecognized until the time of normal puberty (e.g., genetic, chromosomal, and anatomic abnormalities). All causes of secondary amenorrhea also can cause primary amenorrhea.

Disorders of the uterus or outflow tract

Abnormalities of the uterus and outflow tract typically present as primary amenorrhea. In patients with normal pubertal development and a blind vagina, the differential diagnosis includes *obstruction* by a transverse vaginal septum or imperforate hymen; *müllerian agenesis* (Mayer-Rokitansky-Kuster-Hauser syndrome), which has been associated with mutations in the *WNT4* gene; and *androgen insensitivity syndrome* (AIS), which is an X-linked recessive disorder that accounts for ~10% of all cases of primary amenorrhea **(Chap. 11)**. Patients with AIS have a 46,XY karyotype, but because of the lack of androgen receptor responsiveness, those with complete AIS have severe underandrogenization and female external genitalia. The absence of pubic and axillary hair distinguishes them clinically from patients with müllerian agenesis, as does an elevated testosterone level. *Asherman's syndrome* presents as secondary amenorrhea or hypomenorrhea and results from partial or complete obliteration of the uterine cavity by adhesions that prevent normal growth and shedding of the endometrium. Curettage performed for pregnancy complications accounts for >90% of cases; genital tuberculosis is an important cause in regions where it is endemic.

TREATMENT Disorders of the Uterus or Outflow Tract

Obstruction of the outflow tract requires surgical correction. The risk of endometriosis is increased with this condition, perhaps because of retrograde menstrual flow. *Müllerian agenesis* also may require surgical intervention to allow sexual intercourse, although vaginal dilatation is adequate in some patients. Because ovarian function is normal, assisted reproductive techniques can be used with a surrogate carrier. *Androgen resistance syndrome* requires gonadectomy because there is risk of gonadoblastoma in the dysgenetic gonads. Whether this should be performed in early childhood or after completion of breast development is controversial. Estrogen replacement is indicated after gonadectomy, and vaginal dilatation may be required to allow sexual intercourse.

Disorders of ovulation

Once uterus and outflow tract abnormalities have been excluded, other causes of amenorrhea involve disorders of ovulation. The differential diagnosis is based on the results of initial tests, including a pregnancy test, an FSH level (to determine whether the cause is likely to be ovarian or central), and assessment of hyperandrogenism (Fig. 15-2).

Hypogonadotropic hypogonadism

Low estrogen levels in combination with normal or low levels of LH and FSH are seen with anatomic, genetic, or functional abnormalities that interfere with hypothalamic GnRH secretion or normal pituitary responsiveness to GnRH. Although relatively uncommon, tumors and infiltrative diseases should be considered in the differential diagnosis of hypogonadotropic hypogonadism (**Chap. 5**). These disorders may present with primary or secondary amenorrhea. They may occur in association with other features suggestive of hypothalamic or pituitary dysfunction, such as short stature, diabetes

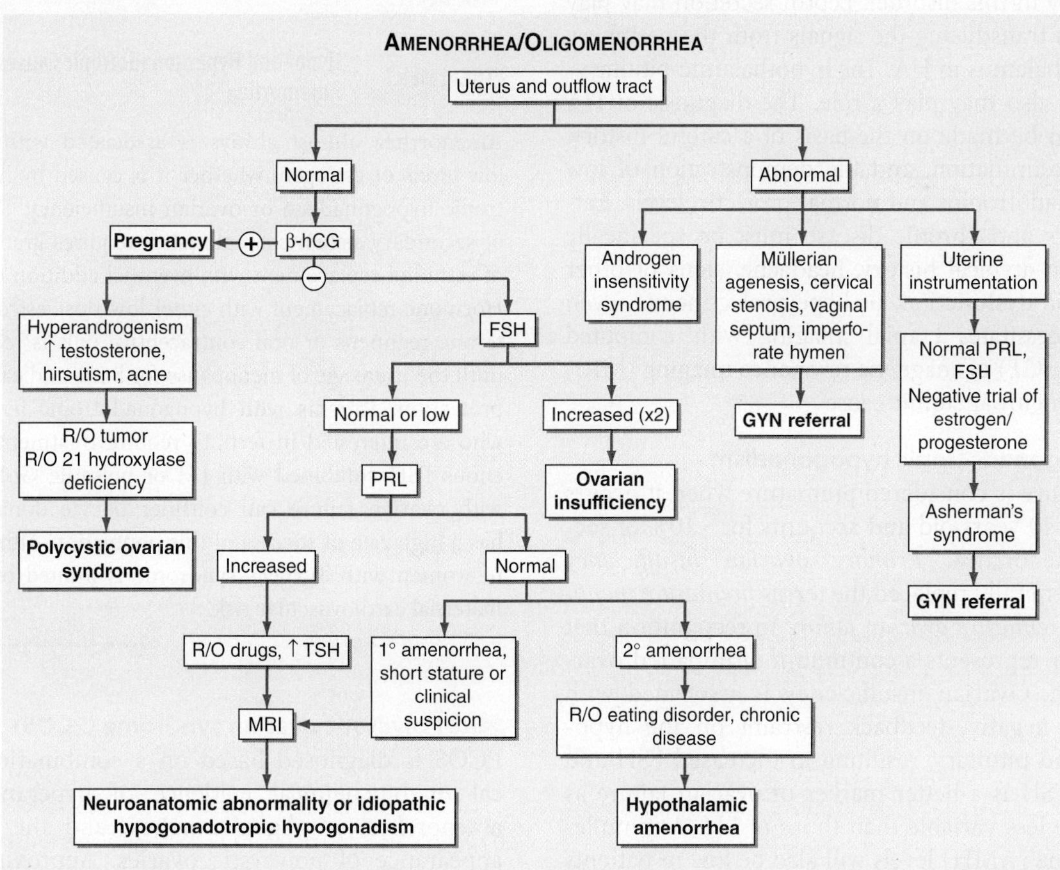

FIGURE 15-2
Algorithm for evaluation of amenorrhea. β-hCG, human chorionic gonadotropin; FSH, follicle-stimulating hormone; GYN, gynecologist; MRI, magnetic resonance imaging; PRL, prolactin; R/O, rule out; TSH, thyroid-stimulating hormone.

insipidus, galactorrhea, and headache. Hypogonadotropic hypogonadism also may be seen after cranial irradiation. In the postpartum period, it may be caused by pituitary necrosis (Sheehan's syndrome) or lymphocytic hypophysitis. Because reproductive dysfunction is commonly associated with hyperprolactinemia from neuroanatomic lesions or medications, prolactin should be measured in all patients with hypogonadotropic hypogonadism **(Chap. 5)**.

Isolated hypogonadotropic hypogonadism (IHH) occurs in women, although it is three times more common in men. IHH generally presents with primary amenorrhea, although 50% have some degree of breast development, and one to two menses have been described in ~10%. IHH is associated with anosmia in about 50% of women (termed Kallmann's syndrome). Genetic causes of IHH have been identified in ~60% of patients **(Chaps. 11 and 13)**.

Functional hypothalamic amenorrhea (HA) is caused by a mismatch between energy expenditure and energy intake. Recent studies suggest that variants in genes associated with IHH may increase susceptibility to these environmental inputs, accounting in part for the clinical variability in this disorder. Leptin secretion may play a key role in transducing the signals from the periphery to the hypothalamus in HA. The hypothalamic-pituitary-adrenal axis also may play a role. The diagnosis of HA generally can be made on the basis of a careful history, a physical examination, and the demonstration of low levels of gonadotropins and normal prolactin levels. Eating disorders and chronic disease must be specifically excluded. An atypical history, headache, signs of other hypothalamic dysfunction, or hyperprolactinemia, even if mild, necessitates cranial imaging with computed tomography (CT) or magnetic resonance imaging (MRI) to exclude a neuroanatomic cause.

Hypergonadotropic hypogonadism

Ovarian failure is considered premature when it occurs in women <40 years old and accounts for ~10% of secondary amenorrhea. *Primary ovarian insufficiency* (POI) has generally replaced the terms *premature menopause* and *premature ovarian failure* in recognition that this disorder represents a continuum of impaired ovarian function. Ovarian insufficiency is associated with the loss of negative-feedback restraint on the hypothalamus and pituitary, resulting in increased FSH and LH levels. FSH is a better marker of ovarian failure as its levels are less variable than those of LH. Antimüllerian hormone (AMH) levels will also be low in patients with POI, but are more frequently used in management of infertility. As with natural menopause, POI may wax and wane, and serial measurements may be necessary to establish the diagnosis.

Once the diagnosis of POI has been established, further evaluation is indicated because of other health problems that may be associated with POI. For example, POI occurs in association with a variety of chromosomal abnormalities, including Turner's syndrome, autoimmune polyglandular failure syndromes, radio- and chemotherapy, and galactosemia. The recognition that early ovarian failure occurs in premutation carriers of the fragile X syndrome is important because of the increased risk of severe mental retardation in male children with *FMR1* mutations. In the majority of cases, a cause for POI is not determined. Although there are increasing reports of genetic mutations in individuals and families with POI, testing for other than chromosomal abnormalities and *FMR1* mutations is not recommended.

Hypergonadotropic hypogonadism occurs rarely in other disorders, such as mutations in the FSH or LH receptors. Aromatase deficiency and 17α-hydroxylase deficiency are associated with decreased estrogen and elevated gonadotropins and with hyperandrogenism and hypertension, respectively. Gonadotropin-secreting tumors in women of reproductive age generally present with high, rather than low, estrogen levels and cause ovarian hyperstimulation or dysfunctional bleeding.

TREATMENT Hypo- and Hypergonadotropic Causes of Amenorrhea

Amenorrhea almost always is associated with chronically low levels of estrogen, whether it is caused by hypogonadotropic hypogonadism or ovarian insufficiency. Development of secondary sexual characteristics requires gradual titration of estradiol replacement with eventual addition of progestin. Hormone replacement with either low-dose estrogen/progesterone regimens or oral contraceptive pills is recommended until the usual age of menopause for bone and cardiovascular protection. Patients with hypogonadotropic hypogonadism who are interested in fertility require treatment with exogenous FSH combined with LH or pulsatile GnRH. Patients with ovarian failure can consider oocyte donation, which has a high rate of success in this population, although its use in women with Turner's syndrome is limited by significant maternal cardiovascular risk.

Polycystic ovarian syndrome (PCOS)

PCOS is diagnosed based on a combination of clinical or biochemical evidence of hyperandrogenism, amenorrhea or oligomenorrhea, and the ultrasound appearance of polycystic ovaries. Approximately half of patients with PCOS are obese, and abnormalities in insulin dynamics are common, as is metabolic syndrome. Symptoms generally begin shortly after menarche and are slowly progressive. Lean oligo-ovulatory patients with PCOS generally have high LH levels in the presence of normal to low levels of FSH and estradiol.

The LH/FSH ratio is less pronounced in obese patients in whom insulin resistance is a more prominent feature.

TREATMENT Polycystic Ovarian Syndrome

A major abnormality in patients with PCOS is the failure of regular, predictable ovulation. Thus, these patients are at risk for the development of dysfunctional bleeding and endometrial hyperplasia associated with unopposed estrogen exposure. Endometrial protection can be achieved with the use of oral contraceptives or progestins (medroxyprogesterone acetate, 5–10 mg, or prometrium, 200 mg daily for 10–14 days of each month). Oral contraceptives are also useful for management of hyperandrogenic symptoms, as are spironolactone and cyproterone acetate (not available in the United States), which function as weak androgen receptor blockers. Management of the associated metabolic syndrome may be appropriate for some patients **(Chap. 22)**. For patients interested in fertility, weight control is a critical first step. Clomiphene citrate is highly effective as a first-line treatment, and there is increasing evidence that the aromatase inhibitor letrozole may also be effective. Exogenous gonadotropins can be used by experienced practitioners; a diagnosis of polycystic ovaries in the presence or absence of cycle abnormalities increases the risk of hyperstimulation.

PELVIC PAIN

The mechanisms that cause pelvic pain are similar to those that cause abdominal pain and include inflammation of the parietal peritoneum, obstruction of hollow viscera, vascular disturbances, and pain originating in the abdominal wall. Pelvic pain may reflect pelvic disease per se but also may reflect extrapelvic disorders that refer pain to the pelvis. In up to 60% of cases, pelvic pain can be attributed to gastrointestinal problems, including appendicitis, cholecystitis, infections, intestinal obstruction, diverticulitis, and inflammatory bowel disease. Urinary tract and musculoskeletal disorders are also common causes of pelvic pain.

APPROACH TO THE PATIENT: Pelvic Pain

As with all types of abdominal pain, the first priority is to identify life-threatening conditions (shock, peritoneal signs) that may require emergent surgical management. The possibility of pregnancy should be identified as soon as possible by menstrual history and/or testing. A thorough history that includes the type, location, radiation, and status with respect to increasing or decreasing severity can help identify the cause of acute pelvic pain. Specific associations with vaginal bleeding, sexual activity, defecation, urination, movement, or eating should be specifically sought. Determination of whether the pain is acute versus chronic and cyclic versus noncyclic will direct further investigation (Table 15-1). However, disorders that cause cyclic pain occasionally may cause noncyclic pain, and the converse is also true.

ACUTE PELVIC PAIN

Pelvic inflammatory disease most commonly presents with bilateral lower abdominal pain. It is generally of recent onset and is exacerbated by intercourse or jarring movements. Fever is present in about half of these patients; abnormal uterine bleeding occurs in about one-third. New vaginal discharge, urethritis, and chills may be present but are less specific signs. *Adnexal pathology* can present acutely and may be due to rupture, bleeding or torsion of cysts, or, much less commonly, neoplasms of the ovary, fallopian tubes, or paraovarian areas. Fever may be present with ovarian torsion. *Ectopic pregnancy* is associated with right- or left-sided lower abdominal pain, with clinical signs generally appearing 6–8 weeks after the last normal menstrual period. Amenorrhea is present in ~75% of cases and vaginal bleeding in ~50% of cases. Orthostatic signs

TABLE 15-1

CAUSES OF PELVIC PAIN

	ACUTE	CHRONIC
Cyclic pelvic pain		Premenstrual symptoms
		Mittelschmerz
		Dysmenorrhea
		Endometriosis
Noncyclic pelvic pain	Pelvic inflammatory disease	Pelvic congestion syndrome
	Ruptured or hemorrhagic ovarian cyst, endometrioma, or ovarian torsion	Adhesions and retroversion of the uterus
	Ectopic pregnancy	Pelvic malignancy
	Endometritis	Vulvodynia
	Acute growth or degeneration of uterine myoma	Chronic pelvic inflammatory disease
	Threatened abortion	Tuberculous salpingitis
		History of sexual abuse

and fever may be present. Risk factors include the presence of known tubal disease, previous ectopic pregnancies, a history of infertility, diethylstilbestrol (DES) exposure of the mother in utero, or a history of pelvic infections. *Threatened abortion* may also present with amenorrhea, abdominal pain, and vaginal bleeding. Although more common than ectopic pregnancy, it is rarely associated with systemic signs. *Uterine pathology* includes endometritis and, less frequently, degenerating leiomyomas (fibroids). Endometritis often is associated with vaginal bleeding and systemic signs of infection. It occurs in the setting of sexually transmitted infections, uterine instrumentation, or postpartum infection.

A sensitive pregnancy test, complete blood count with differential, urinalysis, tests for chlamydial and gonococcal infections, and abdominal ultrasound aid in making the diagnosis and directing further management.

TREATMENT Acute Pelvic Pain

Treatment of acute pelvic pain depends on the suspected etiology but may require surgical or gynecologic intervention. Conservative management is an important consideration for ovarian cysts, if torsion is not suspected, to avoid unnecessary pelvic surgery and the subsequent risk of infertility due to adhesions. Surgical treatment may be required for ectopic pregnancies; however, approximately 35% of ectopic pregnancies are unruptured and may be appropriate for treatment with methotrexate, which is effective in ~90% of cases.

CHRONIC PELVIC PAIN

Some women experience discomfort at the time of ovulation (*mittelschmerz*). The pain can be quite intense but is generally of short duration. The mechanism is thought to involve rapid expansion of the dominant follicle, although it also may be caused by peritoneal irritation by follicular fluid released at the time of ovulation. Many women experience premenstrual symptoms such as breast discomfort, food cravings, and abdominal bloating or discomfort. These moliminal symptoms are a good marker of prior ovulation, although their absence is less helpful.

Dysmenorrhea

Dysmenorrhea refers to the crampy lower abdominal midline discomfort that begins with the onset of menstrual bleeding and gradually decreases over the next 12–72 h. It may be associated with nausea, diarrhea, fatigue, and headache and occurs in 60–93% of adolescents, beginning with the establishment of regular ovulatory cycles. Its prevalence decreases after pregnancy and with the use of oral contraceptives.

Primary dysmenorrhea results from increased stores of prostaglandin precursors, which are generated by sequential stimulation of the uterus by estrogen and progesterone. During menstruation, these precursors are converted to prostaglandins, which cause intense uterine contractions, decreased blood flow, and increased peripheral nerve hypersensitivity, resulting in pain.

Secondary dysmenorrhea is caused by underlying pelvic pathology. *Endometriosis* results from the presence of endometrial glands and stroma outside the uterus. These deposits of ectopic endometrium respond to hormonal stimulation and cause dysmenorrhea, which begins several days before menses. Endometriosis also may be associated with painful intercourse, painful bowel movements, and tender nodules in the uterosacral ligament. Fibrosis and adhesions can produce lateral displacement of the cervix. Transvaginal pelvic ultrasound is part of the initial workup and may detect an endometrioma within the ovary, rectovaginal or bladder nodules, or ureteral involvement. The CA125 level may be increased, but it has low negative predictive value. Definitive diagnosis requires laparoscopy. Symptomatology does not always predict the extent of endometriosis. The prevalence is lower in black and Hispanic women than in Caucasians and Asians. *Other secondary causes* of dysmenorrhea include adenomyosis, a condition caused by the presence of ectopic endometrial glands and stroma within the myometrium. Cervical stenosis may result from trauma, infection, or surgery.

TREATMENT Dysmenorrhea

Local application of heat; dietary dairy intake; use of vitamins B_1, B_6, and E and fish oil; acupuncture; yoga; and exercise are of some benefit for the treatment of dysmenorrhea. Studies of vitamin D_3 are not yet adequate to provide a recommendation. However, nonsteroidal anti-inflammatory drugs (NSAIDs) are the most effective treatment and provide >80% sustained response rates. Ibuprofen, naproxen, ketoprofen, mefanamic acid, and nimesulide are all superior to placebo. Treatment should be started a day before expected menses and generally is continued for 2–3 days. Oral contraceptives also reduce symptoms of dysmenorrhea. The use of tocolytics, antiphosphodiesterase inhibitors, and magnesium has been suggested, but there are insufficient data to recommend them. Failure of response to NSAIDs and/or oral contraceptives is suggestive of a pelvic disorder such as endometriosis, and diagnostic laparoscopy should be considered to guide further treatment.

CHAPTER 16

MENOPAUSE AND POSTMENOPAUSAL HORMONE THERAPY

JoAnn E. Manson ■ Shari S. Bassuk

Menopause is the permanent cessation of menstruation due to loss of ovarian follicular function. It is diagnosed retrospectively after 12 months of amenorrhea. The average age at menopause is 51 years among U.S. women. *Perimenopause* refers to the time period preceding menopause, when fertility wanes and menstrual cycle irregularity increases, until the first year after cessation of menses. The onset of perimenopause precedes the final menses by 2–8 years, with a mean duration of 4 years. Smoking accelerates the menopausal transition by 2 years.

Although the peri- and postmenopausal transitions share many symptoms, the physiology and clinical management of the two differ. Low-dose oral contraceptives have become a therapeutic mainstay in perimenopause, whereas postmenopausal hormone therapy (HT) has been a common method of symptom alleviation after menstruation ceases.

PERIMENOPAUSE

PHYSIOLOGY

Ovarian mass and fertility decline sharply after age 35 and even more precipitously during perimenopause; depletion of primary follicles, a process that begins before birth, occurs steadily until menopause **(Chap. 13)**. In perimenopause, intermenstrual intervals shorten significantly (typically by 3 days) as a result of an accelerated follicular phase. Follicle-stimulating hormone (FSH) levels rise because of altered folliculogenesis and reduced inhibin secretion. In contrast to the consistently high FSH and low estradiol levels seen in menopause, perimenopause is characterized by "irregularly irregular" hormone levels. The propensity for anovulatory cycles can produce a hyperestrogenic, hypoprogestagenic environment that may account for the increased incidence of endometrial hyperplasia or carcinoma, uterine polyps, and leiomyoma observed among women of perimenopausal age. Mean serum levels of selected ovarian and pituitary hormones during the menopausal transition are shown in Fig. 16-1. With transition into menopause, estradiol levels fall markedly, whereas estrone levels are relatively preserved, a pattern reflecting peripheral aromatization of adrenal and ovarian androgens. Levels of FSH increase more than those of luteinizing hormone, presumably because of the loss of inhibin as well as estrogen feedback.

DIAGNOSTIC TESTS

The Stages of Reproductive Aging Workshop +10 (STRAW+10) classification provides a comprehensive framework for the clinical assessment of ovarian aging. As shown in Fig. 16-2, menstrual cycle characteristics are the principal criteria for characterizing the menopausal transition, with biomarker measures as supportive criteria. Because of their extreme intraindividual variability, FSH and estradiol levels are imperfect diagnostic indicators of perimenopause in menstruating women. However, a consistently low FSH level in the early follicular phase (days 2–5) of the menstrual cycle does not support a diagnosis of perimenopause, while levels >25 IU/L in a random blood sample are characteristic of the late menopause transition. FSH measurement can also aid in assessing fertility; levels of <20 IU/L, 20 to <30 IU/L, and ≥30 IU/L measured on day 3 of the cycle indicate a good, fair, and poor likelihood of achieving pregnancy, respectively. Antimüllerian hormone and inhibin B may also be useful for assessing reproductive aging.

SYMPTOMS

Determining whether symptoms that develop in midlife are due to ovarian senescence or to other age-related

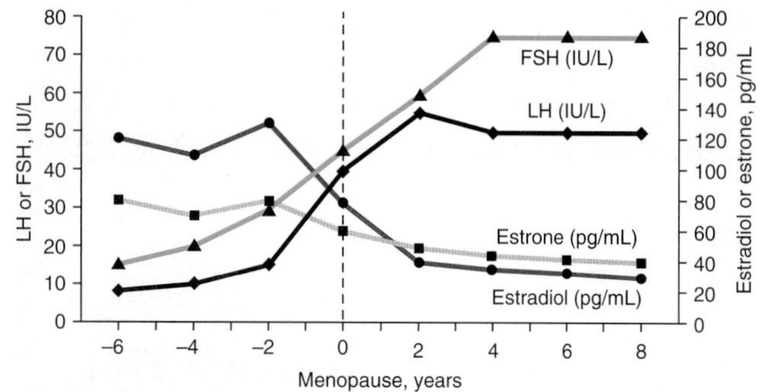

FIGURE 16-1

Mean serum levels of ovarian and pituitary hormones during the menopausal transition. FSH, follicle-stimulating hormone; LH, luteinizing hormone. *(From JL Shifren, I Schiff: J Womens Health Gend Based Med 9 Suppl 1:S3, 2000.)*

changes is difficult. There is strong evidence that the menopausal transition can cause hot flashes, night sweats, irregular bleeding, and vaginal dryness, and there is moderate evidence that it can cause sleep disturbances in some women. There is inconclusive or insufficient evidence that ovarian aging is a major cause of mood swings, depression, impaired memory or concentration, somatic symptoms, urinary incontinence, or sexual dysfunction. In one U.S. study, nearly 60% of women reported hot flashes in the 2 years before their final menses. Symptom intensity, duration, frequency, and effects on quality of life are highly variable.

TREATMENT Perimenopause

PERIMENOPAUSAL THERAPY For women with irregular or heavy menses or hormone-related symptoms that impair quality of life, low-dose combined oral contraceptives are a staple of therapy. Static doses of estrogen and progestin (e.g., 20 μg of ethinyl estradiol and 1 mg of norethindrone acetate daily for 21 days each month) can eliminate vasomotor symptoms and restore regular cyclicity. Oral contraceptives provide other benefits, including protection against ovarian and endometrial cancers and increased bone density, although it is not clear whether use during perimenopause decreases fracture risk later in life. Moreover, the contraceptive benefit is important, given that the unintentional pregnancy rate among women in their forties rivals that of adolescents. Contraindications to oral

	Menarche						FMP (0)			
Stage	−5	−4	−3b	−3a	−2	−1	+1a	+1b	+1c	+2
Terminology	**Reproductive**				**Menopausal transition**		**Postmenopause**			
	Early	Peak	Late		Early	Late	Early			Late
					Perimenopause					
Duration	*Variable*				*Variable*	1–3 years	2 years (1+1)		3–6 years	*Remaining lifespan*
Principal criteria										
Menstrual cycle	Variable to regular	Regular	Regular	Subtle changes in flow/ length	*Variable Length* Persistent ≥7-day difference in length of consecutive cycles	Interval of amenorrhea of ≥60 days				
Supportive criteria										
Endocrine FSH AMH Inhibin B			Low Low	Variable* Low Low	↑ Variable* Low Low	↑ >25 IU/L** Low Low	↑ Variable Low Low		Stabilizes Very low Very low	
Antral follicle count			Low	Low	Low	Low	Very low		Very low	
Descriptive characteristics										
Symptoms						Vasomotor symptoms *Likely*	Vasomotor symptoms *Most likely*			*Increasing symptoms of urogenital atrophy*

*Blood draw on cycle days 2–5 ↑ = elevated.
**Approximate expected level based on assays using current international pituitary standard.

FIGURE 16-2

The Stages of Reproductive Aging Workshop +10 (STRAW +10) staging system for reproductive aging in women. AMH, antimüllerian hormone; FSH, follicle-stimulating hormone. *(From SD Harlow et al: Menopause 14:387, 2012. Reproduced with permission.)*

contraceptive use include cigarette smoking, liver disease, a history of thromboembolism or cardiovascular disease, breast cancer, or unexplained vaginal bleeding. Progestin-only formulations (e.g., 0.35 mg of norethindrone daily) or medroxyprogesterone (Depo-Provera) injections (e.g., 150 mg IM every 3 months) may provide an alternative for the treatment of perimenopausal menorrhagia in women who smoke or have cardiovascular risk factors. Although progestins neither regularize cycles nor reduce the number of bleeding days, they reduce the volume of menstrual flow.

Nonhormonal strategies to reduce menstrual flow include the use of nonsteroidal anti-inflammatory agents such as mefenamic acid (an initial dose of 500 mg at the start of menses, then 250 mg qid for 2–3 days) or, when medical approaches fail, endometrial ablation. It should be noted that menorrhagia requires an evaluation to rule out uterine disorders. Transvaginal ultrasound with saline enhancement is useful for detecting leiomyomata or polyps, and endometrial aspiration can identify hyperplastic changes.

TRANSITION TO MENOPAUSE For sexually active women using contraceptive hormones to alleviate perimenopausal symptoms, the question of when and if to switch to HT must be individualized. Doses of estrogen and progestogen (either synthetic progestins or natural forms of progesterone) in HT are lower than those in oral contraceptives and have not been documented to prevent pregnancy. Although a 1-year absence of spontaneous menses reliably indicates ovulation cessation, it is not possible to assess the natural menstrual pattern while a woman is taking an oral contraceptive. Women willing to switch to a barrier method of contraception should do so; if menses occur spontaneously, oral contraceptive use can be resumed. The average age of final menses among relatives can serve as a guide for when to initiate this process, which can be repeated yearly until menopause has occurred.

MENOPAUSE AND POSTMENOPAUSAL HORMONE THERAPY

One of the most complex health care decisions facing women is whether to use postmenopausal HT. Once prescribed primarily to relieve vasomotor symptoms, HT has been promoted as a strategy to forestall various disorders that accelerate after menopause, including osteoporosis and cardiovascular disease. In 2000, nearly 40% of postmenopausal women age 50–74 in the United States had used HT. This widespread use occurred despite the paucity of conclusive data, until recently, on the health consequences of such therapy. Although many women rely on their health care providers for a definitive answer to the question of whether to use postmenopausal hormones, balancing the benefits and risks for an individual patient is challenging.

Although observational studies suggest that HT prevents cardiovascular and other chronic diseases, the apparent benefits may result at least in part from differences between women who opt to take postmenopausal hormones and women who do not. Those choosing HT tend to be healthier, have greater access to medical care, are more compliant with prescribed treatments, and maintain a more health-promoting lifestyle. Randomized trials, which eliminate these confounding factors, have not consistently confirmed the benefits found in observational studies. Indeed, the largest HT trial to date, the Women's Health Initiative (WHI), which examined more than 27,000 postmenopausal women age 50–79 (mean age, 63) for an average of 5–7 years, was stopped early because of an overall unfavorable benefit-risk ratio in the estrogen-progestin arm and an excess risk of stroke that was not offset by a reduced risk of coronary heart disease (CHD) in the estrogen-only arm.

The following summary offers a decision-making guide based on a synthesis of currently available evidence. Prevention of cardiovascular disease is eliminated from the equation due to lack of evidence for such benefits in recent randomized clinical trials.

BENEFITS AND RISKS OF POSTMENOPAUSAL HORMONE THERAPY

See Table 16-1.

Definite benefits

Symptoms of menopause

Compelling evidence, including data from randomized clinical trials, indicates that estrogen therapy is highly effective for controlling vasomotor and genitourinary symptoms. Alternative approaches, including the use of antidepressants (such as paroxetine, 7.5 mg/d; or venlafaxine, 75–150 mg/d), gabapentin (300–900 mg/d), clonidine (0.1–0.2 mg/d), or vitamin E (400–800 IU/d), or the consumption of soy-based products or other phytoestrogens, may also alleviate vasomotor symptoms, although they are less effective than HT. Paroxetine is the only nonhormonal drug approved by the U.S. Food and Drug Administration for treatment of vasomotor symptoms. Bazedoxifene, an estrogen agonist/antagonist, in combination with conjugated estrogens has also received approval for vasomotor symptom management. For genitourinary symptoms, the efficacy of vaginal estrogen is similar to that of oral or transdermal estrogen; oral ospemifene is an additional option.

Osteoporosis

(See also Chap. 35)

TABLE 16-1

BENEFITS AND RISKS OF POSTMENOPAUSAL HORMONE THERAPY IN THE OVERALL STUDY POPULATION OF WOMEN 50–79 YEARS OF AGE IN THE INTERVENTION PHASE OF THE WOMEN'S HEALTH INITIATIVE (WHI) ESTROGEN-PROGESTIN AND ESTROGEN-ALONE TRIALS[a]

		ESTROGEN-PROGESTIN		ESTROGEN ALONE	
OUTCOME	**EFFECT**	**RELATIVE BENEFIT OR RISK**	**ABSOLUTE BENEFIT OR RISK[b]**	**RELATIVE BENEFIT OR RISK**	**ABSOLUTE BENEFIT OR RISK[b]**
Definite Benefits					
Symptoms of menopause	Definite improvement	↓65–90% decreased risk[c]		↓65–90% decreased risk[c]	
Osteoporosis	Definite increase in bone mineral density and decrease in fracture risk	↓33% decreased risk for hip fracture	6 fewer cases (11 vs. 17) of hip fracture	↓33% decreased risk for hip fracture	6 fewer cases (13 vs. 19) of hip fracture
Definite Risks[h]					
Endometrial cancer	Definite increase in risk with estrogen alone (see below for estrogen-progestin)	See below	See below		4.6 excess cases (observational studies)
Pulmonary embolism	Definite increase in risk	↑98% increased risk	9 excess cases (18 vs. 9)	↑35% increased risk (n.s.)	4 excess cases (14 vs. 10)
Deep vein thrombosis	Definite increase in risk	↑87% increased risk	11.5 excess cases (25 vs. 14)	↑48% increased risk	7.5 excess cases (23 vs. 15)
Breast cancer	Definite increase in risk with long-term use (≥5 years) of estrogen-progestin	↑24% increased risk	8.5 excess cases (43 vs. 35)	↓21% decreased risk (n.s.)	7 fewer cases (28 vs. 35)
Gallbladder disease	Definite increase in risk	↑57% increased risk	47 excess cases (131 vs. 84)	↑55% increased risk	58 excess cases (164 vs. 106)
Probable or Uncertain Risks and Benefits[h]					
Coronary heart disease[d]	Probable increase in risk among older women and women many years past menopause; possible decrease in risk or no effect in younger or recently menopausal women[e]	↑18% increased risk (n.s.)	6 excess cases (41 vs. 35)	No increase in risk	No difference in risk
Myocardial infarction	Significant interaction by age group for estrogen alone, with reduced risk in younger—but not older—women (p for trend by age = .02)	↑24% increased risk (n.s.)	6 excess cases (35 vs. 29)	No increase in risk[e]	No difference in risk[e]
Stroke	Probable increase in risk	↑37% increased risk	9 excess cases (33 vs. 24)	↑35% increased risk	11 excess cases (45 vs. 34)
Ovarian cancer	Probable increase in risk with long-term use (≥5 years)	↑41% increased risk (n.s.)	1 excess cases (5 vs. 4)	Not available	Not available
Endometrial cancer	Probable decrease in risk with estrogen-progestin during long-term follow-up (see above for estrogen alone)	↓33% decreased risk[f]	3 fewer cases (7 vs. 10)	See above	See above

(continued)

TABLE 16-1

BENEFITS AND RISKS OF POSTMENOPAUSAL HORMONE THERAPY IN THE OVERALL STUDY POPULATION OF WOMEN 50–79 YEARS OF AGE IN THE INTERVENTION PHASE OF THE WOMEN'S HEALTH INITIATIVE (WHI) ESTROGEN-PROGESTIN AND ESTROGEN-ALONE TRIALS[a] (CONTINUED)

		ESTROGEN-PROGESTIN		ESTROGEN ALONE	
OUTCOME	**EFFECT**	**RELATIVE BENEFIT OR RISK**	**ABSOLUTE BENEFIT OR RISK[b]**	**RELATIVE BENEFIT OR RISK**	**ABSOLUTE BENEFIT OR RISK[b]**
Urinary incontinence	Probable increase in risk	↑49% increased risk	549 excess cases (1661 vs. 1112)	↑61% increased risk	852 excess cases (2255 vs. 1403)
Colorectal cancer	Probable decrease in risk with estrogen-progestin; possible increase in risk in older women with estrogen alone (p for trend by age = .02 for estrogen alone)	↓38% decreased risk	6.5 fewer cases (10 vs. 17)	No increase or decrease in risk[e]	No difference in risk[e]
Type 2 diabetes	Probable decrease in risk	↓19% decreased risk	16 fewer cases (72 vs. 88)	↓14% decreased risk	21 fewer cases (134 vs. 155)
Dementia (age ≥65)	Increase in risk in older women (but inconsistent data from observational studies and randomized trials)	↑101% increased risk	23 excess cases (46 vs. 23)	↑47% increased risk (n.s.)	15 excess cases (44 vs. 29)
Total mortality	Possible increase in risk among older women and women many years past menopause; possible decrease in risk or no effect in younger or recently menopausal women (p for trend by age <.05 for both trials combined)	No increase in risk	No difference in risk	No increase in risk[e]	No difference in risk[e]
Global index[g]	Probable increase in risk or no effect among older women and women many years past menopause; possible decrease in risk or no effect in younger or recently menopausal women (p for trend by age = 0.02 for estrogen alone)	↑12% increased risk	20.5 excess cases (189 vs. 168)	No increase in risk[e]	No difference in risk[e]

[a]The estrogen-progestin arm of the WHI assessed 5.6 years of conjugated equine estrogen (0.625 mg/d) plus medroxyprogesterone acetate (2.5 mg/d) versus placebo. The estrogen-alone arm of the WHI assessed 7.1 years of conjugated equine estrogen (0.625 mg/d) versus placebo.

[b]Number of cases per 10, 000 women per year.

[c]The WHI was not designed to assess the effect of HT on menopausal symptoms. Data from other randomized trials suggest that HT reduces risk for menopausal symptoms by 65–90%.

[d]*Coronary heart disease* is defined as nonfatal myocardial infarction or coronary death.

[e]There was a significant interaction by age; that is, the association between HT and the specified outcome was different in younger women and older women.

[f]This is the risk reduction that was observed during a cumulative 12-year follow-up period (5.6 years of treatment plus 6.8 years of postintervention observation).

[g]The *global index* is a composite outcome representing the first event for each participant from among the following: coronary heart disease, stroke, pulmonary embolism, breast cancer, colorectal cancer, endometrial cancer (estrogen-progestin arm only), hip fracture, and death. Because participants can experience more than one type of event, the global index cannot be derived by a simple summing of the component events.

[h]Includes some outcomes where results were divergent between the estrogen-progestin arm and the estrogen-alone arm.

Abbreviation: n.s., not statistically significant.

Source: Data from JE Manson et al: JAMA 310:1353, 2013.

Bone density

By reducing bone turnover and resorption rates, estrogen slows the aging-related bone loss experienced by most postmenopausal women. More than 50 randomized trials have demonstrated that postmenopausal estrogen therapy, with or without a progestogen, rapidly increases bone mineral density at the spine by 4–6% and at the hip by 2–3% and that those increases are maintained during treatment.

Fractures

Data from observational studies indicate a 50–80% lower risk of vertebral fracture and a 25–30% lower risk of hip, wrist, and other peripheral fractures among current estrogen users; addition of a progestogen does not appear to modify this benefit. In the WHI, 5–7 years of either combined estrogen-progestin or estrogen-only therapy was associated with a 33% reduction in hip fractures and 25–30% fewer total fractures among a population unselected for osteoporosis. Bisphosphonates (such as alendronate, 10 mg/d or 70 mg once per week; risedronate, 5 mg/d or 35 mg once per week; or ibandronate, 2.5 mg/d or 150 mg once per month or 3 mg every 3 months IV) and raloxifene (60 mg/d), a selective estrogen receptor modulator (SERM), have been shown in randomized trials to increase bone mass density and decrease fracture rates. Other options for treatment of osteoporosis are bazedoxifene in combination with conjugated estrogens and parathyroid hormone (teriparatide, 20 μg/d SC). These agents, unlike estrogen, do not appear to have adverse effects on the endometrium or breast. Increased physical activity, adequate calcium intake (1000–1200 mg/d through diet or supplements in two or three divided doses), and adequate vitamin D intake (600–1000 IU/d) may also reduce the risk of osteoporosis-related fractures. According to the Institute of Medicine's 2011 report, 25-hydroxyvitamin D blood levels of ≥50 nmol/L are sufficient for bone-density maintenance and fracture prevention. The Fracture Risk Assessment (FRAX®) score, an algorithm that combines an individual's bone-density score with age and other risk factors to predict her 10-year risk of hip and major osteoporotic fracture, may be of use in guiding decisions about pharmacologic treatment (see *www.shef.ac.uk/FRAX/*).

Definite risks

Endometrial cancer (with estrogen alone)

A combined analysis of 30 observational studies found a tripling of endometrial cancer risk among short-term users (1–5 years) of unopposed estrogen and a nearly tenfold increased risk among long-term users (≥10 years). These findings are supported by results from the randomized Postmenopausal Estrogen/Progestin Interventions (PEPI) trial, in which 24% of women assigned to unopposed estrogen for 3 years developed atypical endometrial hyperplasia—a premalignant lesion—as opposed to only 1% of women assigned to placebo. Use of a progestogen, which opposes the effects of estrogen on the endometrium, eliminates these risks and may even reduce risk (see later).

Venous thromboembolism

A meta-analysis of observational studies found that current oral estrogen use was associated with a 2.5-fold increase in risk of venous thromboembolism in postmenopausal women. A meta-analysis of randomized trials, including the WHI, found a 2.1-fold increase in risk. Results from the WHI indicate a nearly twofold increase in risk of pulmonary embolism and deep vein thrombosis with estrogen-progestin and a 35–50% increase in these risks with estrogen-only therapy. Transdermal estrogen, taken alone or with certain progestogens (micronized progesterone or pregnane derivatives), appears to be a safer alternative with respect to thrombotic risk.

Breast cancer (with estrogen-progestin)

An increased risk of breast cancer has been found among current or recent estrogen users in observational studies; this risk is directly related to duration of use. In a meta-analysis of 51 case-control and cohort studies, short-term use (<5 years) of postmenopausal HT did not appreciably elevate breast cancer incidence, whereas long-term use (≥5 years) was associated with a 35% increase in risk. In contrast to findings for endometrial cancer, combined estrogen-progestin regimens appear to increase breast cancer risk more than estrogen alone. Data from randomized trials also indicate that estrogen-progestin raises breast cancer risk. In the WHI, women assigned to receive combination hormones for an average of 5.6 years were 24% more likely to develop breast cancer than women assigned to placebo, but 7.1 years of estrogen-only therapy did not increase risk. Indeed, the WHI showed a trend toward a reduction in breast cancer risk with estrogen alone, although it is unclear whether this finding would pertain to formulations of estrogen other than conjugated equine estrogens or to treatment durations of >7 years. In the Heart and Estrogen/Progestin Replacement Study (HERS), 4 years of combination therapy was associated with a 27% increase in breast cancer risk. Although the latter finding was not statistically significant, the totality of evidence strongly implicates estrogen-progestin therapy in breast carcinogenesis.

Some observational data suggest that the length of the interval between menopause onset and HT initiation may influence the association between such therapy and breast cancer risk, with a "gap time" of <3–5 years conferring a higher HT-associated breast cancer risk. (This pattern of findings contrasts with that for

CHD, as discussed later in this chapter.) However, this association remains inconclusive and may be a spurious finding attributable to higher rates of screening mammography and thus earlier cancer detection in HT users than in nonusers, especially in early menopause. Indeed, in the WHI trial, hazard ratios for HT and breast cancer risk did not differ among women 50–59, those 60–69, and those 70–79 years of age at trial entry. (There was insufficient power to examine finer age categories.) Additional research is needed to clarify the issue.

Gallbladder disease

Large observational studies report a two- to threefold increased risk of gallstones or cholecystectomy among postmenopausal women taking oral estrogen. In the WHI, women randomized to estrogen-progestin or estrogen alone were ~55% more likely to develop gallbladder disease than those assigned to placebo. Risks were also increased in HERS. Transdermal HT might be a safer alternative, but further research is needed.

Probable or uncertain risks and benefits

Coronary heart disease/stroke

Until recently, HT had been enthusiastically recommended as a possible cardioprotective agent. In the past three decades, multiple observational studies suggested, in the aggregate, that estrogen use leads to a 35–50% reduction in CHD incidence among postmenopausal women. The biologic plausibility of such an association is supported by data from randomized trials demonstrating that exogenous estrogen lowers plasma low-density lipoprotein (LDL) cholesterol levels and raises high-density lipoprotein (HDL) cholesterol levels by 10–15%. Administration of estrogen also favorably affects lipoprotein(a) levels, LDL oxidation, endothelial vascular function, fibrinogen, and plasminogen activator inhibitor 1. However, estrogen therapy has unfavorable effects on other biomarkers of cardiovascular risk: it boosts triglyceride levels; promotes coagulation via factor VII, prothrombin fragments 1 and 2, and fibrinopeptide A elevations; and raises levels of the inflammatory marker C-reactive protein.

Randomized trials of estrogen or combined estrogen-progestin in women with preexisting cardiovascular disease have not confirmed the benefits reported in observational studies. In HERS (a secondary-prevention trial designed to test the efficacy and safety of estrogen-progestin therapy with regard to clinical cardiovascular outcomes), the 4-year incidence of coronary death and nonfatal myocardial infarction was similar in the active-treatment and placebo groups, and a 50% increase in risk of coronary events was noted during the first year among participants assigned to the active-treatment group. Although it is possible that progestin may mitigate estrogen's benefits, the Estrogen Replacement and Atherosclerosis (ERA) trial indicated that angiographically determined progression of coronary atherosclerosis was unaffected by either opposed or unopposed estrogen treatment. Moreover, no cardiovascular benefit was found in the Papworth Hormone Replacement Therapy Atherosclerosis Study, a trial of transdermal estradiol with and without norethindrone; the Women's Estrogen for Stroke Trial (WEST), a trial of oral 17β-estradiol; or the Estrogen in the Prevention of Reinfarction Trial (ESPRIT), a trial of oral estradiol valerate. Thus, in clinical trials, HT has not proved effective for the secondary prevention of cardiovascular disease in postmenopausal women.

Primary-prevention trials also suggest an early increase in cardiovascular risk and an absence of cardioprotection with postmenopausal HT. In the WHI, women assigned to 5.6 years of estrogen-progestin therapy were 18% more likely to develop CHD (defined in primary analyses as nonfatal myocardial infarction or coronary death) than those assigned to placebo, although this risk elevation was not statistically significant. However, during the trial's first year, there was a significant 80% increase in risk, which diminished in subsequent years (p for trend by time = .03). In the estrogen-only arm of the WHI, no overall effect on CHD was observed during the 7.1 years of the trial or in any specific year of follow-up. This pattern of results was similar to that for the outcome of total myocardial infarction.

However, a closer look at available data suggests that timing of initiation of HT may critically influence the association between such therapy and CHD. Estrogen may slow early stages of atherosclerosis but have adverse effects on advanced atherosclerotic lesions. It has been hypothesized that the prothrombotic and proinflammatory effects of estrogen manifest themselves predominantly among women with subclinical lesions who initiate HT well after the menopausal transition, whereas women with less arterial damage who start HT early in menopause may derive cardiovascular benefit because they have not yet developed advanced lesions. Nonhuman primate data support this concept. Conjugated estrogens had no effect on the extent of coronary artery plaque in cynomolgus monkeys assigned to receive estrogen alone or combined with progestin starting 2 years (~6 years in human terms) after oophorectomy and well after the establishment of atherosclerosis. However, administration of exogenous hormones immediately after oophorectomy, during the early stages of atherosclerosis, reduced the extent of plaque by 70%.

Lending further credence to this hypothesis are results of subgroup analyses of observational and clinical trial data. For example, among women who entered the WHI trial with a relatively favorable cholesterol profile, estrogen with or without progestin led to a 40% lower risk of incident CHD. Among women who entered with a worse cholesterol profile, therapy resulted in a 73% higher risk (p for interaction = .02). The presence or absence of the metabolic syndrome **(Chap. 22)** also strongly influenced the relation between HT and incident CHD. Among women with the metabolic syndrome, HT more than doubled CHD risk, whereas no association was observed among women without the syndrome. Moreover, although there was no association between estrogen-only therapy and CHD in the WHI trial cohort as a whole, such therapy was associated with a CHD risk reduction of 40% among participants age 50–59; in contrast, a risk reduction of only 5% was observed among those age 60–69, and a risk increase of 9% was found among those age 70–79 (p for trend by age = .08). For the outcome of total myocardial infarction, estrogen alone was associated with a borderline-significant 45% reduction and a nonsignificant 24% increase in risk among the youngest and oldest women, respectively (p for trend by age = .02). Estrogen was also associated with lower levels of coronary artery calcified plaque in the younger age group. Although age did not have a similar effect in the estrogen-progestin arm of the WHI, CHD risks increased with years since menopause (p for trend = .08), with a significantly elevated risk among women who were ≥20 years past menopause. For the outcome of total myocardial infarction, estrogen-progestin was associated with a 9% risk reduction among women <10 years past menopause as opposed to a 16% increase in risk among women 10–19 years past menopause and a twofold increase in risk among women >20 years past menopause (p for trend = .01). In the large observational Nurses' Health Study, women who chose to start HT within 4 years of menopause experienced a lower risk of CHD than did nonusers, whereas those who began therapy ≥10 years after menopause appeared to receive little coronary benefit. Observational studies include a high proportion of women who begin HT within 3–4 years of menopause, whereas clinical trials include a high proportion of women ≥12 years past menopause; this difference helps to reconcile some of the apparent discrepancies between the two types of studies.

For the outcome of stroke, WHI participants assigned to estrogen-progestin or estrogen alone were ~35% more likely to suffer a stroke than those assigned to placebo. Whether or not age at initiation of HT influences stroke risk is not well understood. In the WHI and the Nurses' Health Study, HT was associated with an excess risk of stroke in all age groups. Further research is needed on age, time since menopause, and other individual characteristics (including biomarkers) that predict increases or decreases in cardiovascular risk associated with exogenous HT. Furthermore, it remains uncertain whether different doses, formulations, or routes of administration of HT will produce different cardiovascular effects.

Colorectal cancer

Observational studies have suggested that HT reduces risks of colon and rectal cancer, although the estimated magnitudes of the relative benefits have ranged from 8% to 34% in various meta-analyses. In the WHI (the sole trial to examine the issue), estrogen-progestin was associated with a significant 38% reduction in colorectal cancer over a 5.6-year period, although no benefit was seen with 7 years of estrogen-only therapy. However, a modifying effect of age was observed, with a doubling of risk with HT in women age 70–79 but no risk elevation in younger women (p for trend by age = .02).

Cognitive decline and dementia

A meta-analysis of 10 case-control and two cohort studies suggested that postmenopausal HT is associated with a 34% decreased risk of dementia. Subsequent randomized trials (including the WHI), however, have failed to demonstrate any benefit of estrogen or estrogen-progestin therapy on the progression of mild to moderate Alzheimer's disease and/or have indicated a potential adverse effect of HT on the incidence of dementia, at least in women ≥65 years of age. Among women randomized to HT (as opposed to placebo) at age 50–55 in the WHI, no effect on cognition was observed during the postintervention phase. Determining whether timing of initiation of HT influences cognitive outcomes will require further study.

Ovarian cancer and other disorders

On the basis of limited observational and randomized data, it has been hypothesized that HT increases the risk of ovarian cancer and reduces the risk of type 2 diabetes mellitus. Results from the WHI support these hypotheses. The WHI also found that HT use was associated with an increased risk of urinary incontinence and that estrogen-progestin was associated with increased rates of lung cancer mortality.

Endometrial cancer (with estrogen-progestin)

In the WHI, use of estrogen-progestin was associated with a nonsignificant 17% reduction in risk of endometrial cancer. A significant reduction in risk emerged during the postintervention period (see later).

All-cause mortality

In the overall WHI cohort, estrogen with or without progestin was not associated with all-cause mortality. However, there was a trend toward reduced mortality in younger women, particularly with estrogen alone. For women 50–59, 60–69, and 70–79 years of age, relative risks (RRs) associated with estrogen-only therapy were 0.70, 1.01, and 1.21, respectively (p for trend = .04).

Overall benefit-risk profile

Estrogen-progestin was associated with an unfavorable benefit-risk profile (excluding relief from menopausal symptoms) as measured by a "global index"—a composite outcome including CHD, stroke, pulmonary embolism, breast cancer, colorectal cancer, endometrial cancer, hip fracture, and death (Table 16-1)—in the WHI cohort as a whole, and this association did not vary by 10-year age group. Estrogen-only therapy was associated with a neutral benefit-risk profile in the WHI cohort as a whole. However, there was a significant trend toward a more favorable benefit-risk profile among younger women and a less favorable profile among older women, with RRs of 0.84, 0.99, and 1.17 for women 50–59, 60–69, and 70–79 years of age, respectively (p for trend by age = .02).

Changes in health status after discontinuation of hormone therapy

In the WHI, many but not all risks and benefits associated with active use of HT dissipated within 5–7 years after discontinuation of therapy. For estrogen-progestin, an elevated risk of breast cancer persisted (RR = 1.28 [95% confidence interval, 1.11–1.48]) during a cumulative 12-year follow-up period (5.6 years of treatment plus 6.8 years of postintervention observation), but most cardiovascular disease risks became neutral. A reduction in hip fracture risk persisted (RR = 0.81 [0.68–0.97]), and a significant reduction in endometrial cancer risk emerged (RR = 0.67 [0.49–0.91]). For estrogen alone, the reduction in breast cancer risk became statistically significant (RR = 0.79 [0.65–0.97]) during a cumulative 12-year follow-up period (6.8 years of treatment plus 5.1 years of postintervention observation), and significant differences by age group persisted for total myocardial infarction and the global index, with more favorable results for younger women.

APPROACH TO THE PATIENT: Postmenopausal Hormone Therapy

The rational use of postmenopausal HT requires balancing the potential benefits and risks. Figure 16-3 provides one approach to decision making. The clinician should first determine whether the patient has moderate to severe menopausal symptoms—the primary indication for initiation of systemic HT. Systemic HT may also be used to prevent osteoporosis in women at high risk of fracture who cannot tolerate alternative osteoporosis therapies. (Vaginal estrogen or other medications may be used to treat urogenital symptoms in the absence of vasomotor symptoms.) The benefits and risks of such therapy should be reviewed with the patient, giving more emphasis to absolute than to relative measures of effect and pointing out uncertainties in clinical knowledge where relevant. Because chronic disease rates generally increase with age, absolute risks tend to be greater in older women, even when relative risks remain similar. Potential side effects—especially vaginal bleeding that may result from use of the combined estrogen-progestogen formulations recommended for women with an intact uterus—should be noted. The patient's own preference regarding therapy should be elicited and factored into the decision. Contraindications to HT should be assessed routinely and include unexplained vaginal bleeding, active liver disease, venous thromboembolism, history of endometrial cancer (except stage 1 without deep invasion) or breast cancer, and history of CHD, stroke, transient ischemic attack, or diabetes. Relative contraindications include hypertriglyceridemia (>400 mg/dL) and active gallbladder disease; in such cases, transdermal estrogen may be an option. Primary prevention of heart disease should not be viewed as an expected benefit of HT, and an increase in the risk of stroke as well as a small early increase in the risk of coronary artery disease should be considered. Nevertheless, such therapy may be appropriate if the noncoronary benefits of treatment clearly outweigh the risks. A woman who suffers an acute coronary event or stroke while taking HT should discontinue therapy immediately.

Short-term use (<5 years for estrogen-progestogen and <7 years for estrogen alone) is appropriate for relief of menopausal symptoms among women without contraindications to such use. However, such therapy should be avoided by women with an elevated baseline risk of future cardiovascular events. Women who have contraindications for or are opposed to HT may derive benefit from the use of certain antidepressants (including venlafaxine, fluoxetine, or paroxetine), gabapentin, clonidine, soy, or black cohosh and, for genitourinary symptoms, intravaginal estrogen creams or devices, or ospemifene.

Long-term use (≥5 years for estrogen-progestogen and ≥7 years for estrogen alone) is more problematic because a heightened risk of breast cancer must be factored into the decision, especially for estrogen-progestogen. Reasonable candidates for such use include the small percentage of postmenopausal women who have persistent severe vasomotor symptoms along with an increased risk of osteoporosis (e.g., those with osteopenia, a personal or family history of nontraumatic fracture, or a weight below 125 lbs), who also have no personal or family history of breast cancer in a first-degree relative or other contraindications, and who have a strong personal preference for therapy.

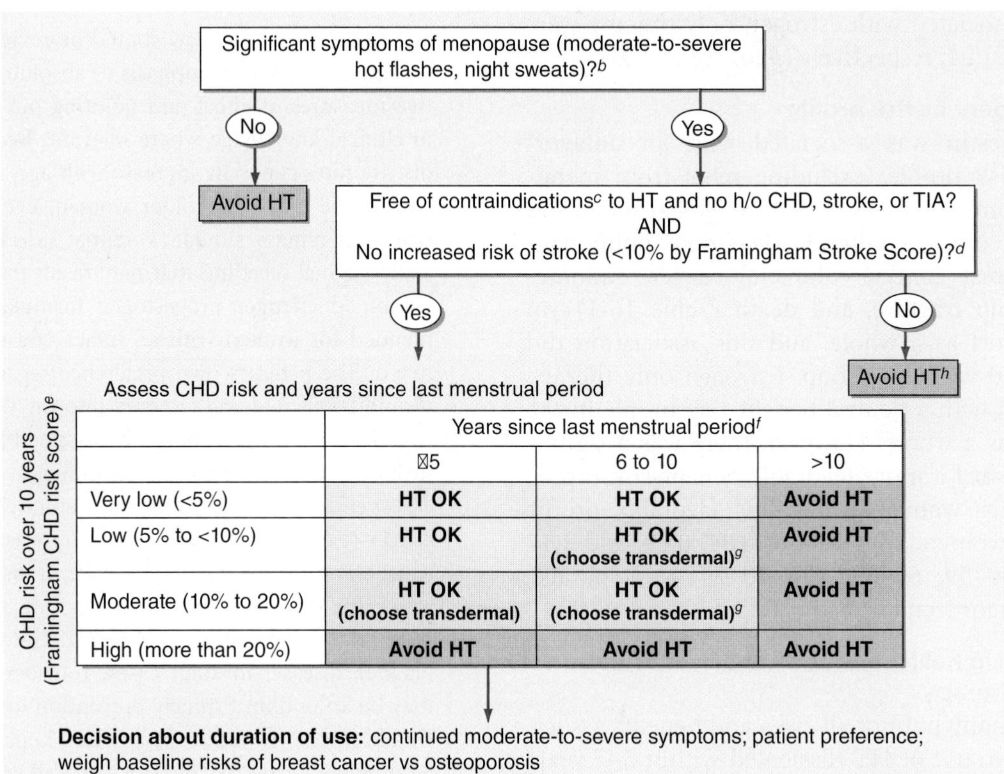

CHD risk over 10 years (Framingham CHD risk score)[e]	Years since last menstrual period[f]		
	≤5	6 to 10	>10
Very low (<5%)	**HT OK**	**HT OK**	**Avoid HT**
Low (5% to <10%)	**HT OK**	**HT OK (choose transdermal)[g]**	**Avoid HT**
Moderate (10% to 20%)	**HT OK (choose transdermal)**	**HT OK (choose transdermal)[g]**	**Avoid HT**
High (more than 20%)	**Avoid HT**	**Avoid HT**	**Avoid HT**

FIGURE 16-3

Chart for identifying appropriate candidates for postmenopausal hormone therapy (HT).

[a]Reassess each step at least once every 6–12 months (assuming the patient's continued preference for HT). [b]Women who are at high risk of osteoporotic fracture but are unable to tolerate alternative preventive medications may also be reasonable candidates for systemic HT even if they do not have moderate to severe vasomotor symptoms. Women who have vaginal dryness without moderate to severe vasomotor symptoms may be candidates for vaginal estrogen. [c]Traditional contraindications are unexplained vaginal bleeding; active liver disease; history of venous thromboembolism due to pregnancy, oral contraceptive use, or an unknown etiology; blood-clotting disorder; history of breast or endometrial cancer; and diabetes. Oral HT should be avoided but transdermal HT may be an option (see *g* below) for other contraindications, including high triglyceride levels (>400 mg/dL); active gallbladder disease; and history of venous thromboembolism due to past immobility, surgery, or bone fracture. [d]Ten-year risk of stroke, based on Framingham Stroke Risk Score (RB *D'Agostino et al: Stroke risk profile: Adjustment for antihypertensive medication. The Framingham Study. Stroke 25:40, 1994*), as modified by JE Manson, SS Bassuk: *Hot Flashes, Hormones & Your Health*. New York, McGraw-Hill, 2007. [e]Ten-year risk of CHD, based on Framingham Coronary Heart Disease Risk Score (*Expert Panel on Detection, Evaluation, and Treatment of High Blood Cholesterol in Adults: JAMA 285:2486, 2001*), as modified by JE Manson, SS Bassuk: *Hot Flashes, Hormones & Your Health*. New York, McGraw-Hill, 2007. [f]Women >10 years past menopause are not good candidates for initiation (first use) of HT. [g]Avoid oral HT. Transdermal HT may be an option because it has a less adverse effect on clotting factors, triglyceride levels, and inflammation factors than oral HT. [h]Consider selective serotonin or serotonin–norepinephrine reuptake inhibitor, gabapentin, clonidine, soy, or another alternative.

Abbreviations: CHD, coronary heart disease; h/o, history of; TIA, transient ischemic attack. *(Adapted from JE Manson, SS Bassuk: Hot Flashes, Hormones & Your Health. New York, McGraw-Hill, 2007. Copyright © 2007 by the President and Fellows of Harvard College. All rights reserved.)*

Poor candidates are women with elevated cardiovascular risk, those at increased risk of breast cancer (e.g., women who have a first-degree relative with breast cancer, susceptibility genes such as *BRCA1* or *BRCA2*, or a personal history of cellular atypia detected by breast biopsy), and those at low risk of osteoporosis. Even for reasonable candidates, strategies to minimize dose and duration of use should be employed. For example, women using HT to relieve intense vasomotor symptoms in early postmenopause should consider discontinuing therapy within 5 years, resuming it only if such symptoms persist. Because of the role of progestogens in increasing breast cancer risk, regimens that employ cyclic rather than continuous progestogen exposure as well as formulations other than medroxyprogesterone acetate should be considered if treatment is extended. For prevention of osteoporosis, alternative therapies such as bisphosphonates or SERMs should be considered. Research on alternative progestogens and androgen-containing preparations has been limited, particularly with respect to long-term safety. Additional research on the effects of these agents on cardiovascular disease, glucose tolerance, and breast cancer will be of particular interest.

In addition to HT, lifestyle choices such as smoking abstention, adequate physical activity, and a healthy diet can play a role in controlling symptoms and preventing chronic disease. An expanding array of pharmacologic options (e.g., bisphosphonates, SERMs, and other agents for osteoporosis; cholesterol-lowering or antihypertensive agents for cardiovascular disease) should also reduce the widespread reliance on hormone use. However, short-term HT may still benefit some women.

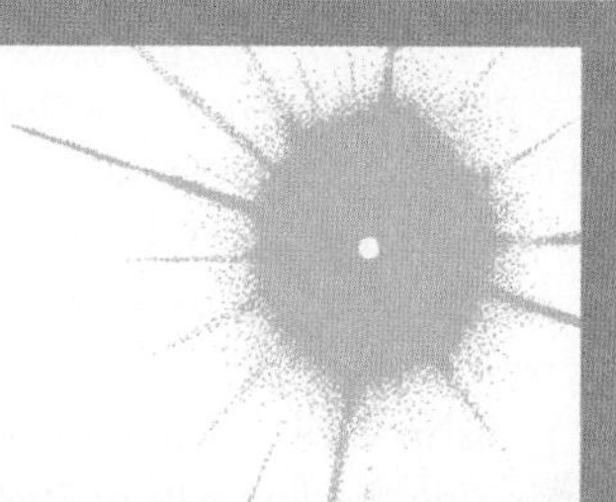

CHAPTER 17
HIRSUTISM

David A. Ehrmann

Hirsutism, which is defined as androgen-dependent excessive male-pattern hair growth, affects approximately 10% of women. Hirsutism is most often idiopathic or the consequence of androgen excess associated with the polycystic ovarian syndrome (PCOS). Less frequently, it may result from adrenal androgen overproduction as occurs in nonclassic congenital adrenal hyperplasia (CAH) (Table 17-1). Rarely, it is a sign of a serious underlying condition. Cutaneous manifestations commonly associated with hirsutism include acne and male-pattern balding (androgenic alopecia). *Virilization* refers to a condition in which androgen levels are sufficiently high to cause additional signs and symptoms, such as deepening of the voice, breast atrophy, increased muscle bulk, clitoromegaly, and increased libido; virilization is an ominous sign that suggests the possibility of an ovarian or adrenal neoplasm.

HAIR FOLLICLE GROWTH AND DIFFERENTIATION

Hair can be categorized as either *vellus* (fine, soft, and not pigmented) or *terminal* (long, coarse, and pigmented). The number of hair follicles does not change over an individual's lifetime, but the follicle size and type of hair can change in response to numerous factors, particularly androgens. Androgens are necessary for terminal hair and sebaceous gland development and mediate differentiation of pilosebaceous units (PSUs) into either a terminal hair follicle or a sebaceous gland. In the former case, androgens transform the vellus hair into a terminal hair; in the latter case, the sebaceous component proliferates and the hair remains vellus.

There are three phases in the cycle of hair growth: (1) *anagen* (growth phase), (2) *catagen* (involution phase), and (3) *telogen* (rest phase). Depending on the body site, hormonal regulation may play an important role in the hair growth cycle. For example, the eyebrows, eyelashes, and vellus hairs are androgen-insensitive, whereas the axillary and pubic areas are sensitive to low levels of androgens. Hair growth on the face, chest, upper abdomen, and back requires higher levels of androgens and is therefore more characteristic of the pattern typically seen in men. Androgen excess in women leads to increased hair growth in most androgen-sensitive sites except in the scalp region, where hair loss occurs because androgens cause scalp hairs to spend less time in the anagen phase.

Although androgen excess underlies most cases of hirsutism, there is only a modest correlation between androgen levels and the quantity of hair growth. This is due to the fact that hair growth from the follicle also depends on local growth factors, and there is variability in end organ (PSU) sensitivity. Genetic factors and ethnic background also influence hair growth. In general, dark-haired individuals tend to be more hirsute than blond or fair individuals. Asians and Native Americans have relatively sparse hair in regions sensitive to high androgen levels, whereas people of Mediterranean descent are more hirsute.

CLINICAL ASSESSMENT

Historic elements relevant to the assessment of hirsutism include the age at onset and rate of progression of hair growth and associated symptoms or signs (e.g., acne). Depending on the cause, excess hair growth typically is first noted during the second and third decades of life. The growth is usually slow but progressive. Sudden development and rapid progression of hirsutism suggest the possibility of an androgen-secreting neoplasm, in which case virilization also may be present.

The age at onset of menstrual cycles (menarche) and the pattern of the menstrual cycle should be ascertained; irregular cycles from the time of menarche onward are more likely to result from ovarian rather than adrenal androgen excess. Associated symptoms

TABLE 17-1

CAUSES OF HIRSUTISM
Gonadal hyperandrogenism
Ovarian hyperandrogenism
Polycystic ovary syndrome/functional ovarian hyperandrogenism
Ovarian steroidogenic blocks
Syndromes of extreme insulin resistance (e.g., lipodystrophy)
Ovarian neoplasms
Adrenal hyperandrogenism
Premature adrenarche
Functional adrenal hyperandrogenism
Congenital adrenal hyperplasia (nonclassic and classic)
Abnormal cortisol action/metabolism
Adrenal neoplasms
Other endocrine disorders
Cushing's syndrome
Hyperprolactinemia
Acromegaly
Peripheral androgen overproduction
Obesity
Idiopathic
Pregnancy-related hyperandrogenism
Hyperreactio luteinalis
Thecoma of pregnancy
Drugs
Androgens
Oral contraceptives containing androgenic progestins
Minoxidil
Phenytoin
Diazoxide
Cyclosporine
True hermaphroditism

such as galactorrhea should prompt evaluation for hyperprolactinemia **(Chap. 5)** and possibly hypothyroidism **(Chap. 7)**. Hypertension, striae, easy bruising, centripetal weight gain, and weakness suggest hypercortisolism (Cushing's syndrome; **Chap. 8**). Rarely, patients with growth hormone excess (i.e., acromegaly) present with hirsutism. Use of medications such as phenytoin, minoxidil, and cyclosporine may be associated with androgen-independent excess hair growth (i.e., hypertrichosis). A family history of infertility and/or hirsutism may indicate disorders such as nonclassic CAH **(Chap. 8)**. Lipodystrophy is often associated with increased ovarian androgen production that occurs as a consequence of insulin resistance. Patients with lipodystrophy have a preponderance of central fat distribution together with scant subcutaneous adipose tissue in the upper and lower extremities.

Physical examination should include measurement of height and weight and calculation of body mass index (BMI). A BMI >25 kg/m^2 is indicative of excess weight for height, and values >30 kg/m^2 are often seen in association with hirsutism, probably the result of increased conversion of androgen precursors to testosterone. Notation should be made of blood pressure, as adrenal causes may be associated with hypertension. Cutaneous signs sometimes associated with androgen excess and insulin resistance include acanthosis nigricans and skin tags. Body fat distribution should also be noted.

An objective clinical assessment of hair distribution and quantity is central to the evaluation in any woman presenting with hirsutism. This assessment permits the distinction between hirsutism and hypertrichosis and provides a baseline reference point to gauge the response to treatment. A simple and commonly used method to grade hair growth is the modified scale of Ferriman and Gallwey (Fig. 17-1), in which each of nine androgen-sensitive sites is graded from 0 to 4. Approximately 95% of white women have a score below 8 on this scale; thus, it is normal for most women to have some hair growth in androgen-sensitive sites. Scores above 8 suggest excess androgen-mediated hair growth, a finding that should be assessed further by means of hormonal evaluation (see below). In racial/ethnic groups that are less likely to manifest hirsutism (e.g., Asian women), additional cutaneous evidence of androgen excess should be sought, including pustular acne and thinning scalp hair.

HORMONAL EVALUATION

Androgens are secreted by the ovaries and adrenal glands in response to their respective tropic hormones: luteinizing hormone (LH) and adrenocorticotropic hormone (ACTH). The principal circulating steroids involved in the etiology of hirsutism are testosterone, androstenedione, and dehydroepiandrosterone (DHEA) and its sulfated form (DHEAS). The ovaries and adrenal glands normally contribute about equally to testosterone production. Approximately half of the total testosterone originates from direct glandular secretion, and the remainder is derived from the peripheral conversion of androstenedione and DHEA **(Chap. 11)**.

Although it is the most important circulating androgen, testosterone is in effect the penultimate androgen in mediating hirsutism; it is converted to the more potent dihydrotestosterone (DHT) by the enzyme 5α-reductase, which is located in the PSU. DHT has a higher affinity for, and slower dissociation from, the androgen receptor. The local production of DHT

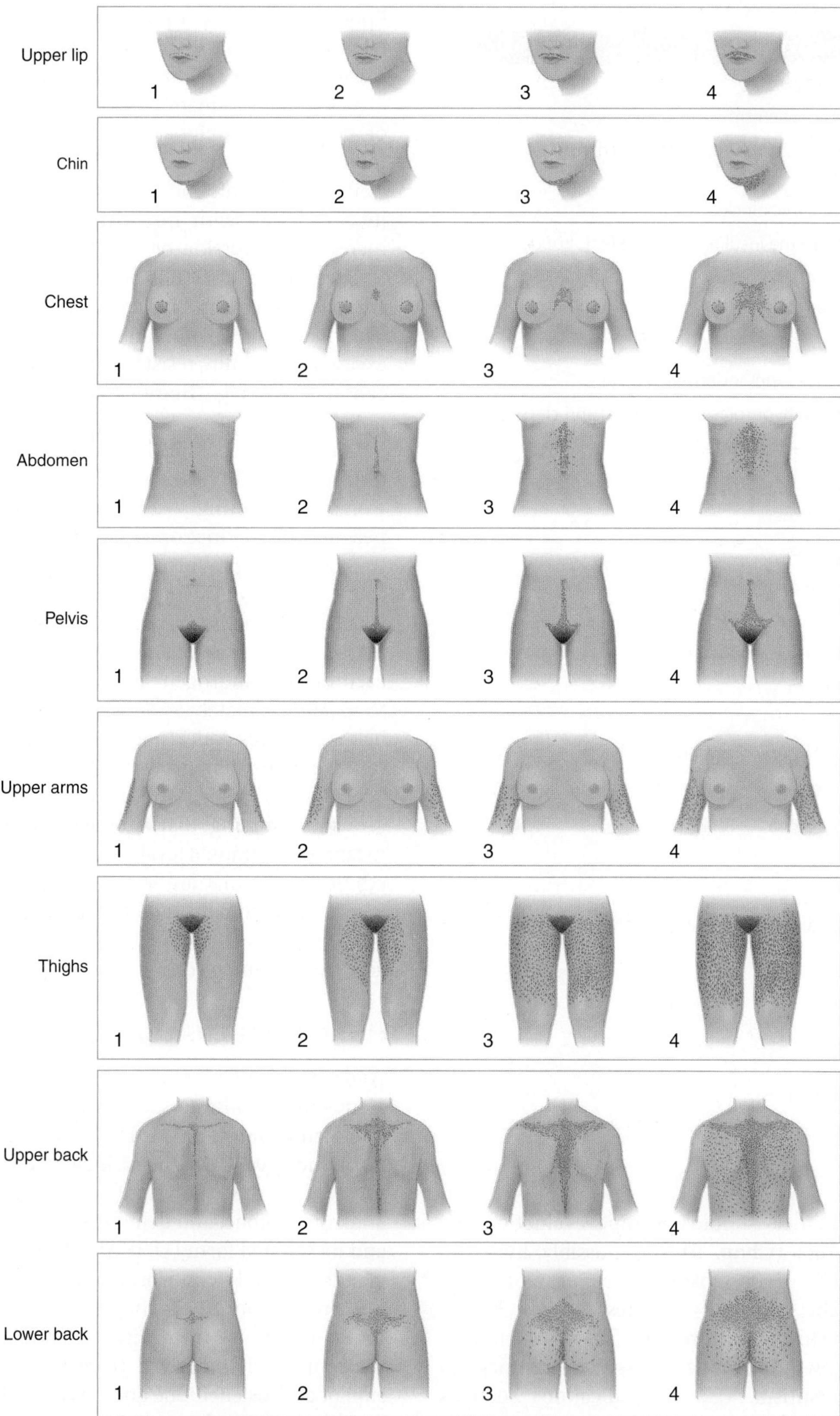

FIGURE 17-1

Hirsutism scoring scale of Ferriman and Gallwey. The nine body areas that have androgen-sensitive areas are graded from 0 (no terminal hair) to 4 (frankly virile) to obtain a total score. A normal hirsutism score is <8. *(Modified from DA Ehrmann et al: Hyperandrogenism, hirsutism, and polycystic ovary syndrome, in LJ DeGroot and JL Jameson [eds], Endocrinology, 5th ed. Philadelphia, Saunders, 2006; with permission.)*

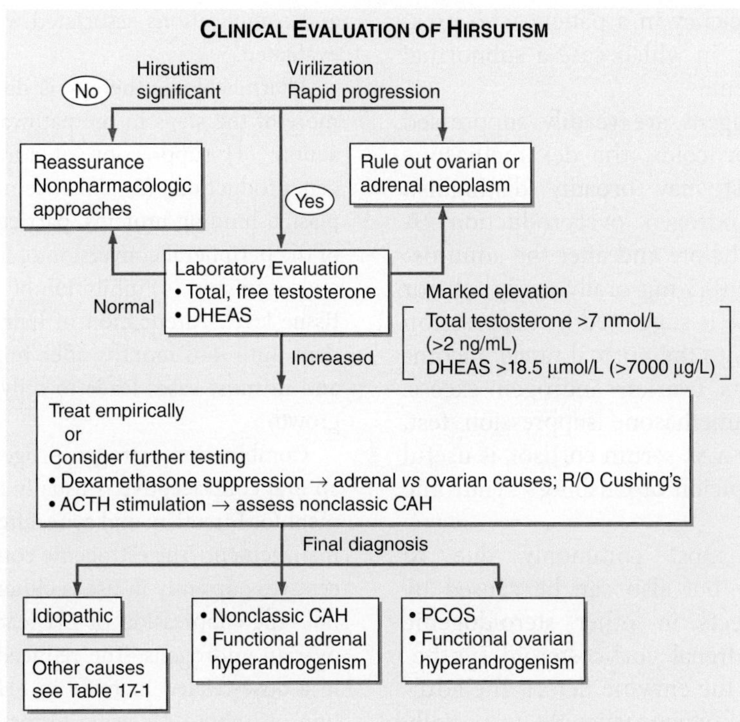

FIGURE 17-2

Algorithm for the evaluation and differential diagnosis of hirsutism. ACTH, adrenocorticotropic hormone; CAH, congenital adrenal hyperplasia; DHEAS, sulfated form of dehydroepiandrosterone; PCOS, polycystic ovarian syndrome.

allows it to serve as the primary mediator of androgen action at the level of the pilosebaceous unit. There are two isoenzymes of 5α-reductase: Type 2 is found in the prostate gland and in hair follicles, and type 1 is found primarily in sebaceous glands.

One approach to the evaluation of hirsutism is depicted in Fig. 17-2. In addition to measuring blood levels of testosterone and DHEAS, it is important to measure the level of free (or unbound) testosterone. The fraction of testosterone that is not bound to its carrier protein, sex hormone–binding globulin (SHBG), is biologically available for conversion to DHT and binding to androgen receptors. Hyperinsulinemia and/or androgen excess decrease hepatic production of SHBG, resulting in levels of total testosterone within the high-normal range, whereas the unbound hormone is elevated more substantially. Although there is a decline in ovarian testosterone production after menopause, ovarian estrogen production decreases to an even greater extent, and the concentration of SHBG is reduced. Consequently, there is an increase in the relative proportion of unbound testosterone, and it may exacerbate hirsutism after menopause.

A baseline plasma total testosterone level >12 nmol/L (>3.5 ng/mL) usually indicates a virilizing tumor, whereas a level >7 nmol/L (>2 ng/mL) is suggestive. A basal DHEAS level >18.5 μmol/L (>7000 μg/L) suggests an adrenal tumor. Although DHEAS has been proposed as a "marker" of predominant adrenal androgen excess, it is not unusual to find modest elevations in DHEAS among women with PCOS. Computed tomography (CT) or magnetic resonance imaging (MRI) should be used to localize an adrenal mass, and transvaginal ultrasound usually suffices to identify an ovarian mass if clinical evaluation and hormonal levels suggest these possibilities.

PCOS is the most common cause of ovarian androgen excess **(Chap. 13)**. An increased ratio of LH to follicle-stimulating hormone (FSH) is characteristic in carefully studied patients with PCOS. However, because of the pulsatile nature of gonadotropin secretion, this finding may be absent in up to half of women with PCOS. Therefore, measurement of plasma LH and FSH is not needed to make a diagnosis of PCOS. Transvaginal ultrasound classically shows enlarged ovaries and increased stroma in women with PCOS. However, cystic ovaries also may be found in women without clinical or laboratory features of PCOS.

It has been suggested that the measurement of circulating levels of antimüllerian hormone (AMH) may help in making the diagnosis of PCOS; however, this remains controversial. AMH levels reflect ovarian reserve and correlate with follicular number. Measurement of AMH can be useful when considering premature ovarian insufficiency in a patient who presents with oligomenorrhea, in which case a subnormal level of AMH will be present.

Because adrenal androgens are readily suppressed by low doses of glucocorticoids, the dexamethasone androgen-suppression test may broadly distinguish ovarian from adrenal androgen overproduction. A blood sample is obtained before and after the administration of dexamethasone (0.5 mg orally every 6 h for 4 days). An adrenal source is suggested by suppression of unbound testosterone into the normal range; incomplete suppression suggests ovarian androgen excess. An overnight 1-mg dexamethasone suppression test, with measurement of 8:00 A.M. serum cortisol, is useful when there is clinical suspicion of Cushing's syndrome **(Chap. 8)**.

Nonclassic CAH is most commonly due to 21-hydroxylase deficiency but also can be caused by autosomal recessive defects in other steroidogenic enzymes necessary for adrenal corticosteroid synthesis **(Chap. 8)**. Because of the enzyme defect, the adrenal gland cannot secrete glucocorticoids (especially cortisol) efficiently. This results in diminished negative feedback inhibition of ACTH, leading to compensatory adrenal hyperplasia and the accumulation of steroid precursors that subsequently are converted to androgen. Deficiency of 21-hydroxylase can be reliably excluded by determining a morning 17-hydroxyprogesterone level <6 nmol/L (<2 μg/L) (drawn in the follicular phase). Alternatively, 21-hydroxylase deficiency can be diagnosed by measurement of 17-hydroxyprogesterone 1 h after the administration of 250 μg of synthetic ACTH (cosyntropin) intravenously.

TREATMENT Hirsutism

Treatment of hirsutism may be accomplished pharmacologically or by mechanical means of hair removal. Nonpharmacologic treatments should be considered in all patients either as the only treatment or as an adjunct to drug therapy.

Nonpharmacologic treatments include (1) bleaching; (2) depilatory (removal from the skin surface), such as shaving and chemical treatments; and (3) epilatory (removal of the hair including the root), such as plucking, waxing, electrolysis, and laser therapy. Despite perceptions to the contrary, shaving does not increase the rate or density of hair growth. Chemical depilatory treatments may be useful for mild hirsutism that affects only limited skin areas, though they can cause skin irritation. Wax treatment removes hair temporarily but is uncomfortable. Electrolysis is effective for more permanent hair removal, particularly in the hands of a skilled electrologist. Laser phototherapy appears to be efficacious for hair removal. It delays hair regrowth and causes permanent hair removal in most patients. The long-term effects and complications associated with laser treatment are being evaluated.

Pharmacologic therapy is directed at interrupting one or more of the steps in the pathway of androgen synthesis and action: (1) suppression of adrenal and/or ovarian androgen production; (2) enhancement of androgen-binding to plasma-binding proteins, particularly SHBG; (3) impairment of the peripheral conversion of androgen precursors to active androgen; and (4) inhibition of androgen action at the target tissue level. Attenuation of hair growth is typically not evident until 4–6 months after initiation of medical treatment and in most cases leads to only a modest reduction in hair growth.

Combination estrogen-progestin therapy in the form of an oral contraceptive is usually the first-line endocrine treatment for hirsutism and acne, after cosmetic and dermatologic management. The estrogenic component of most oral contraceptives currently in use is either ethinyl estradiol or mestranol. The suppression of LH leads to reduced production of ovarian androgens. The reduced androgen levels also result in a dose-related increase in SHBG, thus lowering the fraction of unbound plasma testosterone. Combination therapy also has been demonstrated to decrease DHEAS, perhaps by reducing ACTH levels. Estrogens also have a direct, dose-dependent suppressive effect on sebaceous cell function.

The choice of a specific oral contraceptive should be predicated on the progestational component, as progestins vary in their suppressive effect on SHBG levels and in their androgenic potential. Ethynodiol diacetate has relatively low androgenic potential, whereas progestins such as norgestrel and levonorgestrel are particularly androgenic, as judged from their attenuation of the estrogen-induced increase in SHBG. Norgestimate exemplifies the newer generation of progestins that are virtually nonandrogenic. Drospirenone, an analogue of spironolactone that has both antimineralocorticoid and antiandrogenic activities, has been approved for use as a progestational agent in combination with ethinyl estradiol.

Oral contraceptives are contraindicated in women with a history of thromboembolic disease and women with increased risk of breast or other estrogen-dependent cancers **(Chap. 16)**. There is a relative contraindication to the use of oral contraceptives in smokers and those with hypertension or a history of migraine headaches. In most trials, estrogen-progestin therapy alone improves the extent of acne by a maximum of 50–70%. The effect on hair growth may not be evident for 6 months, and the maximum effect may require 9–12 months owing to the length of the hair growth cycle. Improvements in hirsutism are typically in the range of 20%, but there may be an arrest of further progression of hair growth.

Adrenal androgens are more sensitive than cortisol to the suppressive effects of glucocorticoids. Therefore, glucocorticoids are the mainstay of treatment in patients with CAH. Although glucocorticoids have been reported to restore ovulatory function in some women with PCOS, this effect is highly variable. Because of side effects from excessive glucocorticoids, low doses should be used. Dexamethasone (0.2–0.5 mg) or prednisone (5–10 mg) should be taken at bedtime to achieve maximal suppression by inhibiting the nocturnal surge of ACTH.

Cyproterone acetate is the prototypic antiandrogen. It acts mainly by competitive inhibition of the binding of testosterone and DHT to the androgen receptor. In addition, it may enhance the metabolic clearance of testosterone by inducing hepatic enzymes. Although not available for use in the United States, cyproterone acetate is widely used in Canada, Mexico, and Europe. Cyproterone (50–100 mg) is given on days 1–15 and ethinyl estradiol (50 μg) is given on days 5–26 of the menstrual cycle. Side effects include irregular uterine bleeding, nausea, headache, fatigue, weight gain, and decreased libido.

Spironolactone, which usually is used as a mineralocorticoid antagonist, is also a weak antiandrogen. It is almost as effective as cyproterone acetate when used at high enough doses (100–200 mg daily). Patients should be monitored intermittently for hyperkalemia or hypotension, although these side effects are uncommon. Pregnancy should be avoided because of the risk of feminization of a male fetus. Spironolactone can also cause menstrual irregularity. It often is used in combination with an oral contraceptive, which suppresses ovarian androgen production and helps prevent pregnancy.

Flutamide is a potent nonsteroidal antiandrogen that is effective in treating hirsutism, but concerns about the induction of hepatocellular dysfunction have limited its use. Finasteride is a competitive inhibitor of 5α-reductase type 2. Beneficial effects on hirsutism have been reported, but the predominance of 5α-reductase type 1 in the PSU appears to account for its limited efficacy. Finasteride would also be expected to impair sexual differentiation in a male fetus, and it should not be used in women who may become pregnant.

Eflornithine cream (Vaniqa) has been approved as a novel treatment for unwanted facial hair in women, but long-term efficacy remains to be established. It can cause skin irritation under exaggerated conditions of use. Ultimately, the choice of any specific agent(s) must be tailored to the unique needs of the patient being treated. As noted previously, pharmacologic treatments for hirsutism should be used in conjunction with nonpharmacologic approaches. It is also helpful to review the pattern of female hair distribution in the normal population to dispel unrealistic expectations.

CHAPTER 18
GYNECOLOGIC MALIGNANCIES

Michael V. Seiden

OVARIAN CANCER

INCIDENCE AND PATHOLOGY

Cancer arising in or near the ovary is actually a collection of diverse malignancies. This collection of malignancies, often referred to as "ovary cancer," is the most lethal gynecologic malignancy in the United States and other countries that routinely screen women for cervical neoplasia. In 2014, it was estimated that there were 21,980 cases of ovarian cancer with 14,270 deaths in the United States. The ovary is a complex and dynamic organ and, between the ages of approximately 11 and 50 years, is responsible for follicle maturation associated with egg maturation, ovulation, and cyclical sex steroid hormone production. These complex and linked biologic functions are coordinated through a variety of cells within the ovary, each of which possesses neoplastic potential. By far the most common and most lethal of the ovarian neoplasms arise from the ovarian epithelium or, alternatively, the neighboring specialized epithelium of the fallopian tube, uterine corpus, or cervix. Epithelial tumors may be benign (50%), malignant (33%), or of borderline malignancy (16%). Age influences risk of malignancy; tumors in younger women are more likely benign. The most common of the ovarian epithelial malignancies are serous tumors (50%); tumors of mucinous (25%), endometrioid (15%), clear cell (5%), and transitional cell histology or Brenner tumor (1%) represent smaller proportions of epithelial ovarian tumors. In contrast, stromal tumors arise from the steroid hormone–producing cells and likewise have different phenotypes and clinical presentations largely dependent on the type and quantity of hormone production. Tumors arising in the germ cell are most similar in biology and behavior to testicular tumors in males **(Chap. 12)**.

Tumors may also metastasize to the ovary from breast, colon, appendiceal, gastric, and pancreatic primaries. Bilateral ovarian masses from metastatic mucin-secreting gastrointestinal cancers are termed *Krukenberg tumors*.

OVARIAN CANCER OF EPITHELIAL ORIGIN

Epidemiology and pathogenesis

A female has approximately a 1 in 72 lifetime risk (1.6%) of developing ovarian cancer, with the majority of affected women developing epithelial tumors. Each of the histologic variants of epithelial tumors is distinct with unique molecular features. As a group of malignancies, epithelial tumors of the ovary have a peak incidence in women in their sixties, although age at presentation can range across the extremes of adult life, with cases being reported in women in their twenties to nineties. Each histologic subtype of ovarian cancer likely has its own associated risk factors. Serous cancer, the most common type of epithelial ovarian cancer, is seen with increased frequency in women who are nulliparous or have a history of use of talc agents applied to the perineum; other risk factors include obesity and probably hormone replacement therapy. Protective factors include the use of oral contraceptives, multiparity, and breast-feeding. These protective factors are thought to work through suppression of ovulation and perhaps the associated reduction of ovulation associated inflammation of the ovarian epithelium or, alternatively, the serous epithelium located within the fimbriae of the fallopian tube. Other protective factors, such as fallopian tube ligation, are thought to protect the ovarian epithelium (or perhaps the distal fallopian tube fimbriae) from carcinogens that migrate from the vagina to the tubes and ovarian surface epithelium. Mucinous tumors are more frequent in women with a history of cigarette smoking, whereas endometrioid and clear cell tumors are more frequent in women with a history of endometriosis.

Considerable evidence now suggests that the precursor cell to serous carcinoma of the ovary might actually arise in the fimbria of the fallopian tube with extension or metastasis to the ovarian surface or capture of preneoplastic or neoplastic exfoliating tubal cells into an involuting ovarian follicle around the time of ovulation. Careful histologic and molecular analysis of tubal epithelium demonstrates molecular and histologic abnormalities, termed serous tubular intraepithelial carcinoma (STIC) lesions, in a high proportion of women undergoing risk-reducing salpingo-oophorectomies in the context of high-risk germline mutations in *BRCA1* and *BRCA2*, as well as a modest proportion of women with ovarian cancer in the absence of such mutations.

Genetic risk factors

A variety of genetic syndromes substantially increase a woman's risk of developing ovarian cancer. Approximately 10% of women with ovarian cancer have a germline mutation in one of two DNA repair genes: *BRCA1* (chromosome 17q12-21) or *BRCA2* (chromosome 13q12-13). Individuals inheriting a single copy of a mutant allele have a very high incidence of breast and ovarian cancer. Most of these women have a family history that is notable for multiple cases of breast and/or ovarian cancer, although inheritance through male members of the family can camouflage this genotype through several generations. The most common malignancy in these women is breast carcinoma, although women harboring germline *BRCA1* mutations have a marked increased risk of developing ovarian malignancies in their forties and fifties with a 30–50% lifetime risk of developing ovarian cancer. Women harboring a mutation in *BRCA2* have a lower penetrance of ovarian cancer with perhaps a 20–40% chance of developing this malignancy, with onset typically in their fifties or sixties. Women with a *BRCA2* mutation also are at slightly increased risk of pancreatic cancer. Likewise women with mutations in the DNA mismatch repair genes associated with Lynch syndrome, type 2 (*MSH2, MLH1, MLH6, PMS1, PMS2*) may have a risk of ovarian cancer as high as 1% per year in their forties and fifties. Finally, a small group of women with familial ovarian cancer may have mutations in other *BRCA*-associated genes such as *RAD51*, *CHK2*, and others. Screening studies in this select population suggest that current screening techniques, including serial evaluation of the CA-125 tumor marker and ultrasound, are insufficient at detecting early-stage and curable disease, so women with these germline mutations are advised to undergo prophylactic removal of ovaries and fallopian tubes typically after completing childbearing and ideally before age 35–40 years. Early prophylactic oophorectomy also protects these women from subsequent breast cancer with a reduction of breast cancer risk of approximately 50%.

Presentation

Neoplasms of the ovary tend to be painless unless they undergo torsion. Symptoms are therefore typically related to compression of local organs or due to symptoms from metastatic disease. Women with tumors localized to the ovary do have an increased incidence of symptoms including pelvic discomfort, bloating, and perhaps changes in a woman's typical urinary or bowel pattern. Unfortunately, these symptoms are frequently dismissed by either the woman or her health care team. It is believed that high-grade tumors metastasize early in the neoplastic process. Unlike other epithelial malignancies, these tumors tend to exfoliate throughout the peritoneal cavity and thus present with symptoms associated with disseminated intraperitoneal tumors. The most common symptoms at presentation include a multimonth period of progressive complaints that typically include some combination of heartburn, nausea, early satiety, indigestion, constipation, and abdominal pain. Signs include the rapid increase in abdominal girth due to the accumulation of ascites that typically alerts the patient and her physician that the concurrent gastrointestinal symptoms are likely associated with serious pathology. Radiologic evaluation typically demonstrates a complex adnexal mass and ascites. Laboratory evaluation usually demonstrates a markedly elevated CA-125, a shed mucin (Muc 16) associated with, but not specific for, ovarian cancer. Hematogenous and lymphatic spread are seen but are not the typical presentation. Ovarian cancers are divided into four stages, with stage I tumors confined to the ovary, stage II malignancies confined to the pelvis, and stage III tumors confined to the peritoneal cavity (Table 18-1). These three stages are subdivided, with the most common presentation, stage IIIC, defined as tumors with bulky intraperitoneal disease. About 60% of women present with stage IIIC disease. Stage IV disease includes women with parenchymal metastases (liver, lung, spleen) or, alternatively, abdominal wall or pleural disease. The 40% not presenting with stage IIIC disease are roughly evenly distributed among the other stages, although mucinous and clear cell tumors are overrepresented in stage I tumors.

Screening

Ovarian cancer is the fifth most lethal malignancy in women in the United States. It is curable in early stages, but seldom curable in advanced stages; hence, the development of effective screening strategies is of considerable interest. Furthermore, the ovary is well visualized with a variety of imaging techniques, most notably transvaginal ultrasound. Early-stage

TABLE 18-1

STAGING AND SURVIVAL IN GYNECOLOGIC MALIGNANCIES

STAGE	OVARIAN	5-YEAR SURVIVAL, %	ENDOMETRIAL	5-YEAR SURVIVAL, %	CERVIX	5-YEAR SURVIVAL, %
0	—		—		Carcinoma in situ	100
I	Confined to ovary	90–95	Confined to corpus	89	Confined to uterus	85
II	Confined to pelvis	70–80	Involves corpus and cervix	73	Invades beyond uterus but not to pelvic wall	65
III	Intraabdominal spread	20–50	Extends outside the uterus but not outside the true pelvis or to lymph nodes	52	Extends to pelvic wall and/or lower third of vagina, or hydronephrosis	35
IV	Spread outside abdomen	1–5	Extends outside the true pelvis or involves the bladder or rectum	17	Invades mucosa of bladder or rectum or extends beyond the true pelvis	7

tumors often produce proteins that can be measured in the blood such as CA-125 and HE-4. Nevertheless, the incidence of ovarian cancer in the middle-aged female population is low, with only approximately 1 in 2000 women between the ages of 50 and 60 carrying an asymptomatic and undetected tumor. Thus effective screening techniques must be sensitive but, more importantly, highly specific to minimize the number of false-positive results. Even a screening test with 98% specificity and 50% sensitivity would have a positive predictive value of only about 1%. A large randomized study of active screening versus usual standard care demonstrated that a screening program consisting of six annual CA-125 measurements and four annual transvaginal ultrasounds in a population of women age 55–74 was not effective at reducing death from ovarian cancer and was associated with significant morbidity in the screened arm due to complications associated with diagnostic testing in the screened group. Although ongoing studies are evaluating the utility of alternative screening strategies, currently screening of normal-risk women is not recommended outside of a clinical trial.

TREATMENT Ovarian Cancer

In women presenting with a localized ovarian mass, the principal diagnostic and therapeutic maneuver is to determine if the tumor is benign or malignant and, in the event that the tumor is malignant, whether the tumor arises in the ovary or is a site of metastatic disease. Metastatic disease to the ovary can be seen from primary tumors of the colon, appendix, stomach (Krukenberg tumors), and breast. Typically women undergo a unilateral salpingo-oophorectomy, and if pathology reveals a primary ovarian malignancy, then the procedure is followed by a hysterectomy, removal of the remaining tube and ovary, omentectomy, and pelvic node sampling along with some random biopsies of the peritoneal cavity. This extensive surgical procedure is performed because approximately 30% of tumors that by visual inspection appear to be confined to the ovary have already disseminated to the peritoneal cavity and/or surrounding lymph nodes.

If there is evidence of bulky intraabdominal disease, a comprehensive attempt at maximal tumor cytoreduction is attempted even if it involves partial bowel resection, splenectomy, and in certain cases more extensive upper abdominal surgery. The ability to debulk metastatic ovarian cancer to minimal visible disease is associated with an improved prognosis compared with women left with visible disease. Patients without gross residual disease after resection have a median survival of 39 months, compared with 17 months for those left with macroscopic tumor. Once tumors have been surgically debulked, women receive therapy with a platinum agent, typically a taxane. Debate continues as to whether this therapy should be delivered intravenously or, alternatively, whether some of the therapy should be delivered directly into the peritoneal cavity via a catheter. Three randomized studies have demonstrated improved survival with intraperitoneal therapy, but this approach is still not widely accepted due to technical challenges associated with this delivery route and increased toxicity. In women who present with bulky intraabdominal disease, an alternative approach is to treat with platinum plus a taxane for several cycles before attempting a surgical debulking procedure (neoadjuvant therapy). Subsequent surgical procedures are more effective at leaving the patient without gross residual tumor and appear to be less morbid. Two studies have demonstrated that the neoadjuvant approach is associated with an overall survival that is comparable to the traditional approach of primary surgery followed by chemotherapy.

With optimal debulking surgery and platinum-based chemotherapy (usually carboplatin dosed to an area under the curve [AUC] of 6 plus paclitaxel 175 mg/m^2 by 3-h infusion in 21-day cycles), 70% of women who present with advanced-stage tumors respond, and 40–50% experience a complete remission with normalization of their CA-125, computed tomography (CT) scans, and physical examination. Unfortunately, a small proportion of women who obtain a complete response to therapy will remain in remission. Disease recurs within 1–4 years from the completion of their primary therapy in 75% of the complete responders. CA-125 levels often increase as a first sign of relapse; however, data are not clear that early intervention in relapsing patients influences survival. Recurrent disease is effectively managed, but not cured, with a variety of chemotherapeutic agents. Eventually all women with recurrent disease develop chemotherapy-refractory disease at which point refractory ascites, poor bowel motility, and obstruction or pseudoobstruction due to a tumor-infiltrated aperistaltic bowel are common. Limited surgery to relieve intestinal obstruction, localized radiation therapy to relieve pressure or pain from masses, or palliative chemotherapy may be helpful. Agents with >15% response rates include gemcitabine, topotecan, liposomal doxorubicin, pemetrexed, and bevacizumab. Approximately 10% of ovarian cancers are HER2/neu positive, and trastuzumab may induce responses in this subset.

Five-year survival correlates with the stage of disease: stage I, 85–90%; stage II, 70–80%; stage III, 20–50%; and stage IV, 1–5% (Table 18-1). Low-grade serous tumors are molecularly distinct from high-grade serous tumors and are, in general, poorly responsive to chemotherapy. Targeted therapies focused on inhibiting kinases downstream of *RAS* and *BRAF* are being tested. Patients with tumors of low malignant potential are managed by surgery; chemotherapy and radiation therapy do not improve survival.

OVARIAN SEX CORD AND STROMAL TUMORS

Epidemiology, presentation, and predisposing syndromes

Approximately 7% of ovarian neoplasms are stromal or sex cord tumors, with approximately 1800 cases expected each year in the United States. Ovarian stromal tumors or sex cord tumors are most common in women in their fifties or sixties, but tumors can present in the extremes of age, including the pediatric population. These tumors arise from the mesenchymal components of the ovary, including steroid-producing cells as well as fibroblasts. Essentially all of these tumors are of low malignant potential and present as unilateral solid masses. Three clinical presentations are common: the detection of an abdominal mass; abdominal pain due to ovarian torsion, intratumoral hemorrhage, or rupture; or signs and symptoms due to hormonal production by these tumors.

The most common hormone-producing tumors include thecomas, granulosa cell tumor, or juvenile granulosa tumors in children. These estrogen-producing tumors often present with breast tenderness as well as isosexual precocious pseudopuberty in children, menometrorrhagia, oligomenorrhea, or amenorrhea in premenopausal women, or alternatively as postmenopausal bleeding in older women. In some women, estrogen-associated secondary malignancies, such as endometrial or breast cancer, may present as synchronous malignancies. Alternatively, endometrial cancer may serve as the presenting malignancy with evaluation subsequently identifying a unilateral solid ovarian neoplasm that proves to be an occult granulosa cell tumor. Sertoli-Leydig tumors often present with hirsutism, virilization, and occasionally Cushing's syndrome due to increased production of testosterone, androstenedione, or other 17-ketosteroids. Hormonally inert tumors include fibroma that presents as a solitary mass often in association with ascites and occasionally hydrothorax also known as Meigs' syndrome. A subset of these tumors present in individuals with a variety of inherited disorders that predispose them to mesenchymal neoplasia. Associations include juvenile granulosa cell tumors and perhaps Sertoli-Leydig tumors with Ollier's disease (multiple enchondromatosis) or Maffucci's syndrome, ovarian sex cord tumors with annular tubules with Peutz-Jeghers syndrome, and fibromas with Gorlin's disease. Essentially all granulosa tumors and a minority of juvenile granulosa cell tumors and thecomas have a defined somatic point mutation in the *FOXL2* gene at C134W generated by replacement of cysteine with a guanine at position 402. About 30% of Sertoli-Leydig tumors harbor a mutation in the RNA-processing gene *DICER* in the RNAIIIb domain.

TREATMENT Sex Cord Tumors

The mainstay of treatment for sex cord tumors is surgical resection. Most women present with tumors confined to the ovary. For the small subset of women who present with metastatic disease or develop evidence of tumor recurrence after primary resection, survival is still typically long, often in excess of a decade. Because these tumors are slow growing and relatively refractory to chemotherapy, women with metastatic disease are often debulked because disease is usually peritoneal-based (as with epithelial ovarian cancer). Definitive data that surgical debulking of metastatic or recurrent disease prolongs survival are lacking, but ample data document women who have survived years or, in some cases, decades after resection of recurrent disease. In addition, large peritoneal-based metastases also have a proclivity for hemorrhage, sometimes with catastrophic complications. Chemotherapy is occasionally effective, and women tend to receive regimens designed to treat epithelial or germ cell tumors. Bevacizumab has some activity in clinical trials but is not approved for this specific indication. These tumors often produce high levels of müllerian inhibiting substance (MIS), inhibin, and, in the case of Sertoli-Leydig tumors, α fetoprotein (AFP). These proteins are detectable in serum and can be used as tumor markers to monitor women for recurrent disease because the increase or decrease of these proteins in the serum tends to reflect the changing bulk of systemic tumor.

GERM CELL TUMORS OF THE OVARY

Germ cell tumors, like their counterparts in the testis, are cancers of germ cells. These totipotent cells contain the programming for differentiation to essentially all tissue types, and hence the germ cell tumors include a histologic menagerie of bizarre tumors, including benign teratomas and a variety of malignant tumors, such as immature teratomas, dysgerminomas, yolk sac malignancies, and choriocarcinomas. Benign teratoma (or dermoid cyst) is the most common germ cell neoplasm of the ovary and often presents in young woman. These tumors include a complex mixture of differentiated tissue including tissues from all three germ layers. In older women, these differentiated tumors can develop malignant transformation, most commonly squamous cell carcinomas. Malignant germ cell tumors include dysgerminomas, yolk sac tumors, immature teratomas, and embryonal carcinoma and choriocarcinomas. There are no known genetic abnormalities that unify these tumors. A subset of dysgerminomas harbor mutations in c-*Kit* oncogenes (as seen in gastrointestinal stromal tumors [GIST]), whereas a subset of germ cell tumors have isochromosome 12 abnormalities, as seen in testicular malignancies. In addition, a subset of dysgerminomas is associated with dysgenetic ovaries. Identification of a dysgerminoma arising in genotypic XY gonads is important in that it highlights the need to identify and remove the contralateral gonad due to risk of gonadoblastoma.

Presentation

Germ cell tumors can present at all ages, but the peak age of presentation tends to be in females in their late teens or early twenties. Typically these tumors will become large ovarian masses, which eventually present as palpable low abdominal or pelvic masses. Like sex cord tumors, torsion or hemorrhage may present urgently or emergently as acute abdominal pain. Some of these tumors produce elevated levels of human chorionic gonadotropin (hCG), which can lead to isosexual precocious puberty when tumors present in younger girls. Unlike epithelial ovarian cancer, these tumors have a higher proclivity for nodal or hematogenous metastases. As with testicular tumors, some of these tumors tend to produce AFP (yolk sac tumors) or hCG (embryonal carcinoma, choriocarcinomas, and some dysgerminomas) that are reliable tumor markers.

TREATMENT Germ Cell Tumors

Germ cell tumors typically present in women who are still of childbearing age, and because bilateral tumors are uncommon (except in dysgerminoma, 10–15%), the typical treatment is unilateral oophorectomy or salpingo-oophorectomy. Because nodal metastases to pelvic and para-aortic nodes are common and may affect treatment choices, these nodes should be carefully inspected and, if enlarged, should be resected if possible. Women with malignant germ cell tumors typically receive bleomycin, etoposide, and cisplatin (BEP) chemotherapy. In the majority of women, even those with advanced-stage disease, cure is expected. Close follow-up without adjuvant therapy of women with stage I tumors is reasonable if there is high confidence that the patient and health care team are committed to compulsive and careful follow-up, as chemotherapy at the time of tumor recurrence is likely to be curative.

Dysgerminoma is the ovarian counterpart of testicular seminoma. The 5-year disease-free survival is 100% in early-stage patients and 61% in stage III disease. Although the tumor is highly radiation-sensitive, radiation produces infertility in many patients. BEP chemotherapy is as effective or more so without causing infertility. The use of BEP following incomplete resection is associated with a 2-year disease-free survival rate of 95%. This chemotherapy is now the treatment of choice for dysgerminoma.

FALLOPIAN TUBE CANCER

Transport of the egg to the uterus occurs via transit through the fallopian tube, with the distal ends of these tubes composed of fimbriae that drape about the ovarian surface and capture the egg as it erupts from the ovarian cortex. Fallopian tube malignancies are typically serous tumors. Previous teaching was that these malignancies were rare, but more careful histologic examination suggests that many "ovarian malignancies" might actually arise in the distal fimbria of the fallopian tube (see above). These women often present with adnexal masses, and like ovarian cancer, these tumors spread relatively early throughout the peritoneal cavity and respond to platinum and taxane therapy and have a natural history that is essentially identical to ovarian cancer (Table 18-1).

CERVICAL CANCER

GLOBAL CONSIDERATIONS

Cervical cancer is the second most common and most lethal malignancy in women worldwide likely due to the widespread infection with high-risk strains of human papillomavirus (HPV) and limited utilization of or access to Pap smear screening in many nations throughout the world. Nearly 500,000 cases of cervical cancer are expected worldwide, with approximately 240,000 deaths annually. Cancer incidence is particularly high in women residing in Central and South America, the Caribbean, and southern and eastern Africa. Mortality rate is disproportionately high in Africa. In the United States, 12,360 women were diagnosed with cervical cancer and 4020 women died in 2014. Developed countries have looked at high-technology screening techniques for HPV involving automated polymerase chain reaction in thin preps that identify dysplastic cytology as well as high-risk HPV genetic material. Visual inspection of the cervix coated with acetic acid has demonstrated the ability to reduce mortality from cervical cancer with potential broad applicability in low-resource environments. The development of effective vaccines for high-risk HPV types makes it imperative to determine economical, socially acceptable, and logistically feasible strategies to deliver and distribute this vaccine to girls and boys before their engagement in sexual activity.

HPV INFECTION AND PREVENTIVE VACCINATION

HPV is the primary neoplastic-initiating event in the vast majority of women with invasive cervical cancer. This double-strand DNA virus infects epithelium near the transformation zone of the cervix. More than 60 types of HPV are known, with approximately 20 types having the ability to generate high-grade dysplasia and malignancy. HPV-16 and -18 are the types most frequently associated with high-grade dysplasia and targeted by both U.S. Food and Drug Administration–approved vaccines. The large majority of sexually active adults are exposed to HPV, and most women clear the infection without specific intervention. The 8-kilobase HPV genome encodes seven early genes, most notably *E6* and *E7*, which can bind to *RB* and *p53*, respectively. High-risk types of HPV encode *E6* and *E7* molecules that are particularly effective at inhibiting the normal cell cycle checkpoint functions of these regulatory proteins, leading to immortalization but not full transformation of cervical epithelium. A minority of woman will fail to clear the infection with subsequent HPV integration into the host genome. Over the course of as short as months but more typically years, some of these women develop high-grade dysplasia. The time from dysplasia to carcinoma is likely years to more than a decade and almost certainly requires the acquisition of other poorly defined genetic mutations within the infected and immortalized epithelium.

Risk factors for HPV infection and, in particular, dysplasia include a high number of sexual partners, early age of first intercourse, and history of venereal disease. Smoking is a cofactor; heavy smokers have a higher risk of dysplasia with HPV infection. HIV infection, especially when associated with low CD4+ T cell counts, is associated with a higher rate of high-grade dysplasia and likely a shorter latency period between infection and invasive disease. The administration of highly active antiretroviral therapy reduces the risk of high-grade dysplasia associated with HPV infection.

Currently approved vaccines include the recombinant proteins to the late proteins, L1 and L2, of HPV-16 and -18. Vaccination of women before the initiation of sexual activity dramatically reduces the rate of HPV-16 and -18 infection and subsequent dysplasia. There is also partial protection against other HPV types, although vaccinated women are still at risk for HPV infection and still require standard Pap smear screening. Although no randomized trial data demonstrate the utility of Pap smears, the dramatic drop in cervical cancer incidence and death in developed countries employing wide-scale screening provides strong evidence for its effectiveness. In addition, even visual inspection of the cervix with preapplication of acetic acid using a "see and treat" strategy has demonstrated a 30% reduction in cervical cancer death. The incorporation of HPV testing by polymerase chain reaction or other molecular techniques increases the sensitivity of detecting cervical pathology but at the cost of identifying many women with transient infections who require no specific medical intervention.

CLINICAL PRESENTATIONS

The majority of cervical malignancies are squamous cell carcinomas associated with HPV. Adenocarcinomas are also HPV-related and arise deep in the endocervical canal; they are typically not seen by visual inspection of the cervix and thus are often missed by Pap smear screening. A variety of rarer malignancies including atypical epithelial tumors, carcinoids, small cell carcinomas, sarcomas, and lymphomas have also been reported.

The principal role of Pap smear testing is the detection of asymptomatic preinvasive cervical dysplasia of squamous epithelial lining. Invasive carcinomas often have symptoms or signs including postcoital spotting or intermenstrual cycle bleeding or menometrorrhagia. Foul-smelling or persistent yellow discharge may also be seen. Presentations that include pelvic or sacral pain suggest lateral extension of the tumor into pelvic nerve plexus by either the primary tumor or a pelvic node and are signs of advanced-stage disease. Likewise, flank pain from hydronephrosis from ureteral compression or deep venous thrombosis from iliac vessel compression suggests either extensive nodal disease or direct extension of the primary tumor to the pelvic sidewall. The most common finding of physical exam is a visible tumor on the cervix.

TREATMENT Cervical Cancer

Scans are not part of the formal clinical staging of cervical cancer yet are very useful in planning appropriate therapy. CT can detect hydronephrosis indicative of pelvic sidewall disease but is not accurate at evaluating other pelvic structures. Magnetic resonance imaging (MRI) is more accurate at estimating uterine extension and paracervical extension of disease into soft tissues typically bordered by broad and cardinal ligaments that support the uterus in the central pelvis. Positron emission tomography (PET) scan is the most accurate technique for evaluating the pelvis and more importantly nodal (pelvic, para-aortic, and scalene) sites for disease. This technique seems more prognostic and accurate than CT, MRI, or lymphangiogram, especially in the para-aortic region.

Stage I cervical tumors are confined to the cervix, whereas stage II tumors extend into the upper vagina or paracervical soft tissue (Fig. 18-1). Stage III tumors extend to the lower vagina or the pelvic sidewalls, whereas stage IV tumors invade the bladder or rectum or have spread to distant sites. Very small stage I cervical tumors can be treated with a variety of surgical procedures. In young women desiring to maintain fertility, radical trachelectomy removes the cervix with subsequent anastomosis of the upper vagina to the uterine corpus. Larger cervical tumors confined to the cervix can be treated with either surgical resection or radiation therapy in combination with cisplatin-based chemotherapy with a high chance of cure. Larger tumors that extend regionally down the vagina or into the paracervical soft tissues or the pelvic sidewalls are treated with combination chemotherapy and radiation therapy. The treatment of recurrent or metastatic disease is unsatisfactory due to the relative resistance of these tumors to chemotherapy and currently available biological agents, although bevacizumab, a monoclonal antibody that is said to inhibit tumor-associated angiogenesis, has demonstrated clinically meaningful activity in the management of metastatic disease.

UTERINE CANCER

EPIDEMIOLOGY

Several different tumor types arise in uterine corpus. Most tumors arise in the glandular lining and are endometrial adenocarcinomas. Tumors can also arise in the smooth muscle; most are benign (uterine leiomyoma), with a small minority of tumors being sarcomas. The endometrioid histologic subtype of endometrial cancer is the most common gynecologic malignancy in the United States. In 2014, an estimated 52,630 women were diagnosed with cancer of the uterine corpus, with

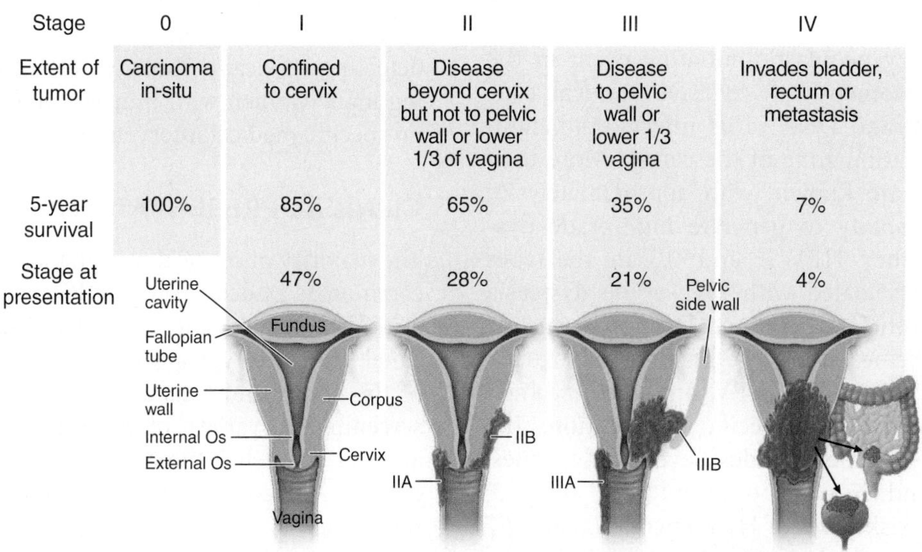

Staging of cervix cancer
Stage
0
I
II
III
IV
Extent of tumor
Carcinoma in-situ
Confined to cervix
Disease beyond cervix but not to pelvic wall or lower 1/3 of vagina
Disease to pelvic wall or lower 1/3 vagina
Invades bladder, rectum or metastasis
5-year survival
100%
85%
65%
35%
7%
Stage at presentation
47%
28%
21%
4%
Uterine cavity
Fundus
Fallopian tube
Uterine wall
Corpus
Internal Os
External Os
Cervix
Vagina
IIA
IIB
IIIA
IIIB
Pelvic side wall

FIGURE 18-1
Anatomic display of the stages of cervix cancer defined by location, extent of tumor, frequency of presentation, and 5-year survival.

8590 deaths from the disease. Development of these tumors is a multistep process, with estrogen playing an important early role in driving endometrial gland proliferation. Relative overexposure to this class of hormones is a risk factor for the subsequent development of endometrioid tumors. In contrast, progestins drive glandular maturation and are protective. Hence, women with high endogenous or pharmacologic exposure to estrogens, especially if unopposed by progesterone, are at high risk for endometrial cancer. Obese women, women treated with unopposed estrogens, or women with estrogen-producing tumors (such as granulosa cell tumors of the ovary) are at higher risk for endometrial cancer. In addition, treatment with tamoxifen, which has antiestrogenic effects in breast tissue but estrogenic effects in uterine epithelium, is associated with an increased risk of endometrial cancer. Events such as the loss of the *PTEN* tumor suppressor gene with activation and often additional mutations in the PIK-3CA/AKT pathways likely serve as secondary events in carcinogenesis. The Cancer Genome Atlas Research Network has demonstrated that endometrioid tumors can be divided into four subgroups: ultramutated, microsatellite instability hypermutated, copy number low, and copy number high subgroups. These groups have different natural histories; therapy for these subgroups may eventually be individualized. Serous tumors of the uterine corpus represent approximately 5–10% of epithelial tumors of the uterine corpus and possess distinct molecular characteristics that are most similar to those seen in serous tumors arising in the ovary or fallopian tube.

Women with a mutation in one of a series of DNA mismatch repair genes associated with the Lynch syndrome, also known as hereditary nonpolyposis colon cancer (HNPCC), are at increased risk for endometrioid endometrial carcinoma. These individuals have germline mutations in *MSH2*, *MLH1*, and in rare cases *PMS1* and *PMS2*, with resulting microsatellite instability and hypermutation. Individuals who carry these mutations typically have a family history of cancer and are at markedly increased risk for colon cancer and modestly increased risk for ovarian cancer and a variety of other tumors. Middle-aged women with HNPCC carry a 4% annual risk of endometrial cancer and a relative overall risk of approximately 200-fold as compared to age-matched women without HNPCC.

PRESENTATIONS

The majority of women with tumors of the uterine corpus present with postmenopausal vaginal bleeding due to shedding of the malignant endometrial lining. Premenopausal women often will present with atypical bleeding between typical menstrual cycles. These signs typically bring a woman to the attention of a health care professional, and hence the majority of women present with early-stage disease with the tumor confined to the uterine corpus. Diagnosis is typically established by endometrial biopsy. Epithelial tumors may spread to pelvic or para-aortic lymph nodes. Pulmonary metastases can appear later in the natural history of this disease but are very uncommon at initial presentation. Serous tumors tend to have patterns of spread much more reminiscent of ovarian cancer with many patients presenting with disseminated peritoneal disease and sometimes ascites. Some women presenting with uterine sarcomas will present with pelvic pain. Nodal metastases are uncommon with sarcomas, which are more likely to present with either intraabdominal disease or pulmonary metastases.

TREATMENT Uterine Cancer

Most women with endometrial cancer have disease that is localized to the uterus (75% are stage I, Table 18-1), and definitive treatment typically involves a hysterectomy with removal of the ovaries and fallopian tubes. The resection of lymph nodes does not improve outcome but does provide prognostic information. Node involvement defines stage III disease, which is present in 13% of patients. Tumor grade and depth of invasion are the two key prognostic variables in early-stage tumors, and women with low-grade and/or minimally invasive tumors are typically observed after definitive surgical therapy. Patients with high-grade tumors or tumors that are deeply invasive (stage IB, 13%) are at higher risk for pelvic recurrence or recurrence at the vaginal cuff, which is typically prevented by vaginal vault brachytherapy.

Women with regional metastases or metastatic disease (3% of patients) with low-grade tumors can be treated with progesterone. Poorly differentiated tumors are typically resistant to hormonal manipulation and thus are treated with chemotherapy. The role of chemotherapy in the adjuvant setting is currently under investigation. Chemotherapy for metastatic disease is delivered with palliative intent. Drugs that effectively target and inhibit signaling of the AKT-mTOR pathway are currently under investigation.

Five-year survival is 89% for stage I, 73% for stage II, 52% for stage III, and 17% for stage IV disease (Table 18-1).

GESTATIONAL TROPHOBLASTIC TUMORS

GLOBAL CONSIDERATIONS

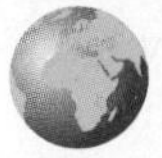

Gestational trophoblastic diseases represent a spectrum of neoplasia from benign hydatidiform mole to choriocarcinoma due to persistent trophoblastic disease associated most commonly with molar pregnancy but occasionally seen after normal gestation. The most common presentations of trophoblastic tumors are partial and complete molar pregnancies. These represent approximately 1 in 1500 conceptions in developed Western countries. The incidence widely varies globally, with areas in Southeast Asia having a much higher incidence of molar pregnancy. Regions with high molar pregnancy rates are often associated with diets low in carotene and animal fats.

RISK FACTORS

Trophoblastic tumors result from the outgrowth or persistence of placental tissue. They arise most commonly in the uterus but can also arise in other sites such as the fallopian tubes due to ectopic pregnancy. Risk factors include poorly defined dietary and environmental factors as well as conceptions at the extremes of reproductive age, with the incidence particularly high in females conceiving younger than age 16 or older than age 50. In older women, the incidence of molar pregnancy might be as high as one in three, likely due to increased risk of abnormal fertilization of the aged ova. Most trophoblastic neoplasms are associated with complete moles, diploid tumors with all genetic material from the paternal donor (known as parental disomy). This is thought to occur when a single sperm fertilizes an enucleate egg that subsequently duplicates the paternal DNA. Trophoblastic proliferation occurs with exuberant villous stroma. If pseudopregnancy extends out past the 12th week, fluid progressively accumulates within the stroma, leading to "hydropic changes." There is no fetal development in complete moles.

Partial moles arise from the fertilization of an egg with two sperm; hence two-thirds of genetic material is paternal in these triploid tumors. Hydropic changes are less dramatic, and fetal development can often occur through late first trimester or early second trimester at which point spontaneous abortion is common. Laboratory findings will include excessively high hCG and high AFP. The risk of persistent gestational trophoblastic disease after partial mole is approximately 5%. Complete and partial moles can be noninvasive or invasive. Myometrial invasion occurs in no more than one in six complete moles and a lower portion of partial moles.

PRESENTATION OF INVASIVE TROPHOBLASTIC DISEASE

The clinical presentation of molar pregnancy is changing in developed countries due to the early detection of pregnancy with home pregnancy kits and the very early use of Doppler and ultrasound to evaluate the early fetus and uterine cavity for evidence of a viable fetus. Thus, in these countries, the majority of women presenting with trophoblastic disease have their moles detected early and have typical symptoms of early pregnancy including nausea, amenorrhea, and breast tenderness. With uterine evacuation of early complete and partial moles, most women experience spontaneous remission of their disease as monitored by serial hCG levels. These women require no chemotherapy. Patients with persistent elevation of hCG or rising hCG after evacuation have persistent or actively growing gestational trophoblastic disease and require therapy. Most series suggest that between 15 and 25% of women will have evidence of persistent gestational trophoblastic disease after molar evacuation.

In women who lack access to prenatal care, presenting symptoms can be life threatening including the development of preeclampsia or even eclampsia. Hyperthyroidism can also be seen. Evacuation of large moles can be associated with life-threatening complications including uterine perforation, volume loss, high-output cardiac failure, and adult respiratory distress syndrome (ARDS).

For women with evidence of rising hCG or radiologic confirmation of metastatic or persistent regional disease, prognosis can be estimated through a variety of scoring algorithms that identify those women at low, intermediate, and high risk for requiring multiagent chemotherapy. In general, women with widely metastatic nonpulmonary disease, very elevated hCG, and prior normal antecedent term pregnancy are considered at high risk and typically require multiagent chemotherapy for cure.

TREATMENT Invasive Trophoblastic Disease

The management for a persistent and rising hCG after evacuation of a molar conception is typically chemotherapy, although surgery can play an important role for disease that is persistently isolated in the uterus (especially if childbearing is complete) or to control hemorrhage. For women wishing to maintain fertility or with metastatic disease, the preferred treatment is chemotherapy. Chemotherapy is guided by the hCG level, which typically drops to undetectable levels with effective therapy. Single-agent treatment with methotrexate or dactinomycin cures 90% of women with low-risk disease. Patients with high-risk disease (high hCG levels, presentation 4 or more months after pregnancy, brain or liver metastases, failure of methotrexate therapy) are typically treated with multiagent chemotherapy (e.g., etoposide, methotrexate, and dactinomycin alternating with cyclophosphamide and vincristine [EMA-CO]), which is typically curative even in women with extensive metastatic disease. Cisplatin, bleomycin, and either etoposide or vinblastine are also active combinations. Survival in high-risk disease exceeds 80%. Cured women may get pregnant again without evidence of increased fetal or maternal complications.

CHAPTER 19

SEXUAL DYSFUNCTION

Kevin T. McVary

Male sexual dysfunction affects 10–25% of middle-aged and elderly men, and female sexual dysfunction occurs with similar frequency. Demographic changes, the popularity of newer treatments, and greater awareness of sexual dysfunction by patients and society have led to increased diagnosis and associated health care expenditures for the management of this common disorder. Because many patients are reluctant to initiate discussion of their sex lives, physicians should address this topic directly to elicit a history of sexual dysfunction.

MALE SEXUAL DYSFUNCTION

PHYSIOLOGY OF MALE SEXUAL RESPONSE

Normal male sexual function requires (1) an intact libido, (2) the ability to achieve and maintain penile erection, (3) ejaculation, and (4) detumescence. *Libido* refers to sexual desire and is influenced by a variety of visual, olfactory, tactile, auditory, imaginative, and hormonal stimuli. Sex steroids, particularly testosterone, act to increase libido. Libido can be diminished by hormonal or psychiatric disorders and by medications.

Penile tumescence leading to erection depends on an increased flow of blood into the lacunar network accompanied by complete relaxation of the arteries and corporal smooth muscle. The microarchitecture of the corpora is composed of a mass of smooth muscle (trabecula) that contains a network of endothelial-lined vessels (lacunar spaces). Subsequent compression of the trabecular smooth muscle against the fibroelastic tunica albuginea causes a passive closure of the emissary veins and accumulation of blood in the corpora. In the presence of a full erection and a competent valve mechanism, the corpora become noncompressible cylinders from which blood does not escape.

The central nervous system (CNS) exerts an important influence by either stimulating or antagonizing spinal pathways that mediate erectile function and ejaculation. The erectile response is mediated by a combination of central (psychogenic) innervation and peripheral (reflexogenic) innervation. Sensory nerves that originate from receptors in the penile skin and glans converge to form the dorsal nerve of the penis, which travels to the S2-S4 dorsal root ganglia via the pudendal nerve. Parasympathetic nerve fibers to the penis arise from neurons in the intermediolateral columns of the S2-S4 sacral spinal segments. Sympathetic innervation originates from the T11 to the L2 spinal segments and descends through the hypogastric plexus.

Neural input to smooth-muscle tone is crucial to the initiation and maintenance of an erection. There is also an intricate interaction between the corporal smooth-muscle cell and its overlying endothelial cell lining (Fig. 19-1). Nitric oxide, which induces vascular relaxation, promotes erection and is opposed by endothelin 1 (ET-1) and Rho kinase, which mediate vascular contraction. Nitric oxide is synthesized from l-arginine by nitric oxide synthase and is released from the nonadrenergic, noncholinergic (NANC) autonomic nerve supply to act postjunctionally on smooth-muscle cells. Nitric oxide increases the production of cyclic 3′,5′-guanosine monophosphate (cyclic GMP), which induces relaxation of smooth muscle (Fig. 19-2). Cyclic GMP is gradually broken down by phosphodiesterase type 5 (PDE-5). Inhibitors of PDE-5, such as the oral medications sildenafil, vardenafil, and tadalafil, maintain erections by reducing the breakdown of cyclic GMP. However, if nitric oxide is not produced at some level, PDE-5 inhibitors are ineffective, as these drugs facilitate, but do not initiate, the initial enzyme cascade. In addition to nitric oxide, vasoactive prostaglandins (PGE_1, $PGF_{2\alpha}$) are synthesized within the cavernosal tissue and increase cyclic AMP levels, also leading to relaxation of cavernosal smooth-muscle cells.

Ejaculation is stimulated by the sympathetic nervous system; this results in contraction of the epididymis, vas

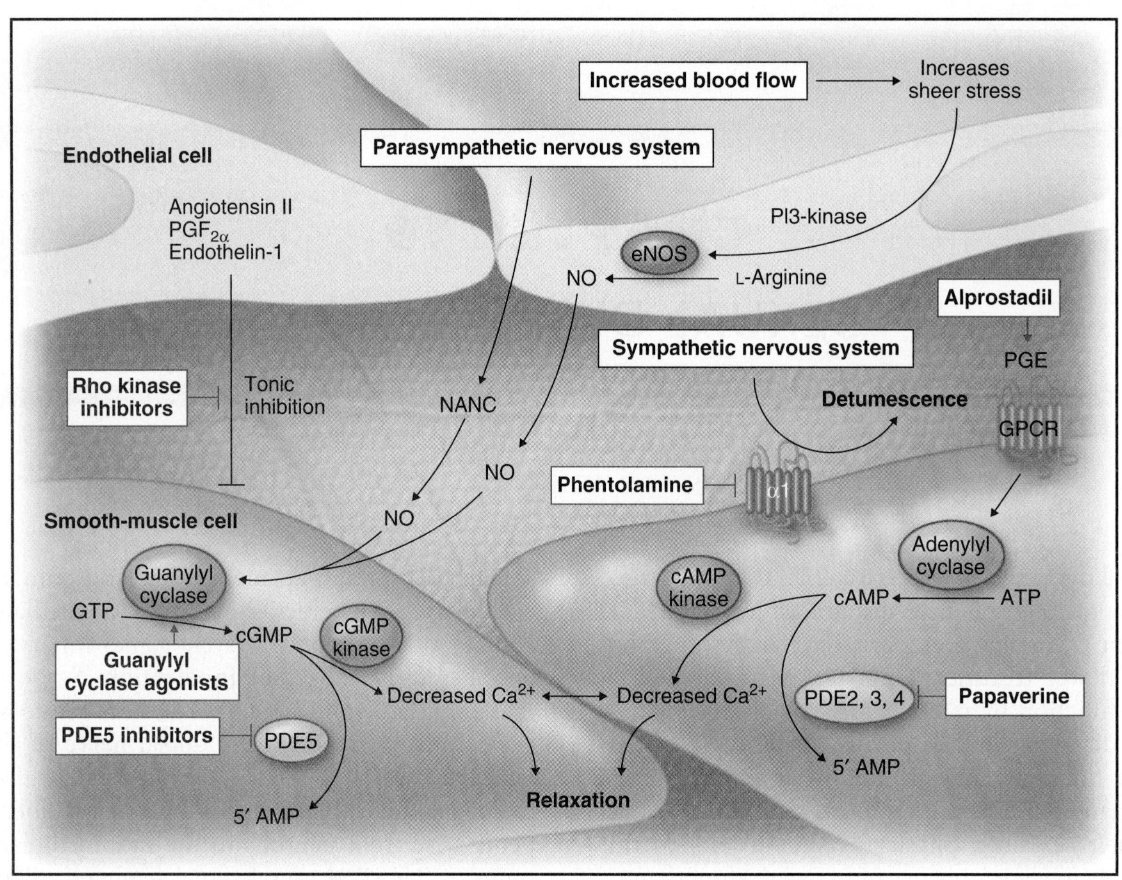

FIGURE 19-1

Pathways that regulate penile smooth-muscle relaxation and erection. *A.* Outflow from the parasympathetic nervous system leads to relaxation of the cavernous sinusoids in two ways, both of which increase the concentration of nitric oxide (NO) in smooth-muscle cells. First, NO is the neurotransmitter in nonadrenergic, noncholinergic (NANC) fibers; second, stimulation of endothelial nitric oxide synthase (eNOS) through cholinergic output causes increased production of NO. The NO produced in the endothelium then diffuses into the smooth-muscle cells and decreases its intracellular calcium concentration through a pathway mediated by cyclic guanosine monophosphate (cGMP), leading to relaxation. A separate mechanism that decreases the intracellular calcium level is mediated by cyclic adenosine monophosphate (cAMP). With increased cavernosal blood flow, as well as increased levels of vascular endothelial growth factor (VEGF), the endothelial release of NO is further sustained through the phosphatidylinositol 3 (PI3) kinase pathway. Active treatments (red boxes) include drugs that affect the cGMP pathway (phosphodiesterase [PDE] type 5 inhibitors and guanylyl cyclase agonists), the cAMP pathway (alprostadil), or both pathways (papaverine), along with neural-tone mediators (phentolamine and Rho kinase inhibitors). Agents that are being developed include guanylyl cyclase agonists (to bypass the need for endogenous NO) and Rho kinase inhibitors (to inhibit tonic contraction of smooth-muscle cells mediated through endothelin). α1, α-adrenergic receptor; GPCR, G-protein–coupled receptor, GTP, guanosine triphosphate; PGE, prostaglandin E; PGF, prostaglandin F. *(K McVary: N Engl J Med 357:2472, 2007; with permission.)*

deferens, seminal vesicles, and prostate, causing seminal fluid to enter the urethra. Seminal fluid emission is followed by rhythmic contractions of the bulbocavernosus and ischiocavernosus muscles, leading to ejaculation. *Premature ejaculation* usually is related to anxiety or a learned behavior and is amenable to behavioral therapy or treatment with medications such as selective serotonin reuptake inhibitors (SSRIs). *Retrograde ejaculation* results when the internal urethral sphincter does not close; it may occur in men with diabetes or after surgery involving the bladder neck.

Detumescence is mediated by norepinephrine from the sympathetic nerves, endothelin from the vascular surface, and smooth-muscle contraction induced by

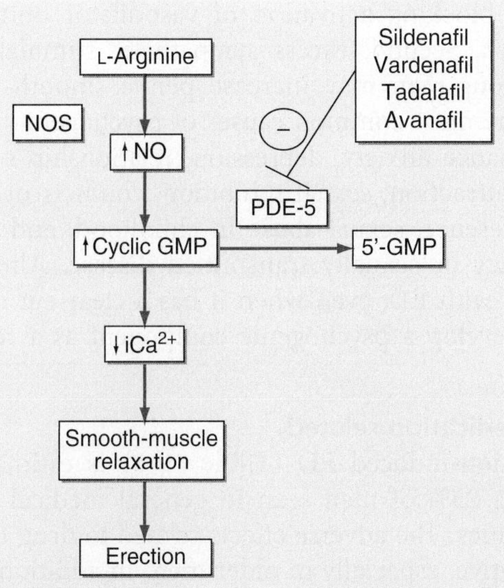

FIGURE 19-2

Biochemical pathways modified by phosphodiesterase type 5 (PDE-5) inhibitors. Sildenafil, vardenafil, tadalafil and avanafil enhance erectile function by inhibiting PDE-5, thereby maintaining high levels of cyclic 3′,5′-guanosine monophosphate (cyclic GMP). iCa^{2+}, intracellular calcium; NO, nitric oxide; NOS, nitric oxide synthase.

postsynaptic α-adrenergic receptors and activation of Rho kinase. These events increase venous outflow and restore the flaccid state. Venous leak can cause premature detumescence and is caused by insufficient relaxation of the corporal smooth muscle rather than a specific anatomic defect. *Priapism* refers to a persistent and painful erection and may be associated with sickle cell anemia, hypercoagulable states, spinal cord injury, or injection of vasodilator agents into the penis.

ERECTILE DYSFUNCTION

Epidemiology

Erectile dysfunction (ED) is not considered a normal part of the aging process. Nonetheless, it is associated with certain physiologic and psychological changes related to age. In the Massachusetts Male Aging Study (MMAS), a community-based survey of men age 40–70, 52% of responders reported some degree of ED. Complete ED occurred in 10% of respondents, moderate ED in 25%, and minimal ED in 17%. The incidence of moderate or severe ED more than doubled between the ages of 40 and 70. In the National Health and Social Life Survey (NHSLS), which included a sample of men and women age 18–59, 10% of men reported being unable to maintain an erection (corresponding to the proportion of men in the MMAS reporting severe ED). Incidence was highest among men in the age group 50–59 (21%) and men who were poor (14%), divorced (14%), and less educated (13%).

The incidence of ED is also higher among men with certain medical disorders, such as diabetes mellitus, obesity, lower urinary tract symptoms secondary to benign prostatic hyperplasia (BPH), heart disease, hypertension, decreased high-density lipoprotein (HDL) levels, and diseases associated with general systemic inflammation (e.g., rheumatoid arthritis). Cardiovascular disease and ED share etiologies as well as pathophysiology (e.g., endothelial dysfunction), and the degree of ED appears to correlate with the severity of cardiovascular disease. Consequently, ED represents a "sentinel symptom" in patients with occult cardiovascular and peripheral vascular disease.

Smoking is also a significant risk factor in the development of ED. Medications used in treating diabetes or cardiovascular disease are additional risk factors (see below). There is a higher incidence of ED among men who have undergone radiation or surgery for prostate cancer and in those with a lower spinal cord injury. Psychological causes of ED include depression, anger, stress from unemployment, and other stress-related causes.

Pathophysiology

ED may result from three basic mechanisms: (1) failure to initiate (psychogenic, endocrinologic, or neurogenic), (2) failure to fill (arteriogenic), and (3) failure to store adequate blood volume within the lacunar network (venoocclusive dysfunction). These categories are not mutually exclusive, and multiple factors contribute to ED in many patients. For example, diminished filling pressure can lead secondarily to venous leak. Psychogenic factors frequently coexist with other etiologic factors and should be considered in all cases. Diabetic, atherosclerotic, and drug-related causes account for >80% of cases of ED in older men.

Vasculogenic

The most common organic cause of ED is a disturbance of blood flow to and from the penis. Atherosclerotic or traumatic arterial disease can decrease flow to the lacunar spaces, resulting in decreased rigidity and an increased time to full erection. Excessive outflow through the veins despite adequate inflow also may contribute to ED. Structural alterations to the fibroelastic components of the corpora may cause a loss of compliance and inability to compress the tunical veins. This condition may result from aging, increased cross-linking of collagen fibers induced by nonenzymatic glycosylation, hypoxemia, or altered synthesis of collagen associated with hypercholesterolemia.

Neurogenic

Disorders that affect the sacral spinal cord or the autonomic fibers to the penis preclude nervous system relaxation of penile smooth muscle, thus leading to ED. In patients with spinal cord injury, the degree of ED depends on the completeness and level of the lesion. Patients with incomplete lesions or injuries to the upper part of the spinal cord are more likely to retain erectile capabilities than are those with complete lesions or injuries to the lower part. Although 75% of patients with spinal cord injuries have some erectile capability, only 25% have erections sufficient for penetration. Other neurologic disorders commonly associated with ED include multiple sclerosis and peripheral neuropathy. The latter is often due to either diabetes or alcoholism. Pelvic surgery may cause ED through disruption of the autonomic nerve supply.

Endocrinologic

Androgens increase libido, but their exact role in erectile function is unclear. Individuals with castrate levels of testosterone can achieve erections from visual or sexual stimuli. Nonetheless, normal levels of testosterone appear to be important for erectile function, particularly in older males. Androgen replacement therapy can improve depressed erectile function when it is secondary to hypogonadism; however, it is not useful for ED when endogenous testosterone levels are normal. Increased prolactin may decrease libido by suppressing gonadotropin-releasing hormone (GnRH), and it also leads to decreased testosterone levels. Treatment of hyperprolactinemia with dopamine agonists can restore libido and testosterone.

Diabetic

ED occurs in 35–75% of men with diabetes mellitus. Pathologic mechanisms are related primarily to diabetes-associated vascular and neurologic complications. Diabetic macrovascular complications are related mainly to age, whereas microvascular complications correlate with the duration of diabetes and the degree of glycemic control **(Chap. 23)**. Individuals with diabetes also have reduced amounts of nitric oxide synthase in both endothelial and neural tissues.

Psychogenic

Two mechanisms contribute to the inhibition of erections in psychogenic ED. First, psychogenic stimuli to the sacral cord may inhibit reflexogenic responses, thereby blocking activation of vasodilator outflow to the penis. Second, excess sympathetic stimulation in an anxious man may increase penile smooth-muscle tone. The most common causes of psychogenic ED are performance anxiety, depression, relationship conflict, loss of attraction, sexual inhibition, conflicts over sexual preference, sexual abuse in childhood, and fear of pregnancy or sexually transmitted disease. Almost all patients with ED, even when it has a clear-cut organic basis, develop a psychogenic component as a reaction to ED.

Medication-related

Medication-induced ED (Table 19-1) is estimated to occur in 25% of men seen in general medical outpatient clinics. The adverse effects related to drug therapy are additive, especially in older men. In addition to the drug itself, the disease being treated is likely to contribute to sexual dysfunction. Among the antihypertensive agents, the thiazide diuretics and beta blockers have been implicated most frequently. Calcium channel blockers and angiotensin converting-enzyme inhibitors are cited less frequently. These drugs may act directly at the corporal level (e.g., calcium channel blockers) or indirectly by reducing pelvic blood pressure, which is important in the development of penile rigidity. α-Adrenergic blockers are less likely to cause ED. Estrogens, GnRH agonists, H_2 antagonists, and spironolactone cause ED by suppressing gonadotropin production or by blocking androgen action. Antidepressant and antipsychotic agents—particularly neuroleptics, tricyclics, and SSRIs—are associated with erectile, ejaculatory, orgasmic, and sexual desire difficulties.

If there is a strong association between the institution of a drug and the onset of ED, alternative medications should be considered. Otherwise, it is often practical to treat the ED without attempting multiple changes in medications, as it may be difficult to establish a causal role for a drug.

APPROACH TO THE PATIENT: Erectile Dysfunction

A good physician-patient relationship helps unravel the possible causes of ED, many of which require discussion of personal and sometimes embarrassing topics. For this reason, a primary care provider is often ideally suited to initiate the evaluation. However, a significant percentage of men experience ED and remain undiagnosed unless specifically questioned about this issue. By far the two most common reasons for underreporting of ED are patient embarrassment and perceptions of physicians' inattention to the disease. Once the topic is initiated by the physician, patients are more willing

TABLE 19-1

DRUGS ASSOCIATED WITH ERECTILE DYSFUNCTION

CLASSIFICATION	DRUGS
Diuretics	Thiazides
	Spironolactone
Antihypertensives	Calcium channel blockers
	Methyldopa
	Clonidine
	Reserpine
	Beta blockers
	Guanethidine
Cardiac/antihyperlipidemics	Digoxin
	Gemfibrozil
	Clofibrate
Antidepressants	Selective serotonin reuptake inhibitors
	Tricyclic antidepressants
	Lithium
	Monoamine oxidase inhibitors
Tranquilizers	Butyrophenones
	Phenothiazines
H_2 antagonists	Ranitidine
	Cimetidine
Hormones	Progesterone
	Estrogens
	Corticosteroids
	GnRH agonists
	5α-Reductase inhibitors
	Cyproterone acetate
Cytotoxic agents	Cyclophosphamide
	Methotrexate
	Roferon-A
Anticholinergics	Disopyramide
	Anticonvulsants
Recreational	Ethanol
	Cocaine
	Marijuana

Abbreviation: GnRH, gonadotropin-releasing hormone.

to discuss their potency issues. A complete medical and sexual history should be taken in an effort to assess whether the cause of ED is organic, psychogenic, or multifactorial (Fig. 19-3).

Both the patient and his sexual partner should be interviewed regarding sexual history. ED should be distinguished from other sexual problems, such as

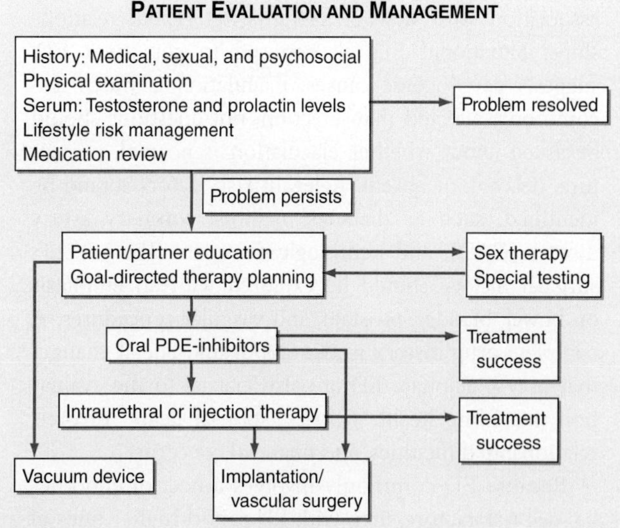

FIGURE 19-3

Algorithm for the evaluation and management of patients with erectile dysfunction. PDE, phosphodiesterase.

premature ejaculation. Lifestyle factors such as sexual orientation, the patient's distress from ED, performance anxiety, and details of sexual techniques should be addressed. Standardized questionnaires are available to assess ED, including the International Index of Erectile Function (IIEF) and the more easily administered Sexual Health Inventory for Men (SHIM), a validated abridged version of the IIEF.

The initial evaluation of ED begins with a review of the patient's medical, surgical, sexual, and psychosocial histories. The history should note whether the patient has experienced pelvic trauma, surgery, or radiation. In light of the increasing recognition of the relationship between lower urinary tract symptoms and ED, it is advisable to evaluate for the presence of symptoms of bladder outlet obstruction. Questions should focus on the onset of symptoms, the presence and duration of partial erections, and the progression of ED. A history of nocturnal or early morning erections is useful for distinguishing physiologic ED from psychogenic ED. Nocturnal erections occur during rapid eye movement (REM) sleep and require intact neurologic and circulatory systems. Organic causes of ED generally are characterized by a gradual and persistent change in rigidity or the inability to sustain nocturnal, coital, or self-stimulated erections. The patient should be questioned about the presence of penile curvature or pain with coitus. It is also important to address libido, as decreased sexual drive and ED are sometimes the earliest signs of endocrine abnormalities (e.g., increased prolactin, decreased testosterone levels). It is useful to ask whether the problem is confined to coitus with one partner or also involves other partners; ED not uncommonly arises in association with new or extramarital sexual relationships. Situational ED, as opposed to consistent ED, suggests psychogenic causes. Ejaculation is much less commonly affected than erection, but questions should be asked about whether ejaculation is normal, premature, delayed, or absent. Relevant risk factors should be identified, such as diabetes mellitus, coronary artery disease (CAD), and neurologic disorders. The patient's surgical history should be explored with an emphasis on bowel, bladder, prostate, and vascular procedures. A complete drug history is also important. Social changes that may precipitate ED are also crucial to the evaluation, including health worries, spousal death, divorce, relationship difficulties, and financial concerns.

Because ED commonly involves a host of endothelial cell risk factors, men with ED report higher rates of overt and silent myocardial infarction. Therefore, ED in an otherwise asymptomatic male warrants consideration of other vascular disorders, including CAD.

The physical examination is an essential element in the assessment of ED. Signs of hypertension as well as evidence of thyroid, hepatic, hematologic, cardiovascular, or renal diseases should be sought. An assessment should be made of the endocrine and vascular systems, the external genitalia, and the prostate gland. The penis should be palpated carefully along the corpora to detect fibrotic plaques. Reduced testicular size and loss of secondary sexual characteristics are suggestive of hypogonadism. Neurologic examination should include assessment of anal sphincter tone, investigation of the bulbocavernosus reflex, and testing for peripheral neuropathy.

Although hyperprolactinemia is uncommon, a serum prolactin level should be measured, as decreased libido and/or ED may be the presenting symptoms of a prolactinoma or another mass lesion of the sella **(Chap. 5)**. The serum testosterone level should be measured, and if it is low, gonadotropins should be measured to determine whether hypogonadism is primary (testicular) or secondary (hypothalamic-pituitary) in origin **(Chap. 11)**. If not performed recently, serum chemistries, complete blood count (CBC), and lipid profiles may be of value, as they can yield evidence of anemia, diabetes, hyperlipidemia, or other systemic diseases associated with ED. Determination of serum prostate-specific antigen (PSA) should be conducted according to recommended clinical guidelines.

Additional diagnostic testing is rarely necessary in the evaluation of ED. However, in selected patients, specialized testing may provide insight into pathologic mechanisms of ED and aid in the selection of treatment options. Optional specialized testing includes (1) studies of nocturnal penile tumescence and rigidity, (2) vascular testing (in-office injection of vasoactive substances, penile Doppler ultrasound, penile angiography, dynamic infusion cavernosography/cavernosometry), (3) neurologic testing (biothesiometry-graded vibratory perception, somatosensory evoked potentials), and (4) psychological diagnostic tests. The information potentially gained from these procedures must be balanced against their invasiveness and cost.

TREATMENT Male Sexual Dysfunction

PATIENT EDUCATION Patient and partner education is essential in the treatment of ED. In goal-directed therapy, education facilitates understanding of the disease, the results of the tests, and the selection of treatment. Discussion of treatment options helps clarify how treatment is best offered and stratify first- and second-line therapies. Patients with high-risk lifestyle issues such as obesity, smoking, alcohol abuse, and recreational drug use should be counseled on the role those factors play in the development of ED.

Therapies currently employed for the treatment of ED include oral PDE-5 inhibitor therapy (most commonly used), injection therapies, testosterone therapy, penile devices, and psychological therapy. In addition, limited data suggest that treatments for underlying risk factors and comorbidities—for example, weight loss, exercise, stress reduction, and smoking cessation—may improve erectile function. Decisions regarding therapy should take into account the preferences and expectations of patients and their partners.

ORAL AGENTS Sildenafil, tadalafil, vardenafil, and avanafil are the only approved and effective oral agents for the treatment of ED. These four medications have markedly improved the management of ED because they are effective for the treatment of a broad range of causes, including psychogenic, diabetic, vasculogenic, post-radical prostatectomy (nerve-sparing procedures), and spinal cord injury. They belong to a class of medications that are selective and potent inhibitors of PDE-5, the predominant phosphodiesterase isoform found in the penis. They are administered in graduated doses and enhance erections after sexual stimulation. The onset of action is approximately 30–120 min, depending on the medication used and other factors, such as recent food intake. Reduced initial doses should be considered for patients who are elderly, are taking concomitant alpha blockers, have renal insufficiency, or are taking medications that inhibit the CYP3A4 metabolic pathway in the liver (e.g., erythromycin, cimetidine, ketoconazole, and possibly itraconazole and mibefradil), as they may increase the serum concentration of the PDE-5 inhibitors (PDE-5i) or promote hypotension.

Initially, there were concerns about the cardiovascular safety of PDE-5i drugs. These agents can act as a mild

TABLE 19-2

CHARACTERISTICS OF PDE-5I MEDICATIONS

DRUG	ONSET OF ACTION	HALF-LIFE	DOSE	ADVERSE EFFECTS	CONTRAINDICATIONS
Sildenafil	T_{max}, 30–120 min Duration, 4 h High-fat meal decreases absorption ETOH may affect efficacy	2–5 h	25–100 mg Starting dose, 50 mg	Headache, flushing, dyspepsia, nasal congestion, altered vision	Nitrates Hypotension Cardiovascular risk factors Retinitis pigmentosa Change dose with some antiretrovirals Should be on stable dose of alpha blockers
Vardenafil	T_{max}, 30–120 min Duration, 4–5 h High-fat meal decreases absorption ETOH may affect efficacy	4.5 h	5–10 mg	Headache, flushing, rhinitis, dyspepsia	Same as sildenafil May have minor prolongation of QT interval Concomitant use of Class I antiarrhythmic
Tadalafil	T_{max}, 30–60 min Duration, 12–36 h Plasma concentration Not affected by food or ETOH	17.5 h	10 mg, 20 mg; 2.5 or 5 mg for daily dose	Headache, dyspepsia, back pain, nasal congestion, myalgia	Same as sildenafil
Avanafil	T_{max}, 30 min Duration, 2 h Plasma concentration not affected by food	3–5 h	50, 100, and 200 mg	Headache, flushing, nasal congestion, nasopharyngitis, back pain	Same as sildenafil

Abbreviations: ETOH, alcohol; T_{max}, time to maximum plasma concentration.

vasodilator, and warnings exist about orthostatic hypotension with concomitant use of alpha blockers. The use of PDE-5i is not contraindicated in men who are also receiving alpha blockers, but they must be stabilized on this blood pressure medication prior to initiating therapy. Concerns also existed that use of PDE-5i would increase cardiovascular events. However, the safety of these drugs has been confirmed in several controlled trials with no increase in myocardial ischemic events or overall mortality compared to the general population.

Several randomized trials have demonstrated the efficacy of this class of medications. There are no compelling data to support the superiority of one PDE-5i over another. Subtle differences between agents have variable clinical relevance (Table 19-2).

Patients may fail to respond to a PDE-5i for several reasons (Table 19-3). Some patients may not tolerate PDE-5i secondary to adverse events from vasodilation in nonpenile tissues expressing PDE-5 or from the inhibition of homologous nonpenile isozymes (i.e., PDE-6 found in the retina). Abnormal vision attributed to the effects of PDE-5i on retinal PDE-6 is of short duration, reported only with sildenafil and not thought to be clinically significant. A more serious concern is the possibility that PDE-5i may cause nonarteritic anterior ischemic optic neuropathy; although data to support that association are limited, it is prudent to avoid the use of these agents in men with a prior history of nonarteritic anterior ischemic optic neuropathy.

Testosterone supplementation combined with a PDE-5i may be beneficial in improving erectile function in hypogonadal men with ED who are unresponsive to PDE-5i alone. These drugs do not affect ejaculation, orgasm, or sexual drive. Side effects associated with PDE-5i include headaches (19%), facial flushing (9%), dyspepsia (6%), and nasal congestion (4%). Approximately 7% of men using sildenafil may experience transient altered color vision (blue halo effect), and 6% of men taking tadalafil may experience loin pain. PDE-5i is contraindicated in men receiving nitrate therapy for cardiovascular disease, including agents delivered by the oral, sublingual, transnasal, and topical routes. These agents can potentiate its hypotensive effect and may result in profound shock. Likewise, amyl/butyl nitrate "poppers" may have a

TABLE 19-3

ISSUES TO CONSIDER IF PATIENTS REPORT FAILURE OF PDE-5I TO IMPROVE ERECTILE DYSFUNCTION

- A trial of medication on at least 6 different days at the maximal dose should be made before declaring patient nonresponsive to PDE-5i use
- Confirm that patient did not take medication after a high-fat meal
- Failure to include physical and psychic stimulation at the time of foreplay to induce endogenous NO
- Unrecognized hypogonadism

Abbreviations: NO, nitric oxide; PDE-5i, phosphodiesterase type 5 inhibitor.

fatal synergistic effect on blood pressure. PDE-5i also should be avoided in patients with congestive heart failure and cardiomyopathy because of the risk of vascular collapse. Because sexual activity leads to an increase in physiologic expenditure (5–6 metabolic equivalents [METS]), physicians have been advised to exercise caution in prescribing any drug for sexual activity to those with active coronary disease, heart failure, borderline hypotension, or hypovolemia and to those on complex antihypertensive regimens.

Although the various forms of PDE-5i have a common mechanism of action, there are a few differences among the four agents (Table 19-2). Tadalafil is unique in its longer half-life, whereas avanafil appears to have the most rapid onset of action. All four drugs are effective for patients with ED of all ages, severities, and etiologies. Although there are pharmacokinetic and pharmacodynamic differences among these agents, clinically relevant differences are not clear.

ANDROGEN THERAPY Testosterone replacement is used to treat both primary and secondary causes of hypogonadism **(Chap. 11)**. Androgen supplementation in the setting of normal testosterone is rarely efficacious in the treatment of ED and is discouraged. Methods of androgen replacement include transdermal patches and gels, parenteral administration of long-acting testosterone esters (enanthate and cypionate), and oral preparations (17 α-alkylated derivatives) **(Chap. 11)**. Oral androgen preparations have the potential for hepatotoxicity and should be avoided.

Men who receive testosterone should be reevaluated after 1–3 months and at least annually thereafter for testosterone levels, erectile function, and adverse effects, which may include gynecomastia, sleep apnea, development or exacerbation of lower urinary tract symptoms or BPH, prostate cancer, lowering of HDL, erythrocytosis, elevations of liver function tests, and reduced fertility. Periodic reevaluation should include measurement of CBC and PSA and digital rectal exam. Therapy should be discontinued in patients who do not respond within 3 months.

VACUUM CONSTRICTION DEVICES Vacuum constriction devices (VCDs) are a well-established noninvasive therapy. They are a reasonable treatment alternative for select patients who cannot take sildenafil or do not desire other interventions. VCDs draw venous blood into the penis and use a constriction ring to restrict venous return and maintain tumescence. Adverse events with VCD include pain, numbness, bruising, and altered ejaculation. Additionally, many patients complain that the devices are cumbersome and that the induced erections have a nonphysiologic appearance and feel.

INTRAURETHRAL ALPROSTADIL If a patient fails to respond to oral agents, a reasonable next choice is intraurethral or self-injection of vasoactive substances. Intraurethral prostaglandin E_1 (alprostadil), in the form of a semisolid pellet (doses of 125–1000 μg), is delivered with an applicator. Approximately 65% of men receiving intraurethral alprostadil respond with an erection when tested in the office, but only 50% achieve successful coitus at home. Intraurethral insertion is associated with a markedly reduced incidence of priapism in comparison to intracavernosal injection.

INTRACAVERNOSAL SELF-INJECTION Injection of synthetic formulations of alprostadil is effective in 70–80% of patients with ED, but discontinuation rates are high because of the invasive nature of administration. Doses range between 1 and 40 μg. Injection therapy is contraindicated in men with a history of hypersensitivity to the drug and men at risk for priapism (hypercoagulable states, sickle cell disease). Side effects include local adverse events, prolonged erections, pain, and fibrosis with chronic use. Various combinations of alprostadil, phentolamine, and/or papaverine sometimes are used.

SURGERY A less frequently used form of therapy for ED involves the surgical implantation of a semirigid or inflatable penile prosthesis. The choice of prosthesis is dependent on patient preference and should take into account body habitus and manual dexterity, which may affect the ability of the patient to manipulate the device. Because of the permanence of prosthetic devices, patients should be advised to first consider less invasive options for treatment. These surgical treatments are invasive, are associated with potential complications, and generally are reserved for treatment of refractory ED. Despite their high cost and invasiveness, penile prostheses are associated with high rates of patient and partner satisfaction.

SEX THERAPY A course of sex therapy may be useful for addressing specific interpersonal factors that may affect sexual functioning. Sex therapy generally consists of in-session discussion and at-home exercises specific to the person and the relationship. Psychosexual therapy involves techniques such as sensate focus (nongenital massage), sensory awareness exercises, correction of misconceptions about sexuality, and interpersonal difficulties therapy (e.g., open communication about sexual issues, physical intimacy scheduling, and behavioral interventions). These approaches may be useful in patients who have psychogenic or social components to their ED, although data from randomized trials are scanty and inconsistent. It is preferable if therapy includes both partners if the patient is involved in an ongoing relationship.

FEMALE SEXUAL DYSFUNCTION

Female sexual dysfunction (FSD) has traditionally included disorders of desire, arousal, pain, and muted orgasm. The associated risk factors for FSD are similar to those in males: cardiovascular disease, endocrine disorders, hypertension, neurologic disorders, and smoking (Table 19-4).

EPIDEMIOLOGY

Epidemiologic data are limited, but the available estimates suggest that as many as 43% of women complain

TABLE 19-4

RISK FACTORS FOR FEMALE SEXUAL DYSFUNCTION
Neurologic disease: stroke, spinal cord injury, parkinsonism
Trauma, genital surgery, radiation
Endocrinopathies: diabetes, hyperprolactinemia
Liver and/or renal failure
Cardiovascular disease
Psychological factors and interpersonal relationship disorders: sexual abuse, life stressors
Medications
Antiandrogens: cimetidine, spironolactone
Antidepressants, alcohol, hypnotics, sedatives
Antiestrogens or GnRH antagonists
Antihistamines, sympathomimetic amines
Antihypertensives: diuretics, calcium channel blockers
Alkylating agents
Anticholinergics

Abbreviation: GnRH, gonadotropin-releasing hormone.

of at least one sexual problem. Despite the recent interest in organic causes of FSD, desire and arousal phase disorders (including lubrication complaints) remain the most common presenting problems when surveyed in a community-based population.

PHYSIOLOGY OF THE FEMALE SEXUAL RESPONSE

The female sexual response requires the presence of estrogens. A role for androgens is also likely but less well established. In the CNS, estrogens and androgens work synergistically to enhance sexual arousal and response. A number of studies report enhanced libido in women during preovulatory phases of the menstrual cycle, suggesting that hormones involved in the ovulatory surge (e.g., estrogens) increase desire.

Sexual motivation is heavily influenced by context, including the environment and partner factors. Once sufficient sexual desire is reached, sexual arousal is mediated by the central and autonomic nervous systems. Cerebral sympathetic outflow is thought to increase desire, and peripheral parasympathetic activity results in clitoral vasocongestion and vaginal secretion (lubrication).

The neurotransmitters for clitoral corporal engorgement are similar to those in the male, with a prominent role for neural, smooth-muscle, and endothelial released nitric oxide (NO). A fine network of vaginal nerves and arterioles promotes a vaginal transudate. The major transmitters of this complex vaginal response are not certain, but roles for NO and vasointestinal polypeptide (VIP) are suspected. Investigators studying the normal female sexual response have challenged the long-held construct of a linear and unmitigated relationship between initial desire, arousal, vasocongestion, lubrication, and eventual orgasm. Caregivers should consider a paradigm of a positive emotional and physical outcome with one, many, or no orgasmic peak and release.

Although there are anatomic differences as well as variation in the density of vascular and neural beds in males and females, the primary effectors of sexual response are strikingly similar. Intact sensation is important for arousal. Thus, reduced levels of sexual functioning are more common in women with peripheral neuropathies (e.g., diabetes). Vaginal lubrication is a transudate of serum that results from the increased pelvic blood flow associated with arousal. Vascular insufficiency from a variety of causes may compromise adequate lubrication and result in dyspareunia. Cavernosal and arteriole smooth-muscle relaxation occurs via increased nitric oxide synthase (NOS) activity and produces engorgement in the clitoris and the surrounding vestibule. Orgasm requires an intact sympathetic outflow tract; hence, orgasmic disorders are common in female patients with spinal cord injuries.

APPROACH TO THE PATIENT: Female Sexual Dysfunction

Many women do not volunteer information about their sexual response. Open-ended questions in a supportive atmosphere are helpful in initiating a discussion of sexual fitness in women who are reluctant to discuss such issues. Once a complaint has been voiced, a comprehensive evaluation should be performed, including a medical history, a psychosocial history, a physical examination, and limited laboratory testing.

The history should include the usual medical, surgical, obstetric, psychological, gynecologic, sexual, and social information. Past experiences, intimacy, knowledge, and partner availability should also be ascertained. Medical disorders that may affect sexual health should be delineated. They include diabetes, cardiovascular disease, gynecologic conditions, obstetric history, depression, anxiety disorders, and neurologic disease. Medications should be reviewed as they may affect arousal, libido, and orgasm. The need for counseling and recognizing life stresses should be identified. The physical examination should assess the genitalia, including the clitoris. Pelvic floor examination may identify prolapse or other disorders. Laboratory studies are needed, especially if menopausal status is uncertain. Estradiol, follicle-stimulating hormone (FSH), and luteinizing hormone (LH) are usually obtained, and dehydroepiandrosterone (DHEA) should be considered as it reflects adrenal androgen secretion. A CBC, liver function assessment, and lipid studies may be useful, if not otherwise obtained. Complicated diagnostic evaluations such as clitoral Doppler ultrasonography and biothesiometry require expensive equipment and are of uncertain utility. It is important for the patient to identify which symptoms are most distressing.

The evaluation of FSD previously occurred mainly in a psychosocial context. However, inconsistencies between diagnostic categories based only on psychosocial considerations and the emerging recognition of organic etiologies have led to a new classification of FSD. This diagnostic scheme is based on four components that are not mutually exclusive: (1) *hypoactive sexual desire*—the persistent or recurrent lack of sexual thoughts and/or receptivity to sexual activity, which causes personal distress; hypoactive sexual desire may result from endocrine failure or may be associated with psychological or emotional disorders; (2) *sexual arousal disorder*—the persistent or recurrent inability to attain or maintain sexual excitement, which causes personal distress; (3) *orgasmic disorder*—the persistent or recurrent loss of orgasmic potential after sufficient sexual stimulation and arousal, which causes personal distress; and (4) *sexual pain disorder*—persistent or recurrent genital pain associated with noncoital sexual stimulation, which causes personal distress. This newer classification emphasizes "personal distress" as a requirement for dysfunction and provides clinicians with an organized framework for evaluation before or in conjunction with more traditional counseling methods.

TREATMENT Female Sexual Dysfunction

GENERAL An open discussion with the patient is important as couples may need to be educated about normal anatomy and physiologic responses, including the role of orgasm, in sexual encounters. Physiologic changes associated with aging and/or disease should be explained. Couples may need to be reminded that clitoral stimulation rather than coital intromission may be more beneficial.

Behavioral modification and nonpharmacologic therapies should be a first step. Patient and partner counseling may improve communication and relationship strains. Lifestyle changes involving known risk factors can be an important part of the treatment process. Emphasis on maximizing physical health and avoiding lifestyles (e.g., smoking, alcohol abuse) and medications likely to produce FSD is important (Table 19-4). The use of topical lubricants may address complaints of dyspareunia and dryness. Contributing medications such as antidepressants may need to be altered, including the use of medications with less impact on sexual function, dose reduction, medication switching, or drug holidays.

HORMONAL THERAPY In postmenopausal women, estrogen replacement therapy may be helpful in treating vaginal atrophy, decreasing coital pain, and improving clitoral sensitivity **(Chap. 16)**. Estrogen replacement in the form of local cream is the preferred method, as it avoids systemic side effects. Androgen levels in women decline substantially before menopause. However, low levels of testosterone or DHEA are not effective predictors of a positive therapeutic outcome with androgen therapy. The widespread use of exogenous androgens is not supported by the literature except in select circumstances (premature ovarian failure or menopausal states) and in secondary arousal disorders.

ORAL AGENTS The efficacy of PDE-5i in FDS has been a marked disappointment in light of the proposed role of nitric oxide–dependent physiology in the normal female sexual response. The use of PDE-5i for FSD should be discouraged pending proof that it is effective.

CLITORAL VACUUM DEVICE In patients with arousal and orgasmic difficulties, the option of using a clitoral vacuum device may be explored. This handheld battery-operated device has a small soft plastic cup that applies a vacuum over the stimulated clitoris. This causes increased cavernosal blood flow, engorgement, and vaginal lubrication.

SECTION IV

DIABETES MELLITUS, OBESITY, LIPOPROTEIN METABOLISM

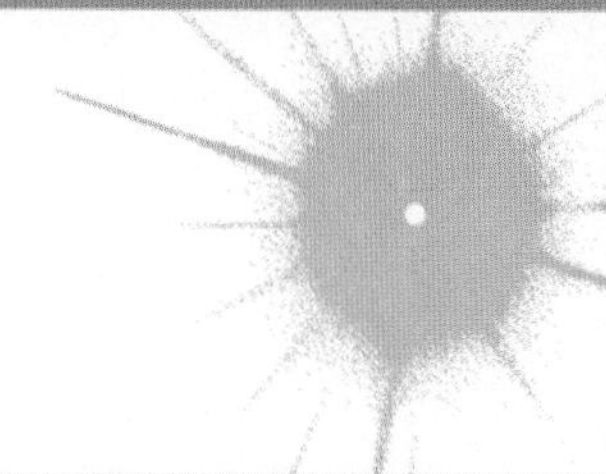

CHAPTER 20
BIOLOGY OF OBESITY

Jeffrey S. Flier ■ Eleftheria Maratos-Flier

In a world where food supplies are intermittent, the ability to store energy in excess of what is required for immediate use is essential for survival. Fat cells, residing within widely distributed adipose tissue depots, are adapted to store excess energy efficiently as triglyceride and, when needed, to release stored energy as free fatty acids for use at other sites. This physiologic system, orchestrated through endocrine and neural pathways, permits humans to survive starvation for as long as several months. However, in the presence of nutritional abundance and a sedentary lifestyle, and influenced importantly by genetic endowment, this system increases adipose energy stores and produces adverse health consequences.

DEFINITION AND MEASUREMENT

Obesity is a state of excess adipose tissue mass. Although often viewed as equivalent to increased body weight, this need not be the case—lean but very muscular individuals may be overweight by numerical standards without having increased adiposity. Body weights are distributed continuously in populations, so that choice of a medically meaningful distinction between lean and obese is somewhat arbitrary. Obesity is therefore defined by assessing its linkage to morbidity or mortality.

Although not a direct measure of adiposity, the most widely used method to gauge obesity is the *body mass index* (BMI), which is equal to weight/height^2 (in kg/m^2) (Fig. 20-1). Other approaches to quantifying obesity include anthropometry (skinfold thickness), densitometry (underwater weighing), computed tomography (CT) or magnetic resonance imaging (MRI), and electrical impedance. Using data from the Metropolitan Life Tables, BMIs for the midpoint of all heights and frames among both men and women range from 19 to 26 kg/m^2; at a similar BMI, women have more body fat than men. Based on data of substantial morbidity, a BMI of 30 is most commonly used as a threshold for obesity in both men and women. Most but not all large-scale epidemiologic studies suggest that all-cause, metabolic, cancer, and cardiovascular morbidity begin to rise (albeit at a slow rate) when BMIs are ≥25. Most authorities use the term *overweight* (rather than obese) to describe individuals with BMIs between 25 and 30. A BMI between 25 and 30 should be viewed as medically significant and worthy of therapeutic intervention in the presence of risk factors that are influenced by adiposity, such as hypertension and glucose intolerance.

The distribution of adipose tissue in different anatomic depots also has substantial implications for morbidity. Specifically, intraabdominal and abdominal subcutaneous fat have more significance than subcutaneous fat present in the buttocks and lower extremities. This distinction is most easily made clinically by determining the waist-to-hip ratio, with a ratio >0.9 in women and >1.0 in men being abnormal. Many of the most important complications of obesity, such as insulin resistance, diabetes, hypertension, hyperlipidemia, and hyperandrogenism in women, are linked more strongly to intraabdominal and/or upper body fat than to overall adiposity **(Chap. 22)**. The mechanism underlying this association is unknown but may relate to the fact that intraabdominal adipocytes are more lipolytically active than those from other depots. Release of free fatty acids into the portal circulation has adverse metabolic actions, especially on the liver. Adipokines and cytokines that are differentially secreted by adipocyte depots may play a role in the systemic complications of obesity.

PREVALENCE

Data from the National Health and Nutrition Examination Surveys (NHANES) show that the percentage of the American adult population with obesity (BMI >30) has increased from 14.5% (between 1976 and 1980) to 35.7% (between 2009 and 2010). As many as 68% of U.S. adults aged ≥20 years were overweight (defined as

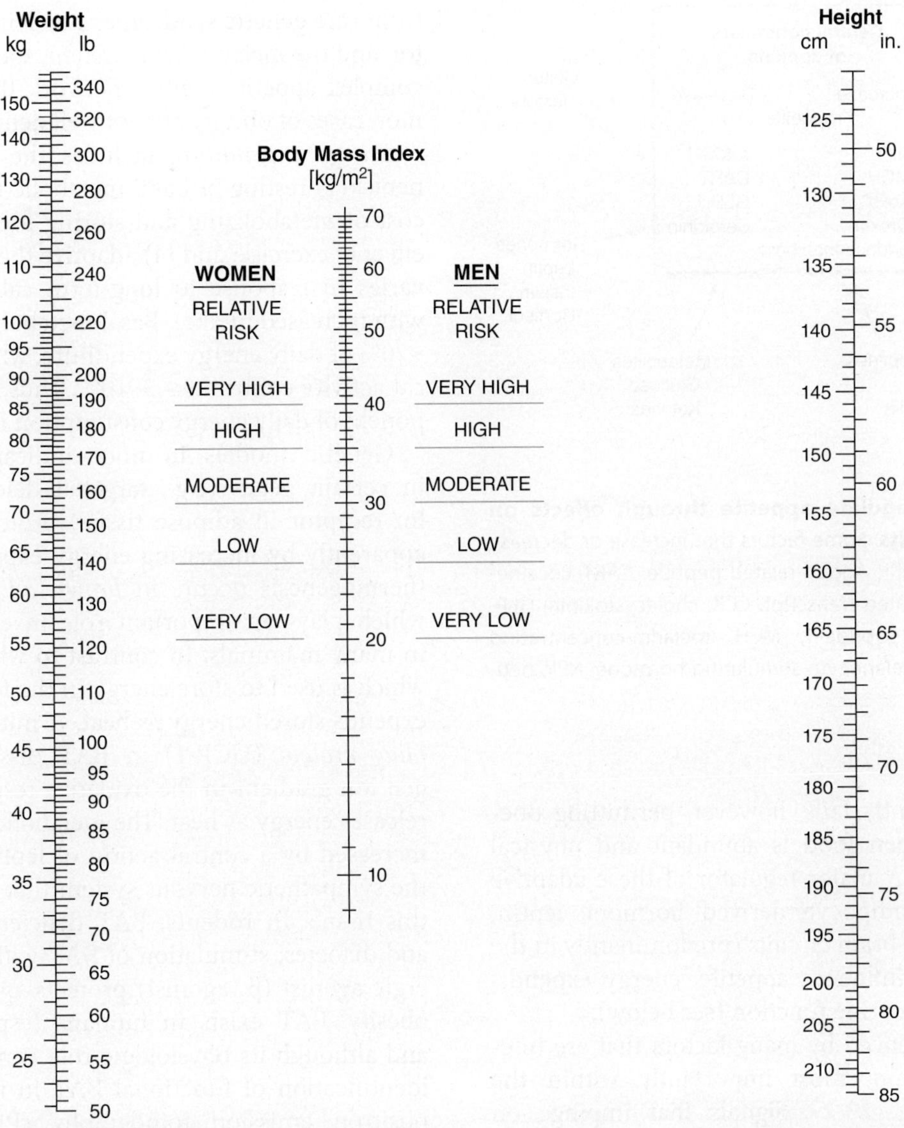

FIGURE 20-1

Nomogram for determining body mass index. To use this nomogram, place a ruler or other straight edge between the body weight (without clothes) in kilograms or pounds located on the left-hand line and the height (without shoes) in centimeters or inches located on the right-hand line. The body mass index is read from the middle of the scale and is in metric units. *(Copyright 1979, George A. Bray, MD; used with permission.)*

BMI >25) between the years of 2007 and 2008. Extreme obesity (BMI ≥40) has also increased and affects 5.7% of the population. The increasing prevalence of medically significant obesity raises great concern. Overall, the prevalence of obesity is comparable in men and women. In women, poverty is associated with increased prevalence. Obesity is more common among blacks and Hispanics. The prevalence in children and adolescents has been rising at a worrisome rate, reaching 15.9% in 2009/2010, but may be leveling off.

PHYSIOLOGIC REGULATION OF ENERGY BALANCE

Substantial evidence suggests that body weight is regulated by both endocrine and neural components that ultimately influence the effector arms of energy intake and expenditure. This complex regulatory system is necessary because even small imbalances between energy intake and expenditure will ultimately have large effects on body weight. For example, a 0.3% positive imbalance over 30 years would result in a 9-kg (20-lb) weight gain. This exquisite regulation of energy balance cannot be monitored easily by calorie-counting in relation to physical activity. Rather, body weight regulation or dysregulation depends on a complex interplay of hormonal and neural signals. Alterations in stable weight by forced overfeeding or food deprivation induce physiologic changes that resist these perturbations: with weight loss, appetite increases and energy expenditure falls; with overfeeding, appetite falls and energy expenditure increases. This latter compensatory

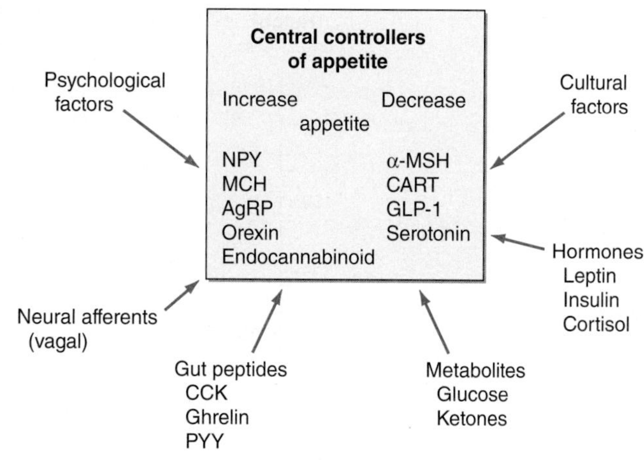

FIGURE 20-2

The factors that regulate appetite through effects on central neural circuits. Some factors that increase or decrease appetite are listed. AgRP, Agouti-related peptide; CART, cocaine- and amphetamine-related transcript; CCK, cholecystokinin; GLP-1, glucagon-related peptide-1; MCH, melanin-concentrating hormone; α-MSH, α-melanocyte-stimulating hormone; NPY, neuropeptide Y.

mechanism frequently fails, however, permitting obesity to develop when food is abundant and physical activity is limited. A major regulator of these adaptive responses is the adipocyte-derived hormone leptin, which acts through brain circuits (predominantly in the hypothalamus) to influence appetite, energy expenditure, and neuroendocrine function (see below).

Appetite is influenced by many factors that are integrated by the brain, most importantly within the hypothalamus (Fig. 20-2). Signals that impinge on the hypothalamic center include neural afferents, hormones, and metabolites. Vagal inputs are particularly important, bringing information from viscera, such as gut distention. Hormonal signals include leptin, insulin, cortisol, and gut peptides. Among the latter is ghrelin, which is made in the stomach and stimulates feeding, and peptide YY (PYY) and cholecystokinin, which is made in the small intestine and signals to the brain through direct action on hypothalamic control centers and/or via the vagus nerve. Metabolites, including glucose, can influence appetite, as seen by the effect of hypoglycemia to induce hunger; however, glucose is not normally a major regulator of appetite. These diverse hormonal, metabolic, and neural signals act by influencing the expression and release of various hypothalamic peptides (e.g., neuropeptide Y [NPY], Agouti-related peptide [AgRP], α-melanocyte-stimulating hormone [α-MSH], and melanin-concentrating hormone [MCH]) that are integrated with serotonergic, catecholaminergic, endocannabinoid, and opioid signaling pathways (see below). Psychological and cultural factors also play a role in the final expression of appetite. Apart from rare genetic syndromes involving leptin, its receptor, and the melanocortin system, specific defects in this complex appetite control network that influence common cases of obesity are not well defined.

Energy expenditure includes the following components: (1) resting or basal metabolic rate; (2) the energy cost of metabolizing and storing food; (3) the thermic effect of exercise; and (4) adaptive thermogenesis, which varies in response to long-term caloric intake (rising with increased intake). Basal metabolic rate accounts for ~70% of daily energy expenditure, whereas active physical activity contributes 5–10%. Thus, a significant component of daily energy consumption is fixed.

Genetic models in mice indicate that mutations in certain genes (e.g., targeted deletion of the insulin receptor in adipose tissue) protect against obesity, apparently by increasing energy expenditure. Adaptive thermogenesis occurs in *brown adipose tissue* (BAT), which plays an important role in energy metabolism in many mammals. In contrast to white adipose tissue, which is used to store energy in the form of lipids, BAT expends stored energy as heat. A mitochondrial *uncoupling protein* (UCP-1) in BAT dissipates the hydrogen ion gradient in the oxidative respiration chain and releases energy as heat. The metabolic activity of BAT is increased by a central action of leptin, acting through the sympathetic nervous system that heavily innervates this tissue. In rodents, BAT deficiency causes obesity and diabetes; stimulation of BAT with a specific adrenergic agonist (β_3 agonist) protects against diabetes and obesity. BAT exists in humans (especially neonates), and although its physiologic role is not yet established, identification of functional BAT in many adults using positron emission tomography (PET) imaging has increased interest in the implications of the tissue for pathogenesis and therapy of obesity. Beige fat cells, recently described, resemble BAT cells in expressing UCP-1. They are scattered through white adipose tissue, and their thermogenic potential is uncertain.

THE ADIPOCYTE AND ADIPOSE TISSUE

Adipose tissue is composed of the lipid-storing adipose cell and a stromal/vascular compartment in which cells including preadipocytes and macrophages reside. Adipose mass increases by enlargement of adipose cells through lipid deposition, as well as by an increase in the number of adipocytes. Obese adipose tissue is also characterized by increased numbers of infiltrating macrophages. The process by which adipose cells are derived from a mesenchymal preadipocyte involves an orchestrated series of differentiation steps mediated by a cascade of specific transcription factors. One of the key transcription factors is *peroxisome proliferator-activated receptor γ* (PPARγ), a nuclear receptor that binds the

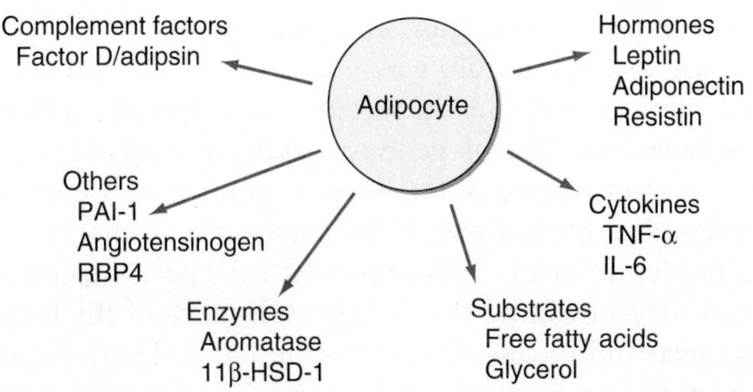

FIGURE 20-3

Factors released by the adipocyte that can affect peripheral tissues. IL-6, interleukin 6; PAI, plasminogen activator inhibitor; RBP4, retinal binding protein 4; TNF, tumor necrosis factor.

thiazolidinedione class of insulin-sensitizing drugs used in the treatment of type 2 diabetes **(Chap. 24)**.

Although the adipocyte has generally been regarded as a storage depot for fat, it is also an endocrine cell that releases numerous molecules in a regulated fashion (Fig. 20-3). These include the energy balance–regulating hormone leptin, cytokines such as tumor necrosis factor (TNF)-α and interleukin (IL)-6, complement factors such as factor D (also known as *adipsin*), prothrombotic agents such as plasminogen activator inhibitor I, and a component of the blood pressure–regulating system, angiotensinogen. Adiponectin, an abundant adipose-derived protein whose levels are reduced in obesity, enhances insulin sensitivity and lipid oxidation and has vascular-protective effects, whereas resistin and RBP4, whose levels are increased in obesity, may induce insulin resistance. These factors, and others not yet identified, play a role in the physiology of lipid homeostasis, insulin sensitivity, blood pressure control, coagulation, and vascular health, and are likely to contribute to obesity-related pathologies.

ETIOLOGY OF OBESITY

Although the molecular pathways regulating energy balance are beginning to be illuminated, the causes of obesity remain elusive. In part, this reflects the fact that obesity is a heterogeneous group of disorders. At one level, the pathophysiology of obesity seems simple: a chronic excess of nutrient intake relative to the level of energy expenditure. However, due to the complexity of the neuroendocrine and metabolic systems that regulate energy intake, storage, and expenditure, it has been difficult to quantitate all the relevant parameters (e.g., food intake and energy expenditure) over time in human subjects.

Role of genes versus environment

Obesity is commonly seen in families, and the heritability of body weight is similar to that for height. Inheritance is usually not Mendelian, however, and it is difficult to distinguish the role of genes and environmental factors. Adoptees more closely resemble their biologic than adoptive parents with respect to obesity, providing strong support for genetic influences. Likewise, identical twins have very similar BMIs whether reared together or apart, and their BMIs are much more strongly correlated than those of dizygotic twins. These genetic effects appear to relate to both energy intake and expenditure. Currently, identified genetic variants, both common and rare, account for less than 5% of the variance of body weight.

Whatever the role of genes, it is clear that the environment plays a key role in obesity, as evidenced by the fact that famine prevents obesity in even the most obesity-prone individual. In addition, the recent increase in the prevalence of obesity in the United States is far too rapid to be due to changes in the gene pool. Undoubtedly, genes influence the susceptibility to obesity in response to specific diets and availability of nutrition. Cultural factors are also important—these relate to both availability and composition of the diet and to changes in the level of physical activity. In industrial societies, obesity is more common among poor women, whereas in underdeveloped countries, wealthier women are more often obese. In children, obesity correlates to some degree with time spent watching television. Although the role of diet composition in obesity continues to generate controversy, it appears that high-fat diets may, when combined with simple, rapidly absorbed carbohydrates, promote obesity. Specific genes are likely to influence the response to specific diets, but these genes are largely unidentified.

Additional environmental factors may contribute to the increasing obesity prevalence. Both epidemiologic correlations and experimental data suggest that sleep deprivation leads to increased obesity. Changes in gut microbiome with capacity to alter energy balance are receiving experimental support from animal studies, and a possible role for obesigenic viral infections continues to receive sporadic attention.

Specific genetic syndromes

For many years, obesity in rodents has been known to be caused by a number of distinct mutations distributed through the genome. Most of these single-gene mutations cause both hyperphagia and diminished energy expenditure, suggesting a physiologic link between these two parameters of energy homeostasis. Identification of the *ob* gene mutation in genetically obese (ob/ob) mice represented a major breakthrough in the field. The ob/ob mouse develops severe obesity, insulin resistance, and hyperphagia, as well as efficient metabolism (e.g., it gets fat even when ingesting the same number of calories as lean litter mates). The product of the *ob* gene is the peptide leptin, a name derived from the Greek

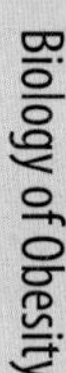

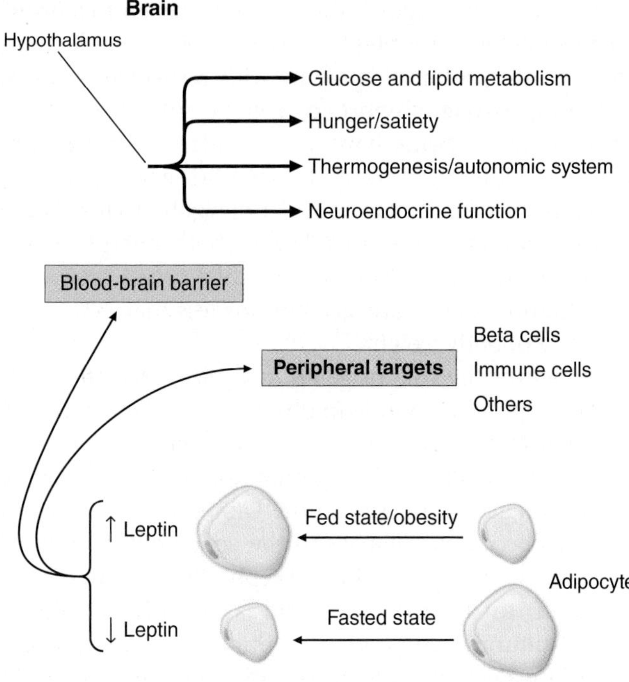

FIGURE 20-4

The physiologic system regulated by leptin. Rising or falling leptin levels act through the hypothalamus to influence appetite, energy expenditure, and neuroendocrine function and through peripheral sites to influence systems such as the immune system.

root *leptos*, meaning thin. Leptin is secreted by adipose cells and acts primarily through the hypothalamus. Its level of production provides an index of adipose energy stores (Fig. 20-4). High leptin levels decrease food intake and increase energy expenditure. Another mouse mutant, db/db, which is resistant to leptin, has a mutation in the leptin receptor and develops a similar syndrome. The *ob* gene is present in humans where it is also expressed in fat. Several families with morbid, early-onset obesity caused by inactivating mutations in either leptin or the leptin receptor have been described, thus demonstrating the biologic relevance of the leptin pathway in humans. Obesity in these individuals begins shortly after birth, is severe, and is accompanied by neuroendocrine abnormalities. The most prominent of these is hypogonadotropic hypogonadism, which is reversed by leptin replacement in the leptin-deficient subset. Central hypothyroidism and growth retardation are seen in the mouse model, but their occurrence in leptin-deficient humans is less clear. Mutations in the leptin or leptin receptor genes do not play a prominent role in common forms of obesity.

Mutations in several other genes cause severe obesity in humans (Table 20-1); each of these syndromes is rare. Mutations in the gene encoding proopiomelanocortin (POMC) cause severe obesity through failure to synthesize α-MSH, a key neuropeptide that inhibits appetite in the hypothalamus. The absence of POMC also causes secondary adrenal insufficiency due to absence of adrenocorticotropic hormone (ACTH), as well as pale skin and red hair due to absence of α-MSH. Proenzyme convertase 1 (PC-1) mutations are thought to cause obesity by preventing synthesis of α-MSH from its precursor peptide, POMC. α-MSH binds to the type 4 melanocortin receptor (MC4R), a key hypothalamic receptor that inhibits eating. Heterozygous

TABLE 20-1

SELECTED OBESITY GENES IN HUMANS AND MICE

GENE	GENE PRODUCT	MECHANISM OF OBESITY	IN HUMAN	IN RODENT
Lep (ob)	Leptin, a fat-derived hormone	Mutation prevents leptin from delivering satiety signal; brain perceives starvation	Yes	Yes
LepR (db)	Leptin receptor	Same as above	Yes	Yes
POMC	Proopiomelanocortin, a precursor of several hormones and neuropeptides	Mutation prevents synthesis of melanocyte-stimulating hormone (MSH), a satiety signal	Yes	Yes
MC4R	Type 4 receptor for MSH	Mutation prevents reception of satiety signal from MSH	Yes	Yes
AgRP	Agouti-related peptide, a neuropeptide expressed in the hypothalamus	Overexpression inhibits signal through *MC4R*	No	Yes
PC-1	Prohormone convertase 1, a processing enzyme	Mutation prevents synthesis of neuropeptide, probably MSH	Yes	No
Fat	Carboxypeptidase E, a processing enzyme	Same as above	No	Yes
Tub	Tub, a hypothalamic protein of unknown function	Hypothalamic dysfunction	No	Yes
TrkB	TrkB, a neurotrophin receptor	Hyperphagia due to uncharacterized hypothalamic defect	Yes	Yes

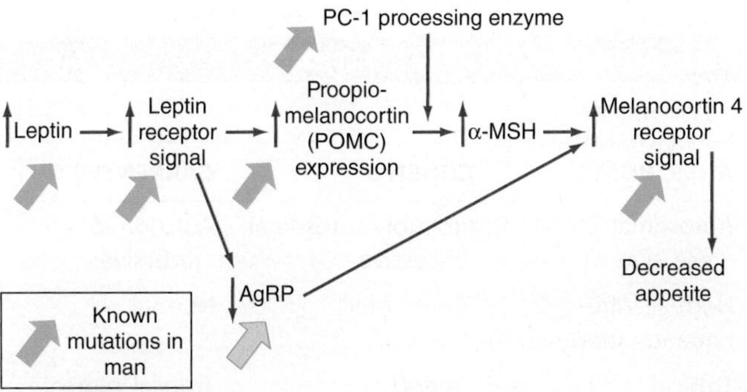

FIGURE 20-5

A central pathway through which leptin acts to regulate appetite and body weight. Leptin signals through proopiomelanocortin (POMC) neurons in the hypothalamus to induce increased production of α-melanocyte-stimulating hormone (α-MSH), requiring the processing enzyme PC-1 (proenzyme convertase 1). α-MSH acts as an agonist on melanocortin-4 receptors to inhibit appetite, and the neuropeptide AgRp (Agouti-related peptide) acts as an antagonist of this receptor. Mutations that cause obesity in humans are indicated by the *solid green arrows*.

loss-of-function mutations of this receptor account for as much as 5% of severe obesity. Loss of function of MRAP2, a protein required for normal MC4R signaling, has been found in rare cases of severe obesity. These six genetic defects define a pathway through which leptin (by stimulating POMC and increasing α-MSH) restricts food intake and limits weight (Fig. 20-5). The results of genomewide association studies to identify genetic loci responsible for obesity in the general population have so far been disappointing. More than 40 replicated loci linked to obesity have been identified, but together they account for less than 3% of interindividual variation in BMI. The most replicated of these is a gene named *FTO*, which is of unknown function, but like many of the other recently described candidates, is expressed in the brain. Because the heritability of obesity is estimated to be 40–70%, it is likely that many more loci remain to be identified. It is possible that epistatic interactions between causative loci or unknown gene-environment interactions explain the poor success at identifying causal loci.

In addition to these human obesity genes, studies in rodents reveal several other molecular candidates for hypothalamic mediators of human obesity or leanness. The *tub* gene encodes a hypothalamic peptide of unknown function; mutation of this gene causes late-onset obesity. The *fat* gene encodes carboxypeptidase E, a peptide-processing enzyme; mutation of this gene is thought to cause obesity by disrupting production of one or more neuropeptides. AgRP is coexpressed with NPY in arcuate nucleus neurons. AgRP antagonizes α-MSH action at MC4 receptors, and its overexpression induces obesity. In contrast, a mouse deficient in the peptide MCH, whose administration causes feeding, is lean.

A number of complex human syndromes with defined inheritance are associated with obesity (Table 20-2). Although specific genes have limited definition at present, their identification will likely enhance our understanding of more common forms of human obesity. In the Prader-Willi syndrome, a multigenic neurodevelopmental disorder, obesity coexists with short stature, mental retardation, hypogonadotropic hypogonadism, hypotonia, small hands and feet, fish-shaped mouth, and hyperphagia. Most patients have reduced expression of imprinted paternally inherited genes encoded in the 15q11-13 chromosomal region. Reduced expression of Snord116, a small nucleolar RNA highly expressed in hypothalamus, may be an important cause of defective hypothalamic function in this disorder. Bardet-Biedl syndrome (BBS) is a genetically heterogeneous disorder characterized by obesity, mental retardation, retinitis pigmentosa, diabetes, renal and cardiac malformations, polydactyly, and hypogonadotropic hypogonadism. At least 12 genetic loci have been identified, and most of the encoded proteins form two multiprotein complexes that are involved in ciliary function and microtubule-based intracellular transport. Some evidence suggests that mutations might disrupt leptin receptor trafficking in key hypothalamic neurons, causing leptin resistance.

Other specific syndromes associated with obesity

Cushing's syndrome

Although obese patients commonly have central obesity, hypertension, and glucose intolerance, they lack other specific stigmata of Cushing's syndrome **(Chap. 8)**. Nonetheless, a potential diagnosis of Cushing's syndrome is often entertained. Cortisol production and urinary metabolites (17OH steroids) may be increased in simple obesity. Unlike in Cushing's syndrome, however, cortisol levels in blood and urine in the basal state and in response to corticotropin-releasing hormone (CRH) or ACTH are normal; the overnight 1-mg dexamethasone suppression test is normal in 90%, with the remainder being normal on a standard 2-day low-dose dexamethasone suppression test. Obesity may be associated with excessive local reactivation of cortisol in fat by 11β-hydroxysteroid dehydrogenase 1, an enzyme that converts inactive cortisone to cortisol.

Hypothyroidism

The possibility of hypothyroidism should be considered, but it is an uncommon cause of obesity; hypothyroidism is easily ruled out by measuring thyroid-stimulating hormone (TSH). Much of the weight gain that occurs in hypothyroidism is due to myxedema **(Chap. 7)**.

Insulinoma

Patients with insulinoma often gain weight as a result of overeating to avoid hypoglycemic symptoms **(Chap. 26)**.

TABLE 20-2

A COMPARISON OF SYNDROMES OF OBESITY—HYPOGONADISM AND MENTAL RETARDATION

	SYNDROME				
FEATURE	**PRADER-WILLI**	**LAURENCE-MOON-BIEDL**	**AHLSTROM'S**	**COHEN'S**	**CARPENTER'S**
Inheritance	Sporadic; two-thirds have defect	Autosomal recessive	Autosomal recessive	Probably autosomal recessive	Autosomal recessive
Stature	Short	Normal; infrequently short	Normal; infrequently short	Short or tall	Normal
Obesity	Generalized	Generalized	Truncal	Truncal	Truncal, gluteal
	Moderate to severe	Early onset, 1–2 years	Early onset, 2–5 years	Mid-childhood, age 5	
	Onset 1–3 years				
Craniofacies	Narrow bifrontal diameter	Not distinctive	Not distinctive	High nasal bridge	Acrocephaly
	Almond-shaped eyes			Arched palate	Flat nasal bridge
	Strabismus			Open mouth	High-arched palate
	V-shaped mouth			Short philtrum	
	High-arched palate				
Limbs	Small hands and feet	Polydactyly	No abnormalities	Hypotonia	Polydactyly
	Hypotonia			Narrow hands and feet	Syndactyly
					Genu valgum
Reproductive status	1° Hypogonadism	1° Hypogonadism	Hypogonadism in males but not in females	Normal gonadal function or hypogonadotropic hypogonadism	2° Hypogonadism
Other features	Enamel hypoplasia			Dysplastic ears	
	Hyperphagia			Delayed puberty	
	Temper tantrums				
	Nasal speech				
Mental retardation	Mild to moderate		Normal intelligence	Mild	Slight

The increased substrate plus high insulin levels promote energy storage in fat. This can be marked in some individuals but is modest in most.

Craniopharyngioma and other disorders involving the hypothalamus

Whether through tumors, trauma, or inflammation, hypothalamic dysfunction of systems controlling satiety, hunger, and energy expenditure can cause varying degrees of obesity **(Chap. 4)**. It is uncommon to identify a discrete anatomic basis for these disorders. Subtle hypothalamic dysfunction is probably a more common cause of obesity than can be documented using currently available imaging techniques. Growth hormone (GH), which exerts lipolytic activity, is diminished in obesity and is increased with weight loss. Despite low GH levels, insulin-like growth factor (IGF) I (somatomedin) production is normal, suggesting that GH suppression may be a compensatory response to increased nutritional supply.

Pathogenesis of common obesity

Obesity can result from increased energy intake, decreased energy expenditure, or a combination of the two. Thus, identifying the etiology of obesity should involve measurements of both parameters. However, it is difficult to perform direct and accurate measurements of energy intake in free-living individuals; and the obese, in particular, often underreport intake. Measurements of chronic energy expenditure are possible using doubly labeled water or metabolic chamber/rooms. In subjects at stable weight and body composition, energy intake equals expenditure. Consequently, these techniques allow assessment of energy intake in free-living individuals. The level of energy expenditure differs in established obesity, during periods of weight gain or loss, and in the pre- or postobese state. Studies that fail to take note of this phenomenon are not easily interpreted.

There is continued interest in the concept of a body weight "set point." This idea is supported by physiologic mechanisms centered around a sensing system in adipose tissue that reflects fat stores and a receptor, or "adipostat," that is in the hypothalamic centers. When fat stores are depleted, the adipostat signal is low, and the hypothalamus responds by stimulating hunger and decreasing energy expenditure to conserve energy. Conversely, when fat stores are abundant, the signal is increased, and the hypothalamus responds by decreasing hunger and increasing energy expenditure. The recent discovery of the *ob* gene, and its product leptin, and the *db* gene, whose product is the leptin receptor, provides important elements of a molecular basis for this physiologic concept (see above).

What is the status of food intake in obesity? (do the obese eat more than the lean?)

This question has stimulated much debate, due in part to the methodologic difficulties inherent in determining food intake. Many obese individuals believe that they eat small quantities of food, and this claim has often been supported by the results of food intake questionnaires. However, it is now established that average energy expenditure increases as individuals get more obese, due primarily to the fact that metabolically active lean tissue mass increases with obesity. Given the laws of thermodynamics, the obese person must therefore eat more than the average lean person to maintain their increased weight. It may be the case, however, that a subset of individuals who are predisposed to obesity have the capacity to become obese initially without an absolute increase in caloric consumption.

What is the state of energy expenditure in obesity?

The average total daily energy expenditure is higher in obese than lean individuals when measured at stable weight. However, energy expenditure falls as weight is lost, due in part to loss of lean body mass and to decreased sympathetic nerve activity. When reduced to near-normal weight and maintained there for a while, (some) obese individuals have lower energy expenditure than (some) lean individuals. There is also a tendency for those who will develop obesity as infants or children to have lower resting energy expenditure rates than those who remain lean. The physiologic basis for variable rates of energy expenditure (at a given body weight and level of energy intake) is essentially unknown.

Another component of thermogenesis, called *nonexercise activity thermogenesis* (NEAT), has been linked to obesity. It is the thermogenesis that accompanies physical activities other than volitional exercise such as the activities of daily living, fidgeting, spontaneous muscle contraction, and maintaining posture. NEAT accounts for about two-thirds of the increased daily energy expenditure induced by overfeeding. The wide variation in fat storage seen in overfed individuals is predicted by the degree to which NEAT is induced. The molecular basis for NEAT and its regulation is unknown.

Leptin in typical obesity

The vast majority of obese persons have increased leptin levels but do not have mutations of either leptin or its receptor. They appear, therefore, to have a form of functional "leptin resistance." Data suggesting that some individuals produce less leptin per unit fat mass than others or have a form of relative leptin deficiency that predisposes to obesity are at present contradictory and unsettled. The mechanism for leptin resistance, and whether it can be overcome by raising leptin levels or combining leptin with other treatments in a subset of obese individuals, is not yet established. Some data suggest that leptin may not effectively cross the blood-brain barrier as levels rise. It is also apparent from animal studies that leptin-signaling inhibitors, such as SOCS3 and PTP1b, are involved in the leptin-resistant state.

PATHOLOGIC CONSEQUENCES OF OBESITY

(See also Chap. 21) Obesity has major adverse effects on health. Obesity is associated with an increase in mortality, with a 50–100% increased risk of death from all causes compared to normal-weight individuals, mostly due to cardiovascular causes. Obesity and overweight together are the second leading cause of preventable death in the United States, accounting for 300,000 deaths per year. Mortality rates rise as obesity increases, particularly when obesity is associated with increased intraabdominal fat (see above). Life expectancy of a moderately obese individual could be shortened by 2–5 years, and a 20- to 30-year-old male with a BMI >45 may lose 13 years of life. It is likely that the degree to which obesity affects particular organ systems is influenced by susceptibility genes that vary in the population.

Insulin resistance and type 2 diabetes mellitus

Hyperinsulinemia and insulin resistance are pervasive features of obesity, increasing with weight gain and diminishing with weight loss **(Chap. 22)**. Insulin resistance is more strongly linked to intraabdominal fat than to fat in other depots. Molecular links between obesity and insulin resistance in fat, muscle, and liver have been sought for many years. Major factors include: (1) insulin itself, by inducing receptor downregulation; (2) free fatty acids that are increased and capable of impairing insulin action; (3) intracellular lipid accumulation; and (4) several circulating peptides produced by adipocytes, including the cytokines TNF-α and IL-6, RBP4, and the "adipokines" adiponectin and resistin, which have altered expression in obese adipocytes and can modify insulin action. Additional mechanisms are obesity-linked inflammation, including infiltration of macrophages into tissues including fat, and induction of the endoplasmic reticulum stress response, which can bring about resistance to insulin action in cells. Despite the prevalence of insulin resistance, most obese individuals do not develop diabetes, suggesting that diabetes requires an interaction between obesity-induced insulin resistance and other factors such as impaired insulin secretion **(Chap. 23)**. Obesity, however, is a major risk factor for diabetes, and as many as 80% of patients with type 2 diabetes mellitus are obese. Weight loss and exercise, even of modest degree, increase insulin sensitivity and often improve glucose control in diabetes.

Reproductive disorders

Disorders that affect the reproductive axis are associated with obesity in both men and women. Male hypogonadism is associated with increased adipose tissue, often distributed in a pattern more typical of females. In men whose weight is >160% ideal body weight (IBW), plasma testosterone and sex hormone–binding globulin (SHBG) are often reduced, and estrogen levels (derived from conversion of adrenal androgens in adipose tissue) are increased **(Chap. 11)**. Gynecomastia may be seen. However, masculinization, libido, potency, and spermatogenesis are preserved in most of these individuals. Free testosterone may be decreased in morbidly obese men whose weight is >200% IBW.

Obesity has long been associated with menstrual abnormalities in women, particularly in women with upper body obesity **(Chap. 13)**. Common findings are increased androgen production, decreased SHBG, and increased peripheral conversion of androgen to estrogen. Most obese women with oligomenorrhea have polycystic ovarian syndrome (PCOS), with its associated anovulation and ovarian hyperandrogenism; 40% of women with PCOS are obese. Most nonobese women with PCOS are also insulin-resistant, suggesting that insulin resistance, hyperinsulinemia, or the combination of the two are causative or contribute to the ovarian pathophysiology in PCOS in both obese and lean individuals. Increasing evidence supports a role for adipokines in mediating a link between obesity and the reproductive dysfunction of PCOS. In obese women with PCOS, weight loss or treatment with insulin-sensitizing drugs often restores normal menses. The increased conversion of androstenedione to estrogen, which occurs to a greater degree in women with lower body obesity, may contribute to the increased incidence of uterine cancer in postmenopausal women with obesity.

Cardiovascular disease

The Framingham Study revealed that obesity was an independent risk factor for the 26-year incidence of cardiovascular disease in men and women (including coronary disease, stroke, and congestive heart failure). The waist-to-hip ratio may be the best predictor of these risks. When the additional effects of hypertension and glucose intolerance associated with obesity are included, the adverse impact of obesity is even more evident. The effect of obesity on cardiovascular mortality in women may be seen at BMIs as low as 25. Obesity, especially abdominal obesity, is associated with an atherogenic lipid profile; with increased low-density lipoprotein cholesterol, very-low-density lipoprotein, and triglyceride; and with decreased high-density lipoprotein cholesterol and decreased levels of the vascular protective adipokine adiponectin **(Chap. 27)**. Obesity is also associated with hypertension. Measurement of blood pressure in the obese requires use of a larger cuff size to avoid artifactual increases. Obesity-induced hypertension is associated with increased peripheral resistance and cardiac output, increased sympathetic nervous system tone, increased salt sensitivity, and insulin-mediated salt retention; it is often responsive to modest weight loss.

Pulmonary disease

Obesity may be associated with a number of pulmonary abnormalities. These include reduced chest wall compliance, increased work of breathing, increased minute ventilation due to increased metabolic rate, and decreased functional residual capacity and expiratory reserve volume. Severe obesity may be associated with obstructive sleep apnea and the "obesity hypoventilation syndrome" with attenuated hypoxic and hypercapnic ventilatory responses. Sleep apnea can be obstructive (most common), central, or mixed and is associated with hypertension. Weight loss (10–20 kg) can bring substantial improvement, as can major weight loss following gastric bypass or restrictive surgery. Continuous positive airway pressure has been used with some success.

Hepatobiliary disease

Obesity is frequently associated with nonalcoholic fatty liver disease (NAFLD), and this association represents one of the most common causes of liver disease in industrialized countries. The hepatic fatty infiltration of NAFLD progresses in a subset to inflammatory nonalcoholic steatohepatitis (NASH) and more rarely to cirrhosis and hepatocellular carcinoma. Steatosis typically improves following weight loss, secondary to diet or bariatric surgery. The mechanism for the association remains unclear. Obesity is associated with enhanced biliary secretion of cholesterol, supersaturation of bile, and a higher incidence of gallstones, particularly cholesterol gallstones. A person 50% above IBW has about a sixfold increased incidence of symptomatic gallstones. Paradoxically, fasting increases supersaturation of bile by decreasing the phospholipid component. Fasting-induced cholecystitis is a complication of extreme diets.

Cancer

Obesity is associated with increased risk of several cancer types, and in addition can lead to poorer treatment outcomes and increased cancer mortality. Obesity in males is associated with higher mortality from cancer of the esophagus, colon, rectum, pancreas, liver, and prostate; obesity in females is associated with higher mortality from cancer of the gallbladder, bile ducts, breasts, endometrium, cervix, and ovaries. Some of the latter may be due to increased rates of conversion of androstenedione to estrone in adipose tissue of obese individuals. Other possible mechanistic links may involve hormones, growth factors, and cytokines whose levels are linked to nutritional state, including insulin, leptin, adiponectin, and IGF-I, as well as activation of signaling pathways linked to both obesity and cancer. It has been estimated that obesity accounts for 14% of cancer deaths in men and 20% in women in the United States.

Bone, joint, and cutaneous disease

Obesity is associated with an increased risk of osteoarthritis, no doubt partly due to the trauma of added weight bearing, but potentially linked as well to activation of inflammatory pathways that could promote synovial pathology. The prevalence of gout may also be increased. One of the skin problems associated with obesity is acanthosis nigricans, manifested by darkening and thickening of the skinfolds on the neck, elbows, and dorsal interphalangeal spaces. Acanthosis reflects the severity of underlying insulin resistance and diminishes with weight loss. Friability of skin may be increased, especially in skinfolds, enhancing the risk of fungal and yeast infections. Finally, venous stasis is increased in the obese.

CHAPTER 21

EVALUATION AND MANAGEMENT OF OBESITY

Robert F. Kushner

More than 66% of U.S. adults are categorized as overweight or obese, and the prevalence of obesity is increasing rapidly in most of the industrialized world. Children and adolescents also are becoming more obese, indicating that the current trends will accelerate over time. Obesity is associated with an increased risk of multiple health problems, including hypertension, type 2 diabetes, dyslipidemia, obstructive sleep apnea, nonalcoholic fatty liver disease, degenerative joint disease, and some malignancies. Thus, it is important for physicians to identify, evaluate, and treat patients for obesity and associated comorbid conditions.

EVALUATION

Physicians should screen all adult patients for obesity and offer intensive counseling and behavioral interventions to promote sustained weight loss. The five main steps in the evaluation of obesity, as described below, are (1) a focused obesity-related history, (2) a physical examination to determine the degree and type of obesity, (3) assessment of comorbid conditions, (4) determination of fitness level, and (5) assessment of the patient's readiness to adopt lifestyle changes.

The obesity-focused history

Information from the history should address the following seven questions:

- What factors contribute to the patient's obesity?
- How is the obesity affecting the patient's health?
- What is the patient's level of risk from obesity?
- What does the patient find difficult about managing weight?
- What are the patient's goals and expectations?
- Is the patient motivated to begin a weight management program?
- What kind of help does the patient need?

Although the vast majority of cases of obesity can be attributed to behavioral factors that affect diet and physical activity patterns, the history may suggest secondary causes that merit further evaluation. Disorders to consider include polycystic ovarian syndrome, hypothyroidism, Cushing's syndrome, and hypothalamic disease. Drug-induced weight gain also should be considered. Common causes include medications for diabetes (insulin, sulfonylureas, thiazolidinediones); steroid hormones; psychotropic agents; mood stabilizers (lithium); antidepressants (tricyclics, monoamine oxidase inhibitors, paroxetine, mirtazapine); and antiepileptic drugs (valproate, gabapentin, carbamazepine). Other medications, such as nonsteroidal anti-inflammatory drugs and calcium channel blockers, may cause peripheral edema but do not increase body fat.

The patient's current diet and physical activity patterns may reveal factors that contribute to the development of obesity and may identify behaviors to target for treatment. This type of historic information is best obtained by the combination of a questionnaire and an interview.

Body mass index (BMI) and waist circumference

Three key anthropometric measurements are important in evaluating the degree of obesity: weight, height, and waist circumference. The BMI, calculated as weight (kg)/height $(m)^2$ or as weight (lbs)/height $(inches)^2$ $\times$ 703, is used to classify weight status and risk of disease (Tables 21-1 and 21-2). BMI provides an estimate of body fat and is related to disease risk. Lower BMI thresholds for overweight and obesity have been proposed for the Asia-Pacific region since this population appears to be at risk for glucose and lipid abnormalities at lower body weights.

Excess abdominal fat, assessed by measurement of waist circumference or waist-to-hip ratio, is independently associated with a higher risk for diabetes mellitus

TABLE 21-1

BODY MASS INDEX (BMI)

BMI	19	20	21	22	23	24	25	26	27	28	29	30	31	32	33	34	35
HEIGHT (INCHES)									**BODY WEIGHT (POUNDS)**								
58	91	96	100	105	110	115	119	124	129	134	138	143	148	153	158	162	167
59	94	99	104	109	114	119	124	128	133	138	143	148	153	158	163	168	173
60	97	102	107	112	118	123	128	133	138	143	148	153	158	163	168	174	179
61	100	106	111	116	122	127	132	137	143	148	153	158	164	169	174	180	185
62	104	109	115	120	126	131	136	142	147	153	158	164	169	175	180	186	191
63	107	113	118	124	130	135	141	146	152	158	163	169	175	180	186	191	197
64	110	116	122	128	134	140	145	151	157	163	169	174	180	186	192	197	204
65	114	120	126	132	138	144	150	156	162	168	174	180	186	192	198	204	210
66	118	124	130	136	142	148	155	161	167	173	179	186	192	198	204	210	216
67	121	127	134	140	146	153	159	166	172	178	185	191	198	204	211	217	223
68	125	131	138	144	151	158	164	171	177	184	190	197	203	210	216	223	230
69	128	135	142	149	155	162	169	176	182	189	196	203	209	216	223	230	236
70	132	139	146	153	160	167	174	181	188	195	202	209	216	222	229	236	243
71	136	143	150	157	165	172	179	186	193	200	208	215	222	229	236	243	250
72	140	147	154	162	169	177	184	191	199	206	213	221	228	235	242	250	258
73	144	151	159	166	174	182	189	197	204	212	219	227	235	242	250	257	265
74	148	155	163	171	179	186	194	202	210	218	225	233	241	249	256	264	272
75	152	160	168	176	184	192	200	208	216	224	232	240	248	256	264	272	279
76	156	164	172	180	189	197	205	213	221	230	238	246	254	263	271	279	287

BMI	36	37	38	39	40	41	42	43	44	45	46	47	48	49	50	51	52	53	54
58	172	177	181	186	191	196	201	205	210	215	220	224	229	234	239	244	248	253	258
59	178	183	188	193	198	203	208	212	217	222	227	232	237	242	247	252	257	262	267
60	184	189	194	199	204	209	215	220	225	230	235	240	245	250	255	261	266	271	276
61	190	195	201	206	211	217	222	227	232	238	243	248	254	259	264	269	275	280	285
62	196	202	207	213	218	224	229	235	240	246	251	256	262	267	273	278	284	289	295
63	203	208	214	220	225	231	237	242	248	254	259	265	270	278	282	287	293	299	304
64	209	215	221	227	232	238	244	250	256	262	267	273	279	285	291	296	302	308	314
65	216	222	228	234	240	246	252	258	264	270	276	282	288	294	300	306	312	318	324
66	223	229	235	241	247	253	260	266	272	278	284	291	297	303	309	315	322	328	334
67	230	236	242	249	255	261	268	274	280	287	293	299	306	312	319	325	331	338	344
68	236	243	249	256	262	269	276	282	289	295	302	308	315	322	328	335	341	348	354
69	243	250	257	263	270	277	284	291	297	304	311	318	324	331	338	345	351	358	365
70	250	257	264	271	278	285	292	299	306	313	320	327	334	341	348	355	362	369	376
71	257	265	272	279	286	293	301	308	315	322	329	338	343	351	358	365	372	379	386
72	265	272	279	287	294	302	309	316	324	331	338	346	353	361	368	375	383	390	397
73	272	280	288	295	302	310	318	325	333	340	348	355	363	371	378	386	393	401	408
74	280	287	295	303	311	319	326	334	342	350	358	365	373	381	389	396	404	412	420
75	287	295	303	311	319	327	335	343	351	359	367	375	383	391	399	407	415	423	431
76	295	304	312	320	328	336	344	353	361	369	377	385	394	402	410	418	426	435	443

TABLE 21-2

CLASSIFICATION OF WEIGHT STATUS AND DISEASE RISK

CLASSIFICATION	BODY MASS INDEX (KG/M²)	OBESITY CLASS	DISEASE RISK
Underweight	<18.5	—	—
Healthy weight	18.5–24.9	—	—
Overweight	25.0–29.9	—	Increased
Obesity	30.0–34.9	I	High
Obesity	35.0–39.9	II	Very high
Extreme obesity	≥40	III	Extremely high

Source: Adapted from the National Institutes of Health, National Heart, Lung, and Blood Institute: Clinical Guidelines on the Identification, Evaluation, and Treatment of Overweight and Obesity in Adults. U.S. Department of Health and Human Services, U.S. Public Health Service, 1998.

and cardiovascular disease. Measurement of the waist circumference is a surrogate for visceral adipose tissue and should be performed in the horizontal plane above the iliac crest (Table 21-3).

Physical fitness

Several prospective studies have demonstrated that physical fitness, reported by questionnaire or measured by a maximal treadmill exercise test, is an important predictor of all-cause mortality rate independent of BMI and body composition. These observations highlight the importance of taking a physical activity and exercise history during examination as well as emphasizing physical activity as a treatment approach.

TABLE 21-3

ETHNIC-SPECIFIC CUTPOINT VALUES FOR WAIST CIRCUMFERENCE

ETHNIC GROUP	WAIST CIRCUMFERENCE
Europeans	
Men	>94 cm (>37 in)
Women	>80 cm (>31.5 in)
South Asians and Chinese	
Men	>90 cm (>35 in)
Women	>80 cm (>31.5 in)
Japanese	
Men	>85 cm (>33.5 in)
Women	>90 cm (>35 in)
Ethnic South and Central Americans	Use South Asian recommendations until more specific data are available.
Sub-Saharan Africans	Use European data until more specific data are available.
Eastern Mediterranean and Middle Eastern (Arab) populations	Use European data until more specific data are available.

Source: From KGMM Alberti et al for the IDF Epidemiology Task Force Consensus Group: Lancet 366:1059, 2005.

Obesity-associated comorbid conditions

The evaluation of comorbid conditions should be based on presentation of symptoms, risk factors, and index of suspicion. For all patients, a fasting lipid panel should be performed (total, low-density lipoprotein, and high-density lipoprotein cholesterol and triglyceride levels) and a fasting blood glucose level and blood pressure determined. Symptoms and diseases that are directly or indirectly related to obesity are listed in Table 21-4. Although individuals vary, the number and severity of organ-specific comorbid conditions usually rise with increasing levels of obesity. Patients at very high absolute risk include those with the following: established coronary heart disease; presence of other atherosclerotic diseases, such as peripheral arterial disease, abdominal aortic aneurysm, and symptomatic carotid artery disease; type 2 diabetes; and sleep apnea.

Assessing the patient's readiness to change

An attempt to initiate lifestyle changes when the patient is not ready usually leads to frustration and may hamper future weight-loss efforts. Assessment includes patient motivation and support, stressful life events, psychiatric status, time availability and constraints, and appropriateness of goals and expectations. Readiness can be viewed as the balance of two opposing forces: (1) motivation, or the patient's desire to change; and (2) resistance, or the patient's resistance to change.

A helpful method to begin a readiness assessment is to use the motivational interviewing technique of "anchoring" the patient's interest and confidence to change on a numerical scale. With this technique, the patient is asked to rate—on a scale from 0 to 10, with 0 being not so important (or confident) and 10 being very important (or confident)—his or her level of interest in and confidence about losing weight at this time. This exercise helps establish readiness to change and also serves as a basis for further dialogue.

TREATMENT Obesity

THE GOAL OF THERAPY The primary goals of treatment are to improve obesity-related comorbid conditions and to reduce the risk of developing future comorbidities. Information obtained from the history, physical examination, and diagnostic tests is used to determine risk and develop a treatment plan (Fig. 21-1). The decision of how aggressively to treat the patient and which modalities to use is determined by the

TABLE 21-4

OBESITY-RELATED ORGAN SYSTEMS REVIEW

CARDIOVASCULAR	RESPIRATORY
Hypertension	Dyspnea
Congestive heart failure	Obstructive sleep apnea
Cor pulmonale	Hypoventilation syndrome
Varicose veins	Pickwickian syndrome
Pulmonary embolism	Asthma
Coronary artery disease	**Gastrointestinal**
Endocrine	Gastroesophageal reflux disease
Metabolic syndrome	Nonalcoholic fatty-liver disease
Type 2 diabetes	Cholelithiasis
Dyslipidemia	Hernias
Polycystic ovarian syndrome	Colon cancer
Musculoskeletal	**Genitourinary**
Hyperuricemia and gout	Urinary stress incontinence
Immobility	Obesity-related glomerulopathy
Osteoarthritis (knees and hips)	Hypogonadism (male)
Low back pain	Breast and uterine cancer
Carpal tunnel syndrome	Pregnancy complications
Psychological	**Neurologic**
Depression/low self-esteem	Stroke
Body image disturbance	Idiopathic intracranial hypertension
Social stigmatization	Meralgia paresthetica
Integument	Dementia
Striae distensae	
Stasis pigmentation of legs	
Lymphedema	
Cellulitis	
Intertrigo, carbuncles	
Acanthosis nigricans	
Acrochordons (skin tags)	
Hidradenitis suppurativa	

patient's risk status, expectations, and available resources. Not all patients who are deemed obese by BMI alone need to be treated, as exemplified by the concepts of obesity paradox or the metabolically healthy obese. However, patients who present with obesity-related comorbidities and who would benefit from weight loss intervention should be managed proactively. Therapy for obesity always begins with lifestyle management and may include pharmacotherapy or surgery, depending on BMI risk category (Table 21-5). Setting an initial weight-loss goal of 8–10% over 6 months is a realistic target.

LIFESTYLE MANAGEMENT Obesity care involves attention to three essential elements of lifestyle: dietary habits, physical activity, and behavior modification. Because obesity is fundamentally a disease of energy imbalance, all patients must learn how and when energy is consumed (diet), how and when energy is expended (physical activity), and how to incorporate this information into their daily lives (behavioral therapy). Lifestyle management has been shown to result in a modest (typically 3–5 kg) weight loss when compared with no treatment or usual care.

Diet Therapy The primary focus of diet therapy is to reduce overall calorie consumption. Guidelines from the National Heart, Lung, and Blood Institute recommend initiating treatment with a calorie deficit of 500–1000 kcal/d compared with the patient's habitual diet. This reduction is consistent with a goal of losing ~1–2 lbs per week. The calorie deficit can

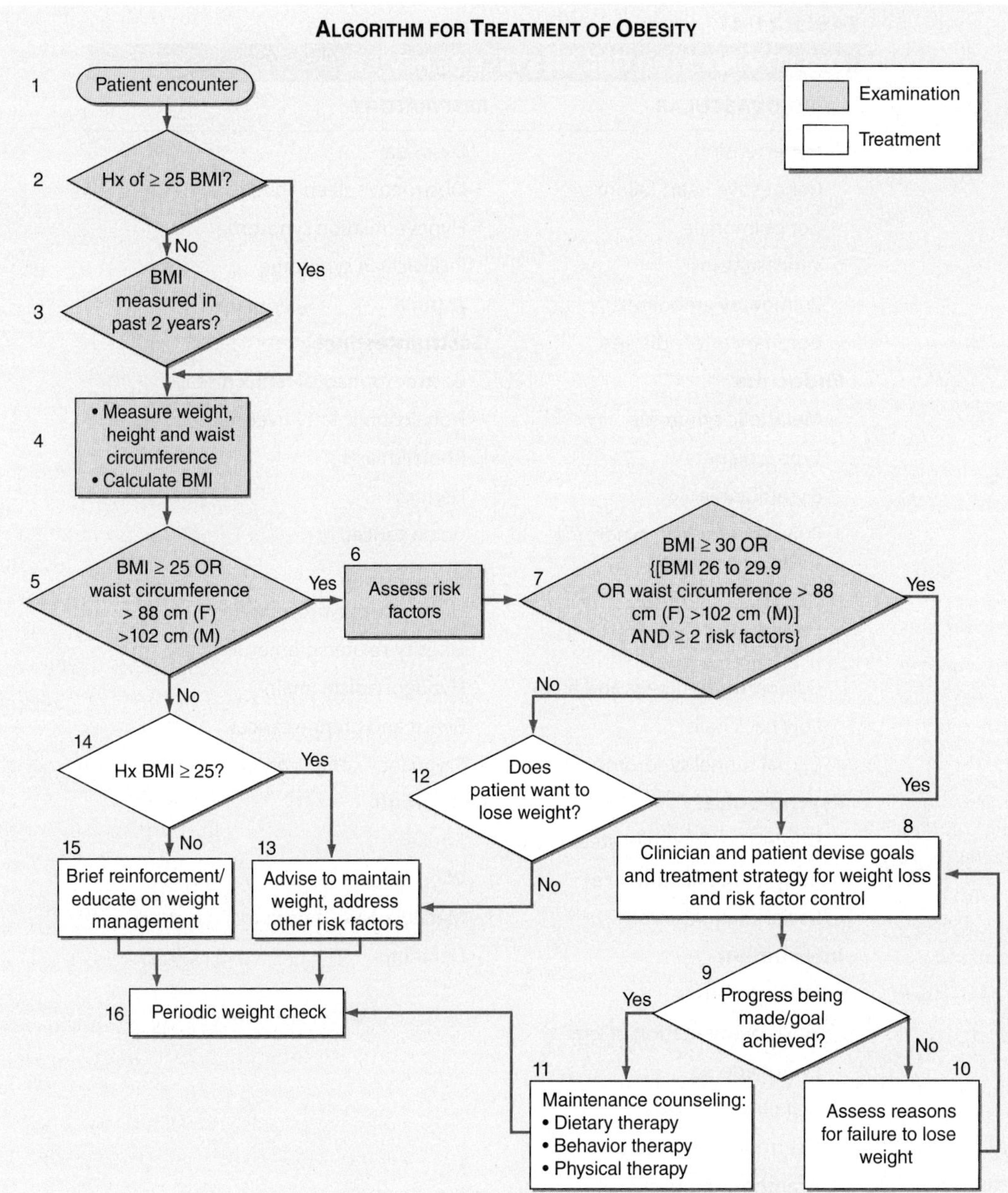

FIGURE 21-1

Algorithm for the treatment of obesity. This algorithm applies only to assessment for overweight and obesity and subsequent decisions based on that assessment. It does not reflect initial overall assessment for other conditions that the physician may wish to perform. BMI, body mass index; Hx, history. *(From the National, Heart, Lung, and Blood Institute: Clinical guidelines on the identification, evaluation, and treatment of overweight and obesity in adults: The evidence report. Washington, DC, US Department of Health and Human Services, 1998.)*

TABLE 21-5

A GUIDE TO OPTING FOR TREATMENT FOR OBESITY

	BMI CATEGORY (KG/M²)				
TREATMENT	**25–26.9**	**27–29.9**	**30–34.9**	**35–39.9**	**≥40**
Diet, exercise, behavioral therapy	With comorbidities	With comorbidities	+	+	+
Pharmacotherapy	—	With comorbidities	+	+	+
Surgery	—	—	—	With comorbidities	+

Source: From the National Heart, Lung, and Blood Institute, North American Association for the Study of Obesity (2000).

be instituted through dietary substitutions or alternatives. Examples include choosing smaller portion sizes, eating more fruits and vegetables, consuming more whole-grain cereals, selecting leaner cuts of meat and skimmed dairy products, reducing consumption of fried foods and other foods with added fats and oils, and drinking water instead of sugar-sweetened beverages. It is important that dietary counseling remain patient centered and that the goals set be practical, realistic, and achievable.

The macronutrient composition of the diet will vary with the patient's preference and medical condition. The 2010 U.S. Department of Agriculture Dietary Guidelines for Americans, which focus on health promotion and risk reduction, can be applied to treatment of overweight or obese patients. The recommendations include maintaining a diet rich in whole grains, fruits, vegetables, and dietary fiber; consuming two servings (8 oz) of fish high in omega 3 fatty acids per week; decreasing sodium intake to <2300 mg/d; consuming 3 cups of milk (or equivalent low-fat or fat-free dairy products) per day; limiting cholesterol intake to <300 mg/d; and keeping total fat intake at 20–35% of daily calories and saturated fat intake at <10% of daily calories. Application of these guidelines to specific calorie goals can be found on the website *www.choosemyplate.gov*. The revised Dietary Reference Intakes for Macronutrients released by the Institute of Medicine recommends that 45–65% of calories come from carbohydrates, 20–35% from fat, and 10–35% from protein. The guidelines also recommend daily fiber intake of 38 g (men) and 25 g (women) for persons over 50 years of age and 30 g (men) and 21 g (women) for those under age 50.

Since portion control is one of the most difficult strategies for patients to manage, the use of pre-prepared products such as meal replacements is a simple and convenient suggestion. Examples include frozen entrees, canned beverages, and bars. Use of meal replacements in the diet has been shown to result in a 7–8% weight loss.

Numerous randomized trials comparing diets of different macronutrient composition (e.g., low-carbohydrate, low-fat, Mediterranean) have shown that weight loss depends primarily on reduction of total caloric intake and adherence to the prescribed diet, not the specific proportions of carbohydrate, fat, and protein in the diet. The macronutrient composition will ultimately be determined by the patient's taste preferences, cooking style, and culture. However, the patient's underlying medical problems are also important in guiding the recommended dietary composition. The dietary prescription will vary according to the patient's metabolic profile and risk factors. A consultation with a registered dietitian for medical nutrition therapy is particularly useful in considering patient preference and treatment of comorbid diseases.

Another dietary approach to consider is based on the concept of *energy density*, which refers to the number of calories (i.e., amount of energy) a food contains per unit of weight. People tend to ingest a constant volume of food regardless of caloric or macronutrient content. Adding water or fiber to a food decreases its energy density by increasing weight without affecting caloric content. Examples of foods with low-energy density include soups, fruits, vegetables, oatmeal, and lean meats. Dry foods and high-fat foods such as pretzels, cheese, egg yolks, potato chips, and red meat have a high-energy density. Diets containing low-energy-dense foods have been shown to control hunger and thus to result in decreased caloric intake and weight loss.

Occasionally, very low-calorie diets (VLCDs) are prescribed as a form of aggressive dietary therapy. The primary purpose of a VLCD is to promote a rapid and significant (13- to 23-kg) short-term weight loss over a 3- to 6-month period. The proprietary formulas designed for this purpose typically supply ≤800 kcal, 50–80 g of protein, and 100% of the recommended daily intake for vitamins and minerals. According to a review by the National Task Force on the Prevention and Treatment of Obesity, indications for initiating a VLCD include the involvement of well-motivated individuals who are moderately to severely obese (BMI, >30 kg/m^2), have failed at more conservative approaches to weight loss, and have a medical condition that would be immediately improved with rapid weight loss. These conditions include poorly controlled type 2 diabetes, hypertriglyceridemia, obstructive sleep apnea, and symptomatic peripheral edema. The risk for gallstone formation increases exponentially at rates of weight loss >1.5 kg/week (3.3 lb/week). Prophylaxis against gallstone formation with ursodeoxycholic acid (600 mg/d) is effective in reducing this risk. Because of the need for close metabolic monitoring, VLCDs usually are prescribed by physicians specializing in obesity care.

Physical Activity Therapy Although exercise alone is only moderately effective for weight loss, the combination of dietary modification and exercise is the most effective behavioral approach for the treatment of obesity. The most important role of exercise appears to be in the maintenance of the weight loss. The 2008 Physical Activity Guidelines for Americans (*www.health.gov/paguidelines*) recommend that adults should engage in 150 min of moderate-intensity or 75 min a week of vigorous-intensity aerobic physical activity per week, performed in episodes of at least 10 min and preferably spread throughout the week. Focusing on simple ways to add physical activity into the normal daily routine through leisure activities, travel, and domestic work should be suggested. Examples include walking, using the stairs, doing housework and yard work, and engaging in sports. Asking the patient to wear a pedometer or accelerometer to monitor total accumulation of steps or kcal expended as part of the activities of daily living is a useful strategy. Step counts are highly correlated with activity level. Studies have demonstrated that lifestyle activities are as effective as structured exercise programs for improving cardiorespiratory fitness and weight loss. A high level of physical activity (>300 min of moderate-intensity activity per week) is often needed to lose weight and sustain weight loss. These exercise recommendations are daunting to most patients and need to be implemented gradually. Consultation with an exercise physiologist or personal trainer may be helpful.

Behavioral Therapy Cognitive behavioral therapy is used to help change and reinforce new dietary and physical activity behaviors. Strategies include self-monitoring techniques (e.g., journaling, weighing, and measuring food and activity); stress management; stimulus control (e.g., using smaller plates, not eating in front of the television or in the car); social support; problem solving; and cognitive restructuring to help patients develop more positive and realistic thoughts about themselves. When recommending any behavioral lifestyle change, the patient should be asked to identify what, when, where, and how the behavioral change will be performed. The patient should keep a record of the anticipated behavioral change so that progress can be reviewed at the next office visit. Because these techniques are time-consuming to implement, their supervision is often undertaken by ancillary office staff, such as a nurse-clinician or registered dietitian.

PHARMACOTHERAPY Adjuvant pharmacologic treatments should be considered for patients with a BMI ≥30 kg/m^2 or—for patients who have concomitant obesity-related diseases and for whom dietary and physical activity therapy has not been successful—a BMI ≥27 kg/m^2. When an anti-obesity medication is prescribed, patients should be actively engaged in a lifestyle program that provides the strategies and skills needed to use the drug effectively, since such support increases total weight loss.

Medications for obesity have traditionally fallen into two major categories: appetite suppressants (*anorexiants*) and gastrointestinal fat blockers. Appetite-suppressing medications have primarily targeted three monoamine receptor systems in the hypothalamus: noradrenergic, dopaminergic, and serotonergic receptors. Two new appetite suppressants were approved by the U.S. Food and Drug Administration (FDA) in 2012: lorcaserin and phentermine/topiramate (PHEN/TPM) extended release. Gastrointestinal fat blockers reduce the absorption of selective macronutrients, such as fat, from the gastrointestinal tract.

Centrally Acting Anorexiant Medications Anorexiants affect *satiety* (the absence of hunger after eating) and hunger (the biologic sensation that prompts eating). By increasing satiety and decreasing hunger, these agents help patients reduce caloric intake without a sense of deprivation. The target site for the actions of anorexiants is the ventromedial and lateral hypothalamic regions in the central nervous system **(Chap. 20)**. The biologic effect of these agents on appetite regulation is produced by augmentation of the neurotransmission of three monoamines: norepinephrine; serotonin (5-hydroxytryptamine, or 5-HT); and, to a lesser degree, dopamine. The classic sympathomimetic adrenergic agents (benzphetamine, phendimetrazine, diethylpropion, mazindol, and phentermine) function by stimulating norepinephrine release or by blocking its reuptake. Among the anorexiants, phentermine has been the most commonly prescribed; there is limited long-term data on its effectiveness. A 2002 review of six randomized, placebo-controlled trials of phentermine for weight control found that patients lost 0.6–6.0 additional kilograms of weight over 2–24 weeks of treatment. The most common side effects of the amphetamine-derived anorexiants are restlessness, insomnia, dry mouth, constipation, and increased blood pressure and heart rate.

PHEN/TPM is a combination drug that contains a catecholamine releaser (phentermine) and an anticonvulsant (topiramate). Topiramate is approved by the FDA as an anticonvulsant for the treatment of epilepsy and for the prophylaxis of migraine headaches. Weight loss was identified as an unintended side effect of topiramate during clinical trials for epilepsy. The mechanism responsible for weight loss is uncertain but is thought to be mediated through the drug's modulation of γ-aminobutyric acid receptors, inhibition of carbonic anhydrase, and antagonism of glutamate. PHEN/TPM has undergone two 1-year pivotal randomized, placebo-controlled, double-blind trials of efficacy and safety: EQUIP and CONQUER. In a third study, SEQUEL, 78% of CONQUER participants continued to receive their blinded treatment for an additional year. All participants received diet and exercise counseling. Participant numbers, eligibility, characteristics, and weight loss outcomes are displayed in Table 21-6. Intention-to-treat 1-year placebo-subtracted weight loss for the PHEN/TPM 15-mg/92-mg dose was 9.3% and 8.6%, respectively, in the EQUIP and CONQUER trials. Clinical and statistical dose-dependent improvements were seen in selected cardiovascular and metabolic outcome measurements that were related to the weight loss. The most common adverse events experienced by the drug-randomized group were paresthesias, dry mouth, constipation, dysgeusia, and insomnia. Because of an increased risk of congenital fetal oral-cleft formation from topiramate, the FDA approval of PHEN/TPM stipulated a Risk Evaluation and Mitigation Strategies requirement to educate prescribers about the need for active birth control among women of childbearing age and a contraindication for use during pregnancy.

Lorcaserin is a selective 5-HT2C receptor agonist with a functional selectivity ~15 times that of 5-HT2A receptors and 100 times that of 5-HT2B receptors. This selectivity is important, since the drug-induced valvulopathy documented with two other serotonergic agents that were removed from the market—fenfluramine and dexfenfluramine—was due to activation of the 5-HT2B receptors expressed on cardiac valvular interstitial cells. By activating the 5-HT2C receptor, lorcaserin is thought to decrease food intake through the pro-opiomelanocortin system of neurons.

Lorcaserin has undergone two randomized, placebo-controlled, double-blind trials for efficacy and safety. Participants were randomized to receive lorcaserin (10 mg bid) or placebo in the BLOOM study and to receive lorcaserin (10 mg bid or qd) or placebo in the BLOSSOM study. All participants received diet and exercise counseling. Participant numbers,

TABLE 21-6

CLINICAL TRIALS FOR WEIGHT LOSS MEDICATIONS[a]

	LORCASERIN		PHEN/TPM[d]	
	BLOOM[b]	BLOSSOM[c]	EQUIP	CONQUER
No. of participants (ITT-LOCF)	3182	4008	1230	2448
Age (years)	18–65	18–65	≥35	27–45
BMI (kg/m^2)	27–45	27–45	18–70	18–70
Comorbid conditions (cardiovascular and metabolic)	≥1	≥1	≥1	≥2
Mean weight loss (%) with treatment vs. placebo	5.8 vs. 2.2	4.8 vs. 2.8	11 vs. 1.6	10.4 vs. 1.8
Placebo-subtracted weight loss (%)	3.6	3.0	9.3	8.6
Categorical change in 5% weight loss with treatment vs. placebo	47.5 vs. 20.3	47.2 vs. 25	67 vs. 17	70 vs. 21
Completion rate (%)	Lorcaserin, 55.4; placebo, 45.1	55.5	59.9	62

[a]Table shows a comparison of two 1-year prospective, randomized, double-blind trials of lorcaserin (BLOOM and BLOSSOM) and phentermine-topiramate extended release (EQUIP and CONQUER).
[b]Lorcaserin dose: 10 mg bid.
[c]Lorcaserin dose: 10 mg bid or qd.
[d]Phentermine-topiramate extended release dose: 15 mg/92 mg.
Abbreviations: BMI, body mass index (see Table 21-1); ITT-LOCF, intention to treat, last observation carried forward; PHEN/TPM, phentermine-topiramate extended release.

eligibility, characteristics, and weight loss outcomes are displayed in Table 21-6. Overweight or obese subjects had at least one coexisting condition (hypertension, dyslipidemia, cardiovascular disease, impaired glucose tolerance, or sleep apnea)—medical conditions that are commonly seen in the office setting. Intention-to-treat 1-year placebo-subtracted weight loss was 3.6% and 3.0%, respectively, in the BLOOM and BLOSSOM trials. Echocardiography was performed at the screening visit and at scheduled time points over the course of the studies. There was no difference in the development of FDA-defined valvulopathy between drug-treated and placebo-treated participants at 1 year or 2 years. Modest statistical improvements consistent with the weight loss were seen in selected cardiovascular and metabolic outcome measurements. The most common adverse events experienced by the drug group were headache, dizziness, and nausea.

In approving both PHEN/TPM and lorcaserin, the FDA introduced a new provision with important clinical relevance: a prescription trial period to assess effectiveness. Response to both medications should be assessed after 3 months of treatment. For lorcaserin, the medication should be discontinued if the patient has not lost at least 5% of body weight by that point. For PHEN/TPM, if the patient has not lost at least 3% of body weight at 3 months, the clinician can either escalate the dose and reassess progress at 6 months or discontinue treatment entirely.

Peripherally Acting Medications Orlistat (Xenical™) is a synthetic hydrogenated derivative of a naturally occurring lipase inhibitor, lipostatin, that is produced by the mold *Streptomyces toxytricini*. This drug is a potent, slowly reversible inhibitor of pancreatic, gastric, and carboxylester lipases and phospholipase A_2, which are required for the hydrolysis of dietary fat into fatty acids and monoacylglycerols. Orlistat acts in the lumen of the stomach and small intestine by forming a covalent bond with the active site of these lipases. Taken at a therapeutic dose of 120 mg tid, orlistat blocks the digestion and absorption of ~30% of dietary fat. After discontinuation of the drug, fecal fat content usually returns to normal within 48–72 h.

Multiple randomized, double-blind, placebo-controlled studies have shown that, after 1 year, orlistat produces a weight loss of ~9–10%, whereas placebo recipients have a 4–6% weight loss. Because orlistat is minimally (<1%) absorbed from the gastrointestinal tract, it has no systemic side effects. The drug's tolerability is related to the malabsorption of dietary fat and the subsequent passage of fat in the feces. Adverse gastrointestinal effects, including flatus with discharge, fecal urgency, fatty/oily stool, and increased defecation, are reported in at least 10% of orlistat-treated patients. These side effects generally are experienced early, diminish as patients control their dietary fat intake, and only infrequently cause patients to withdraw from clinical trials. When taken concomitantly, psyllium mucilloid is helpful in controlling orlistat-induced gastrointestinal side effects. Because serum concentrations of the fat-soluble vitamins D and E and β-carotene may be reduced by orlistat treatment, vitamin supplements are recommended to prevent potential deficiencies. Orlistat was approved for over-the-counter use in 2007.

Antiobesity Drugs in Development Two additional medications are currently in development. Bupropion and naltrexone (Contrave™)—a dopamine and norepinephrine reuptake inhibitor and an opioid receptor antagonist, respectively—are theoretically combined to dampen the motivation/

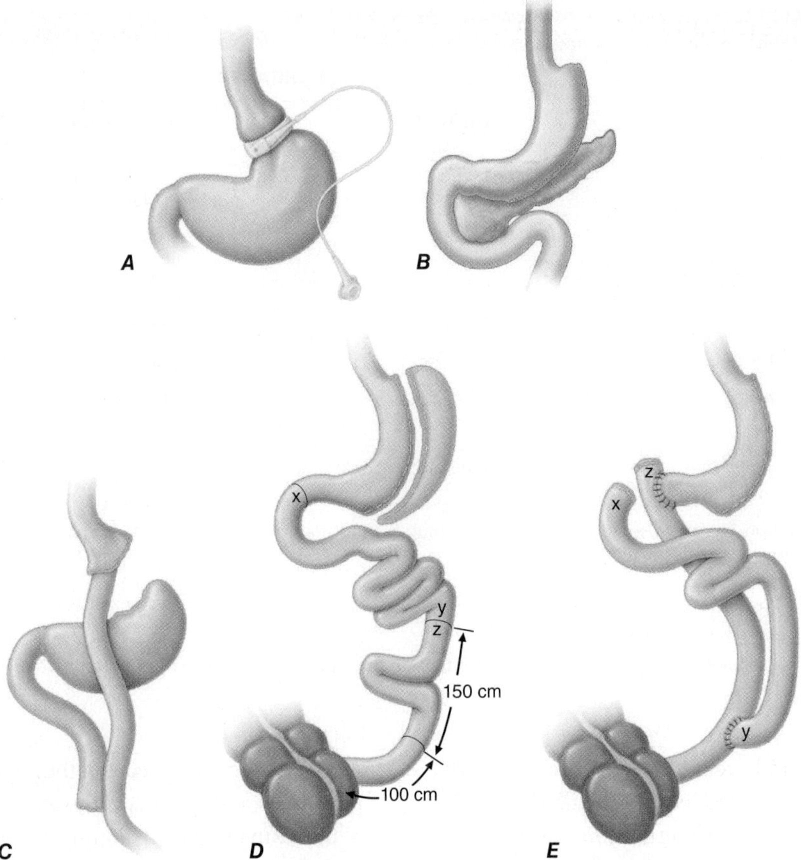

FIGURE 21-2
Bariatric surgical procedures. Examples of operative interventions used for surgical manipulation of the gastrointestinal tract. ***A.*** Laparoscopic adjustable gastric banding. ***B.*** Laparoscopic sleeve gastrectomy. ***C.*** The Roux-en-Y gastric bypass. ***D.*** Biliopancreatic diversion with duodenal switch. ***E.*** Biliopancreatic diversion. *(From ML Kendrick, GF Dakin: Mayo Clin Proc 815:518, 2006; with permission.)*

reinforcement that food brings (dopamine effect) and the pleasure/palatability of eating (opioid effect). In the COR-1 randomized, double-blind, placebo-controlled trial, 1742 enrolled participants, who were 18–65 years of age and had BMIs of 30–45 kg/m^2, were randomized to receive naltrexone (16 mg/d) plus bupropion (360 mg/d), naltrexone (32 mg/d) plus bupropion (360 mg/d), or placebo. Mean change in body weight for the three groups was 5.0%, 6.1%, and 1.3%, respectively. The most common adverse events were nausea, headache, constipation, dizziness, vomiting, and dry mouth. However, the FDA rejected the drug in 2011 because of cardiovascular concerns and concluded that a large-scale study of the long-term cardiovascular effects of naltrexone would be needed before approval could be considered.

Liraglutide, a glucagon-like peptide 1 receptor agonist currently approved for the treatment of type 2 diabetes, has independent weight loss effects via hypothalamic neural activation causing appetite suppression. In a double-blind, placebo-controlled trial, 564 adults with BMIs of 30–40 kg/m^2 were randomized to receive once-daily SC liraglutide (1.2, 1.8, 2.4, or 3.0 mg), placebo, or open-label orlistat (120 mg tid) for 1 year. The liraglutide and placebo recipients were switched to 2.4 mg of liraglutide during the second year and then to 3.0 mg for an additional year. One-year placebo-subtracted mean weight loss was 5.8 kg for liraglutide and 3.8 kg more than those on orlistat. The most common side effects were nausea, vomiting, and change in bowel habits.

SURGERY Bariatric surgery (Fig. 21-2) can be considered for patients with severe obesity (BMI, ≥40 kg/m^2) or for those with moderate obesity (BMI, ≥35 kg/m^2) associated with a serious medical condition. Weight loss surgeries have traditionally been classified into three categories on the basis of anatomic changes: restrictive, restrictive malabsorptive, and malabsorptive. More recently, however, the clinical benefits of bariatric surgery in achieving weight loss and alleviating metabolic comorbidities have been attributed largely to changes in the physiologic responses of gut hormones and in adipose tissue metabolism. Metabolic effects resulting from bypassing the foregut include altered responses of ghrelin, glucagon-like peptide 1, peptide YY3-36, and oxyntonodulin. Additional effects on food intake and body weight control may be attributed to changes in vagal signaling. The loss of fat mass, particularly visceral fat, is associated with multiple metabolic, adipokine, and inflammatory changes that include improved insulin sensitivity and glucose disposal; reduced free fatty acid flux; increased adiponectin levels; and decreased interleukin 6, tumor necrosis factor α, and high-sensitivity C-reactive protein levels.

Restrictive surgeries limit the amount of food the stomach can hold and slow the rate of gastric emptying. *Laparoscopic adjustable gastric banding* is the prototype of this category. The first banding device, the LAP-BAND, was approved for use in the United States in 2001 and the second, the REALIZE band, in 2007. In contrast to previous devices, these bands have diameters that are adjustable by way of their connection to a reservoir that is implanted under the skin. Injection of saline into the reservoir and removal of saline from the reservoir tighten and loosen the band's internal diameter, respectively, thus changing the size of the gastric opening. The mean percentage of total body weight lost at 5 years is estimated at 20–25%. In *laparoscopic sleeve gastrectomy*, the stomach is restricted by stapling and dividing it vertically, removing ~80% of the greater curvature, and leaving a slim banana-shaped remnant stomach along the lesser curvature. Weight loss after this procedure is superior to that after laparoscopic adjustable gastric banding.

The three restrictive-malabsorptive bypass procedures combine the elements of gastric restriction and selective malabsorption. These procedures are Roux-en-Y gastric bypass, biliopancreatic diversion, and biliopancreatic diversion with duodenal switch (Fig. 21-2). Roux-en-Y is the most commonly undertaken and most accepted bypass procedure. It may be performed with an open incision or by laparoscopy.

These procedures generally produce a 30–35% average total body weight loss that is maintained in nearly 60% of patients at 5 years. In general, mean weight loss is greater after the combined restrictive-malabsorptive procedures than after the restrictive procedures. Significant improvement in multiple obesity-related comorbid conditions, including type 2 diabetes, hypertension, dyslipidemia, obstructive sleep apnea, quality of life, and long-term cardiovascular events, has been reported. A meta-analysis of controlled clinical trials comparing bariatric surgery versus no surgery showed that surgery was associated with a reduced odds ratio (OR) risk of global mortality (OR = 0.55), cardiovascular death (OR = 0.58), and all-cause mortality (OR = 0.70).

Among the observed improvements in comorbidities, the prevention and treatment of type 2 diabetes resulting from bariatric surgery has garnered the most attention. Fifteen-year data from the Swedish Obese Subjects study demonstrated a marked reduction (i.e., by 78%) in the incidence of type 2 diabetes development among obese patients who underwent bariatric surgery. Several randomized controlled studies have shown greater weight loss and more improved glycemic control at 1 and 2 years among surgical patients than among patients receiving conventional medical therapy. A retrospective cohort study of more than 4000 adults with diabetes found that, overall, 68.2% of patients experienced an initial complete type 2 diabetes remission within 5 years after surgery. However, among these patients, one-third redeveloped type 2 diabetes within 5 years. The rapid improvement seen in diabetes after restrictive-malabsorptive procedures is thought to be due to surgery-specific, weight-independent effects on glucose homeostasis brought about by alteration of gut hormones.

The mortality rate from bariatric surgery is generally <1% but varies with the procedure, the patient's age and comorbid conditions, and the experience of the surgical team. The most common surgical complications include stomal stenosis or marginal ulcers (occurring in 5–15% of patients) that present as prolonged nausea and vomiting after eating or inability to advance the diet to solid foods. These complications typically are treated by endoscopic balloon dilation and acid suppression therapy, respectively. For patients who undergo laparoscopic adjustable gastric banding, there are no intestinal absorptive abnormalities other than mechanical reduction in gastric size and outflow. Therefore, selective deficiencies are uncommon unless eating habits become unbalanced. In contrast, the restrictive-malabsorptive procedures carry an increased risk for micronutrient deficiencies of vitamin B_{12}, iron, folate, calcium, and vitamin D. Patients with restrictive-malabsorptive procedures require lifelong supplementation with these micronutrients.

CHAPTER 22
THE METABOLIC SYNDROME

Robert H. Eckel

The metabolic syndrome (syndrome X, insulin resistance syndrome) consists of a constellation of metabolic abnormalities that confer increased risk of cardiovascular disease (CVD) and diabetes mellitus. Evolution of the criteria for the metabolic syndrome since the original definition by the World Health Organization in 1998 reflects growing clinical evidence and analysis by a variety of consensus conferences and professional organizations. The major features of the metabolic syndrome include central obesity, hypertriglyceridemia, low levels of high-density lipoprotein (HDL) cholesterol, hyperglycemia, and hypertension (Table 22-1).

EPIDEMIOLOGY

The most challenging feature of the metabolic syndrome to define is waist circumference. Intraabdominal circumference (visceral adipose tissue) is considered most strongly related to insulin resistance and risk of diabetes and CVD, and for any given waist circumference the distribution of adipose tissue between SC and visceral depots varies substantially. Thus, within and between populations, there is a lesser vs. greater risk at the same waist circumference. These differences in populations are reflected in the range of waist circumferences considered to confer risk in different geographic locations (**Table 22-1**).

The prevalence of the metabolic syndrome varies around the world, in part reflecting the age and ethnicity of the populations studied and the diagnostic criteria applied. In general, the prevalence of the metabolic syndrome increases with age. The highest recorded prevalence worldwide is among Native Americans, with nearly 60% of women ages 45–49 and 45% of men ages 45–49 meeting the criteria of the National Cholesterol Education Program and Adult Treatment Panel III (NCEP:ATPIII). In the United States, the metabolic syndrome is less common among African-American men and more common among Mexican-American women. Based on data from the National Health and Nutrition Examination Survey (NHANES) 2003–2006, the age-adjusted prevalence of the metabolic syndrome in U.S. adults without diabetes is 28% for men and 30% for women. In France, studies of a cohort of 30- to 60-year-olds have shown a <10% prevalence for each sex, although 17.5% of people 60–64 years of age are affected. Greater global industrialization is associated with rising rates of obesity, which are expected to increase the prevalence of the metabolic syndrome dramatically, especially as the population ages. Moreover, the rising prevalence and severity of obesity among children is reflected in features of the metabolic syndrome in a younger population.

The frequency distribution of the five components of the syndrome for the U.S. population (NHANES III) is summarized in Fig. 22-1. Increases in waist circumference predominate among women, whereas increases in fasting plasma triglyceride levels (i.e., to >150 mg/dL), reductions in HDL cholesterol levels, and hyperglycemia are more likely in men.

RISK FACTORS

Overweight/Obesity

Although the metabolic syndrome was first described in the early twentieth century, the worldwide overweight/obesity epidemic has recently been the force driving its increasing recognition. Central adiposity is a key feature of the syndrome, and the syndrome's prevalence reflects the strong relationship between waist circumference and increasing adiposity. However, despite the importance of obesity, patients who are of normal weight may also be insulin resistant and may have the metabolic syndrome.

Sedentary lifestyle

Physical inactivity is a predictor of CVD events and the related risk of death. Many components of the

TABLE 22-1

NCEP:ATPIII[a] 2001 AND HARMONIZING DEFINITION CRITERIA FOR THE METABOLIC SYNDROME

NCEP:ATPIII 2001	HARMONIZING DEFINITION[b]		
Three or more of the following: • Central obesity: waist circumference >102 cm (M), >88 cm (F) • Hypertriglyceridemia: triglyceride level ≥150 mg/dL or specific medication • Low HDL[c] cholesterol: <40 mg/dL and <50 mg/dL for men and women, respectively, or specific medication • Hypertension: blood pressure ≥130 mmHg systolic or ≥85 mmHg diastolic or specific medication • Fasting plasma glucose level ≥100 mg/dL or specific medication or previously diagnosed type 2 diabetes	**Three of the following:** • Waist circumference (cm)		
	Men	**Women**	**Ethnicity**
	≥94	≥80	Europid, sub-Saharan African, Eastern and Middle Eastern
	≥90	≥80	South Asian, Chinese, and ethnic South and Central American
	≥85	≥90	Japanese
	• Fasting triglyceride level >150 mg/dL or specific medication • HDL cholesterol level <40 mg/dL and <50 mg/dL for men and women, respectively, or specific medication • Blood pressure >130 mm systolic or >85 mm diastolic or previous diagnosis or specific medication • Fasting plasma glucose level ≥100 mg/dL (alternative indication: drug treatment of elevated glucose levels)		

[a]National Cholesterol Education Program and Adult Treatment Panel III.
[b]In this analysis, the following thresholds for waist circumference were used: white men, ≥94 cm; African-American men, ≥94 cm; Mexican-American men, ≥90 cm; white women, ≥80 cm; African-American women, ≥80 cm; Mexican-American women, ≥80 cm. For participants whose designation was "other race—including multiracial," thresholds that were once based on Europid cutoffs (≥94 cm for men and ≥80 cm for women) and on South Asian cutoffs (≥90 cm for men and ≥80 cm for women) were used. For participants who were considered "other Hispanic," the International Diabetes Federation thresholds for ethnic South and Central Americans were used.
[c]High-density lipoprotein.

metabolic syndrome are associated with a sedentary lifestyle, including increased adipose tissue (predominantly central), reduced HDL cholesterol, and increased triglycerides, blood pressure, and glucose in genetically susceptible persons. Compared with individuals who watch television or videos or use the computer <1 h daily, those who do so for >4 h daily have a twofold increased risk of the metabolic syndrome.

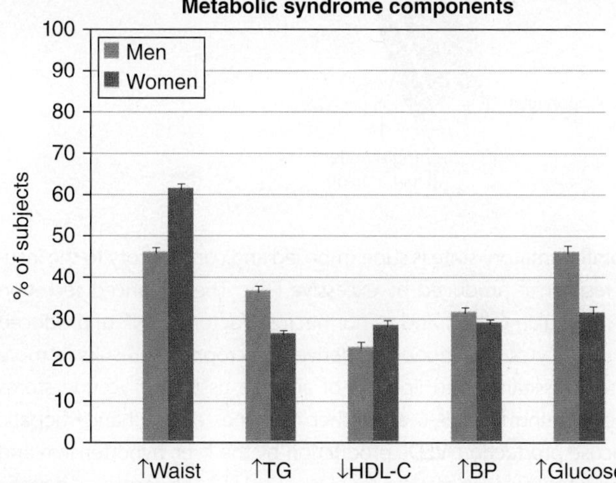

FIGURE 22-1

Prevalence of the metabolic syndrome components, from NHANES 2003–2006. NHANES, National Health and Nutrition Examination Survey; TG, triglyceride; HDL-C, high-density lipoprotein cholesterol; BP, blood pressure. The prevalence of elevated glucose includes individuals with known diabetes mellitus. *(Created from data in ES Ford et al: J Diabetes 2:1753, 2010.)*

Aging

The metabolic syndrome affects nearly 50% of the U.S. population older than age 50, and at >60 years of age women are more often affected than men. The age dependency of the syndrome's prevalence is seen in most populations around the world.

Diabetes mellitus

Diabetes mellitus is included in both the NCEP and the harmonizing definitions of the metabolic syndrome. It is estimated that the great majority (~75%) of patients with type 2 diabetes or impaired glucose tolerance have the metabolic syndrome. The presence of the metabolic syndrome in these populations relates to a higher prevalence of CVD than in patients who have type 2 diabetes or impaired glucose tolerance but do not have this syndrome.

Cardiovascular disease

Individuals with the metabolic syndrome are twice as likely to die of cardiovascular disease as those who do not, and their risk of an acute myocardial infarction or stroke is threefold higher. The approximate prevalence of the metabolic syndrome among patients with coronary heart disease (CHD) is 50%, with a prevalence of ~35% among patients with premature coronary artery disease (before or at age 45) and a particularly high prevalence among women. With appropriate cardiac rehabilitation and changes in lifestyle (e.g., nutrition, physical activity, weight reduction, and—in some cases—pharmacologic therapy), the prevalence of the syndrome can be reduced.

Lipodystrophy

Lipodystrophic disorders in general are associated with the metabolic syndrome. Both genetic lipodystrophy (e.g., Berardinelli-Seip congenital lipodystrophy, Dunnigan familial partial lipodystrophy) and acquired lipodystrophy (e.g., HIV-related lipodystrophy in patients receiving antiretroviral therapy) may give rise to severe insulin resistance and many of the components of the metabolic syndrome.

ETIOLOGY

Insulin resistance

The most accepted and unifying hypothesis to describe the pathophysiology of the metabolic syndrome is insulin resistance, which is caused by an incompletely understood defect in insulin action **(Chap. 23)**. The onset of insulin resistance is heralded by postprandial hyperinsulinemia, which is followed by fasting hyperinsulinemia and ultimately by hyperglycemia.

An early major contributor to the development of insulin resistance is an overabundance of circulating fatty acids (Fig. 22-2). Plasma albumin-bound free fatty acids are derived predominantly from adipose-tissue triglyceride stores released by intracellular lipolytic enzymes.

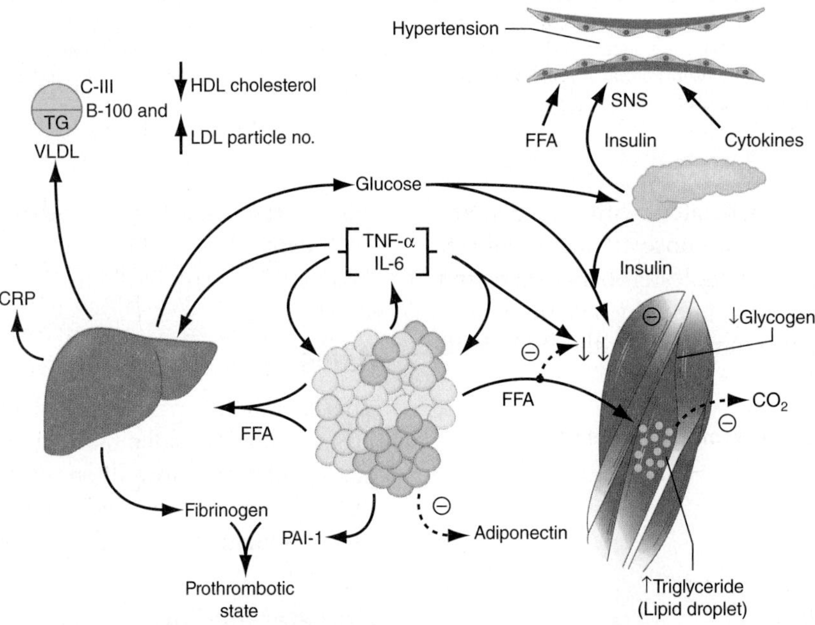

FIGURE 22-2
Pathophysiology of the metabolic syndrome. Free fatty acids (FFAs) are released in abundance from an expanded adipose tissue mass. In the liver, FFAs result in increased production of glucose and triglycerides and secretion of very low density lipoproteins (VLDLs). Associated lipid/lipoprotein abnormalities include reductions in high-density lipoprotein (HDL) cholesterol and an increased low-density lipoprotein (LDL) particle number (no.). FFAs also reduce insulin sensitivity in muscle by inhibiting insulin-mediated glucose uptake. Associated defects include a reduction in glucose partitioning to glycogen and increased lipid accumulation in triglyceride (TG). The increase in circulating glucose, and to some extent FFAs, increases pancreatic insulin secretion, resulting in hyperinsulinemia. Hyperinsulinemia may result in enhanced sodium reabsorption and increased sympathetic nervous system (SNS) activity and contribute to hypertension, as might higher levels of circulating FFAs. The proinflammatory state is superimposed and contributory to the insulin resistance produced by excessive FFAs. The enhanced secretion of interleukin 6 (IL-6) and tumor necrosis factor α (TNF-α) produced by adipocytes and monocyte-derived macrophages results in more insulin resistance and lipolysis of adipose tissue triglyceride stores to circulating FFAs. IL-6 and other cytokines also enhance hepatic glucose production, VLDL production by the liver, hypertension and insulin resistance in muscle. Cytokines and FFAs also increase hepatic production of fibrinogen and adipocyte production of plasminogen activator inhibitor 1 (PAI-1), resulting in a prothrombotic state. Higher levels of circulating cytokines stimulate hepatic production of C-reactive protein (CRP). Reduced production of the anti-inflammatory and insulin-sensitizing cytokine adiponectin is also associated with the metabolic syndrome. *(Modified from RH Eckel et al: Lancet 365:1415, 2005.)*

Fatty acids are also derived from the lipolysis of triglyceride-rich lipoproteins in tissues by lipoprotein lipase. Insulin mediates both antilipolysis and the stimulation of lipoprotein lipase in adipose tissue. Of note, the inhibition of lipolysis in adipose tissue is the most sensitive pathway of insulin action. Thus, when insulin resistance develops, increased lipolysis produces more fatty acids, which further decrease the antilipolytic effect of insulin. Excessive fatty acids enhance substrate availability and create insulin resistance by modifying downstream signaling. Fatty acids impair insulin-mediated glucose uptake and accumulate as triglycerides in both skeletal and cardiac muscle, whereas increased glucose production and triglyceride accumulation take place in the liver.

Leptin resistance has also been raised as a possible pathophysiologic mechanism to explain the metabolic syndrome. Physiologically, leptin reduces appetite, promotes energy expenditure, and enhances insulin sensitivity. In addition, leptin may regulate cardiac and vascular function through a nitric oxide–dependent mechanism. However, when obesity develops, hyperleptinemia ensues, with evidence of leptin resistance in the brain and other tissues resulting in inflammation, insulin resistance, hyperlipidemia, and a plethora of cardiovascular disorders, such as hypertension, atherosclerosis, CHD, and heart failure.

The oxidative stress hypothesis provides a unifying theory for aging and the predisposition to the metabolic syndrome. In studies of insulin-resistant individuals with obesity or type 2 diabetes, the offspring of patients with type 2 diabetes, and the elderly, a defect in mitochondrial oxidative phosphorylation that leads to the accumulation of triglycerides and related lipid molecules in muscle has been identified.

Recently, the gut microbiome has emerged as an important contributor to the development of obesity and related metabolic disorders, including the metabolic syndrome. Although the mechanism remains uncertain, interaction among genetic predisposition, diet, and the intestinal flora is important.

Increased waist circumference

Waist circumference is an important component of the most recent and frequently applied diagnostic criteria for the metabolic syndrome. However, measuring waist circumference does not reliably distinguish increases in SC adipose tissue from those in visceral fat; this distinction requires CT or MRI. With increases in visceral adipose tissue, adipose tissue–derived free fatty acids are directed to the liver. In contrast, increases in abdominal SC fat release lipolysis products into the systemic circulation and avert more direct effects on hepatic metabolism. Relative increases in visceral versus SC adipose tissue with increasing waist circumference in Asians and Asian Indians may explain the greater prevalence of the syndrome in those populations than in African-American men, in whom SC fat predominates. It is also possible that visceral fat is a marker for—but not the source of—excess postprandial free fatty acids in obesity.

Dyslipidemia

In general, free fatty acid flux to the liver is associated with increased production of ApoB-containing, triglyceride-rich, very low-density lipoproteins (VLDLs) **(See also Chap. 27)**. The effect of insulin on this process is complex, but *hypertriglyceridemia* is an excellent marker of the insulin-resistant condition. Not only is hypertriglyceridemia a feature of the metabolic syndrome, but patients with the metabolic syndrome have elevated levels of ApoCIII carried on VLDLs and other lipoproteins. This increase in ApoCIII is inhibitory to lipoprotein lipase, further contributing to hypertriglyceridemia and also associated with more atherosclerotic cardiovascular disease.

The other major lipoprotein disturbance in the metabolic syndrome is a *reduction in HDL cholesterol.* This reduction is a consequence of changes in HDL composition and metabolism. In the presence of hypertriglyceridemia, a decrease in the cholesterol content of HDL is a consequence of reduced cholesteryl ester content of the lipoprotein core in combination with cholesteryl ester transfer protein–mediated alterations in triglyceride that make the particle small and dense. This change in lipoprotein composition also results in increased clearance of HDL from the circulation. These changes in HDL have a relationship to insulin resistance that is probably indirect, occurring in concert with the changes in triglyceride-rich lipoprotein metabolism.

In addition to HDLs, low-density lipoproteins (LDLs) are modified in composition in the metabolic syndrome. With fasting serum triglycerides at >2.0 mM (~180 mg/dL), there is almost always a predominance of small, dense LDLs, which are thought to be more atherogenic although their association with hypertriglyceridemia and low HDLs make their independent contribution to CVD events difficult to assess. Individuals with hypertriglyceridemia often have increases in cholesterol content of both VLDL1 and VLDL2 subfractions and in LDL particle number. Both of these lipoprotein changes may contribute to atherogenic risk in patients with the metabolic syndrome.

Glucose intolerance

Defects in insulin action in the metabolic syndrome lead to impaired suppression of glucose production by the liver and kidney and reduced glucose uptake and metabolism in insulin-sensitive tissues—i.e., muscle and adipose tissue **(See also Chap. 23)**. The relationship between impaired fasting glucose or impaired glucose tolerance and insulin resistance is well supported by studies of humans, nonhuman primates, and rodents. To compensate for defects in insulin action, insulin secretion and/or clearance must be modified so that euglycemia is sustained. Ultimately, this compensatory mechanism fails, usually because of defects in insulin secretion, resulting in progression from impaired fasting glucose and/or impaired glucose tolerance to diabetes mellitus.

Hypertension

The relationship between insulin resistance and hypertension is well established. Paradoxically, under normal physiologic conditions, insulin is a vasodilator with secondary effects on sodium reabsorption in the kidney. However, in the setting of insulin resistance, the vasodilatory effect of insulin is lost but the renal effect on sodium reabsorption is preserved. Sodium reabsorption is increased in whites with the metabolic syndrome but not in Africans or Asians. Insulin also increases the activity of the sympathetic nervous system, an effect that may be preserved in the setting of insulin resistance. Insulin resistance is characterized by pathway-specific impairment in phosphatidylinositol-3-kinase signaling. In the endothelium, this impairment may cause an imbalance between the production of nitric oxide and the secretion of endothelin 1, with a consequent decrease in blood flow. Although these mechanisms are provocative, evaluation of insulin action by measurement of fasting insulin levels or by homeostasis model assessment shows that insulin resistance contributes only partially to the increased prevalence of hypertension in the metabolic syndrome.

Another possible mechanism underlying hypertension in the metabolic syndrome is the vasoactive role of perivascular adipose tissue. Reactive oxygen species released by NADPH oxidase impair endothelial function and result in local vasoconstriction. Other paracrine effects could be mediated by leptin or other proinflammatory cytokines released from adipose tissue, such as tumor necrosis factor α.

Hyperuricemia is another consequence of insulin resistance and is commonly observed in the metabolic syndrome. There is growing evidence not only that uric acid is associated with hypertension but also that reduction of uric acid normalizes blood pressure in hyperuricemic adolescents with hypertension. The mechanism appears to be related to an adverse effect of uric acid on nitric acid synthase in the macula densa of the kidney and stimulation of the renin-angiotensin aldosterone system.

Proinflammatory cytokines

The increases in proinflammatory cytokines—including interleukins 1, 6, and 18; resistin; tumor necrosis factor α; and the systemic biomarker C-reactive protein—reflect overproduction by the expanded adipose tissue mass (Fig. 22-2). Adipose tissue–derived macrophages may be the primary source of proinflammatory cytokines locally and in the systemic circulation. It remains unclear, however, how much of the insulin resistance is caused by the paracrine effects of these cytokines and how much by the endocrine effects.

Adiponectin

Adiponectin is an anti-inflammatory cytokine produced exclusively by adipocytes. Adiponectin enhances insulin sensitivity and inhibits many steps in the inflammatory process. In the liver, adiponectin inhibits the expression of gluconeogenic enzymes and the rate of glucose production. In muscle, adiponectin increases glucose transport and enhances fatty acid oxidation, partially through the activation of AMP kinase. Adiponectin levels are reduced in the metabolic syndrome. The relative contributions of adiponectin deficiency and overabundance of the proinflammatory cytokines are unclear.

CLINICAL FEATURES

Symptoms and signs

The metabolic syndrome typically is not associated with symptoms. On physical examination, waist circumference may be expanded and blood pressure elevated. The presence of either or both of these signs should prompt the clinician to search for other biochemical abnormalities that may be associated with the metabolic syndrome. Less frequently, lipoatrophy or acanthosis nigricans is found on examination. Because these physical findings characteristically are associated with severe insulin resistance, other components of the metabolic syndrome should be expected.

Associated diseases

Cardiovascular disease

The relative risk for new-onset CVD in patients with the metabolic syndrome who do not have diabetes averages 1.5–3 fold. However, an 8-year follow-up of middle-aged participants in the Framingham Offspring Study documented that the population-attributable CVD risk in the metabolic syndrome was 34% among men and only 16% among women. In the same study, both the metabolic syndrome and diabetes predicted ischemic stroke, with greater risk among patients with the metabolic syndrome than among those with diabetes alone (19% vs. 7%) and a particularly large difference among women (27% vs. 5%). Patients with the metabolic syndrome are also at increased risk for peripheral vascular disease.

Type 2 diabetes

Overall, the risk for type 2 diabetes among patients with the metabolic syndrome is increased three- to fivefold. In the Framingham Offspring Study's 8-year follow-up of middle-aged participants, the population-attributable risk for developing type 2 diabetes was 62% among men and 47% among women.

Other associated conditions

In addition to the features specifically associated with the metabolic syndrome, other metabolic alterations accompany insulin resistance. Those alterations include increases in ApoB and ApoCIII, uric acid, prothrombotic factors (fibrinogen, plasminogen activator inhibitor 1), serum viscosity, asymmetric dimethylarginine, homocysteine, white blood cell count, proinflammatory cytokines, C-reactive protein, microalbuminuria, nonalcoholic fatty liver disease and/or nonalcoholic steatohepatitis, polycystic ovary syndrome, and obstructive sleep apnea.

Nonalcoholic fatty liver disease

Fatty liver is a relatively common condition, affecting 25–45% of the U.S. population. However, in nonalcoholic steatohepatitis, triglyceride accumulation and inflammation coexist. Nonalcoholic steatohepatitis is now present in 3–12% of the population of the United States and other Western countries. Of patients with the metabolic syndrome, ~25–60% have nonalcoholic fatty liver disease and up to 35% have nonalcoholic steatohepatitis. As the prevalence of overweight/obesity and the metabolic syndrome increases, nonalcoholic steatohepatitis may become one of the more common causes of end-stage liver disease and hepatocellular carcinoma.

Hyperuricemia

Hyperuricemia reflects defects in insulin action on the renal tubular reabsorption of uric acid and may contribute to hypertension through its effect on the endothelium. An increase in asymmetric dimethylarginine, an endogenous inhibitor of nitric oxide synthase, also relates to endothelial dysfunction. In addition, microalbuminuria may be caused by altered endothelial pathophysiology in the insulin-resistant state.

Polycystic ovary syndrome

Polycystic ovary syndrome is highly associated with insulin resistance (50–80%) and the metabolic syndrome, with a prevalence of the syndrome between 40% and 50% **(See also Chap. 13)**. Women with polycystic ovary syndrome are two to four times more likely to have the metabolic syndrome than are women without polycystic ovary syndrome.

Obstructive sleep apnea

Obstructive sleep apnea is commonly associated with obesity, hypertension, increased circulating cytokines, impaired glucose tolerance, and insulin resistance. With these associations, it is not surprising that individuals with obstructive sleep apnea frequently have the metabolic syndrome. Moreover, when biomarkers of insulin resistance are compared between patients with obstructive sleep apnea and weight-matched controls, insulin resistance is found to be more severe in those with apnea. Continuous positive airway pressure treatment improves insulin sensitivity in patients with obstructive sleep apnea.

DIAGNOSIS

The diagnosis of the metabolic syndrome relies on fulfillment of the criteria listed in Table 22-1, as assessed using tools at the bedside and in the laboratory. The medical history should include evaluation of symptoms for obstructive sleep apnea in all patients and polycystic ovary syndrome in premenopausal women. Family history will help determine risk for CVD and diabetes mellitus. Blood pressure and waist circumference measurements provide information necessary for the diagnosis.

Laboratory tests

Measurement of fasting lipids and glucose is needed in determining whether the metabolic syndrome is present. The measurement of additional biomarkers associated with insulin resistance can be individualized. Such tests might include those for ApoB, high-sensitivity C-reactive protein, fibrinogen, uric acid, urinary microalbumin, and liver function. A sleep study should be performed if symptoms of obstructive sleep apnea are present. If polycystic ovary syndrome is suspected on the basis of clinical features and anovulation, testosterone, luteinizing hormone, and follicle-stimulating hormone should be measured.

TREATMENT The Metabolic Syndrome

LIFESTYLE Obesity is the driving force behind the metabolic syndrome **(See also Chap. 21)**. Thus, weight reduction is the primary approach to the disorder. With weight reduction, improvement in insulin sensitivity is often accompanied by favorable modifications in many components of the metabolic syndrome. In general, recommendations for weight loss include a combination of caloric restriction, increased physical activity, and behavior modification. Caloric restriction is the most important component, whereas increases in physical activity are important for maintenance of weight loss. Some but not all evidence suggests that the addition of exercise to caloric restriction may promote greater weight loss from the visceral depot. The tendency for weight regain after successful weight reduction underscores the need for long-lasting behavioral changes.

Diet Before prescribing a weight-loss diet, it is important to emphasize that it has taken the patient a long time to develop an expanded fat mass; thus, the correction need not occur quickly. Given that ~3500 kcal = 1 lb of fat, ~500-kcal restriction daily equates to weight reduction of 1 lb per week. Diets restricted in carbohydrate typically provide a rapid initial weight loss. However, after 1 year, the amount of weight reduction is minimally reduced or no different from that with caloric restriction alone. Thus, adherence to the diet is more important than which diet is chosen. Moreover, there is concern about low-carbohydrate diets enriched in saturated fat, particularly for patients at risk for CVD. Therefore, a high-quality dietary pattern—i.e., a diet enriched in fruits, vegetables, whole grains, lean poultry, and fish—should be encouraged to maximize overall health benefit.

Physical Activity Before a physical activity recommendation is provided to patients with the metabolic syndrome, it is important to ensure that the increased activity does not incur risk. Some high-risk patients should undergo formal cardiovascular evaluation before initiating an exercise program. For an inactive participant, gradual increases in physical activity should be encouraged to enhance adherence and avoid injury. Although increases in physical activity can lead to modest weight reduction, 60–90 min of daily activity is required to achieve this goal. Even if an overweight or obese adult is unable to undertake this level of activity, a significant health benefit will follow from at least 30 min of moderate-intensity activity daily. The caloric value of 30 min of a variety of activities can be found at *www.heart.org/HEARTORG/GettingHealthy/WeightManagement/LosingWeight/Losing-Weight_UCM_307904_Article.jsp*. Of note, a variety of routine activities, such as gardening, walking, and housecleaning, require moderate caloric expenditure. Thus, physical activity need not be defined solely in terms of formal exercise such as jogging, swimming, or tennis.

Behavior Modification Behavioral treatment typically includes recommendations for dietary restriction and more physical activity, resulting in weight loss that benefits metabolic health. The subsequent challenge is the duration of the program because weight regain so often follows successful weight reduction. Long-term outcomes may be enhanced by a variety of methods, such as the Internet, social media, and telephone follow-up to maintain contact between providers and patients.

Obesity In some patients with the metabolic syndrome, treatment options need to extend beyond lifestyle intervention (**See also Chap. 21**). Weight-loss drugs come in two major classes: appetite suppressants and absorption inhibitors. Appetite suppressants approved by the U.S. Food and Drug Administration include phentermine (for short-term use [3 months] only) as well as the more recent additions phentermine/topiramate and lorcaserin, which are approved without restrictions on the duration of therapy. In clinical trials, the phentermine/topiramate combination has resulted in ~10% weight loss in 50% of patients. Side effects include palpitations, headache, paresthesias, constipation, and insomnia. Lorcaserin results in less weight loss—typically ~5% beyond placebo—but can cause headache and nasopharyngitis. Orlistat inhibits fat absorption by ~30% and is moderately effective compared with placebo (~5% more weight loss). Orlistat has been shown to reduce the incidence of type 2 diabetes, an effect that was especially evident among patients with impaired glucose tolerance at baseline. This drug is often difficult of take because of oily leakage per rectum.

Metabolic or bariatric surgery is an option for patients with the metabolic syndrome who have a body mass index >40 kg/m^2, or >35 kg/m^2 with comorbidities. An evolving application for metabolic surgery includes patients with a body mass index as low as 30 kg/m^2 and type 2 diabetes. Gastric bypass or vertical sleeve gastrectomy results in dramatic weight reduction and improvement in the features of the metabolic syndrome. A survival benefit with gastric bypass has also been realized.

LDL CHOLESTEROL The rationale for the NCEP:ATPIII's development of criteria for the metabolic syndrome was to go beyond LDL cholesterol in identifying and reducing the risk of CVD (**See also Chap. 27**). The working assumption by the panel was that LDL cholesterol goals had already been achieved and that increasing evidence supports a linear reduction in CVD events as a result of progressive lowering of LDL cholesterol with statins. For patients with the metabolic syndrome and diabetes, a statin should be prescribed. For those patients with diabetes and known CVD, the current evidence supports a maximum of penultimate dose of a potent statin (e.g., atorvastatin or rosuvastatin). For those patients with the metabolic syndrome but without diabetes, a score that predicts a 10-year CVD risk exceeding 7.5% should also take a statin. With a 10-year risk of <7.5%, use of statin therapy is not evidence based.

Diets restricted in saturated fats (<7% of calories) and *trans*-fats (as few as possible) should be applied aggressively. Although less evidence exists, dietary cholesterol should also be restricted. If LDL cholesterol remains elevated, pharmacologic intervention is needed. Treatment with statins, which lower LDL cholesterol by 15–60%, is evidence based and is the first-choice medication intervention. Of note, for each doubling of the statin dose, LDL cholesterol is further lowered by only ~6%. Hepatotoxicity (more than a threefold increase in hepatic aminotransferases) is rare, and myopathy is seen in ~10% of patients. The cholesterol absorption inhibitor ezetimibe is well tolerated and should be the second-choice medication intervention. Ezetimibe typically reduces LDL cholesterol by 15–20%. The bile acid sequestrants cholestyramine, colestipol, and colesevalam may be more effective than ezetimibe but, because they can increase triglyceride levels, must be used with caution in patients with the metabolic syndrome. In general, bile sequestrants should not be administered when fasting triglyceride levels are >250 mg/dL. Side effects include gastrointestinal symptoms (palatability, bloating, belching, constipation, anal irritation). Nicotinic acid has modest LDL cholesterol–lowering capabilities (<20%). Fibrates are best employed to lower LDL cholesterol when both LDL cholesterol and triglycerides are elevated. Fenofibrate may be more effective than gemfibrozil in this setting.

TRIGLYCERIDES The NCEP:ATPIII has focused on non-HDL cholesterol rather than on triglycerides **(See also Chap. 27)**. However, a fasting triglyceride value of <150 mg/dL is recommended. In general, the response of fasting triglycerides relates to the amount of weight reduction achieved: a weight reduction of >10% is necessary to lower fasting triglyceride levels.

A fibrate (gemfibrozil or fenofibrate) is the drug of choice to lower fasting triglyceride levels, which are typically reduced by 30–45%. Concomitant administration with drugs metabolized by the 3A4 cytochrome P450 system (including some statins) increases the risk of myopathy. In these cases, fenofibrate may be preferable to gemfibrozil. In the Veterans Affairs HDL Intervention Trial, gemfibrozil was administered to men with known CHD and levels of HDL cholesterol <40 mg/dL. A coronary disease event and mortality rate benefit was experienced predominantly among men with hyperinsulinemia and/or diabetes, many of whom were identified retrospectively as having the metabolic syndrome. Of note, the degree of triglyceride lowering in this trial did not predict benefit. Although levels of LDL cholesterol did not change, a decrease in LDL particle number correlated with benefit. Several additional clinical trials have not shown clear evidence that fibrates reduce CVD risk; however, post hoc analyses of several studies demonstrated that patients with baseline triglyceride levels >200 mg/dL and HDL cholesterol levels <35 mg/dL did benefit.

Other drugs that lower triglyceride levels include statins, nicotinic acid, and—in high doses—omega-3 fatty acids. For this purpose, an intermediate or high dose of the "more potent" statins (atorvastatin, rosuvastatin) is needed. The effect of nicotinic acid on fasting triglycerides is dose related and ~20–35%, an effect that is less pronounced than that of fibrates. In patients with the metabolic syndrome and diabetes, nicotinic acid may increase fasting glucose levels. Omega-3 fatty acid preparations that include high doses of docosahexaenoic acid plus eicosapentaenoic acid (~1.5–4.5 g/d) or eicosapentaenoic acid alone lower fasting triglyceride levels by ~30–40%. No drug interactions with fibrates or statins occur, and the main side effect of their use is eructation with a fishy taste. This taste can be partially blocked by ingestion of the nutraceutical after freezing. Clinical trials of nicotinic acid or high-dose omega-3 fatty acids in patients with the metabolic syndrome have not been reported.

HDL CHOLESTEROL Very few lipid-modifying compounds increase HDL cholesterol levels **(See also Chap. 27)**. Statins, fibrates, and bile acid sequestrants have modest effects (5–10%), whereas ezetimibe and omega-3 fatty acids have no effect. Nicotinic acid is the only currently available drug with predictable HDL cholesterol-raising properties. The response is dose related, and nicotinic acid can increase HDL cholesterol by ~30% above baseline. After several trials of nicotinic acid versus placebo in statin-treated patients, there is still no evidence that raising HDL with nicotinic acid beneficially affects CVD events in patients with or without the metabolic syndrome.

BLOOD PRESSURE The direct relationship between blood pressure and all-cause mortality rate has been well established in studies comparing patients with hypertension (>140/90 mmHg), patients with pre-hypertension (>120/80 mmHg but <140/90 mmHg), and individuals with normal blood pressure (<120/80 mmHg). In patients who have the metabolic syndrome without diabetes, the best choice for the initial antihypertensive medication is an angiotensin-converting enzyme (ACE) inhibitor or an angiotensin II receptor blocker, as these two classes of drugs appear to reduce the incidence of new-onset type 2 diabetes. In all patients with hypertension, a sodium-restricted dietary pattern enriched in fruits and vegetables, whole grains, and low-fat dairy products should be advocated. Home monitoring of blood pressure may assist in maintaining good blood-pressure control.

IMPAIRED FASTING GLUCOSE In patients with the metabolic syndrome and type 2 diabetes, aggressive glycemic control may favorably modify fasting levels of triglycerides and/or HDL cholesterol **(See also Chap. 23)**. In patients with impaired fasting glucose who do not have diabetes, a lifestyle intervention that includes weight reduction, dietary fat restriction, and increased physical activity has been shown to reduce the incidence of type 2 diabetes. Metformin also reduces the incidence of diabetes, although the effect is less pronounced than that of lifestyle intervention.

INSULIN RESISTANCE Several drug classes (biguanides, thiazolidinediones [TZDs]) increase insulin sensitivity **(See also Chap. 24)**. Because insulin resistance is the primary pathophysiologic mechanism for the metabolic syndrome, representative drugs in these classes reduce its prevalence. Both metformin and TZDs enhance insulin action in the liver and suppress endogenous glucose production. TZDs, but not metformin, also improve insulin-mediated glucose uptake in muscle and adipose tissue. Benefits of both drugs have been seen in patients with nonalcoholic fatty liver disease and polycystic ovary syndrome, and the drugs have been shown to reduce markers of inflammation.

CHAPTER 23

DIABETES MELLITUS: DIAGNOSIS, CLASSIFICATION, AND PATHOPHYSIOLOGY

Alvin C. Powers

Diabetes mellitus (DM) refers to a group of common metabolic disorders that share the phenotype of hyperglycemia. Several distinct types of DM are caused by a complex interaction of genetics and environmental factors. Depending on the etiology of the DM, factors contributing to hyperglycemia include reduced insulin secretion, decreased glucose utilization, and increased glucose production. The metabolic dysregulation associated with DM causes secondary pathophysiologic changes in multiple organ systems that impose a tremendous burden on the individual with diabetes and on the health care system. In the United States, DM is the leading cause of end-stage renal disease (ESRD), nontraumatic lower extremity amputations, and adult blindness. It also predisposes to cardiovascular diseases. With an increasing incidence worldwide, DM will be likely a leading cause of morbidity and mortality in the future.

CLASSIFICATION

DM is classified on the basis of the pathogenic process that leads to hyperglycemia, as opposed to earlier criteria such as age of onset or type of therapy (Fig. 23-1). There are two broad categories of DM, designated type 1 and type 2 (Table 23-1). However, there is increasing recognition of other forms of diabetes in which the pathogenesis is better understood. These other forms of diabetes may share features of type 1 and/or type 2 DM. Both type 1 and type 2 DM are preceded by a phase of abnormal glucose homeostasis as the pathogenic processes progress. Type 1 DM is the result of complete or near-total insulin deficiency. Type 2 DM is a heterogeneous group of disorders characterized by variable degrees of insulin resistance, impaired insulin secretion, and increased glucose production. Distinct genetic and metabolic defects in insulin action and/or secretion give rise to the common phenotype of hyperglycemia in type 2 DM and have important potential therapeutic implications now that pharmacologic agents are available to target specific metabolic derangements. Type 2 DM is preceded by a period of abnormal glucose homeostasis classified as impaired fasting glucose (IFG) or impaired glucose tolerance (IGT).

Two features of the current classification of DM merit emphasis from previous classifications. First, the terms *insulin-dependent diabetes mellitus* (IDDM) and *non-insulin-dependent diabetes mellitus* (NIDDM) are obsolete. Because many individuals with type 2 DM eventually require insulin treatment for control of glycemia, the use of the term NIDDM generated considerable confusion. A second difference is that age or treatment modality is not a criterion. Although type 1 DM most commonly develops before the age of 30, an autoimmune beta cell destructive process can develop at any age. It is estimated that between 5 and 10% of individuals who develop DM after age 30 years have type 1 DM. Although type 2 DM more typically develops with increasing age, it is now being diagnosed more frequently in children and young adults, particularly in obese adolescents.

OTHER TYPES OF DM

Other etiologies for DM include specific genetic defects in insulin secretion or action, metabolic abnormalities that impair insulin secretion, mitochondrial abnormalities, and a host of conditions that impair glucose tolerance (**Table 23-1**). *Maturity-onset diabetes of the young* (MODY) and *monogenic diabetes* are subtypes of DM characterized by autosomal dominant inheritance, early onset of hyperglycemia (usually <25 years; sometimes in neonatal period), and impaired insulin secretion (discussed below). Mutations in the insulin receptor cause a group of rare disorders characterized by severe insulin resistance.

DM can result from pancreatic exocrine disease when the majority of pancreatic islets are destroyed. Cystic fibrosis–related DM is an important consideration in that patient population. Hormones that antagonize insulin

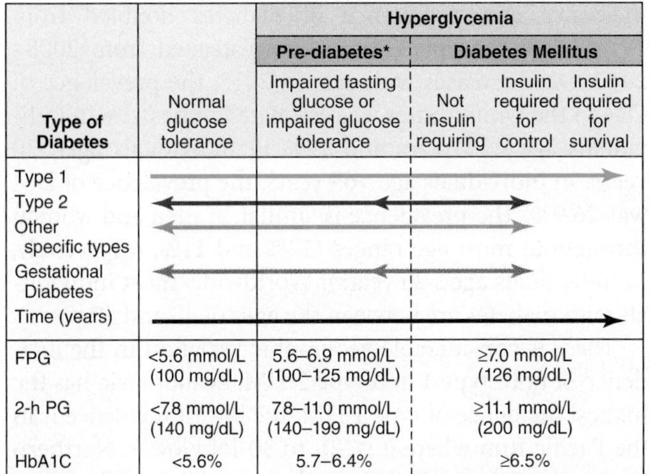

Hyperglycemia
Pre-diabetes*
Diabetes Mellitus
Type of Diabetes
Normal glucose tolerance
Impaired fasting glucose or impaired glucose tolerance
Not insulin requiring
Insulin required for control
Insulin required for survival
Type 1
Type 2
Other specific types
Gestational Diabetes
Time (years)
FPG
<5.6 mmol/L (100 mg/dL)
5.6–6.9 mmol/L (100–125 mg/dL)
≥7.0 mmol/L (126 mg/dL)
2-h PG
<7.8 mmol/L (140 mg/dL)
7.8–11.0 mmol/L (140–199 mg/dL)
≥11.1 mmol/L (200 mg/dL)
HbA1C
<5.6%
5.7–6.4%
≥6.5%

FIGURE 23-1

Spectrum of glucose homeostasis and diabetes mellitus (DM). The spectrum from normal glucose tolerance to diabetes in type 1 DM, type 2 DM, other specific types of diabetes, and gestational DM is shown from left to right. In most types of DM, the individual traverses from normal glucose tolerance to impaired glucose tolerance to overt diabetes (these should be viewed not as abrupt categories but as a spectrum). *Arrows* indicate that changes in glucose tolerance may be bidirectional in some types of diabetes. For example, individuals with type 2 DM may return to the impaired glucose tolerance category with weight loss; in gestational DM, diabetes may revert to impaired glucose tolerance or even normal glucose tolerance after delivery. The fasting plasma glucose (FPG), the 2-h plasma glucose (PG) after a glucose challenge, and the hemoglobin A_{1c} (HbA_{1c}) for the different categories of glucose tolerance are shown at the lower part of the figure. These values do not apply to the diagnosis of gestational DM. Some types of DM may or may not require insulin for survival. *Some use the term *increased risk for diabetes* or *intermediate hyperglycemia* (World Health Organization) rather than *prediabetes. (Adapted from the American Diabetes Association, 2014.)*

action can also lead to DM. Thus, DM is often a feature of endocrinopathies such as acromegaly and Cushing's disease. Viral infections have been implicated in pancreatic islet destruction but are an extremely rare cause of DM. A form of acute onset of type 1 diabetes, termed *fulminant diabetes*, has been noted in Japan and may be related to viral infection of islets.

GESTATIONAL DIABETES MELLITUS

Glucose intolerance developing during pregnancy is classified as gestational diabetes mellitus (GDM). Insulin resistance is related to the metabolic changes of late pregnancy, and the increased insulin requirements may lead to IGT or diabetes. GDM occurs in ~7% (range 1–14%) of pregnancies in the United States; most women revert to normal glucose tolerance postpartum but have a substantial risk (35–60%) of developing DM in the next 10–20 years. The International Association of the Diabetes and Pregnancy Study Groups and

TABLE 23-1

ETIOLOGIC CLASSIFICATION OF DIABETES MELLITUS

I. Type 1 diabetes (beta cell destruction, usually leading to absolute insulin deficiency)
   A. Immune-mediated
   B. Idiopathic
II. Type 2 diabetes (may range from predominantly insulin resistance with relative insulin deficiency to a predominantly insulin secretory defect with insulin resistance)
III. Other specific types of diabetes
   A. Genetic defects of beta cell development or function characterized by mutations in:
      1. Hepatocyte nuclear transcription factor (HNF) 4α (MODY 1)
      2. Glucokinase (MODY 2)
      3. HNF-1α (MODY 3)
      4. Insulin promoter factor-1 (IPF-1; MODY 4)
      5. HNF-1β (MODY 5)
      6. NeuroD1 (MODY 6)
      7. Mitochondrial DNA
      8. Subunits of ATP-sensitive potassium channel
      9. Proinsulin or insulin
      10. Other pancreatic islet regulators/proteins such as *KLF11, PAX4, BLK, GATA4, GATA6, SLC2A2* (GLUT2), *RFX6, GLIS3*
   B. Genetic defects in insulin action
      1. Type A insulin resistance
      2. Leprechaunism
      3. Rabson-Mendenhall syndrome
      4. Lipodystrophy syndromes
   C. Diseases of the exocrine pancreas—pancreatitis, pancreatectomy, neoplasia, cystic fibrosis, hemochromatosis, fibrocalculous pancreatopathy, mutations in carboxyl ester lipase
   D. Endocrinopathies—acromegaly, Cushing's syndrome, glucagonoma, pheochromocytoma, hyperthyroidism, somatostatinoma, aldosteronoma
   E. Drug- or chemical-induced—glucocorticoids, vacor (a rodenticide), pentamidine, nicotinic acid, diazoxide, β-adrenergic agonists, thiazides, calcineurin and mTOR inhibitors, hydantoins, asparaginase, α-interferon, protease inhibitors, antipsychotics (atypicals and others), epinephrine
   F. Infections—congenital rubella, cytomegalovirus, coxsackievirus
   G. Uncommon forms of immune-mediated diabetes—"stiff-person" syndrome, anti-insulin receptor antibodies
   H. Other genetic syndromes sometimes associated with diabetes—Wolfram's syndrome, Down's syndrome, Klinefelter's syndrome, Turner's syndrome, Friedreich's ataxia, Huntington's chorea, Laurence-Moon-Biedl syndrome, myotonic dystrophy, porphyria, Prader-Willi syndrome
IV. Gestational diabetes mellitus (GDM)

Abbreviation: MODY, maturity-onset diabetes of the young.
Source: Adapted from American Diabetes Association: Diabetes Care 37(Suppl 1):S14, 2014.

the American Diabetes Association (ADA) recommend that diabetes diagnosed at the initial prenatal visit should be classified as "overt" diabetes rather than

GDM. With the rising rates of obesity, the number of women being diagnosed with GDM or overt diabetes is rising worldwide.

EPIDEMIOLOGY AND GLOBAL CONSIDERATIONS

The worldwide prevalence of DM has risen dramatically over the past two decades, from an estimated 30 million cases in 1985 to 382 million in 2013 (Fig. 23-2). Based on current trends, the International Diabetes Federation projects that 592 million individuals will have diabetes by the year 2035 (see *http://www.idf.org/*). Although the prevalence of both type 1 and type 2 DM is increasing worldwide, the prevalence of type 2 DM is rising much more rapidly, presumably because of increasing obesity, reduced activity levels as countries become more industrialized, and the aging of the population. In 2013, the prevalence of diabetes in individuals from age 20–79 ranged from 23 to 37% in the 10 countries with the highest prevalence (Tuvalu, Federated States of Micronesia, Marshall Islands, Kiribati, Vanuatu, Cook Islands, Saudi Arabia, Nauru, Kuwait, and Qatar, in descending order of prevalence). The countries with the greatest number of individuals with diabetes in 2013 are China (98.4 million), India (65.1 million), United States (24.4 million), Brazil (11.9 million), and the Russian Federation (10.9 million). Up to 80% of individuals with diabetes live in low-income or medium-income countries. In the most recent estimate for the United States (2012), the Centers for Disease Control and Prevention (CDC) estimated that 9.3% of the population had diabetes (~28% of the individuals with diabetes were undiagnosed; globally, it is estimated that 50% of individuals may be undiagnosed). The CDC estimated that the incidence and prevalence of diabetes doubled from 1990–2008, but appears to have plateaued from 2008–2012. DM increases with age. In 2012, the prevalence of DM in the United Sates was estimated to be 0.2% in individuals age <20 years and 12% in individuals age >20 years. In individuals age >65 years, the prevalence of DM was 26.9%. The prevalence is similar in men and women throughout most age ranges (14% and 11%, respectively, in individuals age >20 years). Worldwide, most individuals with diabetes are between the ages of 40 and 59 years.

There is considerable geographic variation in the incidence of both type 1 and type 2 DM. Scandinavia has the highest incidence of type 1 DM; the lowest incidence is in the Pacific Rim where it is 20- to 30-fold lower. Northern Europe and the United States have an intermediate rate. Much of the increased risk of type 1 DM is believed to reflect the frequency of high-risk human leukocyte antigen (HLA) alleles among ethnic groups in different geographic locations. The prevalence of type 2 DM and its harbinger, IGT, is highest in certain Pacific islands and the Middle East and intermediate in countries such as India and the United States. This variability is likely due to genetic, behavioral, and environmental factors. DM prevalence also varies among different ethnic populations within a given country, with indigenous populations usually having a greater incidence of diabetes than the general population of the country. For example, the CDC estimated that the age-adjusted prevalence of DM in the United States (age >20 years; 2010–2012) was 8% in non-Hispanic whites, 9% in Asian Americans, 13% in Hispanics, 13% in non-Hispanic blacks, and 16% in American-Indian and Alaskan native populations. The onset of type 2 DM occurs, on average, at an earlier age in ethnic groups other than non-Hispanic whites. In Asia, the prevalence of diabetes is increasing rapidly, and the diabetes phenotype appears to be somewhat different

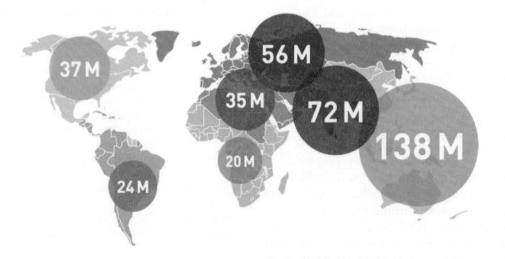

FIGURE 23-2

Worldwide prevalence of diabetes mellitus. Global estimate is 382 million individuals with diabetes. Regional estimates of the number of individuals with diabetes (20–79 years of age) are shown (2013). *(Used with permission from the IDF Diabetes Atlas, the International Diabetes Federation, 2013.)*

from that in the United States and Europe, with an onset at a lower body mass index (BMI) and younger age, greater visceral adiposity, and reduced insulin secretory capacity.

Diabetes is a major cause of mortality, but several studies indicate that diabetes is likely underreported as a cause of death. In the United States, diabetes was listed as the seventh leading cause of death in 2010. A recent estimate suggested that diabetes was responsible for almost 5.1 million deaths or 8% of deaths worldwide in 2013. In 2013, it was estimated that \$548 billion or 11% of health care expenditures worldwide were spent on individuals with diabetes.

DIAGNOSIS

Glucose tolerance is classified into three broad categories: normal glucose homeostasis, DM, or impaired glucose homeostasis. Glucose tolerance can be assessed using the fasting plasma glucose (FPG), the response to oral glucose challenge, or the hemoglobin A_{1c} (HbA_{1c}). An FPG <5.6 mmol/L (100 mg/dL), a plasma glucose <140 mg/dL (7.8 mmol/L) following an oral glucose challenge, and an HbA_{1c} <5.7% are considered to define normal glucose tolerance. The International Expert Committee with members appointed by the ADA, the European Association for the Study of Diabetes, and the International Diabetes Federation have issued diagnostic criteria for DM (Table 23-2) based on the following premises: (1) the FPG, the response to an oral glucose challenge (oral glucose tolerance test [OGTT]), and HbA_{1c} differ among individuals, and (2) DM is defined as the level of glycemia at which diabetes-specific complications occur rather than on deviations from a population-based mean. For example, the prevalence of retinopathy in Native Americans (Pima Indian population) begins to increase at an FPG >6.4 mmol/L (116 mg/dL) (Fig. 23-3).

TABLE 23-2

CRITERIA FOR THE DIAGNOSIS OF DIABETES MELLITUS

- Symptoms of diabetes plus random blood glucose concentration ≥11.1 mmol/L (200 mg/dL)[a] *or*
- Fasting plasma glucose ≥7.0 mmol/L (126 mg/dL)[b] *or*
- Hemoglobin A_{1c} ≥ 6.5%[c] *or*
- 2-h plasma glucose ≥11.1 mmol/L (200 mg/dL) during an oral glucose tolerance test[d]

[a]Random is defined as without regard to time since the last meal.
[b]Fasting is defined as no caloric intake for at least 8 h.
[c]Hemoglobin A_{1c} test should be performed in a laboratory using a method approved by the National Glycohemoglobin Standardization Program and correlated to the reference assay of the Diabetes Control and Complications Trial. Point-of-care hemoglobin A_{1c} should not be used for diagnostic purposes.
[d]The test should be performed using a glucose load containing the equivalent of 75 g anhydrous glucose dissolved in water, not recommended for routine clinical use.

Note: In the absence of unequivocal hyperglycemia and acute metabolic decompensation, these criteria should be confirmed by repeat testing on a different day.

Source: Adapted from American Diabetes Association: Diabetes Care 37(Suppl 1):S14, 2014.

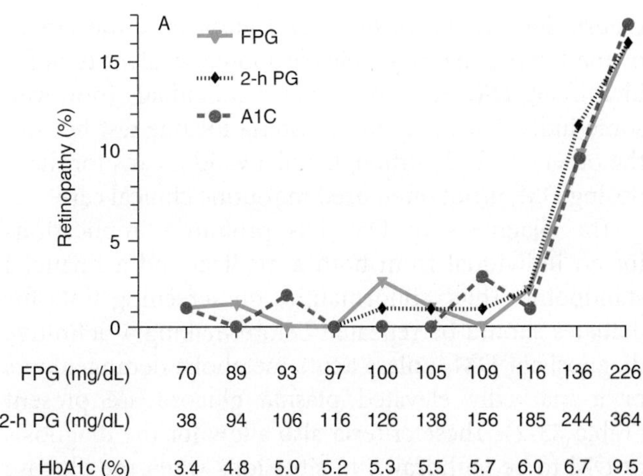

FIGURE 23-3

Relationship of diabetes-specific complication and glucose tolerance. This figure shows the incidence of retinopathy in Pima Indians as a function of the fasting plasma glucose (FPG), the 2-h plasma glucose after a 75-g oral glucose challenge (2-h PG), or the hemoglobin A_{1c} (HbA_{1c}). Note that the incidence of retinopathy greatly increases at a fasting plasma glucose >116 mg/dL, a 2-h plasma glucose of 185 mg/dL, or an HbA_{1c} >6.5%. (Blood glucose values are shown in mg/dL; to convert to mmol/L, divide value by 18.) *(Copyright 2002, American Diabetes Association. From Diabetes Care 25[Suppl 1]: S5–S20, 2002.)*

An FPG ≥7.0 mmol/L (126 mg/dL), a glucose ≥11.1 mmol/L (200 mg/dL) 2 h after an oral glucose challenge, or an HbA_{1c} ≥6.5% warrants the diagnosis of DM (Table 23-2). A random plasma glucose concentration ≥11.1 mmol/L (200 mg/dL) accompanied by classic symptoms of DM (polyuria, polydipsia, weight loss) is also sufficient for the diagnosis of DM (Table 23-2).

Abnormal glucose homeostasis (Fig. 23-1) is defined as (1) FPG = 5.6–6.9 mmol/L (100–125 mg/dL), which is defined as *impaired fasting glucose* (IFG); (2) plasma glucose levels between 7.8 and 11 mmol/L (140 and 199 mg/dL) following an oral glucose challenge, which is termed *impaired glucose tolerance* (IGT); or (3) HbA_{1c} of 5.7–6.4%. An HbA_{1c} of 5.7–6.4%, IFG, and IGT do not identify the same individuals, but individuals in all three groups are at greater risk of progressing to type 2 DM, have an increased risk of cardiovascular disease, and should be counseled about ways to decrease these risks (see below). Some use the terms *prediabetes*, *increased risk of diabetes*, or *intermediate hyperglycemia* (World Health Organization) for this category. These values for the fasting plasma glucose, the glucose following an oral glucose challenge, and HbA_{1c} are continuous variables and not discrete categories. The current criteria for the diagnosis of DM emphasize the HbA_{1c} or the FPG as the most reliable and convenient tests for identifying DM in asymptomatic individuals (however, some individuals may meet criteria for one test but not the other). OGTT, although still a valid means for diagnosing DM, is not often used in routine clinical care.

The diagnosis of DM has profound implications for an individual from both a medical and a financial standpoint. Thus, abnormalities on screening tests for diabetes should be repeated before making a definitive diagnosis of DM, unless acute metabolic derangements or a markedly elevated plasma glucose are present (Table 23-2). These criteria also allow for the diagnosis of DM to be withdrawn in situations when the glucose intolerance reverts to normal.

SCREENING

Widespread use of the FPG or the HbA_{1c} as a screening test for type 2 DM is recommended because (1) a large number of individuals who meet the current criteria for DM are asymptomatic and unaware that they have the disorder, (2) epidemiologic studies suggest that type 2 DM may be present for up to a decade before diagnosis, (3) some individuals with type 2 DM have one or more diabetes-specific complications at the time of their diagnosis, (4) treatment of type 2 DM may favorably alter the natural history of DM, diagnosis of prediabetes should spur efforts for diabetes prevention. The ADA recommends screening all individuals >45 years every 3 years and screening individuals at an earlier age if they are overweight (BMI >25 kg/m^2 or ethnically relevant definition for overweight) and have one additional risk factor for diabetes (Table 23-3). In contrast to type 2 DM, a long asymptomatic period of hyperglycemia is rare prior to the diagnosis of type 1 DM. A number of immunologic markers for type 1 DM are becoming available (discussed below), but their routine use outside a clinical trial is discouraged, pending the identification of clinically beneficial interventions for individuals at high risk for developing type 1 DM.

TABLE 23-3

RISK FACTORS FOR TYPE 2 DIABETES MELLITUS

- Family history of diabetes (i.e., parent or sibling with type 2 diabetes)
- Obesity (BMI ≥25 kg/m^2 or ethnically relevant definition for overweight)
- Physical inactivity
- Race/ethnicity (e.g., African American, Latino, Native American, Asian American, Pacific Islander)
- Previously identified with IFG, IGT, or an hemoglobin A_{1c} of 5.7–6.4%
- History of GDM or delivery of baby >4 kg (9 lb)
- Hypertension (blood pressure ≥140/90 mmHg)
- HDL cholesterol level <35 mg/dL (0.90 mmol/L) and/or a triglyceride level >250 mg/dL (2.82 mmol/L)
- Polycystic ovary syndrome or acanthosis nigricans
- History of cardiovascular disease

Abbreviations: BMI, body mass index; GDM, gestational diabetes mellitus; HDL, high-density lipoprotein; IFG, impaired fasting glucose; IGT, impaired glucose tolerance.

Source: Adapted from American Diabetes Association: Diabetes Care 37(Suppl 1):S14, 2014.

REGULATION OF GLUCOSE HOMEOSTASIS

OVERALL REGULATION OF GLUCOSE HOMEOSTASIS

Glucose homeostasis reflects a balance between hepatic glucose production and peripheral glucose uptake and utilization. Insulin is the most important regulator of this metabolic equilibrium, but neural input, metabolic signals, and other hormones (e.g., glucagon) result in integrated control of glucose supply and utilization (Fig. 23-4). The organs that regulate glucose and lipids communicate by neural and humoral mechanisms with fat and muscle producing adipokines, myokines, and metabolites that influence liver function. In the fasting state, low insulin levels increase glucose production by promoting hepatic gluconeogenesis and glycogenolysis and reduce glucose uptake in insulin-sensitive tissues (skeletal muscle and fat), thereby promoting mobilization of stored precursors such as amino acids and free fatty acids (lipolysis). Glucagon, secreted by pancreatic alpha cells when blood glucose or insulin levels are low, stimulates glycogenolysis and gluconeogenesis by the liver and renal medulla (**Chap. 26**). Postprandially, the glucose load elicits a rise in insulin and fall in glucagon,

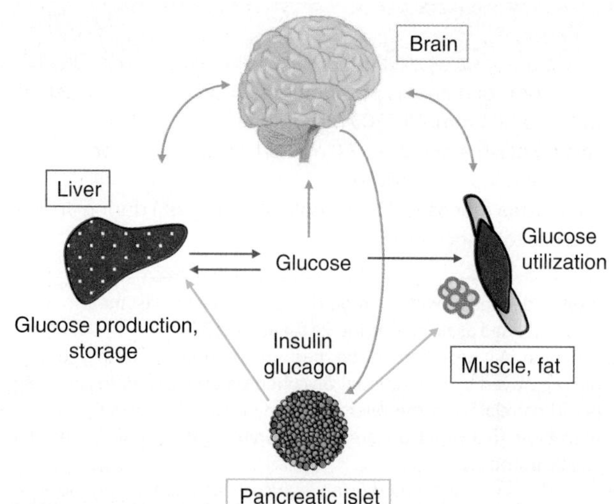

FIGURE 23-4

Regulation of glucose homeostasis. The organs shown contribute to glucose utilization, production, or storage. See text for a description of the communications (*arrows*), which can be neural or humoral.

leading to a reversal of these processes. Insulin, an anabolic hormone, promotes the storage of carbohydrate and fat and protein synthesis. The major portion of postprandial glucose is used by skeletal muscle, an effect of insulin-stimulated glucose uptake. Other tissues, most notably the brain, use glucose in an insulin-independent fashion. Factors secreted by skeletal myocytes (irisin), adipocytes (leptin, resistin, adiponectin, etc.), and bone also influence glucose homeostasis.

INSULIN BIOSYNTHESIS

Insulin is produced in the beta cells of the pancreatic islets. It is initially synthesized as a single-chain 86-amino-acid precursor polypeptide, preproinsulin. Subsequent proteolytic processing removes the amino-terminal signal peptide, giving rise to proinsulin. Proinsulin is structurally related to insulin-like growth factors I and II, which bind weakly to the insulin receptor. Cleavage of an internal 31-residue fragment from proinsulin generates the C peptide and the A (21 amino acids) and B (30 amino acids) chains of insulin, which are connected by disulfide bonds. The mature insulin molecule and C peptide are stored together and co-secreted from secretory granules in the beta cells. Because C peptide is cleared more slowly than insulin, it is a useful marker of insulin secretion and allows discrimination of endogenous and exogenous sources of insulin in the evaluation of hypoglycemia **(Chaps. 26 and 28)**. Pancreatic beta cells co-secrete islet amyloid polypeptide (IAPP) or amylin, a 37-amino-acid peptide, along with insulin. The role of IAPP in normal physiology is incompletely defined, but it is the major component of the amyloid fibrils found in the islets of patients with type 2 diabetes, and an analogue is sometimes used in treating type 1 and type 2 DM. Human insulin is produced by recombinant DNA technology; structural alterations at one or more amino acid residues modify its physical and pharmacologic characteristics **(Chap. 24)**.

INSULIN SECRETION

Glucose is the key regulator of insulin secretion by the pancreatic beta cell, although amino acids, ketones, various nutrients, gastrointestinal peptides, and neurotransmitters also influence insulin secretion. Glucose levels >3.9 mmol/L (70 mg/dL) stimulate insulin synthesis, primarily by enhancing protein translation and processing. Glucose stimulation of insulin secretion begins with its transport into the beta cell by a facilitative glucose transporter (Fig. 23-5). Glucose phosphorylation by glucokinase is the rate-limiting step that controls glucose-regulated insulin secretion. Further metabolism of glucose-6-phosphate via glycolysis generates ATP, which inhibits the activity of an ATP-sensitive K^+ channel. This channel consists of two separate proteins: one is the binding site for certain oral hypoglycemics (e.g., sulfonylureas, meglitinides); the other is an inwardly rectifying K^+ channel protein (Kir6.2). Inhibition of this K^+ channel induces beta cell membrane depolarization, which opens voltage-dependent calcium channels (leading to an influx of calcium) and stimulates insulin secretion. Insulin secretory profiles reveal a pulsatile pattern of hormone release, with small secretory bursts occurring about every 10 min, superimposed upon greater amplitude oscillations of about 80–150 min. Incretins are released from neuroendocrine cells of the gastrointestinal tract following food ingestion and amplify glucose-stimulated insulin secretion and suppress glucagon secretion. Glucagon-like peptide 1 (GLP-1), the most potent incretin, is released from L cells in the small intestine and stimulates insulin secretion only when the blood glucose is above the fasting level. Incretin analogues or pharmacologic agents that prolong the activity of endogenous GLP-1 enhance insulin secretion.

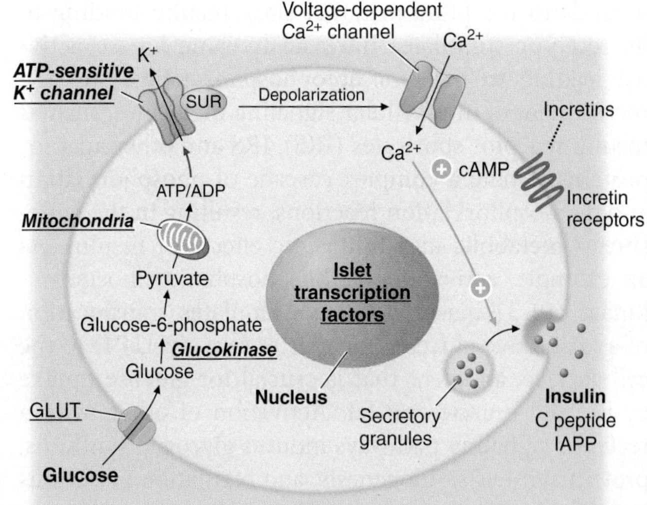

FIGURE 23-5

Mechanisms of glucose-stimulated insulin secretion and abnormalities in diabetes. Glucose and other nutrients regulate insulin secretion by the pancreatic beta cell. Glucose is transported by a glucose transporter (GLUT1 and/or GLUT2 in humans, GLUT2 in rodents); subsequent glucose metabolism by the beta cell alters ion channel activity, leading to insulin secretion. The SUR receptor is the binding site for some drugs that act as insulin secretagogues. Mutations in the events or proteins underlined are a cause of monogenic forms of diabetes. ADP, adenosine diphosphate; ATP, adenosine triphosphate; cAMP, cyclic adenosine monophosphate; IAPP, islet amyloid polypeptide or amylin; SUR, sulfonylurea receptor.

INSULIN ACTION

Once insulin is secreted into the portal venous system, ~50% is removed and degraded by the liver. Unextracted insulin enters the systemic circulation where it binds to receptors in target sites. Insulin binding to its receptor stimulates intrinsic tyrosine kinase activity, leading to receptor autophosphorylation and the recruitment of intracellular signaling molecules, such as insulin receptor substrates (IRS). IRS and other adaptor proteins initiate a complex cascade of phosphorylation and dephosphorylation reactions, resulting in the widespread metabolic and mitogenic effects of insulin. As an example, activation of the phosphatidylinositol-3′-kinase (PI-3-kinase) pathway stimulates translocation of a facilitative glucose transporter (e.g., GLUT4) to the cell surface, an event that is crucial for glucose uptake by skeletal muscle and fat. Activation of other insulin receptor signaling pathways induces glycogen synthesis, protein synthesis, lipogenesis, and regulation of various genes in insulin-responsive cells.

PATHOGENESIS

TYPE 1 DM

Type 1 DM is the result of interactions of genetic, environmental, and immunologic factors that ultimately lead to the destruction of the pancreatic beta cells and insulin deficiency. Type 1 DM, which can develop at any age, develops most commonly before 20 years of age. Worldwide, the incidence of type 1 DM is increasing at the rate of 3–4% per year for uncertain reasons. Type 1 DM results from autoimmune beta cell destruction, and most, but not all, individuals have evidence of islet-directed autoimmunity. Some individuals who have the clinical phenotype of type 1 DM lack immunologic markers indicative of an autoimmune process involving the beta cells and the genetic markers of type 1 DM. These individuals are thought to develop insulin deficiency by unknown, nonimmune mechanisms and may be ketosis prone; many are African American or Asian in heritage. The temporal development of type 1 DM is shown schematically as a function of beta cell mass in Fig. 23-6. Individuals with a genetic susceptibility are thought to have normal beta cell mass at birth but begin to lose beta cells secondary to autoimmune destruction that occurs over months to years. This autoimmune process is thought to be triggered by an infectious or environmental stimulus and to be sustained by a beta cell–specific molecule. In the majority of patients, immunologic markers appear after the triggering event but before diabetes becomes clinically overt. Beta cell mass then begins to decrease, and insulin secretion progressively declines, although normal glucose tolerance is maintained. The rate of decline in beta cell mass varies widely among individuals, with some patients progressing rapidly to clinical diabetes and others evolving more slowly. Features of diabetes do not become evident until a majority of beta cells are destroyed (70–80%). At this point, residual functional beta cells exist but are insufficient in number to maintain glucose tolerance. The events that trigger the transition from glucose intolerance to frank diabetes are often associated with increased insulin requirements, as might occur during infections or puberty. After the initial clinical presentation of type 1 DM, a "honeymoon" phase may ensue during which time glycemic control is achieved with modest doses of insulin or, rarely, insulin is not needed. However, this fleeting phase of endogenous insulin production from residual beta cells disappears and the individual becomes insulin deficient. Many individuals with long-standing type 1 DM produce a small amount of insulin (as reflected by C-peptide production), and some individuals with more than 50 years of type 1 DM have insulin-positive cells in the pancreas at autopsy.

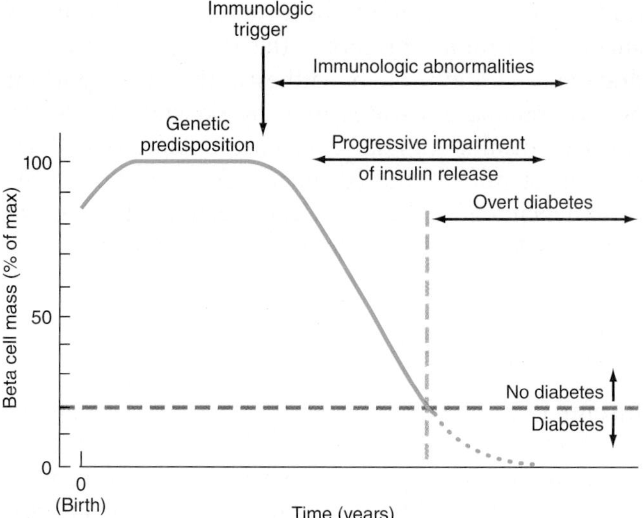

FIGURE 23-6

Temporal model for development of type 1 diabetes. Individuals with a genetic predisposition are exposed to a trigger that initiates an autoimmune process, resulting in a gradual decline in beta cell mass. The downward slope of the beta cell mass varies among individuals and may not be continuous. This progressive impairment in insulin release results in diabetes when ~80% of the beta cell mass is destroyed. A "honeymoon" phase may be seen in the first 1 or 2 years after the onset of diabetes and is associated with reduced insulin requirements. *(Adapted from ER Kaufman: Medical Management of Type 1 Diabetes, 6th ed. American Diabetes Association, Alexandria, VA, 2012.)*

GENETIC CONSIDERATIONS

Susceptibility to type 1 DM involves multiple genes. The concordance of type 1 DM in identical twins ranges between 40 and 60%, indicating that additional modifying factors are likely involved in determining whether diabetes develops. The major susceptibility gene for type 1 DM is located in the HLA region on chromosome 6. Polymorphisms in the HLA complex account for 40–50% of the genetic risk of developing type 1 DM. This region contains genes that encode the class II major histocompatibility complex (MHC) molecules, which present antigen to helper T cells and thus are involved in initiating the immune response. The ability of class II MHC molecules to present antigen is dependent on the amino acid composition of their antigen-binding sites. Amino acid substitutions may influence the specificity of the immune response by altering the binding affinity of different antigens for class II molecules.

Most individuals with type 1 DM have the HLA DR3 and/or DR4 haplotype. Refinements in genotyping of HLA loci have shown that the haplotypes DQA1*0301, DQB1*0302, and DQB1*0201 are most strongly associated with type 1 DM. These haplotypes are present in 40% of children with type 1 DM as compared to 2% of the normal U.S. population. However, most individuals with predisposing haplotypes do not develop diabetes.

In addition to MHC class II associations, genome association studies have identified at least 20 different genetic loci that contribute susceptibility to type 1 DM (polymorphisms in the promoter region of the insulin gene, the CTLA-4 gene, interleukin 2 receptor, *CTLA4*, and PTPN22, etc.). Genes that confer protection against the development of the disease also exist. The haplotype DQA1*0102, DQB1*0602 is extremely rare in individuals with type 1 DM (<1%) and appears to provide protection from type 1 DM.

Although the risk of developing type 1 DM is increased tenfold in relatives of individuals with the disease, the risk is relatively low: 3–4% if the parent has type 1 DM and 5–15% in a sibling (depending on which HLA haplotypes are shared). Hence, most individuals with type 1 DM do not have a first-degree relative with this disorder.

Pathophysiology

Although other islet cell types (alpha cells [glucagon-producing], delta cells [somatostatin-producing], or PP cells [pancreatic polypeptide-producing]) are functionally and embryologically similar to beta cells and express most of the same proteins as beta cells, they are spared from the autoimmune destruction. Pathologically, the pancreatic islets have a modest infiltration of lymphocytes (a process termed *insulitis*). After beta cells are destroyed, it is thought that the inflammatory process abates and the islets become atrophic. Studies of the autoimmune process in humans and in animal models of type 1 DM (NOD mouse and BB rat) have identified the following abnormalities in the humoral and cellular arms of the immune system: (1) islet cell autoantibodies; (2) activated lymphocytes in the islets, peripancreatic lymph nodes, and systemic circulation; (3) T lymphocytes that proliferate when stimulated with islet proteins; and (4) release of cytokines within the insulitis. Beta cells seem to be particularly susceptible to the toxic effect of some cytokines (tumor necrosis factor α [TNF-α], interferon γ, and interleukin 1 [IL-1]). The precise mechanisms of beta cell death are not known but may involve formation of nitric oxide metabolites, apoptosis, and direct CD8+ T cell cytotoxicity. The islet destruction is mediated by T lymphocytes rather than islet autoantibodies, as these antibodies do not generally react with the cell surface of islet cells and are not capable of transferring DM to animals. Efforts to suppress the autoimmune process at the time of diagnosis of diabetes have largely been ineffective or only temporarily effective in slowing beta cell destruction.

Pancreatic islet molecules targeted by the autoimmune process include insulin, glutamic acid decarboxylase (GAD; the biosynthetic enzyme for the neurotransmitter GABA), ICA-512/IA-2 (homology with tyrosine phosphatases), and a beta cell–specific zinc transporter (ZnT-8). Most of the autoantigens are not beta cell–specific, which raises the question of how the beta cells are selectively destroyed. Current theories favor initiation of an autoimmune process directed at one beta cell molecule, which then spreads to other islet molecules as the immune process destroys beta cells and creates a series of secondary autoantigens. The beta cells of individuals who develop type 1 DM do not differ from beta cells of normal individuals because islets transplanted from a genetically identical twin are destroyed by a recurrence of the autoimmune process of type 1 DM.

Immunologic markers

Islet cell autoantibodies (ICAs) are a composite of several different antibodies directed at pancreatic islet molecules such as GAD, insulin, IA-2/ICA-512, and ZnT-8, and serve as a marker of the autoimmune process of type 1 DM. Assays for autoantibodies to GAD-65 are commercially available. Testing for ICAs can be useful in classifying the type of DM as type 1 and in identifying nondiabetic individuals at risk for developing type 1 DM. ICAs are present in the majority of individuals (>85%) diagnosed with new-onset type 1 DM, in a significant minority of individuals with newly diagnosed type 2 DM (5–10%), and occasionally in individuals with GDM (<5%). ICAs are present in 3–4% of first-degree relatives of individuals with type 1 DM. In combination with impaired insulin secretion after IV glucose tolerance testing, they predict a >50% risk of developing type 1 DM within 5 years. At present, the measurement of ICAs in nondiabetic individuals is a research tool because no treatments have been demonstrated to prevent the occurrence or progression to type 1 DM.

Environmental factors

Numerous environmental events have been proposed to trigger the autoimmune process in genetically susceptible individuals; however, none have been conclusively linked to diabetes. Identification of an environmental trigger has been difficult because the event may precede the onset of DM by several years (Fig. 23-6). Putative environmental triggers include viruses (coxsackie, rubella, enteroviruses most prominently), bovine milk proteins, and nitrosourea compounds. There is increasing interest in the microbiome and type 1 diabetes.

Prevention of type 1 DM

A number of interventions have prevented diabetes in animal models. None of these interventions have been successful in preventing type 1 DM in humans. For example, the Diabetes Prevention Trial–Type 1 concluded that administering insulin (IV or PO) to individuals at high risk for developing type 1 DM did not prevent type 1 DM. This is an area of active clinical investigation.

TYPE 2 DM

Insulin resistance and abnormal insulin secretion are central to the development of type 2 DM. Although the primary defect is controversial, most studies support the view that insulin resistance precedes an insulin secretory defect but that diabetes develops only when insulin secretion becomes inadequate. Type 2 DM likely encompasses a range of disorders with common phenotype of hyperglycemia. Most of our current understanding (and the discussion below) of the pathophysiology and genetics is based on studies of individuals of European descent. It is becoming increasing apparent that DM in other ethnic groups (Asian, African, and Latin American) has a somewhat different, but yet undefined, pathophysiology. In general, Latinos have greater insulin resistance and East Asians and South Asians have more beta cell dysfunction, but both defects are present in both populations. East and South Asians appear to develop type 2 DM at a younger age and a lower BMI. In some groups, DM that is ketosis prone (often obese) or ketosis-resistant (often lean) is seen.

GENETIC CONSIDERATIONS

Type 2 DM has a strong genetic component. The concordance of type 2 DM in identical twins is between 70 and 90%. Individuals with a parent with type 2 DM have an increased risk of diabetes; if both parents have type 2 DM, the risk approaches 40%. Insulin resistance, as demonstrated by reduced glucose utilization in skeletal muscle, is present in many nondiabetic, first-degree relatives of individuals with type 2 DM. The disease is polygenic and multifactorial, because in addition to genetic susceptibility, environmental factors (such as obesity, nutrition, and physical activity) modulate the phenotype. The in utero environment also contributes, and either increased or reduced birth weight increases the risk of type 2 DM in adult life. The genes that predispose to type 2 DM are incompletely identified, but recent genome-wide association studies have identified a large number of genes that convey a relatively small risk for type 2 DM (>70 genes, each with a relative risk of 1.06–1.5). Most prominent is a variant of the transcription factor 7–like 2 gene that has been associated with type 2 DM in several populations and with IGT in one population at high risk for diabetes. Genetic polymorphisms associated with type 2 DM have also been found in the genes encoding the peroxisome proliferator–activated receptor γ, inward rectifying potassium channel, zinc transporter, IRS, and calpain 10. The mechanisms by which these genetic loci increase the susceptibility to type 2 DM are not clear, but most are predicted to alter islet function or development or insulin secretion. Although the genetic susceptibility to type 2 DM is under active investigation (it is estimated that <10% of genetic risk is determined by loci identified thus far), it is currently not possible to use a combination of known genetic loci to predict type 2 DM.

Pathophysiology

Type 2 DM is characterized by impaired insulin secretion, insulin resistance, excessive hepatic glucose production, and abnormal fat metabolism. Obesity, particularly visceral or central (as evidenced by the hip-waist ratio), is very common in type 2 DM (≥80% of patients are obese). In the early stages of the disorder, glucose tolerance remains near-normal, despite insulin resistance, because the pancreatic beta cells compensate by increasing insulin output (Fig. 23-7). As insulin resistance and compensatory hyperinsulinemia progress, the pancreatic islets in certain individuals are unable to sustain the hyperinsulinemic state. IGT, characterized by elevations in postprandial glucose, then develops. A further decline in insulin secretion and an increase in hepatic glucose production lead to overt diabetes with fasting hyperglycemia. Ultimately, beta cell failure ensues. Although both insulin resistance and impaired insulin secretion contribute to the pathogenesis of type 2 DM, the relative contribution of each varies from individual to individual.

Metabolic Abnormalities

Abnormal muscle and fat metabolism

Insulin resistance, the decreased ability of insulin to act effectively on target tissues (especially muscle, liver, and fat), is a prominent feature of type 2 DM and results

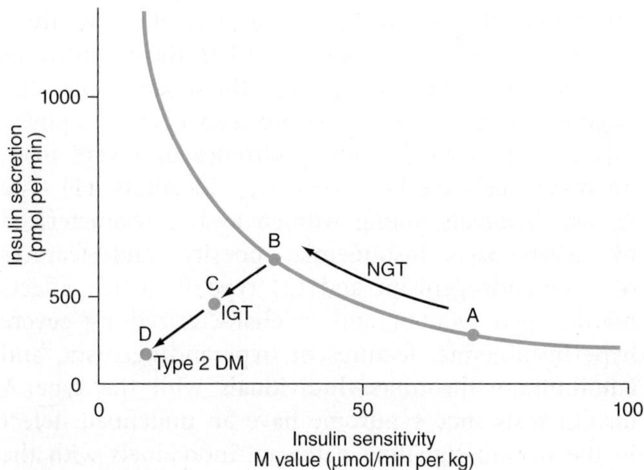

FIGURE 23-7

Metabolic changes during the development of type 2 diabetes mellitus (DM). Insulin secretion and insulin sensitivity are related, and as an individual becomes more insulin resistant (by moving from point A to point B), insulin secretion increases. A failure to compensate by increasing the insulin secretion results initially in impaired glucose tolerance (IGT; point C) and ultimately in type 2 DM (point D). NGT, normal glucose tolerance. *(Adapted from SE Kahn: J Clin Endocrinol Metab 86:4047, 2001; RN Bergman, M Ader: Trends Endocrinol Metab 11:351, 2000.)*

from a combination of genetic susceptibility and obesity. Insulin resistance is relative, however, because supranormal levels of circulating insulin will normalize the plasma glucose. Insulin dose-response curves exhibit a rightward shift, indicating reduced sensitivity, and a reduced maximal response, indicating an overall decrease in maximum glucose utilization (30–60% lower than in normal individuals). Insulin resistance impairs glucose utilization by insulin-sensitive tissues and increases hepatic glucose output; both effects contribute to the hyperglycemia. Increased hepatic glucose output predominantly accounts for increased FPG levels, whereas decreased peripheral glucose usage results in postprandial hyperglycemia. In skeletal muscle, there is a greater impairment in nonoxidative glucose usage (glycogen formation) than in oxidative glucose metabolism through glycolysis. Glucose metabolism in insulin-independent tissues is not altered in type 2 DM.

The precise molecular mechanism leading to insulin resistance in type 2 DM has not been elucidated. Insulin receptor levels and tyrosine kinase activity in skeletal muscle are reduced, but these alterations are most likely secondary to hyperinsulinemia and are not a primary defect. Therefore, "postreceptor" defects in insulin-regulated phosphorylation/dephosphorylation appear to play the predominant role in insulin resistance. Abnormalities include the accumulation of lipid within skeletal myocytes, which may impair mitochondrial oxidative phosphorylation and reduce insulin-stimulated mitochondrial ATP production. Impaired fatty acid oxidation and lipid accumulation within skeletal myocytes also may generate reactive oxygen species such as lipid peroxides. Of note, not all insulin signal transduction pathways are resistant to the effects of insulin (e.g., those controlling cell growth and differentiation using the mitogenic-activated protein kinase pathway). Consequently, hyperinsulinemia may increase the insulin action through these pathways, potentially accelerating diabetes-related conditions such as atherosclerosis.

The obesity accompanying type 2 DM, particularly in a central or visceral location, is thought to be part of the pathogenic process **(Chap. 20)**. In addition to these white fat depots, humans now are recognized to have brown fat, which has much greater thermogenic capacity. Efforts are under way to increase the activity or quantity of brown fat (e.g., a myokine, irisin, may convert white to brown fat). The increased adipocyte mass leads to increased levels of circulating free fatty acids and other fat cell products. For example, adipocytes secrete a number of biologic products (nonesterified free fatty acids, retinol-binding protein 4, leptin, TNF-α, resistin, IL-6, and adiponectin). In addition to regulating body weight, appetite, and energy expenditure, adipokines also modulate insulin sensitivity. The increased production of free fatty acids and some adipokines may cause insulin resistance in skeletal muscle and liver. For example, free fatty acids impair glucose utilization in skeletal muscle, promote glucose production by the liver, and impair beta cell function. In contrast, the production by adipocytes of adiponectin, an insulin-sensitizing peptide, is reduced in obesity, and this may contribute to hepatic insulin resistance. Adipocyte products and adipokines also produce an inflammatory state and may explain why markers of inflammation such as IL-6 and C-reactive protein are often elevated in type 2 DM. In addition, inflammatory cells have been found infiltrating adipose tissue. Inhibition of inflammatory signaling pathways such as the nuclear factor-κB (NF-κB) pathway appears to reduce insulin resistance and improve hyperglycemia in animal models and is being tested in humans.

Impaired insulin secretion

Insulin secretion and sensitivity are interrelated (Fig. 23-7). In type 2 DM, insulin secretion initially increases in response to insulin resistance to maintain normal glucose tolerance. Initially, the insulin secretory defect is mild and selectively involves glucose-stimulated insulin secretion, including a greatly reduced first secretory phase. The response to other nonglucose secretagogues, such as arginine, is preserved, but overall beta function is reduced by as much as 50% at the onset of type 2 DM. Abnormalities in proinsulin processing are reflected by increased secretion of proinsulin in type 2 DM. Eventually, the insulin secretory defect is progressive.

The reason(s) for the decline in insulin secretory capacity in type 2 DM is unclear. The assumption is that a second genetic defect—superimposed upon insulin resistance—leads to beta cell failure. Beta cell mass is decreased by approximately 50% in individuals with long-standing type 2 DM. Islet amyloid polypeptide or amylin, co-secreted by the beta cell, forms the amyloid fibrillar deposit found in the islets of individuals with long-standing type 2 DM. Whether such islet amyloid deposits are a primary or secondary event is not known. The metabolic environment of diabetes may also negatively impact islet function. For example, chronic hyperglycemia paradoxically impairs islet function ("glucose toxicity") and leads to a worsening of hyperglycemia. Improvement in glycemic control is often associated with improved islet function. In addition, elevation of free fatty acid levels ("lipotoxicity") and dietary fat may also worsen islet function. Reduced GLP-1 action may contribute to the reduced insulin secretion.

Increased hepatic glucose and lipid production

In type 2 DM, insulin resistance in the liver reflects the failure of hyperinsulinemia to suppress gluconeogenesis, which results in fasting hyperglycemia and decreased glycogen storage by the liver in the postprandial state. Increased hepatic glucose production occurs early in the course of diabetes, although likely after the onset of insulin secretory abnormalities and insulin resistance in skeletal muscle. As a result of insulin resistance in adipose tissue, lipolysis and free fatty acid flux from adipocytes are increased, leading to increased lipid (very-low-density lipoprotein [VLDL] and triglyceride) synthesis in hepatocytes. This lipid storage or steatosis in the liver may lead to nonalcoholic fatty liver disease and abnormal liver function tests. This is also responsible for the dyslipidemia found in type 2 DM (elevated triglycerides, reduced high-density lipoprotein [HDL], and increased small dense low-density lipoprotein [LDL] particles).

Insulin resistance syndromes

The insulin resistance condition comprises a spectrum of disorders, with hyperglycemia representing one of the most readily diagnosed features. The *metabolic syndrome*, the *insulin resistance syndrome*, and *syndrome X* are terms used to describe a constellation of metabolic derangements that includes insulin resistance, hypertension, dyslipidemia (decreased HDL and elevated triglycerides), central or visceral obesity, type 2 DM or IGT/IFG, and accelerated cardiovascular disease. This syndrome is discussed in **Chap. 22**.

A number of relatively rare forms of severe insulin resistance include features of type 2 DM or IGT (Table 23-1). Mutations in the insulin receptor that interfere with binding or signal transduction are a rare cause of insulin resistance. Acanthosis nigricans and signs of hyperandrogenism (hirsutism, acne, and oligomenorrhea in women) are also common physical features. Two distinct syndromes of severe insulin resistance have been described in adults: (1) type A, which affects young women and is characterized by severe hyperinsulinemia, obesity, and features of hyperandrogenism; and (2) type B, which affects middle-aged women and is characterized by severe hyperinsulinemia, features of hyperandrogenism, and autoimmune disorders. Individuals with the type A insulin resistance syndrome have an undefined defect in the insulin-signaling pathway; individuals with the type B insulin resistance syndrome have autoantibodies directed at the insulin receptor. These receptor autoantibodies may block insulin binding or may stimulate the insulin receptor, leading to intermittent hypoglycemia.

Polycystic ovary syndrome (PCOS) is a common disorder that affects premenopausal women and is characterized by chronic anovulation and hyperandrogenism **(Chap. 13)**. Insulin resistance is seen in a significant subset of women with PCOS, and the disorder substantially increases the risk for type 2 DM, independent of the effects of obesity.

Prevention

Type 2 DM is preceded by a period of IGT or IFG, and a number of lifestyle modifications and pharmacologic agents prevent or delay the onset of DM. Individuals with prediabetes or increased risk of diabetes should be referred to a structured program to reduce body weight and increase physical activity as well as being screened for cardiovascular disease. The Diabetes Prevention Program (DPP) demonstrated that intensive changes in lifestyle (diet and exercise for 30 min/d five times/week) in individuals with IGT prevented or delayed the development of type 2 DM by 58% compared to placebo. This effect was seen in individuals regardless of age, sex, or ethnic group. In the same study, metformin prevented or delayed diabetes by 31% compared to placebo. The lifestyle intervention group lost 5–7% of their body weight during the 3 years of the study. Studies in Finnish and Chinese populations noted similar efficacy of diet and exercise in preventing or delaying type 2 DM. A number of agents, including α-glucosidase inhibitors, metformin, thiazolidinediones, GLP-1 receptor pathway modifiers, and orlistat, prevent or delay type 2 DM but are not approved for this purpose. Individuals with a strong family history of type 2 DM and individuals with IFG or IGT should be strongly encouraged to maintain a normal BMI and engage in regular physical activity. Pharmacologic therapy for individuals with prediabetes is currently controversial because its cost-effectiveness and safety profile are not known.

The ADA has suggested that metformin be considered in individuals with both IFG and IGT who are at very high risk for progression to diabetes (age <60 years, BMI ≥35 kg/m^2, family history of diabetes in first-degree relative, and women with a history of GDM). Individuals with IFG, IGT, or an HbA$_{1c}$ of 5.7–6.4% should be monitored annually to determine if diagnostic criteria for diabetes are present.

GENETICALLY DEFINED, MONOGENIC FORMS OF DIABETES MELLITUS RELATED TO REDUCED INSULIN SECRETION

Several monogenic forms of DM have been identified. More than 10 different variants of MODY, caused by mutations in genes encoding islet-enriched transcription factors or glucokinase (Fig. 23-5; Table 23-1), are transmitted as autosomal dominant disorders. MODY 1, MODY 3, and MODY 5 are caused by mutations in hepatocyte nuclear transcription factor (HNF) 4α, HNF-1α, and HNF-1β, respectively. As their names imply, these transcription factors are expressed in the liver but also in other tissues, including the pancreatic islets and kidney. These factors most likely affect islet development or the expression of genes important in glucose-stimulated insulin secretion or the maintenance of beta cell mass. For example, individuals with an HNF-1α mutation (MODY 3) have a progressive decline in glycemic control but may respond to sulfonylureas. In fact, some of these patients were initially thought to have type 1 DM but were later shown to respond to a sulfonylurea, and insulin was discontinued. Individuals with a HNF-1β mutation have progressive impairment of insulin secretion and hepatic insulin resistance, and require insulin treatment (minimal response to sulfonylureas). These individuals often have other abnormalities such as renal cysts, mild pancreatic exocrine insufficiency, and abnormal liver function tests. Individuals with MODY 2, the result of mutations in the glucokinase gene, have mild-to-moderate, stable hyperglycemia that does not respond to oral hypoglycemic agents. Glucokinase catalyzes the formation of glucose-6-phosphate from glucose, a reaction that is important for glucose sensing by the beta cells (**Fig. 23-5**) and for glucose utilization by the liver. As a result of glucokinase mutations, higher glucose levels are required to elicit insulin secretory responses, thus altering the set point for insulin secretion. Studies of populations with type 2 DM suggest that mutations in MODY-associated genes are an uncommon (<5%) cause of type 2 DM. Mutations in mitochondrial DNA are associated with diabetes and deafness.

Transient or permanent neonatal diabetes (onset <12 months of age) occurs. Permanent neonatal diabetes may be caused by several genetic mutations, usually requires treatment with insulin, and phenotypically is similar to type 1 DM. Mutations in the ATP-sensitive potassium channel subunits (Kir6.2 and ABCC8) and the insulin gene (interfere with proinsulin folding and processing) (Fig. 23-5) are the major causes of permanent neonatal diabetes. Although these activating mutations in the ATP-sensitive potassium channel subunits impair glucose-stimulated insulin secretion, these individuals may respond to sulfonylureas and can be treated with these agents. These mutations are often associated with a spectrum of neurologic dysfunction. MODY 4 is a rare variant caused by mutations in the insulin promoter factor (IPF) 1, a transcription factor that regulates pancreatic development and insulin gene transcription. Homozygous inactivating mutations cause pancreatic agenesis, whereas heterozygous mutations may result in DM. Mutations in the transcription factor of *GATA6* are the most common cause of pancreatic agenesis. Homozygous glucokinase mutations cause a severe form of neonatal diabetes.

APPROACH TO THE PATIENT: Diabetes Mellitus

Once the diagnosis of DM is made, attention should be directed to symptoms related to diabetes (acute and chronic) and classifying the type of diabetes. DM and its complications produce a wide range of symptoms and signs; those secondary to acute hyperglycemia may occur at any stage of the disease, whereas those related to chronic hyperglycemia begin to appear during the second decade of hyperglycemia (**Chap. 25**). Individuals with previously undetected type 2 DM may present with chronic complications of DM at the time of diagnosis. The history and physical examination should assess for symptoms or signs of acute hyperglycemia and should screen for the chronic complications and conditions associated with DM.

HISTORY A complete medical history should be obtained with special emphasis on DM-relevant aspects such as weight, family history of DM and its complications, risk factors for cardiovascular disease, exercise, smoking, and ethanol use. Symptoms of hyperglycemia include polyuria, polydipsia, weight loss, fatigue, weakness, blurry vision, frequent superficial infections (vaginitis, fungal skin infections), and slow healing of skin lesions after minor trauma. Metabolic derangements relate mostly to hyperglycemia (osmotic diuresis) and to the catabolic state of the patient (urinary loss of glucose and calories, muscle breakdown due to protein degradation and decreased protein synthesis). Blurred vision results from changes in the water content of the lens and resolves as the hyperglycemia is controlled.

In a patient with established DM, the initial assessment should also include special emphasis on prior diabetes care, including the type of therapy, prior HbA_{1c} levels, self-monitoring blood glucose results, frequency of hypoglycemia, presence of DM-specific complications, and assessment of the patient's knowledge about diabetes, exercise, and nutrition. Diabetes-related complications may afflict several organ systems, and an individual patient may exhibit some, all, or none of the symptoms related to the complications of DM **(Chap. 25)**. In addition, the presence of DM-related comorbidities should be sought (cardiovascular disease, hypertension, dyslipidemia). Pregnancy plans should be ascertained in women of childbearing age.

PHYSICAL EXAMINATION In addition to a complete physical examination, special attention should be given to DM-relevant aspects such as weight or BMI, retinal examination, orthostatic blood pressure, foot examination, peripheral pulses, and insulin injection sites. Blood pressure >140/80 mmHg is considered hypertension in individuals with diabetes. Because periodontal disease is more frequent in DM, the teeth and gums should also be examined.

An annual foot examination should (1) assess blood flow, sensation (vibratory sensation [128-MHz tuning fork at the base of the great toe], the ability to sense touch with a monofilament [5.07, 10-g monofilament], pinprick sensation, testing for ankle reflexes, and vibration perception threshold using a biothesiometer), ankle reflexes, and nail care; (2) look for the presence of foot deformities such as hammer or claw toes and Charcot foot; and (3) identify sites of potential ulceration. The ADA recommends annual screening for distal symmetric neuropathy beginning with the initial diagnosis of diabetes and annual screening for autonomic neuropathy 5 years after diagnosis of type 1 DM and at the time of diagnosis of type 2 DM. This includes testing for loss of protective sensation (LOPS) using monofilament testing plus one of the following tests: vibration, pinprick, ankle reflexes, or vibration perception threshold (using a biothesiometer). If the monofilament test or one of the other tests is abnormal, the patient is diagnosed with LOPS and counseled accordingly **(Chap. 25)**.

CLASSIFICATION OF DM IN AN INDIVIDUAL PATIENT The etiology of diabetes in an individual with new-onset disease can usually be assigned on the basis of clinical criteria. Individuals with type 1 DM tend to have the following characteristics: (1) onset of disease prior to age 30 years; (2) lean body habitus; (3) requirement of insulin as the initial therapy; (4) propensity to develop ketoacidosis; and (5) an increased risk of other autoimmune disorders such as autoimmune thyroid disease, adrenal insufficiency, pernicious anemia, celiac disease, and vitiligo. In contrast, individuals with type 2 DM often exhibit the following features: (1) develop diabetes after the age of 30 years; (2) are usually obese (80% are obese, but elderly individuals may be lean); (3) may not require insulin therapy initially; and (4) may have associated conditions such as insulin resistance, hypertension, cardiovascular disease, dyslipidemia, or PCOS. In type 2 DM, insulin resistance is often associated with abdominal obesity (as opposed to hip and thigh obesity) and hypertriglyceridemia. Although most individuals diagnosed with type 2 DM are older, the age of diagnosis is declining, and there is a marked increase among overweight children and adolescents. Some individuals with phenotypic type 2 DM present with diabetic ketoacidosis but lack autoimmune markers and may be later treated with oral glucose-lowering agents rather than insulin (this clinical picture is sometimes referred to as *ketosis-prone type 2 DM*). On the other hand, some individuals (5–10%) with the phenotypic appearance of type 2 DM do not have absolute insulin deficiency but have autoimmune markers (GAD and other ICA autoantibodies) suggestive of type 1 DM (termed *latent autoimmune diabetes of the adult*). Such individuals are more likely to be <50 years of age, thinner, and have a personal or family history of other autoimmune disease than individuals with type 2 DM. They are much more likely to require insulin treatment within 5 years. Monogenic forms of diabetes (discussed above) should be considered in those with diabetes onset at <30 years of age, an autosomal pattern of diabetes inheritance, and the lack of nearly complete insulin deficiency. Despite recent advances in the understanding of the pathogenesis of diabetes, it remains difficult to categorize some patients unequivocally. Individuals who deviate from the clinical profile of type 1 and type 2 DM, or who have other associated defects such as deafness, pancreatic exocrine disease, and other endocrine disorders, should be classified accordingly (Table 23-1).

LABORATORY ASSESSMENT The laboratory assessment should first determine whether the patient meets the diagnostic criteria for DM (Table 23-2) and then assess the degree of glycemic control **(Chap. 24)**. In addition to the standard laboratory evaluation, the patient should be screened for DM-associated conditions (e.g., albuminuria, dyslipidemia, thyroid dysfunction).

The classification of the type of DM may be facilitated by laboratory assessments. Serum insulin or C-peptide measurements often do not distinguish type 1 from type 2 DM, but a low C-peptide level confirms a patient's need for insulin. Many individuals with new-onset type 1 DM retain some C-peptide production. Measurement of islet cell antibodies at the time of diabetes onset may be useful if the type of DM is not clear based on the characteristics described above.

CHAPTER 24

DIABETES MELLITUS: MANAGEMENT AND THERAPIES

Alvin C. Powers

OVERALL GOALS

The goals of therapy for type 1 or type 2 diabetes mellitus (DM) are to (1) eliminate symptoms related to hyperglycemia, (2) reduce or eliminate the long-term microvascular and macrovascular complications of DM **(Chap. 25)**, and (3) allow the patient to achieve as normal a lifestyle as possible. To reach these goals, the physician should identify a target level of glycemic control for each patient, provide the patient with the educational and pharmacologic resources necessary to reach this level, and monitor/treat DM-related complications. Symptoms of diabetes usually resolve when the plasma glucose is <11.1 mmol/L (200 mg/dL), and thus most DM treatment focuses on achieving the second and third goals. This chapter first reviews the ongoing treatment of diabetes in the outpatient setting and then discusses the treatment of severe hyperglycemia, as well as the treatment of diabetes in hospitalized patients.

The care of an individual with either type 1 or type 2 DM requires a multidisciplinary team. Central to the success of this team are the patient's participation, input, and enthusiasm, all of which are essential for optimal diabetes management. Members of the health care team include the primary care provider and/or the endocrinologist or diabetologist, a certified diabetes educator, a nutritionist, and a psychologist. In addition, when the complications of DM arise, subspecialists (including neurologists, nephrologists, vascular surgeons, cardiologists, ophthalmologists, and podiatrists) with experience in DM-related complications are essential.

ONGOING ASPECTS OF COMPREHENSIVE DIABETES CARE

A number of names are sometimes applied to different approaches to diabetes care, such as intensive insulin therapy, intensive glycemic control, and "tight control." The current chapter, and other sources, uses the term *comprehensive diabetes care* to emphasize the fact that optimal diabetes therapy involves more than plasma glucose management and medications. Although glycemic control is central to optimal diabetes therapy, comprehensive diabetes care of both type 1 and type 2 DM should also detect and manage DM-specific complications **(Chap. 25)** and modify risk factors for DM-associated diseases. The key elements of comprehensive diabetes care are summarized in Table 24-1. In addition to the physical aspects of DM, social, family, financial, cultural, and employment-related issues may impact diabetes care. The International Diabetes Federation (IDF), recognizing that resources available for diabetes care vary widely throughout the world, has issued guidelines for "recommended care" (a well-developed service base and with health care funding systems consuming a significant part of their national wealth), "limited care" (health care settings with very limited resources), and "comprehensive care" (health care settings with considerable resources). This chapter provides guidance for this comprehensive level of diabetes care. The treatment goals for patients with diabetes are summarized in Table 24-2 and should be individualized.

DETECTION AND PREVENTION OF COMPLICATIONS RELATED TO DIABETES

The morbidity and mortality rates of DM-related complications **(Chap. 25)** can be greatly reduced by timely and consistent surveillance procedures (Table 24-1). These screening procedures are indicated for all individuals with DM, but many individuals with diabetes do not receive comprehensive diabetes care. A comprehensive eye examination should be performed by

TABLE 24-1

GUIDELINES FOR ONGOING, COMPREHENSIVE MEDICAL CARE FOR PATIENTS WITH DIABETES

- Optimal and individualized glycemic control
- Self-monitoring of blood glucose (individualized frequency)
- HbA_{1c} testing (2–4 times/year)
- Patient education in diabetes management (annual); diabetes-self management education and support
- Medical nutrition therapy and education (annual)
- Eye examination (annual or biannual; **Chap. 25**)
- Foot examination (1–2 times/year by physician; daily by patient; **Chap. 25**)
- Screening for diabetic nephropathy (annual; **Chap. 25**)
- Blood pressure measurement (quarterly)
- Lipid profile and serum creatinine (estimate GFR) (annual; **Chap. 25**)
- Influenza/pneumococcal/hepatitis B immunizations
- Consider antiplatelet therapy **(Chap. 25)**

Abbreviations: GFR, glomerular filtration rate; HbA_{1c}, hemoglobin A_{1c}.

a qualified optometrist or ophthalmologist. Because many individuals with type 2 DM have had asymptomatic diabetes for several years before diagnosis, the American Diabetes Association (ADA) recommends the following ophthalmologic examination schedule: (1) individuals with type 1 DM should have an initial eye examination within 5 years of diagnosis, (2) individuals with type 2 DM should have an initial eye examination at the time of diabetes diagnosis, (3) women with DM who are pregnant or contemplating pregnancy should have an eye examination prior to conception and during the first trimester, and (4) if eye exam is normal, repeat examination in 2–3 years is appropriate.

TABLE 24-2

TREATMENT GOALS FOR ADULTS WITH DIABETES[a]

INDEX	GOAL
Glycemic control[b]	
HbA_{1c}	<7.0%[c]
Preprandial capillary plasma glucose	4.4–7.2 mmol/L (80–130 mg/dL)
Peak postprandial capillary plasma glucose[d]	<10.0 mmol/L (<180 mg/dL)
Blood pressure	<140/90 mmHg[e]
Lipids[f]	
Low-density lipoprotein	<2.6 mmol/L (100 mg/dL)[g]
High-density lipoprotein	>1 mmol/L (40 mg/dL) in men
	>1.3 mmol/L (50 mg/dL) in women
Triglycerides	<1.7 mmol/L (150 mg/dL)

[a]As recommended by the American Diabetes Association; goals should be individualized for each patient (see text). Goals may be different for certain patient populations. [b]HbA_{1c} is primary goal. [c]Diabetes Control and Complications Trial–based assay. [d]1–2 h after beginning of a meal. [e]Goal of <130/80 mmHg may be appropriate for younger individuals [f]In decreasing order of priority. Recent guidelines from the American College of Cardiology and American Heart Association no longer advocate specific LDL and HDL goals **(see Chap. 25)**. [g]Goal of <1.8 mmol/L (70 mg/dL) may be appropriate for individuals with cardiovascular disease.

Abbreviation: HbA_{1c}, hemoglobin A_{1c}.

Source: Adapted from American Diabetes Association: Diabetes Care 38(Suppl 1):S1, 2015.

PATIENT EDUCATION ABOUT DM, NUTRITION, AND EXERCISE

The patient with type 1 or type 2 DM should receive education about nutrition, exercise, care of diabetes during illness, and medications to lower the plasma glucose. Along with improved compliance, patient education allows individuals with DM to assume greater responsibility for their care. Patient education should be viewed as a continuing process with regular visits for reinforcement; it should not be a process that is completed after one or two visits to a nurse educator or nutritionist. The ADA refers to education about the individualized management plan for the patient as diabetes self-management education (DSME) and diabetes self-management support (DSMS). DSME and DSMS are ways to improve the patient's knowledge, skills, and abilities necessary for diabetes self-care and should also emphasize psychosocial issues and emotional wellbeing. More frequent contact between the patient and the diabetes management team (e.g., electronic, telephone) improves glycemic control.

Diabetes education

The diabetes educator is a health care professional (nurse, dietician, or pharmacist) with specialized patient education skills who is certified in diabetes education (e.g., American Association of Diabetes Educators). Education topics important for optimal diabetes care include self-monitoring of blood glucose; urine ketone monitoring (type 1 DM); insulin administration; guidelines for diabetes management during illnesses; prevention and management of hypoglycemia **(Chap. 26)**; foot and skin care; diabetes management before, during, and after exercise; and risk factor–modifying activities.

Psychosocial aspects

Because the individual with DM can face challenges that affect many aspects of daily life, psychosocial assessment and treatment are a critical part of providing comprehensive diabetes care. The individual with DM must accept that he or she may develop complications related to DM. Even with considerable effort, normoglycemia can be an elusive goal, and solutions to worsening glycemic control may not be easily identifiable. The patient should view him- or herself as an essential member of the diabetes care team and not as someone who is cared for by the diabetes management team. Emotional stress may provoke a change in behavior so that individuals no longer adhere to a dietary, exercise, or therapeutic regimen. This can lead to the appearance of either hyper- or hypoglycemia. Eating disorders, including binge eating disorders, bulimia, and anorexia nervosa, appear to occur more frequently in individuals with type 1 or type 2 DM.

Nutrition

Medical nutrition therapy (MNT) is a term used by the ADA to describe the optimal coordination of caloric intake with other aspects of diabetes therapy (insulin, exercise, weight loss). Primary prevention measures of MNT are directed at preventing or delaying the onset of type 2 DM in high-risk individuals (obese or with prediabetes) by promoting weight reduction. Medical treatment of obesity is a rapidly evolving area and is discussed in **Chap. 21**. Secondary prevention measures of MNT are directed at preventing or delaying diabetes-related complications in diabetic individuals by improving glycemic control. Tertiary prevention measures of MNT are directed at managing diabetes-related complications (cardiovascular disease, nephropathy) in diabetic individuals. MNT in patients with diabetes and cardiovascular disease should incorporate dietary principles used in nondiabetic patients with cardiovascular disease. Although the recommendations for all three types of MNT overlap, this chapter emphasizes secondary prevention measures of MNT. Pharmacologic approaches that facilitate weight loss and bariatric surgery should be considered in selected patients **(Chaps. 20 and 21)**.

In general, the components of optimal MNT are similar for individuals with type 1 or type 2 DM and similar to those for the general population (fruits, vegetables, fiber-containing foods, and low fat; Table 24-3). MNT education is an important component of comprehensive diabetes care and should be reinforced by regular patient education. Historically, nutrition education imposed restrictive, complicated regimens on the patient. Current practices have greatly changed, although many patients and health care providers still view the diabetic diet as monolithic and static. For example, MNT now includes foods with sucrose and seeks to modify other risk factors such as hyperlipidemia and hypertension rather than focusing exclusively on weight loss in individuals with type 2 DM. The *glycemic index* is an estimate of the postprandial rise in the blood glucose when a certain amount of that food is consumed. Consumption of foods with a low glycemic index appears to reduce postprandial glucose excursions and improve glycemic control. Reduced-calorie and nonnutritive sweeteners are useful. Currently, evidence does not support supplementation of the diet with vitamins, antioxidants (vitamin C and E), or micronutrients (chromium) in patients with diabetes.

TABLE 24-3

NUTRITIONAL RECOMMENDATIONS FOR ADULTS WITH DIABETES OR PREDIABETES[a]

Weight loss diet (in prediabetes and type 2 DM)
- Hypocaloric diet that is low-carbohydrate

Fat in diet (optimal % of diet is not known; should be individualized)
- Minimal *trans* fat consumption
- Mediterranean-style diet rich in monounsaturated fatty acids may be better

Carbohydrate in diet (optimal % of diet is not known; should be individualized)
- Monitor carbohydrate intake in regard to calories
- Sucrose-containing foods may be consumed with adjustments in insulin dose, but minimize intake
- Amount of carbohydrate determined by estimating grams of carbohydrate in diet (type 1 DM)
- Use glycemic index to predict how consumption of a particular food may affect blood glucose
- Fructose preferred over sucrose or starch

Protein in diet (optimal % of diet is not known; should be individualized)

Other components
- Dietary fiber, vegetable, fruits, whole grains, dairy products, and sodium intake as advised for general population
- Nonnutrient sweeteners
- Routine supplements of vitamins, antioxidants, or trace elements not advised

[a]See text for differences for patients with type 1 or type 2 diabetes.
Source: Adapted from American Diabetes Association: Diabetes Care 37(Suppl 1):S14, 2014.

The goal of MNT in the individual with type 1 DM is to coordinate and match the caloric intake, both temporally and quantitatively, with the appropriate amount of insulin. MNT in type 1 DM and self-monitoring of blood glucose must be integrated to define the optimal insulin regimen. The ADA encourages patients and providers to use carbohydrate counting or exchange systems to estimate the nutrient content of a meal or snack. Based on the patient's estimate of the carbohydrate content of a meal, an insulin-to-carbohydrate ratio determines the bolus insulin dose for a meal or snack. MNT must be flexible enough to allow for exercise, and the insulin regimen must allow for deviations in caloric intake. An important component of MNT in type 1 DM is to minimize the weight gain often associated with intensive diabetes management.

The goals of MNT in type 2 DM should focus on weight loss and address the greatly increased prevalence of cardiovascular risk factors (hypertension, dyslipidemia, obesity) and disease in this population. The majority of these individuals are obese, and weight loss is strongly encouraged and should remain an important goal. Hypocaloric diets and modest weight loss (5–7%) often result in rapid and dramatic glucose lowering in individuals with new-onset type 2 DM. Nevertheless, numerous studies document that long-term weight loss is uncommon. MNT for type 2 DM should emphasize modest caloric reduction (low-carbohydrate) and increased physical activity. Increased consumption of soluble, dietary fiber may improve glycemic control in individuals with type 2 DM. Weight loss and exercise improve insulin resistance.

Exercise

Exercise has multiple positive benefits including cardiovascular risk reduction, reduced blood pressure, maintenance of muscle mass, reduction in body fat, and weight loss. For individuals with type 1 or type 2 DM, exercise is also useful for lowering plasma glucose (during and following exercise) and increasing insulin sensitivity. In patients with diabetes, the ADA recommends 150 min/week (distributed over at least 3 days) of moderate aerobic physical activity with no gaps longer than 2 days. The exercise regimen should also include resistance training.

Despite its benefits, exercise presents challenges for individuals with DM because they lack the normal glucoregulatory mechanisms (normally, insulin falls and glucagon rises during exercise). Skeletal muscle is a major site for metabolic fuel consumption in the resting state, and the increased muscle activity during vigorous, aerobic exercise greatly increases fuel requirements. Individuals with type 1 DM are prone to either hyperglycemia or hypoglycemia during exercise, depending on the preexercise plasma glucose, the circulating insulin level, and the level of exercise-induced catecholamines. If the insulin level is too low, the rise in catecholamines may increase the plasma glucose excessively, promote ketone body formation, and possibly lead to ketoacidosis. Conversely, if the circulating insulin level is excessive, this relative hyperinsulinemia may reduce hepatic glucose production (decreased glycogenolysis, decreased gluconeogenesis) and increase glucose entry into muscle, leading to hypoglycemia.

To avoid exercise-related hyper- or hypoglycemia, individuals with type 1 DM should (1) monitor blood glucose before, during, and after exercise; (2) delay exercise if blood glucose is >14 mmol/L (250 mg/dL) and ketones are present; (3) if the blood glucose is <5.6 mmol/L (100 mg/dL), ingest carbohydrate before exercising; (4) monitor glucose during exercise and ingest carbohydrate to prevent hypoglycemia; (5) decrease insulin doses (based on previous experience) before exercise and inject insulin into a nonexercising area; and (6) learn individual glucose responses to different types of exercise and increase food intake for up to 24 h after exercise, depending on intensity and duration of exercise. In individuals with type 2 DM, exercise-related hypoglycemia is less common but can occur in individuals taking either insulin or insulin secretagogues.

Despite asymptomatic cardiovascular disease appearing at a younger age in both type 1 and type 2 DM, routine screening for coronary artery disease has not been shown to be effective and is not recommended **(Chap. 25)**. Untreated proliferative retinopathy is a relative contraindication to vigorous exercise, because this may lead to vitreous hemorrhage or retinal detachment.

MONITORING THE LEVEL OF GLYCEMIC CONTROL

Optimal monitoring of glycemic control involves plasma glucose measurements by the patient and an assessment of long-term control by the physician (measurement of hemoglobin A_{1c} [HbA_{1c}] and review of the patient's self-measurements of plasma glucose). These measurements are complementary: the patient's measurements provide a picture of short-term glycemic control, whereas the HbA_{1c} reflects average glycemic control over the previous 2–3 months.

Self-monitoring of blood glucose

Self-monitoring of blood glucose (SMBG) is the standard of care in diabetes management and allows the patient to monitor his or her blood glucose at any time. In SMBG, a small drop of blood and an easily detectable enzymatic reaction allow measurement of the capillary plasma glucose. Many glucose monitors can rapidly and accurately measure glucose (calibrated to provide plasma glucose value even though blood glucose is measured) in small amounts of blood (3–10 μL) obtained from the fingertip; alternative testing sites (e.g., forearm) are less reliable, especially when the blood glucose is changing rapidly (postprandially). A large number of blood glucose monitors are available, and the certified diabetes educator is critical in helping the patient select the optimal device and learn to use it properly. By combining glucose measurements with diet history, medication changes, and exercise history, the diabetes management team and patient can improve the treatment program.

The frequency of SMBG measurements must be individualized and adapted to address the goals of diabetes care. Individuals with type 1 DM or individuals with type 2 DM taking multiple insulin injections each day should routinely measure their plasma glucose three or more times per day to estimate and select mealtime boluses of short-acting insulin and to modify long-acting insulin doses. Most individuals with type 2 DM require less frequent monitoring, although the optimal frequency of SMBG has not been clearly defined. Individuals with type 2 DM who are taking insulin should use SMBG more frequently than those on oral agents. Individuals with type 2 DM who are on oral medications should use SMBG as a means of assessing the efficacy of their medication and the impact of diet. Because plasma glucose levels fluctuate less in these individuals, one to two SMBG measurements per day (or fewer in patients who are on oral agents or are diet-controlled) may be sufficient. Most measurements in individuals with type 1 or type 2 DM should be performed prior to a meal and supplemented with postprandial measurements to assist in reaching postprandial glucose targets (Table 24-2).

Devices for continuous glucose monitoring (CGM) have been approved by the U.S. Food and Drug Administration (FDA), and others are in various stages of development. These devices do not replace the need for traditional glucose measurements and require calibration with SMBG. This rapidly evolving technology requires substantial expertise on the part of the diabetes management team and the patient. Current CGM systems measure the glucose in interstitial fluid, which is in equilibrium with the blood glucose. These devices provide useful short-term information about the patterns of glucose changes as well as an enhanced ability to detect hypoglycemic episodes. Alarms notify the patient if the blood glucose falls into the hypoglycemic range. Clinical experience with these devices is rapidly growing, and they are most useful in individuals with hypoglycemia unawareness, individuals with frequent hypoglycemia, or those who have not achieved glycemic targets despite major efforts. The utility of CGM in the intensive care unit (ICU) setting remains to be determined.

Assessment of long-term glycemic control

Measurement of glycated hemoglobin (HbA1c) is the standard method for assessing long-term glycemic control. When plasma glucose is consistently elevated, there is an increase in nonenzymatic glycation of hemoglobin; this alteration reflects the glycemic history over the previous 2–3 months, because erythrocytes have an average life span of 120 days (glycemic level in the preceding month contributes about 50% to the HbA_{1c} value). Measurement of HbA_{1c} at the "point of care" allows for more rapid feedback and may therefore assist in adjustment of therapy.

HbA_{1c} should be measured in all individuals with DM during their initial evaluation and as part of their comprehensive diabetes care. As the primary predictor of long-term complications of DM, the HbA_{1c} should mirror, to a certain extent, the short-term measurements of SMBG. These two measurements are complementary in that recent intercurrent illnesses may impact the SMBG measurements but not the HbA_{1c}. Likewise, postprandial and nocturnal hyperglycemia may not be detected by the SMBG of fasting and preprandial capillary plasma glucose but will be reflected in the HbA_{1c}. In standardized assays, the HbA_{1c} approximates the following mean plasma glucose values: an HbA_{1c} of 6% = 7.0 mmol/L (126 mg/dL), 7% = 8.6 mmol/L (154 mg/dL), 8% = 10.2 mmol/L (183 mg/dL), 9% = 11.8 mmol/L (212 mg/dL), 10% = 13.4 mmol/L (240 mg/dL), 11% = 14.9 mmol/L (269 mg/dL), and 12% = 16.5 mmol/L (298 mg/dL). In patients achieving their glycemic goal, the ADA recommends measurement of the HbA_{1c} at least twice per year. More frequent testing (every 3 months) is warranted when glycemic control is inadequate or when therapy has changed. Laboratory standards for the HbA_{1c} test have been established and should be correlated to the reference assay of the Diabetes Control and Complications Trial (DCCT). Clinical conditions such hemoglobinopathies, anemias, reticulocytosis, transfusions, and uremia may interfere with the HbA_{1c} result. The degree of glycation of other proteins, such as albumin, can be used as an alternative indicator of glycemic control when the HbA_{1c} is inaccurate. The fructosamine assay (measuring glycated albumin) reflects the glycemic status over the prior 2 weeks.

PHARMACOLOGIC TREATMENT OF DIABETES

Comprehensive care of type 1 and type 2 DM requires an emphasis on nutrition, exercise, and monitoring of glycemic control but also usually involves glucose-lowering medication(s). This chapter discusses classes of such medications but does not describe every glucose-lowering agent available worldwide. The initial step is to select an individualized, glycemic goal for the patient.

ESTABLISHMENT OF TARGET LEVEL OF GLYCEMIC CONTROL

Because the complications of DM are related to glycemic control, normoglycemia or near-normoglycemia is the desired, but often elusive, goal for most patients. Normalization or near-normalization of the plasma glucose for long periods of time is extremely difficult, as demonstrated by the DCCT and United Kingdom Prospective Diabetes Study (UKPDS). Regardless of the level of hyperglycemia, improvement in glycemic control will lower the risk of diabetes-specific complications **(Chap. 25)**.

The target for glycemic control (as reflected by the HbA_{1c}) must be individualized, and the goals of therapy should be developed in consultation with the patient after considering a number of medical, social, and lifestyle issues. The ADA calls this a *patient-centered approach*, and other organizations such as the IDF and

American Association of Clinical Endocrinologists (AACE) also suggest an individualized glycemic goal. Important factors to consider include the patient's age and ability to understand and implement a complex treatment regimen, presence and severity of complications of diabetes, known cardiovascular disease (CVD), ability to recognize hypoglycemic symptoms, presence of other medical conditions or treatments that might affect survival or the response to therapy, lifestyle and occupation (e.g., possible consequences of experiencing hypoglycemia on the job), and level of support available from family and friends.

In general, the ADA suggests that the goal is to achieve an HbA_{1c} as close to normal as possible without significant hypoglycemia. In most individuals, the target HbA_{1c} should be <7% (Table 24-2) with a more stringent target for some patients. For instance, the HbA_{1c} goal in a young adult with type 1 DM may be 6.5%. A higher HbA_{1c} goal may be appropriate for the very young or old or in individuals with limited life span or comorbid conditions. For example, an appropriate HbA_{1c} goal in elderly individuals with multiple, chronic illnesses and impaired activities of daily living might be 8.0 or 8.5%. A major consideration is the frequency and severity of hypoglycemia, because this becomes more common with a more stringent HbA_{1c} goal.

More stringent glycemic control (HbA_{1c} of ≤6%) is not beneficial, and may be detrimental, in patients with type 2 DM and a high risk of CVD. Large clinical trials (UKPDS, Action to Control Cardiovascular Risk in Diabetes [ACCORD], Action in Diabetes and Vascular Disease: Preterax and Diamicron MR Controlled Evaluation [ADVANCE], Veterans Affairs Diabetes Trial [VADT]; **Chap. 25**) have examined glycemic control in type 2 DM in individuals with low risk of CVD, with high risk of CVD, or with established CVD and have found that more intense glycemic control is not beneficial and, in some patient populations, may have a negative impact on some outcomes. These divergent outcomes stress the need for individualized glycemic goals based on the following general guidelines: (1) early in the course of type 2 diabetes when the CVD risk is lower, improved glycemic control likely leads to improved cardiovascular outcome, but this benefit occurs more than a decade after the period of improved glycemic control; (2) intense glycemic control in individuals with established CVD or at high risk for CVD is not advantageous, and may be deleterious, over a follow-up of 3–5 years; an HbA_{1c} goal <7.0% is not appropriate in this population; (3) hypoglycemia in such high-risk populations (elderly, CVD) should be avoided; and (4) improved glycemic control reduces microvascular complications of diabetes **(Chap. 25)** even if it does not improve macrovascular complications like CVD.

TYPE 1 DIABETES MELLITUS

General aspects

The ADA recommendations for fasting and bedtime glycemic goals and HbA_{1c} targets are summarized in Table 24-2. The goal is to design and implement insulin regimens that mimic physiologic insulin secretion. Because individuals with type 1 DM partially or completely lack endogenous insulin production, administration of basal insulin is essential for regulating glycogen breakdown, gluconeogenesis, lipolysis, and ketogenesis. Likewise, insulin replacement for meals should be appropriate for the carbohydrate intake and promote normal glucose utilization and storage.

Intensive management

Intensive diabetes management has the goal of achieving euglycemia or near-normal glycemia. This approach requires multiple resources, including thorough and continuing patient education, comprehensive recording of plasma glucose measurements and nutrition intake by the patient, and a variable insulin regimen that matches glucose intake and insulin dose. Insulin regimens usually include multiple-component insulin regimens, multiple daily injections (MDIs), or insulin infusion devices (each discussed below).

The benefits of intensive diabetes management and improved glycemic control include a reduction in the microvascular complications of DM and a reduction in diabetes-related complications. From a psychological standpoint, the patient experiences greater control over his or her diabetes and often notes an improved sense of well-being, greater flexibility in the timing and content of meals, and the capability to alter insulin dosing with exercise. In addition, intensive diabetes management prior to and during pregnancy reduces the risk of fetal malformations and morbidity. Intensive diabetes management is encouraged in newly diagnosed patients with type 1 DM because it may prolong the period of C-peptide production, which may result in better glycemic control and a reduced risk of serious hypoglycemia. Although intensive management confers impressive benefits, it is also accompanied by significant personal and financial costs and is therefore not appropriate for all individuals.

Insulin preparations

Current insulin preparations are generated by recombinant DNA technology and consist of the amino acid sequence of human insulin or variations thereof. In the United States, most insulin is formulated as U-100 (100 units/mL). Regular insulin formulated as U-500 (500 units/mL) is available and sometimes useful in patients with severe insulin resistance. Human insulin

TABLE 24-4

PROPERTIES OF INSULIN PREPARATIONS[a]

PREPARATION	TIME OF ACTION		
	ONSET, H	**PEAK, H**	**EFFECTIVE DURATION, H**
Short-acting			
Aspart	<0.25	0.5–1.5	2–4
Glulisine	<0.25	0.5–1.5	2–4
Lispro	<0.25	0.5–1.5	2–4
Regular	0.5–1.0	2–3	3–6
Long-acting			
Detemir	1–4	—[b]	12-24[c]
Glargine	2–4	—[b]	20-24
NPH	2–4	4–10	10–16
Insulin combinations[d]			
75/25–75% protamine lispro, 25% lispro	<0.25	Dual[e]	10–16
70/30–70% protamine aspart, 30% aspart	<0.25	Dual[e]	15–18
50/50–50% protamine lispro, 50% lispro	<0.25	Dual[e]	10–16
70/30–70% NPH, 30% regular	0.5–1	Dual[e]	10–16

[a]Insulin preparations available in the United States; others are available in the United Kingdom and Europe.
[b]Glargine and detemir have minimal peak activity.
[c]Duration is dose-dependent (shorter at lower doses).
[d]Other insulin combinations are available
[e]Dual: two peaks—one at 2–3 h and the second one several hours later.
Source: Adapted from FR Kaufman: Medical Management of Type 1 Diabetes, 6th edition. Alexandria, VA: American Diabetes Association, 2012.

has been formulated with distinctive pharmacokinetics or genetically modified to more closely mimic physiologic insulin secretion. Insulins can be classified as short-acting or long-acting (Table 24-4). For example, one short-acting insulin formulation, insulin lispro, is an insulin analogue in which the 28th and 29th amino acids (lysine and proline) on the insulin B chain have been reversed by recombinant DNA technology. Insulin aspart and insulin glulisine are genetically modified insulin analogues with properties similar to lispro. All three of the insulin analogues have full biologic activity but less tendency for self-aggregation, resulting in more rapid absorption and onset of action and a shorter duration of action. These characteristics are particularly advantageous for allowing entrainment of insulin injection and action to rising plasma glucose levels following meals. The shorter duration of action also appears to be associated with a decreased number of hypoglycemic episodes, primarily because the decay of insulin action corresponds to the decline in plasma glucose after a meal. Thus, insulin aspart, lispro, or glulisine is preferred over regular insulin for prandial coverage. Insulin glargine is a long-acting biosynthetic human insulin that differs from normal insulin in that asparagine is replaced by glycine at amino acid 21, and two arginine residues are added to the C terminus of the B chain. Compared to neutral protamine Hagedorn (NPH) insulin, the onset of insulin glargine action is later, the duration of action is longer (~24 h), and there is a less pronounced peak. A lower incidence of hypoglycemia, especially at night, has been reported with insulin glargine when compared to NPH insulin. The most recent evidence does not support an association between glargine and increased cancer risk. Insulin detemir has a fatty acid side chain that prolongs its action by slowing absorption and catabolism. Twice-daily injections of glargine or detemir are sometimes required to provide 24-h coverage. Regular and NPH insulin have the native insulin amino acid sequence.

Basal insulin requirements are provided by long-acting (NPH insulin, insulin glargine, or insulin detemir) insulin formulations. These are usually prescribed with short-acting insulin in an attempt to mimic physiologic insulin release with meals. Although mixing of NPH and short-acting insulin formulations is common practice, this mixing may alter the insulin absorption profile (especially the short-acting insulins). For example, lispro absorption is delayed by mixing with NPH. The alteration in insulin absorption when the patient mixes different insulin formulations should not prevent mixing insulins. However, the following guidelines should be followed: (1) mix the different insulin formulations in the syringe immediately before injection (inject within 2 min after mixing); (2) do not store insulin as a mixture; (3) follow the same routine in terms of insulin mixing and administration to standardize the physiologic response to injected insulin; and (4) do not mix insulin glargine or detemir with other insulins. The miscibility of some insulins allows for the production of combination insulins that contain 70% NPH and 30% regular (70/30), or equal mixtures of NPH and regular (50/50). By including the insulin analogue mixed with protamine, several combinations have a short-acting and long-acting profile (Table 24-4). Although more convenient for the patient (only two injections/day), combination insulin formulations do not allow independent adjustment of short-acting and long-acting activity. Several insulin formulations are available as insulin "pens," which may be more convenient for some patients. Insulin delivery by inhalation has recently been approved but is not yet available. Other insulins, such as one with a duration of action of several days, are under development but are not currently available in the United States.

Insulin regimens

Representations of the various insulin regimens that may be used in type 1 DM are illustrated in Fig. 24-1. Although the insulin profiles are depicted as "smooth," symmetric curves, there is considerable patient-to-patient variation in the peak and duration. In all regimens, long-acting insulins (NPH, glargine, or detemir) supply basal insulin, whereas regular, insulin aspart, glulisine, or lispro insulin provides prandial insulin. Short-acting insulin analogues should be injected just before (<10 min) or just after a meal; regular insulin is given 30–45 min prior to a meal. Sometimes short-acting insulin analogues are injected just after a meal (gastroparesis, unpredictable food intake).

A shortcoming of current insulin regimens is that injected insulin immediately enters the systemic circulation, whereas endogenous insulin is secreted into the portal venous system. Thus, exogenous insulin administration exposes the liver to subphysiologic insulin levels. No insulin regimen reproduces the precise insulin secretory pattern of the pancreatic islet. However, the most physiologic regimens entail more frequent insulin injections, greater reliance on short-acting insulin, and more frequent capillary plasma glucose measurements. In general, individuals with type 1 DM require 0.5–1 U/kg per day of insulin divided into multiple doses, with ~50% of the insulin given as basal insulin.

Multiple-component insulin regimens refer to the combination of basal insulin and bolus insulin (preprandial short-acting insulin). The timing and dose of short-acting, preprandial insulin are altered to accommodate the SMBG results, anticipated food intake, and physical activity. Such regimens offer the patient with type 1 diabetes more flexibility in terms of lifestyle and the best chance for achieving near normoglycemia. One such regimen, shown in Fig. 24-1B, consists of basal insulin with glargine or detemir and preprandial lispro, glulisine, or insulin aspart. The insulin aspart, glulisine, or lispro dose is based on individualized algorithms that integrate the preprandial glucose and the anticipated carbohydrate intake. To determine the meal component of the preprandial insulin dose, the patient uses an

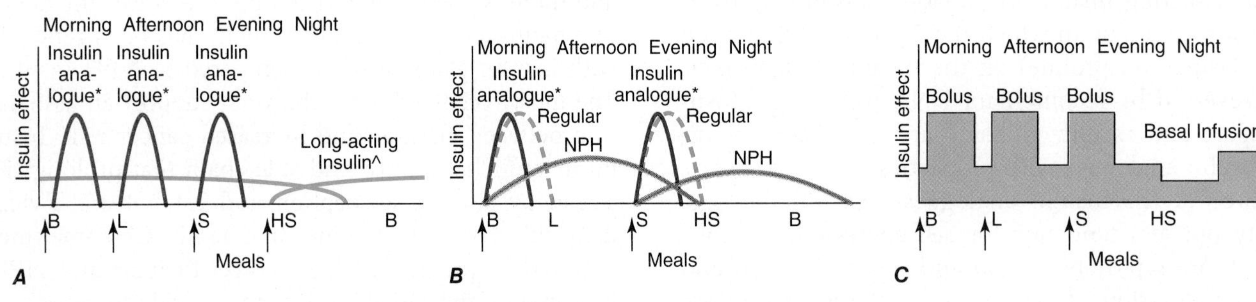

FIGURE 24-1

Representative insulin regimens for the treatment of diabetes. For each panel, the *y*-axis shows the amount of insulin effect and the *x*-axis shows the time of day. B, breakfast; HS, bedtime; L, lunch; S, supper. *Lispro, glulisine, or insulin aspart can be used. The time of insulin injection is shown with a *vertical arrow*. The type of insulin is noted above each insulin curve. ***A.*** Multiple-component insulin regimen consisting of long-acting insulin (^glargine or detemir) to provide basal insulin coverage and three shots of glulisine, lispro, or insulin aspart to provide glycemic coverage for each meal. ***B.*** Injection of two shots of long-acting insulin (NPH) and short-acting insulin analogue (glulisine, lispro, insulin aspart [*solid red line*], or regular insulin [*green dashed line*]). Only one formulation of short-acting insulin is used. ***C.*** Insulin administration by insulin infusion device is shown with the basal insulin and a bolus injection at each meal. The basal insulin rate is decreased during the evening and increased slightly prior to the patient awakening in the morning. Glulisine, lispro, or insulin aspart is used in the insulin pump. *(Adapted from H Lebovitz [ed]: Therapy for Diabetes Mellitus. American Diabetes Association, Alexandria, VA, 2004.)*

insulin-to-carbohydrate ratio (a common ratio for type 1 DM is 1–1.5 units/10 g of carbohydrate, but this must be determined for each individual). To this insulin dose is added the supplemental or correcting insulin based on the preprandial blood glucose (one formula uses 1 unit of insulin for every 2.7 mmol/L [50 mg/dL] over the preprandial glucose target; another formula uses [body weight in kg] × [blood glucose – desired glucose in mg/dL]/1500). An alternative multiple-component insulin regimen consists of bedtime NPH insulin, a small dose of NPH insulin at breakfast (20–30% of bedtime dose), and preprandial short-acting insulin. Other variations of this regimen are in use but have the disadvantage that NPH has a significant peak, making hypoglycemia more common. Frequent SMBG (more than three times per day) is absolutely essential for these types of insulin regimens.

In the past, one commonly used regimen consisted of twice-daily injections of NPH mixed with a short-acting insulin before the morning and evening meals (Fig. 24-1B). Such regimens usually prescribe two-thirds of the total daily insulin dose in the morning (with about two-thirds given as long-acting insulin and one-third as short-acting) and one-third before the evening meal (with approximately one-half given as long-acting insulin and one-half as short-acting). The drawback to such a regimen is that it forces a rigid schedule on the patient, in terms of daily activity and the content and timing of meals. Although it is simple and effective at avoiding severe hyperglycemia, it does not generate near-normal glycemic control in individuals with type 1 DM. Moreover, if the patient's meal pattern or content varies or if physical activity is increased, hyperglycemia or hypoglycemia may result. Moving the long-acting insulin from before the evening meal to bedtime may avoid nocturnal hypoglycemia and provide more insulin as glucose levels rise in the early morning (so-called dawn phenomenon). The insulin dose in such regimens should be adjusted based on SMBG results with the following general assumptions: (1) the fasting glucose is primarily determined by the prior evening long-acting insulin; (2) the pre-lunch glucose is a function of the morning short-acting insulin; (3) the pre-supper glucose is a function of the morning long-acting insulin; and (4) the bedtime glucose is a function of the pre-supper, short-acting insulin. This is not an optimal regimen for the patient with type 1 DM, but is sometimes used for patients with type 2 DM.

Continuous SC insulin infusion (CSII) is a very effective insulin regimen for the patient with type 1 DM (Fig. 24-1C). To the basal insulin infusion, a preprandial insulin ("bolus") is delivered by the insulin infusion device based on instructions from the patient, who uses an individualized algorithm incorporating the preprandial plasma glucose and anticipated carbohydrate intake. These sophisticated insulin infusion devices can accurately deliver small doses of insulin (microliters per hour) and have several advantages: (1) multiple basal infusion rates can be programmed to accommodate nocturnal versus daytime basal insulin requirement; (2) basal infusion rates can be altered during periods of exercise; (3) different waveforms of insulin infusion with meal-related bolus allow better matching of insulin depending on meal composition; and (4) programmed algorithms consider prior insulin administration and blood glucose values in calculating the insulin dose. These devices require instruction by a health professional with considerable experience with insulin-infusion devices and very frequent patient interactions with the diabetes management team. Insulin-infusion devices present unique challenges, such as infection at the infusion site, unexplained hyperglycemia because the infusion set becomes obstructed, or diabetic ketoacidosis if the pump becomes disconnected. Because most physicians use lispro, glulisine, or insulin aspart in CSII, the extremely short half-life of these insulins quickly leads to insulin deficiency if the delivery system is interrupted. Essential to the safe use of infusion devices is thorough patient education about pump function and frequent SMBG. Efforts to create a closed-loop system in which data from continuous glucose measurement regulate the insulin infusion rate are under way.

Other agents that improve glucose control

The role of amylin, a 37-amino-acid peptide co-secreted with insulin from pancreatic beta cells, in normal glucose homeostasis is uncertain. However, based on the rationale that patients who are insulin deficient are also amylin deficient, an analogue of amylin (pramlintide) was created and found to reduce postprandial glycemic excursions in type 1 and type 2 diabetic patients taking insulin. Pramlintide injected just before a meal slows gastric emptying and suppresses glucagon but does not alter insulin levels. Pramlintide is approved for insulin-treated patients with type 1 and type 2 DM. Addition of pramlintide produces a modest reduction in the HbA_{1c} and seems to dampen meal-related glucose excursions. In type 1 DM, pramlintide is started as a 15-μg SC injection before each meal and titrated up to a maximum of 30–60 μg as tolerated. In type 2 DM, pramlintide is started as a 60-μg SC injection before each meal and may be titrated up to a maximum of 120 μg. The major side effects are nausea and vomiting, and dose escalations should be slow to limit these side effects. Because pramlintide slows gastric emptying, it may influence absorption of other medications and should not be used in combination with other drugs that slow GI motility. The short-acting insulin given before the meal should initially be reduced to avoid hypoglycemia and then titrated as the effects of the pramlintide become evident. α-Glucosidase inhibitors are sometimes used with insulin in type 1 DM.

TYPE 2 DIABETES MELLITUS

General aspects

The goals of glycemia-controlling therapy for type 2 DM are similar to those in type 1 DM. Whereas glycemic control tends to dominate the management of type 1 DM, the care of individuals with type 2 DM must also include attention to the treatment of conditions associated with type 2 DM (e.g., obesity, hypertension, dyslipidemia, CVD) and detection/management of DM-related complications (Fig. 24-2). Reduction in cardiovascular risk is of paramount importance because this is the leading cause of mortality in these individuals.

Type 2 DM management should begin with MNT (discussed above). An exercise regimen to increase insulin sensitivity and promote weight loss should also be instituted. Pharmacologic approaches to the management of type 2 DM include oral glucose-lowering agents, insulin, and other agents that improve glucose control; most physicians and patients prefer oral glucose-lowering agents as the initial choice. Any therapy that improves glycemic control reduces "glucose toxicity" to beta cells and improves endogenous insulin secretion. However, type 2 DM is a progressive disorder and ultimately requires multiple therapeutic agents and often insulin in most patients.

Glucose-lowering agents

Advances in the therapy of type 2 DM have generated oral glucose-lowering agents that target different pathophysiologic processes in type 2 DM. Based on their mechanisms of action, glucose-lowering agents are subdivided into agents that increase insulin secretion, reduce glucose production, increase insulin sensitivity, enhance GLP-1 action, or promote urinary excretion of glucose (Table 24-5). Glucose-lowering agents other than insulin (with the exception of amylin analogue and α-glucosidase inhibitors) are ineffective in type 1 DM and should not be used for glucose management of severely ill individuals with type 2 DM. Insulin is sometimes the initial glucose-lowering agent in type 2 DM.

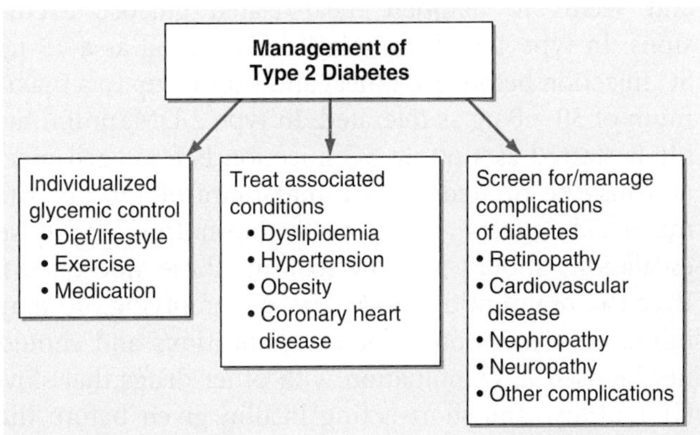

FIGURE 24-2
Essential elements in comprehensive care of type 2 diabetes.

Biguanides

Metformin, representative of this class of agents, reduces hepatic glucose production and improves peripheral glucose utilization slightly (Table 24-5). Metformin activates AMP-dependent protein kinase and enters cells through organic cation transporters (polymorphisms of these may influence the response to metformin). Recent evidence indicates that metformin's mechanism for reducing hepatic glucose production is to antagonize glucagon's ability to generate cAMP in hepatocytes. Metformin reduces fasting plasma glucose (FPG) and insulin levels, improves the lipid profile, and promotes modest weight loss. An extended-release form is available and may have fewer gastrointestinal side effects (diarrhea, anorexia, nausea, metallic taste). Because of its relatively slow onset of action and gastrointestinal symptoms with higher doses, the initial dose should be low and then escalated every 2–3 weeks based on SMBG measurements. Metformin is effective as monotherapy and can be used in combination with other oral agents or with insulin. The major toxicity of metformin, lactic acidosis, is very rare and can be prevented by careful patient selection. Vitamin B_{12} levels are ~30% lower during metformin treatment. Metformin should not be used in patients with renal insufficiency (glomerular filtration rate [GFR] <60 mL/min), any form of acidosis, unstable congestive heart failure (CHF), liver disease, or severe hypoxemia. Some feel that that these guidelines are too restrictive and prevent individuals with mild to moderate renal impairment from being safely treated with metformin. The National Institute for Health and Clinical Excellence in the United Kingdom suggests that metformin be used at a GFR >30 mL/min, with a reduced dose when the GFR is <45 mL/min. Metformin should be discontinued in hospitalized patients, in patients who can take nothing orally, and in those receiving radiographic contrast material. Insulin should be used until metformin can be restarted.

Insulin secretagogues—agents that affect the ATP-sensitive K^+ channel

Insulin secretagogues stimulate insulin secretion by interacting with the ATP-sensitive potassium channel on the beta cell **(Chap. 23)**. These drugs are most effective in individuals with type 2 DM of relatively recent onset (<5 years) who have residual endogenous insulin production. First-generation sulfonylureas

TABLE 24-5

AGENTS USED FOR TREATMENT OF TYPE 1 OR TYPE 2 DIABETES

	MECHANISM OF ACTION	EXAMPLES[a]	HBA_{1C} REDUCTION (%)[b]	AGENT-SPECIFIC ADVANTAGES	AGENT-SPECIFIC DISADVANTAGES	CONTRAINDICATIONS
Oral						
Biguanides[c*]	↓ Hepatic glucose production	Metformin	1–2	Weight neutral, do not cause hypoglycemia, inexpensive, extensive experience, ↓ CV events	Diarrhea, nausea, lactic acidosis	Serum creatinine >1.5 mg/dL (men) >1.4 mg/dL (women) (see text), CHF, radiographic contrast studies, hospitalized patients, acidosis
α-Glucosidase inhibitors[c**]	↓ GI glucose absorption	Acarbose, miglitol, voglibose	0.5–0.8	Reduce postprandial glycemia	GI flatulence, liver function tests	Renal/liver disease
Dipeptidyl peptidase IV inhibitors[c***]	Prolong endogenous GLP-1 action	Alogliptin, Anagliptin, Gemigliptin, linagliptin, saxagliptin, sitagliptin, teneligliptin, vildagliptin	0.5–0.8	Well tolerated, do not cause hypoglycemia		Reduced dose with renal disease; one associated with increase heart failure risk; possible association with ACE inhibitor–induced angioedema
Insulin secretagogues: Sulfonylureas[c*]	↑ Insulin secretion	Glibornuride, gliclazide, glimepiride, glipizide, gliquidone, glyburide, glyclopyramide	1–2	Short onset of action, lower postprandial glucose, inexpensive	Hypoglycemia, weight gain	Renal/liver disease
Insulin secretagogues: Nonsulfonylureas[c***]	↑ Insulin secretion	Nateglinide, repaglinide, mitiglinide	0.5–1.0	Short onset of action, lower postprandial glucose	Hypoglycemia	Renal/liver disease
Sodium-glucose co-transporter 2 inhibitors***	↑ Urinary glucose excretion	Canagliflozin, dapagliflozin, empagliflozin	0.5–1.0	Insulin secretion and action independent	Urinary and vaginal infections, dehydration, exacerbate tendency to hyperkalemia	Limited clinical experience; moderate renal insufficiency
Thiazolidinediones[c***]	↓ Insulin resistance, ↑ glucose utilization	Rosiglitazone, pioglitazone	0.5–1.4	Lower insulin requirements	Peripheral edema, CHF, weight gain, fractures, macular edema	CHF, liver disease
Parenteral						
Amylin agonists[c,d***]	Slow gastric emptying, ↓ glucagon	Pramlintide	0.25–0.5	Reduce postprandial glycemia, weight loss	Injection, nausea, ↑ risk of hypoglycemia with insulin	Agents that also slow GI motility
GLP-1 receptor agonists[c***]	↑ Insulin, ↓ glucagon, slow gastric emptying, satiety	Exenatide, liraglutide, dulaglutide	0.5–1.0	Weight loss, do not cause hypoglycemia	Injection, nausea, ↑ risk of hypoglycemia with insulin secretagogues	Renal disease, agents that also slow GI motility; medullary carcinoma of thyroid

(continued)

TABLE 24-5

AGENTS USED FOR TREATMENT OF TYPE 1 OR TYPE 2 DIABETES (CONTINUED)

	MECHANISM OF ACTION	EXAMPLES[a]	HBA$_{1C}$ REDUCTION (%)[b]	AGENT-SPECIFIC ADVANTAGES	AGENT-SPECIFIC DISADVANTAGES	CONTRAINDICATIONS
Insulin[c,d]****	↑ Glucose utilization, ↓ hepatic glucose production, and other anabolic actions	See text and Table 24-4	Not limited	Known safety profile	Injection, weight gain, hypoglycemia	
Medical nutrition therapy and physical activity[c]*	↓ Insulin resistance, ↑ insulin secretion	Low-calorie, low-fat diet, exercise	1–3	Other health benefits	Compliance difficult, long-term success low	

[a]Examples are approved for use in at least one country, but may not be available in the United States or all countries. Examples may not include all agents in the class. [b]HbA*1c* reduction (absolute) depends partly on starting HbA$_{1c}$. [c]Used for treatment of type 2 diabetes. [d]Used in conjunction with insulin for treatment of type 1 diabetes. Cost of agent: *low, **moderate, ***high, ****variable.

Note: Some agents used to treat type 2 DM are not included in table (see text).

Abbreviations: ACE, angiotensin-converting enzyme; CHF, congestive heart failure; CV, cardiovascular; GI, gastrointestinal; HbA$_{1c}$, hemoglobin A$_{1c}$.

(chlorpropamide, tolazamide, tolbutamide) have a longer half-life, a greater incidence of hypoglycemia, and more frequent drug interactions, and are no longer used. Second-generation sulfonylureas have a more rapid onset of action and better coverage of the postprandial glucose rise, but the shorter half-life of some agents may require more than once-a-day dosing. Sulfonylureas reduce both fasting and postprandial glucose and should be initiated at low doses and increased at 1- to 2-week intervals based on SMBG. In general, sulfonylureas increase insulin acutely and thus should be taken shortly before a meal; with chronic therapy, though, the insulin release is more sustained. Glimepiride and glipizide can be given in a single daily dose and are preferred over glyburide, especially in the elderly. Repaglinide, nateglinide, and mitiglinide are not sulfonylureas but also interact with the ATP-sensitive potassium channel. Because of their short half-life, these agents are given with each meal or immediately before to reduce meal-related glucose excursions.

Insulin secretagogues, especially the longer acting ones, have the potential to cause hypoglycemia, especially in elderly individuals. Hypoglycemia is usually related to delayed meals, increased physical activity, alcohol intake, or renal insufficiency. Individuals who ingest an overdose of some agents develop prolonged and serious hypoglycemia and should be monitored closely in the hospital **(Chap. 26)**. Most sulfonylureas are metabolized in the liver to compounds (some of which are active) that are cleared by the kidney. Thus, their use in individuals with significant hepatic or renal dysfunction is not advisable. Weight gain, a common side effect of sulfonylurea therapy, results from the increased insulin levels and improvement in glycemic control. Some sulfonylureas have significant drug interactions with alcohol and some medications including warfarin, aspirin, ketoconazole, α-glucosidase inhibitors, and fluconazole. A related isoform of ATP-sensitive potassium channels is present in the myocardium and the brain. All of these agents except glyburide have a low affinity for this isoform. Despite concerns that this agent might affect the myocardial response to ischemia and observational studies suggesting that sulfonylureas increase cardiovascular risk, studies have not shown an increased cardiac mortality with glyburide or other agents in this class.

Insulin secretagogues—agents that enhance GLP-1 receptor signaling

"Incretins" amplify glucose-stimulated insulin secretion **(Chap. 23)**. Agents that either act as a GLP-1 receptor agonist or enhance endogenous GLP-1 activity are approved for the treatment of type 2 DM (Table 24-5). Agents in this class do not cause hypoglycemia because of the glucose-dependent nature of incretin-stimulated insulin secretion (unless there is concomitant use of an agent that can lead to hypoglycemia—sulfonylureas, etc.). Exenatide, a synthetic version of a peptide initially identified in the saliva of the Gila monster (exendin-4), is an analogue of GLP-1. Unlike native GLP-1, which has a half-life of >5 min, differences in the exenatide amino acid sequence render it resistant to the enzyme that degrades GLP-1 (dipeptidyl peptidase IV [DPP-IV]). Thus, exenatide has prolonged GLP-1-like action and binds to GLP-1 receptors found in islets, the gastrointestinal tract, and the brain. Liraglutide, another

GLP-1 receptor agonist, is almost identical to native GLP-1 except for an amino acid substitution and addition of a fatty acyl group (coupled with a γ-glutamic acid spacer) that promote binding to albumin and plasma proteins and prolong its half-life. GLP-1 receptor agonists increase glucose-stimulated insulin secretion, suppress glucagon, and slow gastric emptying. These agents do not promote weight gain; in fact, most patients experience modest weight loss and appetite suppression. Treatment with these agents should start at a low dose to minimize initial side effects (nausea being the limiting one). GLP-1 receptor agonists, available in twice daily, daily, and weekly injectable formulations, can be used as combination therapy with metformin, sulfonylureas, and thiazolidinediones. Some patients taking insulin secretagogues may require a reduction in those agents to prevent hypoglycemia. The major side effects are nausea, vomiting, and diarrhea. Some formulations carry a black box warning from the FDA because of an increased risk of thyroid C-cell tumors in rodents and are contraindicated in individuals with medullary carcinoma of the thyroid or multiple endocrine neoplasia. Because GLP-1 receptor agonists slow gastric emptying, they may influence the absorption of other drugs. Whether GLP-1 receptor agonists enhance beta cell survival, promote beta cell proliferation, or alter the natural history of type 2 DM is not known. Other GLP-1 receptor agonists and formulations are under development.

DPP-IV inhibitors inhibit degradation of native GLP-1 and thus enhance the incretin effect. DPP-IV, which is widely expressed on the cell surface of endothelial cells and some lymphocytes, degrades a wide range of peptides (not GLP-1 specific). DPP-IV inhibitors promote insulin secretion in the absence of hypoglycemia or weight gain and appear to have a preferential effect on postprandial blood glucose. The levels of GLP-1 action in the patient are greater with the GLP-1 receptor agonists than with DPP-IV inhibitors. DPP-IV inhibitors are used either alone or in combination with other oral agents in type 2 DM. Reduced doses should be given to patients with renal insufficiency. Initial concerns about the pancreatic side effects of GLP-1 receptor agonists and DPP-IV inhibitors (pancreatitis, possible premalignant lesions) appear to be unfounded.

α-Glucosidase inhibitors

α-Glucosidase inhibitors reduce postprandial hyperglycemia by delaying glucose absorption; they do not affect glucose utilization or insulin secretion **(Table 24-5)**. Postprandial hyperglycemia, secondary to impaired hepatic and peripheral glucose disposal, contributes significantly to the hyperglycemic state in type 2 DM. These drugs, taken just before each meal, reduce glucose absorption by inhibiting the enzyme that cleaves oligosaccharides into simple sugars in the intestinal lumen. Therapy should be initiated at a low dose with the evening meal and increased to a maximal dose over weeks to months. The major side effects (diarrhea, flatulence, abdominal distention) are related to increased delivery of oligosaccharides to the large bowel and can be reduced somewhat by gradual upward dose titration. α-Glucosidase inhibitors may increase levels of sulfonylureas and increase the incidence of hypoglycemia. Simultaneous treatment with bile acid resins and antacids should be avoided. These agents should not be used in individuals with inflammatory bowel disease, gastroparesis, or a serum creatinine >177 μmol/L (2 mg/dL). This class of agents is not as potent as other oral agents in lowering the HbA_{1c} but is unique because it reduces the postprandial glucose rise even in individuals with type 1 DM. If hypoglycemia from other diabetes treatments occurs while taking these agents, the patient should consume glucose because the degradation and absorption of complex carbohydrates will be retarded.

Thiazolidinediones

Thiazolidinediones (Table 24-5) reduce insulin resistance by binding to the PPAR-γ (peroxisome proliferator–activated receptor γ) nuclear receptor (which forms a heterodimer with the retinoid X receptor). The PPAR-γ receptor is found at highest levels in adipocytes but is expressed at lower levels in many other tissues. Agonists of this receptor regulate a large number of genes, promote adipocyte differentiation, reduce hepatic fat accumulation, and promote fatty acid storage. Thiazolidinediones promote a redistribution of fat from central to peripheral locations. Circulating insulin levels decrease with use of the thiazolidinediones, indicating a reduction in insulin resistance. Although direct comparisons are not available, the two currently available thiazolidinediones appear to have similar efficacy. The prototype of this class of drugs, troglitazone, was withdrawn from the U.S. market after reports of hepatotoxicity and an association with an idiosyncratic liver reaction that sometimes led to hepatic failure. Although rosiglitazone and pioglitazone do not appear to induce the liver abnormalities seen with troglitazone, the FDA recommends measurement of liver function tests prior to initiating therapy.

Rosiglitazone raises low-density lipoprotein (LDL), high-density lipoprotein (HDL), and triglycerides slightly. Pioglitazone raises HDL to a greater degree and LDL a lesser degree but lowers triglycerides. The clinical significance of the lipid changes with these agents is not known and may be difficult to ascertain because most patients with type 2 DM are also treated with a statin.

Thiazolidinediones are associated with weight gain (2–3 kg), a small reduction in the hematocrit, and a mild increase in plasma volume. Peripheral edema and CHF are more common in individuals treated with these agents. These agents are contraindicated in patients with liver disease or CHF (class III or IV). The FDA has issued an alert that rare patients taking these agents may experience a worsening of diabetic macular edema. An increased risk of fractures has been noted in women taking these agents. Thiazolidinediones have been shown to induce ovulation in premenopausal women with polycystic ovary syndrome. Women should be warned about the risk of pregnancy because the safety of thiazolidinediones in pregnancy is not established.

Concerns about increased cardiovascular risk associated with rosiglitazone led to considerable restrictions on its use and to the FDA issuing a "black box" warning in 2007. However, based on new information, the FDA has revised its guidelines and categorizes rosiglitazone similar to other drugs for type 2 DM. Because of a possible increased risk of bladder cancer, pioglitazone is part of an ongoing FDA safety review.

Sodium-glucose co-transporter 2 inhibitors (SLGT2)

These agents (Table 24-5) lower the blood glucose by selectively inhibiting this co-transporter, which is expressed almost exclusively in the proximal, convoluted tubule in the kidney. This inhibits glucose reabsorption, lowers the renal threshold for glucose, and leads to increased urinary glucose excretion. Thus, the glucose-lowering effect is insulin independent and not related to changes in insulin sensitivity or secretion. Because these agents are the newest class to treat type 2 DM (Table 24-5), clinical experience is limited. Due to the increased urinary glucose, urinary or vaginal infections are more common, and the diuretic effect can lead to reduced intravascular volume. As part of the FDA approval of canagliflozin in 2013, postmarketing studies for cardiovascular outcomes and for monitoring bladder and urinary cancer risk are under way.

Other therapies for type 2 DM

Bile acid–binding resins

Evidence indicates that bile acids, by signaling through nuclear receptors, may have a role in metabolism. Bile acid metabolism is abnormal in type 2 DM. The bile acid–binding resin colesevelam has been approved for the treatment of type 2 DM (already approved for treatment of hypercholesterolemia). Because bile acid–binding resins are minimally absorbed into the systemic circulation, how bile acid–binding resins lower blood glucose is not known. The most common side effects are gastrointestinal (constipation, abdominal pain, and nausea). Bile acid–binding resins can increase plasma triglycerides and should be used cautiously in patients with a tendency for hypertriglyceridemia. The role of this class of drugs in the treatment of type 2 DM is not yet defined.

Bromocriptine

A formulation of the dopamine receptor agonist bromocriptine (Cycloset) has been approved by the FDA for the treatment of type 2 DM. However, its role in the treatment of type 2 DM is uncertain.

Insulin therapy in type 2 DM

Insulin should be considered as the initial therapy in type 2 DM, particularly in lean individuals or those with severe weight loss, in individuals with underlying renal or hepatic disease that precludes oral glucose-lowering agents, or in individuals who are hospitalized or acutely ill. Insulin therapy is ultimately required by a substantial number of individuals with type 2 DM because of the progressive nature of the disorder and the relative insulin deficiency that develops in patients with long-standing diabetes. Both physician and patient reluctance often delay the initiation of insulin therapy, but glucose control and patient well-being are improved by insulin therapy in patients who have not reached the glycemic target.

Because endogenous insulin secretion continues and is capable of providing some coverage of mealtime caloric intake, insulin is usually initiated in a single dose of long-acting insulin (0.3–0.4 U/kg per day), given in the evening (NPH) or just before bedtime (NPH, glargine, detemir). Because fasting hyperglycemia and increased hepatic glucose production are prominent features of type 2 DM, bedtime insulin is more effective in clinical trials than a single dose of morning insulin. Glargine given at bedtime has less nocturnal hypoglycemia than NPH insulin. Some physicians prefer a relatively low, fixed starting dose of long-acting insulin (5–15 units) or a weight-based dose (0.2 units/kg). The insulin dose may then be adjusted in 10% increments as dictated by SMBG results. Both morning and bedtime long-acting insulin may be used in combination with oral glucose-lowering agents. Initially, basal insulin may be sufficient, but often prandial insulin coverage with multiple insulin injections is needed as diabetes progresses (see insulin regimens used for type 1 DM). Other insulin formulations that have a combination of short-acting and long-acting insulin (Table 24-4) are sometimes used in patients with type 2 DM because of convenience but do not allow independent adjustment of short-acting and long-acting insulin dose and often do not achieve the same degree of glycemic control as basal/bolus regimens. In selected patients with type 2 DM, insulin-infusion devices may be considered.

Choice of initial glucose-lowering agent

The level of hyperglycemia and the patient's individualized goal (see "Establishment of Target Level of Glycemic Control") should influence the initial choice of therapy. Assuming that maximal benefit of MNT and increased physical activity has been realized, patients with mild to moderate hyperglycemia (FPG <11.1–13.9 mmol/L [200–250 mg/dL]) often respond well to a single, oral glucose-lowering agent. Patients with more severe hyperglycemia (FPG >13.9 mmol/L [250 mg/dL]) may respond partially but are unlikely to achieve normoglycemia with oral monotherapy. A stepwise approach that starts with a single agent and adds a second agent to achieve the glycemic target can be used (see "Combination therapy with glucose-lowering agents," below). Insulin can be used as initial therapy in individuals with severe hyperglycemia (FPG <13.9–16.7 mmol/L [250–300 mg/dL]) or in those who are symptomatic from the hyperglycemia. This approach is based on the rationale that more rapid glycemic control will reduce "glucose toxicity" to the islet cells, improve endogenous insulin secretion, and possibly allow oral glucose-lowering agents to be more effective. If this occurs, the insulin may be discontinued.

Insulin secretagogues, biguanides, α-glucosidase inhibitors, thiazolidinediones, GLP-1 receptor agonists, DPP-IV inhibitors, SLGT2 inhibitors, and insulin are approved for monotherapy of type 2 DM. Although each class of oral glucose-lowering agents has advantages and disadvantages (Table 24-5), certain generalizations apply: (1) insulin secretagogues, biguanides, GLP-1 receptor agonists, and thiazolidinediones improve glycemic control to a similar degree (1–2% reduction in HbA_{1c}) and are more effective than α-glucosidase inhibitors, DPP-IV inhibitors, and SLGT2 inhibitors; (2) assuming a similar degree of glycemic improvement, no clinical advantage to one class of drugs has been demonstrated; any therapy that improves glycemic control is likely beneficial; (3) insulin secretagogues, GLP-1 receptor agonists, DPP-IV inhibitors, α-glucosidase inhibitors, and SLGT2 inhibitors begin to lower the plasma glucose immediately, whereas the glucose-lowering effects of the biguanides and thiazolidinediones are delayed by weeks; (4) not all agents are effective in all individuals with type 2 DM; (5) biguanides, α-glucosidase inhibitors, GLP-1 receptor agonists, DPP-IV inhibitors, thiazolidinediones, and SLGT2 inhibitors do not directly cause hypoglycemia; (6) most individuals will eventually require treatment with more than one class of oral glucose-lowering agents or insulin, reflecting the progressive nature of type 2 DM; and (7) durability of glycemic control is slightly less for glyburide compared to metformin or rosiglitazone.

Considerable clinical experience exists with metformin and sulfonylureas because they have been available for several decades. It is assumed that the α-glucosidase inhibitors, GLP-1 agonists, DPP-IV inhibitors, thiazolidinediones, and SLGT2 inhibitors will reduce DM-related complications by improving glycemic control, but long-term data are not yet available. The thiazolidinediones are theoretically attractive because they target a fundamental abnormality in type 2 DM, namely insulin resistance. However, all of these agents are currently more costly than metformin and sulfonylureas.

Treatment algorithms by several professional societies (ADA/European Association for the Study of Diabetes [EASD], IDF, AACE) suggest metformin as initial therapy because of its efficacy, known side effect profile, and low cost (Fig. 24-3). Metformin's advantages are that it promotes mild weight loss, lowers insulin levels, and improves the lipid profile slightly. Based on SMBG results and the HbA_{1c}, the dose of metformin should be increased until the glycemic target is achieved or maximum dose is reached. If metformin is not tolerated, then initial therapy with an insulin secretagogue or DPP-IV inhibitor is reasonable.

Combination therapy with glucose-lowering agents

A number of combinations of therapeutic agents are successful in type 2 DM (metformin + second oral agent, metformin + GLP-1 receptor agonist, or metformin + insulin), and the dosing of agents in combination is the same as when the agents are used alone. Because mechanisms of action of the first and second

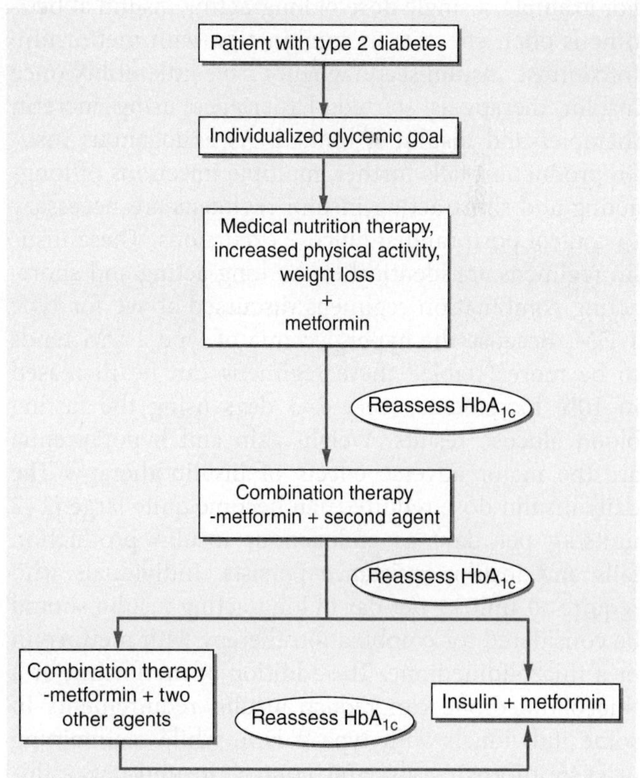

FIGURE 24-3

Glycemic management of type 2 diabetes. See text for discussion of treatment of severe hyperglycemia or symptomatic hyperglycemia. Agents that can be combined with metformin include insulin secretagogues, thiazolidinediones, α-glucosidase inhibitors, DPP-IV inhibitors, GLP-1 receptor agonists, SLGT2 inhibitors, and insulin. HbA_{1c}, hemoglobin HbA_{1c}.

agents should be different, the effect on glycemic control is usually additive. There are little data to support the choice of one combination over another combination. Medication costs vary considerably (Table 24-5), and this often factors into medication choice. Several fixed-dose combinations of oral agents are available, but evidence that they are superior to titration of single agent to a maximum dose and then addition of a second agent is lacking. If adequate control is not achieved with the combination of two agents (based on reassessment of the HbA_{1c} every 3 months), a third oral agent or basal insulin should be added (Fig. 24-3). Treatment approaches vary considerably from country to country. For example, α-glucosidase inhibitors are used commonly in South Asian patients (Indian), but infrequently in the United States or Europe. Whether this reflects an underlying difference in the disease or physician preference is not clear.

Treatment with insulin becomes necessary as type 2 DM enters the phase of relative insulin deficiency (as seen in long-standing DM) and is signaled by inadequate glycemic control with one or two oral glucose-lowering agents. Insulin alone or in combination should be used in patients who fail to reach the glycemic target. For example, a single dose of long-acting insulin at bedtime is often effective in combination with metformin. In contrast, insulin secretagogues have little utility once insulin therapy is started. Experience using incretin therapies and insulin is limited. As endogenous insulin production falls further, multiple injections of long-acting and short-acting insulin regimens are necessary to control postprandial glucose excursions. These insulin regimens are identical to the long-acting and short-acting combination regimens discussed above for type 1 DM. Because the hyperglycemia of type 2 DM tends to be more "stable," these regimens can be increased in 10% increments every 2–3 days using the fasting blood glucose results. Weight gain and hypoglycemia are the major adverse effects of insulin therapy. The daily insulin dose required can become quite large (1–2 units/kg per day) as endogenous insulin production falls and insulin resistance persists. Individuals who require >1 unit/kg per day of long-acting insulin should be considered for combination therapy with metformin or a thiazolidinedione. The addition of metformin or a thiazolidinedione can reduce insulin requirements in some individuals with type 2 DM, while maintaining or even improving glycemic control. Insulin plus a thiazolidinedione promotes weight gain and is associated with peripheral edema. Addition of a thiazolidinedione to a patient's insulin regimen may necessitate a reduction in the insulin dose to avoid hypoglycemia. Patients requiring large doses of insulin (>200 units/day) can be treated with a more concentrated form of insulin, U-500.

EMERGING THERAPIES

Whole pancreas transplantation (performed concomitantly with a renal transplant) may normalize glucose tolerance and is an important therapeutic option in type 1 DM with end-stage renal disease, although it requires substantial expertise and is associated with the side effects of immunosuppression. Pancreatic islet transplantation has been plagued by limitations in pancreatic islet supply and graft survival and remains an area of clinical investigation. Many individuals with long-standing type 1 DM still produce very small amounts of insulin or have insulin-positive cells within the pancreas. This suggests that beta cells may slowly regenerate but are quickly destroyed by the autoimmune process. Thus, efforts to suppress the autoimmune process and to stimulate beta cell regeneration are being tested both at the time of diagnosis and in years after the diagnosis of type 1 DM. Closed-loop pumps that infuse the appropriate amount of insulin in response to changing glucose levels are potentially feasible now that CGM technology has been developed. Bi-hormonal pumps that deliver both insulin and glucagon are under development. New therapies under development for type 2 DM include activators of glucokinase, inhibitors of 11 β-hydroxysteroid dehydrogenase-1, GPR40 agonists, monoclonal antibodies to reduce inflammation, and salsalate.

Bariatric surgery for obese individuals with type 2 DM has shown considerable promise, sometimes with dramatic resolution of the diabetes or major reductions in the needed dose of glucose-lowering therapies **(Chap. 21)**. Several large, unblinded clinical trials have demonstrated a much greater efficacy of bariatric surgery compared to medical management in the treatment of type 2 DM; the durability of the diabetes reversal or improvement is uncertain. The ADA clinical guidelines state that bariatric surgery should be considered in individuals with DM and a body mass index >35 kg/m^2.

ADVERSE EFFECTS OF THERAPY FOR DIABETES MELLITUS

As with any therapy, the benefits of efforts directed toward glycemic control must be balanced against the risks of treatment (Table 24-5). Side effects of intensive treatment include an increased frequency of serious hypoglycemia, weight gain, increased economic costs, and greater demands on the patient. In the DCCT, quality of life was very similar in the intensive and standard therapy groups. The most serious complication of therapy for DM is hypoglycemia, and its treatment with oral glucose or glucagon injection is discussed in **Chap. 26.** Severe, recurrent hypoglycemia warrants examination of treatment regimen and glycemic goal for the individual patient. Weight gain occurs with most (insulin, insulin secretagogues, thiazolidinediones) but not all (metformin, α-glucosidase inhibitors, GLP-1 receptor agonists, DPP-IV inhibitors) therapies. The weight gain is partially due to the anabolic effects of insulin and the reduction in glucosuria. As a result of recent controversies about the optimal glycemic goal and concerns about safety, the FDA now requires information about the cardiovascular safety profile as part of its evaluation of new treatments for type 2 DM.

ACUTE DISORDERS RELATED TO SEVERE HYPERGLYCEMIA

Individuals with type 1 or type 2 DM and severe hyperglycemia (>16.7 mmol/L [300 mg/dL]) should be assessed for clinical stability, including mentation and hydration. Depending on the patient and the rapidity and duration of the severe hyperglycemia, an individual may require more intense and rapid therapy to lower the blood glucose. However, many patients with poorly controlled diabetes and hyperglycemia have few symptoms. The physician should assess if the patient is stable or if diabetic ketoacidosis or a hyperglycemic hyperosmolar state should be considered. Ketones, an indicator of diabetic ketoacidosis, should be measured in individuals with type 1 DM when the plasma glucose is >16.7 mmol/L (300 mg/dL), during a concurrent illness, or with symptoms such as nausea, vomiting, or abdominal pain. Blood measurement of β-hydroxybutyrate is preferred over urine testing with nitroprusside-based assays that measure only acetoacetate and acetone.

Diabetic ketoacidosis (DKA) and hyperglycemic hyperosmolar state (HHS) are acute, severe disorders directly related to diabetes. DKA was formerly considered a hallmark of type 1 DM, but also occurs in individuals who lack immunologic features of type 1 DM and who can sometimes subsequently be treated with oral glucose-lowering agents (these obese individuals with type 2 DM are often of Hispanic or African-American descent). HHS is primarily seen in individuals with type 2 DM. Both disorders are associated with absolute or relative insulin deficiency, volume depletion, and acid-base abnormalities. DKA and HHS exist along a continuum of hyperglycemia, with or without ketosis. The metabolic similarities and differences in DKA and HHS are highlighted in Table 24-6. Both disorders are associated with potentially serious complications if not promptly diagnosed and treated.

TABLE 24-6

LABORATORY VALUES IN DIABETIC KETOACIDOSIS (DKA) AND HYPERGLYCEMIC HYPEROSMOLAR STATE (HHS) (REPRESENTATIVE RANGES AT PRESENTATION)

	DKA	HHS
Glucose,[a] mmol/L (mg/dL)	13.9–33.3 (250–600)	33.3–66.6 (600–1200)
Sodium, meq/L	125–135	135–145
Potassium[a,b]	Normal to ↑	Normal
Magnesium[a]	Normal	Normal
Chloride[a]	Normal	Normal
Phosphate[a,b]	Normal	Normal
Creatinine	Slightly ↑	Moderately ↑
Osmolality (mOsm/mL)	300–320	330–380
Plasma ketones[a]	++++	+/–
Serum bicarbonate,[a] meq/L	<15	Normal to slightly ↓
Arterial pH	6.8–7.3	>7.3
Arterial Pco_2,[a] mmHg	20–30	Normal
Anion gap[a](Na – [Cl + HCO_3])	↑	Normal to slightly ↑

[a]Large changes occur during treatment of DKA. [b]Although plasma levels may be normal or high at presentation, total-body stores are usually depleted.

DIABETIC KETOACIDOSIS

Clinical features

The symptoms and physical signs of DKA are listed in Table 24-7 and usually develop over 24 h. DKA may be the initial symptom complex that leads to a diagnosis of type 1 DM, but more frequently, it occurs in individuals with established diabetes. Nausea and vomiting are often prominent, and their presence in an individual with diabetes warrants laboratory evaluation for DKA. Abdominal pain may be severe and can resemble acute pancreatitis or ruptured viscus. Hyperglycemia leads to glucosuria, volume depletion, and tachycardia. Hypotension can occur because of volume depletion in combination with peripheral vasodilatation. Kussmaul

TABLE 24-7

MANIFESTATIONS OF DIABETIC KETOACIDOSIS

Symptoms	Physical Findings
Nausea/vomiting	Tachycardia
Thirst/polyuria	Dehydration/hypotension
Abdominal pain	Tachypnea/Kussmaul respirations/respiratory distress
Shortness of breath	Abdominal tenderness (may resemble acute pancreatitis or surgical abdomen)
Precipitating events	Lethargy/obtundation/cerebral edema/possibly coma
Inadequate insulin administration	
Infection (pneumonia/UTI/gastroenteritis/sepsis)	
Infarction (cerebral, coronary, mesenteric, peripheral)	
Drugs (cocaine)	
Pregnancy	

Abbreviation: UTI, urinary tract infection.

respirations and a fruity odor on the patient's breath (secondary to metabolic acidosis and increased acetone) are classic signs of the disorder. Lethargy and central nervous system depression may evolve into coma with severe DKA but should also prompt evaluation for other reasons for altered mental status (e.g., infection, hypoxemia). Cerebral edema, an extremely serious complication of DKA, is seen most frequently in children. Signs of infection, which may precipitate DKA, should be sought on physical examination, even in the absence of fever. Tissue ischemia (heart, brain) can also be a precipitating factor. Omission of insulin because of an eating disorder, mental health disorders, or an unstable psychosocial environment may sometimes be a factor precipitating DKA.

Pathophysiology

DKA results from relative or absolute insulin deficiency combined with counterregulatory hormone excess (glucagon, catecholamines, cortisol, and growth hormone). Both insulin deficiency and glucagon excess, in particular, are necessary for DKA to develop. The decreased ratio of insulin to glucagon promotes gluconeogenesis, glycogenolysis, and ketone body formation in the liver, as well as increases in substrate delivery from fat and muscle (free fatty acids, amino acids) to the liver. Markers of inflammation (cytokines, C-reactive protein) are elevated in both DKA and HHS

The combination of insulin deficiency and hyperglycemia reduces the hepatic level of fructose-2,6-bisphosphate, which alters the activity of phosphofructokinase and fructose-1,6-bisphosphatase. Glucagon excess decreases the activity of pyruvate kinase, whereas insulin deficiency increases the activity of phosphoenolpyruvate carboxykinase. These changes shift the handling of pyruvate toward glucose synthesis and away from glycolysis. The increased levels of glucagon and catecholamines in the face of low insulin levels promote glycogenolysis. Insulin deficiency also reduces levels of the GLUT4 glucose transporter, which impairs glucose uptake into skeletal muscle and fat and reduces intracellular glucose metabolism.

Ketosis results from a marked increase in free fatty acid release from adipocytes, with a resulting shift toward ketone body synthesis in the liver. Reduced insulin levels, in combination with elevations in catecholamines and growth hormone, increase lipolysis and the release of free fatty acids. Normally, these free fatty acids are converted to triglycerides or very-low-density lipoprotein (VLDL) in the liver. However, in DKA, hyperglucagonemia alters hepatic metabolism to favor ketone body formation, through activation of the enzyme carnitine palmitoyltransferase I. This enzyme is crucial for regulating fatty acid transport into the mitochondria, where beta oxidation and conversion to ketone bodies occur. At physiologic pH, ketone bodies exist as ketoacids, which are neutralized by bicarbonate. As bicarbonate stores are depleted, metabolic acidosis ensues. Increased lactic acid production also contributes to the acidosis. The increased free fatty acids increase triglyceride and VLDL production. VLDL clearance is also reduced because the activity of insulin-sensitive lipoprotein lipase in muscle and fat is decreased. Hypertriglyceridemia may be severe enough to cause pancreatitis.

DKA is often precipitated by increased insulin requirements, as occurs during a concurrent illness (Table 24-7). Failure to augment insulin therapy often compounds the problem. Complete omission or inadequate administration of insulin by the patient or health care team (in a hospitalized patient with type 1 DM) may precipitate DKA. Patients using insulin-infusion devices with short-acting insulin may develop DKA, because even a brief interruption in insulin delivery (e.g., mechanical malfunction) quickly leads to insulin deficiency.

Laboratory abnormalities and diagnosis

The timely diagnosis of DKA is crucial and allows for prompt initiation of therapy. DKA is characterized by hyperglycemia, ketosis, and metabolic acidosis (increased anion gap) along with a number of secondary metabolic derangements (Table 24-6). Occasionally, the serum glucose is only minimally elevated. Serum bicarbonate is frequently <10 mmol/L, and arterial pH ranges between 6.8 and 7.3, depending on the severity of the acidosis. Despite a total-body potassium deficit, the serum potassium at presentation may be mildly elevated, secondary to the acidosis. Total-body stores of sodium, chloride, phosphorus, and magnesium are reduced in DKA but are not accurately reflected by their levels in the serum because of hypovolemia and hyperglycemia. Elevated blood urea nitrogen (BUN) and serum creatinine levels reflect intravascular volume depletion. Interference from acetoacetate may falsely elevate the serum creatinine measurement. Leukocytosis, hypertriglyceridemia, and hyperlipoproteinemia are commonly found as well. Hyperamylasemia may suggest a diagnosis of pancreatitis, especially when accompanied by abdominal pain. However, in DKA the amylase is usually of salivary origin and thus is not diagnostic of pancreatitis. Serum lipase should be obtained if pancreatitis is suspected.

The measured serum sodium is reduced as a consequence of the hyperglycemia (1.6-mmol/L [1.6-meq] reduction in serum sodium for each 5.6-mmol/L [100-mg/dL] rise in the serum glucose). A normal serum sodium in the setting of DKA indicates a more profound water deficit. In "conventional" units, the calculated serum osmolality ($2 \times$ [serum sodium + serum potassium] + plasma glucose [mg/dL]/18 + BUN/2.8) is mildly to moderately elevated, although to a lesser degree than that found in HHS (see below).

In DKA, the ketone body, β-hydroxybutyrate, is synthesized at a threefold greater rate than acetoacetate; however, acetoacetate is preferentially detected by a commonly used ketosis detection reagent (nitroprusside). Serum ketones are present at significant levels (usually positive at serum dilution of ≥1:8). The nitroprusside tablet, or stick, is often used to detect urine ketones; certain medications such as captopril or penicillamine may cause false-positive reactions. Serum or plasma assays for β-hydroxybutyrate are preferred because they more accurately reflect the true ketone body level.

The metabolic derangements of DKA exist along a spectrum, beginning with mild acidosis with moderate hyperglycemia evolving into more severe findings. The degree of acidosis and hyperglycemia do not necessarily correlate closely because a variety of factors determine the level of hyperglycemia (oral intake, urinary glucose loss). Ketonemia is a consistent finding in DKA and distinguishes it from simple hyperglycemia. The differential diagnosis of DKA includes starvation ketosis, alcoholic ketoacidosis (bicarbonate usually >15 meq/L), and other forms of increased anion-gap acidosis.

TREATMENT Diabetic Ketoacidosis

The management of DKA is outlined in Table 24-8. After initiating IV fluid replacement and insulin therapy, the agent or event that precipitated the episode of DKA should be sought and aggressively treated. If the patient is vomiting or has altered mental status, a nasogastric tube should be inserted to prevent aspiration of gastric contents. Central to successful treatment of DKA is careful monitoring and frequent reassessment to ensure that the patient and the metabolic derangements are improving. A comprehensive flow sheet should record chronologic changes in vital signs, fluid intake and output, and laboratory values as a function of insulin administered.

After the initial bolus of normal saline, replacement of the sodium and free water deficit is carried out over the next 24 h (fluid deficit is often 3–5 L). When hemodynamic stability and adequate urine output are achieved, IV fluids should be switched to 0.45% saline depending on the calculated volume deficit. The change to 0.45% saline helps to reduce the trend toward hyperchloremia later in the course of DKA. Alternatively, initial use of lactated Ringer's IV solution may reduce the hyperchloremia that commonly occurs with normal saline.

A bolus of IV (0.1 units/kg) short-acting insulin should be administered immediately (Table 24-8), and subsequent treatment should provide continuous and adequate levels of circulating insulin. IV administration is preferred (0.1 units/kg of regular insulin per hour) because it ensures rapid distribution and allows adjustment of the infusion rate as the patient responds to therapy. In mild episodes of DKA, short-acting insulin can be used SC. IV insulin should be continued until the acidosis resolves and the patient is metabolically stable. As the acidosis and insulin resistance associated with DKA resolve, the insulin infusion rate can be decreased (to 0.05–0.1 units/kg per hour). Long-acting insulin, in combination with SC short-acting insulin, should be administered as soon as the patient resumes eating, because this facilitates transition to an outpatient insulin regimen and reduces length of hospital stay. It is crucial to continue the insulin infusion until adequate insulin levels are achieved by administering long-acting insulin by the SC route. Even

TABLE 24-8

MANAGEMENT OF DIABETIC KETOACIDOSIS

1. Confirm diagnosis (↑ plasma glucose, positive serum ketones, metabolic acidosis).
2. Admit to hospital; intensive care setting may be necessary for frequent monitoring or if pH <7.00 or unconscious.
3. Assess:
   Serum electrolytes (K^+, Na^+, Mg^{2+}, Cl^-, bicarbonate, phosphate)
   Acid-base status—pH, HCO_3^-, Pco_2, β-hydroxybutyrate
   Renal function (creatinine, urine output)
4. Replace fluids: 2–3 L of 0.9% saline over first 1–3 h (10–20 mL/kg per hour); subsequently, 0.45% saline at 250–500 mL/h; change to 5% glucose and 0.45% saline at 150–250 mL/h when plasma glucose reaches 250 mg/dL (13.9 mmol/L).
5. Administer short-acting insulin: IV (0.1 units/kg), then 0.1 units/kg per hour by continuous IV infusion; increase two- to threefold if no response by 2–4 h. If the initial serum potassium is <3.3 mmol/L (3.3 meq/L), do not administer insulin until the potassium is corrected.
6. Assess patient: What precipitated the episode (noncompliance, infection, trauma, pregnancy, infarction, cocaine)? Initiate appropriate workup for precipitating event (cultures, CXR, ECG).
7. Measure capillary glucose every 1–2 h; measure electrolytes (especially K^+, bicarbonate, phosphate) and anion gap every 4 h for first 24 h.
8. Monitor blood pressure, pulse, respirations, mental status, fluid intake and output every 1–4 h.
9. Replace K^+: 10 meq/h when plasma K^+ <5.0–5.2 meq/L (or 20–30 meq/L of infusion fluid), ECG normal, urine flow and normal creatinine documented; administer 40–80 meq/h when plasma K^+ <3.5 meq/L or if bicarbonate is given. If initial serum potassium is >5.2 mmol/L (5.2 meq/L), do not supplement K^+ until the potassium is corrected.
10. See text about bicarbonate or phosphate supplementation.
11. Continue above until patient is stable, glucose goal is 8.3–13.9 mmol/L (150–250 mg/dL), and acidosis is resolved. Insulin infusion may be decreased to 0.05–0.1 units/kg per hour.
12. Administer long-acting insulin as soon as patient is eating. Allow for a 2–4 hour overlap in insulin infusion and SC insulin injection.

Abbreviations: CXR, chest x-ray; ECG, electrocardiogram.
Source: Adapted from M Sperling, in Therapy for Diabetes Mellitus and Related Disorders, American Diabetes Association, Alexandria, VA, 1998; and AE Kitabchi et al: Diabetes Care 32:1335, 2009.

relatively brief periods of inadequate insulin administration in this transition phase may result in DKA relapse.

Hyperglycemia usually improves at a rate of 4.2–5.6 mmol/L (75–100 mg/dL) per hour as a result of insulin-mediated glucose disposal, reduced hepatic glucose release, and rehydration. The latter reduces catecholamines, increases urinary glucose loss, and expands the intravascular volume. The decline in the plasma glucose within the first 1–2 h may be more rapid and is mostly related to volume expansion. When the plasma glucose reaches 13.9 mmol/L (250 mg/dL), glucose should be added to the 0.45% saline infusion to maintain the plasma glucose in the 8.3–13.9 mmol/L (150–250 mg/dL) range, and the insulin infusion should be continued. Ketoacidosis begins to resolve as insulin reduces lipolysis, increases peripheral ketone body use, suppresses hepatic ketone body formation, and promotes bicarbonate regeneration. However, the acidosis and ketosis resolve more slowly than hyperglycemia. As ketoacidosis improves, β-hydroxybutyrate is converted to acetoacetate. Ketone body levels may appear to increase if measured by laboratory assays that use the nitroprusside reaction, which only detects acetoacetate and acetone. The improvement in acidosis and anion gap, a result of bicarbonate regeneration and decline in ketone bodies, is reflected by a rise in the serum bicarbonate level and the arterial pH. Depending on the rise of serum chloride, the anion gap (but not bicarbonate) will normalize. A hyperchloremic acidosis (serum bicarbonate of 15–18 mmol/L [15–18 meq/L]) often follows successful treatment and gradually resolves as the kidneys regenerate bicarbonate and excrete chloride.

Potassium stores are depleted in DKA (estimated deficit 3–5 mmol/kg [3–5 meq/kg]). During treatment with insulin and fluids, various factors contribute to the development of hypokalemia. These include insulin-mediated potassium transport into cells, resolution of the acidosis (which also promotes potassium entry into cells), and urinary loss of potassium salts of organic acids. Thus, potassium repletion should commence as soon as adequate urine output and a normal serum potassium are documented. If the initial serum potassium level is elevated, then potassium repletion should be delayed until the potassium falls into the normal range. Inclusion of 20–40 meq of potassium in each liter of IV fluid is reasonable, but additional potassium supplements may also be required. To reduce the amount of chloride administered, potassium phosphate or acetate can be substituted for the chloride salt. The goal is to maintain the serum potassium at >3.5 mmol/L (3.5 meq/L).

Despite a bicarbonate deficit, bicarbonate replacement is not usually necessary. In fact, theoretical arguments suggest that bicarbonate administration and rapid reversal of acidosis may impair cardiac function, reduce tissue oxygenation, and promote hypokalemia. The results of most clinical trials do not support the routine use of bicarbonate replacement, and one study in children found that bicarbonate use was associated with an increased risk of cerebral edema. However, in the presence of severe acidosis (arterial pH <7.0), the ADA advises bicarbonate (50 mmol [meq/L] of sodium bicarbonate in 200 mL of sterile water with 10 meq/L KCl per hour for 2 h until the pH is >7.0). Hypophosphatemia may result from increased glucose usage, but randomized clinical trials have not demonstrated that phosphate replacement is beneficial in DKA. If the serum phosphate is <0.32 mmol/L (1 mg/dL), then phosphate supplement should be considered and the serum calcium monitored. Hypomagnesemia may develop during DKA therapy and may also require supplementation.

With appropriate therapy, the mortality rate of DKA is low (<1%) and is related more to the underlying or precipitating event, such as infection or myocardial infarction. Venous thrombosis, upper gastrointestinal bleeding, and acute respiratory distress syndrome occasionally complicate DKA. The major nonmetabolic complication of DKA therapy is cerebral edema, which most often develops in children as DKA is resolving. The etiology of and optimal therapy for cerebral edema are not well established, but overreplacement of free water should be avoided.

Following treatment, the physician and patient should review the sequence of events that led to DKA to prevent future recurrences. Foremost is patient education about the symptoms of DKA, its precipitating factors, and the management of diabetes during a concurrent illness. During illness or when oral intake is compromised, patients should (1) frequently measure the capillary blood glucose; (2) measure urinary ketones when the serum glucose is >16.5 mmol/L (300 mg/dL); (3) drink fluids to maintain hydration; (4) continue or increase insulin; and (5) seek medical attention if dehydration, persistent vomiting, or uncontrolled hyperglycemia develop. Using these strategies, early DKA can be prevented or detected and treated appropriately on an outpatient basis.

HYPERGLYCEMIC HYPEROSMOLAR STATE

Clinical features

The prototypical patient with HHS is an elderly individual with type 2 DM, with a several-week history of polyuria, weight loss, and diminished oral intake that culminates in mental confusion, lethargy, or coma. The physical examination reflects profound dehydration and hyperosmolality and reveals hypotension, tachycardia, and altered mental status. Notably absent are symptoms of nausea, vomiting, and abdominal pain and the Kussmaul respirations characteristic of DKA. HHS is often precipitated by a serious, concurrent illness such as myocardial infarction or stroke. Sepsis, pneumonia, and other serious infections are frequent precipitants and should be sought. In addition, a debilitating condition (prior stroke or dementia) or social situation that compromises water intake usually contributes to the development of the disorder.

Pathophysiology

Relative insulin deficiency and inadequate fluid intake are the underlying causes of HHS. Insulin deficiency increases hepatic glucose production (through glycogenolysis and gluconeogenesis) and impairs glucose utilization in skeletal muscle (see above discussion of DKA). Hyperglycemia induces an osmotic diuresis that leads to intravascular volume depletion, which is exacerbated by inadequate fluid replacement. The absence of ketosis in HHS is not understood. Presumably, the insulin deficiency is only relative and less severe than in DKA. Lower levels of counterregulatory hormones and free fatty acids have been found in HHS than in DKA in some studies. It is also possible that the liver is less capable of ketone body synthesis or that the insulin/glucagon ratio does not favor ketogenesis.

Laboratory abnormalities and diagnosis

The laboratory features in HHS are summarized in Table 24-6. Most notable are the marked hyperglycemia (plasma glucose may be >55.5 mmol/L [1000 mg/dL]), hyperosmolality (>350 mosmol/L), and prerenal azotemia. The measured serum sodium may be normal or slightly low despite the marked hyperglycemia. The corrected serum sodium is usually increased (add 1.6 meq to measured sodium for each 5.6-mmol/L [100-mg/dL] rise in the serum glucose). In contrast to DKA, acidosis and ketonemia are absent or mild. A small anion-gap metabolic acidosis may be present secondary to increased lactic acid. Moderate ketonuria, if present, is secondary to starvation.

TREATMENT Hyperglycemic Hyperosmolar State

Volume depletion and hyperglycemia are prominent features of both HHS and DKA. Consequently, therapy of these disorders shares several elements (Table 24-8). In both disorders, careful monitoring of the patient's fluid status, laboratory values, and insulin infusion rate is crucial. Underlying or precipitating problems should be aggressively sought and treated. In HHS, fluid losses and dehydration are usually more pronounced than in DKA due to the longer duration of the illness. The patient with HHS is usually older, more likely to have mental status changes, and more likely to have a life-threatening precipitating event with accompanying comorbidities. Even with proper treatment, HHS has a substantially higher mortality rate than DKA (up to 15% in some clinical series).

Fluid replacement should initially stabilize the hemodynamic status of the patient (1–3 L of 0.9% normal saline over the first 2–3 h). Because the fluid deficit in HHS is accumulated over a period of days to weeks, the rapidity of reversal of the hyperosmolar state must balance the need for free water repletion with the risk that too rapid a reversal may worsen neurologic function. If the serum sodium is >150 mmol/L (150 meq/L), 0.45% saline should be used. After hemodynamic stability is achieved, the IV fluid administration is directed at reversing the free water deficit using hypotonic fluids (0.45% saline initially, then 5% dextrose in water [D_5W]). The calculated free water deficit (which averages 9–10 L) should be reversed over the next 1–2 days (infusion rates of 200–300 mL/h of hypotonic solution). Potassium repletion is usually necessary and should be dictated by repeated measurements of the serum potassium. In patients taking diuretics, the potassium deficit can be quite large and may be accompanied by magnesium deficiency. Hypophosphatemia may occur during therapy and can be improved by using KPO_4 and beginning nutrition.

As in DKA, rehydration and volume expansion lower the plasma glucose initially, but insulin is also required. A reasonable regimen for HHS begins with an IV insulin bolus of 0.1 unit/kg followed by IV insulin at a constant infusion rate of 0.1 unit/kg per hour. If the serum glucose does not fall, increase the insulin infusion rate by twofold. As in DKA, glucose should be added to IV fluid when the plasma glucose falls to 13.9 mmol/L (250 mg/dL), and the insulin infusion rate should be decreased to 0.05–0.1 unit/kg per hour. The insulin infusion should be continued until the patient has resumed eating and can be transferred to a SC insulin regimen. The patient should be discharged from the hospital on insulin, although some patients can later switch to oral glucose-lowering agents.

MANAGEMENT OF DIABETES IN A HOSPITALIZED PATIENT

Virtually all medical and surgical subspecialties are involved in the care of hospitalized patients with diabetes. Hyperglycemia, whether in a patient with known diabetes or in someone without known diabetes, appears to be a predictor of poor outcome in hospitalized patients. General anesthesia, surgery, infection, or concurrent illness raises the levels of counterregulatory hormones (cortisol, growth hormone, catecholamines, and glucagon) and cytokines that may lead to transient insulin resistance and hyperglycemia. These factors increase insulin requirements by increasing glucose production and impairing glucose utilization and thus may worsen glycemic control. The concurrent illness or surgical procedure may lead to variable insulin absorption and also prevent the patient with DM from eating normally and, thus, may promote hypoglycemia. Glycemic control should be assessed on admission using the HbA_{1c}. Electrolytes, renal function, and intravascular volume status should be assessed as well. The high prevalence of CVD in individuals with DM (especially in type 2 DM) may necessitate preoperative cardiovascular evaluation **(Chap. 25)**.

The goals of diabetes management during hospitalization are near-normoglycemia, avoidance of hypoglycemia, and transition back to the outpatient diabetes treatment regimen. Upon hospital admission, frequent glycemic monitoring should begin, as should planning for diabetes management after discharge. Glycemic control appears to improve the clinical outcomes in a variety of settings, but optimal glycemic goals for the hospitalized patient are incompletely defined. In a number of cross-sectional studies of patients with diabetes, a greater degree of hyperglycemia was associated with worse cardiac, neurologic, and infectious outcomes. In some studies, patients who do not have preexisting diabetes but who develop modest blood glucose elevations during their hospitalization appear to benefit from achieving near-normoglycemia using insulin treatment. However, a large randomized clinical trial (Normoglycemia in Intensive Care Evaluation Survival Using Glucose Algorithm Regulation [NICE-SUGAR]) of individuals in the ICU (most of whom were receiving mechanical ventilation) found an increased mortality rate and a greater number of episodes of severe hypoglycemia with very strict glycemic control (target blood glucose of 4.5–6 mmol/L or 81–108 mg/dL) compared to individuals with a more moderate glycemic goal (mean blood glucose of 8 mmol/L or 144 mg/dL). Currently, most data suggest that very strict blood glucose control in acutely ill patients likely worsens outcomes and increases the frequency of hypoglycemia. The ADA suggests the following glycemic goals for hospitalized patients: (1) in critically ill patients: glucose of 7.8–10.0 mmol/L or 140–180 mg/dL; (2) in non–critically ill patients: premeal glucose <7.8 mmol/L (140 mg/dL) and at other times blood glucose <10 mmol/L (180 mg/dL).

Critical aspects for optimal diabetes care in the hospital include the following. (1) A hospital system approach to treatment of hyperglycemia and prevention of hypoglycemia is needed. Inpatient diabetes management teams consisting of nurse practitioners and physicians are increasingly common. (2) Diabetes treatment plans should focus on the transition from the ICU and the transition from the inpatient to outpatient setting. (3) Adjustment of the discharge treatment regimen of patients whose diabetes was poorly controlled on admission (as reflected by the HbA_{1c}) is necessary.

The physician caring for an individual with diabetes in the perioperative period, during times of infection or serious physical illness, or simply when the patient is fasting for a diagnostic procedure must monitor the plasma glucose vigilantly, adjust the diabetes treatment regimen, and provide glucose infusion as needed. Hypoglycemia is frequent in hospitalized patients, and many of these episodes are avoidable. Hospital systems should have a diabetes management protocol to avoid inpatient hypoglycemia. Measures to reduce or prevent hypoglycemia include frequent glucose monitoring and anticipating potential modifications of insulin/glucose administration because of changes in the clinical situation or treatment (e.g., tapering of glucocorticoids) or interruption of enteral or parenteral infusions or PO intake.

Depending on the severity of the patient's illness and the hospital setting, the physician can use either an insulin infusion or SC insulin. Insulin infusions are preferred in the ICU or in a clinically unstable setting. The absorption of SC insulin may be variable in such situations. Insulin infusions can also effectively control plasma glucose in the perioperative period and when the patient is unable to take anything by mouth. Regular insulin is used rather than insulin analogues for IV insulin infusion because it is less expensive and equally effective. The physician must consider carefully the clinical setting in which an insulin infusion will be used, including whether adequate ancillary personnel are available to monitor the plasma glucose frequently and whether they can adjust the insulin infusion rate to maintain the plasma glucose within the optimal range. Insulin-infusion algorithms should integrate the insulin sensitivity of the patient, frequent blood glucose monitoring, and the trend of changes in the blood glucose to determine the insulin-infusion rate. Insulin-infusion algorithms jointly developed and implemented by nursing and physician staff are advised. Because of the short half-life of IV regular insulin, it is necessary to administer long-acting insulin prior to discontinuation of the insulin infusion (2–4 h before the infusion is stopped) to avoid a period of insulin deficiency.

In patients who are not critically ill or not in the ICU, basal or "scheduled" insulin is provided by SC, long-acting insulin supplemented by prandial and/or "corrective" insulin using a short-acting insulin (insulin analogues preferred). The use of "sliding scale," short-acting insulin alone, where no insulin is given unless the blood glucose is elevated, is inadequate for inpatient glucose management and should not be used. The short-acting, preprandial insulin dose should include coverage for food consumption (based on anticipated carbohydrate intake) plus a corrective or supplemental insulin based on the patient's insulin sensitivity and the blood glucose. For example, if the patient is thin (and likely insulin-sensitive), a corrective insulin supplement might be 1 unit for each 2.7 mmol/L (50 mg/dL) over the glucose target. If the patient is obese and insulin-resistant, then the insulin supplement might be 2 units for each 2.7 mmol/L (50 mg/dL) over the glucose target. It is critical to individualize the regimen and adjust the basal or "scheduled" insulin dose frequently, based on the corrective insulin required. A consistent carbohydrate diabetes meal plan for hospitalized patients provides a predictable amount of carbohydrate for a particular meal each day (but not necessarily the same amount for breakfast, lunch, and supper). The hospital diet should be determined by a nutritionist; terms such as *ADA diet* or *low-sugar diet* are no longer used.

Individuals with type 1 DM who are undergoing general anesthesia and surgery or who are seriously ill should receive continuous insulin, either through an IV insulin infusion or by SC administration of a reduced dose of long-acting insulin. Short-acting insulin alone is insufficient. Prolongation of a surgical procedure or delay in the recovery room is not uncommon and may result in periods of insulin deficiency leading to DKA. Insulin infusion is the preferred method for managing patients with type 1 DM in the perioperative period or when serious concurrent illness is present (0.5–1.0 units/h of regular insulin). If the diagnostic or surgical procedure is brief and performed under local or regional anesthesia, a reduced dose of SC, long-acting insulin may suffice (30–50% reduction, with short-acting insulin withheld or reduced). This approach facilitates the transition back to long-acting insulin after the procedure. Glucose may be infused to prevent hypoglycemia. The blood glucose should be monitored frequently during the illness or in the perioperative period.

Individuals with type 2 DM can be managed with either an insulin infusion or SC long-acting insulin (25–50% reduction depending on clinical setting) plus preprandial, short-acting insulin. Oral glucose-lowering agents should be discontinued upon admission and are not useful in regulating the plasma glucose in clinical situations where the insulin requirements and glucose intake are changing rapidly. Moreover, these oral agents may be dangerous if the patient is fasting (e.g., hypoglycemia with sulfonylureas). Metformin should be withheld when radiographic contrast media will be given or if unstable CHF, acidosis, or declining renal function is present.

SPECIAL CONSIDERATIONS IN DIABETES MELLITUS

TOTAL PARENTERAL NUTRITION

Total parenteral nutrition (TPN) greatly increases insulin requirements. In addition, individuals not previously known to have DM may become hyperglycemic during TPN and require insulin treatment. IV insulin infusion is the preferred treatment for hyperglycemia, and rapid titration to the required insulin dose is done most efficiently using a separate insulin infusion. After the total insulin dose has been determined, insulin may be added directly to the TPN solution or, preferably, given as a separate infusion or subcutaneously. Often, individuals receiving either TPN or enteral nutrition receive their caloric loads continuously and not at "meal times"; consequently, SC insulin regimens must be adjusted.

GLUCOCORTICOIDS

Glucocorticoids increase insulin resistance, decrease glucose utilization, increase hepatic glucose production, and impair insulin secretion. These changes lead to a worsening of glycemic control in individuals with DM and may precipitate diabetes in other individuals ("steroid-induced diabetes"). The effects of glucocorticoids on glucose homeostasis are dose-related, usually reversible, and most pronounced in the postprandial period. If the FPG is near the normal range, oral diabetes agents (e.g., sulfonylureas, metformin) may be sufficient to reduce hyperglycemia. If the FPG is >11.1 mmol/L (200 mg/dL), oral agents are usually not efficacious and insulin therapy is required. Short-acting insulin may be required to supplement long-acting insulin in order to control postprandial glucose excursions.

REPRODUCTIVE ISSUES

Reproductive capacity in either men or women with DM appears to be normal. Menstrual cycles may be associated with alterations in glycemic control in women with DM. Pregnancy is associated with marked insulin resistance; the increased insulin requirements often precipitate DM and lead to the diagnosis of gestational diabetes mellitus (GDM). Glucose, which at high levels is a teratogen to the developing fetus, readily crosses the placenta, but insulin does not. Thus, hyperglycemia from the maternal circulation may stimulate insulin secretion in the fetus. The anabolic and growth effects of insulin may result in macrosomia. GDM complicates ~7% (range 1–14%) of pregnancies. The incidence of GDM is greatly increased in certain ethnic groups, including African Americans and Latinas, consistent with a similar increased risk of type 2 DM. Current recommendations advise screening for glucose intolerance between weeks 24 and 28 of pregnancy in women with increased risk for GDM (≥25 years; obesity; family history of DM; member of an ethnic group such as Latina, Native American, Asian American, African American, or Pacific Islander). Therapy for GDM is similar to that for individuals with pregnancy-associated diabetes and involves MNT and insulin, if hyperglycemia persists. Oral glucose-lowering agents are not approved for use during pregnancy, but studies using metformin or glyburide have shown efficacy and have not found toxicity. However, many physicians use insulin to treat GDM. With current practices, the morbidity and mortality rates of the mother with GDM and the fetus are not different from those in the nondiabetic population. Individuals who develop GDM are at marked increased risk for developing type 2 DM in the future and should be screened periodically for DM. Most individuals with GDM revert to normal glucose tolerance after delivery, but some will continue to have overt diabetes or impairment of glucose tolerance after delivery. In addition, children of women with GDM appear to be at risk for obesity and glucose intolerance and have an increased risk of diabetes beginning in the later stages of adolescence.

Pregnancy in individuals with known DM requires meticulous planning and adherence to strict treatment regimens. Intensive diabetes management and normalization of the HbA_{1c} are essential for individuals with existing DM who are planning pregnancy. The most crucial period of glycemic control is soon after fertilization. The risk of fetal malformations is increased 4–10 times in individuals with uncontrolled DM at the time of conception, and normal plasma glucose during the preconception period and throughout the periods of organ development in the fetus should be the goal.

LIPODYSTROPHIC DM

Lipodystrophy, or the loss of subcutaneous fat tissue, may be generalized in certain genetic conditions such as leprechaunism. Generalized lipodystrophy is associated with severe insulin resistance and is often accompanied by acanthosis nigricans and dyslipidemia. Localized lipodystrophy associated with insulin injections has been reduced considerably by the use of human insulin.

Protease inhibitors and lipodystrophy

Protease inhibitors used in the treatment of HIV disease have been associated with a centripetal accumulation of fat (visceral and abdominal area), accumulation of fat in the dorsocervical region, loss of extremity fat, decreased insulin sensitivity (elevations of the fasting insulin level and reduced glucose tolerance on IV glucose tolerance testing), and dyslipidemia. Although many aspects of the physical appearance of these individuals resemble Cushing's syndrome, increased cortisol levels do not account for this appearance. The possibility remains that this is related to HIV infection by some undefined mechanism, because some features of the syndrome were observed before the introduction of protease inhibitors. Therapy for HIV-related lipodystrophy is not well established.

CHAPTER 25

DIABETES MELLITUS: COMPLICATIONS

Alvin C. Powers

Diabetes-related complications affect many organ systems and are responsible for the majority of morbidity and mortality associated with the disease. Strikingly, in the United States, diabetes is the leading cause of new blindness in adults, renal failure, and nontraumatic lower extremity amputation. Diabetes-related complications usually do not appear until the second decade of hyperglycemia. Because type 2 diabetes mellitus (DM) often has a long asymptomatic period of hyperglycemia before diagnosis, many individuals with type 2 DM have complications at the time of diagnosis. Fortunately, many of the diabetes-related complications can be prevented or delayed with early detection, aggressive glycemic control, and efforts to minimize the risks of complications.

Diabetes-related complications can be divided into vascular and nonvascular complications and are similar for type 1 and type 2 DM (Table 25-1). The vascular complications of DM are further subdivided into microvascular (retinopathy, neuropathy, nephropathy) and macrovascular complications (coronary heart disease [CHD], peripheral arterial disease [PAD], cerebrovascular disease). Microvascular complications are diabetes-specific, whereas macrovascular complications are similar to those in nondiabetics but occur at greater frequency in individuals with diabetes. Nonvascular complications include gastroparesis, infections, skin changes, and hearing loss. Whether type 2 DM increases the risk of dementia or impaired cognitive function is not clear.

GLYCEMIC CONTROL AND COMPLICATIONS

The microvascular complications of both type 1 and type 2 DM result from chronic hyperglycemia (Fig. 25-1). Evidence implicating a causative role for chronic hyperglycemia in the development of macrovascular complications is less conclusive. CHD events and mortality rate are two to four times greater in patients with type 2 DM and correlate with fasting and postprandial plasma glucose levels as well the hemoglobin A_{1c} (HbA_{1c}). Other factors such as dyslipidemia and hypertension also play important roles in macrovascular complications.

The Diabetes Control and Complications Trial (DCCT) provided definitive proof that reduction in chronic hyperglycemia can prevent many complications of type 1 DM (Fig. 25-1). This large multicenter clinical trial randomized more than 1400 individuals with type 1 DM to either intensive or conventional diabetes management and prospectively evaluated the development of diabetes-related complications during a mean follow-up of 6.5 years. Individuals in the intensive diabetes management group received multiple administrations of insulin each day (injection or pump) along with extensive educational, psychological, and medical support. Individuals in the conventional diabetes management group received twice-daily insulin injections and quarterly nutritional, educational, and clinical evaluation. The goal in the former group was normoglycemia; the goal in the latter group was prevention of symptoms of diabetes. Individuals in the intensive diabetes management group achieved a substantially lower HbA_{1c} (7.3%) than individuals in the conventional diabetes management group (9.1%). After the DCCT results were reported in 1993, study participants continue to be followed in the Epidemiology of Diabetes Intervention and Complications (EDIC) trial, which recently completed 30 years of follow-up (DCCT + EDIC). At the end of the DCCT phase, study participants in both intensive and conventional arms were offered intensive therapy. However, during the subsequent follow-up of more than 18 years, the initial separation in glycemic control disappeared with both arms maintaining a mean HbA_{1c} of 8.0%.

The DCCT phase demonstrated that improvement of glycemic control reduced nonproliferative and proliferative retinopathy (47% reduction), microalbuminuria

TABLE 25-1

DIABETES-RELATED COMPLICATIONS
Microvascular
Eye disease
Retinopathy (nonproliferative/proliferative)
Macular edema
Neuropathy
Sensory and motor (mono- and polyneuropathy)
Autonomic
Nephropathy (albuminuria and declining renal function)
Macrovascular
Coronary heart disease
Peripheral arterial disease
Cerebrovascular disease
Other
Gastrointestinal (gastroparesis, diarrhea)
Genitourinary (uropathy/sexual dysfunction)
Dermatologic
Infectious
Cataracts
Glaucoma
Cheiroarthropathy[a]
Periodontal disease
Hearing loss
Other comorbid conditions associated with diabetes (relationship to hyperglycemia is uncertain): depression, obstructive sleep apnea, fatty liver disease, hip fracture, osteoporosis (in type 1 diabetes), cognitive impairment or dementia, low testosterone in men

[a]Thickened skin and reduced joint mobility.

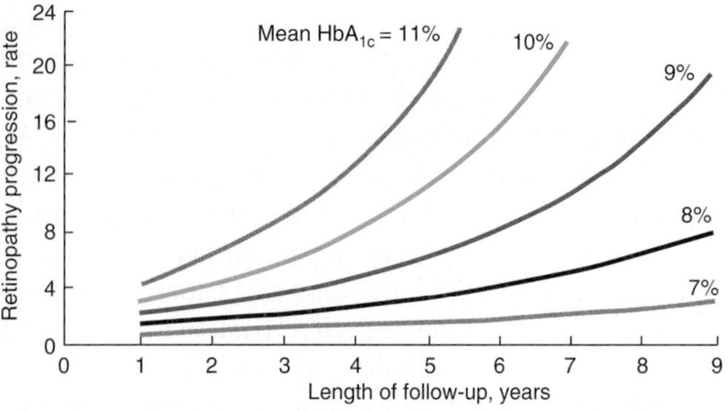

FIGURE 25-1

Relationship of glycemic control and diabetes duration to diabetic retinopathy. The progression of retinopathy in individuals in the Diabetes Control and Complications Trial is graphed as a function of the length of follow-up with different curves for different hemoglobin A_{1c} (HbA_{1c}) values. *(Adapted from The Diabetes Control and Complications Trial Research Group: Diabetes 44:968, 1995.)*

(39% reduction), clinical nephropathy (54% reduction), and neuropathy (60% reduction). Improved glycemic control also slowed the progression of early diabetic complications. During the DCCT phase, weight gain (4.6 kg) and severe hypoglycemia (requiring assistance of another person to treat) were more common in the intensive therapy group. The benefits of an improvement in glycemic control occurred over the entire range of HbA_{1c} values **(Fig. 25-1)**, indicating that at any HbA_{1c} level, an improvement in glycemic control is beneficial. The results of the DCCT predicted that individuals in the intensive diabetes management group would gain 7.7 additional years of vision, 5.8 additional years free from end-stage renal disease (ESRD), and 5.6 years free from lower extremity amputations. If all complications of DM were combined, individuals in the intensive diabetes management group would experience 15.3 more years of life without significant microvascular or neurologic complications of DM, compared to individuals who received standard therapy. This translates into an additional 5.1 years of life expectancy for individuals in the intensive diabetes management group. The 30-year follow-up data in the intensively treated group show a continued reduction in retinopathy, nephropathy, and cardiovascular disease. For example, individuals in the intensive therapy group had a 42–57% reduction in cardiovascular events (nonfatal myocardial infarction [MI], stroke, or death from a cardiovascular event) at a mean follow-up of 17 years, even though their subsequent glycemic control was the same as those in the conventional diabetes management group from years 6.5–17. During the EDIC phase, less than 1% of the cohort had become blind, lost a limb to amputation, or required dialysis.

The United Kingdom Prospective Diabetes Study (UKPDS) studied the course of >5000 individuals with type 2 DM for >10 years. This study used multiple treatment regimens and monitored the effect of intensive glycemic control and risk factor treatment on the development of diabetic complications. Newly diagnosed individuals with type 2 DM were randomized to (1) intensive management using various combinations of insulin, a sulfonylurea, or metformin or (2) conventional therapy using dietary modification and pharmacotherapy with the goal of symptom prevention. In addition, individuals were randomly assigned to different antihypertensive regimens. Individuals in the intensive treatment arm achieved an HbA_{1c} of 7%, compared to a 7.9% HbA_{1c} in the standard treatment group. The UKPDS demonstrated that each percentage point reduction in HbA_{1c} was associated with a 35% reduction in microvascular complications. As in the DCCT, there was a continuous relationship between glycemic control and development of complications. Improved glycemic control also reduced the cardiovascular event rate in the follow-up period of >10 years.

One of the major findings of the UKPDS was that strict blood pressure control significantly reduced both macro- and microvascular complications. In fact, the beneficial effects of blood pressure control were greater than the beneficial effects of glycemic control. Lowering blood pressure to moderate goals (144/82 mmHg) reduced the risk of DM-related death, stroke, microvascular endpoints, retinopathy, and heart failure (risk reductions between 32 and 56%).

Similar reductions in the risks of retinopathy and nephropathy were also seen in a small trial of lean Japanese individuals with type 2 DM randomized to either intensive glycemic control or standard therapy with insulin (Kumamoto study). These results demonstrate the effectiveness of improved glycemic control in individuals of different ethnicity and, presumably, a different etiology of DM (i.e., phenotypically different from those in the DCCT and UKPDS). The Action to Control Cardiovascular Risk in Diabetes (ACCORD) and Action in Diabetes and Vascular Disease: Preterax and Diamicron MR Controlled Evaluation (ADVANCE) trials also found that improved glycemic control reduced microvascular complications.

Thus, these large clinical trials in type 1 and type 2 DM indicate that chronic hyperglycemia plays a causative role in the pathogenesis of diabetic microvascular complications. In both the DCCT and the UKPDS, cardiovascular events were reduced at follow-up of >10 years, even though the improved glycemic control was not maintained. The positive impact of a period of improved glycemic control on later disease has been termed a *legacy effect* or *metabolic memory*.

A summary of the features of diabetes-related complications includes the following. (1) Duration and degree of hyperglycemia correlate with complications. (2) Intensive glycemic control is beneficial in all forms of DM. (3) Blood pressure control is critical, especially in type 2 DM. (4) Survival in patients with type 1 DM is improving, and diabetes-related complications are declining. (5) Not all individuals with diabetes develop diabetes-related complications. Other incompletely defined factors appear to modulate the development of complications. For example, despite long-standing DM, some individuals never develop nephropathy or retinopathy. Many of these patients have glycemic control that is indistinguishable from those who develop microvascular complications, suggesting a genetic susceptibility for developing particular complications.

MECHANISMS OF COMPLICATIONS

Although chronic hyperglycemia is an important etiologic factor leading to complications of DM, the mechanism(s) by which it leads to such diverse cellular and organ dysfunction is unknown. An emerging hypothesis is that hyperglycemia leads to epigenetic changes that influence gene expression in affected cells. For example, this may explain the legacy effect or metabolic memory mentioned above.

Four theories, which are not mutually exclusive, on how hyperglycemia might lead to the chronic complications of DM include the following pathways. (1) Increased intracellular glucose leads to the formation of advanced glycosylation end products, which bind to a cell surface receptor, via the nonenzymatic glycosylation of intra- and extracellular proteins, leading to cross-linking of proteins, accelerated atherosclerosis, glomerular dysfunction, endothelial dysfunction, and altered extracellular matrix composition. (2) Hyperglycemia increases glucose metabolism via the sorbitol pathway related to the enzyme aldose reductase. However, testing of this theory in humans, using aldose reductase inhibitors, has not demonstrated beneficial effects. (3) Hyperglycemia increases the formation of diacylglycerol, leading to activation of protein kinase C, which alters the transcription of genes for fibronectin, type IV collagen, contractile proteins, and extracellular matrix proteins in endothelial cells and neurons. (4) Hyperglycemia increases the flux through the hexosamine pathway, which generates fructose-6-phosphate, a substrate for O-linked glycosylation and proteoglycan production, leading to altered function by glycosylation of proteins such as endothelial nitric oxide synthase or by changes in gene expression of transforming growth factor β (TGF-β) or plasminogen activator inhibitor-1.

Growth factors may play an important role in some diabetes-related complications, and their production is increased by most of these proposed pathways. Vascular endothelial growth factor A (VEGF-A) is increased locally in diabetic proliferative retinopathy and decreases after laser photocoagulation. TGF-β is increased in diabetic nephropathy and stimulates basement membrane production of collagen and fibronectin by mesangial cells. A possible unifying mechanism is that hyperglycemia leads to increased production of reactive oxygen species or superoxide in the mitochondria; these compounds may activate all four of the pathways described above. Although hyperglycemia serves as the initial trigger for complications of diabetes, it is still unknown whether the same pathophysiologic processes are operative in all complications or whether some pathways predominate in certain organs.

OPHTHALMOLOGIC COMPLICATIONS OF DIABETES MELLITUS

DM is the leading cause of blindness between the ages of 20 and 74 in the United States. The gravity of this problem is highlighted by the finding that individuals with DM are 25 times more likely to become legally blind than individuals without DM. Severe vision loss is primarily the result of progressive diabetic retinopathy

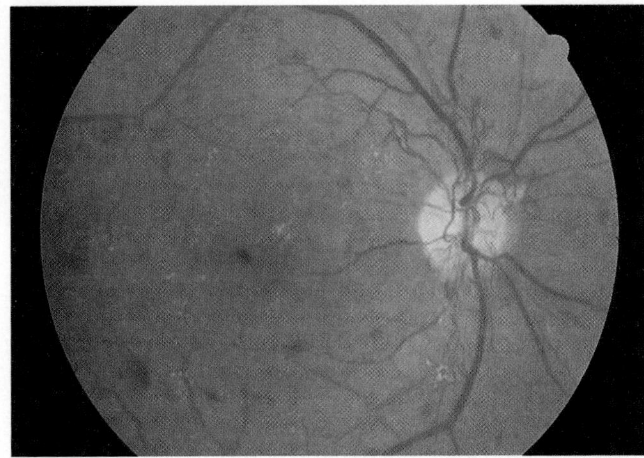

FIGURE 25-2
Diabetic retinopathy results in scattered hemorrhages, yellow exudates, and neovascularization. This patient has neovascular vessels proliferating from the optic disc, requiring urgent panretinal laser photocoagulation.

and clinically significant macular edema. Diabetic retinopathy is classified into two stages: nonproliferative and proliferative. Nonproliferative diabetic retinopathy usually appears late in the first decade or early in the second decade of the disease and is marked by retinal vascular microaneurysms, blot hemorrhages, and cotton-wool spots (Fig. 25-2). Mild nonproliferative retinopathy may progress to more extensive disease, characterized by changes in venous vessel caliber, intraretinal microvascular abnormalities, and more numerous microaneurysms and hemorrhages. The pathophysiologic mechanisms invoked in nonproliferative retinopathy include loss of retinal pericytes, increased retinal vascular permeability, alterations in retinal blood flow, and abnormal retinal microvasculature, all of which can lead to retinal ischemia. A new concept is that the pathology involves inflammatory processes in the retinal neurovascular unit, which consists of neurons, glia, astrocytes, Muüller cells, and specialized vasculature.

The appearance of neovascularization in response to retinal hypoxemia is the hallmark of proliferative diabetic retinopathy **(Fig. 25-2)**. These newly formed vessels appear near the optic nerve and/or macula and rupture easily, leading to vitreous hemorrhage, fibrosis, and ultimately retinal detachment. Not all individuals with nonproliferative retinopathy go on to develop proliferative retinopathy, but the more severe the nonproliferative disease, the greater the chance of evolution to proliferative retinopathy within 5 years. This creates an important opportunity for early detection and treatment of diabetic retinopathy. Clinically significant macular edema can occur in the context of nonproliferative or proliferative retinopathy. Fluorescein angiography and optical coherence tomography are useful to detect macular edema, which is associated with a 25% chance of moderate visual loss over the next 3 years. Duration of DM and degree of glycemic control are the best predictors of the development of retinopathy; hypertension and nephropathy are also risk factors. Nonproliferative retinopathy is found in many individuals who have had DM for >20 years. Although there is genetic susceptibility for retinopathy, it confers less influence than either the duration of DM or the degree of glycemic control.

TREATMENT Diabetic Retinopathy

The most effective therapy for diabetic retinopathy is prevention. Intensive glycemic and blood pressure control will delay the development or slow the progression of retinopathy in individuals with either type 1 or type 2 DM. Paradoxically, during the first 6–12 months of improved glycemic control, established diabetic retinopathy may transiently worsen. Fortunately, this progression is temporary, and in the long term, improved glycemic control is associated with less diabetic retinopathy. Individuals with known retinopathy may be candidates for prophylactic laser photocoagulation when initiating intensive therapy. Once advanced retinopathy is present, improved glycemic control imparts less benefit, although adequate ophthalmologic care can prevent most blindness.

Regular, comprehensive eye examinations are essential for all individuals with DM (see Table 24-1). Most diabetic eye disease can be successfully treated if detected early. Routine, nondilated eye examinations by the primary care provider or diabetes specialist are inadequate to detect diabetic eye disease, which requires an ophthalmologist for optimal care of these disorders. Laser photocoagulation is very successful in preserving vision. Proliferative retinopathy is usually treated with panretinal laser photocoagulation, whereas macular edema is treated with focal laser photocoagulation and anti-vascular endothelial growth factor therapy (ocular injection). Aspirin therapy (650 mg/d) does not appear to influence the natural history of diabetic retinopathy.

RENAL COMPLICATIONS OF DIABETES MELLITUS

Diabetic nephropathy is the leading cause of chronic kidney disease (CKD), ESRD, and CKD requiring renal replacement therapy. Furthermore, the prognosis of diabetic patients on dialysis is poor, with survival comparable to many forms of cancer. Albuminuria in individuals with DM is associated with an increased risk of cardiovascular disease. Individuals with diabetic nephropathy commonly have diabetic retinopathy.

Like other microvascular complications, the pathogenesis of diabetic nephropathy is related to chronic hyperglycemia. The mechanisms by which chronic hyperglycemia leads to diabetic nephropathy, although incompletely defined, involve the effects of soluble factors (growth factors, angiotensin II, endothelin, advanced glycation end products [AGEs]), hemodynamic alterations in the renal microcirculation (glomerular hyperfiltration or hyperperfusion, increased glomerular capillary pressure), and structural changes in the glomerulus (increased extracellular matrix, basement membrane thickening, mesangial expansion, fibrosis). Some of these effects may be mediated through angiotensin II receptors. Smoking accelerates the decline in renal function. Because only 20–40% of patients with diabetes develop diabetic nephropathy, additional genetic or environmental susceptibility factors remain unidentified. Known risk factors include race and a family history of diabetic nephropathy.

Diabetic nephropathy and ESRD secondary to DM develop more commonly in African Americans, Native Americans, and Hispanic individuals with diabetes.

The natural history of diabetic nephropathy is characterized by a fairly predictable sequence of events that was initially defined for individuals with type 1 DM but appears to be similar in type 2 DM (Fig. 25-3). Glomerular hyperperfusion and renal hypertrophy occur in the first years after the onset of DM and are associated with an increase of the glomerular filtration rate (GFR). During the first 5 years of DM, thickening of the glomerular basement membrane, glomerular hypertrophy, and mesangial volume expansion occur as the GFR returns to normal. After 5–10 years of type 1 DM, many individuals begin to excrete small amounts of albumin in the urine. The American Diabetes Association (ADA) recently suggested that the terms previously used to refer to increased urinary protein (microalbuminuria as defined as 30–299 mg/d in a 24-h collection or 30–299 μg/mg creatinine in a spot collection or macroalbuminuria as defined as >300 mg/24 h) be replaced by the phrases "persistent albuminuria (30–299 mg/24 h)" and "persistent albuminuria (≥300 mg/24 h)" to better reflect the continuous nature of albumin excretion in the urine as risk factor for nephropathy and cardiovascular disease (CVD). This chapter uses the terms *microalbuminuria* and *macroalbuminuria*. Although the appearance of microalbuminuria in type 1 DM is an important risk factor for progression to macroalbuminuria, only ~50% of individuals progress to macroalbuminuria over the next 10 years. In some individuals with type 1 diabetes and microalbuminuria of short duration, the microalbuminuria regresses. Microalbuminuria is also a risk factor for CVD. Once macroalbuminuria is present, there is a steady decline in GFR, and ~50% of individuals reach ESRD in 7–10 years. Once macroalbuminuria develops, blood pressure rises slightly and the pathologic changes are likely irreversible.

The nephropathy that develops in type 2 DM differs from that of type 1 DM in the following respects: (1) microalbuminuria or macroalbuminuria may be present when type 2 DM is diagnosed, reflecting its long asymptomatic period; (2) hypertension more commonly accompanies microalbuminuria or macroalbuminuria in type 2 DM; and (3) microalbuminuria may be less predictive of diabetic nephropathy and likelihood of progression to macroalbuminuria in type 2 DM, in large part due to increased CV mortality in this population. Finally, it should be noted that albuminuria in type 2 DM may be secondary to factors unrelated to DM, such as hypertension, congestive heart failure (CHF), prostate disease, or infection.

As part of comprehensive diabetes care **(Chap. 24)**, albuminuria should be detected at an early stage when effective therapies can be instituted. Because some individuals with type 1 or type 2 DM have a decline in GFR in the absence of albuminuria, annual measurement of the serum creatinine to estimate GFR should also be performed. An annual microalbuminuria measurement (albumin-to-creatinine ratio in spot urine) is advised in individuals with type 1 or type 2 DM (Fig. 25-4). The urine protein measurement in a routine urinalysis does not detect these low levels of albumin excretion. Screening for albuminuria should commence 5 years after the onset of type 1 DM and at the time of diagnosis of type 2 DM.

Type IV renal tubular acidosis (hyporeninemic hypoaldosteronism) may occur in type 1 or 2 DM.

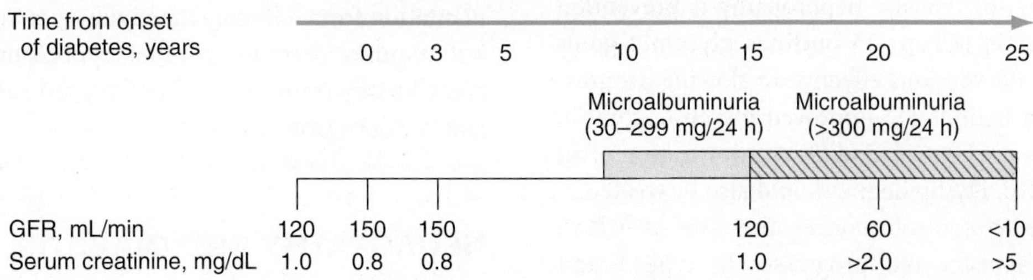

FIGURE 25-3

Time course of development of diabetic nephropathy. The relationship of time from onset of diabetes, the glomerular filtration rate (GFR), and the serum creatinine are shown. *(Adapted from RA DeFranzo, in Therapy for Diabetes Mellitus and Related Disorders, 3rd ed. American Diabetes Association, Alexandria, VA, 1998.)*

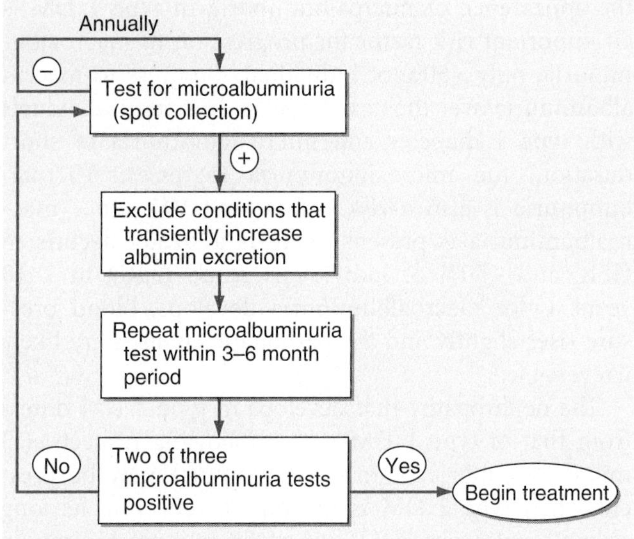

FIGURE 25-4

Screening for microalbuminuria should be performed in patients with type 1 diabetes for ≥5 years, in patients with type 2 diabetes, and during pregnancy. Non-diabetes-related conditions that might increase microalbuminuria are urinary tract infection, hematuria, heart failure, febrile illness, severe hyperglycemia, severe hypertension, and vigorous exercise. *(Adapted from RA DeFranzo, in Therapy for Diabetes Mellitus and Related Disorders, 3rd ed. American Diabetes Association, Alexandria, VA, 1998.)*

These individuals develop a propensity to hyperkalemia and acidemia, which may be exacerbated by medications (especially angiotensin-converting enzyme [ACE] inhibitors, angiotensin receptor blockers [ARBs], and spironolactone). Patients with DM are predisposed to radiocontrast-induced nephrotoxicity. Risk factors for radiocontrast-induced nephrotoxicity are preexisting nephropathy and volume depletion. Individuals with DM undergoing radiographic procedures with contrast dye should be well hydrated before and after dye exposure, and the serum creatinine should be monitored for 24–48 h following the procedure. Metformin should be held if indicated.

TREATMENT Diabetic Nephropathy

The optimal therapy for diabetic nephropathy is prevention by control of glycemia **(Chap. 24 outlines glycemic goals and approaches)**. Interventions effective in slowing progression of albuminuria include (1) improved glycemic control, (2) strict blood pressure control, and (3) administration of an ACE inhibitor or ARB. Dyslipidemia should also be treated.

Improved glycemic control reduces the rate at which microalbuminuria appears and progresses in type 1 and type 2 DM. However, once macroalbuminuria is present, it is unclear whether improved glycemic control will slow progression of renal disease. During the later phase of declining renal function, insulin requirements may fall as the kidney is a site of insulin degradation. As the GFR decreases with progressive nephropathy, the use and dose of glucose-lowering agents should be reevaluated (see Table 24-5). Some glucose-lowering medications (sulfonylureas and metformin) are contraindicated in advanced renal insufficiency.

Many individuals with type 1 or type 2 DM develop hypertension. Numerous studies in both type 1 and type 2 DM demonstrate the effectiveness of strict blood pressure control in reducing albumin excretion and slowing the decline in renal function. Blood pressure should be maintained at <140/90 mmHg in diabetic individuals.

Either ACE inhibitors or ARBs should be used to reduce the albuminuria and the associated decline in GFR that accompanies it in individuals with type 1 or type 2 DM (see "Hypertension," below). Although direct comparisons of ACE inhibitors and ARBs are lacking, most experts believe that the two classes of drugs are equivalent in patient with diabetes. ARBs can be used as an alternative in patients who develop ACE inhibitor–associated cough or angioedema. After 2–3 months of therapy in patients with microalbuminuria, the drug dose is increased until the maximum tolerated dose is reached. Recent studies do not show benefit of intervention prior to onset of microalbuminuria. The combination of an ACE inhibitor and an ARB is not recommended and appears to be detrimental. If use of either ACE inhibitors or ARBs is not possible or the blood pressure is not controlled, then, diuretics, calcium channel blockers (nondihydropyridine class), or beta blockers should be used. These salutary effects are mediated by reducing intraglomerular pressure and inhibition of angiotensin-driven sclerosing pathways, in part through inhibition of TGF-β-mediated pathways.

The ADA does not suggest restriction of protein intake in diabetic individuals with albuminuria because studies have failed to show benefit.

Nephrology consultation should be considered when albuminuria appears and again when the estimated GFR is <60 mL/min per 1.743 m^2. As compared with nondiabetic individuals, hemodialysis in patients with DM is associated with more frequent complications, such as hypotension (due to autonomic neuropathy or loss of reflex tachycardia), more difficult vascular access, and accelerated progression of retinopathy. Complications of atherosclerosis are the leading cause of death in diabetic individuals with nephropathy and hyperlipidemia should be treated aggressively. Renal transplantation from a living related donor is the preferred therapy but requires chronic immunosuppression. Combined pancreas-kidney transplant offers the promise of normoglycemia and freedom from dialysis.

NEUROPATHY AND DIABETES MELLITUS

Diabetic neuropathy occurs in ~50% of individuals with long-standing type 1 and type 2 DM. It may manifest as polyneuropathy, mononeuropathy, and/or autonomic neuropathy. As with other complications of DM, the development of neuropathy correlates with the duration of diabetes and glycemic control. Additional risk factors are body mass index (BMI) (the greater the BMI, the greater the risk of neuropathy) and smoking. The presence of CVD, elevated triglycerides, and hypertension is also associated with diabetic peripheral neuropathy. Both myelinated and unmyelinated nerve fibers are lost. Because the clinical features of diabetic neuropathy are similar to those of other neuropathies, the diagnosis of diabetic neuropathy should be made only after other possible etiologies are excluded.

Polyneuropathy/mononeuropathy

The most common form of diabetic neuropathy is distal symmetric polyneuropathy. It most frequently presents with distal sensory loss and pain, but up to 50% of patients do not have symptoms of neuropathy. Hyperesthesia, paresthesia, and dysesthesia also may occur. Any combination of these symptoms may develop as neuropathy progresses. Symptoms may include a sensation of numbness, tingling, sharpness, or burning that begins in the feet and spreads proximally. Neuropathic pain develops in some of these individuals, occasionally preceded by improvement in their glycemic control. Pain typically involves the lower extremities, is usually present at rest, and worsens at night. Both an acute (lasting <12 months) and a chronic form of painful diabetic neuropathy have been described. The acute form is sometimes treatment-related, occurring in the context of improved glycemic control. As diabetic neuropathy progresses, the pain subsides and eventually disappears, but a sensory deficit in the lower extremities persists. Physical examination reveals sensory loss, loss of ankle deep-tendon reflexes, and abnormal position sense.

Diabetic polyradiculopathy is a syndrome characterized by severe disabling pain in the distribution of one or more nerve roots. It may be accompanied by motor weakness. Intercostal or truncal radiculopathy causes pain over the thorax or abdomen. Involvement of the lumbar plexus or femoral nerve may cause severe pain in the thigh or hip and may be associated with muscle weakness in the hip flexors or extensors (diabetic amyotrophy). Fortunately, diabetic polyradiculopathies are usually self-limited and resolve over 6–12 months.

Mononeuropathy (dysfunction of isolated cranial or peripheral nerves) is less common than polyneuropathy in DM and presents with pain and motor weakness in the distribution of a single nerve. Mononeuropathies can occur at entrapment sites such as carpal tunnel or be noncompressive. A vascular etiology for noncompressive mononeuropathies has been suggested, but the pathogenesis is unknown. Involvement of the third cranial nerve is most common and is heralded by diplopia. Physical examination reveals ptosis and ophthalmoplegia with normal pupillary constriction to light. Sometimes other cranial nerves, such as IV, VI, or VII (Bell's palsy), are affected. Peripheral mononeuropathies or simultaneous involvement of more than one nerve (mononeuropathy multiplex) may also occur.

Autonomic neuropathy

Individuals with long-standing type 1 or 2 DM may develop signs of autonomic dysfunction involving the cholinergic, noradrenergic, and peptidergic (peptides such as pancreatic polypeptide, substance P, etc.) systems. DM-related autonomic neuropathy can involve multiple systems, including the cardiovascular, gastrointestinal, genitourinary, sudomotor, and metabolic systems. Autonomic neuropathies affecting the cardiovascular system cause a resting tachycardia and orthostatic hypotension. Reports of sudden death have also been attributed to autonomic neuropathy. Gastroparesis and bladder-emptying abnormalities are often caused by the autonomic neuropathy seen in DM (discussed below). Hyperhidrosis of the upper extremities and anhidrosis of the lower extremities result from sympathetic nervous system dysfunction. Anhidrosis of the feet can promote dry skin with cracking, which increases the risk of foot ulcers. Autonomic neuropathy may reduce counterregulatory hormone release (especially catecholamines), leading to an inability to sense hypoglycemia appropriately (hypoglycemia unawareness; **Chap. 26**), thereby subjecting the patient to the risk of severe hypoglycemia and complicating efforts to improve glycemic control.

TREATMENT Diabetic Neuropathy

Treatment of diabetic neuropathy is less than satisfactory. Improved glycemic control should be aggressively pursued and will improve nerve conduction velocity, but symptoms of diabetic neuropathy may not necessarily improve. Efforts to improve glycemic control in long-standing diabetes may be confounded by autonomic neuropathy and hypoglycemia unawareness. Risk factors for neuropathy such as hypertension and hypertriglyceridemia should be treated. Avoidance of neurotoxins (alcohol) and smoking, supplementation with vitamins for possible deficiencies (B_{12}, folate), and symptomatic treatment are the mainstays of therapy. Loss of sensation in the foot places the patient at risk for ulceration and its sequelae; consequently, prevention of such problems is of paramount importance. Patients with symptoms or signs of neuropathy should check their feet daily and take precautions (footwear) aimed at preventing calluses or ulcerations. If foot deformities are present, a podiatrist should be involved.

Chronic, painful diabetic neuropathy is difficult to treat but may respond to duloxetine, amitriptyline, gabapentin, valproate, pregabalin, or opioids. Two agents, duloxetine and pregabalin, have been approved by the U.S. Food and Drug Administration (FDA) for pain associated with diabetic neuropathy, but no treatments are satisfactory. No direct comparisons of agents are available, and it is reasonable to switch agents if there is no response or if side effects develop. Referral to a pain management center may be necessary. Because the pain of acute diabetic neuropathy may resolve over time, medications may be discontinued as progressive neuronal damage from DM occurs.

Therapy of orthostatic hypotension secondary to autonomic neuropathy is also challenging. A variety of agents have limited success (fludrocortisone, midodrine, clonidine, octreotide, and yohimbine), but each has significant side effects. Nonpharmacologic maneuvers (adequate salt intake, avoidance of dehydration and diuretics, and lower extremity support hose) may offer some benefit.

GASTROINTESTINAL/GENITOURINARY DYSFUNCTION

Long-standing type 1 and 2 DM may affect the motility and function of the gastrointestinal (GI) and genitourinary systems. The most prominent GI symptoms are delayed gastric emptying (gastroparesis) and altered small- and large-bowel motility (constipation or diarrhea). Gastroparesis may present with symptoms of anorexia, nausea, vomiting, early satiety, and abdominal bloating. Microvascular complications (retinopathy and neuropathy) are usually present. Nuclear medicine scintigraphy after ingestion of a radiolabeled meal may document delayed gastric emptying, but may not correlate well with the patient's symptoms. Noninvasive "breath tests" following ingestion of a radiolabeled meal have been developed, but are not yet validated. Although parasympathetic dysfunction secondary to chronic hyperglycemia is important in the development of gastroparesis, hyperglycemia itself also impairs gastric emptying. Nocturnal diarrhea, alternating with constipation, is a feature of DM-related GI autonomic neuropathy. In type 1 DM, these symptoms should also prompt evaluation for celiac sprue because of its increased frequency. Esophageal dysfunction in long-standing DM may occur but is usually asymptomatic.

Diabetic autonomic neuropathy may lead to genitourinary dysfunction including cystopathy and female sexual dysfunction (reduced sexual desire, dyspareunia, reduced vaginal lubrication). Symptoms of diabetic cystopathy begin with an inability to sense a full bladder and a failure to void completely. As bladder contractility worsens, bladder capacity and the postvoid residual increase, leading to symptoms of urinary hesitancy, decreased voiding frequency, incontinence, and recurrent urinary tract infections. Diagnostic evaluation includes cystometry and urodynamic studies.

Erectile dysfunction and retrograde ejaculation are very common in DM and may be one of the earliest signs of diabetic neuropathy **(Chap. 19)**. Erectile dysfunction, which increases in frequency with the age of the patient and the duration of diabetes, may occur in the absence of other signs of diabetic autonomic neuropathy.

TREATMENT Gastrointestinal/Genitourinary Dysfunction

Current treatments for these complications of DM are inadequate. Improved glycemic control should be a primary goal, because some aspects (neuropathy, gastric function) may improve. Smaller, more frequent meals that are easier to digest (liquid) and low in fat and fiber may minimize symptoms of gastroparesis. Metoclopramide has been used but is now restricted in both the United States and Europe and not advised for long-term use. Gastric electrical stimulatory devices are available but not approved. Diabetic diarrhea in the absence of bacterial overgrowth is treated symptomatically.

Diabetic cystopathy should be treated with scheduled voiding or self-catheterization. Drugs that inhibit type 5 phosphodiesterase are effective for erectile dysfunction, but their efficacy in individuals with DM is slightly lower than in the nondiabetic population **(Chap. 19)**. Sexual dysfunction in women may be improved with use of vaginal lubricants, treatment of vaginal infections, and systemic or local estrogen replacement.

CARDIOVASCULAR MORBIDITY AND MORTALITY

CVD is increased in individuals with type 1 or type 2 DM. The Framingham Heart Study revealed a marked increase in PAD, coronary artery disease, MI, and CHF (risk increase from one- to fivefold) in DM. In addition, the prognosis for individuals with diabetes who have coronary artery disease or MI is worse than for nondiabetics. CHD is more likely to involve multiple vessels in individuals with DM. In addition to CHD, cerebrovascular disease is increased in individuals with DM (threefold increase in stroke). Thus, after controlling for all known cardiovascular risk factors, type 2 DM increases the cardiovascular death rate twofold in men and fourfold in women.

The American Heart Association has designated DM as a "CHD risk equivalent," and type 2 DM patients without a prior MI have a similar risk for coronary artery–related events as nondiabetic individuals who have had a prior MI. However, the cardiovascular risk assessment in type 2 DM should encompass a more nuanced approach. Cardiovascular risk is lower and not equivalent in a younger individual with a brief duration of type 2 DM compared to an older individual with long-standing type 2DM. Because of the extremely high prevalence of underlying CVD in individuals with diabetes (especially in type 2 DM), evidence of atherosclerotic vascular disease (e.g., cardiac stress test) should be sought in an individual with diabetes who has symptoms suggestive of cardiac ischemia or peripheral or carotid arterial disease. The screening of asymptomatic individuals with diabetes for CHD, even with a risk-factor scale, is not recommended because recent studies have not shown a clinical benefit. The absence of chest pain ("silent ischemia") is common in individuals with diabetes, and a thorough cardiac evaluation should be considered prior to major surgical procedures.

The increase in cardiovascular morbidity and mortality rates in diabetes appears to relate to the synergism of hyperglycemia with other cardiovascular risk factors. Risk factors for macrovascular disease in diabetic individuals include dyslipidemia, hypertension, obesity, reduced physical activity, and cigarette smoking. Additional risk factors more prevalent in the diabetic population include microalbuminuria, macroalbuminuria, an elevation of serum creatinine, abnormal platelet function and endothelial dysfunction The possibility of atherogenic potential of insulin is suggested by the data in nondiabetic individuals showing higher serum insulin levels (indicative of insulin resistance) in association with greater risk of cardiovascular morbidity and mortality. However, treatment with insulin and the sulfonylureas did not increase the risk of CVD in individuals with type 2 DM.

TREATMENT Cardiovascular Disease

In general, the treatment of coronary disease is not different in the diabetic individual. Revascularization procedures for CHD, including percutaneous coronary interventions (PCI) and coronary artery bypass grafting (CABG), may be less efficacious in the diabetic individual. Initial success rates of PCI in diabetic individuals are similar to those in the nondiabetic population, but diabetic patients have higher rates of restenosis and lower long-term patency and survival rates in older studies.

Aggressive cardiovascular risk modification in all individuals with DM and glycemic control should be individualized, as discussed in **Chap. 24**. In patients with known CHD and type 2 DM, an ACE inhibitor (or ARB), a statin, and acetylsalicylic acid (ASA; aspirin) should be considered. Past trepidation about using beta blockers in individuals who have diabetes should not prevent use of these agents because they clearly benefit diabetic patients after MI. In patients with CHF, thiazolidinediones should not be used **(Chap. 24)**. However, metformin can be used in patients with stable CHF if the renal function is normal.

Antiplatelet therapy reduces cardiovascular events in individuals with DM who have CHD and is recommended. Current recommendations by the ADA include the use of aspirin for primary prevention of coronary events in diabetic individuals with an increased 10-year cardiovascular risk >10% (at least one risk factor such as hypertension, smoking, family history, albuminuria, or dyslipidemia in men >50 years or women >60 years of age). ASA is not recommended for primary prevention in those with a 10-year cardiovascular risk <10%. The aspirin dose is the same as in nondiabetic individuals.

Cardiovascular risk factors

Dyslipidemia

Individuals with DM may have several forms of dyslipidemia **(Chap. 27)**. Because of the additive cardiovascular risk of hyperglycemia and hyperlipidemia, lipid abnormalities should be assessed aggressively and treated as part of comprehensive diabetes care **(Chap. 24)**. The most common pattern of dyslipidemia is hypertriglyceridemia and reduced high-density lipoprotein (HDL) cholesterol levels. DM itself does not increase levels of low-density lipoprotein (LDL), but the small dense LDL particles found in type 2 DM are more atherogenic because they are more easily glycated and susceptible to oxidation.

Almost all treatment studies of diabetic dyslipidemia have been performed in individuals with type 2 DM because of the greater frequency of dyslipidemia in this form of diabetes. Interventional studies have shown that the beneficial effects of LDL reduction with statins are similar in the diabetic and nondiabetic populations. Large prospective trials of primary and secondary intervention for CHD have included some individuals with type 2 DM, and subset analyses have consistently found that reductions in LDL reduce cardiovascular events and morbidity in individuals with DM. No prospective studies have addressed similar questions in individuals with type 1 DM. Because the frequency of CVD is low in children and young adults with diabetes, assessment of cardiovascular risk should be incorporated into the guidelines discussed below.

Based on the guidelines provided by the ADA, priorities in the treatment of dyslipidemia are as follows: (1) lower the LDL cholesterol, (2) raise the HDL cholesterol, and (3) decrease the triglycerides. A treatment strategy depends on the pattern of lipoprotein abnormalities. Initial therapy for all forms of dyslipidemia should include dietary changes, as well as the same lifestyle modifications recommended in the nondiabetic population (smoking cessation, blood pressure control, weight loss, increased physical activity). The dietary recommendations for individuals with DM include increased monounsaturated fat and carbohydrates and reduced saturated fats and cholesterol **(Chap. 27)**. According to guidelines of the ADA, the target lipid values in diabetic individuals (age >40 years) without CVD should be as follows: LDL <2.6 mmol/L (100 mg/dL); HDL >1 mmol/L (40 mg/dL) in men and >13 mmol/L (50 mg/dL) in women; and triglycerides <1.7 mmol/L (150 mg/dL). In patients >40 years, the ADA recommends addition of a statin, regardless of the LDL level, in patients with CHD and those without CHD who have CHD risk factors. Recently released guidelines by the American College of Cardiology (ACC) and American Heart Association (AHA) differ slightly and recommend that diabetic individuals aged 40–75 without CHD and a LDL of 70–189 mg/dl receive "moderate" intensity statin therapy. Improvement in glycemic control will lower triglycerides and have a modest beneficial effect by raising HDL.

If the patient is known to have CHD, the ADA recommends an LDL goal of <18 mmol/L (70 mg/dL) as an "option" (in keeping with evidence that such a goal is beneficial in nondiabetic individuals with CHD [**Chap. 27**]). The ACC/AHA guidelines do not advocate a specific LDL for statin therapy. HMG-CoA reductase inhibitors are the agents of choice for lowering LDL. Combination therapy with an HMG-CoA reductase inhibitor and a fibrate or another lipid-lowering agent (ezetimibe, niacin) may be considered but increases the possibility of side effects such as myositis and has not been shown to be beneficial. Nicotinic acid effectively raises HDL and can be used in patients with diabetes, but may worsen glycemic control and increase insulin resistance and has not been shown to provide additional benefit beyond statin therapy alone. Bile acid–binding resins should not be used if hypertriglyceridemia is present. In large clinical trials, statin usage is associated with a mild increase in the risk of developing type 2 DM. This risk is greatest in individuals with other risk factors for type 2 DM (**Chap. 23**). However, the cardiovascular benefits of statin use outweigh the mildly increased risk of diabetes.

Hypertension

Hypertension can accelerate other complications of DM, particularly CVD, nephropathy, and retinopathy. In targeting a goal of blood pressure of <140/80 mmHg, therapy should first emphasize lifestyle modifications such as weight loss, exercise, stress management, and sodium restriction. The BP goal should be individualized. In some younger individuals, the provider may target a blood pressure of <130/80 mmHg. Realizing that more than one agent is usually required to reach the blood pressure goal, the ADA recommends that all patients with diabetes and hypertension be treated with an ACE inhibitor or an ARB. Subsequently, agents that reduce cardiovascular risk (beta blockers, thiazide diuretics, and calcium channel blockers) should be incorporated into the regimen. ACE inhibitors and ARBs are likely equivalent in most patients with diabetes and renal disease. Serum potassium and renal function should be monitored.

Because of the high prevalence of atherosclerotic disease in individuals with type 2 DM, the possibility of renovascular hypertension should be considered when the blood pressure is not readily controlled.

LOWER EXTREMITY COMPLICATIONS

DM is the leading cause of nontraumatic lower extremity amputation in the United States. Foot ulcers and infections are also a major source of morbidity in individuals with DM. The reasons for the increased incidence of these disorders in DM involve the interaction of several pathogenic factors: neuropathy, abnormal foot biomechanics, PAD, and poor wound healing. The peripheral sensory neuropathy interferes with normal protective mechanisms and allows the patient to sustain major or repeated minor trauma to the foot, often without knowledge of the injury. Disordered proprioception causes abnormal weight bearing while walking and subsequent formation of callus or ulceration. Motor and sensory neuropathy lead to abnormal foot muscle mechanics and to structural changes in the foot (hammer toe, claw toe deformity, prominent metatarsal heads, Charcot joint). Autonomic neuropathy results in anhidrosis and altered superficial blood flow in the foot, which promote drying of the skin and fissure formation. PAD and poor wound healing impede resolution of minor breaks in the skin, allowing them to enlarge and to become infected.

Many individuals with type 2 DM develop a foot ulcer (great toe or metatarsophalangeal areas are most common), and a significant subset who develop an ulceration will ultimately undergo amputation (14–24% risk with that ulcer or subsequent ulceration). Risk factors for foot ulcers or amputation include male sex, diabetes for >10 years, peripheral neuropathy, abnormal structure of foot (bony abnormalities, callus, thickened nails), PAD, smoking, history of previous ulcer or amputation, visual impairment, and poor glycemic control. Large calluses are often precursors to or overlie ulcerations.

TREATMENT Lower Extremity Complications

The optimal therapy for foot ulcers and amputations is prevention through identification of high-risk patients, education of the patient, and institution of measures to prevent ulceration. High-risk patients should be identified during the routine, annual foot examination performed on all patients with DM (see "Ongoing Aspects of Comprehensive Diabetes Care" in **Chap. 24**). If the monofilament test or one of the other tests is abnormal, the patient is diagnosed with loss of protective sensation (LOPS; **Chap. 23**). Providers should consider screening for asymptomatic PAD in individuals >50 years of age who have diabetes and other risk factors using ankle-brachial index testing in high-risk individuals. Patient education should emphasize (1) careful selection of footwear, (2) daily inspection of the feet to detect early signs of poor-fitting footwear or minor trauma, (3) daily foot hygiene to keep the skin clean and moist, (4) avoidance of self-treatment of foot abnormalities and high-risk behavior (e.g., walking barefoot), and (5) prompt consultation with a health care provider if an abnormality arises. Patients at high risk for ulceration or amputation may benefit from evaluation by a foot care specialist. Calluses and nail deformities should be treated by a podiatrist. Interventions directed at risk factor modification include orthotic shoes and devices, callus management, nail care, and prophylactic measures to reduce increased skin pressure from abnormal bony architecture. Attention to other risk factors for vascular disease (smoking, dyslipidemia, hypertension) and improved glycemic control are also important.

Despite preventive measures, foot ulceration and infection are common and represent a serious problem. Due to the multifactorial pathogenesis of lower extremity ulcers, management of these lesions is multidisciplinary and often demands expertise in orthopedics, vascular surgery, endocrinology, podiatry, and infectious diseases. The plantar surface of the foot is the most common site of ulceration. Ulcers may be primarily neuropathic (no accompanying infection) or may have surrounding cellulitis or osteomyelitis. Cellulitis without ulceration is also frequent and should be treated with antibiotics that provide broad-spectrum coverage, including anaerobes (see below).

An infected ulcer is a clinical diagnosis, because superficial culture of any ulceration will likely find multiple possible bacterial species. The infection surrounding the foot ulcer is often the result of multiple organisms, with aerobic gram-positive cocci (staphylococci including MRSA, Group A and B streptococci) being most common and with aerobic gram-negative bacilli and/or obligate anaerobes as co-pathogens.

Gas gangrene may develop in the absence of clostridial infection. Cultures taken from the surface of the ulcer are not helpful; a culture from the debrided ulcer base or from purulent drainage or aspiration of the wound is the most helpful. Wound depth should be determined by inspection and probing with a blunt-tipped sterile instrument. Plain radiographs of the foot should be performed to assess the possibility of osteomyelitis in chronic ulcers that have not responded to therapy. Magnetic resonance imaging (MRI) is the most specific modality, with nuclear medicine scans and labeled white cell studies as alternatives. Surgical debridement is often necessary.

Osteomyelitis is best treated by a combination of prolonged antibiotics (IV, then oral) and/or possibly debridement of infected bone. The possible contribution of vascular insufficiency should be considered in all patients. Peripheral arterial bypass procedures are often effective in promoting wound healing and in decreasing the need for amputation of the ischemic limb.

A consensus statement from the ADA identified six interventions with demonstrated efficacy in diabetic foot wounds: (1) off-loading, (2) debridement, (3) wound dressings, (4) appropriate use of antibiotics, (5) revascularization, and (6) limited amputation. Off-loading is the complete avoidance of weight bearing on the ulcer, which removes the mechanical trauma that retards wound healing. Bed rest and a variety of orthotic devices or contact casting limit weight bearing on wounds or pressure points. Surgical debridement is important and effective, but clear efficacy of other modalities for wound cleaning (enzymes, soaking, whirlpools) is lacking. Dressings such as hydrocolloid dressings promote wound healing by creating a moist environment and protecting the wound. Antiseptic agents should be avoided. Topical antibiotics are of limited value. Referral for physical therapy, orthotic evaluation, and rehabilitation should occur once the infection is controlled.

Mild or non-limb-threatening infections can be treated with oral antibiotics directed predominantly at methicillin-susceptible staphylococci and streptococci (e.g., dicloxacillin, cephalosporin, amoxicillin/clavulanate). However the increasing prevalence of MRSA often requires the use of clindamycin, doxycycline, or trimethoprim-sulfamethoxazole. Trimethoprim-sulfamethoxazole exhibits less reliable coverage of streptococci than the β-lactams, and diabetic patients may develop adverse effects including acute kidney injury and hyperkalemia. Surgical debridement of necrotic tissue, local wound care (avoidance of weight bearing over the ulcer), and close surveillance for progression of infection are crucial. More severe infections require IV antibiotics as well as bed rest and local wound care. Urgent surgical debridement may be required. Optimization of glycemic control should be a goal. IV antibiotics should provide broad-spectrum coverage directed toward *Staphylococcus aureus*, including MRSA, streptococci, gram-negative aerobes, and anaerobic bacteria. Initial antimicrobial regimens include vancomycin plus a β-lactam/β-lactamase inhibitor or carbapenem or vancomycin plus a combination of quinolone plus metronidazole. Daptomycin, ceftaroline, or linezolid may be substituted for vancomycin. If the infection surrounding the ulcer is not improving with IV antibiotics, reassessment of antibiotic coverage and reconsideration of the need for surgical debridement or revascularization are indicated. With clinical improvement, oral antibiotics and local wound care can be continued on an outpatient basis with close follow-up.

INFECTIONS

Individuals with DM have a greater frequency and severity of infection. The reasons for this include incompletely defined abnormalities in cell-mediated immunity and phagocyte function associated with hyperglycemia, as well as diminished vascularization. Hyperglycemia aids the colonization and growth of a variety of organisms (*Candida* and other fungal species). Many common infections are more frequent and severe in the diabetic population, whereas several rare infections are seen almost exclusively in the diabetic population. Examples of this latter category include rhinocerebral mucormycosis, emphysematous infections of the gallbladder and urinary tract, and "malignant" or invasive otitis externa. Invasive otitis externa is usually secondary to *P. aeruginosa* infection in the soft tissue surrounding the external auditory canal, usually begins with pain and discharge, and may rapidly progress to osteomyelitis and meningitis. These infections should be sought, in particular, in patients presenting with severe hyperglycemia **(Chap. 24)**.

Pneumonia, urinary tract infections, and skin and soft tissue infections are all more common in the diabetic population. In general, the organisms that cause pulmonary infections are similar to those found in the nondiabetic population; however, gram-negative organisms, *S. aureus*, and *Mycobacterium tuberculosis* are more frequent pathogens. Urinary tract infections (either lower tract or pyelonephritis) are the result of common bacterial agents such as *Escherichia coli*, although several yeast species (*Candida* and *Torulopsis glabrata*) are commonly observed. Complications of urinary tract infections include emphysematous pyelonephritis and emphysematous cystitis. Bacteriuria occurs frequently in individuals with diabetic cystopathy. Susceptibility to furunculosis, superficial candidal infections, and vulvovaginitis are increased. Poor glycemic control is a common denominator in individuals with these infections. Diabetic individuals have an increased rate of colonization of *S. aureus* in the skinfolds and nares. Diabetic patients also have a greater risk of postoperative wound infections.

DERMATOLOGIC MANIFESTATIONS

The most common skin manifestations of DM are xerosis and pruritus and are usually relieved by skin moisturizers. Protracted wound healing and skin ulcerations are also frequent complications. Diabetic dermopathy, sometimes termed *pigmented pretibial papules*, or "diabetic skin spots," begins as an erythematous macule or papule that evolves into an area of circular hyperpigmentation. These lesions result from minor mechanical trauma in the pretibial region and are more common in elderly men with DM. Bullous diseases, such as bullosa diabeticorum (shallow ulcerations or erosions in the pretibial region), are also seen. *Necrobiosis lipoidica diabeticorum* is an uncommon disorder, accompanying diabetes in predominantly young women. This usually begins in the pretibial region as an erythematous plaque or papules that gradually enlarge, darken, and develop irregular margins, with atrophic centers and central ulceration. They are often painful. Vitiligo occurs at increased frequency in individuals with type 1 DM. *Acanthosis nigricans* (hyperpigmented velvety plaques seen on the neck, axilla, or extensor surfaces) is sometimes a feature of severe insulin resistance and accompanying diabetes. Generalized or localized *granuloma annulare* (erythematous plaques on the extremities or trunk) and *scleredema* (areas of skin thickening on the back or neck at the site of previous superficial infections) are more common in the diabetic population. *Lipoatrophy* and *lipohypertrophy* can occur at insulin injection sites but are now unusual with the use of human insulin.

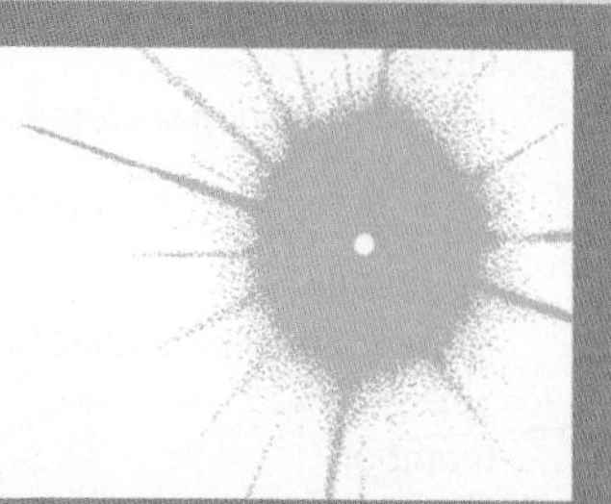

CHAPTER 26

HYPOGLYCEMIA

Philip E. Cryer ■ Stephen N. Davis

Hypoglycemia is most commonly caused by drugs used to treat diabetes mellitus or by exposure to other drugs, including alcohol. However, a number of other disorders, including critical organ failure, sepsis and inanition, hormone deficiencies, non-β-cell tumors, insulinoma, and prior gastric surgery, can cause hypoglycemia (Table 26-1). Hypoglycemia is most convincingly documented by *Whipple's triad:* (1) symptoms consistent with hypoglycemia, (2) a low plasma glucose concentration measured with a precise method (not a glucose monitor), and (3) relief of symptoms after the plasma glucose level is raised. The lower limit of the fasting plasma glucose concentration is normally ~70 mg/dL (~3.9 mmol/L), but lower venous glucose levels occur normally, late after a meal, during pregnancy, and during prolonged fasting (>24 h). Hypoglycemia can cause serious morbidity; if severe and prolonged, it can be fatal. It should be considered in any patient with episodes of confusion, an altered level of consciousness, or a seizure.

SYSTEMIC GLUCOSE BALANCE AND GLUCOSE COUNTERREGULATION

Glucose is an obligate metabolic fuel for the brain under physiologic conditions. The brain cannot synthesize glucose or store more than a few minutes' supply as glycogen and therefore requires a continuous supply of glucose from the arterial circulation. As the arterial plasma glucose concentration falls below the physiologic range, blood-to-brain glucose transport becomes insufficient to support brain energy metabolism and function. However, redundant glucose counterregulatory mechanisms normally prevent or rapidly correct hypoglycemia.

Plasma glucose concentrations are normally maintained within a relatively narrow range—roughly 70–110 mg/dL (3.9–6.1 mmol/L) in the fasting state, with transient higher excursions after a meal—despite wide variations in exogenous glucose delivery from meals and in endogenous glucose utilization by, for example, exercising muscle. Between meals and during fasting, plasma glucose levels are maintained by endogenous glucose production, hepatic glycogenolysis, and hepatic (and renal) gluconeogenesis (Fig. 26-1). Although hepatic glycogen stores are usually sufficient to maintain plasma glucose levels for ~8 h, this period can be shorter if glucose demand is increased by exercise or if glycogen stores are depleted by illness or starvation.

Gluconeogenesis normally requires low insulin levels and the presence of anti-insulin (counterregulatory) hormones together with a coordinated supply of precursors from muscle and adipose tissue to the liver (and kidneys). Muscle provides lactate, pyruvate, alanine, glutamine, and other amino acids. Triglycerides in adipose tissue are broken down into fatty acids and glycerol, which is a gluconeogenic precursor. Fatty acids provide an alternative oxidative fuel to tissues other than the brain (which requires glucose).

Systemic glucose balance—maintenance of the normal plasma glucose concentration—is accomplished by a network of hormones, neural signals, and substrate effects that regulate endogenous glucose production and glucose utilization by tissues other than the brain (**Chap. 23**). Among the regulatory factors, insulin plays a dominant role (Table 26-2; Fig. 26-1). As plasma glucose levels decline within the physiologic range in the fasting state, pancreatic β-cell insulin secretion decreases, thereby increasing hepatic glycogenolysis and hepatic (and renal) gluconeogenesis. Low insulin levels also reduce glucose utilization in peripheral tissues, inducing lipolysis and proteolysis and consequently releasing gluconeogenic precursors. Thus, a decrease in insulin secretion is the first defense against hypoglycemia.

TABLE 26-1

CAUSES OF HYPOGLYCEMIA IN ADULTS

Ill or Medicated Individual
1. Drugs
Insulin or insulin secretagogue
Alcohol
Others
2. Critical illness
Hepatic, renal or cardiac failure
Sepsis
Inanition
3. Hormone deficiency
Cortisol
Glucagon and epinephrine (in insulin-deficient diabetes)
4. Non–islet cell tumor
Seemingly Well Individual
5. Endogenous hyperinsulinism
Insulinoma
Functional β-cell disorders (nesidioblastosis)
Noninsulinoma pancreatogenous hypoglycemia
Post–gastric bypass hypoglycemia
Insulin autoimmune hypoglycemia
Antibody to insulin
Antibody to insulin receptor
Insulin secretagogue
Other
6. Accidental, surreptitious, or malicious hypoglycemia

Source: From PE Cryer et al: J Clin Endocrinol Metab 94:709, 2009. ©The Endocrine Society, 2009.

As plasma glucose levels decline just below the physiologic range, glucose counterregulatory (plasma glucose–raising) hormones are released (Table 26-2; Fig. 26-1). Among these, pancreatic α-cell glucagon, which stimulates hepatic glycogenolysis, plays a primary role. Glucagon is the second defense against hypoglycemia. Adrenomedullary epinephrine, which stimulates hepatic glycogenolysis and gluconeogenesis (and renal gluconeogenesis), is not normally critical. However, it becomes critical when glucagon is deficient. Epinephrine is the third defense against hypoglycemia. When hypoglycemia is prolonged beyond ~4 h, cortisol and growth hormone also support glucose production and restrict glucose utilization to a limited amount (~20% compared to epinephrine). Thus cortisol and growth hormone play no role in defense against acute hypoglycemia.

As plasma glucose levels fall further, symptoms prompt behavioral defense against hypoglycemia, including the ingestion of food (Table 26-2; Fig. 26-1). The normal glycemic thresholds for these responses to decreasing plasma glucose concentrations are shown in Table 26-2. However, these thresholds are dynamic. They shift to higher-than-normal glucose levels in people with poorly controlled diabetes, who can experience symptoms of hypoglycemia when their glucose levels decline toward the normal range (*pseudohypoglycemia*). On the other hand, thresholds shift to lower-than-normal glucose levels in people with recurrent

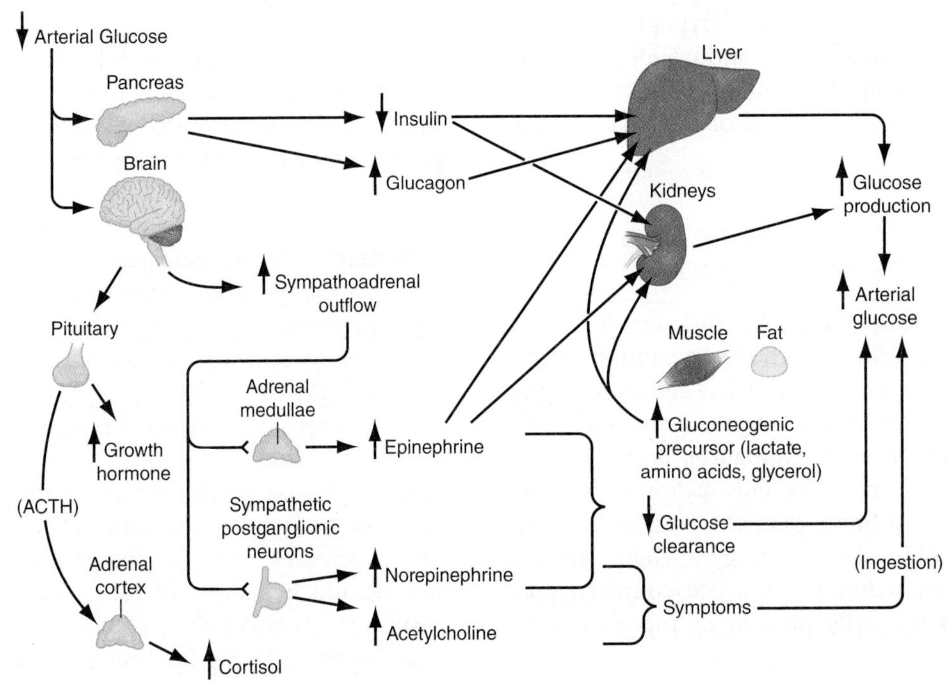

FIGURE 26-1

Physiology of glucose counterregulation: mechanisms that normally prevent or rapidly correct hypoglycemia. In insulin-deficient diabetes, the key counterregulatory responses—suppression of insulin and increases in glucagon—are lost, and stimulation of sympathoadrenal outflow is attenuated. ACTH, adrenocorticotropic hormone.

TABLE 26-2

PHYSIOLOGIC RESPONSES TO DECREASING PLASMA GLUCOSE CONCENTRATIONS

RESPONSE	GLYCEMIC THRESHOLD, MMOL/L (MG/DL)	PHYSIOLOGIC EFFECTS	ROLE IN PREVENTION OR CORRECTION OF HYPOGLYCEMIA (GLUCOSE COUNTERREGULATION)
↓ Insulin	4.4–4.7 (80–85)	↑ R_a (↓ R_d)	Primary glucose regulatory factor/first defense against hypoglycemia
↑ Glucagon	3.6–3.9 (65–70)	↑ R_a	Primary glucose counterregulatory factor/second defense against hypoglycemia
↑ Epinephrine	3.6–3.9 (65–70)	↑ R_a, ↓ R_c	Third defense against hypoglycemia, critical when glucagon is deficient
↑ Cortisol and growth hormone	3.6–3.9 (65–70)	↑ R_a, ↓ R_c	Involved in defense against prolonged hypoglycemia; not critical
Symptoms	2.8–3.1 (50–55)	Recognition of hypoglycemia	Prompt behavioral defense against hypoglycemia (food ingestion)
↓ Cognition	<2.8 (<50)	—	Compromises behavioral defense against hypoglycemia

Note: R_a, rate of glucose appearance, glucose production by the liver and kidneys; R_c, rate of glucose clearance, glucose utilization relative to the ambient plasma glucose by insulin-sensitive tissues; R_d, rate of glucose disappearance, glucose utilization by insulin-sensitive tissues such as skeletal muscle. R_d by the brain is not altered by insulin, glucagon, epinephrine, cortisol, or growth hormone.

Source: From PE Cryer, in S Melmed et al (eds): *Williams Textbook of Endocrinology*, 12th ed. New York, Elsevier, 2012.

hypoglycemia; e.g., patients with aggressively treated diabetes or an insulinoma have symptoms at glucose levels lower than those that cause symptoms in healthy individuals.

Clinical manifestations

Neuroglycopenic manifestations of hypoglycemia are the direct result of central nervous system glucose deprivation. These features include behavioral changes, confusion, fatigue, seizure, loss of consciousness, and, if hypoglycemia is severe and prolonged, death. Neurogenic (or autonomic) manifestations of hypoglycemia result from the perception of physiologic changes caused by the central nervous system–mediated sympathoadrenal discharge that is triggered by hypoglycemia. They include *adrenergic* symptoms (mediated largely by norepinephrine released from sympathetic postganglionic neurons but perhaps also by epinephrine released from the adrenal medullae), such as palpitations, tremor, and anxiety, as well as *cholinergic* symptoms (mediated by acetylcholine released from sympathetic postganglionic neurons), such as sweating, hunger, and paresthesias. Clearly, these are nonspecific symptoms. Their attribution to hypoglycemia requires that the corresponding plasma glucose concentration be low and that the symptoms resolve after the glucose level is raised (as delineated by Whipple's triad).

Common signs of hypoglycemia include diaphoresis and pallor. Heart rate and systolic blood pressure are typically increased but may not be raised in an individual who has experienced repeated, recent episodes of hypoglycemia. Neuroglycopenic manifestations are often observable. Transient focal neurologic deficits occur occasionally. Permanent neurologic deficits are rare.

Etiology and pathophysiology

Hypoglycemia is most commonly a result of the treatment of diabetes. This topic is therefore addressed before other causes of hypoglycemia are considered.

HYPOGLYCEMIA IN DIABETES

Impact and frequency

Hypoglycemia is the limiting factor in the glycemic management of diabetes mellitus. First, it causes recurrent morbidity in most people with type 1 diabetes (T1DM) and in many with advanced type 2 diabetes (T2DM), and it is sometimes fatal. Second, it precludes maintenance of euglycemia over a lifetime of diabetes and thus full realization of the well-established microvascular benefits of glycemic control. Third, it causes a vicious cycle of recurrent hypoglycemia by producing hypoglycemia-associated autonomic failure—i.e., the clinical syndromes of defective glucose counterregulation and of hypoglycemia unawareness (see later).

Hypoglycemia is a fact of life for people with T1DM. They suffer an average of two episodes of symptomatic hypoglycemia per week and at least one episode of severe, at least temporarily disabling hypoglycemia each year. An estimated 6–10% of people with T1DM die as a result of hypoglycemia. The incidence of hypoglycemia is lower in T2DM than in T1DM. However, its prevalence in insulin-requiring T2DM is surprisingly high. Recent studies investigating insulin-pump or multiple-injection therapies have revealed a hypoglycemia prevalence approaching 70%. In fact, as patients with T2DM outnumber those with T1DM by ten- to twentyfold, the prevalence of hypoglycemia is now greater in T2DM. Insulin, a sulfonylurea, or a glinide can cause hypoglycemia in T2DM. Metformin, thiazolidinediones, α-glucosidase inhibitors, glucagon-like peptide 1 (GLP-1) receptor agonists, and dipeptidyl peptidase IV (DPP-IV) inhibitors should not cause hypoglycemia. However, they increase the risk when combined with one of the sulfonylureas or glinides, or with insulin. Notably, the frequency of hypoglycemia approaches that in T1DM as persons with T2DM develop absolute insulin deficiency and require more complex treatment with insulin.

Conventional risk factors

The conventional risk factors for hypoglycemia in diabetes are identified on the basis of the premise that relative or absolute insulin excess is the sole determinant of risk. Relative or absolute insulin excess occurs when (1) insulin (or insulin secretagogue) doses are excessive, ill-timed, or of the wrong type; (2) the influx of exogenous glucose is reduced (e.g., during an overnight fast or after missed meals or snacks); (3) insulin-independent glucose utilization is increased (e.g., during exercise); (4) sensitivity to insulin is increased (e.g., with improved glycemic control, in the middle of the night, late after exercise, or with increased fitness or weight loss); (5) endogenous glucose production is reduced (e.g., after alcohol ingestion); and (6) insulin clearance is reduced (e.g., in renal failure). However, these conventional risk factors alone explain a minority of episodes; other factors are typically involved.

Hypoglycemia-associated autonomic failure (HAAF)

While marked insulin excess alone can cause hypoglycemia, iatrogenic hypoglycemia in diabetes is typically the result of the interplay of relative or absolute therapeutic insulin excess and compromised physiologic and behavioral defenses against falling plasma glucose concentrations (Table 26-2; Fig. 26-2). Defective glucose counterregulation compromises physiologic defense (particularly decrements in insulin and increments in glucagon and epinephrine), and hypoglycemia unawareness compromises behavioral defense (ingestion of carbohydrate).

Defective glucose counterregulation

In the setting of absolute endogenous insulin deficiency, insulin levels do not decrease as plasma glucose levels fall; the first defense against hypoglycemia is lost. Furthermore, probably because the decrement in intraislet insulin is normally a signal to stimulate glucagon secretion, glucagon levels do not increase as plasma glucose levels fall further; a second defense against hypoglycemia is lost. Finally, the increase in epinephrine levels, a third defense against hypoglycemia, in response to a given level of hypoglycemia is typically attenuated. The glycemic threshold for the sympathoadrenal (adrenomedullary epinephrine and sympathetic neural norepinephrine) response is shifted to lower plasma glucose concentrations. That shift is typically the result of recent antecedent iatrogenic hypoglycemia. In the setting of absent decrements in insulin and of absent increments in glucagon, the attenuated increment in epinephrine causes the clinical syndrome of defective glucose counterregulation. Affected patients are at ≥25-fold greater risk of severe iatrogenic hypoglycemia during aggressive glycemic therapy for their diabetes than are patients with normal epinephrine responses. This functional—and potentially reversible—disorder is distinct from classic diabetic autonomic neuropathy—a structural and irreversible disorder.

Hypoglycemia unawareness

The attenuated sympathoadrenal response (largely the reduced sympathetic neural response) to hypoglycemia causes the clinical syndrome of *hypoglycemia unawareness*—i.e., loss of the warning adrenergic and cholinergic symptoms that previously allowed the patient to recognize developing hypoglycemia and therefore to abort the episode by ingesting carbohydrates. Affected patients are at a sixfold increased risk of severe iatrogenic hypoglycemia during aggressive glycemic therapy of their diabetes.

HAAF in diabetes

The concept of HAAF in diabetes posits that recent antecedent iatrogenic hypoglycemia (or sleep or prior exercise) causes both defective glucose counterregulation (by reducing the epinephrine response to a given level of subsequent hypoglycemia in the setting of absent insulin and glucagon responses) and hypoglycemia unawareness (by reducing the sympathoadrenal response to a given level of subsequent hypoglycemia). These impaired responses create a vicious cycle of recurrent iatrogenic hypoglycemia (Fig. 26-2). Hypoglycemia unawareness and, to some extent, the reduced epinephrine component of defective glucose counterregulation are reversible by as little as 2–3 weeks of scrupulous avoidance of hypoglycemia in most affected patients.

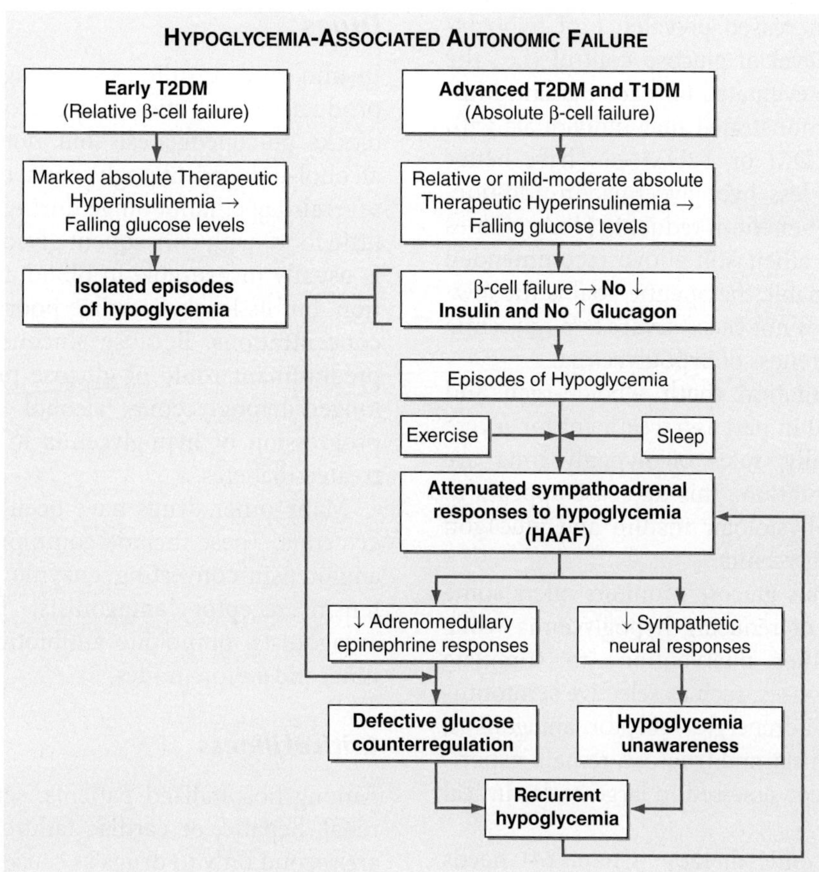

FIGURE 26-2

Hypoglycemia-associated autonomic failure (HAAF) in insulin-deficient diabetes. T1DM, type 1 diabetes mellitus; T2DM, type 2 diabetes mellitus. *(Modified from PE Cryer: Hypoglycemia in Diabetes. Pathophysiology, Prevalence, and Prevention, 2nd ed. © American Diabetes Association, 2012.)*

On the basis of this pathophysiology, additional risk factors for hypoglycemia in diabetes include (1) absolute insulin deficiency, indicating that insulin levels will not decrease and glucagon levels will not increase as plasma glucose levels fall; (2) a history of severe hypoglycemia or of hypoglycemia unawareness, implying recent antecedent hypoglycemia, as well as prior exercise or sleep, indicating that the sympathoadrenal response will be attenuated; and (3) lower hemoglobin A_{1c} (HbA_{1c}) levels or lower glycemic goals that, all other factors being equal, increase the probability of recent antecedent hypoglycemia.

Hypoglycemia risk factor reduction

Several recent multicenter, randomized, controlled trials investigating the potential benefits of tight glucose control in either inpatient or outpatient settings have reported a high prevalence of severe hypoglycemia. In the NICE-SUGAR study, attempts to control in-hospital plasma glucose values towards physiologic levels resulted in increased mortality risk. The ADVANCE and ACCORD studies and the Veterans Affairs Diabetes Trial (VADT) also found a significant incidence of severe hypoglycemia among T2DM patients. Severe hypoglycemia with accompanying serious cardiovascular morbidity and mortality also occurred in the standard (e.g., not receiving intensified treatment) control group in both the ACCORD study and the VADT. Thus, severe hypoglycemia can and does occur at HbA_{1c} values of 8–9% in both T1DM and T2DM. Somewhat surprisingly, all three studies found little or no benefit of intensive glucose control to reduce macrovascular events in T2DM. In fact, the ACCORD study was ended early because of the increased mortality rate in the intensive glucose control arm. Whether iatrogenic hypoglycemia was the cause of the increased mortality risk is not known. In light of these findings, some new recommendations and paradigms have been formulated. Whereas there is little debate regarding the need to reduce hyperglycemia in the hospital, the glycemic maintenance goals have been modified to lie between 140 and 180 mg/dL. Accordingly, the benefits of insulin therapy and reduced hyperglycemia can be obtained while the prevalence of hypoglycemia is reduced.

Similarly, evidence exists that intensive glucose control can reduce the prevalence of microvascular disease in both T1DM and T2DM. These benefits need to be weighed against the increased prevalence of hypoglycemia. Certainly, the level of glucose control (i.e., the HbA_{1c} level) should be evaluated for each patient. Multicenter trials have demonstrated that individuals with recently diagnosed T1DM or T2DM can have better glycemic control with less hypoglycemia. In addition, there is still long-term benefit in reducing HbA_{1c} values from higher to lower, albeit still above recommended levels. Perhaps a reasonable therapeutic goal is the lowest HbA_{1c} level that does not cause severe hypoglycemia and that preserves awareness of hypoglycemia.

Pancreatic transplantation (both whole-organ and islet-cell) has been used in part as a treatment for severe hypoglycemia. Generally, rates of hypoglycemia are reduced after transplantation. This decrease appears to be due to increased physiologic insulin and glucagon responses during hypoglycemia.

The use of continuous glucose monitors offers some promise as a method of reducing hypoglycemia while improving HbA_{1c}. Other interventions to stimulate counterregulatory responses, such as selective serotonin-reuptake inhibitors, β-adrenergic receptor antagonists, opiate receptor antagonists, and fructose, remain experimental and have not been assessed in large-scale clinical trials.

Thus, intensive glycemic therapy **(Chap. 24)** needs to be applied along with the patient's education and empowerment, frequent self-monitoring of blood glucose, flexible insulin (and other drug) regimens (including the use of insulin analogues, both short- and longer-acting), individualized glycemic goals, and ongoing professional guidance, support, and consideration of both the conventional risk factors and those indicative of compromised glucose counterregulation. Given a history of hypoglycemia unawareness, a 2- to 3-week period of scrupulous avoidance of hypoglycemia is indicated.

HYPOGLYCEMIA WITHOUT DIABETES

There are many causes of hypoglycemia (Table 26-1). Because hypoglycemia is common in insulin- or insulin secretagogue–treated diabetes, it is often reasonable to assume that a clinically suspicious episode is the result of hypoglycemia. On the other hand, because hypoglycemia is rare in the absence of relevant drug-treated diabetes, it is reasonable to conclude that a hypoglycemic disorder is present only in patients in whom Whipple's triad can be demonstrated.

Particularly when patients are ill or medicated, the initial diagnostic focus should be on the possibility of drug involvement and then on critical illnesses, hormone deficiency, or non–islet cell tumor hypoglycemia. In the absence of any of these etiologic factors and in a seemingly well individual, the focus should shift to possible endogenous hyperinsulinism or accidental, surreptitious, or even malicious hypoglycemia.

Drugs

Insulin and insulin secretagogues suppress glucose production and stimulate glucose utilization. Ethanol blocks gluconeogenesis but not glycogenolysis. Thus, alcohol-induced hypoglycemia typically occurs after a several-day ethanol binge during which the person eats little food, with consequent glycogen depletion. Ethanol is usually measurable in blood at the time of presentation, but its levels correlate poorly with plasma glucose concentrations. Because gluconeogenesis becomes the predominant route of glucose production during prolonged hypoglycemia, alcohol can contribute to the progression of hypoglycemia in patients with insulin-treated diabetes.

Many other drugs have been associated with hypoglycemia. These include commonly used drugs such as angiotensin-converting enzyme inhibitors and angiotensin receptor antagonists, β-adrenergic receptor antagonists, quinolone antibiotics, indomethacin, quinine, and sulfonamides.

Critical illness

Among hospitalized patients, serious illnesses such as renal, hepatic, or cardiac failure; sepsis; and inanition are second only to drugs as causes of hypoglycemia.

Rapid and extensive hepatic destruction (e.g., toxic hepatitis) causes fasting hypoglycemia because the liver is the major site of endogenous glucose production. The mechanism of hypoglycemia in patients with cardiac failure is unknown. Hepatic congestion and hypoxia may be involved. Although the kidneys are a source of glucose production, hypoglycemia in patients with renal failure is also caused by the reduced clearance of insulin and the reduced mobilization of gluconeogenic precursors in renal failure.

Sepsis is a relatively common cause of hypoglycemia. Increased glucose utilization is induced by cytokine production in macrophage-rich tissues such as the liver, spleen, and lung. Hypoglycemia develops if glucose production fails to keep pace. Cytokine-induced inhibition of gluconeogenesis in the setting of nutritional glycogen depletion, in combination with hepatic and renal hypoperfusion, may also contribute to hypoglycemia.

Hypoglycemia can be seen with starvation, perhaps because of loss of whole-body fat stores and subsequent depletion of gluconeogenic precursors (e.g., amino acids), necessitating increased glucose utilization.

Hormone deficiencies

Neither cortisol nor growth hormone is critical to the prevention of hypoglycemia, at least in adults. Nonetheless, hypoglycemia can occur with prolonged fasting in patients with primary adrenocortical failure (Addison's disease) or hypopituitarism. Anorexia and weight loss are typical features of chronic cortisol deficiency and likely result in glycogen depletion. Cortisol deficiency is associated with impaired gluconeogenesis and low levels of gluconeogenic precursors; these associations suggest that substrate-limited gluconeogenesis, in the setting of glycogen depletion, is the cause of hypoglycemia. Growth hormone deficiency can cause hypoglycemia in young children. In addition to extended fasting, high rates of glucose utilization (e.g., during exercise or in pregnancy) or low rates of glucose production (e.g., after alcohol ingestion) can precipitate hypoglycemia in adults with previously unrecognized hypopituitarism.

Hypoglycemia is not a feature of the epinephrine-deficient state that results from bilateral adrenalectomy when glucocorticoid replacement is adequate, nor does it occur during pharmacologic adrenergic blockade when other glucoregulatory systems are intact. Combined deficiencies of glucagon and epinephrine play a key role in the pathogenesis of iatrogenic hypoglycemia in people with insulin-deficient diabetes, as discussed earlier. Otherwise, deficiencies of these hormones are not usually considered in the differential diagnosis of a hypoglycemic disorder.

Non-β-cell tumors

Fasting hypoglycemia, often termed *non–islet cell tumor hypoglycemia*, occurs occasionally in patients with large mesenchymal or epithelial tumors (e.g., hepatomas, adrenocortical carcinomas, carcinoids). The glucose kinetic patterns resemble those of hyperinsulinism (see next), but insulin secretion is suppressed appropriately during hypoglycemia. In most instances, hypoglycemia is due to overproduction of an incompletely processed form of insulin-like growth factor II ("big IGF-II") that does not complex normally with circulating binding proteins and thus more readily gains access to target tissues. The tumors are usually apparent clinically, plasma ratios of IGF-II to IGF-I are high, and free IGF-II levels (and levels of pro-IGF-II [1–21]) are elevated. Curative surgery is seldom possible, but reduction of tumor bulk may ameliorate hypoglycemia. Therapy with a glucocorticoid, a growth hormone, or both has also been reported to alleviate hypoglycemia. Hypoglycemia attributed to ectopic IGF-I production has been reported but is rare.

Endogenous hyperinsulinism

Hypoglycemia due to endogenous hyperinsulinism can be caused by (1) a primary β-cell disorder—typically a β-cell tumor (*insulinoma*), sometimes multiple insulinomas, or a functional β-cell disorder with β-cell hypertrophy or hyperplasia; (2) an antibody to insulin or to the insulin receptor; (3) a β-cell secretagogue such as a sulfonylurea; or perhaps (4) ectopic insulin secretion, among other very rare mechanisms. None of these causes is common.

The fundamental pathophysiologic feature of endogenous hyperinsulinism caused by a primary β-cell disorder or an insulin secretagogue is the failure of insulin secretion to fall to very low levels during hypoglycemia. This feature is assessed by measurement of plasma insulin, C-peptide (the connecting peptide that is cleaved from proinsulin to produce insulin), proinsulin, and glucose concentrations during hypoglycemia. Insulin, C-peptide, and proinsulin levels need not be high relative to normal, euglycemic values; rather, they are inappropriately high in the setting of a low plasma glucose concentration. Critical diagnostic findings are a plasma insulin concentration ≥3 μU/mL (≥18 pmol/L), a plasma C-peptide concentration ≥0.6 ng/mL (≥0.2 nmol/L), and a plasma proinsulin concentration ≥5.0 pmol/L when the plasma glucose concentration is <55 mg/dL (<3.0 mmol/L) with symptoms of hypoglycemia. A low plasma β-hydroxybutyrate concentration (≤2.7 mmol/L) and an increment in plasma glucose level of >25 mg/dL (>1.4 mmol/L) after IV administration of glucagon (1.0 mg) indicate increased insulin (or IGF) actions.

The diagnostic strategy is (1) to measure plasma glucose, insulin, C-peptide, proinsulin, and β-hydroxybutyrate concentrations and to screen for circulating oral hypoglycemic agents during an episode of hypoglycemia and (2) to assess symptoms during the episode and seek their resolution following correction of hypoglycemia by IV injection of glucagon (i.e., to document Whipple's triad). This is straightforward if the patient is hypoglycemic when seen. Since endogenous hyperinsulinemic disorders usually, but not invariably, cause fasting hypoglycemia, a diagnostic episode may develop after a relatively short outpatient fast. Serial sampling during an inpatient diagnostic fast of up to 72 h or after a mixed meal is more problematic. An alternative is to give patients a detailed list of the required measurements and ask them to present to an emergency room, with the list, during a symptomatic episode. Obviously, a normal plasma glucose concentration during a symptomatic episode indicates that the symptoms are not the result of hypoglycemia.

An *insulinoma*—an insulin-secreting pancreatic islet β-cell tumor—is the prototypical cause of endogenous hyperinsulinism and therefore should be sought in patients with a compatible clinical syndrome. However, insulinoma is not the only cause of endogenous hyperinsulinism. Some patients with fasting endogenous hyperinsulinemic hypoglycemia have diffuse islet involvement with β-cell hypertrophy and sometimes hyperplasia. This pattern is commonly referred to as *nesidioblastosis*, although β-cells budding from ducts are not invariably found. Other patients have a similar islet pattern but with postprandial hypoglycemia, a disorder termed *noninsulinoma pancreatogenous hypoglycemia*. Postgastric bypass postprandial hypoglycemia, which most often follows Roux-en-Y gastric bypass, is also characterized by diffuse islet involvement and endogenous hyperinsulinism. Some have suggested that exaggerated GLP-1 responses to meals cause hyperinsulinemia and hypoglycemia, but the relevant pathogenesis has not been clearly established. If medical treatments with agents such as an α-glucosidase inhibitor, diazoxide, or octreotide fail, partial pancreatectomy may be required. Autoimmune hypoglycemias include those caused by an antibody to insulin that binds postmeal insulin and then gradually disassociates, with consequent late postprandial hypoglycemia. Alternatively, an insulin receptor antibody can function as an agonist. The presence of an insulin secretagogue, such as a sulfonylurea or a glinide, results in a clinical and biochemical pattern similar to that of an insulinoma but can be distinguished by the presence of the circulating secretagogue. Finally, there are reports of very rare phenomena such as ectopic insulin secretion, a gain-of-function insulin receptor mutation, and exercise-induced hyperinsulinemia.

Insulinomas are uncommon, with an estimated yearly incidence of 1 in 250, 000. Because more than 90% of insulinomas are benign, they are a treatable cause of potentially fatal hypoglycemia. The median age at presentation is 50 years in sporadic cases, but the tumor usually presents in the third decade when it is a component of multiple endocrine neoplasia type 1 **(Chap. 29)**. More than 99% of insulinomas are within the substance of the pancreas, and the tumors are usually small (<2.0 cm in diameter in 90% of cases). Therefore, they come to clinical attention because of hypoglycemia rather than mass effects. CT or MRI detects ~70–80% of insulinomas. These methods detect metastases in the roughly 10% of patients with a malignant insulinoma. Transabdominal ultrasound often identifies insulinomas, and endoscopic ultrasound has a sensitivity of ~90%. Somatostatin receptor scintigraphy is thought to detect insulinomas in about half of patients. Selective pancreatic arterial calcium injections, with the endpoint of a sharp increase in hepatic venous insulin levels, regionalize insulinomas with high sensitivity, but this invasive procedure is seldom necessary except to confirm endogenous hyperinsulinism in the diffuse islet disorders. Intraoperative pancreatic ultrasonography almost invariably localizes insulinomas that are not readily palpable by the surgeon. Surgical resection of a solitary insulinoma is generally curative. Diazoxide, which inhibits insulin secretion, or the somatostatin analogue octreotide can be used to treat hypoglycemia in patients with unresectable tumors; everolimus, an mTOR (mammalian target of rapamycin) inhibitor, is promising.

ACCIDENTAL, SURREPTITIOUS, OR MALICIOUS HYPOGLYCEMIA

Accidental ingestion of an insulin secretagogue (e.g., as the result of a pharmacy or other medical error) or even accidental administration of insulin can occur. Factitious hypoglycemia, caused by surreptitious or even malicious administration of insulin or an insulin secretagogue, shares many clinical and laboratory features with insulinoma. It is most common among health care workers, patients with diabetes or their relatives, and people with a history of other factitious illnesses. However, it should be considered in all patients being evaluated for hypoglycemia of obscure cause. Ingestion of an insulin secretagogue causes hypoglycemia with increased C-peptide levels, whereas exogenous insulin causes hypoglycemia with low C-peptide levels reflecting suppression of insulin secretion.

Analytical error in the measurement of plasma glucose concentrations is rare. On the other hand, glucose monitors used to guide treatment of diabetes are not quantitative instruments, particularly at low glucose levels, and should not be used for the definitive diagnosis of hypoglycemia. Even with a quantitative method, low measured glucose concentrations can be artifactual—e.g., the result of continued glucose metabolism by the formed elements of the blood ex vivo, particularly in the presence of leukocytosis, erythrocytosis, or thrombocytosis or with delayed separation of the serum from the formed elements (pseudohypoglycemia).

INBORN ERRORS OF METABOLISM CAUSING HYPOGLYCEMIA

Nondiabetic hypoglycemia also results from inborn errors of metabolism. Such hypoglycemia most commonly occurs in infancy but can also occur in adulthood. Cases in adults can be classified into those resulting in fasting hypoglycemia, postprandial hypoglycemia, and exercise-induced hypoglycemia.

Fasting hypoglycemia

Although rare, disorders of glycogenolysis can result in fasting hypoglycemia. These disorders include glycogen storage disease (GSD) of types 0, I, III, and IV and Fanconi-Bickel syndrome. Patients with GSD types I and III characteristically have high blood lactate levels before and after meals, respectively. Both groups have hypertriglyceridemia, but ketones are high in GSD type III. Defects in fatty acid oxidation also result in fasting hypoglycemia. These defects can include (1) defects in the carnitine cycle; (2) fatty-acid β-oxidation disorders; (3) electron transfer disturbances; and (4) ketogenesis disorders. Finally, defects in gluconeogenesis (fructose-1, 6-biphosphatase) have been reported to result in recurrent hypoglycemia and lactic acidosis.

Postprandial hypoglycemia

Inborn errors of metabolism resulting in postprandial hypoglycemia are also rare. These errors include (1) glucokinase, SUR1, and Kir6.2 potassium channel mutations; (2) congenital disorders of glycosylation; and (3) inherited fructose intolerance.

Exercise-induced hypoglycemia

Exercise-induced hypoglycemia, by definition, follows exercise. It results in hyperinsulinemia caused by increased activity of monocarboxylate transporter 1 in β cells.

APPROACH TO THE PATIENT: Hypoglycemia

In addition to the recognition and documentation of hypoglycemia as well as its treatment (often on an urgent basis), diagnosis of the hypoglycemic mechanism is critical for the selection of therapy that prevents, or at least minimizes, recurrent hypoglycemia.

RECOGNITION AND DOCUMENTATION Hypoglycemia is suspected in patients with typical symptoms; in the presence of confusion, an altered level of consciousness, or a seizure; or in a clinical setting in which hypoglycemia is known to occur. Blood should be drawn, whenever possible, before the administration of glucose to allow documentation of a low plasma glucose concentration. Convincing documentation of hypoglycemia requires the fulfillment of Whipple's triad. Thus, the ideal time to measure the plasma glucose level is during a symptomatic episode. A normal glucose level excludes hypoglycemia as the cause of the symptoms. A low glucose level confirms that hypoglycemia is the cause of the symptoms, provided the latter resolve after the glucose level is raised. When the cause of the hypoglycemic episode is obscure, additional measurements—made while the glucose level is low and before treatment—should include plasma insulin, C-peptide, proinsulin, and β-hydroxybutyrate levels; also critical are screening for circulating oral hypoglycemic agents and assessment of symptoms before and after the plasma glucose concentration is raised.

When the history suggests prior hypoglycemia and no potential mechanism is apparent, the diagnostic strategy is to evaluate the patient as just described and assess for Whipple's triad during and after an episode of hypoglycemia. On the other hand, while it cannot be ignored, a distinctly low plasma glucose concentration measured in a patient without corresponding symptoms raises the possibility of an artifact (pseudohypoglycemia).

DIAGNOSIS OF THE HYPOGLYCEMIC MECHANISM In a patient with documented hypoglycemia, a plausible hypoglycemic mechanism can often be deduced from the history, physical examination, and available laboratory data (Table 26-1). Drugs, particularly alcohol or agents used to treat diabetes, should be the first consideration—even in the absence of known use of a relevant drug—given the possibility of surreptitious, accidental, or malicious drug administration. Other considerations include evidence of a relevant critical illness, hormone deficiencies (less commonly), and a non-β-cell tumor that can be pursued diagnostically (rarely). Absent one of these mechanisms in an otherwise seemingly well individual, the physician should consider endogenous hyperinsulinism and proceed with measurements and assessment of symptoms during spontaneous hypoglycemia or under conditions that might elicit hypoglycemia.

URGENT TREATMENT If the patient is able and willing, oral treatment with glucose tablets or glucose-containing fluids, candy, or food is appropriate. A reasonable initial dose is 20 g of glucose. If the patient is unable or unwilling (because of neuroglycopenia) to take carbohydrates orally, parenteral therapy is necessary. IV administration of glucose (25 g) should be followed by a glucose infusion guided by serial plasma glucose measurements. If IV therapy is not practical, SC or IM glucagon (1.0 mg in adults) can be used, particularly in patients with T1DM. Because it acts by stimulating glycogenolysis, glucagon is ineffective in glycogen-depleted individuals (e.g., those with alcohol-induced hypoglycemia). Glucagon also stimulates insulin secretion and is therefore less useful in T2DM. The somatostatin analogue octreotide can be used to suppress insulin secretion in sulfonylurea-induced hypoglycemia. These treatments raise plasma glucose concentrations only transiently, and patients should therefore be urged to eat as soon as is practical to replete glycogen stores.

PREVENTION OF RECURRENT HYPOGLYCEMIA Prevention of recurrent hypoglycemia requires an understanding of the hypoglycemic mechanism. Offending drugs can be discontinued or their doses reduced. Hypoglycemia caused by a sulfonylurea can persist for hours or even days. Underlying critical illnesses can often be treated. Cortisol and growth hormone can be replaced if levels are deficient. Surgical, radiotherapeutic, or chemotherapeutic reduction of a non–islet cell tumor can alleviate hypoglycemia even if the tumor cannot be cured; glucocorticoid or growth hormone administration also may reduce hypoglycemic episodes in such patients. Surgical resection of an insulinoma is curative; medical therapy with diazoxide or octreotide can be used if resection is not possible and in patients with a nontumor β-cell disorder. Partial pancreatectomy may be necessary in the latter patients. The treatment of autoimmune hypoglycemia (e.g., with glucocorticoid or immunosuppressive drugs) is problematic, but these disorders are sometimes self-limited. Failing these treatments, frequent feedings and avoidance of fasting may be required. Administration of uncooked cornstarch at bedtime or even an overnight intragastric infusion of glucose may be necessary for some patients.

CHAPTER 27

DISORDERS OF LIPOPROTEIN METABOLISM

Daniel J. Rader ■ Helen H. Hobbs

Lipoproteins are complexes of lipids and proteins that are essential for transport of cholesterol, triglycerides, and fat-soluble vitamins. Previously, lipoprotein disorders were the purview of specialized lipidologists, but the demonstration that lipid-lowering therapy significantly reduces the clinical complications of atherosclerotic cardiovascular disease (ASCVD) has brought the diagnosis and treatment of these disorders into the domain of the internist. The number of individuals who are candidates for lipid-lowering therapy continues to increase. Therefore, the appropriate diagnosis and management of lipoprotein disorders is of critical importance in the practice of medicine. This chapter reviews normal lipoprotein physiology, the pathophysiology of disorders of lipoprotein metabolism, the effects of diet and other environmental factors that influence lipoprotein metabolism, and the practical approaches to the diagnosis and management of lipoprotein disorders.

LIPOPROTEIN METABOLISM

LIPOPROTEIN CLASSIFICATION AND COMPOSITION

Lipoproteins are large macromolecular complexes composed of lipids and proteins that transport poorly soluble lipids (primarily triglycerides, cholesterol, and fat-soluble vitamins) through body fluids (plasma, interstitial fluid, and lymph) to and from tissues. Lipoproteins play an essential role in the absorption of dietary cholesterol, long-chain fatty acids, and fat-soluble vitamins; the transport of triglycerides, cholesterol, and fat-soluble vitamins from the liver to peripheral tissues; and the transport of cholesterol from peripheral tissues to the liver and intestine.

Lipoproteins contain a core of hydrophobic lipids (triglycerides and cholesteryl esters) surrounded by a shell of hydrophilic lipids (phospholipids, unesterified cholesterol) and proteins (called apolipoproteins) that interact with body fluids. The plasma lipoproteins are divided into five major classes based on their relative density (Fig. 27-1 and Table 27-1): chylomicrons, very-low-density lipoproteins (VLDLs), intermediate-density lipoproteins (IDLs), low-density lipoproteins (LDLs), and high-density lipoproteins (HDLs). Each lipoprotein class comprises a family of particles that vary in density, size, and protein composition. Because lipid is less dense than water, the density of a lipoprotein particle is primarily determined by the amount of lipid per particle. Chylomicrons are the most lipid-rich and therefore least dense lipoprotein particles, whereas HDLs have the least lipid and are therefore the most dense lipoproteins. In addition to their density, lipoprotein particles can be classified according to their size, determined either by nondenaturing gel electrophoresis or by nuclear magnetic resonance profiling. There is a strong inverse relationship between density and size, with the largest particles being the most buoyant (chylomicrons) and the smallest particles being the most dense (HDL).

The proteins associated with lipoproteins, called *apolipoproteins* (Table 27-2), are required for the assembly, structure, function, and metabolism of lipoproteins. Apolipoproteins activate enzymes important in lipoprotein metabolism and act as ligands for cell surface receptors. ApoB is a very large protein and is the major structural protein of chylomicrons, VLDLs, IDLs, and LDLs; one molecule of apoB, either apoB-48 (chylomicron) or apoB-100 (VLDL, IDL, or LDL), is present on each lipoprotein particle. The human liver synthesizes apoB-100, and the intestine makes apoB-48, which is derived from the same gene by mRNA editing. HDLs have different apolipoproteins that define this lipoprotein class, most importantly apoA-I, which is synthesized in the liver and intestine and is found on virtually all HDL particles. ApoA-II is the second most abundant HDL apolipoprotein and is on approximately two-thirds of the HDL particles. ApoC-I, apoC-II, and

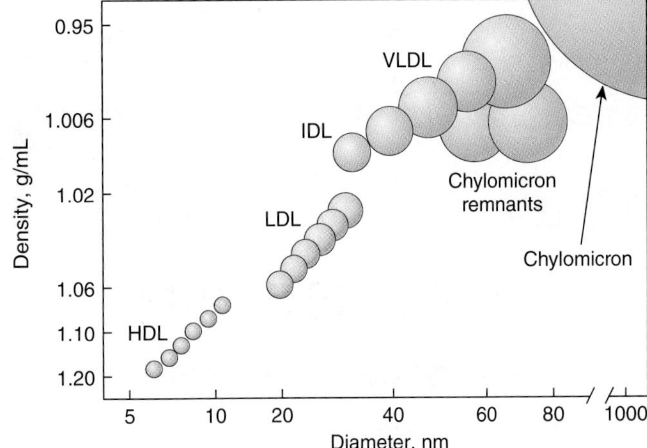

FIGURE 27-1

The density and size distribution of the major classes of lipoprotein particles. Lipoproteins are classified by density and size, which are inversely related. HDL, high-density lipoprotein; IDL, intermediate-density lipoprotein; LDL, low-density lipoprotein; VLDL, very-low-density lipoprotein.

apoC-III participate in the metabolism of triglyceride-rich lipoproteins. ApoE also plays a critical role in the metabolism and clearance of triglyceride-rich particles. Most apolipoproteins, other than apoB, exchange actively among lipoprotein particles in the blood. Apolipoprotein(a) [apo(a)] is a distinctive apolipoprotein and is discussed more below.

TRANSPORT OF INTESTINALLY DERIVED DIETARY LIPIDS BY CHYLOMICRONS

One critical role of lipoproteins is the efficient transport of dietary lipids from the intestine to tissues that require fatty acids for energy or store and metabolize lipids (Fig. 27-2). Dietary triglycerides are hydrolyzed by lipases within the intestinal lumen and emulsified with bile acids to form micelles. Dietary cholesterol, fatty acids, and fat-soluble vitamins are absorbed in the proximal small intestine. Cholesterol and retinol are esterified (by the addition of a fatty acid) in the enterocyte to form cholesteryl esters and retinyl esters, respectively. Longer-chain fatty acids (>12 carbons) are incorporated into triglycerides and packaged with apoB-48, cholesteryl esters, retinyl esters, phospholipids, and cholesterol to form chylomicrons. Nascent chylomicrons are secreted into the intestinal lymph and delivered via the thoracic duct directly to the systemic circulation, where they are extensively processed by peripheral tissues before reaching the liver. The particles encounter lipoprotein lipase (LPL), which is anchored to a glycosylphosphatidylinositol-anchored protein, GPIHBP1, that is attached to the endothelial surfaces of capillaries in adipose tissue, heart, and skeletal muscle (Fig. 27-2). The triglycerides of chylomicrons are hydrolyzed by LPL, and free fatty acids are released. ApoC-II, which is transferred to circulating chylomicrons from HDL, acts as a required cofactor for LPL in this reaction. The released free fatty acids are taken up

TABLE 27-1

MAJOR LIPOPROTEIN CLASSES

LIPOPROTEIN	DENSITY, G/ML[a]	SIZE, NM[b]	ELECTROPHORETIC MOBILITY[c]	APOLIPOPROTEINS: MAJOR	APOLIPOPROTEINS: OTHER	OTHER CONSTITUENTS
Chylomicrons	0.930	75–1200	Origin	ApoB-48	A-I, A-V, C-I, C-II, C-III, E	Retinyl esters
Chylomicron remnants	0.930–1.006	30–80	Slow pre-β	ApoB-48	A-I, A-V, C-I, C-II, C-III, E	Retinyl esters
VLDL	0.930–1.006	30–80	Pre-β	ApoB-100	A-I, A-II, A-V, C-I, C-II, C-III, E	Vitamin E
IDL	1.006–1.019	25–35	Slow pre-β	ApoB-100	C-I, C-II, C-III, E	Vitamin E
LDL	1.019–1.063	18–25	β	ApoB-100		Vitamin E
HDL	1.063–1.210	5–12	α	ApoA-I	A-II, A-IV, A-V, C-III, E	LCAT, CETP, paroxonase
Lp(a)	1.050–1.120	25	Pre-β	ApoB-100	Apo(a)	Oxidized phospholipids

[a]The density of the particle is determined by ultracentrifugation.
[b]The size of the particle is measured using gel electrophoresis.
[c]The electrophoretic mobility of the particle on agarose gel electrophores reflects the size and surface charge of the particle, with β being the position of LDL and α being the position of HDL.

Note: All of the lipoprotein classes contain phospholipids, esterified and unesterified cholesterol, and triglycerides to varying degrees.

Abbreviations: CETP, cholesteryl ester transfer protein; HDL, high-density lipoprotein; IDL, intermediate-density lipoprotein; LCAT, lecithin-cholesterol acyltransferase; LDL, low-density lipoprotein; Lp(a), lipoprotein A; VLDL, very-low-density lipoprotein.

TABLE 27-2

MAJOR APOLIPOPROTEINS

APOLIPOPROTEIN	PRIMARY SOURCE	LIPOPROTEIN ASSOCIATION	FUNCTION
ApoA-I	Intestine, liver	HDL, chylomicrons	Structural protein for HDL Activates LCAT
ApoA-II	Liver	HDL, chylomicrons	Structural protein for HDL
ApoA-IV	Intestine, liver	HDL, chylomicrons	Unknown
ApoA-V	Liver	VLDL, chylomicrons	Promotes LPL-mediated triglyceride lipolysis
Apo(a)	Liver	Lp(a)	Unknown
ApoB-48	Intestine	Chylomicrons, chylomicron remnants	Structural protein for chylomicrons
ApoB-100	Liver	VLDL, IDL, LDL, Lp(a)	Structural protein for VLDL, LDL, IDL, Lp(a) Ligand for binding to LDL receptor
ApoC-I	Liver	Chylomicrons, VLDL, HDL	Unknown
ApoC-II	Liver	Chylomicrons, VLDL, HDL	Cofactor for LPL
ApoC-III	Liver, intestine	Chylomicrons, VLDL, HDL	Inhibits LPL activity and lipoprotein binding to receptors
ApoE	Liver	Chylomicron remnants, IDL, HDL	Ligand for binding to LDL receptor and other receptors

Abbreviations: HDL, high-density lipoprotein; IDL, intermediate-density lipoprotein; LCAT, lecithin-cholesterol acyltransferase; LDL, low-density lipoprotein; Lp(a), lipoprotein A; LPL, lipoprotein lipase; VLDL, very-low-density lipoprotein.

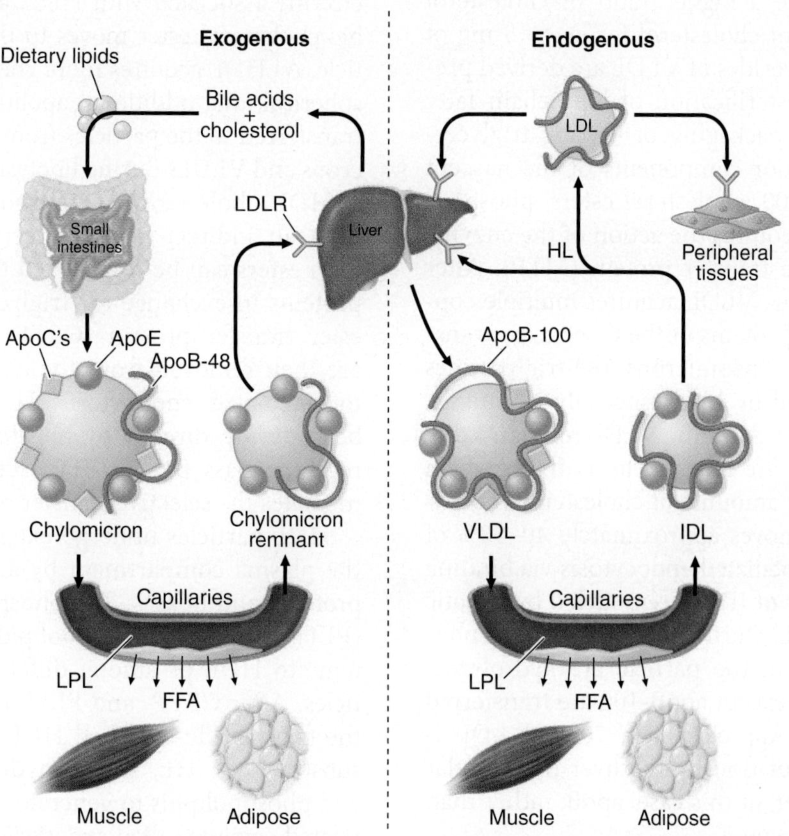

FIGURE 27-2

The exogenous and endogenous lipoprotein metabolic pathways. The exogenous pathway transports dietary lipids to the periphery and the liver. The endogenous pathway transports hepatic lipids to the periphery. FFA, free fatty acid; HL, hepatic lipase; IDL, intermediate-density lipoprotein; LDL, low-density lipoprotein; LDLR, low-density lipoprotein receptor; LPL, lipoprotein lipase; VLDL, very-low-density lipoprotein.

by adjacent myocytes or adipocytes and either oxidized to generate energy or reesterified and stored as triglyceride. Some of the released free fatty acids bind albumin before entering cells and are transported to other tissues, especially the liver. The chylomicron particle progressively shrinks in size as the hydrophobic core is hydrolyzed and the hydrophilic lipids (cholesterol and phospholipids) and apolipoproteins on the particle surface are transferred to HDL, creating chylomicron remnants.

Chylomicron remnants are rapidly removed from the circulation by the liver through a process that requires apoE as a ligand for receptors in the liver. Consequently, few, if any, chylomicrons or chylomicron remnants are generally present in the blood after a 12-h fast, except in patients with certain disorders of lipoprotein metabolism.

TRANSPORT OF HEPATICALLY DERIVED LIPIDS BY VLDL AND LDL

Another key role of lipoproteins is the transport of hepatic lipids from the liver to the periphery (Fig. 27-2). VLDL particles resemble chylomicrons in protein composition but contain apoB-100 rather than apoB-48 and have a higher ratio of cholesterol to triglyceride (~1 mg of cholesterol for every 5 mg of triglyceride). The triglycerides of VLDL are derived predominantly from the esterification of long-chain fatty acids in the liver. The packaging of hepatic triglycerides with the other major components of the nascent VLDL particle (apoB-100, cholesteryl esters, phospholipids, and vitamin E) requires the action of the enzyme microsomal triglyceride transfer protein (MTP). After secretion into the plasma, VLDL acquires multiple copies of apoE and apolipoproteins of the C series by transfer from HDL. As with chylomicrons, the triglycerides of VLDL are hydrolyzed by LPL, especially in muscle, heart, and adipose tissue. After the VLDL remnants dissociate from LPL, they are referred to as IDLs, which contain roughly similar amounts of cholesterol and triglyceride. The liver removes approximately 40–60% of IDL by LDL receptor–mediated endocytosis via binding to apoE. The remainder of IDL is remodeled by hepatic lipase (HL) to form LDL. During this process, phospholipids and triglyceride in the particle are hydrolyzed, and all apolipoproteins except apoB-100 are transferred to other lipoproteins. Approximately 70% of LDL is removed from the circulation by the liver in a similar manner as IDL; however, in this case, apoB, rather than apoE, binds the LDL receptor.

Lp(a) is a lipoprotein similar to LDL in lipid and protein composition, but it contains an additional protein called apolipoprotein(a) [apo(a)]. Apo(a) is synthesized in the liver and attached to apoB-100 by a disulfide linkage. The major site of clearance of Lp(a) is the liver, but the uptake pathway is not known.

HDL METABOLISM AND REVERSE CHOLESTEROL TRANSPORT

All nucleated cells synthesize cholesterol, but only hepatocytes and enterocytes can effectively excrete cholesterol from the body, into either the bile or the gut lumen. In the liver, cholesterol is secreted into the bile, either directly or after conversion to bile acids. Cholesterol in peripheral cells is transported from the plasma membranes of peripheral cells to the liver and intestine by a process termed "reverse cholesterol transport" that is facilitated by HDL (Fig. 27-3).

Nascent HDL particles are synthesized by the intestine and the liver. Newly secreted apoA-I rapidly acquires phospholipids and unesterified cholesterol from its site of synthesis (intestine or liver) via efflux promoted by the membrane protein ATP-binding cassette protein A1 (ABCA1). This process results in the formation of discoidal HDL particles, which then recruit additional unesterified cholesterol from cells or circulating lipoproteins. Within the HDL particle, the cholesterol is esterified by lecithin-cholesterol acyltransferase (LCAT), a plasma enzyme associated with HDL, and the more hydrophobic cholesteryl ester moves to the core of the HDL particle. As HDL acquires more cholesteryl ester, it becomes spherical, and additional apolipoproteins and lipids are transferred to the particles from the surfaces of chylomicrons and VLDLs during lipolysis.

HDL cholesterol is transported to hepatocytes by both an indirect and a direct pathway. HDL cholesteryl esters can be transferred to apoB-containing lipoproteins in exchange for triglyceride by the cholesteryl ester transfer protein (CETP). The cholesteryl esters are then removed from the circulation by LDL receptor–mediated endocytosis. HDL cholesterol can also be taken up directly by hepatocytes via the scavenger receptor class B1 (SR-B1), a cell surface receptor that mediates the selective transfer of lipids to cells.

HDL particles undergo extensive remodeling within the plasma compartment by a variety of lipid transfer proteins and lipases. The phospholipid transfer protein (PLTP) transfers phospholipids from other lipoproteins to HDL or among different classes of HDL particles. After CETP- and PLTP-mediated lipid exchange, the triglyceride-enriched HDL becomes a much better substrate for HL, which hydrolyzes the triglycerides and phospholipids to generate smaller HDL particles. A related enzyme called *endothelial lipase* hydrolyzes HDL phospholipids, generating smaller HDL particles that are catabolized faster. Remodeling of HDL influences the metabolism, function, and plasma concentrations of HDL.

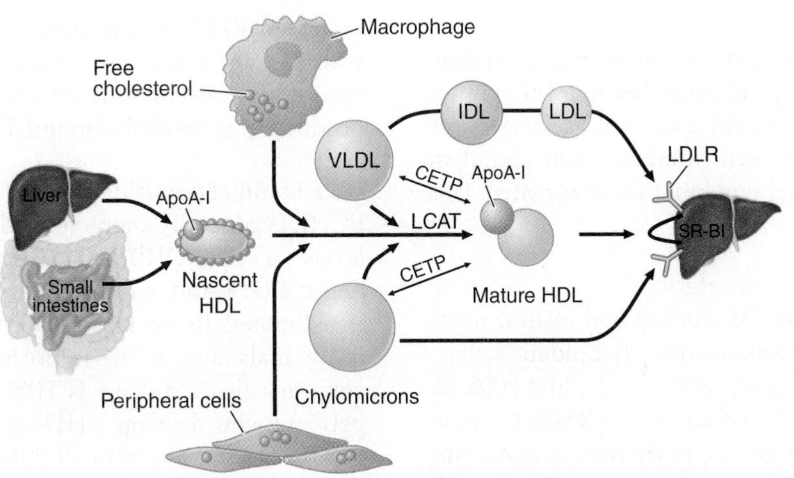

FIGURE 27-3
High-density lipoprotein (HDL) metabolism and reverse cholesterol transport. This pathway transports excess cholesterol from the periphery back to the liver for excretion in the bile. The liver and the intestine produce nascent HDLs. Free cholesterol is acquired from macrophages and other peripheral cells and esterified by lecithin-cholesterol acyltransferase (LCAT), forming mature HDLs. HDL cholesterol can be selectively taken up by the liver via SR-BI (scavenger receptor class BI). Alternatively, HDL cholesteryl ester can be transferred by cholesteryl ester transfer protein (CETP) from HDLs to very-low-density lipoproteins (VLDLs) and chylomicrons, which can then be taken up by the liver. IDL, intermediate-density lipoprotein; LDL, low-density lipoprotein; LDLR, low-density lipoprotein receptor.

DISORDERS OF ELEVATED CHOLESTEROL AND TRIGLYCERIDES

Disorders of lipoprotein metabolism are collectively referred to as "dyslipidemias." Dyslipidemias are generally characterized clinically by increased plasma levels of cholesterol, triglycerides, or both, variably accompanied by reduced levels of HDL cholesterol. Because plasma lipids are commonly screened (see below), dyslipidemia is frequently seen in clinical practice. The majority of patients with dyslipidemia have some combination of genetic predisposition (often polygenic) and environmental contribution (lifestyle, medical condition, or drug). Many, but not all, patients with dyslipidemia are at increased risk for ASCVD, the primary reason for making the diagnosis, as intervention may reduce this risk. In addition, patients with substantially elevated levels of triglycerides may be at risk for acute pancreatitis and require intervention to reduce this risk.

Although literally hundreds of proteins influence lipoprotein metabolism and may interact to produce dyslipidemia in an individual patient, there are a limited number of discrete "nodes" that regulate lipoprotein metabolism. These include: (1) assembly and secretion of triglyceride-rich VLDLs by the liver; (2) lipolysis of triglyceride-rich lipoproteins by LPL; (3) receptor-mediated uptake of apoB-containing lipoproteins by the liver; (4) cellular cholesterol metabolism in the hepatocyte and the enterocyte; and (5) neutral lipid transfer and phospholipid hydrolysis in the plasma. The following discussion will focus on these regulatory nodes, recognizing that in many cases these nodes interact with and influence each other.

DYSLIPIDEMIA CAUSED BY EXCESSIVE HEPATIC SECRETION OF VLDL

Excessive production of VLDL by the liver is one of the most common causes of dyslipidemia. Individuals with excessive hepatic VLDL production usually have elevated fasting triglycerides and low levels of HDL cholesterol (HDL-C), with variable elevations in LDL cholesterol (LDL-C) but usually elevated plasma levels of apoB. A cluster of other metabolic risk factors are often found in association with VLDL overproduction, including obesity, glucose intolerance, insulin resistance, and hypertension (the so-called metabolic syndrome, **Chap. 22**). Some of the major factors that drive hepatic VLDL secretion include obesity, insulin resistance, a high-carbohydrate diet, alcohol use, exogenous estrogens, and genetic predisposition.

Secondary causes of VLDL overproduction

High-carbohydrate diet

Dietary carbohydrates are converted to fatty acids in the liver. Some of the newly synthesized fatty acids are esterified forming triglycerides (TGs) and secreted as constituents of VLDL. Thus, excessive intake of calories as carbohydrates, which is frequent in Western societies, leads to increased hepatic VLDL-TG secretion.

Alcohol

Regular alcohol consumption inhibits hepatic oxidation of free fatty acids, thus promoting hepatic TG synthesis and VLDL secretion. Regular alcohol use also raises plasma levels of HDL-C and should be considered in patients with the unusual combination of elevated TGs and elevated HDL-C.

Obesity and insulin resistance

(See also Chaps. 21 and 23) Obesity and insulin resistance are frequently accompanied by dyslipidemia characterized by elevated plasma levels of TG, low HDL-C, variable levels of LDL-C, and increased levels of small dense LDL. The increase in adipocyte mass and accompanying decreased insulin sensitivity associated with obesity have multiple effects on lipid metabolism, with one of the major effects being excessive hepatic VLDL production. More free fatty acids are delivered from the expanded and insulin-resistant adipose tissue to the liver, where they are reesterified in hepatocytes to form TGs, which are packaged into VLDLs for secretion into the circulation. In addition, the increased insulin levels promote increased fatty acid synthesis in the liver. In insulin-resistant patients who progress to type 2 diabetes mellitus, dyslipidemia remains common, even when the patient is under relatively good glycemic control. In addition to increased VLDL production, insulin resistance can also result in decreased LPL activity, resulting in reduced catabolism of chylomicrons and VLDLs and more severe hypertriglyceridemia (see below).

Nephrotic syndrome

Nephrotic syndrome is a classic cause of excessive VLDL production. The molecular mechanism of VLDL overproduction remains poorly understood but has been attributed to the effects of hypoalbuminemia leading to increased hepatic protein synthesis. Effective treatment of the underlying renal disease often normalizes the lipid profile, but most patients with chronic nephrotic syndrome require lipid-lowering drug therapy.

Cushing's syndrome

(See also Chap. 8) Endogenous or exogenous glucocorticoid excess is associated with increased VLDL synthesis and secretion and hypertriglyceridemia. Patients with Cushing's syndrome frequently have dyslipidemia especially characterized by hypertriglyceridemia and low HDL-C, although elevations in plasma levels of LDL-C can also be seen.

Primary (genetic) causes of VLDL overproduction

Genetic variation influences hepatic VLDL production. A number of genes have been identified in which common and low-frequency variants likely contribute to increased VLDL production, likely involving interactions with diet and other environmental factors. The best recognized inherited condition associated with VLDL overproduction is familial combined hyperlipidemia.

Familial combined hyperlipidemia (FCHL)

FCHL is generally characterized by elevations in plasma levels of TGs (VLDL) and LDL-C (including small dense LDL) and reduced plasma levels of HDL-C. It is estimated to occur in approximately 1 in 100–200 individuals and is an important cause of premature coronary heart disease (CHD); approximately 20% of patients who develop CHD under age 60 have FCHL. FCHL can manifest in childhood but is usually not fully expressed until adulthood. The disease clusters in families, with affected family members typically have one of three possible phenotypes: (1) elevated plasma levels of LDL-C, (2) elevated plasma levels of TGs due to elevation in VLDL, or (3) elevated plasma levels of both LDL-C and TG. The lipoprotein profile can switch among these three phenotypes in the same individual over time and may depend on factors such as diet, exercise, weight, and insulin sensitivity. Patients with FCHL almost always have significantly elevated plasma levels of apoB. The levels of apoB are disproportionately high relative to the plasma LDL-C concentration, indicating the presence of small, dense LDL particles, which are characteristic of this syndrome.

Individuals with this phenotype generally share the same metabolic defect, namely overproduction of VLDL by the liver. The molecular etiology of this condition remains poorly understood, and no single gene has been identified in which mutations cause this disorder. It is likely that defects in a combination of genes can cause the condition, suggesting that a more appropriate term for the disorder might be *polygenic combined hyperlipidemia.*

The presence of a mixed dyslipidemia (plasma TG levels between 200 and 600 mg/dL and total cholesterol levels between 200 and 400 mg/dL, usually with HDL-C levels <40 mg/dL in men and <50 mg/dL in women) and a family history of mixed dyslipidemia and/or premature CHD strongly suggests the diagnosis. Individuals with this phenotype should be treated aggressively due to significantly increased risk of premature CHD. Decreased dietary intake of simple carbohydrates, aerobic exercise, and weight loss can all have beneficial effects on the lipid profile. Patients with diabetes should be aggressively treated to maintain good glucose control. Most patients with FCHL require lipid-lowering drug therapy, starting with statins, to reduce lipoprotein levels and lower the risk of cardiovascular disease.

Lipodystrophy

Lipodystrophy is a condition in which the generation of adipose tissue generally or in certain fat depots is impaired. Lipodystrophies are often associated with insulin resistance and elevated plasma levels of VLDL and chylomicrons due to increased fatty acid synthesis and VLDL production, as well as reduced clearance of TG-rich particles. This disorder can be especially difficult to control. Patients with congenital generalized lipodystrophy are very rare and have nearly complete absence of subcutaneous fat, accompanied by profound insulin resistance and leptin deficiency, and accumulation of TGs in multiple tissues including the liver. Some patients with generalized lipodystrophy have been treated successfully with leptin administration. Partial lipodystrophy is somewhat more common and can be caused by mutations in several different genes, most notably lamin A. Partial lipodystrophy is usually characterized by increased truncal fat accompanied by markedly reduced or absent subcutaneous fat in the extremities and buttocks. These patients generally have insulin resistance, often quite severe, accompanied by type 2 diabetes, hepatosteatosis, and dyslipidemia. The dyslipidemia is usually characterized by elevated TGs and cholesterol and can be difficult to manage clinically. Patients with partial lipodystrophy are at substantially increased risk of atherosclerotic vascular disease and should therefore be treated aggressively for their dyslipidemia with statins and, if necessary, additional lipid-lowering therapies.

DYSLIPIDEMIA CAUSED BY IMPAIRED LIPOLYSIS OF TRIGLYCERIDE-RICH LIPOPROTEINS

Impaired lipolysis of the TGs in TG-rich lipoproteins (TRLs) also commonly contributes to dyslipidemia. As noted above, LPL is the key enzyme responsible for hydrolyzing the TGs in chylomicrons and VLDL. LPL is synthesized and secreted into the extracellular space from adipocytes, myocytes, and cardiomyocytes. It is then transported from the subendothelial to the vascular endothelial surfaces by GPIHPB1. LPL is also synthesized in macrophages. Individuals with impaired LPL activity, whether secondary or due to a primary genetic disorder, have elevated fasting TGs and low levels of HDL-C, usually without elevation in LDL-C or apoB. Insulin resistance, in addition to causing excessive VLDL production, can also cause impaired LPL activity and lipolysis. A number of common and low-frequency genetic variants have been described that influence LPL activity, and single-gene Mendelian disorders that reduce LPL activity have also been described (Table 27-3).

Secondary causes of impaired lipolysis of TRLs

Obesity and insulin resistance

(See also Chaps. 20, 21, and 23) In addition to hepatic overproduction of VLDL, as discussed above, obesity, insulin resistance, and type 2 diabetes have been reported to be associated with variably reduced LPL activity. This may be due in part to the effects of tissue insulin resistance leading to reduced transcription of LPL in skeletal muscle and adipose, as well as to increased production of the LPL inhibitor apoC-III by the liver. This reduction in LPL activity often contributes to the dyslipidemia seen in these patients.

Primary (genetic) causes and genetic predisposition to impaired lipolysis of TRLs

Familial chylomicronemia syndrome

As noted above, LPL is required for the hydrolysis of TGs in chylomicrons and VLDLs, and apoC-II is a cofactor for LPL. Genetic deficiency or inactivity of either protein results in impaired lipolysis and profound elevations in plasma chylomicrons. These patients can also have elevated plasma levels of VLDL, but chylomicronemia predominates. The fasting plasma is turbid, and if left at 4°C (39.2°F) for a few hours, the chylomicrons float to the top and form a creamy supernatant. In these disorders, collectively called the *familial chylomicronemia syndrome*, fasting TG levels are almost invariably >1000 mg/dL. Fasting cholesterol levels are also elevated but to a lesser degree.

LPL deficiency has autosomal recessive inheritance and has a frequency of approximately 1 in 1 million in the population. *ApoC-II deficiency* is also recessive in inheritance pattern and is even less common than LPL deficiency. Multiple different mutations in the LPL and *APOC2* genes cause these diseases. Obligate LPL heterozygotes often have mild-to-moderate elevations in plasma TG levels, whereas individuals heterozygous for mutation in apoC-II do not have hypertriglyceridemia.

Both LPL and apoC-II deficiency usually present in childhood with recurrent episodes of severe abdominal pain due to acute pancreatitis. On funduscopic examination, the retinal blood vessels are opalescent (lipemia retinalis). Eruptive xanthomas, which are small, yellowish-white papules, often appear in clusters on the back, buttocks, and extensor surfaces of the arms and legs. These typically painless skin lesions may become pruritic. Hepatosplenomegaly results from the uptake of circulating chylomicrons by reticuloendothelial cells in the liver and spleen. For unknown reasons, some patients with persistent and pronounced chylomicronemia never develop pancreatitis, eruptive xanthomas, or hepatosplenomegaly. Premature CHD is not generally a feature of familial chylomicronemia syndromes.

The diagnoses of LPL and apoC-II deficiency are established enzymatically in specialized laboratories by assaying TG lipolytic activity in postheparin plasma. Blood is sampled after an IV heparin injection to

TABLE 27-3

PRIMARY HYPERLIPOPROTEINEMIAS CAUSED BY KNOWN SINGLE-GENE MUTATIONS

GENETIC DISORDER	PROTEIN (GENE) DEFECT	LIPOPROTEINS ELEVATED	CLINICAL FINDINGS	GENETIC TRANSMISSION	ESTIMATED INCIDENCE
Hypertriglyceridemia					
Lipoprotein lipase deficiency	LPL (*LPL*)	Chylomicrons, VLDL	Eruptive xanthomas, hepatosplenomegaly, pancreatitis	AR	~1/1,000,000
Familial apoC-II deficiency	ApoC-II (*APOC2*)	Chylomicrons, VLDL	Eruptive xanthomas, hepatosplenomegaly, pancreatitis	AR	<1/1,000,000
ApoA-V deficiency	ApoA-V (*APOA5*)	Chylomicrons, VLDL	Eruptive xanthomas, hepatosplenomegaly, pancreatitis	AR	<1/1,000,000
GPIHBP1 deficiency	*GPIHBP1*	Chylomicrons	Eruptive xanthomas, pancreatitis	AR	<1/1,000,000
Combined Hyperlipidemia					
Familial hepatic lipase deficiency	Hepatic lipase (*LIPC*)	VLDL remnants, HDL	Pancreatitis, CHD	AR	<1/1,000,000
Familial dysbetalipoproteinemia	ApoE (*APOE*)	Chylomicron remnants, VLDL remnants	Palmar and tuberoeruptive xanthomas, CHD, PVD	AR	~1/10,000
Hypercholesterolemia					
Familial hypercholesterolemia	LDL receptor (*LDLR*)	LDL	Tendon xanthomas, CHD	AD	~1/250 to 1/500
Familial defective apoB-100	ApoB-100 (*APOB*)	LDL	Tendon xanthomas, CHD	AD	<~1/1500
Autosomal dominant hypercholesterolemia, type 3	PCSK9 (*PCSK9*)	LDL	Tendon xanthomas, CHD	AD	<1/1,000,000
Autosomal recessive hypercholesterolemia	ARH (*LDLRAP*)	LDL	Tendon xanthomas, CHD	AR	<1/1,000,000
Sitosterolemia	*ABCG5* or *ABCG8*	LDL	Tendon xanthomas, CHD	AR	<1/1,000,000

Abbreviations: AD, autosomal dominant; apo, apolipoprotein; AR, autosomal recessive; ARH, autosomal recessive hypercholesterolemia; CHD, coronary heart disease; LDL, low-density lipoprotein; LPL, lipoprotein lipase; PVD, peripheral vascular disease; VLDL, very-low density lipoprotein.

release the endothelial-bound LPL. LPL activity is profoundly reduced in both LPL and apoC-II deficiency; in patients with apoC-II deficiency, it normalizes after the addition of normal plasma (providing a source of apoC-II). Molecular sequencing of the genes can be used to confirm the diagnosis.

The major therapeutic intervention in familial chylomicronemia syndrome is dietary fat restriction (to as little as 15 g/d) with fat-soluble vitamin supplementation. Consultation with a registered dietician familiar with this disorder is essential. Caloric supplementation with medium-chain TGs, which are absorbed directly into the portal circulation, can be useful, but there is uncertainty about their hepatic safety with prolonged use. If dietary fat restriction alone is not successful in resolving the chylomicronemia, fish oils have been effective in some patients. In patients with apoC-II deficiency, apoC-II can be provided by infusing fresh-frozen plasma to resolve the chylomicronemia in the acute setting. Management of patients with familial chylomicronemia syndrome is particularly challenging during pregnancy when VLDL production is increased. A gene therapy approach, called alipogene tiparvovec, is approved for LPL deficiency in Europe; it involves multiple intramuscular injections of an adeno-associated viral vector encoding a gain-of-function LPL variant, leading to skeletal myocyte expression of LPL.

APOA-V deficiency

Another apolipoprotein, ApoA-V, facilitates the association of VLDL and chylomicrons with LPL and promotes their hydrolysis. Individuals harboring loss-of-function mutations in both *APOA5* alleles develop hyperchylomicronemia. Heterozygosity for variants in *APOA5* that reduce its function contributes to the polygenic basis of hypertriglyceridemia.

GPIHBP1 deficiency

Homozygosity for mutations that interfere with GPIHBP1 synthesis or folding cause severe hypertriglyceridemia by compromising the transport of LPL to the vascular endothelium. The frequency of chylomicronemia due to mutations in GHIHBP1 has not been established but appears to be very rare.

Familial hypertriglyceridemia (FHTG)

FHTG is characterized by elevated fasting TGs without a clear secondary cause, average to below average LDL-C levels, low HDL-C levels, and a family history of hypertriglyceridemia. Plasma LDL-C levels are often reduced due to defective conversion of TG-rich particles to LDL. In contrast to FCHL, apoB levels are not elevated. The identification of other first-degree relatives with hypertriglyceridemia is useful in making the diagnosis. Unlike in FCHL, this condition is not generally associated with a significantly increased risk of CHD. However, if the hypertriglyceridemia is exacerbated by environmental factors, medical conditions, or drugs, the TGs can rise to a level at which acute pancreatitis is a risk. Indeed, management of patients with this condition is mostly geared toward reduction of TGs to prevent pancreatitis.

Individuals with this phenotype generally have reduced lipolysis of TRLs, although overproduction of VLDL by the liver can also contribute. No single gene has been identified in which mutations cause this disorder, whereas combinations of gene variants have been shown to cause this phenotype. A more appropriate term for this condition might be *polygenic hypertriglyceridemia.*

It is important to consider and rule out secondary causes of the hypertriglyceridemia as discussed above. Increased intake of simple carbohydrates, obesity, insulin resistance, alcohol use, estrogen treatment, and certain medications can exacerbate this phenotype. Patients who are at high risk for CHD due to other risk factors should be treated with statin therapy. In patients who are otherwise not at high risk for CHD, lipid-lowering drug therapy can frequently be avoided with appropriate dietary and lifestyle changes. Patients with plasma TG levels >500 mg/dL after a trial of diet and exercise should be considered for drug therapy with a fibrate or fish oil to reduce TGs in order to prevent pancreatitis.

DYSLIPIDEMIA CAUSED BY IMPAIRED HEPATIC UPTAKE OF APOB-CONTAINING LIPOPROTEINS

Impaired uptake of LDL and remnant lipoproteins by the liver is another common cause of dyslipidemia. As discussed above, the LDL receptor is the major receptor responsible for uptake of LDL and remnant particles by the liver. Downregulation of LDL receptor activity or genetic variation that reduces the activity of the LDL receptor pathway leads to elevations in LDL-C. One major factor that reduces LDL receptor activity is a diet high in saturated and *trans* fats. Other medical conditions that reduce LDL receptor activity include hypothyroidism and estrogen deficiency. In addition, genetic variation in a number of genes influences LDL clearance, and mutations in some of these genes cause several discrete Mendelian disorders of elevated LDL-C (Table 27-3).

Secondary causes of impaired hepatic uptake of lipoproteins

Hypothyroidism

(See also Chap. 7) Hypothyroidism is associated with elevated plasma LDL-C levels due primarily to a reduction in hepatic LDL receptor function and delayed clearance of LDL. Thyroid hormone increases hepatic expression of the LDL receptor. Hypothyroid patients also frequently have increased levels of circulating IDL, and some patients with hypothyroidism also have mild hypertriglyceridemia. Because hypothyroidism is often subtle and therefore easily overlooked, all patients presenting with elevated plasma levels of LDL-C, especially if there has been an unexplained increase in LDL-C, should be screened for hypothyroidism. Thyroid replacement therapy usually ameliorates the hypercholesterolemia; if not, the patient probably has a primary lipoprotein disorder and may require lipid-lowering drug therapy with a statin.

Chronic kidney disease

Chronic kidney disease (CKD) is often associated with mild hypertriglyceridemia (<300 mg/dL) due to the accumulation of VLDLs and remnant lipoproteins in the circulation. TG lipolysis and remnant clearance are both reduced in patients with renal failure. Because the risk of ASCVD is increased in end-stage renal disease, subjects with hyperlipidemia, they should usually be aggressively treated with lipid-lowering agents, even though there is inadequate data at present to indicate that this population benefits from LDL-lowering therapy.

Patients with solid organ transplants often have increased lipid levels due to the effect of the drugs required for immunosuppression. These patients can present a difficult clinical management problem, since statins should be used cautiously in these patients due to untoward muscle-related side effects.

Primary (genetic) causes of impaired hepatic uptake of lipoproteins

Genetic variation contributes substantially to elevated LDL-C levels in the general population. It has been estimated that at least 50% of variation in LDL-C is genetically determined. Many patients with elevated LDL-C have *polygenic hypercholesterolemia* characterized by hypercholesterolemia in the absence of secondary causes of hypercholesterolemia (other than dietary factors) or a primary Mendelian disorder. In patients who are genetically predisposed to higher LDL-C levels, diet plays a key role; indeed increased saturated and *trans* fats in the diet shifts the entire distribution of LDL levels in the population to the right. Inheritance of several variants that together elevate LDL-C, coupled with diet, is generally the cause of this condition; <10% of first-degree relatives themselves have hypercholesterolemia. However, single-gene (Mendelian) causes of elevated LDL-C are relatively common and should be considered in the differential diagnosis of elevated LDL-C.

Familial hypercholesterolemia (FH)

FH, also known as autosomal dominant hypercholesterolemia (ADH) type 1, is an autosomal co-dominant disorder characterized by elevated plasma levels of LDL-C in the absence of hypertriglyceridemia. FH is caused by loss-of-function mutations in the gene encoding the LDL receptor. The reduction in LDL receptor activity in the liver results in a reduced rate of clearance of LDL from the circulation. The plasma level of LDL increases to a level such that the rate of LDL production equals the rate of LDL clearance by residual LDL receptor as well as non-LDL receptor mechanisms. More than 1600 different mutations have been reported in association with FH. The elevated levels of LDL-C in FH are primarily due to delayed removal of LDL from the blood; in addition, because the removal of IDL is also delayed, the production of LDL from IDL is also increased. Individuals with two mutated LDL receptor alleles (FH homozygotes, or compound heterozygotes) have much higher LDL-C levels than those with one mutant allele (FH heterozygotes).

Heterozygous FH is caused by the inheritance of one mutant LDL receptor allele. The population frequency of heterozygous FH due to LDL receptor mutations was originally estimated to be 1 in 500 individuals, but recent data suggest it may be as high as approximately 1 in 250 individuals, making it one of the most common single-gene disorders in humans. FH has a higher prevalence in certain founder populations, such as South African Afrikaners, Christian Lebanese, and French Canadians. Heterozygous FH is characterized by elevated plasma levels of LDL-C (usually 200–400 mg/dL) and normal levels of TGs. Patients with heterozygous FH have hypercholesterolemia from birth, and disease recognition is usually based on detection of hypercholesterolemia on routine screening, the appearance of tendon xanthomas, or the development of symptomatic cardiovascular disease. Inheritance is dominant, meaning that the condition was inherited from one parent and ~50% of the patient's siblings can be expected to have hypercholesterolemia. The family history is frequently positive for premature CHD on the side of the family from which the mutation was inherited. Physical findings in many, but not all, patients with heterozygous FH include corneal arcus and tendon xanthomas particularly involving the dorsum of the hands and the Achilles tendons. Untreated heterozygous FH is associated with a markedly increased risk of cardiovascular disease. Untreated men with heterozygous FH have an ~50% chance of having a myocardial infarction before age 60 years, and women with heterozygous FH are at substantially increased risk as well. The age of onset of cardiovascular disease is highly variable and depends on the specific molecular defect, the level of LDL-C, and coexisting cardiovascular risk factors. FH heterozygotes with elevated plasma levels of Lp(a) (see below) appear to be at greater risk for cardiovascular disease.

No definitive diagnostic test for heterozygous FH is available, except in certain founder populations where selected mutations predominate. Most LDL receptor mutations are private and require sequencing of the LDL receptor gene for identification. Sequencing for clinical diagnosis is available but not standard of care and is rarely performed in the United States, because the clinical utility of identifying the specific mutation has not been demonstrated. A family history of hypercholesterolemia and/or premature coronary disease is supportive of the diagnosis. Secondary causes of significant hypercholesterolemia such as hypothyroidism, nephrotic syndrome, and obstructive liver disease should be excluded.

Heterozygous FH patients should be aggressively treated to lower plasma levels of LDL-C, starting in childhood. Initiation of a diet low in saturated and *trans* fats is recommended, but heterozygous FH patients virtually always require lipid-lowering drug therapy for effective control of their LDL-C levels. Statins are effective in heterozygous FH and are clearly the drug class of choice, and usually a more potent member of the class. However, some heterozygous FH patients cannot achieve adequate control of their LDL-C levels even with high-dose statin therapy and require additional drugs; a cholesterol absorption inhibitor and/or a bile acid sequestrant are the next-line classes of drugs. Currently, heterozygous FH patients whose LDL-C levels remain markedly elevated (>200 mg/dL with cardiovascular disease [CVD] or >300 mg/dL without CVD) on maximally tolerated drug therapy are candidates for LDL apheresis, a physical method of purging the blood of LDL in which the LDL particles are selectively removed from the circulation; LDL apheresis is usually performed every 2 weeks. A new class of drugs known as PCSK9 inhibitors is under clinical development and has the potential to effectively control LDL-C levels in the vast majority of patients with heterozygous FH who are inadequately controlled on a statin alone or who are statin intolerant.

Homozygous FH is caused by mutations in both alleles of the LDL receptor and therefore much rarer than heterozygous FH. Patients with homozygous FH have been classified into those patients with virtually no detectable LDL receptor activity (*receptor negative*) and those patients with markedly reduced but detectable LDL receptor activity (*receptor defective*). LDL-C levels in patients with homozygous FH range from about 400 to >1000 mg/dL, with receptor-defective patients at the lower end and receptor-negative patients at the higher end of the range. TGs are usually normal. Many patients with homozygous FH, particularly receptor-negative patients, present in childhood with cutaneous xanthomas on the hands, wrists, elbows, knees, heels, or buttocks. The devastating consequence of homozygous FH is accelerated ASCVD, which often presents in childhood or early adulthood. Atherosclerosis often develops first in the aortic root, where it can cause aortic valvular or supravalvular stenosis, and typically extends into the coronary ostia, which become stenotic. Symptoms can be atypical, and sudden death is not uncommon. Untreated, receptor-negative patients with homozygous FH rarely survive beyond the second decade; patients with receptor-defective LDL receptor defects have a better prognosis but almost invariably develop clinically apparent atherosclerotic vascular disease by age 30, and often much sooner. Carotid and femoral disease develops later in life and is usually not clinically significant.

Homozygous FH should be suspected in a child or young adult with LDL >400 mg/dL without secondary cause. Cutaneous xanthomas, evidence of CVD, and hypercholesterolemia in both parents all are supportive of the diagnosis. Although the specific mutations in the LDL receptor can usually be identified by DNA sequencing, this is not generally performed, and the diagnosis is usually made on clinical grounds.

Patients with homozygous FH must be treated aggressively to delay the onset and progression of CVD. Receptor defective patients sometimes respond to statins and other LDL-lowering drug classes such as a cholesterol absorption inhibitor or a bile acid sequestrant, which upregulate the LDL receptor activity. Two drugs that reduce the hepatic production of VLDL and thus LDL, a small-molecule inhibitor of the microsomal TG transfer protein (MTP) and an antisense oligonucleotide to apoB, are approved in the United States for the treatment of adults with homozygous FH and can be considered. PCSK9 inhibitors, which work through increasing LDL receptor availability, appear to have some benefit in receptor-defective patients and are under clinical development. LDL apheresis is used to lower plasma LDL levels in these patients and can promote regression of xanthomas as well as slow the progression of atherosclerosis. Because the liver is quantitatively the most important tissue for removing circulating LDLs via the LDL receptor, liver transplantation is effective in decreasing plasma LDL-C levels in this disorder but is infrequently used because of the associated problems with immunosuppression.

Familial defective APOB-100 (FDB)

FDB, also known as autosomal dominant hypercholesterolemia (ADH) type 2, is a dominantly inherited disorder that clinically resembles heterozygous FH with elevated LDL-C levels and normal TGs. FDB is caused by mutations in the gene encoding apoB-100, specifically in LDL receptor–binding domain of apoB-100. Several different mutations have been identified, but a single mutation predominates: substitution of glutamine for arginine at position 3500. The mutation results in a reduction in the affinity of LDL binding to the LDL receptor, so LDL is removed from the circulation at a reduced rate. FDB is less common than FH but is more prevalent in individuals of central European descent; the Lancaster County (United States) Amish are a founder population in which the prevalence of FDB is as high as 1 in 10 individuals. FDB is characterized by elevated plasma LDL-C levels with normal TGs; tendon xanthomas can be seen, although not as frequently as in FH, and there is an associated increase in risk of CHD. Patients with FDB cannot be clinically distinguished from patients with heterozygous FH, although patients with FDB tend to have somewhat lower plasma levels of LDL-C than FH heterozygotes, presumably due to the fact that IDL clearance is not impaired in this disorder. Homozygotes for FDB mutations have higher LDL-C levels than FDB heterozygotes but are not as severely affected as homozygous FH patients. The apoB-100 gene mutations can be detected directly through sequencing of the receptor-binding region of the apoB gene or genotyping for the most common mutation, but genetic diagnosis is not generally performed because there is no direct implication for clinical management. As with FH, patients are treated with statins first and, if necessary, with additional classes of LDL-lowering drugs.

Autosomal dominant hypercholesterolemia due to mutations in PCSK9 (ADH-PCSK9 or ADH3)

ADH-PCSK9, also known as autosomal dominant hypercholesterolemia (ADH) type 3, is a very rare autosomal dominant disorder caused by gain-of-function mutations in proprotein convertase subtilisin/kexin type 9 (PCSK9). PCSK9 is a secreted protein that binds to the LDL receptor, targeting it for degradation. Normally, after LDL binds to the LDL receptor, it is internalized along with the receptor, and in the low pH of the endosome, the LDL receptor dissociates from the LDL and recycles to the cell surface. When PCSK9 binds the receptor, the complex is internalized and the receptor is directed to the lysosome, rather than to the cell surface. The missense mutations in PCSK9 that cause hypercholesterolemia enhance the activity of PCSK9. As a consequence, the number of hepatic LDL receptors is reduced. Patients with ADH-PCSK9 are similar clinically to patients with FH. They may be particularly responsive to PCSK9 inhibitors in clinical development. Loss-of-function mutations in PCSK9 cause low LDL-C levels (see below).

Autosomal recessive hypercholesterolemia (ARH)

ARH is a very rare disorder that is mostly seen in individuals of Sardinian descent. The disease is caused by mutations in a protein, ARH (also called LDLR adaptor protein, LDLRAP), which is required for LDL receptor–mediated endocytosis in the liver. ARH binds to the cytoplasmic domain of the LDL receptor and links the receptor to the endocytic machinery. In the absence of LDLRAP, LDL binds to the extracellular domain of the LDL receptor, but the lipoprotein-receptor complex fails to be internalized. ARH, like homozygous FH, is characterized by hypercholesterolemia, tendon xanthomas, and premature coronary artery disease (CAD). The levels of plasma LDL-C tend to be intermediate between the levels present in FH homozygotes and FH heterozygotes, and CAD is not usually symptomatic until the third decade. LDL receptor function in cultured fibroblasts is normal or only modestly reduced in ARH, whereas LDL receptor function in lymphocytes and the liver is negligible. Unlike FH homozygotes, the hyperlipidemia responds to treatment with statins, but these patients usually require additional therapy to lower plasma LDL-C to acceptable levels.

Sitosterolemia

Sitosterolemia is a rare autosomal recessive disease that can result in severe hypercholesterolemia, tendon xanthomas, and premature ASCVD. Sitosterolemia is caused by loss-of-function mutations in either of two members of the ATP-binding cassette (ABC) half transporter family, *ABCG5* and *ABCG8*. These genes are expressed in enterocytes and hepatocytes. The proteins heterodimerize to form a functional complex that transports plant sterols such as sitosterol and campesterol, and animal sterols, predominantly cholesterol, across the biliary membrane of hepatocytes into the bile and across the intestinal luminal surface of enterocytes into the gut lumen. In normal individuals, <5% of dietary plant sterols are absorbed by the proximal small intestine. The small amounts of plant sterols that enter the circulation are preferentially excreted into the bile. Thus, levels of plant sterols are kept very low in tissues. In sitosterolemia, the intestinal absorption of sterols is increased and biliary and fecal excretion of the sterols is reduced, resulting in increased plasma and tissue levels of both plant sterols and cholesterol. The increase in hepatic sterol levels results in transcriptional suppression of the expression of the LDL receptor, resulting in reduced uptake of LDL and substantially increased LDL-C levels. In addition to the usual clinical picture of hypercholesterolemia (i.e., tendon xanthomas and premature ASCVD), these patients also have anisocytosis and poikilocytosis of erythrocytes and megathrombocytes due to the incorporation of plant sterols into cell membranes. Episodes of hemolysis and splenomegaly are a distinctive clinical feature of this disease compared to other genetic forms of hypercholesterolemia and can be a clue to the diagnosis.

Sitosterolemia should be suspected in a patient with severe hypercholesterolemia without a family history of such or who responds dramatically to dietary therapy and/or ezetimibe but not statins. Sitosterolemia can be diagnosed by a laboratory finding of a substantial increase in the plasma level of sitosterol and/or other plant sterols. It is important to make the diagnosis, because bile acid sequestrants and cholesterol-absorption inhibitors are the most effective agents to reduce LDL-C and plasma plant sterol levels in these patients.

Cholesteryl ester storage disease (CESD)

CESD, also known as *lysosomal acid lipase deficiency*, is an autosomal recessive disorder characterized by elevated LDL-C, usually in association with low HDL-C, together with progressive fatty liver ultimately leading to hepatic fibrosis. Plasma TG levels can also be mild to moderately increased in this disorder. The most severe form of this disorder, Wolman's disease, presents in infancy and is rapidly fatal. Both Wolman's disease and CESD are caused by loss-of-function variants in both alleles of the gene encoding lysosomal acid lipase (LAL; gene name *LIPA*). LAL is responsible for hydrolyzing neutral lipids, particularly TGs and cholesteryl esters, after delivery to the lysosome by cell-surface receptors such as the LDL receptor. It is particularly important in the liver, which clears large amounts of lipoproteins from the circulation. Genetic deficiency of LAL results in accumulation of neutral lipid in the hepatocytes, leading to hepatosplenomegaly, microvesicular steatosis, and ultimately fibrosis and end-stage liver disease. The etiology of the elevated LDL-C levels is uncertain; one study suggested that VLDL production is increased, but impaired LDL receptor–mediated clearance of LDL is also likely.

CESD should be particularly suspected in nonobese patients with elevated LDL-C, low HDL-C, and evidence of fatty liver in the absence of overt insulin resistance. The diagnosis can be made with a dried blood spot assay of LAL activity and confirmed by DNA genotyping for the most common mutation, followed if necessary by sequencing of the gene to find the second mutation. Liver biopsy is required to assess the degree of inflammation and fibrosis. It is important to make the diagnosis because it has implications for liver monitoring and potentially for therapeutic approaches under development.

Familial dysbetalipoproteinemia (FDBL)

FDBL (also known as *type III hyperlipoproteinemia*) is usually a recessive disorder characterized by a mixed hyperlipidemia (elevated cholesterol and TGs) due to the accumulation of remnant lipoprotein particles (chylomicron remnants and VLDL remnants, or IDL). ApoE is present in multiple copies on chylomicron remnants and IDL, and mediates their removal via hepatic lipoprotein receptors (Fig. 27-2). FDBL is due to genetic variants of apoE, most commonly apoE2, that result in an apoE protein with reduced ability to bind lipoprotein receptors. The *APOE* gene is polymorphic in sequence, resulting in the expression of three common isoforms: apoE3, which is the most common; and apoE2 and apoE4, which both differ from apoE3 by a single amino acid. Although associated with slightly higher LDL-C levels and increased CHD risk, the apoE4 allele is not associated with FDBL. Individuals who carry one or two apoE4 alleles have an increased risk of Alzheimer's disease. ApoE2 has a lower affinity for the LDL receptor; therefore, chylomicron remnants and IDL containing apoE2 are removed from plasma at a slower rate. Individuals who are homozygous for the E2 allele (the E2/E2 genotype) comprise the most common subset of patients with FDBL.

Approximately 0.5% of the general population are apoE2/E2 homozygotes, but only a small minority of these individuals actually develop hyperlipidemia characteristic of FDBL. In most cases, an additional, sometimes identifiable, factor precipitates the development of hyperlipoproteinemia. The most common precipitating factors are a high-fat diet, diabetes mellitus, obesity, hypothyroidism, renal disease, HIV infection, estrogen deficiency, alcohol use, or certain drugs. The disease seldom presents in women before menopause. Other mutations in apoE can cause a dominant form of FDBL where the hyperlipidemia is fully manifest in the heterozygous state, but these mutations are very rare.

Patients with FDBL usually present in adulthood with hyperlipidemia, xanthomas, or premature coronary or peripheral vascular disease. In FDBL, in contrast to other disorders of elevated TGs, the plasma levels of cholesterol and TG are often elevated to a similar degree, and the level of HDL-C is usually normal or reduced. Two distinctive types of xanthomas, tuberoeruptive and palmar, are seen in FDBL patients. Tuberoeruptive xanthomas begin as clusters of small papules on the elbows, knees, or buttocks and can grow to the size of small grapes. Palmar xanthomas (alternatively called *xanthomata striata palmaris*) are orange-yellow discolorations of the creases in the palms and wrists. Both of these xanthoma types are virtually pathognomonic for FDBL. Subjects with FDBL have premature ASCVD and tend to have more peripheral vascular disease than is typically seen in FH.

The definitive diagnosis of FDBL can be made either by the documentation of very high levels of remnant lipoproteins or by identification of the apoE2/E2 genotype. A variety of methods are used to identify remnant lipoproteins in the plasma, including "β-quantification" by ultracentrifugation (ratio of directly measured VLDL-C to total plasma TG >0.30), lipoprotein electrophoresis (broad β band), or nuclear magnetic resonance lipoprotein profiling. The Friedewald formula for calculation of LDL-C is not valid in FDBL because the VLDL particles are depleted in TG and enriched in cholesterol. The plasma levels of LDL-C are actually low in this disorder due to defective metabolism of VLDL to LDL. DNA-based methods (apoE genotyping) can be performed to confirm homozygosity for apoE2. However, absence of the apoE2/E2 genotype does not strictly rule out the diagnosis of FDBL, because other mutations in apoE can (rarely) cause this condition.

Because FDBL is associated with increased risk of premature ASCVD, it should be treated aggressively. Other metabolic conditions that can worsen the hyperlipidemia (see above) should be managed. Patients with FDBL are typically diet-responsive and can respond favorably to weight reduction and to low-cholesterol, low-fat diets. Alcohol intake should be curtailed. Pharmacologic therapy is often required, and statins are the first line in management. In the event of statin intolerance or insufficient control of hyperlipidemia, cholesterol absorption inhibitors, fibrates, and niacin are also effective in the treatment of FDBL.

Hepatic lipase deficiency

Hepatic lipase (HL; gene name *LIPC*) is a member of the same gene family as LPL and hydrolyzes TGs and phospholipids in remnant lipoproteins and HDL. Hydrolysis of lipids in remnant particles by HL contributes to their hepatic uptake via an apoE-mediated process. HL deficiency is a very rare autosomal recessive disorder characterized by elevated plasma levels of cholesterol and TGs (mixed hyperlipidemia) due to the accumulation of lipoprotein remnants, accompanied by elevated plasma level of HDL-C. The diagnosis is confirmed by measuring HL activity in postheparin plasma and/or confirmation of loss-of-function mutations in both alleles of HL/*LIPC*. Due to the small number of patients with HL deficiency, the association of this genetic defect with ASCVD is not entirely clear, although anecdotally patients with HL deficiency who have premature CVD have been described. As with FDBL, statin therapy is recommended to reduce remnant lipoproteins and cardiovascular risk.

Additional secondary causes of dyslipidemia

Many of the secondary causes of dyslipidemia (Table 27-4) have been described above. Additional considerations are discussed here.

Liver disorders

Because the liver is the principal site of formation and clearance of lipoproteins, liver disorders can affect plasma lipid levels in a variety of ways. Hepatitis due to infection, drugs, or alcohol is often associated with increased VLDL synthesis and mild to moderate hypertriglyceridemia. Severe hepatitis and liver failure are associated with dramatic reductions in plasma cholesterol and TGs due to reduced lipoprotein biosynthetic capacity.

Cholestasis is associated with hypercholesterolemia, which can be very severe. A major pathway by which cholesterol is excreted from the body is via secretion into bile, either directly or after conversion to bile acids, and cholestasis blocks this critical excretory pathway. In cholestasis, free cholesterol, coupled with phospholipids, is secreted into the plasma as a constituent of a lamellar particle called *LP-X*. The particles can deposit in skinfolds, producing lesions resembling those seen in patients with FDBL (xanthomata strata palmaris). Planar and eruptive xanthomas can also be seen in patients with cholestasis.

Drugs

Many drugs have an impact on lipid metabolism and can result in significant alterations in the lipoprotein profile (Table 27-4). Estrogen administration is associated with

TABLE 27-4

SECONDARY CAUSES OF DYSLIPIDEMIA

LDL		HDL		VLDL		CHYLOMICRONS	LP(A)
ELEVATED	**REDUCED**	**ELEVATED**	**REDUCED**	**ELEVATED**	**IDL ELEVATED**	**ELEVATED**	**ELEVATED**
Hypothyroidism	Severe liver disease	Alcohol	Smoking	Obesity	Multiple myeloma	Autoimmune disease	Chronic kidney disease Nephrotic syndrome
Nephrotic syndrome Cholestasis	Malabsorption Malnutrition Gaucher's disease	Exercise Exposure to chlorinated hydrocarbons	DM type 2 Obesity Malnutrition	DM type 2 Glycogen storage disease	Monoclonal gammopathy	DM type 2	Inflammation Menopause
Acute intermittent porphyria	Chronic infectious disease	Drugs: estrogen	Gaucher's disease	Nephrotic syndrome Hepatitis Alcohol	Autoimmune disease		Orchidectomy
Anorexia nervosa Hepatoma Drugs: thiazides, cyclosporin, carbamazepine	Hyperthyroidism Drugs: niacin toxicity		Cholesteryl ester storage disease Drugs: anabolic steroids, beta blockers	Renal failure Sepsis Stress Cushing's syndrome Pregnancy Acromegaly Lipodystrophy Drugs: estrogen, beta blockers, glucocorticoids, bile acid binding resins, retinoic acid	Hypothyroidism		Hypothyroidism Acromegaly Drugs: growth hormone, isotretinoin

Abbreviations: DM, diabetes mellitus; HDL, high-density lipoprotein; IDL, intermediate-density lipoprotein; LDL, low-density lipoprotein; Lp(a), lipoprotein A; VLDL, very-low-density lipoprotein.

increased VLDL and HDL synthesis, resulting in elevated plasma levels of both TGs and HDL-C. This lipoprotein pattern is distinctive because the levels of plasma TG and HDL-C are typically inversely related. Plasma TG levels should be monitored when birth control pills or postmenopausal estrogen therapy is initiated to ensure that the increase in VLDL production does not lead to severe hypertriglyceridemia. Use of low-dose preparations of estrogen or the estrogen patch can minimize the effect of exogenous estrogen on lipids.

INHERITED CAUSES OF LOW LEVELS OF ApoB-CONTAINING LIPOPROTEINS

Plasma concentrations of LDL-C <60 mg/dL are unusual. Although in some cases LDL-C levels in this range may be reflective of malnutrition or serious chronic illness, LDL-C <60 mg/dL in an otherwise healthy individual suggests an inherited condition. The major inherited causes of low LDL-C are reviewed here.

Abetalipoproteinemia

The synthesis and secretion of apoB-containing lipoproteins in the enterocytes of the proximal small bowel and in the hepatocytes of the liver involve a complex series of events that coordinate the coupling of various lipids with apoB-48 and apoB-100, respectively. Abetalipoproteinemia is a rare autosomal recessive disease caused by loss-of-function mutations in the gene encoding microsomal TG transfer protein (MTP; gene name *MTTP*), a protein that transfers lipids to nascent chylomicrons and VLDLs in the intestine and liver, respectively. Plasma levels of cholesterol and TG are extremely low in this disorder, and chylomicrons, VLDLs, LDLs, and apoB are undetectable in plasma. The parents of patients with abetalipoproteinemia (obligate heterozygotes) have normal plasma lipid and apoB levels. Abetalipoproteinemia usually presents in early childhood with diarrhea and failure to thrive due to fat malabsorption. The initial neurologic manifestations are loss of deep tendon reflexes, followed by decreased distal lower extremity vibratory and proprioceptive sense, dysmetria, ataxia, and the development of a spastic gait, often by the third or fourth decade. Patients with abetalipoproteinemia also develop a progressive pigmented retinopathy presenting with decreased night and color vision, followed by reductions in daytime visual acuity and ultimately progressing to near-blindness. The presence of spinocerebellar degeneration and pigmented retinopathy in this disease has resulted in some patients with abetalipoproteinemia being misdiagnosed as having Friedreich's ataxia.

Most of the clinical manifestations of abetalipoproteinemia result from defects in the absorption and transport of fat-soluble vitamins. Vitamin E and retinyl esters are normally transported from enterocytes to the liver by chylomicrons, and vitamin E is dependent on VLDL for transport out of the liver and into the circulation. As a consequence of the inability of these patients to secrete apoB-containing particles, patients with abetalipoproteinemia are markedly deficient in vitamin E and are also mildly to moderately deficient in vitamins A and K. Patients with abetalipoproteinemia should be referred to specialized centers for confirmation of the diagnosis and appropriate therapy. Treatment consists of a low-fat, high-caloric, vitamin-enriched diet accompanied by large supplemental doses of vitamin E. It is imperative that treatment be initiated as soon as possible to prevent development of neurologic sequelae, which can progress even with appropriate therapy. New therapies for this serious disease are needed.

Familial hypobetalipoproteinemia (FHBL)

FHBL generally refers to a condition of low total cholesterol, LDL-C, and apoB due to mutations in apoB. Most of the mutations causing FHBL result in a truncated apoB protein, resulting in impaired assembly and secretion of chylomicrons from enterocytes and VLDL from the liver. Mutations that result in VLDL particles containing a truncated apoB protein are cleared from the circulation at an accelerated rate, which also contributes to patients with this disorder having low levels of LDL-C and apoB. Individuals heterozygous for these mutations usually have LDL-C levels <60–80 mg/dL and also tend to have lower levels of plasma TG. Many FHBL patients have elevated levels of hepatic fat (due to reduced VLDL export) and sometimes have increased levels of liver transaminases, although it appears that these patients infrequently develop associated inflammation and fibrosis.

Mutations in both apoB alleles cause homozygous FHBL, an extremely rare disorder resembling abetalipoproteinemia with nearly undetectable LDL-C and apoB. The neurologic defects in this form of hypobetalipoproteinemia tend to be less severe than is typically seen in abetalipoproteinemia. Homozygous hypobetalipoproteinemia can be distinguished from abetalipoproteinemia by examining the inheritance pattern of the plasma LDL-C level. The levels of LDL-C and apoB are normal in the parents of patients with abetalipoproteinemia and low in those of patients with homozygous hypobetalipoproteinemia.

PCSK9 deficiency

Another inherited cause of low LDL-C results from loss-of-function mutations in PCSK9. PCSK9 is a secreted protein that binds to the extracellular domain of the LDL receptor in the liver and promotes the degradation of the receptor. Heterozygosity for nonsense mutations in PCSK9 that interfere with the synthesis of the protein are associated with increased hepatic LDL receptor activity and reduced plasma levels of LDL-C. Such mutations are particularly frequent in individuals of African descent. Individuals who are heterozygous for a loss-of-function mutation in PCSK9 have an ~30–40% reduction in plasma levels of LDL-C and have a substantial protection from CHD relative to those without a PCSK9 mutation, presumably due to having lower plasma cholesterol levels since birth. This observation led to the development of PCSK9 inhibitors as a new strategy for reducing LDL-C levels and cardiovascular risk. Homozygotes for these nonsense mutations have been reported and have extremely low LDL-C levels (<20 mg/dL) but appear otherwise healthy. A sequence variation of somewhat higher frequency (R46L) is found predominantly in individuals of European descent. This mutation impairs, but does not completely destroy, PCSK9 function. As a consequence, the plasma levels of LDL-C in individuals carrying this mutation are more modestly reduced (~15–20%); individuals with these mutations have a 45% reduction in ASCVD risk.

DISORDERS OF REDUCED HDL CHOLESTEROL

Low levels of HDL-C are very commonly encountered in clinical practice. Low HDL-C is an important independent predictor of increased cardiovascular risk and has been used regularly in standardized risk calculators, including the most recent one from the American Heart Association (AHA)/American College of Cardiology (ACC). However, it remains very uncertain whether low HDL-C is directly causal for the development of ASCVD. HDL metabolism is strongly influenced by TRLs, insulin resistance, and inflammation, among other environmental and medical factors. Thus the HDL-C measurement integrates a number of cardiovascular risk factors, potentially explaining its strong inverse association with ASCVD.

The majority of patients with low HDL-C have some combination of genetic predisposition and secondary factors. Variants in dozens of genes have been shown to influence HDL-C levels. Even more important quantitatively, obesity and insulin resistance have strong suppressive effects on HDL-C, and low HDL-C in these conditions is widely observed. Furthermore, the vast majority of patients with elevated TGs have reduced levels of HDL-C. Most patients with low HDL-C who have been studied in detail have accelerated catabolism of HDL and its associated apoA-I as the physiologic basis for the low HDL-C. Importantly, although HDL-C remains an important biomarker for assessing cardiovascular risk, it is not currently a direct target of intervention for raising the level in order to reduce cardiovascular risk. Certain therapeutic approaches in clinical development, such as inhibitors of CETP (see below), have the potential to change this paradigm.

INHERITED CAUSES OF VERY LOW LEVELS OF HDL-C

Mutations in genes encoding proteins that play critical roles in HDL synthesis and catabolism can result in reductions in plasma levels of HDL-C. Unlike the genetic forms of hypercholesterolemia, which are invariably associated with premature coronary atherosclerosis, genetic forms of hypoalphalipoproteinemia (low HDL-C) are often not associated with clearly increased risk of ASCVD.

Gene deletions in the APOA5-A1-C3-A4 locus and coding mutations in APOA1

Complete genetic deficiency of apoA-I due to a complete deletion of the *APOA1* gene results in the virtual absence of circulating HDL and appears to increase the risk of premature ASCVD. The genes encoding *APOA5*, *APOA1*, *APOC3*, and *APOA4* are clustered together on chromosome 11. Some patients with no apoA-I have genomic deletions that include other genes in the cluster. ApoA-I is required for LCAT activity. In the absence of LCAT, free cholesterol levels increase in both plasma (not HDL) and in tissues. The free cholesterol can form deposits in the cornea and in the skin, resulting in corneal opacities and planar xanthomas. Premature CHD is associated with apoA-I deficiency.

Missense and nonsense mutations in the apoA-I gene are present in some patients with low plasma levels of HDL-C (usually 15–30 mg/dL), but are a rare cause of low plasma HDL-C levels. Most individuals with low plasma HDL-C levels due to missense mutations in apoA-I do not appear to have premature CHD. Patients who are heterozygous for an Arg173Cys substitution in apoA-I (so-called apoA-I_{Milano}) have very low plasma levels of HDL-C due to impaired LCAT activation and accelerated clearance of the HDL particles containing the abnormal apoA-I. Despite having very low plasma levels of HDL-C, these individuals do not have an increased risk of premature CHD.

A few selected missense mutations in apoA-I and apoA-II promote the formation of amyloid fibrils, which can cause systemic amyloidosis.

Tangier disease (ABCA1 deficiency)

Tangier disease is a rare autosomal co-dominant form of extremely low plasma HDL-C levels that is caused by mutations in the gene encoding ABCA1, a cellular transporter that facilitates efflux of unesterified cholesterol and phospholipids from cells to apoA-I (Fig. 27-3). ABCA1 in the liver and intestine rapidly lipidates the apoA-I secreted from the basolateral membranes of these tissues. In the absence of ABCA1, the nascent, poorly lipidated apoA-I is immediately cleared from the circulation. Thus, patients with Tangier disease have extremely low circulating plasma levels of HDL-C (<5 mg/dL) and apoA-I (<5 mg/dL). Cholesterol accumulates in the reticuloendothelial system of these patients, resulting in hepatosplenomegaly and pathognomonic enlarged, grayish yellow or orange tonsils. An intermittent peripheral neuropathy (mononeuritis multiplex) or a sphingomyelia-like neurologic disorder can also be seen in this disorder. Tangier disease is probably associated with some increased risk of premature atherosclerotic disease, although the association is not as robust as might be anticipated, given the very low levels of HDL-C and apoA-I in these patients. Patients with Tangier disease also have low plasma levels of LDL-C, which may attenuate the atherosclerotic risk. Obligate heterozygotes for ABCA1 mutations have moderately reduced plasma HDL-C levels (15–30 mg/dL), and their risk of premature CHD remains uncertain.

Familial LCAT deficiency

This rare autosomal recessive disorder is caused by mutations in LCAT, an enzyme synthesized in the liver and secreted into the plasma, where it circulates associated with lipoproteins (Fig. 27-3). As reviewed above, the enzyme is activated by apoA-I and mediates the esterification of cholesterol to form cholesteryl esters. Consequently, in familial LCAT deficiency, the proportion of free cholesterol in circulating lipoproteins is greatly increased (from ~25% to >70% of total plasma cholesterol). Deficiency in this enzyme interferes with the maturation of HDL particles and results in rapid catabolism of circulating apoA-I.

Two genetic forms of familial LCAT deficiency have been described in humans: complete deficiency (also called *classic LCAT deficiency*) and partial deficiency (also called *fish-eye disease*). Progressive corneal opacification due to the deposition of free cholesterol in the cornea, very low plasma levels of HDL-C (usually <10 mg/dL), and variable hypertriglyceridemia are characteristic of both disorders. In partial LCAT deficiency, there are no other known clinical sequelae. In contrast, patients with complete LCAT deficiency have hemolytic anemia and progressive renal insufficiency that eventually leads to end-stage renal disease. Remarkably, despite the extremely low plasma levels of HDL-C and apoA-I, premature ASCVD is not a consistent feature of either LCAT deficiency or fish eye disease. The diagnosis can be confirmed in a specialized laboratory by assaying plasma LCAT activity or by sequencing the *LCAT* gene.

Primary hypoalphalipoproteinemia

The condition of low plasma levels of HDL-C (the "alpha lipoprotein") is referred to as *hypoalphalipoproteinemia*. Primary hypoalphalipoproteinemia is defined as a plasma HDL-C level below the tenth percentile in the setting of relatively normal cholesterol and TG levels, no apparent secondary causes of low plasma HDL-C, and no clinical signs of LCAT deficiency or Tangier disease. This syndrome is often referred to as *isolated low HDL*. A family history of low HDL-C facilitates the diagnosis of an inherited condition, which may follow an autosomal dominant pattern. The metabolic etiology of this disease appears to be primarily accelerated catabolism of HDL and its apolipoproteins. Some of these patients may have ABCA1 mutations and therefore technically have heterozygous Tangier disease. Several kindreds with primary hypoalphalipoproteinemia and an increased incidence of premature CHD have been described, although it is not clear if the low HDL-C level is the cause of the accelerated atherosclerosis in these families. Association of hypoalphalipoproteinemia with premature CHD may depend on the specific nature of the gene defect or the underlying metabolic defect that either directly or indirectly causes the low plasma HDL-C level.

INHERITED CAUSES OF VERY HIGH LEVELS OF HDL-C

CETP deficiency

Loss-of-function mutations in both alleles of the gene encoding CETP cause substantially elevated HDL-C levels (usually >150 mg/dL). As noted above, CETP transfers cholesteryl esters from HDL to apoB-containing lipoproteins (Fig. 27-3). Absence of this transfer activity results in an increase in the cholesteryl ester content of HDL and a reduction in plasma levels of LDL-C. The large, cholesterol-rich HDL particles circulating in these patients are cleared at a reduced rate. CETP deficiency was first diagnosed in Japanese persons and is rare outside of Japan. The relationship of CETP deficiency to ASCVD remains unresolved. Heterozygotes for CETP deficiency have only modestly elevated HDL-C levels. Based on the phenotype of high HDL-C in CETP deficiency, pharmacologic inhibition of CETP is under development as a new therapeutic approach to both raise HDL-C levels and lower LDL-C levels, but whether it will reduce risk of ASCVD remains to be determined.

SCREENING, DIAGNOSIS, AND MANAGEMENT OF DISORDERS OF LIPOPROTEIN METABOLISM

SCREENING

Plasma lipid and lipoprotein levels should be measured in all adults, preferably after a 12-h overnight fast. In most clinical laboratories, the total cholesterol and TGs in the plasma are measured enzymatically, and then the cholesterol in the supernatant is measured after precipitation of apoB-containing lipoproteins to determine the HDL-C. The LDL-C is then estimated using the following equation:

LDL-C = total cholesterol – (TG/5) – HDL-C

(The VLDL cholesterol content is estimated by dividing the plasma TG by 5, reflecting the ratio of TG to cholesterol in VLDL particles.) This formula (the Friedewald formula) is reasonably accurate if test results are obtained on fasting plasma and if the TG level does not exceed ~200 mg/dL; by convention it cannot be used if the TG level is >400 mg/dL. LDL-C can be directly measured by a number of methods. Further evaluation and treatment are based primarily on the clinical assessment of absolute cardiovascular risk using risk calculators such as the AHA/ACC risk calculator based on a large amount of observational data.

DIAGNOSIS

A critical first step in managing a lipoprotein disorder is to attempt to determine the class or classes of lipoproteins that are increased or decreased in the patient. Once the hyperlipidemia is accurately classified, efforts should be directed to rule out any possible secondary causes of the hyperlipidemia (Table 27-4). Although many patients with hyperlipidemia have a primary (i.e., genetic) cause of their lipid disorder, secondary factors frequently contribute to the hyperlipidemia. A careful social, medical, and family history should be obtained. A fasting glucose should be obtained in the initial workup of all subjects with an elevated TG level. Nephrotic syndrome and chronic renal insufficiency should be excluded by obtaining urine protein and serum creatinine. Liver function tests should be performed to rule out hepatitis and cholestasis. Hypothyroidism should be ruled out by measuring serum thyroid-stimulating hormone.

Once secondary causes have been ruled out, attempts should be made to diagnose the primary lipid disorder because the underlying genetic defect can provide important prognostic information regarding the risk of developing CHD, the response to drug therapy, and the management of other family members. Obtaining the correct diagnosis often requires a detailed family medical history, lipid analyses in family members, and sometimes specialized testing.

Severe hypertriglyceridemia

If the fasting plasma TG level is >1000 mg/dL, the patient has chylomicronemia. If the cholesterol-to-TG ratio is >10, familial chylomicronemia syndrome must be considered, and LPL activity measured in postheparin plasma can help with making that diagnosis. Most adults with chylomicronemia also have elevated VLDL levels. These individuals usually do not have a Mendelian disorder but instead are genetically predisposed and have secondary factors (diet, obesity, glucose intolerance, alcohol ingestion, estrogen therapy) that contribute to the hyperlipidemia. Such patients are a risk of acute pancreatitis and should be treated to reduce their TG levels and thus their risk of pancreatitis.

Severe hypercholesterolemia

If the levels of LDL-C are very high (greater than a ninety-fifth percentile for age and sex), it is likely that the patient has a genetic cause of hypercholesterolemia. At present, there is no compelling reason to perform molecular studies to further refine the molecular diagnosis because the clinical management is not affected. Recessive forms of severe hypercholesterolemia are rare, but if a patient with severe hypercholesterolemia has parents with normal cholesterol levels, ARH, sitosterolemia, and CESD should be considered. Patients with more moderate hypercholesterolemia that does not segregate in families as a monogenic trait are likely to have polygenic hypercholesterolemia.

Combined hyperlipidemia

The most common errors in the diagnosis of lipid disorders involve patients with combined hyperlipidemia. Elevations in the plasma levels of both cholesterol and TGs are seen in patients with increased plasma levels of VLDL and LDL or of remnant lipoproteins. A β-quantification to determine the VLDL cholesterol/TG ratio in plasma (see discussion of FDBL) or a direct measurement of the plasma LDL-C should be performed at least once prior to initiation of lipid-lowering therapy to determine if the hyperlipidemia is due to the accumulation of remnants or to an increase in both LDL and VLDL. Measurement of plasma apoB levels can help identify patients with FCHL who may require more aggressive treatment.

APPROACH TO THE PATIENT: Lipoprotein Disorders

The major goals in the clinical management of lipoprotein disorders are: (1) prevention of acute pancreatitis in patients with severe hypertriglyceridemia; and (2) prevention of CVD and related cardiovascular events.

MANAGEMENT OF SEVERE HYPERTRIGLYCERIDEMIA TO PREVENT PANCREATITIS Although the observational relationship between severe hypertriglyceridemia, particularly chylomicronemia, and acute pancreatitis is well-established, there has never been a clinical trial designed or powered to prove that intervention to reduce TGs reduces the risk of pancreatitis. Nevertheless, it is generally considered appropriate medical practice to intervene in patients with TGs >500 mg/dL in order to reduce the risk of pancreatitis. It remains controversial whether individuals with severe hypertriglyceridemia are at increased risk for ASCVD.

Lifestyle Modifying the lifestyle of the patient with severe hypertriglyceridemia often is associated with a significant reduction in plasma TG level. Patients who drink alcohol should be encouraged to decrease or preferably eliminate their intake. Patients with severe hypertriglyceridemia often benefit from a formal dietary consultation with a dietician intimately familiar with counseling patients on the dietary management of high TGs. Dietary fat intake should be restricted to reduce the formation of chylomicrons in the intestine. The excessive intake of simple carbohydrates should be discouraged because insulin drives TG production in the liver. Aerobic exercise and even increase in regular physical activity can have a positive effect in reducing TG levels and should be strongly encouraged. For patients who are overweight, weight loss can help to reduce TG levels. In extreme cases, bariatric surgery has been shown to not only produce effective weight loss but also substantially reduce plasma TG levels.

Pharmacologic Therapy for Severe Hypertriglyceridemia Despite the above interventions, however, many patients with severe hypertriglyceridemia require pharmacologic therapy (Table 27-5). Patients who persist in having fasting TG >500 mg/dL despite active lifestyle management are candidates for pharmacologic therapy. There are three classes of drugs that are used for management of these patients: fibrates, omega-3 fatty acids (fish oils), and niacin. In addition, statins can reduce plasma TG levels and also reduce ASCVD risk.

Fibrates Fibric acid derivatives, or fibrates, are agonists of PPARα, a nuclear receptor involved in the regulation of lipid metabolism. Fibrates stimulate LPL activity (enhancing TG hydrolysis), reduce apoC-III synthesis (enhancing lipoprotein remnant clearance), promote β-oxidation of fatty acids, and may reduce VLDL TG production. Fibrates are a first-line therapy for severe hypertriglyceridemia (>500 mg/dL). This class of therapeutic agents sometimes lowers but more often raises the plasma level of LDL-C in individuals with severe hypertriglyceridemia. Fibrates are generally well tolerated, but are associated with an increase in the incidence of gallstones. Fibrates can cause myopathy, especially when combined with other lipid-lowering therapy (statins, niacin), and can raise creatinine. Fibrates should be used with caution in patients with CKD. Importantly, fibrates can potentiate the effect of warfarin and certain oral hypoglycemic agents, so the anticoagulation status and plasma glucose levels should be closely monitored in patients on these agents.

Omega 3 Fatty Acids (Fish Oils) Omega-3 fatty acids, or omega-3 polyunsaturated fatty acids (n-3 PUFAs), commonly known as fish oils, are present in high concentration in fish and in flaxseed. The most widely used n-3 PUFAs for the treatment of hyperlipidemias are the two active molecules in fish oil: eicosapentaenoic acid (EPA) and docosahexaenoic acid (DHA). n-3 PUFAs have been concentrated into tablets and in doses of 3–4 g/d are effective at lowering fasting TG levels. Fish oils are a reasonable consideration for first-line therapy in patients with severe hypertriglyceridemia (>500 mg/dL) to prevent pancreatitis. Fish oils can cause an increase in plasma LDL-C levels in some patients. In general, fish oils are well tolerated, with the major side effect being dyspepsia. They appear to be safe, at least at doses up to 3–4 g, but can be associated with a prolongation in the bleeding time.

Nicotinic Acid Nicotinic acid, or niacin, is a B-complex vitamin that has been used as a lipid-modifying agent for more than five decades. Niacin suppresses lipolysis in the adipocyte through its effect on the niacin receptor GPR109A and has other effects on hepatic lipid metabolism that are poorly understood. Niacin reduces plasma TG and LDL-C levels and also raises the plasma concentration of HDL-C. Because it has a number of side effects and can be difficult to use, it is at best a third-line agent for the management of severe hypertriglyceridemia. Niacin therapy is generally started at lower doses and gradually titrated up to higher doses. The most frequent side effect of niacin is cutaneous flushing, which is mediated by activating GPR109A in the skin. Niacin can cause dyspepsia and can exacerbate esophageal reflux and peptic ulcer disease. Mild elevations in transaminases occur in up to 15% of patients treated with any form of niacin. Niacin can raise plasma levels of uric acid and precipitate gouty attacks in susceptible patients. Acanthosis nigricans, a dark-colored coarse skin lesion, and maculopathy are infrequent side effects of niacin.

MANAGEMENT OF CHOLESTEROL TO PREVENT CARDIOVASCULAR DISEASE In contrast to hypertriglyceridemia and pancreatitis, there are abundant and compelling data that intervention to reduce LDL-C substantially reduces the risk of CVD, including myocardial infarction and stroke, as well as total mortality. Thus, it is imperative that patients with

TABLE 27-5

SUMMARY OF THE MAJOR APPROVED DRUGS USED FOR THE TREATMENT OF DYSLIPIDEMIA

DRUG	MAJOR INDICATIONS	STARTING DOSE	MAXIMAL DOSE	MECHANISM	COMMON SIDE EFFECTS
HMG-CoA reductase inhibitors (statins)	Elevated LDL-C; increased CV risk			↓ Cholesterol synthesis, ↑ Hepatic LDL receptors, ↓ VLDL production	Myalgias, arthralgias, elevated transaminases, dyspepsia
Lovastatin		20–40 mg daily	80 mg daily		
Pravastatin		40–80 mg daily	80 mg daily		
Simvastatin		20–40 mg daily	80 mg daily		
Fluvastatin		20–40 mg daily	80 mg daily		
Atorvastatin		20–40 mg daily	80 mg daily		
Rosuvastatin		5–20 mg daily	40 mg daily		
Pitavastatin		1–2 mg daily	4 mg daily		
Cholesterol absorption inhibitor	Elevated LDL-C			↓ Cholesterol absorption, ↑ LDL receptors	Elevated transaminases
Ezetimibe		10 mg daily	10 mg daily		
Bile acid sequestrants	Elevated LDL-C			↑ Bile acid excretion and ↑ LDL receptors	Bloating, constipation, elevated triglycerides
Cholestyramine		4 g daily	32 g daily		
Colestipol		5 g daily	40 g daily		
Colesevelam		3750 mg daily	4375 mg daily		
MTP inhibitor Lomitapide	HoFH	5 mg daily	60 mg daily	↓ VLDL production	Nausea, diarrhea, increased hepatic fat
ApoB inhibitor Mipomersen	HoFH	200 mg SC weekly	200 mg SC weekly	↓ VLDL production	Injection site reactions, flu-like symptoms, increased hepatic fat
Nicotinic acid	Elevated LDL-C, elevated TG			↓ VLDL production	Cutaneous flushing, GI upset, elevated glucose, uric acid, and elevated liver function tests
Immediate-release		100 mg tid	1 g tid		
Sustained-release		250 mg bid	1.5 g bid		
Extended-release		500 mg qhs	2 g qhs		
Fibric acid derivatives	Elevated TG			↑ LPL, ↓ VLDL synthesis	Dyspepsia, myalgia, gallstones, elevated transaminases
Gemfibrozil		600 mg bid	600 mg bid		
Fenofibrate		145 mg qd	145 mg qd		
Omega-3 fatty acids Omega-3 acid ethyl esters	Elevated TG	4 g daily	4 g daily	↑ TG catabolism	Dyspepsia, fishy odor to breath
Icosapent ethyl		4 g daily	4 g daily		

Abbreviations: GI, gastrointestinal; HDL-C, high-density lipoprotein cholesterol; HoFH, homozygous familial hypercholesterolemia; LDL, low-density lipoprotein; LDL-C, LDL-cholesterol; LPL, lipoprotein lipase; TG, triglyceride; VLDL, very-low-density lipoprotein.

hypercholesterolemia be assessed for cardiovascular risk and for the need for intervention. It is also worth noting that patients at high risk for CVD who have plasma LDL-C levels in the "normal" or average range also benefit from intervention to reduce LDL-C levels.

Lifestyle The first approach to a patient with hypercholesterolemia and high cardiovascular risk is to make any necessary lifestyle changes. In obese patients, efforts should be made to reduce body weight to the ideal level. Patients should receive dietary counseling to reduce the content of saturated fats, *trans* fats, and cholesterol in the diet. Regular aerobic exercise has relatively little impact on reducing plasma LDL-C levels, although it has cardiovascular benefits independent of LDL lowering.

Pharmacologic Therapy for Hypercholesterolemia The decision to use LDL-lowering drug therapy (Table 27-5)—with a statin being first-line therapy—depends on the level of LDL-C as well as the level of cardiovascular risk. In general, patients with a Mendelian disorder of elevated LDL-C such as FH must be treated to reduce the very high lifetime risk of CVD, and treatment should be initiated as early as possible in adulthood or, in some cases, during childhood.

Otherwise, the decision to initiate LDL-lowering drug therapy is generally determined by the level of cardiovascular risk. In patients with established CVD, statin therapy is well supported by clinical trial data and should be used regardless of the LDL-C level. For patients >40 years old without clinical CVD, the AHA/ACC risk calculator *(http://my.americanheart.org/professional/StatementsGuidelines/PreventionGuidelines/Prevention-Guidelines_UCM_457698_SubHomePage.jsp)* can be used to determine the 10-year absolute risk for CVD, and current guidelines suggest that a 10-year risk >7.5% merits consideration of statin therapy regardless of plasma LDL-C level. For younger patients, the assessment of lifetime risk of CVD may help inform the decision to start a statin.

HMG-CoA Reductase Inhibitors (Statins) Statins inhibit HMG-CoA reductase, a key enzyme in cholesterol biosynthesis. By inhibiting cholesterol biosynthesis, statins lead to increased hepatic LDL receptor activity and accelerated clearance of circulating LDL, resulting in a dose-dependent reduction in plasma levels of LDL-C. The magnitude of LDL lowering associated with statin treatment varies widely among individuals, but once a patient is on a statin, the doubling of the statin dose produces an ~6% further reduction in the level of plasma LDL-C. The statins currently available differ in their LDL-C–reducing potency (Table 27-5). Currently, there is no convincing evidence that any of the different statins confer an advantage that is independent of the effect on LDL-C. Statins also reduce plasma TGs in a dose-dependent fashion, which is roughly proportional to their LDL-C–lowering effects (if the TGs are <400 mg/dL). Statins have a modest HDL-raising effect (5–10%) that is not generally dose-dependent.

Statins are well tolerated and can be taken in tablet form once a day. Potential side effects include dyspepsia, headaches, fatigue, and muscle or joint pains. Severe myopathy and even rhabdomyolysis occur rarely with statin treatment. The risk of statin-associated myopathy is increased by the presence of older age, frailty, renal insufficiency, and coadministration of drugs that interfere with the metabolism of statins, such as erythromycin and related antibiotics, antifungal agents, immunosuppressive drugs, and fibric acid derivatives (particularly gemfibrozil). Severe myopathy can usually be avoided by careful patient selection, avoidance of interacting drugs, and instructing the patient to contact the physician immediately in the event of unexplained muscle pain. In the event of muscle symptoms, the plasma creatine kinase (CK) level should be obtained to differentiate myopathy from myalgia. Serum CK levels need not be monitored on a routine basis in patients taking statins, because an elevated CK in the absence of symptoms does not predict the development of myopathy and does not necessarily suggest the need for discontinuing the drug.

Another consequence of statin therapy can be elevation in liver transaminases (alanine aminotransferase [ALT] and aspartate aminotransferase [AST]). They should be checked before starting therapy, at 2–3 months, and then annually. Substantial (greater than three times the upper limit of normal) elevation in transaminases is relatively rare, and mild-to-moderate (one to three times normal) elevation in transaminases in the absence of symptoms need not mandate discontinuing the medication. Severe clinical hepatitis associated with statins is exceedingly rare, and the trend is toward less frequent monitoring of transaminases in patients taking statins. The statin-associated elevation in liver enzymes resolves upon discontinuation of the medication.

Statins appear to be remarkably safe. Meta-analyses of large randomized controlled clinical trials with statins do not suggest an increase in any major noncardiac diseases except type 2 diabetes. A small excess percentage of those taking statins will develop diabetes but the benefits associated with the reduction in cardiovascular events outweigh the increase in incidence of diabetes. Statins are the drug class of choice for LDL-C reduction and are by far the most widely used class of lipid-lowering drugs.

Cholesterol Absorption Inhibitors Cholesterol within the lumen of the small intestine is derived from the diet (about one-third) and the bile (about two-thirds) and is actively absorbed by the enterocyte through a process that involves the protein NPC1L1. Ezetimibe (Table 27-5) is a cholesterol absorption inhibitor that binds directly to and inhibits NPC1L1 and blocks the intestinal absorption of cholesterol. Ezetimibe (10 mg) inhibits cholesterol absorption by almost 60%, resulting in a reduction in delivery of dietary sterols in the liver and an increase in hepatic LDL receptor expression. The mean reduction in plasma LDL-C on ezetimibe (10 mg) is 18%, and the effect is additive when used in combination with a statin. Effects on TG and HDL-C levels are negligible. When used in combination with a statin, monitoring of liver transaminases is recommended. The only roles for ezetimibe in monotherapy are in patients who do not tolerate statins and in sitosterolemia.

Bile Acid Sequestrants (Resins) Bile acid sequestrants bind bile acids in the intestine and promote their excretion rather than reabsorption in the ileum. To maintain the bile acid pool size, the liver diverts cholesterol to bile acid synthesis. The decreased hepatic intracellular cholesterol content results in upregulation of the LDL receptor and enhanced LDL clearance from the plasma. Bile acid sequestrants, including cholestyramine, colestipol, and colesevelam (Table 27-5), primarily reduce plasma LDL-C levels but can cause an increase in plasma TGs. Therefore, patients with hypertriglyceridemia generally should not be treated with bile acid–binding resins. Cholestyramine and colestipol are insoluble resins that must be suspended in liquids. Colesevelam is available as tablets but generally requires up to six to seven tablets per day for effective LDL-C lowering. Most side effects of resins are limited to the gastrointestinal tract and include bloating and constipation. Because bile acid sequestrants are not systemically absorbed, they are very safe and the cholesterol-lowering drug of choice in children and in women of childbearing age who are lactating, pregnant, or could become pregnant. They are effective in combination with statins and in combination with ezetimibe and are particularly useful with one or both of these drugs for patients with severe hypercholesterolemia or those with statin intolerance.

Specialized Drugs For Homozygous FH Two "orphan" drugs are approved specifically for the management of homozygous FH. They include a small-molecule inhibitor of MTP, called lomitapide, and an antisense oligonucleotide against apoB, called mipomersen. These drugs reduce VLDL production and LDL-C levels in homozygous FH patients. Due to their mechanism of action, each drug causes an increase in hepatic fat, the long-term consequences of which are unknown. In addition, lomitapide is associated with gastrointestinal-related side effects, and mipomersen is associated with skin reactions and flu-like symptoms.

LDL Apheresis Patients who remain severely hypercholesterolemic despite optimally tolerated drug therapy are candidates for LDL apheresis. In this process, the patient's plasma is passed over a column that selectively removes the LDL, and the LDL-depleted plasma is returned to the patient. Patients on maximally tolerated combination drug therapy who have CHD and a plasma LDL-C level >200 mg/dL or no CHD and a plasma LDL-C level >300 mg/dL are candidates for every-other-week LDL apheresis and should be referred to a specialized lipid center.

SECTION V

DISORDERS AFFECTING MULTIPLE ENDOCRINE SYSTEMS

CHAPTER 28

ENDOCRINE TUMORS OF THE GASTROINTESTINAL TRACT AND PANCREAS

Robert T. Jensen

GENERAL FEATURES OF GASTROINTESTINAL NEUROENDOCRINE TUMORS

Gastrointestinal (GI) neuroendocrine tumors (NETs) are tumors derived from the diffuse neuroendocrine system of the GI tract; that system is composed of amine- and acid-producing cells with different hormonal profiles, depending on the site of origin. The tumors historically are divided into GI-NETs (in the GI tract) (also frequently called *carcinoid tumors*) and pancreatic neuroendocrine tumors (pNETs), although newer pathologic classifications have proposed that they all be classified as GI-NETs. The term *GI-NET* has been proposed to replace the term *carcinoid*; however, the term *carcinoid* is widely used, and many are not familiar with this change. Accordingly, this chapter will use the term *GI-NETs* (carcinoids). These tumors originally were classified as APUDomas (for *a*mine *p*recursor *u*ptake and *d*ecarboxylation), as were pheochromocytomas, melanomas, and medullary thyroid carcinomas, because they share certain cytochemical features as well as various pathologic, biologic, and molecular features (Table 28-1). It was originally proposed that APUDomas had a similar embryonic origin from neural crest cells, but it is now known the peptide-secreting cells are not of neuroectodermal origin. Nevertheless, the concept of APUDomas is useful because these tumors have important similarities as well as some differences (Table 28-1). In this section, the areas of similarity between pNETs and GI-NETs (carcinoids) will be discussed together, and areas in which there are important differences will be discussed separately.

CLASSIFICATION/PATHOLOGY/TUMOR BIOLOGY OF NETs

NETs generally are composed of monotonous sheets of small round cells with uniform nuclei, and mitoses are uncommon. They can be identified tentatively on routine histology; however, these tumors are now recognized principally by their histologic staining patterns due to shared cellular proteins. Historically, silver staining was used, and tumors were classified as showing an argentaffin reaction if they took up and reduced silver or as being argyrophilic if they did not reduce it. Currently, immunocytochemical localization of chromogranins (A, B, C), neuron-specific enolase, and synaptophysin, which are all neuroendocrine cell markers, is used (Table 28-1). Chromogranin A is the most widely used.

Ultrastructurally, these tumors possess electron-dense neurosecretory granules and frequently contain small clear vesicles that correspond to synaptic vesicles of neurons. NETs synthesize numerous peptides, growth factors, and bioactive amines that may be ectopically secreted, giving rise to a specific clinical syndrome (Table 28-2). The diagnosis of the specific syndrome requires the clinical features of the disease (Table 28-2) and cannot be made from the immunocytochemistry results alone. The presence or absence of a specific clinical syndrome also cannot be predicted from the immunocytochemistry alone (Table 28-1). Furthermore, pathologists cannot distinguish between benign and malignant NETs unless metastasis or invasion is present.

GI-NETs (carcinoids) frequently are classified according to their anatomic area of origin (i.e., foregut, midgut, hindgut) because tumors with similar areas

TABLE 28-1

GENERAL CHARACTERISTICS OF GASTROINTESTINAL NEUROENDOCRINE TUMORS (GI-NETs [CARCINOIDS], PANCREATIC NEUROENDOCRINE TUMORS [pNETs])

A. Share general neuroendocrine cell markers (identification used for diagnosis)
   1. Chromogranins (A, B, C) are acidic monomeric soluble proteins found in the large secretory granules. Chromogranin A is the most widely used.
   2. Neuron-specific enolase (NSE) is the γ-γ dimer of the enzyme enolase and is a cytosolic marker of neuroendocrine differentiation.
   3. Synaptophysin is an integral membrane glycoprotein of 38,000 molecular weight found in small vesicles of neurons and neuroendocrine tumors.
B. Pathologic similarities
   1. All are APUDomas showing *a*mine *p*recursor *u*ptake and *d*ecarboxylation.
   2. Ultrastructurally, they have dense-core secretory granules (>80 nm).
   3. Histologically, they generally appear similar with few mitoses and uniform nuclei.
   4. Frequently synthesize multiple peptides/amines, which can be detected immunocytochemically but may not be secreted.
   5. Presence or absence of clinical syndrome or type cannot be predicted by immunocytochemical studies.
   6. Histologic classifications (grading, TNM classification) have prognostic significance. Only invasion or metastases establish malignancy.
C. Similarities of biologic behavior
   1. Generally slow growing, but some are aggressive.
   2. Most are well-differentiated tumors having low proliferative indices.
   3. Secrete biologically active peptides/amines, which can cause clinical symptoms.
   4. Generally have high densities of somatostatin receptors, which are used for both localization and treatment.
   5. Most (>70%) secrete chromogranin A, which is frequently used as a tumor marker.
D. Similarities/differences in molecular abnormalities
   1. Similarities
      a. Uncommon—mutations in common oncogenes (*ras, jun, fos,* etc).
      b. Uncommon—mutations in common tumor-suppressor genes (*p53*, retinoblastoma).
      c. Alterations at MEN 1 locus (11q13) (frequently foregut, less commonly mid/hindgut NETs) and $p16^{INK4a}$ (9p21) occur in a proportion (10–45%).
      d. Methylation of various genes occurs in 40–87% (*ras*-associated domain family I, p14, p16, O^6-methylguanine methyltransferases, retinoic acid receptor β).
   2. Differences
      a. pNETs—loss of 1p (21%), 3p (8–47%), 3q (8–41%), 11q (21–62%), 6q (18–68%), Y (45%). Gains at 17q (10–55%), 7q (16–68%), 4q (33%), 18 (up to 45%).
      b. GI-NETs (carcinoids)—loss of 18q (38–88%), >18p (33–43%), >9p, 16q21 (21–23%). Gains at 17q, 19p (57%), 4q (33%), 14q (20%), 5 (up to 36%).
      c. pNETs: *ATRX/DAXX* mutations in 43%, MEN 1 mutations in 44%, mTor mutations (14%); uncommon in midgut GI-NETs (0–2%).

Abbreviations: *ATRX,* alpha-thalassemia X-lined mental retardation protein; *DAXX,* death domain associated protein; *MEN 1,* multiple endocrine neoplasia type 1; TNM, tumor, node, metastasis.

of origin share functional manifestations, histochemistry, and secretory products (Table 28-3). Foregut tumors generally have a low serotonin (5-HT) content; are argentaffin-negative but argyrophilic; occasionally secrete adrenocorticotropic hormone (ACTH) or 5-hydroxytryptophan (5-HTP), causing an atypical carcinoid syndrome (Fig. 28-1); are often multihormonal; and may metastasize to bone. They uncommonly produce a clinical syndrome due to the secreted products. Midgut carcinoids are argentaffin-positive, have a high serotonin content, most frequently cause the typical carcinoid syndrome when they metastasize (Table 28-3, Fig. 28-1), release serotonin and tachykinins (substance P, neuropeptide K, substance K), rarely secrete 5-HTP or ACTH, and less commonly metastasize to bone. Hindgut carcinoids (rectum, transverse and descending colon) are argentaffin-negative, are often argyrophilic, rarely contain serotonin or cause the carcinoid syndrome (Fig. 28-1, Table 28-3), rarely secrete 5-HTP or ACTH, contain numerous peptides, and may metastasize to bone.

pNETs can be classified into nine well-established specific functional syndromes (Table 28-2), six additional very rare specific functional syndromes (less than five cases described), five possible specific functional syndromes (pNETs secreting calcitonin, neurotensin, pancreatic polypeptide, ghrelin) (Table 28-2), and nonfunctional pNETs. Other functional hormonal syndromes due to nonpancreatic tumors (usually intraabdominal in location) have been described only rarely and are not included in (Table 28-2). These include secretion by intestinal and ovarian tumors of peptide tyrosine tyrosine (PYY), which results in altered

TABLE 28-2

GASTROINTESTINAL NEUROENDOCRINE TUMOR SYNDROMES

NAME	BIOLOGICALLY ACTIVE PEPTIDE(S) SECRETED	INCIDENCE (NEW CASES/10^6 POPULATION/ YEAR)	TUMOR LOCATION	MALIGNANT, %	ASSOCIATED WITH MEN 1, %	MAIN SYMPTOMS/ SIGNS
I. Established Specific Functional Syndromes						
A. Carcinoid syndrome due to GI-NET						
Carcinoid syndrome	Serotonin, possibly tachykinins, motilin, prostaglandins	0.5–2	Midgut (75–87%) Foregut (2–33%) Hindgut (1–8%) Unknown (2–15%)	95–100	Rare	Diarrhea (32–84%) Flushing (63–75%) Pain (10–34%) Asthma (4–18%) Heart disease (11–41%)
B. Well-established functional pNET syndromes						
Zollinger-Ellison syndrome	Gastrin	0.5–1.5	Duodenum (70%) Pancreas (25%) Other sites (5%)	60–90	20–25	Pain (79–100%) Diarrhea (30–75%) Esophageal symptoms (31–56%)
Insulinoma	Insulin	1–2	Pancreas (>99%)	<10	4–5	Hypoglycemic symptoms (100%)
VIPoma (Verner-Morrison syndrome, pancreatic cholera, WDHA)	Vasoactive intestinal peptide	0.05–0.2	Pancreas (90%, adult) Other (10%, neural, adrenal, periganglionic)	40–70	6	Diarrhea (90–100%) Hypokalemia (80–100%) Dehydration (83%)
Glucagonoma	Glucagon	0.01–0.1	Pancreas (100%)	50–80	1–20	Rash (67–90%) Glucose intolerance (38–87%) Weight loss (66–96%)
Somatostatinoma	Somatostatin	Rare	Pancreas (55%) Duodenum/jejunum (44%)	>70	45	Diabetes mellitus (63–90%) Cholelithiasis (65–90%) Diarrhea (35–90%)
GRFoma	Growth hormone–releasing hormone	Unknown	Pancreas (30%) Lung (54%) Jejunum (7%) Other (13%)	>60	16	Acromegaly (100%)
ACTHoma	ACTH	Rare	Pancreas (4–16% all ectopic Cushing's)	>95	Rare	Cushing's syndrome (100%)
pNET causing carcinoid syndrome	Serotonin, ?tachykinins	Rare (43 cases)	Pancreas (<1% all carcinoids)	60–88	Rare	Same as carcinoid syndrome above
pNET causing hypercalcemia	PTHrP Others unknown	Rare	Pancreas (rare cause of hypercalcemia)	84	Rare	Abdominal pain due to hepatic metastases

(continued)

TABLE 28-2

GASTROINTESTINAL NEUROENDOCRINE TUMOR SYNDROMES (CONTINUED)

NAME	BIOLOGICALLY ACTIVE PEPTIDE(S) SECRETED	INCIDENCE (NEW CASES/10^6 POPULATION/ YEAR)	TUMOR LOCATION	MALIGNANT, %	ASSOCIATED WITH MEN 1, %	MAIN SYMPTOMS/ SIGNS
II. Rare Specific Functional Syndromes						
pNET secreting renin	Renin	Rare	Pancreas	Unknown	No	Hypertension
pNET secreting luteinizing hormone	Luteinizing hormone	Rare	Pancreas	Unknown	No	Anovulation, virilization (female); reduced libido (male)
pNET secreting erythropoietin	Erythropoietin	Rare	Pancreas	100	No	Polycythemia
pNET secreting IGF-II	Insulin-like growth factor II	Rare	Pancreas	Unknown	No	Hypoglycemia
pNET secreting GLP-1	Glucagon-like peptide-1	Rare	Pancreas	Unknown	No	Hypoglycemia, diabetes
pNET secreting enteroglucagon	Enteroglucagon	Rare	Pancreas, small intestine	Unknown	Rare	Small intestinal hypertrophy, intestinal stasis, malabsorption
III. Possible Specific Functional pNET Syndromes						
pNET secreting calcitonin	Calcitonin	Rare	Pancreas (rare cause of hypercalcitonemia)	>80	16	Diarrhea (50%)
pNET secreting neurotensin	Neurotensin	Rare	Pancreas (100%)	Unknown	No	Motility disturbances, vascular symptoms
pNET secreting pancreatic polypeptide (PPoma)	Pancreatic polypeptide	1–2	Pancreas	>60	18–44	Watery diarrhea
pNET secreting ghrelin	Ghrelin	Rare	Pancreas	Unknown	No	Effects on appetite, body weight
IV. Nonfunctional Syndrome pNET						
PPoma/nonfunctional[a]	None	1–2	Pancreas (100%)	>60	18–44	Weight loss (30–90%) Abdominal mass (10–30%) Pain (30–95%)

Abbreviations: ACTH, adrenocorticotropic hormone; GRFoma, growth hormone–releasing factor secreting pancreatic endocrine tumor; IGF-II, insulin-like growth factor II; MEN, multiple endocrine neoplasia; pNET, pancreatic neuroendocrine tumor; PPoma, tumor secreting pancreatic polypeptide; PTHrP, parathyroid hormone–related peptide; VIPoma, tumor secreting vasoactive intestinal peptide; WDHA, *w*atery *d*iarrhea, *h*ypokalemia, and *a*chlorhydria syndrome.

[a]Pancreatic polypeptide–secreting tumors (PPomas) are listed in two places because most authorities classify these as not associated with a specific hormonal syndrome (nonfunctional); however, rare cases of watery diarrhea proposed to be due to PPomas have been reported.

motility and constipation, and ovarian tumors secreting renin or aldosterone causing alterations in blood pressure or somatostatin causing diabetes or reactive hypoglycemia. Each of the functional syndromes listed in Table 28-2 is associated with symptoms due to the specific hormone released. In contrast, nonfunctional pNETs release no products that cause a specific clinical syndrome. "Nonfunctional" is a misnomer in the strict sense because those tumors frequently ectopically secrete a number of peptides (pancreatic polypeptide [PP], chromogranin A, ghrelin,

TABLE 28-3

GI-NET (CARCINOID) LOCATION, FREQUENCY OF METASTASES, AND ASSOCIATION WITH THE CARCINOID SYNDROME

	LOCATION (% OF TOTAL)	INCIDENCE OF METASTASES	INCIDENCE OF CARCINOID SYNDROME
Foregut			
Esophagus	<0.1	—	—
Stomach	4.6	10	9.5
Duodenum	2.0	—	3.4
Pancreas	0.7	71.9	20
Gallbladder	0.3	17.8	5
Bronchus, lung, trachea	27.9	5.7	13
Midgut			
Jejunum	1.8	{58.4	9
Ileum	14.9		9
Meckel's diverticulum	0.5	—	13
Appendix	4.8	38.8	<1
Colon	8.6	51	5
Liver	0.4	32.	—
Ovary	1.0	2 32	50
Testis	<0.1	—	50
Hindgut			
Rectum	13.6	3.9	—

Abbreviation: GI-NET, gastrointestinal neuroendocrine tumor.
Source: Location is from the PAN-SEER data (1973–1999), and incidence of metastases is from the SEER data (1992–1999), reported by IM Modlin et al: Cancer 97:934, 2003. Incidence of carcinoid syndrome is from 4349 cases studied from 1950–1971, reported by JD Godwin: Cancer 36:560, 1975.

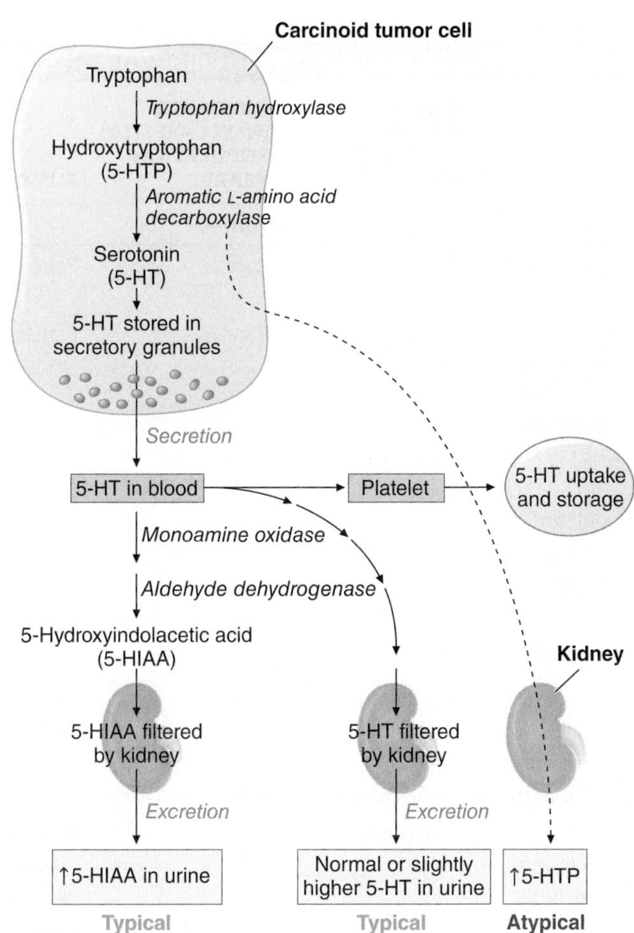

FIGURE 28-1
Synthesis, secretion, and metabolism of serotonin (5-HT) in patients with typical and atypical carcinoid syndromes. 5-HIAA, 5-hydroxyindolacetic acid.

neurotensin, α subunits of human chorionic gonadotropin, and neuron-specific enolase); however, they cause no specific clinical syndrome. The symptoms caused by nonfunctional pNETs are entirely due to the tumor per se. pNETs frequently ectopically secrete PP (60–85%), neurotensin (30–67%), calcitonin (30–42%), and to a lesser degree, ghrelin (5–65%). Whereas a few studies have proposed their secretion can cause a specific functional syndrome, most studies support the conclusion that their ectopic secretion is not associated with a specific clinical syndrome, and thus they are listed in Table 28-2 as possible clinical syndromes. Because a large proportion of nonfunctional pNETs (60–90%) secrete PP, these tumors are often referred to as PPomas (Table 28-2).

GI-NETs (carcinoids) can occur in almost any GI tissue (Table 28-3); however, at present, most (70%) have their origin in one of three sites: bronchus, jejunoileum, or colon/rectum. In the past, GI-NET (carcinoids) most frequently were reported in the appendix (i.e., 40%); however, the bronchus/lung, rectum, and small intestine are now the most common sites. Overall, the GI tract is the most common site for these tumors, accounting for 64%, with the respiratory tract a distant second at 28%. Both race and sex can affect the frequency as well as the distribution of GI-NETs (carcinoids). African Americans have a higher incidence of carcinoids. Race is particularly important for rectal carcinoids, which are found in 41% of Asians/Pacific Islanders with NETs compared to 32% of American Indians/Alaskan natives, 26% of African Americans, and 12% of white Americans. Females have a lower incidence of small intestinal and pancreatic carcinoids.

The term *pancreatic neuroendocrine* or *endocrine tumor*, although widely used and therefore retained here, is also a misnomer, strictly speaking, because these tumors can occur either almost entirely in the pancreas (insulinomas, glucagonomas, nonfunctional pNETs, pNETs causing hypercalcemia) or at both pancreatic and extrapancreatic sites (gastrinomas, VIPomas [vasoactive intestinal peptide], somatostatinomas, GRFomas [growth hormone–releasing factor]). pNETs are also called islet cell tumors; however, the use of this term is discouraged because it is not established that they originate from the islets, and many can occur at extrapancreatic sites.

Whereas the classification of GI neuroendocrine tumors into foregut, midgut, or hindgut is widely used and generally useful because the NETs within these areas have many similarities, they also have marked differences, particularly in biologic behavior, and it has not proved useful for prognostic purposes. More general classifications have been developed that allow NETs with similar features in different locations to be compared, have proven prognostic value, and are widely used. New classification systems have been developed for both GI-NETs (carcinoids) and pNETs by the World Health Organization (WHO), European Neuroendocrine Tumor Society (ENETS), and the American Joint Committee on Cancer/International Union Against Cancer (AJCC/UICC). Although there are some differences between these different classification systems, each uses similar information, and it is now recommended that the basic data underlying the classification be included in all standard pathology reports. These classification systems divide NETs from all sites into those that are well differentiated (low grade [G1] or intermediate grade [G2]) and those that are poorly differentiated (high grade [G3] divided into either small-cell carcinoma or large-cell neuroendocrine carcinoma). In these classification systems, both pNETs and GI-NETs (carcinoids) are classified as neuroendocrine tumors, and the old term of carcinoid is equivalent to well-differentiated neuroendocrine tumors of the GI tract. These classification systems are based on not only the differentiation of the NET, but also a grading system assessing proliferative indices (Ki-67 and the mitotic count). NETs are considered low grade (ENETS G1) if the Ki-67 is <3% and the mitotic count is <2 mitoses/high-power field (HPF), intermediate grade (ENETS G2) if the Ki-67 is 3–20% and the mitotic count is 2–20 mitoses/HPF, and high grade (ENETS G3) if the Ki-67 is >20% and the mitotic count is >20 mitoses/HPF. In addition to the grading system, a TNM classification has been proposed that is based on the level of tumor invasion, tumor size, and tumor extent (see Table 28-4 for an example with pNETs and appendiceal GI-NETs [carcinoids]). Because of the proven prognostic value of these classification and grading systems, as well as the fact that NETs with different classifications/grades respond differently to treatments, the systems are now essential for the management of all NETs.

In addition to these classification/grading systems, a number of other factors have been identified that provide important prognostic information that can guide treatment (Table 28-5).

TABLE 28-4

COMPARISON OF THE CRITERIA FOR THE TUMOR CATEGORY IN THE ENETS AND SEVENTH EDITION AJCC TNM CLASSIFICATIONS OF PANCREATIC AND APPENDICEAL NETs

	ENETS TNM	AJCC/UICC TNM
pNETs		
T1	Confined to pancreas, <2 cm	Confined to pancreas, <2 cm
T2	Confined to pancreas, 2–4 cm	Confined to pancreas, >2 cm
T3	Confined to pancreas, >4 cm, or invasion of duodenum or bile duct	Peripancreatic spread, but without major vascular invasion (truncus coeliacus, superior mesenteric artery)
T4	Invasion of adjacent organs or major vessels	Major vascular invasion
Appendiceal NETs		
T1	≤1 cm; invasion of muscularis propria	T1a, ≤1 cm; T1b, >1–2 cm
T2	≤2 cm and <3 mm invasion of subserosa/mesoappendix	>2–4 cm or invasion of cecum
T3	>2 cm or >3 mm invasion of subserosa/mesoappendix	>4 cm or invasion of ileum
T4	Invasion of peritoneum/other organs	Invasion of peritoneum/other organs

Abbreviations: AJCC, American Joint Committee on Cancer; ENETS, European Neuroendocrine Tumor Society; NET, neuroendocrine tumor; pNET, pancreatic neuroendocrine tumor; TNM, tumor, node, metastasis; UICC, International Union Against Cancer.

Source: Modified from DS Klimstra: Semin Oncol 40:23, 2013 and G Kloppel et al: Virchow Arch 456:595, 2010.

The exact incidence of GI-NETs (carcinoids) or pNETs varies according to whether only symptomatic tumors or all tumors are considered. The incidence of clinically significant carcinoids is 7–13 cases/million population per year, whereas any malignant carcinoids at autopsy are reported in 21–84 cases/million population per year. The incidence of GI-NETs (carcinoids) is approximately 25–50 cases per million in the United States, which makes them less common than adenocarcinomas of the GI tract. However, their incidence has increased sixfold in the last 30 years. In an analysis of 35,825 GI-NETs (carcinoids) (2004) from the U.S. Surveillance, Epidemiology, and End Results (SEER) database, their incidence was 5.25/100,000 per year, and the 29-year prevalence was 35/100,000. Clinically significant pNETs have a prevalence of 10 cases/million population, with insulinomas, gastrinomas, and

TABLE 28-5

PROGNOSTIC FACTORS IN NEUROENDOCRINE TUMORS

I. Both GI-NETs (carcinoids) and pNETs

Symptomatic presentation ($p < .05$)
Presence of liver metastases ($p < .001$)
Extent of liver metastases ($p < .001$)
Presence of lymph node metastases ($p < .001$)
Development of bone or extrahepatic metastases ($p < .01$)
Depth of invasion ($p < .001$)
Rapid rate of tumor growth
Elevated serum alkaline phosphatase levels ($p = .003$)
Primary tumor site ($p < .001$)
Primary tumor size ($p < .005$)
High serum chromogranin A level ($p < .01$)
Presence of one or more circulating tumor cells ($p < .001$)
Various histologic features
- Tumor differentiation ($p < .001$)
- High growth indices (high Ki-67 index, PCNA expression)
- High mitotic counts ($p < .001$)
- Necrosis present
- Presence of cytokeratin 19 ($p < .02$)
- Vascular or perineural invasion
- Vessel density (low microvessel density, increased lymphatic density)
- High CD10 metalloproteinase expression (in series with all grades of NETs)
- Flow cytometric features (i.e., aneuploidy)
- High VEGF expression (in low-grade or well-differentiated NETs only)

WHO, ENETS, AJCC/UICC, and grading classification
Presence of a pNET rather than GI-NET associated with poorer prognosis ($p = .0001$)
Older age ($p < .01$)

II. GI-NETs (Carcinoids)

Location of primary: appendix < lung, rectum < small intestine < pancreas
Presence of carcinoid syndrome
Laboratory results (urinary 5-HIAA levels [$p < .01$], plasma neuropeptide K [$p < .05$], serum chromogranin A [$p < .01$])
Presence of a second malignancy
Male sex ($p < .001$)
Molecular findings (TGF-α expression [$p < .05$], chr 16q LOH or gain chr 4p [$p < .05$])
WHO, ENETS, AJCC/UICC, and grading classification
Molecular findings (gain in chr 14, loss of 3p13 [ileal carcinoid], upregulation of Hoxc6)

III. pNETs

Location of primary: duodenal (gastrinoma) better than pancreatic
Ha-*ras* oncogene or p53 overexpression
Female gender
MEN 1 syndrome absent
Presence of nonfunctional tumor (some studies, not all)
WHO, ENETS, AJCC/UICC, and grading classification
Various histologic features: IHC positivity for c-KIT, low cyclin B1 expression ($p < .01$), loss of PTEN or of tuberous sclerosis-2 IHC, expression of fibroblast growth factor-13
Laboratory findings (increased chromogranin A in some studies; gastrinomas—increased gastrin level)
Molecular findings (increased HER2/*neu* expression [$p = .032$], chr 1q, 3p, 3q, or 6q LOH [$p = .0004$], EGF receptor overexpression [$p = .034$], gains in chr 7q, 17q, 17p, 20q; alterations in the VHL gene [deletion, methylation]; presence of FGFR4-G388R single-nucleotide polymorphism)

Abbreviations: 5-HIAA, 5-hydroxyindoleacetic acid; AJCC, American Joint Committee on Cancer; chr, chromosome; EGF, epidermal growth factor; FGFR, fibroblast growth factor receptor; GI-NET, gastrointestinal neuroendocrine tumor; IHC, immunohistochemistry; Ki-67, proliferation-associated nuclear antigen recognized by Ki-67 monoclonal antibody; LOH, loss of heterozygosity; MEN, multiple endocrine neoplasia; NET, neuroendocrine tumors; PCNA, proliferating cell nuclear antigen; pNET, pancreatic neuroendocrine tumor; PTEN, phosphatase and tensin homologue deleted from chromosome 10; TGF-α, transforming growth factor α; TNM, tumor, node, metastasis; UICC, International Union Against Cancer; VEGF, vascular endothelial growth factor; WHO, World Health Organization.

nonfunctional pNETs having an incidence of 0.5–2 cases/million population per year (Table 28-2). pNETs account for 1–10% of all tumors arising in the pancreas and 1.3% of tumors in the SEER database, which consists primarily of malignant tumors. VIPomas are 2–8 times less common, glucagonomas are 17–30 times less common, and somatostatinomas are the least common. In autopsy studies, 0.5–1.5% of all cases have a pNET; however, in less than 1 in 1000 cases was a functional tumor thought to occur.

Both GI-NETs (carcinoids) and pNETs commonly show malignant behavior (Tables 28-2 and 28-3). With pNETs, except for insulinomas in which <10% are malignant, 50–100% in different series are malignant. With GI-NETs (carcinoids), the percentage showing malignant behavior varies in different locations (Table 28-3). For the three most common sites of occurrence, the incidence of metastases varies greatly from the jejunoileum (58%), lung/bronchus (6%), and rectum (4%) (Table 28-3). With both GI-NETs (carcinoids) and pNETs, a number of factors (Table 28-5) are important prognostic factors in determining survival and the aggressiveness of the tumor. Patients with pNETs (excluding insulinomas) generally have a poorer prognosis than do patients with GI-NETs (carcinoids). The presence of liver metastases is the single most important prognostic factor in single and multivariate analyses for both GI-NETs (carcinoids) and pNETs. Particularly important in the development of liver metastases is the size of the primary tumor. For example, with small intestinal carcinoids, which are the most common cause of the carcinoid syndrome due to metastatic disease in the liver (Table 28-2), metastases occur in 15–25% if the tumor is <1 cm in diameter, 58–80% if it is 1–2 cm in diameter, and >75% if it is >2 cm in diameter. Similar data exist for gastrinomas and other pNETs; the size of the primary tumor is an independent predictor of the development of liver metastases. The presence of lymph node metastases or extrahepatic metastases; the depth of invasion; the rapid rate of growth; various histologic features (differentiation, mitotic rates, growth indices, vessel density, vascular endothelial growth factor [VEGF], and CD10 metalloproteinase expression); necrosis; presence of cytokeratin; elevated serum alkaline phosphatase levels; older age; presence of circulating tumor cells; and flow cytometric results, such as the presence of aneuploidy, are all important prognostic factors for the development of metastatic disease (Table 28-5). For patients with GI-NETs (carcinoids), additional associations with a worse prognosis include the development of the carcinoid syndrome (especially the development of carcinoid heart disease), male sex, the presence of a symptomatic tumor or greater increases in a number of tumor markers (5-hydroxyindolacetic acid [5-HIAA], neuropeptide K, chromogranin A), and the presence of various molecular features. With pNETs or gastrinomas, a worse prognosis is associated with female sex, overexpression of the Ha-*ras* oncogene or p53, the absence of multiple endocrine neoplasia type 1 (MEN 1), higher levels of various tumor markers (i.e., chromogranin A, gastrin), and presence of various histologic features (immunohistochemistry for c-KIT, low cyclin B1, loss of PTEN/TSC-2, expression of fibroblast growth factor-13) and various molecular features (Table 28-5). The TNM classification systems and the grading systems (G1–G3) have important prognostic value.

A number of diseases due to various genetic disorders are associated with an increased incidence of NETs (Table 28-6). Each one is caused by a loss of a possible tumor-suppressor gene. The most important is MEN 1, which is an autosomal dominant disorder due to a

TABLE 28-6

GENETIC SYNDROMES ASSOCIATED WITH AN INCREASED INCIDENCE OF NEUROENDOCRINE TUMORS (NETS) (GI-NETS [CARCINOIDS] OR PNETS)

SYNDROME	LOCATION OF GENE MUTATION AND GENE PRODUCT	NETs SEEN/ FREQUENCY
Multiple endocrine neoplasia type 1 (MEN 1)	11q13 (encodes 610-amino-acid protein, menin)	80–100% develop pNETS (microscopic), 20–80% (clinical): (nonfunctional > gastrinoma > insulinoma) GI-NETs (Carcinoids): gastric (13–30%), bronchial/thymic (8%)
von Hippel–Lindau disease	3q25 (encodes 213-amino-acid protein)	12–17% develop pNETS (almost always nonfunctional)
von Recklinghausen's disease (neurofibromatosis 1 [NF-1])	17q11.2 (encodes 2485-amino-acid protein, neurofibromin)	0–10% develop pNETs, primarily duodenal somatostatinomas (usually nonfunctional) Rarely insulinoma, gastrinoma
Tuberous sclerosis	9q34 (TSCI) (encodes 1164-amino-acid protein, hamartin), 16p13 (TSC2) (encodes 1807-amino-acid protein, tuberin)	Uncommonly develop pNETS (nonfunctional and functional [insulinoma, gastrinoma])

Abbreviations: GI, gastrointestinal; PNETs, pancreatic neuroendocrine tumors.

defect in a 10-exon gene on 11q13, which encodes for a 610-amino-acid nuclear protein, menin **(Chap. 29)**. Patients with MEN 1 develop hyperparathyroidism due to parathyroid hyperplasia in 95–100% of cases, pNETs in 80–100%, pituitary adenomas in 54–80%, adrenal adenomas in 27–36%, bronchial carcinoids in 8%, thymic carcinoids in 8%, gastric carcinoids in 13–30% of patients with Zollinger-Ellison syndrome, skin tumors (angiofibromas [88%], collagenomas [72%]), central nervous system (CNS) tumors (meningiomas [<8%]), and smooth-muscle tumors (leiomyomas, leiomyosarcomas [1–7%]). Among patients with MEN 1, 80–100% develop nonfunctional pNETs (most are microscopic with 0–13% large/symptomatic), and functional pNETs occur in 20–80% in different series, with a mean of 54% developing Zollinger-Ellison syndrome, 18% insulinomas, 3% glucagonomas, 3% VIPomas, and <1% GRFomas or somatostatinomas. MEN 1 is present in 20–25% of all patients with Zollinger-Ellison syndrome, 4% of patients with insulinomas, and a low percentage (<5%) of patients with other pNETs.

Three phacomatoses associated with NETs are von Hippel–Lindau disease (VHL), von Recklinghausen's disease (neurofibromatosis type 1 [NF-1]), and tuberous sclerosis (Bourneville's disease) (Table 28-6). VHL is an autosomal dominant disorder due to defects on chromosome 3p25, which encodes for a 213-amino-acid protein that interacts with the elongin family of proteins as a transcriptional regulator **(Chaps. 9, and 29)**. In addition to cerebellar hemangioblastomas, renal cancer, and pheochromocytomas, 10–17% develop a pNET. Most are nonfunctional, although insulinomas and VIPomas have been reported. Patients with NF-1 (von Recklinghausen's disease) have defects in a gene on chromosome 17q11.2 that encodes for a 2845-amino-acid protein, neurofibromin, which functions in normal cells as a suppressor of the *ras* signaling cascade. Up to 10% of these patients develop an upper GI-NET (carcinoid), characteristically in the periampullary region (54%). Many are classified as somatostatinomas because they contain somatostatin immunocytochemically; however, they uncommonly secrete somatostatin and rarely produce a clinical somatostatinoma syndrome. NF-1 has rarely been associated with insulinomas and Zollinger-Ellison syndrome. NF-1 accounts for 48% of all duodenal somatostastinomas and 23% of all ampullary GI-NETs (carcinoids). Tuberous sclerosis is caused by mutations that alter either the 1164-amino-acid protein hamartin (TSC1) or the 1807-amino-acid protein tuberin (TSC2). Both hamartin and tuberin interact in a pathway related to phosphatidylinositol 3-kinases and mammalian target of rapamycin (mTOR) signaling cascades. A few cases including nonfunctional and functional pNETs (insulinomas and gastrinomas) have been reported in these patients (**Table 28-6**). Mahvash disease is associated with the development of α-cell hyperplasia, hyperglucagonemia, and the development of NF pNETs and is due to a homozygous P86S mutation of the human glucagon receptor.

Mutations in common oncogenes (*ras, myc, fos, src, jun*) or common tumor-suppressor genes (*p53*, retinoblastoma susceptibility gene) are not commonly found in either pNETs or GI-NETs (carcinoids) (Table 28-1). However, frequent (70%) gene amplifications in *MDM2, MDM4,* and *WIPI* inactivating the p53 pathway are noted in well-differentiated pNETs, and the retinoblastoma pathway is altered in the majority of pNETs. In addition to these genes, additional alterations that may be important in their pathogenesis include changes in the *MEN1* gene, *p16/MTS1* tumor-suppressor gene, and *DPC4/Smad4* gene; amplification of the HER-2/*neu* protooncogene; alterations in transcription factors (Hoxc6 [GI carcinoids]), growth factors, and their receptors; methylation of a number of genes that probably results in their inactivation; and deletions of unknown tumor-suppressor genes as well as gains in other unknown genes (Table 28-1). The clinical antitumor activity of everolimus, an mTOR inhibitor, and sunitinib, a tyrosine kinase inhibitor (PDGFR, VEGFR1, VEGFR2, c-KIT, FLT-3), support the importance of the mTOR-AKT pathway and tyrosine kinase receptors in mediating growth of malignant NETs (especially pNETs). The importance of the mTOR pathway in pNET growth is further supported by the finding that a single-nucleotide polymorphism (FGFR4-G388R, in fibroblast growth factor receptor 4) affects selectivity to the mTOR inhibitor and can result in significantly higher risk of advanced pNET stage and liver metastases (Table 28-5). Comparative genomic hybridization, genome-wide allelotyping studies, and genome-wide single-nucleotide polymorphism analyses have shown that chromosomal losses and gains are common in pNETs and GI-NETs (carcinoids), but they differ between these two NETs, and some have prognostic significance (Table 28-5). Mutations in the *MEN1* gene are probably particularly important. Loss of heterozygosity at the MEN 1 locus on chromosome 11q13 is noted in 93% of sporadic pNETs (i.e., in patients without MEN 1) and in 26–75% of sporadic GI-NETs (carcinoids). Mutations in the *MEN1* gene are reported in 31–34% of sporadic gastrinomas. Exomic sequencing of sporadic pNETs found that the most frequently altered gene was *MEN1*, occurring in 44% of patients, followed by mutations in 43% of patients in genes encoding for two subunits of a transcription/chromatin remodeling complex consisting of DAXX (death-domain-associated protein) and ATRX (α-thalassemia/mental retardation syndrome X-linked) and in 15% of patients in the mTOR pathway. The presence of a number of these molecular alterations in pNETs or GI-NETs (carcinoids) correlates with tumor growth, tumor size, and disease extent or invasiveness and may have prognostic significance (Table 28-5).

GI-NETs (CARCINOIDS) AND CARCINOID SYNDROME

CHARACTERISTICS OF THE MOST COMMON GI-NETs (CARCINOIDS)

Appendiceal NETs (Carcinoids)

Appendiceal NETs (carcinoids) occur in 1 in every 200–300 appendectomies, usually in the appendiceal tip, have an incidence of 0.15/100,000 per year, comprise 2–5% of all GI-NETs (carcinoids), and comprise 32–80% of all appendiceal tumors. Most (i.e., >90%) are <1 cm in diameter without metastases in older studies, but more recently, 2–35% have had metastases (Table 28-3). In the SEER data of 1570 appendiceal carcinoids, 62% were localized, 27% had regional metastases, and 8% had distant metastases. The risk of metastases increases with size, with those <1 cm having a 0 to <10% risk of metastases and those >2 cm having a 25–44% risk. Besides tumor size, other important prognostic factors for metastases include basal location, invasion of mesoappendix, poor differentiation, advanced stage or WHO/ENETS classification, older age, and positive resection margins. The 5-year survival is 88–100% for patients with localized disease, 78–100% for patients with regional involvement, and 12–28% for patients with distal metastases. In patients with tumors <1 cm in diameter, the 5-year survival is 95–100%, whereas it is 29% if tumors are >2 cm in diameter. Most tumors are well-differentiated G1 tumors (87%) (Table 28-4), with the remainder primarily well-differentiated G2 tumors (13%); poorly differentiated G3 tumors are uncommon (<1%). Their percentage of the total number of carcinoids decreased from 43.9% (1950–1969) to 2.4% (1992–1999). Appendiceal goblet cell (GC) NETs (carcinoids)/carcinomas are a rare subtype (<5%) that are mixed adeno-neuroendocrine carcinomas. They are malignant and are thought to comprise a distinct entity; they frequently present with advanced disease and are recommended to be treated as adenocarcinomas, not carcinoid tumors.

SMALL INTESTINAL NETs (CARCINOIDS)

Small intestinal (SI) NETs (carcinoids) have a reported incidence of 0.67/100,000 in the United States, 0.32/100,000 in England, and 1.12/100,000 in Sweden and comprise >50% of all SI tumors. There is a male predominance (1.5:1), and race affects frequency, with a lower frequency in Asians and greater frequency in African Americans. The mean age of presentation is 52–63 years, with a wide range (1–93 years). Familial SI carcinoid families exist but are very uncommon. These are frequently multiple; 9–18% occur in the jeunum, 70–80% are present in the ileum, and 70% occur within 6 cm (2.4 in.) of the ileocecal valve. Forty percent are <1 cm in diameter, 32% are 1–2 cm, and 29% are >2 cm. They are characteristically well differentiated; however, they are generally invasive, with 1.2% being intramucosal in location, 27% penetrating the submucosa, and 20% invading the muscularis propria. Metastases occur in a mean of 47–58% (range 20–100%). Liver metastases occur in 38%, to lymph nodes in 37% and more distant in 20–25%. They characteristically cause a marked fibrotic reaction, which can lead to intestinal obstruction. Tumor size is an important variable in the frequency of metastases. However, even small NETs (carcinoids) of the small intestine (<1 cm) have metastases in 15–25% of cases, whereas the proportion increases to 58–100% for tumors 1–2 cm in diameter. Carcinoids also occur in the duodenum, with 31% having metastases. Duodenal tumors <1 cm virtually never metastasize, whereas 33% of those >2 cm had metastases. SI NETs (carcinoids) are the most common cause (60–87%) of the carcinoid syndrome and are discussed in a later section (Table 28-7). Important prognostic factors are listed in (Table 28-5), and particularly important are the tumor extent, proliferative index by grading, and stage (Table 28-4). The overall survival at 5 years is 55–75%; however, it varies markedly with disease extent, being 65–90% with localized disease, 66–72% with regional involvement, and 36–43% with distant disease.

Rectal NETs (Carcinoids)

Rectal NETs (carcinoids) comprise 27% of all GI-NETs (carcinoids) and 16% of all NETs and are increasing in frequency. In the U.S. SEER data, they currently have an incidence of 0.86/100,000 per year (up from 0.2/100,000 per year in 1973) and represent 1–2% of all rectal tumors. They are found in approximately 1 in every 1500/2500 proctoscopies/colonoscopies or 0.05–0.07% of individuals undergoing these procedures. Nearly all occur between 4 and 13 cm above the dentate line. Most are small, with 66–80% being <1 cm in diameter, and rarely metastasize (5%). Tumors between 1 and 2 cm can metastasize in 5–30%, and those >2 cm, which are uncommon, in >70%. Most invade only to the submucosa (75%), with 2.1% confined to the mucosa, 10% to the muscular layer, and 5% to adjacent structures. Histologically, most are well differentiated (98%) with 72% ENETS/WHO grade G1 and 28% grade G2 (Table 28-4). Overall survival is 88%; however, it is very

TABLE 28-7
CLINICAL CHARACTERISTICS IN PATIENTS WITH CARCINOID SYNDROME

	PERCENTAGE (RANGE)	
	AT PRESENTATION	DURING COURSE OF DISEASE
Symptoms/signs		
Diarrhea	32–93%	68–100%
Flushing	23–100%	45–96%
Pain	10%	34%
Asthma/wheezing	4–14%	3–18%
Pellagra	0–7%	0–5%
None	12%	22%
Carcinoid heart disease present	11–40%	14–41%
Demographics		
Male	46–59%	46–61%
Age		
Mean	57 yrs	59.2 yrs
Range	25–79 yrs	18–91 yrs
Tumor location		
Foregut	5–14%	0–33%
Midgut	57–87%	60–100%
Hindgut	1–7%	0–8%
Unknown	2–21%	0–26%

much dependent of the stage, with 5-year survival of 91% for localized disease, 36–49% for regional disease, and 20–32% for distant disease. Risk factors are listed in Table 28-5 and particularly include tumor size, depth of invasion, presence of metastases, differentiation, and recent TNM classification and grade.

Bronchial NETs (Carcinoids)

Bronchial NETs (carcinoids) comprise 25–33% of all well-differentiated NETs and 90% of all the poorly differentiated NETs found, likely due to a strong association with smoking. Their incidence ranges from 0.2 to 2/100,000 per year in the United States and European countries and is increasing at a rate of 6% per year. They are slightly more frequent in females and in whites compared with those of Hispanic/Asian/African descent, and are most commonly seen in the sixth decade of life, with a younger age of presentation for typical carcinoids (45 years) compared to atypical carcinoids (55 years).

A number of different classifications of bronchial GI-NETs (carcinoids) have been proposed. In some studies, they are classified into four categories: typical carcinoid (also called bronchial carcinoid tumor, Kulchitsky cell carcinoma I [KCC-I]), atypical carcinoid (also called well-differentiated neuroendocrine carcinoma [KC-II]), intermediate small-cell neuroendocrine carcinoma, and small-cell neuroendocarcinoma (KC-III). Another proposed classification includes three categories of lung NETs: benign or low-grade malignant (typical carcinoid), low-grade malignant (atypical carcinoid), and high-grade malignant (poorly differentiated carcinoma of the large-cell or small-cell type). The WHO classification includes four general categories: typical carcinoid, atypical carcinoid, large-cell neuroendocrine carcinoma, and small-cell carcinoma. The ratio of typical to atypical carcinoids is 8–10:1, with the typical carcinoids comprising 1–2% of lung tumors, atypical 0.1–0.2%, large-cell neuroendocrine tumors 0.3%, and small-cell lung cancer 9.8% of all lung tumors. These different categories of lung NETs have different prognoses, varying from excellent for typical carcinoid to poor for small-cell neuroendocrine carcinomas. The occurrence of large-cell and small-cell lung carcinoids, but not typical or atypical lung carcinoids, is related to tobacco use. The 5-year survival is very much influenced by the classification of the tumor, with survival of 92–100% for patients with a typical carcinoid, 61–88% with an atypical carcinoid, 13–57% with a large-cell neuroendocrine tumor, and 5% with a small-cell lung cancer.

Gastric NET (Carcinoids)

Gastric NETs (carcinoids) account for 3 of every 1000 gastric neoplasms and 1.3–2% of all carcinoids, and their relative frequency has increased three- to fourfold over the last five decades (2.2% in 1950 to 9.6% in 2000–2007, SEER data). At present, it is unclear whether this increase is due to better detection with the increased use of upper GI endoscopy or to a true increase in incidence. Gastric NETs (carcinoids) are classified into three different categories, and this has important implications for pathogenesis, prognosis, and treatment. Each originates from gastric enterochromaffin-like (ECL) cells, one of the six types of gastric neuroendocrine cells, in the gastric mucosa. Two subtypes are associated with hypergastrinemic states, either chronic atrophic gastritis (type I) (80% of all gastric NETs [carcinoids]) or Zollinger-Ellison syndrome, which is almost always a part of the MEN 1 syndrome (type II) (6% of all cases). These tumors generally pursue a benign course, with type I uncommonly (<10%) associated with metastases, whereas type II tumors are slightly more aggressive, with 10–30% associated with metastases. They are usually multiple, small, and infiltrate only to the submucosa. The third subtype of gastric NETs (carcinoids) (type III) (sporadic) occurs without hypergastrinemia (14–25% of all gastric carcinoids) and has an aggressive course, with 54–66% developing metastases. Sporadic carcinoids are usually single, large tumors; 50% have atypical histology, and they can be a cause of the carcinoid syndrome. Five-year survival is 99–100% in patients with type I, 60–90% in patients with type II, and 50% in patients with type III gastric NETs (carcinoids).

CLINICAL PRESENTATION OF NETs (CARCINOIDS)

GI/Lung NET (Carcinoid) without the carcinoid syndrome

The age of patients at diagnosis ranges from 10 to 93 years, with a mean age of 63 years for the small intestine and 66 years for the rectum. The presentation is diverse and is related to the site of origin and the extent of malignant spread. In the appendix, NETs (carcinoids) usually are found incidentally during surgery for suspected appendicitis. SI NETs (carcinoids) in the jejunoileum present with periodic abdominal pain (51%), intestinal obstruction with ileus/invagination (31%), an abdominal tumor (17%), or GI bleeding (11%). Because of the vagueness of the symptoms, the diagnosis usually is delayed approximately 2 years from onset of the symptoms, with a range up to 20 years. Duodenal, gastric, and rectal NETs (carcinoids) are most frequently found by chance at endoscopy. The most common symptoms of rectal carcinoids are melena/bleeding (39%), constipation (17%), and diarrhea (12%). Bronchial NETs (carcinoids) frequently are discovered as a lesion on a chest radiograph, and 31% of the patients are asymptomatic. Thymic NETs (carcinoids) present as anterior mediastinal masses, usually on chest radiograph or computed tomography (CT) scan. Ovarian and testicular NETs (carcinoids) usually present as masses discovered on physical examination or ultrasound. Metastatic NETs (carcinoids) in the liver frequently presents as hepatomegaly in a patient who may have minimal symptoms and nearly normal liver function test results.

GI-NETs (CARCINOIDS) WITH SYSTEMIC SYMPTOMS DUE TO SECRETED PRODUCTS

GI/lung NETs (carcinoids) immunocytochemically can contain numerous GI peptides: gastrin, insulin, somatostatin, motilin, neurotensin, tachykinins (substance K, substance P, neuropeptide K), glucagon, gastrin-releasing peptide, vasoactive intestinal peptide (VIP), PP, ghrelin, other biologically active peptides (ACTH, calcitonin, growth hormone), prostaglandins, and bioactive amines (serotonin). These substances may or may not be released in sufficient amounts to cause symptoms. In various studies of patients with GI-NETs (carcinoids), elevated serum levels of PP were found in 43%, motilin in 14%, gastrin in 15%, and VIP in 6%. Foregut NETs (carcinoids) are more likely to produce various GI peptides than are midgut NETs (carcinoids). Ectopic ACTH production causing Cushing's syndrome is seen increasingly with foregut carcinoids (respiratory tract primarily) and, in some series, has been the most common cause of the ectopic ACTH syndrome, accounting for 64% of all cases. Acromegaly due to growth hormone–releasing factor release occurs with foregut NETs (carcinoids), as does the somatostatinoma syndrome, but rarely occurs with duodenal NETs (carcinoids). The most common systemic syndrome with GI-NETs (carcinoids) is the carcinoid syndrome, which is discussed in detail in the next section.

CARCINOID SYNDROME

Clinical features

The cardinal features from a number of series at presentation as well as during the disease course are shown in Table 28-7. Flushing and diarrhea are the two most common symptoms, occurring in a mean of 69–70% of patients initially and in up to 78% of patients during the course of the disease. The characteristic flush is of sudden onset; it is a deep red or violaceous erythema of the upper body, especially the neck and face, often associated with a feeling of warmth and occasionally associated with pruritus, lacrimation, diarrhea, or facial edema. Flushes may be precipitated by stress; alcohol; exercise; certain foods, such as cheese; or certain agents, such as catecholamines, pentagastrin, and serotonin reuptake inhibitors. Flushing episodes may be brief, lasting 2–5 min, especially initially, or may last hours, especially later in the disease course. Flushing usually is associated with metastatic midgut NETs (carcinoids) but can also occur with foregut NETs (carcinoids). With bronchial NETs (carcinoids), the flushes frequently are prolonged for hours to days, reddish in color, and associated with salivation, lacrimation, diaphoresis, diarrhea, and hypotension. The flush associated with gastric NETs (carcinoids) can also be reddish in color, but with a patchy distribution over the face and neck, although the classic flush seen with midgut NETs (carcinoids) can also be seen with gastric NETs (carcinoids). It may be provoked by food and have accompanying pruritus.

Diarrhea usually occurs with flushing (85% of cases). The diarrhea usually is described as watery, with 60% of patients having <1 L/d of diarrhea. Steatorrhea is present in 67%, and in 46%, it is >15 g/d (normal <7 g). Abdominal pain may be present with the diarrhea or independently in 10–34% of cases.

Cardiac manifestations occur initially in 11–40% (mean 26%) of patients with carcinoid syndrome and in 14–41% (mean 30%) at some time in the disease course. The cardiac disease is due to the formation of fibrotic plaques (composed of smooth-muscle cells, myofibroblasts, and elastic tissue) involving the endocardium, primarily on the right side, although lesions on the left side also occur occasionally, especially if a patent foramen ovale exists. The dense fibrous deposits are most commonly on the ventricular aspect of the tricuspid valve and less commonly on the pulmonary valve cusps. They can result in constriction of the valves, and pulmonic stenosis is usually predominant, whereas the tricuspid valve is often fixed open, resulting in regurgitation predominating. Overall, in patients with carcinoid heart disease, 90–100% have tricuspid insufficiency, 43–59% have tricuspid stenosis, 50–81% have pulmonary insufficiency, 25–59% have pulmonary stenosis, and 11% (0–25%) left-side lesions. Up to 80% of patients with cardiac lesions develop heart failure. Lesions on the left side are much less extensive, occur in 30% at autopsy, and most frequently affect the mitral valve. Up to 80% of patients with cardiac lesions have evidence of heart failure. At diagnosis in various series, 27–43% of patients are in New York Heart Association class I, 30–40% are in class II, 13–31% are in class III, and 3–12% are in class IV. At present, carcinoid heart disease is reported to be decreasing in frequency and severity, with mean occurrence in 20% of patients and occurrence in as few as 3–4% in some reports. Whether this decrease is due to the widespread use of somatostatin analogues, which control the release of bioactive agents thought involved in mediating the heart disease, is unclear.

Other clinical manifestations include wheezing or asthma-like symptoms (8–18%), pellagra-like skin lesions (2–25%), and impaired cognitive function. A variety of noncardiac problems due to increased fibrous tissue have been reported, including retroperitoneal fibrosis causing urethral obstruction, Peyronie's disease of the penis, intraabdominal fibrosis, and occlusion of the mesenteric arteries or veins.

Pathobiology

Carcinoid syndrome occurred in 8% of 8876 patients with GI-NETs (carcinoids), with a rate of 1.7–18.4% in different studies. It occurs only when sufficient concentrations of products secreted by the tumor reach the systemic circulation. In 91–100% of cases, this occurs after distant metastases to the liver. Rarely, primary GI-NETs (carcinoids) with nodal metastases with extensive retroperitoneal invasion, pNETs (carcinoids) with retroperitoneal lymph nodes, or NETs (carcinoids) of the lung or ovary with direct access to the systemic circulation can cause the carcinoid syndrome without hepatic metastases. All GI-NETs (carcinoids) do not have the same propensity to metastasize and cause the carcinoid syndrome (Table 28-3). Midgut NETs (carcinoids) account for 57–67% of cases of carcinoid syndrome, foregut NETs (carcinoids) for 0–33%, hindgut for 0–8%, and an unknown primary location for 2–26% (Tables 28-3 and 28-7).

One of the main secretory products of GI-NETs (carcinoids) involved in the carcinoid syndrome is serotonin (5-HT) (Fig. 28-1), which is synthesized from tryptophan. Up to 50% of dietary tryptophan can be used in this synthetic pathway by tumor cells, and this can result in inadequate supplies for conversion to niacin; hence, some patients (2.5%) develop pellagra-like lesions. Serotonin has numerous biologic effects, including stimulating intestinal secretion with inhibition of absorption, stimulating increases in intestinal motility, and stimulating fibrogenesis. In various studies, 56–88% of all GI-NETs (carcinoids) were associated with serotonin overproduction; however, 12–26% of the patients did not have the carcinoid syndrome. In one study, platelet serotonin was elevated in 96% of patients with midgut NETs (carcinoids), 43% with foregut tumors, and 0% with hindgut tumors. In 90–100% of patients with the carcinoid syndrome, there is evidence of serotonin overproduction. Serotonin is thought to be predominantly responsible for the diarrhea. Patients with the carcinoid syndrome have increased colonic motility with a shortened transit time and possibly a secretory/absorptive alteration that is compatible with the known actions of serotonin in the gut mediated primarily through 5-HT_3 and, to a lesser degree, 5-HT_4 receptors. Serotonin receptor antagonists (especially 5-HT_3 antagonists) relieve the diarrhea in many, but not all, patients. A tryptophan 5-hydroxylase inhibitor, LX-1031, which inhibits serotonin synthesis in peripheral tissues, is reported to cause a 44% decrease in bowel movement frequency and a 20% improvement in stool form in patients with the carcinoid syndrome. Additional studies suggest that tachykinins may be important mediators of diarrhea in some patients. In one study, plasma tachykinin levels correlated with symptoms of diarrhea. Serotonin does not appear to be involved in the flushing because serotonin receptor antagonists do not relieve flushing. In patients with gastric carcinoids, the characteristic red, patchy pruritic flush is thought due to histamine release because H_1 and H_2 receptor antagonists can prevent it. Numerous studies have shown that tachykinins (substance P, neuropeptide K) are stored in GI-NETs (carcinoids) and released during flushing. However, some studies have demonstrated that octreotide can relieve the flushing induced by pentagastrin in these patients without altering the stimulated increase in plasma substance

P, suggesting that other mediators must be involved in the flushing. A correlation between plasma tachykinin levels (but not substance P levels) and flushing has been reported. Prostaglandin release could be involved in mediating either the diarrhea or flush, but conflicting data exist. Both histamine and serotonin may be responsible for the wheezing as well as the fibrotic reactions involving the heart, causing Peyronie's disease and intraabdominal fibrosis.

The exact mechanism of the heart disease remains unclear, although increasing evidence supports a central role for serotonin. Patients with heart disease have higher plasma levels of neurokinin A, substance P, plasma atrial natriuretic peptide (ANP), pro-brain natriuretic peptide, chromogranin A, and activin A as well as higher urinary 5-HIAA excretion.

The valvular heart disease caused by the appetite-suppressant drug dexfenfluramine is histologically indistinguishable from that observed in carcinoid disease. Furthermore, ergot-containing dopamine receptor agonists used for Parkinson's disease (pergolide, cabergoline) cause valvular heart disease that closely resembles that seen in the carcinoid syndrome. Furthermore, in animal studies, the formation of valvular plaques/fibrosis occurs after prolonged treatment with serotonin as well as in animals with a deficiency of the 5-HIAA transporter gene, which results in an inability to inactivate serotonin. Metabolites of fenfluramine, as well as the dopamine receptor agonists, have high affinity for serotonin receptor subtype 5-HT_{2B} receptors, whose activation is known to cause fibroblast mitogenesis. Serotonin receptor subtypes 5-$HT_{1B,1D,2A,2B}$ normally are expressed in human heart valve interstitial cells. High levels of 5-HT_{2B} receptors are known to occur in heart valves and occur in cardiac fibroblasts and cardiomyocytes. Studies of cultured interstitial cells from human cardiac valves have demonstrated that these valvulopathic drugs induce mitogenesis by activating 5-HT_{2B} receptors and stimulating upregulation of transforming growth factor β and collagen biosynthesis. These observations support the conclusion that serotonin overproduction by GI-NETs (carcinoids) is important in mediating the valvular changes, possibly by activating 5-HT_{2B} receptors in the endocardium. Both the magnitude of serotonin overproduction and prior chemotherapy are important predictors of progression of the heart disease, whereas patients with high plasma levels of ANP have a worse prognosis. Plasma connective tissue growth factor levels are elevated in many fibrotic conditions; elevated levels occur in patients with carcinoid heart disease and correlate with the presence of right ventricular dysfunction and the extent of valvular regurgitation in patients with GI-NETs (carcinoids).

Patients may develop either a typical or, rarely, an atypical carcinoid syndrome (Fig. 28-1). In patients with the typical form, which characteristically is caused by midgut NETs (carcinoids), the conversion of tryptophan to 5-HTP is the rate-limiting step (Fig. 28-1). Once 5-HTP is formed, it is rapidly converted to 5-HT and stored in secretory granules of the tumor or in platelets. A small amount remains in plasma and is converted to 5-HIAA, which appears in large amounts in the urine. These patients have an expanded serotonin pool size, increased blood and platelet serotonin, and increased urinary 5-HIAA. Some GI-NETs (carcinoids) cause an atypical carcinoid syndrome that is thought to be due to a deficiency in the enzyme dopa decarboxylase; thus, 5-HTP cannot be converted to 5-HT (serotonin), and 5-HTP is secreted into the bloodstream (Fig. 28-1). In these patients, plasma serotonin levels are normal but urinary levels may be increased because some 5-HTP is converted to 5-HT in the kidney. Characteristically, urinary 5-HTP and 5-HT are increased, but urinary 5-HIAA levels are only slightly elevated. Foregut carcinoids are the most likely to cause an atypical carcinoid syndrome; however, they also can cause a typical carcinoid syndrome.

One of the most immediate life-threatening complications of the carcinoid syndrome is the development of a carcinoid crisis. This is more common in patients who have intense symptoms or have greatly increased urinary 5-HIAA levels (i.e., >200 mg/d). The crisis may occur spontaneously; however, it is usually provoked by procedures such as anesthesia, chemotherapy, surgery, biopsy, endoscopy, or radiologic examinations such as during biopsies, hepatic artery embolization, and vessel catheterization. It can be provoked by stress or procedures as mild as repeated palpation of the tumor during physical examination. Patients develop intense flushing, diarrhea, abdominal pain, cardiac abnormalities including tachycardia, hypertension, or hypotension, and confusion or stupor. If not adequately treated, this can be a terminal event.

DIAGNOSIS OF THE CARCINOID SYNDROME AND GI-NETs (CARCINOIDS)

The diagnosis of carcinoid syndrome relies on measurement of urinary or plasma serotonin or its metabolites in the urine. The measurement of 5-HIAA is used most frequently. False-positive elevations may occur if the patient is eating serotonin-rich foods such as bananas, pineapples, walnuts, pecans, avocados, or hickory nuts or is taking certain medications (cough syrup containing guaifenesin, acetaminophen, salicylates, serotonin reuptake inhibitors, or L-dopa). The normal range for daily urinary 5-HIAA excretion is 2–8 mg/d. Serotonin overproduction was noted in 92% of patients with carcinoid syndrome in one study, and in another study, 5-HIAA had 73% sensitivity and 100% specificity for carcinoid syndrome. Serotonin overproduction is *not* synonymous with the presence of clinical carcinoid syndrome because 12–26% of patients with serotonin overproduction do not have clinical evidence of the carcinoid syndrome.

Most physicians use only the urinary 5-HIAA excretion rate; however, plasma and platelet serotonin levels, if available, may provide additional information. Platelet serotonin levels are more sensitive than urinary 5-HIAA but are not generally available. A single plasma 5-HIAA determination was found to correlate with the 24-h urinary values, raising the possibility that this could replace the standard urinary collection because of its greater convenience and avoidance of incomplete or improper collections. Because patients with foregut NETs (carcinoids) may produce an atypical carcinoid syndrome, if this syndrome is suspected and the urinary 5-HIAA is minimally elevated or normal, other urinary metabolites of tryptophan, such as 5-HTP and 5-HT, should be measured (Fig. 28-1).

Flushing occurs in a number of other diseases, including systemic mastocytosis, chronic myeloid leukemia with increased histamine release, menopause, reactions to alcohol or glutamate, and side effects of chlorpropamide, calcium channel blockers, and nicotinic acid. None of these conditions cause increased urinary 5-HIAA.

The diagnosis of carcinoid tumor can be suggested by the carcinoid syndrome, recurrent abdominal symptoms in a healthy-appearing individual, or the discovery of hepatomegaly or hepatic metastases associated with minimal symptoms. Ileal NETs (carcinoids), which make up 25% of all clinically detected carcinoids, should be suspected in patients with bowel obstruction, abdominal pain, flushing, or diarrhea.

Serum chromogranin A levels are elevated in 56–100% of patients with GI-NETs (carcinoids), and the level correlates with tumor bulk. Serum chromogranin A levels are not specific for GI-NETs (carcinoids) because they are also elevated in patients with pNETs and other NETs. Furthermore, a major problem is caused by potent acid antisecretory drugs such as proton pump inhibitors (omeprazole and related drugs) because they almost invariably cause elevation of plasma chromogranin A levels; the elevation occurs rapidly (3–5 days) with continued use, and the elevated levels overlap with the levels seen in many patients with NETs. Plasma neuron-specific enolase levels are also used as a marker of GI-NETs (carcinoids) but are less sensitive than chromogranin A, being increased in only 17–47% of patients. Newer markers have been proposed including pancreastatin (a chromogranin A breakdown product) and activin A. The former is not affected by proton pump inhibitors; however, its sensitivity and specificity are not established. Plasma activin elevations are reported to correlate with the presence of cardiac disease with a sensitivity of 87% and specificity of 57%.

TREATMENT Carcinoid Syndrome and Nonmetastatic Gastrointestinal Neuroendocrine Tumors (Carcinoids)

CARCINOID SYNDROME Treatment includes avoiding conditions that precipitate flushing, dietary supplementation with nicotinamide, treatment of heart failure with diuretics, treatment of wheezing with oral bronchodilators, and control of the diarrhea with antidiarrheal agents such as loperamide and diphenoxylate. If patients still have symptoms, serotonin receptor antagonists or somatostatin analogues (Fig. 28-2) are the drugs of choice.

There are 14 subclasses of serotonin receptors, and antagonists for many are not available. The 5-HT_1 and 5-HT_2 receptor antagonists methysergide, cyproheptadine, and ketanserin have all been used to control the diarrhea but usually do not decrease flushing. The use of methysergide is limited because it can cause or enhance retroperitoneal fibrosis. Ketanserin diminishes diarrhea in 30–100% of patients. 5-HT_3 receptor antagonists (ondansetron, tropisetron, alosetron) can control diarrhea and nausea in up to 100% of patients and occasionally ameliorate the flushing. A combination of histamine H_1 and H_2 receptor antagonists (i.e., diphenhydramine and cimetidine or ranitidine) may control flushing in patients with foregut carcinoids. The tryptophan 5-hydoxylase inhibitor telotristat etiprate decreased bowel frequency in 44% and improved stool consistency in 20%.

Synthetic analogues of somatostatin (octreotide, lanreotide) are now the most widely used agents to control the symptoms of patients with carcinoid syndrome (Fig. 28-2). These drugs are effective at relieving symptoms and decreasing urinary 5-HIAA levels in patients with this syndrome. Octreotide-LAR and lanreotide-SR/autogel (Somatuline) (sustained-release formulations allowing monthly injections) control symptoms in 74% and 68% of patients, respectively, with carcinoid syndrome and show a biochemical response in 51% and 64%, respectively. Patients with mild to moderate symptoms usually are treated initially with octreotide 100 μg SC every 8 h and then begun on the long-acting monthly depot forms (octreotide-LAR or lanreotide-autogel). Forty percent of patients escape control after a median time of 4 months, and the depot dosage may have to be increased as well as supplemented with the shorter-acting formulation, SC octreotide. Pasireotide (SOM230) is a somatostatin analogue with broader selectivity (high-affinity somatostatin receptors [sst_1, sst_2, sst_3, sst_5]) than octreotide/lanreotide (sst_2, sst_5). In a phase II study of patients with refractory carcinoid syndrome, pasireotide controlled symptoms in 27%.

Carcinoid heart disease is associated with a decreased mean survival (3.8 years), and therefore, it should be sought for and carefully assessed in all patients with carcinoid

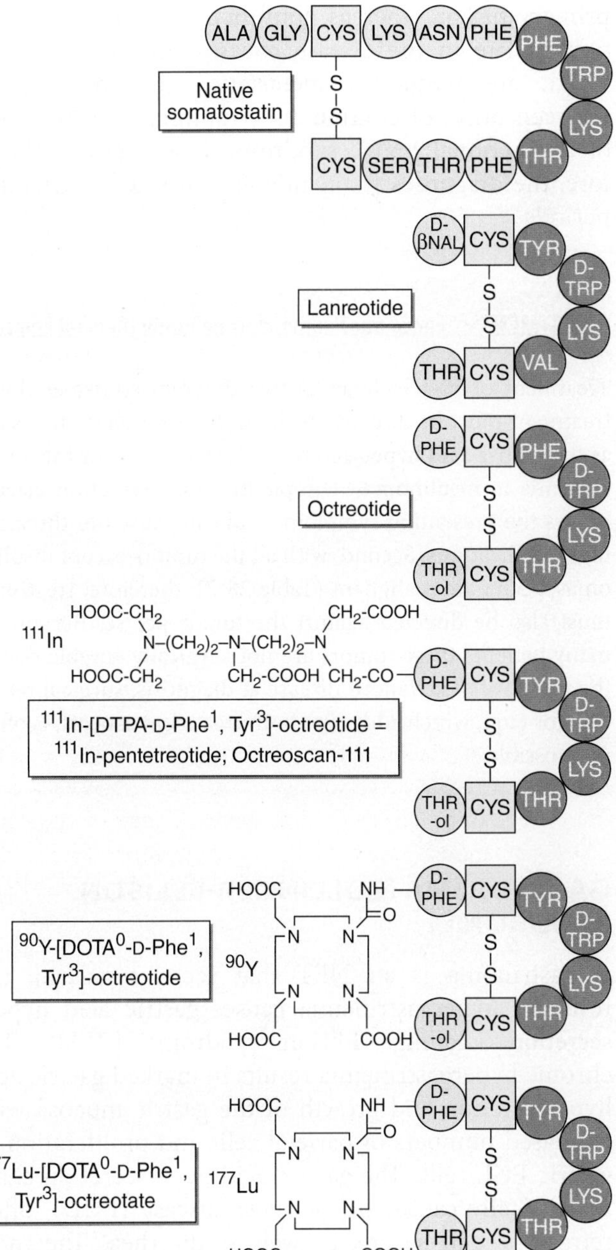

FIGURE 28-2
Structure of somatostatin and synthetic analogues used for diagnostic or therapeutic indications.

syndrome. Transthoracic echocardiography remains a key element in establishing the diagnosis of carcinoid heart disease and determining the extent and type of cardiac abnormalities. Treatment with diuretics and somatostatin analogues can reduce the negative hemodynamic effects and secondary heart failure. It remains unclear whether long-term treatment with these drugs will decrease the progression of carcinoid heart disease. Balloon valvuloplasty for stenotic valves or cardiac valve surgery may be required.

In patients with carcinoid crises, somatostatin analogues are effective at both treating the condition and preventing their development during known precipitating events such as surgery, anesthesia, chemotherapy, and stress. It is recommended that octreotide 150–250 μg SC every 6 to 8 h be used 24–48 h before anesthesia and then continued throughout the procedure.

Currently, sustained-release preparations of both octreotide (octreotide-LAR [long-acting release], 10, 20, 30 mg) and lanreotide (lanreotide-PR [prolonged release, lanreotide-autogel], 60, 90, 120 mg) are available and widely used because their use greatly facilitates long-term treatment. Octreotide-LAR (30 mg/month) gives a plasma level ≥1 ng/mL for 25 days, whereas this requires three to six injections a day of the non-sustained-release form. Lanreotide-autogel (Somatuline) is given every 4–6 weeks.

Short-term side effects occur in up to one-half of patients. Pain at the injection site and side effects related to the GI tract (59% discomfort, 15% nausea, diarrhea) are the most common. They are usually short-lived and do not interrupt treatment. Important long-term side effects include gallstone formation, steatorrhea, and deterioration in glucose tolerance. The overall incidence of gallstones/biliary sludge in one study was 52%, with 7% having symptomatic disease that required surgical treatment.

Interferon α is reported to be effective in controlling symptoms of the carcinoid syndrome either alone or combined with hepatic artery embolization. With interferon α alone, the clinical response rate is 30–70%, and with interferon α with hepatic artery embolization, diarrhea was controlled for 1 year in 43% and flushing was controlled in 86%. Side effects develop in almost all patients, with the most frequent being a flu-like syndrome (80–100%), followed by anorexia and fatigue, even though these frequently improve with continued treatment. Other more severe side effects include bone marrow toxicity, hepatotoxicity, autoimmune disorders, and rarely CNS side effects (depression, mental disorders, visual problems).

Hepatic artery embolization alone or with chemotherapy (chemoembolization) has been used to control the symptoms of carcinoid syndrome. Embolization alone is reported to control symptoms in up to 76% of patients, and chemoembolization (5-fluorouracil, doxorubicin, cisplatin, mitomycin) controls symptoms in 60–75% of patients. Hepatic artery embolization can have major side effects, including nausea, vomiting, pain, and fever. In two studies, 5–7% of patients died from complications of hepatic artery occlusion.

Other drugs have been used successfully in small numbers of patients to control the symptoms of carcinoid syndrome. Parachlorophenylanine can inhibit tryptophan hydroxylase and therefore the conversion of tryptophan to 5-HTP. However, its severe side effects, including psychiatric disturbances, make it intolerable for long-term use. α-Methyldopa inhibits the conversion of 5-HTP to 5-HT, but its effects are only partial.

Peptide radioreceptor therapy (using radiotherapy with radiolabeled somatostatin analogues), the use of radiolabeled microspheres, and other methods for treatment of advanced metastatic disease may facilitate control of the carcinoid syndrome and are discussed in a later section dealing with treatment of advanced disease.

GI-NETs (CARCINOIDS) (NONMETASTATIC) Surgery is the only potentially curative therapy. Because with most GI-NETs (carcinoids), the probability of metastatic disease increases with increasing size, the extent of surgical resection is determined accordingly. With appendiceal NETs (carcinoids) <1 cm, simple appendectomy was curative in 103 patients followed for up to 35 years. With rectal NETs (carcinoids) <1 cm, local resection is curative. With SI NETs (carcinoids) <1 cm, there is not complete agreement. Because 15–69% of SI NETs (carcinoids) this size have metastases in different studies, some recommend a wide resection with en bloc resection of the adjacent lymph-bearing mesentery. If the tumor is >2 cm for rectal, appendiceal, or SI NETs (carcinoids), a full cancer operation should be done. This includes a right hemicolectomy for appendiceal NETs (carcinoids), an abdominoperineal resection or low anterior resection for rectal NETs (carcinoids), and an en bloc resection of adjacent lymph nodes for SI NETs (carcinoids). For appendiceal NETs (carcinoids) 1–2 cm in diameter, a simple appendectomy is proposed by some, whereas others favor a formal right hemicolectomy. For 1–2 cm rectal NETs (carcinoids), it is recommended that a wide, local, full-thickness excision be performed.

With type I or II gastric NETs (carcinoids), which are usually <1 cm, endoscopic removal is recommended. In type I or II gastric carcinoids, if the tumor is >2 cm or if there is local invasion, some recommend total gastrectomy, whereas others recommend antrectomy in type I to reduce the hypergastrinemia, which has led to regression of the carcinoids in a number of studies. For types I and II gastric NETs (carcinoids) of 1–2 cm, there is no agreement, with some recommending endoscopic treatment followed by chronic somatostatin treatment and careful follow-up and others recommending surgical treatment. With type III gastric NETs (carcinoids) >2 cm, excision and regional lymph node clearance are recommended. Most tumors <1 cm are treated endoscopically.

Resection of isolated or limited hepatic metastases may be beneficial and will be discussed in a later section on treatment of advanced disease.

PANCREATIC NEUROENDOCRINE TUMORS

Functional pNETs usually present clinically with symptoms due to the hormone-excess state (Table 28-2). Only late in the course of the disease does the tumor per se cause prominent symptoms such as abdominal pain. In contrast, all the symptoms due to nonfunctional pNETs are due to the tumor per se. The overall result of this is that some functional pNETs may present with severe symptoms with a small or undetectable primary tumor, whereas nonfunctional tumors usually present late in the disease course with large tumors, which are frequently metastatic. The mean delay between onset of continuous symptoms and diagnosis of a functional pNET syndrome is 4–7 years. Therefore, the diagnoses frequently are missed for extended periods.

TREATMENT Pancreatic Neuroendocrine Tumor (General Points)

Treatment of pNETs requires two different strategies. First, treatment must be directed at the hormone-excess state such as the gastric acid hypersecretion in gastrinomas or the hypoglycemia in insulinomas. Ectopic hormone secretion usually causes the presenting symptoms and can cause life-threatening complications. Second, with all the tumors except insulinomas, >50% are malignant (Table 28-2); therefore, treatment must also be directed against the tumor per se. Because in many patients these tumors are not surgically curable due to the presence of advanced disease at diagnosis, surgical resection for cure, which addresses both treatment aspects, is often not possible.

GASTRINOMA (ZOLLINGER-ELLISON SYNDROME)

A gastrinoma is an NET that secretes gastrin; the resultant hypergastrinemia causes gastric acid hypersecretion (Zollinger-Ellison syndrome [ZES]). The chronic hypergastrinemia results in marked gastric acid hypersecretion and growth of the gastric mucosa with increased numbers of parietal cells and proliferation of gastric ECL cells. The gastric acid hypersecretion characteristically causes peptic ulcer disease (PUD), often refractory and severe, as well as diarrhea. The most common presenting symptoms are abdominal pain (70-100%), diarrhea (37-73%), and gastroesophageal reflux disease (GERD) (30-35%); 10-20% of patients have diarrhea only. Although peptic ulcers may occur in unusual locations, most patients have a typical duodenal ulcer. Important observations that should suggest this diagnosis include PUD with diarrhea; PUD in an unusual location or with multiple ulcers; PUD refractory to treatment or persistent; PUD associated with prominent gastric folds; PUD associated with findings suggestive of MEN 1 (endocrinopathy, family history of ulcer or endocrinopathy, nephrolithiases); and PUD without *Helicobacter pylori* present. *H. pylori* is present in >90% of idiopathic peptic ulcers but is present in <50% of patients with gastrinomas. Chronic unexplained diarrhea also should suggest ZES.

Approximately 20-25% of patients with ZES have MEN 1 (MEN1/ZES), and in most cases, hyperparathyroidism is present before the ZES develops. These patients are treated differently from those without MEN 1 (sporadic ZES); therefore, MEN 1 should be sought in all patients with ZES by family history and by measuring plasma ionized calcium and prolactin levels and plasma hormone levels (parathormone, growth hormone).

Most gastrinomas (50–90%) in sporadic ZES are present in the duodenum, followed by the pancreas (10–40%) and other intraabdominal sites (mesentery, lymph nodes, biliary tract, liver, stomach, ovary). Rarely, the tumor may involve extraabdominal sites (heart, lung cancer). In MEN 1/ZES the gastrinomas are also usually in the duodenum (70–90%), followed by the pancreas (10–30%), and are almost always multiple. About 60–90% of gastrinomas are malignant (Table 28-2) with metastatic spread to lymph nodes and liver. Distant metastases to bone occur in 12–30% of patients with liver metastases.

Diagnosis

The diagnosis of ZES requires the demonstration of inappropriate fasting hypergastrinemia, usually by demonstrating hypergastrinemia occurring with an increased basal gastric acid output (BAO) (hyperchlorhydria). More than 98% of patients with ZES have fasting hypergastrinemia, although in 40–60% the level may be elevated less than tenfold. Therefore, when the diagnosis is suspected, a fasting gastrin is usually the initial test performed. It is important to remember that potent gastric acid suppressant drugs such as proton pump inhibitors (PPIs) (omeprazole, esomeprazole, pantoprazole, lansoprazole, rabeprazole) can suppress acid secretion sufficiently to cause hypergastrinemia; because of their prolonged duration of action, these drugs have to be tapered or frequently discontinued for a week before the gastrin determination. Withdrawal of PPIs should be performed carefully because PUD complications can rapidly develop in some patients and is best done in consultation with GI units with experience in this area. The widespread use of PPIs can confound the diagnosis of ZES by raising a false-positive diagnosis by causing hypergastrinemia in a patient being treated with idiopathic PUD (without ZES) and lead to a false-negative diagnosis because at routine doses used to treat patients with idiopathic PUD, PPIs control symptoms in most ZES patients and thus mask the diagnosis. If ZES is suspected and the gastrin level is elevated, it is important to show that it is increased when gastric pH is ≤2.0 because physiologically hypergastrinemia secondary to achlorhydria (atrophic gastritis, pernicious anemia) is one of the most common causes of hypergastrinemia. Nearly all ZES patients have a fasting pH ≤2 when off antisecretory drugs. If the fasting gastrin is >1000 pg/mL (increased tenfold) and the pH is ≤2.0, which occurs in 40–60% of patients with ZES, the diagnosis of ZES is established after the possibility of retained antrum syndrome has been ruled out by history. In patients with hypergastrinemia with fasting gastrins <1000 pg/mL (<10-fold increased) and gastric pH ≤2.0, other conditions, such as *H. pylori* infections, antral G-cell hyperplasia/hyperfunction, gastric outlet obstruction, and, rarely, renal failure, can masquerade as ZES. To establish the diagnosis in this group, a determination of BAO and a secretin provocative test should be done. In patients with ZES without previous gastric acid–reducing surgery, the BAO is usually (>90%) elevated (i.e., >15 mEq/h). The secretin provocative test is usually positive, with the criterion of a >120-pg/mL increase over the basal level having the highest sensitivity (94%) and specificity (100%). Unfortunately the diagnosis of ZES is becoming increasing more difficult. This is due not only to the widespread use of PPIs (leading to false-positive results as well as masking ZES presentation), but also recent studies demonstrate than many of the commercial gastrin kits that are used by most laboratories to measure fasting serum gastrin levels are not reliable. In one study, 7 of the 12 tested commercial gastrin kits inaccurately assessed the true serum concentration of gastrin primarily because the antibodies used had inappropriate specificity for the different circulating forms of gastrin and were not adequately validated. Both underestimation and overestimation of fasting serum gastrin levels occurred using these commercial kits. To circumvent this problem, it is either necessary to use one of the five reliable kits identified or, alternatively, to refer the patient to a center with expertise in making the diagnosis in your area, or if this is not possible, to contact such a center and use the gastrin assay they recommend. An accurate gastrin assay is essential for accurate measurement of fasting serum gastrin level as well as for assessing gastrin levels during the secretin provocative test, and thus, the diagnosis of ZES cannot reliably be made without one.

TREATMENT Zollinger-Ellison Syndrome

Gastric acid hypersecretion in patients with ZES can be controlled in almost every case by oral gastric antisecretory drugs. Because of their long duration of action and potency, which allows dosing once or twice a day, the PPIs (H^+, K^+-ATPase inhibitors) are the drugs of choice. Histamine H_2-receptor antagonists are also effective, although more frequent dosing (q 4–8 h) and high doses are required. In patients with MEN 1/ZES with hyperparathyroidism, correction of the hyperparathyroidism increases the sensitivity to gastric antisecretory drugs and decreases the basal acid output. Long-term treatment with PPIs (>15 years) has proved to be safe and effective, without development of tachyphylaxis. Although patients with ZES, especially those with MEN 1/ZES, more frequently develop gastric NETs (carcinoids), no data suggest that the long-term use of PPIs increases this risk in these patients. With long-term PPI use in ZES patients, vitamin B_{12} deficiency can develop; thus, vitamin B_{12} levels should be assessed during follow-up. Epidemiologic studies suggest that long-term PPI use may be associated with an increased incidence of bone fractures; however, at present, there is no such report in ZES patients.

With the increased ability to control acid hypersecretion, more than 50% of patients who are not cured (>60% of patients) will die from tumor-related causes. At presentation, careful imaging studies are essential to localize the extent of the tumor to determine the appropriate treatment. A third of patients present with hepatic metastases, and in <15% of those patients, the disease is limited, so that surgical resection may be possible. Surgical short-term cure is possible in 60% of all patients without MEN 1/ZES or liver metastases (40% of all patients) and in 30% of patients long term. In patients with MEN 1/ZES, long-term surgical cure is rare because the tumors are multiple, frequently with lymph node metastases. Surgical studies demonstrate that successful resection of the gastrinoma not only decreases the chances of developing liver metastases but also increases the disease-related survival rate. Therefore, all patients with gastrinomas without MEN 1/ZES or a medical condition that limits life expectancy should undergo surgery by a surgeon experienced in the treatment of these disorders.

INSULINOMAS

An insulinoma is an NET of the pancreas that is thought to be derived from beta cells that ectopically secrete insulin, which results in hypoglycemia. The average age of occurrence is 40–50 years old. The most common clinical symptoms are due to the effect of the hypoglycemia on the CNS (neuroglycemic symptoms) and include confusion, headache, disorientation, visual difficulties, irrational behavior, and even coma. Also, most patients have symptoms due to excess catecholamine release secondary to the hypoglycemia, including sweating, tremor, and palpitations. Characteristically, these attacks are associated with fasting.

Insulinomas are generally small (>90% are <2 cm) and usually not multiple (90%); only 5–15% are malignant, and they almost invariably occur only in the pancreas, distributed equally in the pancreatic head, body, and tail.

Insulinomas should be suspected in all patients with hypoglycemia, especially when there is a history suggesting that attacks are provoked by fasting, or with a family history of MEN 1. Insulin is synthesized as proinsulin, which consists of a 21-amino-acid α chain and a 30-amino-acid β chain connected by a 33-amino-acid connecting peptide (C peptide). In insulinomas, in addition to elevated plasma insulin levels, elevated plasma proinsulin levels are found, and C-peptide levels are elevated.

Diagnosis

The diagnosis of insulinoma requires the demonstration of an elevated plasma insulin level at the time of hypoglycemia. A number of other conditions may cause fasting hypoglycemia, such as the inadvertent or surreptitious use of insulin or oral hypoglycemic agents, severe liver disease, alcoholism, poor nutrition, and other extrapancreatic tumors. Furthermore, postprandial hypoglycemia can be caused by a number of conditions that confuse the diagnosis of insulinoma. Particularly important here is the increased occurrence of hypoglycemia after gastric bypass surgery for obesity, which is now widely performed. A new entity, insulinomatosis, was described that can cause hypoglycemia and mimic insulinomas. It occurs in 10% of patients with persistent hyperinsulinemic hypoglycemia and is characterized by the occurrence of multiple macro-/microadenomas expressing insulin, and it is not clear how to distinguish this entity from insulinoma preoperatively. The most reliable test to diagnose insulinoma is a fast up to 72 h with serum glucose, C-peptide, proinsulin, and insulin measurements every 4–8 h. If at any point the patient becomes symptomatic or glucose levels are persistently below <2.2 mmol/L (40 mg/dL), the test should be terminated, and repeat samples for the above studies should be obtained before glucose is given. Some 70–80% of patients will develop hypoglycemia during the first 24 h, and 98% by 48 h. In nonobese normal subjects, serum insulin levels should decrease to <43 pmol/L (<6 μU/mL) when blood glucose decreases to <2.2 mmol/L (<40 mg/dL) and the ratio of insulin to glucose is <0.3 (in mg/dL). In addition to having an insulin level >6 μU/mL when blood glucose is <40 mg/dL, some investigators also require an elevated C-peptide and serum proinsulin level, an insulin/glucose ratio >0.3, and a decreased plasma β-hydroxybutyrate level for the diagnosis of insulinomas. Surreptitious use of insulin or hypoglycemic agents may be difficult to distinguish from insulinomas. The combination of proinsulin levels (normal in exogenous insulin/hypoglycemic agent users), C-peptide levels (low in exogenous insulin users), antibodies to insulin (positive in exogenous insulin users), and measurement of sulfonylurea levels in serum or plasma will allow the correct diagnosis to be made. The diagnosis of insulinoma has been complicated by the introduction of specific insulin assays that do not also interact with proinsulin, as do many of the older radioimmunoassays (RIAs), and therefore give lower plasma insulin levels. The increased use of these specific insulin assays has resulted in increased numbers of patients with insulinomas having lower plasma insulin values (<6 μU/mL) than levels proposed to be characteristic of insulinomas by RIA. In these patients, the assessment of proinsulin and C-peptide levels at the time of hypoglycemia is particularly helpful for establishing the correct diagnosis. An elevated proinsulin level when the fasting glucose level is <45 mg/dL is sensitive and specific.

TREATMENT Insulinomas

Only 5–15% of insulinomas are malignant; therefore, after appropriate imaging (see below), surgery should be performed. In different studies, 75–100% of patients are cured by surgery. Before surgery, the hypoglycemia can be controlled by frequent small meals and the use of diazoxide (150–800 mg/d). Diazoxide is a benzothiadiazide whose hyperglycemic effect is attributed to inhibition of insulin release. Its side effects are sodium retention and GI symptoms such as nausea. Approximately 50–60% of patients respond to diazoxide. Other agents effective in some patients to control the hypoglycemia include verapamil and diphenylhydantoin. Long-acting somatostatin analogues such as octreotide and lanreotide are acutely effective in 40% of patients. However, octreotide must be used with care because it inhibits growth hormone secretion and can alter plasma glucagon levels; therefore, in some patients, it can worsen the hypoglycemia.

For the 5–15% of patients with malignant insulinomas, these drugs or somatostatin analogues are used initially. In a small number of patients with insulinomas, some with malignant tumors, mammalian target of rapamycin (mTOR) inhibitors (everolimus, rapamycin) are reported to control the hypoglycemia. If they are not effective, various antitumor treatments such as hepatic arterial embolization, chemoembolization, chemotherapy, and peptide receptor radiotherapy have been used (see below).

Insulinomas, which are usually benign (>90%) and intrapancreatic in location, are increasingly resected using a laparoscopic approach, which has lower morbidity rates. This approach requires that the insulinoma be localized on preoperative imaging studies.

GLUCAGONOMAS

A glucagonoma is NET of the pancreas that secretes excessive amounts of glucagon, which causes a distinct syndrome characterized by dermatitis, glucose intolerance or diabetes, and weight loss. Glucagonomas principally occur between 45 and 70 years of age. The tumor is clinically heralded by a characteristic dermatitis (migratory necrolytic erythema) (67–90%), accompanied by glucose intolerance (40–90%), weight loss (66–96%), anemia (33–85%), diarrhea (15–29%), and thromboembolism (11–24%). The characteristic rash usually starts as an annular erythema at intertriginous and periorificial sites, especially in the groin or buttock. It subsequently becomes raised, and bullae form; when the bullae rupture, eroded areas form. The lesions can wax and wane. The development of a similar rash in patients receiving glucagon therapy suggests that the rash is a direct effect of the hyperglucagonemia. A characteristic laboratory finding is hypoaminoacidemia, which occurs in 26–100% of patients.

Glucagonomas are generally large tumors at diagnosis (5–10 cm). Some 50–80% occur in the pancreatic tail. From 50 to 82% have evidence of metastatic spread at presentation, usually to the liver. Glucagonomas are rarely extrapancreatic and usually occur singly.

Two new entities have been described that can also cause hyperglucagonemia and may mimic glucagonomas. Mahvash disease is due to a homozygous P86S mutation of the human glucagon receptor. It is associated with the development of α-cell hyperplasia, hyperglucagonemia, and the development of nonfunctioning pNETs. A second disease called *glucagon cell adenomatosis* can mimic glucagonoma syndrome clinically and is characterized by the presence of hyperplastic islets staining positive for glucagon instead of a single glucagonoma.

Diagnosis

The diagnosis is confirmed by demonstrating an increased plasma glucagon level. Characteristically, plasma glucagon levels exceed 1000 pg/mL (normal is <150 pg/mL) in 90%; 7% are between 500 and 1000 pg/mL, and 3% are <500 pg/mL. A trend toward lower levels at diagnosis has been noted in the last decade. A plasma glucagon level >1000 pg/mL is considered diagnostic of glucagonoma. Other diseases causing increased plasma glucagon levels include cirrhosis, diabetic ketoacidosis, celiac disease, renal insufficiency, acute pancreatitis, hypercorticism, hepatic insufficiency, severe stress, and prolonged fasting or familial hyperglucagonemia, as well as danazol treatment. With the exception of cirrhosis, these disorders do not increase plasma glucagon >500 pg/mL.

Necrolytic migratory erythema is not pathognomonic for glucagonoma and occurs in myeloproliferative disorders, hepatitis B infection, malnutrition, short-bowel syndrome, inflammatory bowel disease, zinc deficiency, and malabsorption disorders.

TREATMENT Glucagonomas

In 50–80% of patients, hepatic metastases are present, and so curative surgical resection is not possible. Surgical debulking in patients with advanced disease or other antitumor treatments may be beneficial (see below). Long-acting somatostatin analogues such as octreotide and lanreotide improve the skin rash in 75% of patients and may improve the weight loss, pain, and diarrhea, but usually do not improve the glucose intolerance.

SOMATOSTATINOMA SYNDROME

The somatostatinoma syndrome is due to an NET that secretes excessive amounts of somatostatin, which causes a distinct syndrome characterized by diabetes mellitus, gallbladder disease, diarrhea, and steatorrhea. There is no general distinction in the literature between a tumor that contains somatostatin-like immunoreactivity (somatostatinoma) and does (11–45%) or does not (55–90%) produce a clinical syndrome (somatostatinoma syndrome) by secreting somatostatin. In a review of 173 cases of somatostatinomas, only 11% were associated with the somatostatinoma syndrome. The mean age is 51 years. Somatostatinomas occur primarily in the pancreas and small intestine, and the frequency of the symptoms and occurrence of the somatostatinoma syndrome differ in each. Each of the usual symptoms is more common in pancreatic than in intestinal somatostatinomas: diabetes mellitus (95% vs 21%), gallbladder disease (94% vs 43%), diarrhea (92% vs 38%), steatorrhea (83% vs 12%), hypochlorhydria (86% vs 12%), and weight loss (90% vs 69%). The somatostatinoma syndrome occurs in 30–90% of pancreatic and 0–5% of SI somatostatinomas. In various series, 43% of all duodenal NETs contain somatostatin; however, the somatostatinoma syndrome is rarely present (<2%). Somatostatinomas occur in the pancreas in 56–74% of cases, with the primary location being the pancreatic head. The tumors are usually solitary (90%) and large (mean size 4.5 cm). Liver metastases are common, being present in 69–84% of patients. Somatostatinomas are rare in patients with MEN 1, occurring in only 0.65%.

Somatostatin is a tetradecapeptide that is widely distributed in the CNS and GI tract, where it functions as a neurotransmitter or has paracrine and autocrine actions. It is a potent inhibitor of many processes, including release of almost all hormones, acid secretion, intestinal and pancreatic secretion, and intestinal absorption. Most of the clinical manifestations are directly related to these inhibitory actions.

Diagnosis

In most cases, somatostatinomas have been found by accident either at the time of cholecystectomy or during endoscopy. The presence of psammoma bodies in a duodenal tumor should particularly raise suspicion. Duodenal somatostatin-containing tumors are increasingly associated with von Recklinghausen's disease (NF-1) (Table 28-6). Most of these tumors (>98%) do not cause the somatostatinoma syndrome. The diagnosis of the somatostatinoma syndrome requires the demonstration of elevated plasma somatostatin levels.

TREATMENT Somatostatinomas

Pancreatic tumors are frequently (70–92%) metastatic at presentation, whereas 30–69% of SI somatostatinomas have metastases. Surgery is the treatment of choice for those without widespread hepatic metastases. Symptoms in patients with the somatostatinoma syndrome are also improved by octreotide treatment.

VIPOMAS

VIPomas are NETs that secrete excessive amounts of vasoactive intestinal peptide (VIP), which causes a distinct syndrome characterized by large-volume diarrhea, hypokalemia, and dehydration. This syndrome also is called Verner-Morrison syndrome, pancreatic cholera, and WDHA syndrome for *w*atery *d*iarrhea, *h*ypokalemia, and *a*chlorhydria, which some patients develop. The mean age of patients with this syndrome is 49 years; however, it can occur in children, and when it does, it is usually caused by a ganglioneuroma or ganglioneuroblastoma.

The principal symptoms are large-volume diarrhea (100%) severe enough to cause hypokalemia (80–100%), dehydration (83%), hypochlorhydria (54–76%), and flushing (20%). The diarrhea is secretory in nature, persisting during fasting, and is almost always >1 L/d and in 70% is >3 L/d. In a number of studies, the diarrhea was intermittent initially in up to half the patients. Most patients do not have accompanying steatorrhea (16%), and the increased stool volume is due to increased excretion of sodium and potassium, which, with the anions, accounts for the osmolality of the stool. Patients frequently have hyperglycemia (25–50%) and hypercalcemia (25–50%).

VIP is a 28-amino-acid peptide that is an important neurotransmitter, ubiquitously present in the CNS and GI tract. Its known actions include stimulation of SI chloride secretion as well as effects on smooth-muscle contractility, inhibition of acid secretion, and vasodilatory effects, which explain most features of the clinical syndrome.

In adults, 80–90% of VIPomas are pancreatic in location, with the rest due to VIP-secreting pheochromocytomas, intestinal carcinoids, and rarely ganglioneuromas. These tumors are usually solitary, 50–75% are in the pancreatic tail, and 37–68% have hepatic metastases at diagnosis. In children <10 years old, the syndrome is usually due to ganglioneuromas or ganglioblastomas and is less often malignant (10%).

Diagnosis

The diagnosis requires the demonstration of an elevated plasma VIP level and the presence of large-volume diarrhea. A stool volume <700 mL/d is proposed to exclude the diagnosis of VIPoma. When the patient fasts, a number of diseases can be excluded that can cause marked diarrhea because the high volume of diarrhea is not sustained during the fast. Other diseases that can produce a secretory large-volume diarrhea include gastrinomas, chronic laxative abuse, carcinoid syndrome, systemic mastocytosis, rarely medullary thyroid cancer, diabetic diarrhea, sprue, and AIDS. Among these conditions, only VIPomas caused a marked increase in plasma VIP. Chronic surreptitious use of laxatives/diuretics can be particularly difficult to detect clinically. Hence, in a patient with unexplained chronic diarrhea, screens for laxatives should be performed; they will detect many, but not all, laxative abusers. Elevated plasma levels of VIP should not be the only basis of the diagnosis of VIPomas because they can occur with some diarrheal states including inflammatory bowel disease, post small bowel resection, and radiation enteritis. Furthermore, nesidioblastosis can mimic VIPomas by causing elevated plasma VIP levels, diarrhea, and even false-positive location in the pancreatic region on somatostatin receptor scintigraphy.

TREATMENT VIPomas

The most important initial treatment in these patients is to correct their dehydration, hypokalemia, and electrolyte losses with fluid and electrolyte replacement. These patients may require 5 L/d of fluid and >350 mEq/d of potassium. Because 37–68% of adults with VIPomas have metastatic disease in the liver at presentation, a significant number of patients cannot be cured surgically. In these patients, long-acting somatostatin analogues such as octreotide and lanreotide are the drugs of choice.

Octreotide/lanreotide will control the diarrhea short- and long-term in 75–100% of patients. In nonresponsive patients, the combination of glucocorticoids and octreotide/lanreotide has proved helpful in a small number of patients. Other drugs reported to be helpful in small numbers of patients include prednisone (60–100 mg/d), clonidine, indomethacin, phenothiazines, loperamide, lidamidine, lithium, propranolol, and metoclopramide. Treatment of advanced disease with cytoreductive surgery, embolization, chemoembolization, chemotherapy, radiotherapy, radiofrequency ablation, and peptide receptor radiotherapy may be helpful (see below).

NONFUNCTIONAL PANCREATIC NEUROENDOCRINE TUMORS (NF-pNETs)

NF-pNETs are NETs that originate in the pancreas and either secrete no products or their products do not cause a specific clinical syndrome. Their symptoms are due entirely to the tumor per se. NF-pNETs secrete chromogranin A (90–100%), chromogranin B (90–100%), α-HCG (human chorionic gonadotropin) (40%), neuron-specific enolase (31%), and β-HCG (20%), and because 40–90% secrete PP, they are also often called PPomas. Because the symptoms are due to the tumor mass, patients with NF-pNETs usually present late in the disease course with invasive tumors and hepatic metastases (64–92%), and the tumors are usually large (72% >5 cm). NF-pNETs are usually solitary except in patients with MEN 1, in which case they are multiple. They occur primarily in the pancreatic head. Even though these tumors do not cause a functional syndrome, immunocytochemical studies show that they synthesize numerous peptides and cannot be distinguished from functional pNETs by immunocytochemistry. In MEN 1, 80–100% of patients have microscopic NF-pNETs, but they become large or symptomatic in a minority (0–13%) of cases. In VHL, 12–17% develop NF-pNETs, and in 4%, they are ≥3 cm in diameter.

The most common symptoms are abdominal pain (30–80%), jaundice (20–35%), and weight loss, fatigue, or bleeding; 10–35% are found incidentally. The average time from the beginning of symptoms to diagnosis is 5 years.

Diagnosis

The diagnosis is established by histologic confirmation in a patient without either the clinical symptoms or the elevated plasma hormone levels of one of the established syndromes. The principal difficulty in diagnosis is to distinguish an NF-pNET from a nonendocrine pancreatic tumor, which is more common, as well as from a functional pNET. Even though chromogranin A levels are elevated in almost every patient, this is not specific for this disease as it can be found in functional pNETs, GI-NETs (carcinoids), and other neuroendocrine disorders. Plasma PP elevations should strongly suggest the diagnosis in a patient with a pancreatic mass because it is usually normal in patients with pancreatic adenocarcinomas. Elevated plasma PP is not diagnostic of this tumor because it is elevated in a number of other conditions, such as chronic renal failure, old age, inflammatory conditions, alcohol abuse, pancreatitis, hypoglycemia, postprandially, and diabetes. A positive somatostatin receptor scan in a patient with a pancreatic mass should suggest the presence of pNET/NF-pNET rather than a nonendocrine tumor.

TREATMENT Nonfunctional Pancreatic Neuroendocrine Tumors (NF-pNETs)

Overall survival in patients with sporadic NF-pNET is 30–63% at 5 years, with a median survival of 6 years. Unfortunately, surgical curative resection can be considered only in a minority of these patients because 64–92% present with diffuse metastatic disease. Treatment needs to be directed against the tumor per se using the various modalities discussed below for advanced disease. The treatment of NF-pNETs in either MEN 1 patients or patients with VHL is controversial. Most recommend surgical resection for any tumor >2–3 cm in diameter; however, there is no consensus on smaller NF-pNETs in these inherited disorders, with most recommending careful surveillance of these patients. The treatment of small sporadic, asymptomatic NF-pNETs (≤2 cm) is also controversial. Most of these are low- or intermediate-grade lesions, and <7% are malignant. Some advocate a nonoperative approach with careful, regular follow-up, whereas other recommend an operative approach with specially consideration for a laparoscopic surgical approach.

GRFOMAS

GRFomas are NETs that secrete excessive amounts of growth hormone–releasing factor (GRF) that cause acromegaly. GRF is a 44-amino-acid peptide, and 25–44% of pNETs have GRF immunoreactivity, although it is uncommonly secreted. GRFomas are lung tumors in 47–54% of cases, pNETs in 29–30%, and SI carcinoids in 8–10%; up to 12% occur at other sites. Patients have a mean age of 38 years, and the symptoms usually are due to either acromegaly or the tumor per se. The acromegaly caused by GRFomas is indistinguishable from classic acromegaly. The pancreatic tumors are usually large (>6 cm), and liver metastases are present in 39%. They should be suspected in any patient with acromegaly and an abdominal tumor, a patient with MEN 1 with acromegaly, or a patient without a pituitary adenoma with acromegaly or associated with hyperprolactinemia, which occurs in 70% of GRFomas. GRFomas are an uncommon cause of acromegaly. GRFomas occur in <1% of MEN 1 patients. The diagnosis is established by performing plasma assays for GRF and growth hormone. Most GRFomas have a plasma GRF level >300 pg/mL (normal <5 pg/mL men, <10 pg/mL women). Patients with GRFomas also have increased plasma levels of insulin-like growth factor type I (IGF-I) similar to those in classic acromegaly. Surgery is the treatment of choice if diffuse metastases are not present. Long-acting somatostatin analogues such as octreotide and lanreotide are the agents of choice, with 75–100% of patients responding.

OTHER RARE PANCREATIC NEUROENDOCRINE TUMOR SYNDROMES

Cushing's syndrome (ACTHoma) due to a pNET occurs in 4–16% of all ectopic Cushing's syndrome cases. It occurs in 5% of cases of sporadic gastrinomas, almost invariably in patients with hepatic metastases, and is an independent poor prognostic factor. Paraneoplastic hypercalcemia due to pNETs releasing parathyroid hormone–related peptide (PTHrP), a PTH-like material, or unknown factor, is rarely reported. The tumors are usually large, and liver metastases are usually present. Most (88%) appear to be due to release of PTHrP. pNETs occasionally can cause the carcinoid syndrome. A number of very rare pNET syndromes involving a few cases (less than five) have been described; these include a renin-producing pNET in a patient presenting with hypertension; pNETs secreting luteinizing hormone, resulting in masculinization or decreased libido; a pNET secreting erythropoietin, resulting in polycythemia; pNETs secreting IGF-II, causing hypoglycemia; and pNETs secreting enteroglucagon, causing small intestinal hypertrophy, colonic/SI stasis, and malabsorption (Table 28-2). A number of other possible functional pNETs have been proposed, but most authorities classify these as unclear or as a nonfunctional pNET because in each case numerous patients have been described with similar plasma hormone elevations that do not cause any symptoms. These include pNETs secreting calcitonin, neurotensin (neurotensinoma), PP (PPoma), and ghrelin (Table 28-2).

TUMOR LOCALIZATION

Localization of the primary tumor and knowledge of the extent of the disease are essential to the proper management of all GI-NETs (carcinoids) and pNETs. Without proper localization studies, it is not possible to determine whether the patient is a candidate for surgical resection (curative or cytoreductive) or requires antitumor treatment, to determine whether the patient is responding to antitumor therapies, or to appropriately classify/stage the patient's disease to assess prognosis.

Numerous tumor localization methods are used in both types of NETs, including cross-sectional imaging studies (CT, magnetic resonance imaging [MRI], transabdominal ultrasound), selective angiography, somatostatin receptor scintigraphy (SRS), and positron emission tomography. In pNETs, endoscopic ultrasound (EUS) and functional localization by measuring venous hormonal gradients are also reported to be useful. Bronchial carcinoids are usually detected by standard chest radiography and assessed by CT. Rectal, duodenal, colonic, and gastric carcinoids are usually detected by GI endoscopy. Because of their wide availability, CT and MRI are generally initially used to determine the location of the primary NETs and the extent of disease. NETs are hypervascular tumors, and with both MRI and CT, contrast enhancement is essential for maximal sensitivity, and it is recommended that generally triple-phase scanning be used. The ability of cross-sectional imaging and, to a lesser extent, SRS to detect NETs is a function of NET size. With CT and MRI, <10% of tumors <1 cm in diameter are detected, 30–40% of tumors 1–3 cm are detected, and >50% of tumors >3 cm are detected. Many primary GI-NETs (carcinoids) are small, as are insulinomas and duodenal gastrinomas, and are frequently not detected by cross-sectional imaging, whereas most other pNETs present late in the course of their disease and are large (>4 cm). Selective angiography is more sensitive, localizing 60–90% of all NETs; however, it is now used infrequently. For detecting liver metastases, CT and MRI are more sensitive than ultrasound, and with recent improvements, 5–25% of patients with liver metastases will be missed by CT and/or MRI.

pNETs, as well as GI-NETs (carcinoids), frequently (>80%) overexpress high-affinity somatostatin receptors in both the primary tumors and the metastases. Of the five types of somatostatin receptors (sst_{1-5}), radiolabeled octreotide binds with high affinity to sst_2 and sst_5, has a lower affinity for sst_3, and has a very low affinity for sst_1 and sst_4. Between 80 and 100% of GI-NETs (carcinoids) and pNETs possess sst_2, and many also have the other four sst subtypes. Interaction with these receptors can be used to treat these tumors as well as to localize NETs by using radiolabeled somatostatin analogues (SRS). In the United States, [^{111}In-DTPA-D-Phe^1]octreotide (octreoscan) is generally used with gamma camera detection using single-photon emission computed tomography (SPECT) imaging. Numerous studies, primarily in Europe, using gallium-68-labeled somatostatin analogues and positron emission tomography (PET) detection, demonstrate even greater sensitivity than with SRS with ^{111}In-labeled somatostatin analogues. Although not yet approved in the United States, there are a number of centers starting to use this approach. Because of its sensitivity and ability to localize tumor throughout the body, SRS is the initial imaging modality of choice for localizing both the primary tumor and metastatic NETs. SRS localizes tumor in 73–95% of patients with GI-NETs (carcinoids) and in 56–100% of patients with pNETs, except insulinomas. Insulinomas are usually small and have low densities of sst receptors, resulting in SRS being positive in only 12–50% of patients with insulinomas. SRS identifies >90–95% of patients with liver metastases due to NETs. Figure 28-3 shows an example of the increased sensitivity of SRS in a patient with a GI-NET (carcinoid) tumor. The CT scan showed a single liver metastasis, whereas the SRS demonstrated three metastases in the liver in multiple locations. Occasional false-positive responses with SRS can occur (12% in one study) because numerous other normal tissues as well as diseases can have high densities of sst receptors, including granulomas (sarcoid, tuberculosis, etc.), thyroid diseases (goiter, thyroiditis), and activated lymphocytes

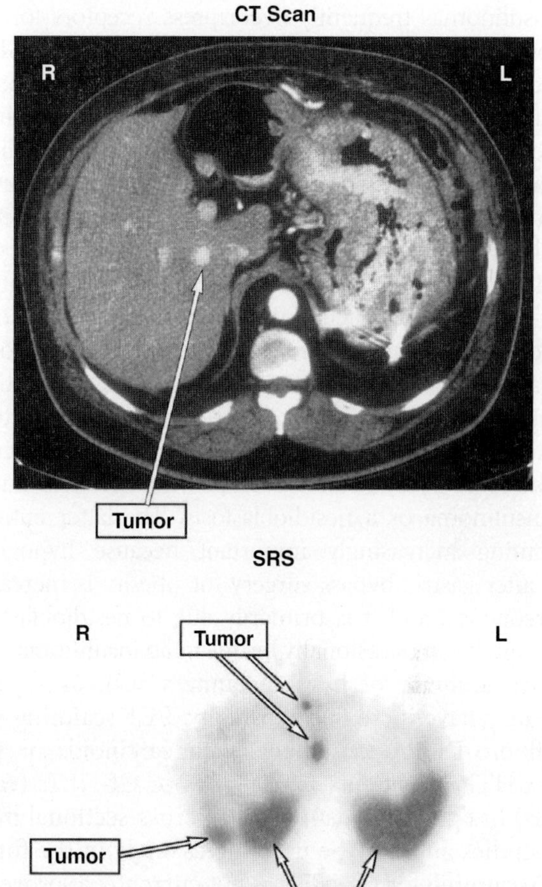

FIGURE 28-3
Ability of computed tomography (CT) scanning (*top*) or somatostatin receptor scintigraphy (SRS) (*bottom*) to localize metastatic carcinoid in the liver.

(lymphomas, wound infections). If liver metastases are identified by SRS, to plan the proper treatment, either a CT or an MRI (with contrast enhancement) is recommended to assess the size and exact location of the metastases because SRS does not provide information on tumor size. For pNETs in the pancreas, EUS is highly sensitive, localizing 77–100% of insulinomas, which occur almost exclusively within the pancreas. Endoscopic ultrasound is less sensitive for extrapancreatic tumors. It is increasingly used in patients with MEN 1, and to a lesser extent VHL, to detect small pNETs not seen with other modalities or for serial pNET assessments to determine size changes or rapid growth in patients in whom surgery is deferred. EUS with cytologic evaluation also is used frequently to distinguish an NF-pNET from a pancreatic adenocarcinoma or another nonendocrine pancreatic tumor. Not infrequently patients present with liver metastases due to an NET and the primary site is unclear. Occult small intestinal NETs (carcinoids) are increasingly detected by double-balloon enteroscopy or capsule endoscopy.

Insulinomas frequently overexpress receptors for glucagon-like peptide-1 (GLP-1), and radiolabeled GLP-1 analogues have been developed that can detect occult insulinomas not localized by other imaging modalities. Functional localization by measuring hormonal gradients is now uncommonly used with gastrinomas (after intra-arterial secretin injections) but is still frequently used in insulinoma patients in whom other imaging studies are negative (assessing hepatic vein insulin concentrations post-intra-arterial calcium injections). Functional localization measuring hormone gradients in insulinomas or gastrin gradients in gastrinoma is a sensitive method, being positive in 80–100% of patients. The intra-arterial calcium test may also allow differentiation of the cause of the hypoglycemia and indicate whether it is due to an insulinoma or a nesidioblastosis. The latter entity is becoming increasingly important because hypoglycemia after gastric bypass surgery for obesity is increasing in frequency, and it is primarily due to nesidioblastosis, although it can occasionally be due to an insulinoma.

PET and use of hybrid scanners such as CT and SRS may have increased sensitivity. PET scanning with ^{18}F-fluoro-DOPA in patients with carcinoids or with ^{11}C-5-HTP in patients with pNETs or GI-NETs (carcinoids) has greater sensitivity than cross-sectional imaging studies and may be used increasingly in the future. PET scanning for GI-NETs is not currently approved in the United States.

TREATMENT Advanced Disease (Diffuse Metastatic Disease)

The single most important prognostic factor for survival is the presence of liver metastases (Fig. 28-4). For patients with foregut carcinoids without hepatic metastases, the 5-year survival in one study was 95%, and with distant metastases, it was 20% (Fig. 28-4). With gastrinomas, the 5-year survival without liver metastases is 98%; with limited metastases in one hepatic lobe, it is 78%; and with diffuse metastases, 16% (Fig. 28-4). In a large study of 156 patients (67 pNETs, rest carcinoids), the overall 5-year survival rate was 77%; it was 96% without liver metastases, 73% with liver metastases, and 50% with distant disease. Another very important prognostic factor is whether the NET is well-differentiated (G1/G2) or poorly differentiated (<1% of all NETs) (G3). Well-differentiated NETs have a 5-year survival of 50–80%, whereas poorly differentiated NETs have a 5-year survival of only 0–15%.

Therefore, treatment for advanced metastatic disease is an important challenge. A number of different modalities are reported to be effective, including cytoreductive surgery (surgically or by radiofrequency ablation [RFA]), treatment with chemotherapy, somatostatin analogues, interferon α, hepatic embolization alone or with chemotherapy (chemoembolization), molecular targeted therapy, radiotherapy with radiolabeled beads/microspheres, peptide radioreceptor therapy (PRRT), and liver transplantation.

SPECIFIC ANTITUMOR TREATMENTS Cytoreductive surgery is considered if either all of the visible metastatic disease or at last 90% is thought resectable; however, unfortunately, this is possible in only the 9–22% of patients who present with limited hepatic metastases. Although no randomized studies have proven that it extends life, results from a number of studies suggest that it may increase survival; therefore, it is recommended, if possible. RFA can be applied to NET liver metastases if they are limited in number (usually less than five) and size (usually <3.5 cm in diameter). It can be used at the time of surgery (either general or laparoscopic) or using radiologic guidance.

Response rates are >80%, the responses can last up to 3 years, the morbidity rate is low, and this procedure may be particularly helpful in patients with functional pNETs that are difficult to control medically. Although RFA has not been established in a controlled trial, both the European and North American Neuroendocrine Tumor Society guidelines (ENETS, NANETS) state it can be an effective antitumor treatment for both refractory functional syndromes and for palliative treatment.

Chemotherapy plays a different role in the treatment of patients with pNETs and GI-NETs (carcinoids). Chemotherapy continues to be widely used in the treatment of patients with advanced pNETs with moderate success (response rates 20–70%); however, in general, its results in patients with metastatic GI-NETs (carcinoids) has been disappointing, with response rates of 0–30% with various two- and three-drug combinations, and thus, it is infrequently used in these patients. An important distinction in patients with pNETs is whether the tumor is well differentiated (G1/G2) or poorly differentiated (G3). The chemotherapeutic approach is different for these two groups. The current regimen of choice for patients with well-differentiated pNETs is the combination of streptozotocin and doxorubicin with or without 5-fluorouracil. Streptozotocin is a glucosamine nitrourea compound originally found to have cytotoxic effects on pancreatic islets, and later in studies with doxorubicin with or without 5-fluorouracil, it produced response rates of 20–45% in advanced pNETs. Streptozotocin causes considerable morbidity, with 70–100% of patients developing side effects (most prominent being nausea/vomiting in 60–100% or leukopenia/thrombocytopenia) and 15–40% of patients developing some degree of renal dysfunction (proteinuria in 40–50%, decreased creatine clearance). The combination of temozolomide (TMZ) with capecitabine produces partial response rates as high as 70% in patients with advance pNETs and a 2-year survival of 92%. The use of TMZ or another alkylating agent in advanced pNETs is supported by studies that show low levels of the DNA repair enzyme O^6-methylguanine DNA methyltransferase in pNETs, but not in GI-NETs (carcinoids), which

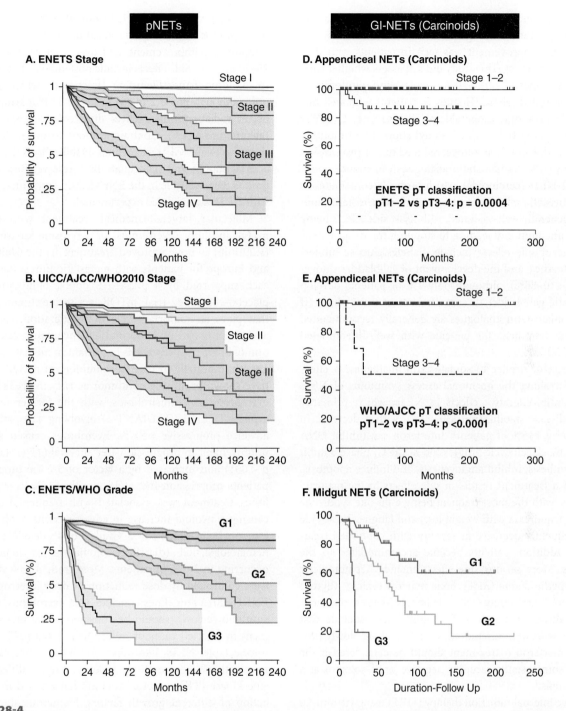

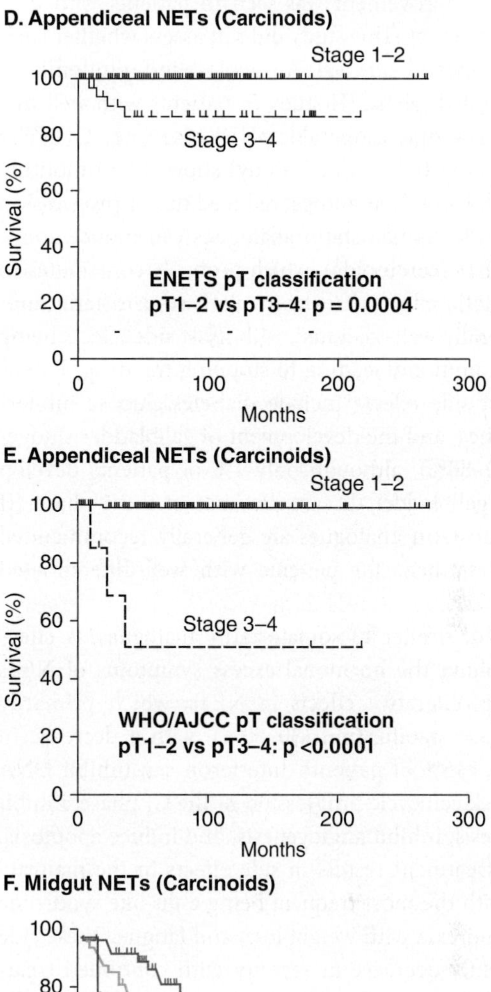

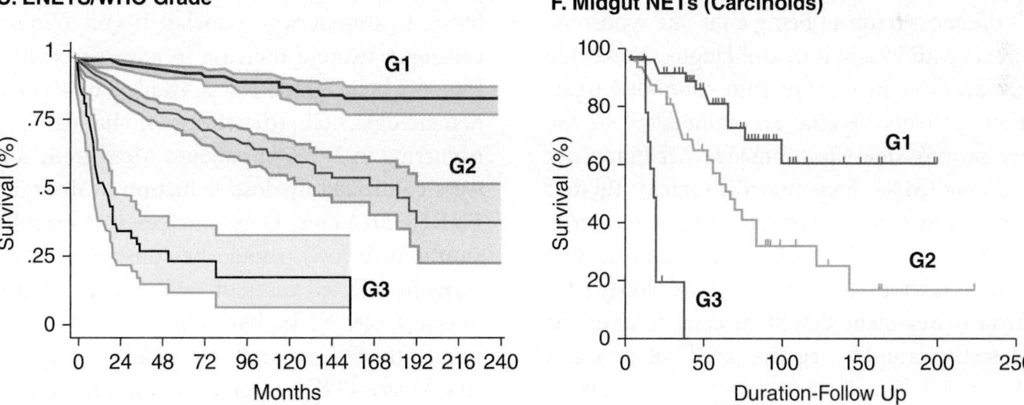

FIGURE 28-4

Survival (Kaplan-Meier plots) of patients with pancreatic neuroendocrine tumors (pNETs; n = 1072) (*A–C*) or gastrointestinal neuroendocrine tumors (GI-NETs; carcinoids) (appendix, n = 138; midgut, n = 238) (*D–F*) stratified according to recent proposed classification and grading systems. *(Panels A–C are drawn from data in G Rindi et al: J Natl Cancer Inst 104:764, 2012; panels D and E are drawn from data in M Volante et al: Am J Surg Pathol 37:606, 2013; and panel F is drawn from data in MS Khan: Br J Cancer 108:1838, 2013.)*

increases the sensitivity of pNETs to TMZ. In poorly differentiated NETs (G3), chemotherapy with a cisplatin-based regimen with etoposide or other agents (vincristine, paclitaxel) is the recommended treatment, with response rates of 40–70%; however, responses are generally short-lived (<12 months). This chemotherapy regimen can be associated with significant toxicity including GI toxicities (nausea, vomiting), myelosuppression, and renal toxicity.

In addition to the effectiveness in controlling the functional hormonal state, long-acting somatostatin analogues such as octreotide and lanreotide are increasingly used for their antiproliferative effects. Whereas somatostatin analogues rarely decrease tumor size (i.e., 0–17%), these drugs have tumoristatic effects, stopping additional growth in 26–95% of patients with NETs. In a randomized, double-blind study in patients with metastatic midgut carcinoids

(PROMID study) octreotide-LAR demonstrated a marked lengthening of time to progression (14.3 vs 6 months, $p = .000072$). This improvement was seen in patients with limited liver involvement. This study did not assess whether such treatment will extend survival. A double-blind, randomized, placebo-controlled, phase III study in patients with well-differentiated, metastatic, inoperable pNETs (45%) or GI-NETs (carcinoids) (55%) (CLARINET study) showed that monthly treatment with lanreotide-autogel reduced tumor progression or death by 53%. Somatostatin analogues can induce apoptosis in GI-NETs (carcinoids), which probably contributes to their tumoristatic effects. Treatment with somatostatin analogues is generally well-tolerated, with most side effects being mild and uncommonly leading to stopping the drug. Potential long-term side effects include diabetes/glucose intolerance, steatorrhea, and the development of gallbladder sludge/gallstones (10–80%), although only 1% of patients develop symptomatic gallbladder disease. Because of these phase III studies, somatostatin analogues are generally recommended as first-line treatment for patients with well-differentiated metastatic NETs.

Interferon α, similar to somatostatin analogues, is effective at controlling the hormonal excess symptoms of NETs and has antiproliferative effects in NETs, which primarily result in disease stabilization (30–80%), with a decrease in tumor size in <15% of patients. Interferon can inhibit DNA synthesis, block cell cycle progression in the G_1 phase, inhibit protein synthesis, inhibit angiogenesis, and induce apoptosis. Interferon α treatment results in side effects in the majority of patients, with the most frequent being a flu-like syndrome (80–100%), anorexia with weight loss, and fatigue. These side effects frequently decrease in severity with continued treatment. In addition, patients become accommodated to the symptoms. More serious side effects include hepatotoxicity (31%), hyperlipidemia (31%), bone marrow toxicity, thyroid disease (19%), and rarely CNS side effects (depression, mental/visual disorders). ENETS 2012 guidelines conclude that in patients with well-differentiated NETs that are slowly progressive, interferon α treatment should be considered if the tumor is somatostatin receptor negative or if somatostatin treatment fails.

Selective internal radiation therapy (SIRT) using yttrium-90 (^{90}Y) glass or resin microspheres is a relatively newer approach being evaluated in patients with unresectable NET liver metastases, with approximately 500 NET patients treated. The treatment requires careful evaluation for vascular shunting before treatment and a pretreatment angiogram to evaluate placement of the catheter and is generally is reserved for patients without extrahepatic metastatic disease and with adequate hepatic reserve. One of two types of ^{90}Y microspheres are used: either microspheres with a 20- to 60-μm diameter and 50 Bq/sphere (SIR-Spheres) or glass microspheres (TheraSpheres) with a 20- to 30-μm diameter and 2500 Bq/sphere. The ^{90}Y-microspheres are delivered to the liver by intra-arterial injection from percutaneously placed catheters. In four studies involving metastatic NETs, the response rate varied from 50–61% (partial or complete), tumor stabilization occurred in 22–41%, 60–100% had symptomatic improvement, and overall survival varied from 25–70 months. Side effects include postembolization syndrome (pain, fever, nausea/vomiting [frequent]), which is usually mild, although grade 2 (43%) or grade 3 (1%) symptoms can occur; radiation-induced liver disease (<1%); and radiation pneumonitis (<1%). Contraindications to use include excess shunting to the GI tract or lung, inability to isolate the liver arterial supply, and inadequate liver reserve. Because of the limited data available in the ENETS 2012 guidelines, treatment with SIRTs is considered experimental.

Molecular targeted medical treatment with either an mTOR inhibitor (everolimus) or a tyrosine kinase inhibitor (sunitinib) is now approved treatment in the United States and Europe for patients with metastatic unresectable pNET, each supported by a phase III, double-blind, prospective, placebo-controlled trial. mTOR is a serine-threonine kinase that plays an important role in proliferation, cell growth, and apoptosis in both normal and neoplastic cells. Activation of the mTOR cascade is important in mediating NET cell growth, especially in pNETs. A number of mTOR inhibitors have shown promising antitumor activity in NETs including everolimus and temsirolimus, with the former undergoing a phase III trial (RADIANT-3) involving 410 patients with advance progressive pNETs. Everolimus caused significant improvement in progression-free survival (11 vs 4.6 months, $p < .001$) and increased by a factor of 3.7 the proportion of patients progression-free at 18 months (37% vs 9%). Everolimus treatment was associated with frequent side effects, causing a twofold increase in adverse events, with the most frequent being grade 1 or 2. Grade 3 or 4 side effects included hematologic, GI (diarrhea), stomatitis, or hypoglycemia occurring in 3–7% of patients. Most grade 3 or 4 side effects were controlled by dose reduction or drug interruption. The ENETS 2012 guidelines conclude that everolimus, similar to sunitinib (below), should be considered as a first-line treatment in selected cases of well-differentiated pNETs that are unresectable. NETs, like other normal and neoplastic cells, frequently possess multiple types of the 20 different tyrosine kinase (TK) receptors that are known and mediate the action of different growth factors. Numerous studies demonstrate that TK receptors in normal and neoplastic tissues as well as NETs are especially important in mediating cell growth, angiogenesis, differentiation, and apoptosis. Whereas a number of TK inhibitors show antiproliferative activity in NETs only sunitinib has undergone a phase III controlled trial. Sunitinib is an orally active small-molecule inhibitor of TK receptors (PDGFRs, VEGFR-1, VEGFR-2, c-KIT, FLT-3). In a phase III study in which 171 patients with progressive, metastatic, nonresectable pNETs were treated with sunitinib (37.5 mg/d) or placebo, sunitinib treatment caused a doubling of progression-free survival (11.4 vs 4.5 months, $p < .001$), an increase in objective tumor response rate (9% vs 0%, $p = .007$), and an increase in overall survival. Sunitinib treatment was associated with an overall threefold increase in side effects, although most were grade 1 or 2. The most frequent grade 3 or 4 side effects were neutropenia (12%) and hypertension (9.6%), which were controlled by dose reduction or temporary interruption. There is no consensus regarding the order of sunitinib or everolimus use in patients with advanced, well-differentiated, progressive pNETs.

PRRT for NETs involves treatment with radiolabeled somatostatin analogues. The success of this approach is based on the finding that somatostatin receptors (sst) are overexpressed or ectopically expressed by 60–100% of all NETs, which allows the targeting of cytotoxic, radiolabeled somatostatin receptor ligands.

Three different radionuclides are being used. High doses of [^{111}In-DTPA-d-Phe^{1}]octreotide, which emits γ-rays, internal conversion, and Auger electrons; ^{90}yttrium, which emits high-energy β-particles coupled by a DOTA chelating group to octreotide or octreotate; and ^{177}lutetium-coupled analogues, which emit both, are all in clinical studies. At present, the ^{177}lutetium-coupled analogues are the most widely used. ^{111}Indium-, ^{90}yttrium-, and ^{177}lutetium-labeled compounds caused tumor stabilization in 41–81%, 44–88%, and 23–40%, respectively, and a decrease in tumor size in 8–30%, 6–37%, and 38%, respectively, of patients with advanced metastatic NETs. In one large study involving 504 patients with malignant NETs, ^{177}lutetium-labeled analogues produced a reduction of tumor size of >50% in 30% of patients (2% complete) and tumor stabilization in 51% of patients. An effect on survival has not been established. At present, PRRT is not approved for use in either the United States or Europe, but because of the above promising results, a large phase III study is now being conducted in both the United States and Europe. The ENETS 2012, NANETS 2010, Nordic 2010, and European Society for Medical Oncology (ESMO) guidelines list PRRT as an experimental or investigational treatment at present.

The use of liver transplantation has been abandoned for treatment of most metastatic tumors to the liver. However, for metastatic NETs, it is still a consideration. Among 213 European patients with NETs (50% functional NETs) who had liver transplantation from 1982 to 2009, the overall 5-year survival was 52% and disease free-survival was 30%. In various studies, the postoperative mortality rate is 10–14%. These results are similar to the United Network for Organ Sharing data in the United States in which 150 NET patients had liver transplants and the 5-year survival was 49%. In various studies, important prognostic factors for a poor outcome include a major resection performed in addition at the time of the liver transplant; poor tumor differentiation; hepatomegaly; age >45 years; a primary NET in the duodenum or pancreas; the presence of extrahepatic metastatic disease or extensive liver involvement (>50%); Ki-67 proliferative index >10%; and abnormal E-cadherin staining. The ENETS 2012 guidelines conclude that liver transplantation should be viewed as providing palliative care, with cure an exception, and recommend it be reserved for patients with life-threatening hormonal disturbances refractory to other treatments or for selected patients with a nonfunctional tumor with diffuse liver metastatic disease refractory to all other treatments.

CHAPTER 29

MULTIPLE ENDOCRINE NEOPLASIA

Rajesh V. Thakker

Multiple endocrine neoplasia (MEN) is characterized by a predilection for tumors involving two or more endocrine glands. Four major forms of MEN are recognized and referred to as MEN types 1–4 (MEN 1–4) (Table 29-1). Each type of MEN is inherited as an autosomal dominant syndrome or may occur sporadically; that is, without a family history. However, this distinction between familial and sporadic forms is often difficult because family members with the disease may have died before symptoms developed. In addition to MEN 1–4, at least six other syndromes are associated with multiple endocrine and other organ neoplasias (MEONs) (Table 29-2). These MEONs include the hyperparathyroidism-jaw tumor syndrome, Carney complex, von Hippel-Lindau disease **(Chap. 9)**, neurofibromatosis type 1, Cowden's syndrome, and McCune-Albright syndrome **(Chap. 36)**; all of these are inherited as autosomal dominant disorders, except for McCune-Albright syndrome, which is caused by mosaic expression of a postzygotic somatic cell mutation (Table 29-2).

A diagnosis of a MEN or MEON syndrome may be established in an individual by one of three criteria: (1) clinical features (two or more of the associated tumors [or lesions] in an individual); (2) familial pattern (one of the associated tumors [or lesions] in a first-degree relative of a patient with a clinical diagnosis of the syndrome); and (3) genetic analysis (a germline mutation in the associated gene in an individual, who may be clinically affected or asymptomatic). Mutational analysis in MEN and MEON syndromes is helpful in clinical practice to: (1) confirm the clinical diagnosis; (2) identify family members who harbor the mutation and require screening for relevant tumor detection and early/appropriate treatment; and (3) identify the ~50% of family members who do not harbor the germline mutation and can, therefore, be alleviated of the anxiety of developing associated tumors. This latter aspect also helps to reduce health care costs by reducing the need for unnecessary biochemical and radiologic investigations.

MULTIPLE ENDOCRINE NEOPLASIA TYPE 1

Clinical manifestations

MEN type 1 (MEN 1), which is also referred to as Wermer's syndrome, is characterized by the triad of tumors involving the parathyroids, pancreatic islets, and anterior pituitary. In addition, adrenal cortical tumors, carcinoid tumors usually of the foregut, meningiomas, facial angiofibromas, collagenomas, and lipomas may also occur in some patients with MEN 1. Combinations of the affected glands and their pathologic features (e.g., hyperplastic adenomas of the parathyroid glands) may differ in members of the same family and even between identical twins. In addition, a nonfamilial (e.g., sporadic) form occurs in 8–14% of patients with MEN 1, and molecular genetic studies have confirmed the occurrence of de novo mutations of the *MEN1* gene in approximately 10% of patients with MEN 1. The prevalence of MEN 1 is approximately 0.25% based on randomly chosen postmortem studies but is 1–18% among patients with primary hyperparathyroidism, 16–38% among patients with pancreatic islet tumors, and <3% among patients with pituitary tumors. The disorder affects all age groups, with a reported age range of 5 to 81 years, with clinical and biochemical manifestations developing in the vast majority by the fifth decade. The clinical manifestations of MEN 1 are related to the sites of tumors and their hormonal products. In the absence of treatment, endocrine tumors are associated with an earlier mortality in patients with MEN 1, with a 50% probability of death by the age of 50 years. The cause of death is usually a malignant tumor, often from a pancreatic neuroendocrine tumor (NET) or foregut carcinoid. In addition, the treatment outcomes of patients with MEN 1–associated tumors are not as successful

TABLE 29-1
MULTIPLE ENDOCRINE NEOPLASIA (MEN) SYNDROMES

TYPE (CHROMOSOMAL LOCATION)	TUMORS (ESTIMATED PENETRANCE)	GENE AND MOST FREQUENTLY MUTATED CODONS
MEN 1 (11q13)	Parathyroid adenoma (90%) Enteropancreatic tumor (30–70%) • Gastrinoma (>50%) • Insulinoma (10–30%) • Nonfunctioning and PPoma (20–55%) • Glucagonoma (<3%) • VIPoma (<1%) Pituitary adenoma (15–50%) • Prolactinoma (60%) • Somatotrophinoma (25%) • Corticotropinoma (<5%) • Nonfunctioning (<5%) Associated tumors • Adrenal cortical tumor (20–70%) • Pheochromocytoma (<1%) • Bronchopulmonary NET (2%) • Thymic NET (2%) • Gastric NET (10%) • Lipomas (>33%) • Angiofibromas (85%) • Collagenomas (70%) • Meningiomas (8%)	*MEN1* 83/84, 4-bp del (≈4%) 119, 3-bp del (≈3%) 209-211, 4-bp del (≈8%) 418, 3-bp del (≈4%) 514-516, del or ins (≈7%) Intron 4 ss (≈10%)
MEN 2 (10 cen-10q11.2)		
MEN 2A	MTC (90%)	*RET*
	Pheochromocytoma (>50%)	634, e.g., Cys → Arg (~85%)
	Parathyroid adenoma (10–25%)	
MTC only	MTC (100%)	*RET* 618, missense (>50%)
MEN 2B (also known as MEN 3)	MTC (>90%)	*RET* 918, Met → Thr (>95%)
	Pheochromocytoma (>50%)	
	Associated abnormalities (40–50%) • Mucosal neuromas • Marfanoid habitus • Medullated corneal nerve fibers • Megacolon	
MEN 4 (12p13)	Parathyroid adenoma[a] Pituitary adenoma[a] Reproductive organ tumors[a] (e.g., testicular cancer, neuroendocrine cervical carcinoma) ?Adrenal + renal tumors[a]	*CDKN1B*; no common mutations identified to date

[a]Insufficient numbers reported to provide prevalence information.
Note: Autosomal dominant inheritance of the MEN syndromes has been established.
Abbreviations: del, deletion; ins, insertion; MTC, medullary thyroid cancer; NET, neuroendocrine tumor; PPoma, pancreatic polypeptide–secreting tumor; VIPoma, vasoactive intestinal polypeptide–secreting tumor.
Source: Reproduced from RV Thakker et al: J Clin Endocrinol Metab 97:2990, 2012.

as those in patients with non–MEN 1 tumors. This is because MEN 1–associated tumors, with the exception of pituitary NETs, are usually multiple, making it difficult to achieve a successful surgical cure. Occult metastatic disease is also more prevalent in MEN 1, and the tumors may be larger, more aggressive, and resistant to treatment.

Parathyroid tumors

(See also Chap. 34) Primary hyperparathyroidism occurs in approximately 90% of patients and is the most common feature of MEN 1. Patients may have asymptomatic hypercalcemia or vague symptoms associated with hypercalcemia (e.g., polyuria, polydipsia,

TABLE 29-2

MULTIPLE ENDOCRINE AND OTHER ORGAN NEOPLASIA SYNDROMES (MEONs)

DISEASE[a]	GENE PRODUCT	CHROMOSOMAL LOCATION
Hyperparathyroid-ism-jaw tumor (HPT-JT)	Parafibromin	1q31.2
Carney complex		
CNC1	PPKAR1A	17q24.2
CNC2	?[b]	2p16
von Hippel-Lindau disease (VHL)	pVHL (elongin)	3p25
Neurofibromatosis type 1 (NF1)	Neurofibromin	17q11.2
Cowden's syndrome (CWD)		
CWD1	PTEN	10q23.31
CWD2	SDHB	1p36.13
CWD3	SDHD	11q23.1
CWD4	KLLN	10q23.31
CWD5	PIK3CA	3q26.32
CWD6	AKT1	14q32.33
McCune-Albright syndrome (MAS)	Gsα	20q13.32

[a]The inheritance for these disorders is autosomal dominant, except MAS, which is due to mosaicism that results from the postzygotic somatic cell mutation of the *GNAS1* gene, encoding Gsα.
[b]?, unknown.

constipation, malaise, or dyspepsia). Nephrolithiasis and osteitis fibrosa cystica (less commonly) may also occur. Biochemical investigations reveal hypercalcemia, usually in association with elevated circulating parathyroid hormone (PTH) (Table 29-3). The hypercalcemia is usually mild, and severe hypercalcemia or parathyroid cancer is a rare occurrence. Additional differences in the primary hyperparathyroidism of patients with MEN 1, as opposed to those without MEN 1, include an earlier age at onset (20–25 years vs 55 years) and an equal male-to-female ratio (1:1 vs 1:3). Preoperative imaging (e.g., neck ultrasound with ^{99m}Tc-sestamibi parathyroid scintigraphy) is of limited benefit because all parathyroid glands may be affected, and neck exploration may be required irrespective of preoperative localization studies.

TREATMENT Parathyroid Tumors

Surgical removal of the abnormally overactive parathyroids in patients with MEN 1 is the definitive treatment. However, it is controversial whether to perform subtotal (e.g., removal of 3.5 glands) or total parathyroidectomy with or without autotransplantation of parathyroid tissue in the forearm, and whether surgery should be performed at an early or late stage. Minimally invasive parathyroidectomy is not recommended because all four parathyroid glands are usually affected with multiple adenomas or hyperplasia. Surgical experience should be taken into account given the variability in pathology in MEN 1. Calcimimetics (e.g., cinacalcet), which act via the calcium-sensing receptor, have been used to treat primary hyperparathyroidism in some patients when surgery is unsuccessful or contraindicated.

TABLE 29-3

BIOCHEMICAL AND RADIOLOGICAL SCREENING IN MULTIPLE ENDOCRINE NEOPLASIA TYPE 1

TUMOR	AGE TO BEGIN (YEARS)	BIOCHEMICAL TEST (PLASMA OR SERUM) ANNUALLY	IMAGING TEST (TIME INTERVAL)
Parathyroid	8	Calcium, PTH	None
Pancreatic NETs			
Gastrinoma	20	Gastrin (± gastric pH)	None
Insulinoma	5	Fasting glucose, insulin	None
Other pancreatic NET	<10	Chromogranin A; pancreatic polypeptide, glucagon, vasoactive intestinal peptide	MRI, CT, or EUS (annually)
Anterior pituitary	5	Prolactin, IGF-I	MRI (every 3 years)
Adrenal	<10	None unless symptoms or signs of functioning tumor and/or tumor >1 cm identified on imaging	MRI or CT (annually with pancreatic imaging)
Thymic and bronchial carcinoid	15	None	CT or MRI (every 1–2 years)

Abbreviations: CT, computed tomography; EUS, endoscopic ultrasound; IGF-I, insulin-like growth factor I; MRI, magnetic resonance imaging; PTH, parathyroid hormone.
Source: Reproduced from RV Thakker et al: J Clin Endocrinol Metab 97:2990, 2012.

Pancreatic tumors

(See also Chap. 28) The incidence of pancreatic islet cell tumors, which are NETs, in patients with MEN 1 ranges from 30 to 80% in different series. Most of these tumors (Table 29-1) produce excessive amounts of hormone (e.g., gastrin, insulin, glucagon, vasoactive intestinal polypeptide [VIP]) and are associated with distinct clinical syndromes, although some are nonfunctioning or nonsecretory. These pancreatic islet cell tumors have an earlier age at onset in patients with MEN 1 than in patients without MEN 1.

Gastrinoma

Gastrin-secreting tumors (gastrinomas) are associated with marked gastric acid production and recurrent peptic ulcerations, a combination referred to as the Zollinger-Ellison syndrome. Gastrinomas occur more often in patients with MEN 1 who are older than age 30 years. Recurrent severe multiple peptic ulcers, which may perforate, and cachexia are major contributors to the high mortality. Patients with Zollinger-Ellison syndrome may also suffer from diarrhea and steatorrhea. The diagnosis is established by demonstration of an elevated fasting serum gastrin concentration in association with increased basal gastric acid secretion (Table 29-3). However, the diagnosis of Zollinger-Ellison syndrome may be difficult in hypercalcemic MEN 1 patients, because hypercalcemia can also cause hypergastrinemia. Ultrasonography, endoscopic ultrasonography, computed tomography (CT), nuclear magnetic resonance imaging (MRI), selective abdominal angiography, venous sampling, and somatostatin receptor scintigraphy are helpful in localizing the tumor prior to surgery. Gastrinomas represent more than 50% of all pancreatic NETs in patients with MEN 1, and approximately 20% of patients with gastrinomas will be found to have MEN 1. Gastrinomas, which may also occur in the duodenal mucosa, are the major cause of morbidity and mortality in patients with MEN 1. Most MEN 1 gastrinomas are malignant and metastasize before a diagnosis is established.

TREATMENT Gastrinoma

Medical treatment of patients with MEN 1 and Zollinger-Ellison syndrome is directed toward reducing basal acid output to <10 mmol/L. Parietal cell H^+-K^+-adenosine triphosphatase (ATPase) inhibitors (e.g., omeprazole or lansoprazole) reduce acid output and are the drugs of choice for gastrinomas. Some patients may also require additional treatment with the histamine H_2 receptor antagonists, cimetidine or ranitidine. The role of surgery in the treatment of gastrinomas in patients with MEN 1 is controversial. The goal of surgery is to reduce the risk of distant metastatic disease and improve survival. For a nonmetastatic gastrinoma situated in the pancreas, surgical excision is often effective. However, the risk of hepatic metastases increases with tumor size, such that 25–40% of patients with pancreatic NETs >4 cm develop hepatic metastases, and 50–70% of patients with tumors 2–3 cm in size have lymph node metastases. Survival in MEN 1 patients with gastrinomas <2.5 cm in size is 100% at 15 years, but 52% at 15 years, if metastatic disease is present. The presence of lymph node metastases does not appear to adversely affect survival. Surgery for gastrinomas that are >2–2.5 cm has been recommended, because the disease-related survival in these patients is improved following surgery. In addition, duodenal gastrinomas, which occur more frequently in patients with MEN 1, have been treated successfully with surgery. However, in most patients with MEN 1, gastrinomas are multiple or extrapancreatic, and with the exception of duodenal gastrinomas, surgery is rarely successful. For example, the results of one study revealed that only ~15% of patients with MEN 1 were free of disease immediately after surgery, and at 5 years, this number had decreased to ~5%; the respective outcomes in patients without MEN 1 were better, at 45% and 40%. Given these findings, most specialists recommend a nonsurgical management for gastrinomas in MEN 1, except as noted earlier for smaller, isolated lesions. Treatment of disseminated gastrinomas is difficult. Chemotherapy with streptozotocin and 5-fluorouracil; hormonal therapy with octreotide or lanreotide, which are human somatostatin analogues; hepatic artery embolization; administration of human leukocyte interferon; and removal of all resectable tumor have been successful in some patients.

Insulinoma

These β islet cell insulin-secreting tumors represent 10–30% of all pancreatic tumors in patients with MEN 1. Patients with an insulinoma present with hypoglycemic symptoms (e.g., weakness, headaches, sweating, faintness, seizures, altered behavior, weight gain) that typically develop after fasting or exertion and improve after glucose intake. The most reliable test is a supervised 72-h fast. Biochemical investigations reveal increased plasma insulin concentrations in association with hypoglycemia (Table 29-3). Circulating concentrations of C peptide and proinsulin, which are also increased, are useful in establishing the diagnosis. It also is important to demonstrate the absence of sulfonylureas in plasma and urine samples obtained during the investigation of hypoglycemia (Table 29-3). Surgical success is greatly enhanced by preoperative localization by endoscopic ultrasonography, CT scanning, or celiac axis angiography. Additional localization methods may include preoperative and perioperative percutaneous transhepatic portal venous sampling, selective intraarterial stimulation with hepatic venous sampling, and intraoperative direct pancreatic ultrasonography.

Insulinomas occur in association with gastrinomas in 10% of patients with MEN 1, and the two tumors may arise at different times. Insulinomas occur more often in patients with MEN 1 who are younger than 40 years, and some arise in individuals younger than 20 years. In contrast, in patients without MEN 1, insulinomas generally occur in those older than 40 years. Insulinomas may be the first manifestation of MEN 1 in 10% of patients, and approximately 4% of patients with insulinomas will have MEN 1.

TREATMENT Insulinoma

Medical treatment, which consists of frequent carbohydrate meals and diazoxide or octreotide, is not always successful, and surgery is the optimal treatment. Surgical treatment, which ranges from enucleation of a single tumor to a distal pancreatectomy or partial pancreatectomy, has been curative in many patients. Chemotherapy may include streptozotocin, 5-fluorouracil, and doxorubicin. Hepatic artery embolization has been used for metastatic disease.

Glucagonoma

These glucagon-secreting pancreatic NETs occur in <3% of patients with MEN 1. The characteristic clinical manifestations of a skin rash (necrolytic migratory erythema), weight loss, anemia, and stomatitis may be absent. The tumor may have been detected in an asymptomatic patient with MEN 1 undergoing pancreatic imaging or by the finding of glucose intolerence and hyperglucagonemia.

TREATMENT Glucagonoma

Surgical removal of the glucagonoma is the treatment of choice. However, treatment may be difficult because approximately 50–80% of patients have metastases at the time of diagnosis. Medical treatment with somatostatin analogues (e.g., octreotide or lanreotide) or chemotherapy with streptozotocin and 5-fluorouracil has been successful in some patients, and hepatic artery embolization has been used to treat metastatic disease.

Vasoactive intestinal peptide (VIP) tumors (VIPomas)

VIPomas have been reported in only a few patients with MEN 1. This clinical syndrome is characterized by watery diarrhea, hypokalemia, and achlorhydria and is also referred to as the Verner-Morrison syndrome, the WDHA (watery diarrhea, hypokalemia, and achlorhydria) syndrome, or the VIPoma syndrome. The diagnosis is established by excluding laxative and diuretic abuse, by confirming a stool volume in excess of 0.5–1.0 L/d during a fast, and by documenting a markedly increased plasma VIP concentration.

TREATMENT VIPomas

Surgical management of VIPomas, which are mostly located in the tail of the pancreas, can be curative. However, in patients with unresectable tumor, somatostatin analogues, such as octreotide and lanreotide, may be effective. Streptozotocin with 5-fluorouracil may be beneficial, along with hepatic artery embolization for the treatment of metastases.

Pancreatic polypeptide-secreting tumors (PPomas) and nonfunctioning pancreatic NETs

PPomas are found in a large number of patients with MEN 1. No pathologic sequelae of excessive polypeptide (PP) secretion are apparent, and the clinical significance of PP is unknown. Many PPomas may have been unrecognized or classified as nonfunctioning pancreatic NETs, which likely represent the most common enteropancreatic NET associated with MEN 1 (Fig. 29-1). The absence of both a clinical syndrome and specific biochemical abnormalities may result in a delayed diagnosis of nonfunctioning pancreatic NETs, which are associated with a worse prognosis than other functioning tumors, including insulinoma and gastrinoma. The optimum screening method and its timing interval for nonfunctioning pancreatic NETs remain to be established. At present, endoscopic ultrasound likely represents the most sensitive method of detecting small pancreatic tumors, but somatostatin receptor scintography is the most reliable method for detecting metastatic disease (Table 29-3).

TREATMENT PPomas and Nonfunctioning Pancreatic NETs

The management of nonfunctioning pancreatic NETs in the asymptomatic patient is controversial. One recommendation is to undertake surgery irrespective of tumor size after biochemical assessment is complete. Alternatively, other experts recommend surgery based on tumor size, using either >1 cm or >3 cm at different centers. Pancreatoduodenal surgery is successful in removing the tumors in 80% of patients, but more than 40% of patients develop complications, including diabetes mellitus, frequent steatorrhea, early and late dumping syndromes, and other gastrointestinal symptoms. However, ~50–60% of patients treated surgically survive >5 years. When considering these recommendations, it is important to consider that occult metastatic disease (e.g., tumors not detected by imaging investigations) is likely to be present in a substantial proportion of these patients at the time of presentation. Inhibitors of tyrosine kinase receptors (TKRs) and of the mammalian target of rapamycin (mTOR) signaling pathway have been reported to be effective in treating pancreatic NETs and in doubling the progression-free survival time.

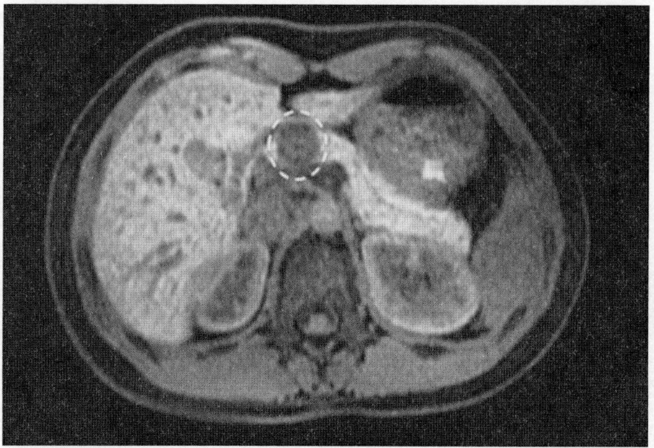

A

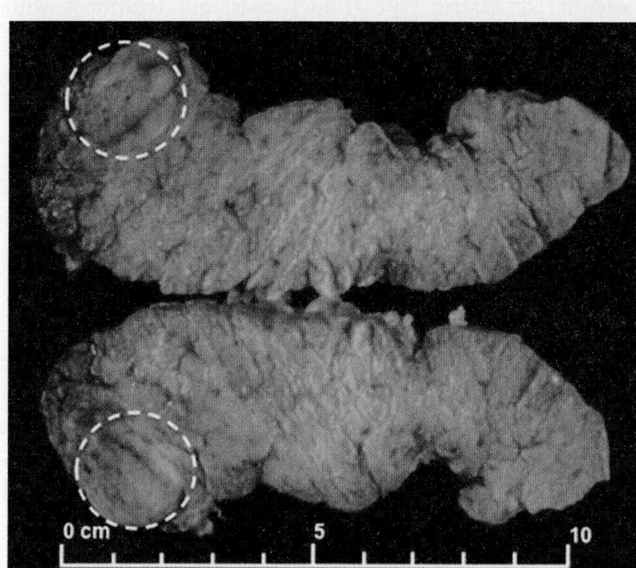

B

FIGURE 29-1

Pancreatic nonfunctioning neuroendocrine tumor (NET) in a 14-year-old patient with multiple endocrine neoplasia type 1 (MEN 1). ***A.*** An abdominal magnetic resonance imaging scan revealed a low-intensity >2.0 cm (anteroposterior maximal diameter) tumor within the neck of pancreas. There was no evidence of invasion of adjacent structures or metastases. The tumor is indicated by *white dashed circle*. ***B.*** The pancreatic NET was removed by surgery, and macroscopic examination confirmed the location of the tumor (*white dashed circles*) in the neck of the pancreas. Immunohistochemistry showed the tumor to immunostain for chromogranin A, but not gastrointestinal peptides or menin, thereby confirming that it was a nonsecreting NET due to loss of menin expression. *(Part A adapted with permission from PJ Newey et al: J Clin Endocrinol Metab 10:3640, 2009.)*

Other pancreatic NETs

NETs secreting growth hormone–releasing hormone (GHRH), GHRHomas, have been reported rarely in patients with MEN 1. It is estimated that ~33% of patients with GHRHomas have other MEN 1–related tumors. GHRHomas may be diagnosed by demonstrating elevated serum concentrations of growth hormone and GHRH. More than 50% of GHRHomas occur in the lung, 30% occur in the pancreas, and 10% are found in the small intestine. Somatostatinomas secrete somatostatin, a peptide that inhibits the secretion of a variety of hormones, resulting in hyperglycemia, cholelithiasis, low acid output, steatorrhea, diarrhea, abdominal pain, anemia, and weight loss. Although 7% of pancreatic NETs secrete somatostatin, the clinical features of somatostatinoma syndrome are unusual in patients with MEN 1.

Pituitary tumors

(See also Chap. 5) Pituitary tumors occur in 15–50% of patients with MEN 1 (Table 29-1). These occur as early as 5 years of age or as late as the ninth decade. MEN 1 pituitary adenomas are more frequent in women than men and significantly are macroadenomas (i.e., diameter >1 cm). Moreover, about one-third of these pituitary tumors show invasive features such as infiltration of tumor cells into surrounding normal juxtatumoral pituitary tissue. However, no specific histologic parameters differentiate between MEN 1 and non–MEN 1 pituitary tumors. Approximately 60% of MEN 1–associated pituitary tumors secrete prolactin, <25% secrete growth hormone, 5% secrete adrenocorticotropic hormone (ACTH), and the remainder appear to be nonfunctioning, with some secreting glycoprotein subunits (Table 29-1). However, pituitary tumors derived from MEN 1 patients may exhibit immunoreactivity to several hormones. In particular, there is a greater frequency of somatolactotrope tumors. Prolactinomas are the first manifestation of MEN 1 in ~15% of patients, whereas somatotrope tumors occur more often in patients older than 40 years of age. Fewer than 3% of patients with anterior pituitary tumors will have MEN 1. Clinical manifestations are similar to those in patients with sporadic pituitary tumors without MEN 1 and depend on the hormone secreted and the size of the pituitary tumor. Thus, patients may have symptoms of hyperprolactinemia (e.g., amenorrhea, infertility, and galactorrhea in women, or impotence and infertility in men) or have features of acromegaly or Cushing's disease. In addition, enlarging pituitary tumors may compress adjacent structures such as the optic chiasm or normal pituitary tissue, causing visual disturbances and/or hypopituitarism. In asymptomatic patients with MEN 1, periodic biochemical monitoring of serum prolactin and insulin-like growth factor I (IGF-I) levels, as well as MRI of the pituitary, can lead to early identification of pituitary tumors (Table 29-3). In patients with abnormal results, hypothalamic-pituitary testing should characterize the nature of the pituitary lesion and its effects on the secretion of other pituitary hormones.

TREATMENT Pituitary Tumors

Treatment of pituitary tumors in patients with MEN 1 consists of therapies similar to those used in patients without MEN 1 and includes appropriate medical therapy (e.g., bromocriptine or cabergoline for prolactinoma; or octreotide or lanreotide for somatotrope tumors) or selective transsphenoidal adenomectomy, if feasible, with radiotherapy reserved for residual unresectable tumor tissue. Pituitary tumors in MEN 1 patients may be more aggressive and less responsive to medical or surgical treatments.

Associated tumors

Patients with MEN 1 may also develop carcinoid tumors, adrenal cortical tumors, facial angiofibromas, collagenomas, thyroid tumors, and lipomatous tumors.

Carcinoid tumors

(See also Chap. 28) Carcinoid tumors occur in more than 3% of patients with MEN 1 (Table 29-1). The carcinoid tumor may be located in the bronchi, gastrointestinal tract, pancreas, or thymus. At the time of diagnosis, most patients are asymptomatic and do not have clinical features of the carcinoid syndrome. Importantly, no hormonal or biochemical abnormality (e.g., plasma chromogranin A) is consistently observed in individuals with thymic or bronchial carcinoid tumors. Thus, screening for these tumors is dependent on radiologic imaging. The optimum method for screening has not been established. CT and MRI are sensitive for detecting thymic and bronchial tumors (Table 29-3), although repeated CT scanning raises concern about exposure to repeated doses of ionizing radiation. Octreotide scintigraphy may also reveal some thymic and bronchial carcinoids, although there is insufficient evidence to recommend its routine use. Gastric carcinoids, of which the type II gastric enterochromaffin-like (ECL) cell carcinoids (ECLomas) are associated with MEN 1 and Zollinger-Ellison syndrome, may be detected incidentally at the time of gastric endoscopy for dyspeptic symptoms in MEN 1 patients. These tumors, which may be found in >10% of MEN 1 patients, are usually multiple and smaller than 1.5 cm. Bronchial carcinoids in patients with MEN 1 occur predominantly in women (male-to-female ratio, 1:4). In contrast, thymic carcinoids in European patients with MEN 1 occur predominantly in men (male-to-female ratio, 20:1), with cigarette smokers having a higher risk for these tumors; thymic carcinoids in Japanese patients with MEN 1 have a less marked sex difference (male-to-female ratio 2:1). The course of thymic carcinoids in MEN 1 appears to be particularly aggressive. The presence of thymic tumors in patients with MEN 1 is associated with a median survival after diagnosis of approximately 9.5 years, with 70% of patients dying as a direct result of the tumor.

TREATMENT Carcinoid Tumors

If resectable, surgical removal of carcinoid tumors is the treatment of choice. For unresectable tumors and those with metastatic disease, treatment with radiotherapy or chemotherapeutic agents (e.g., cisplatin, etoposide) may be used. In addition, somatostatin analogues, such as octreotide or lanreotide, have resulted in symptom improvement and regression of some tumors. Little is known about the malignant potential of gastric type II ECLomas, but treatment with somatostatin analogues, such as octreotide or lanreotide, has resulted in regression of these ECLomas.

Adrenocortical tumors

(See also Chap. 8) Asymptomatic adrenocortical tumors occur in 20–70% of patients with MEN 1 depending on the radiologic screening methods used (Table 29-1). Most of these tumors, which include cortical adenomas, hyperplasia, multiple adenomas, nodular hyperplasia, cysts, and carcinomas, are nonfunctioning. Indeed, <10% of patients with enlarged adrenal glands have hormonal hypersecretion, with primary hyperaldosteronism and ACTH-independent Cushing's syndrome being encountered most commonly. Occasionally, hyperandrogenemia may occur in association with adrenocortical carcinoma. Pheochromocytoma in association with MEN 1 is rare. Biochemical investigation (e.g., plasma renin and aldosterone concentrations, low-dose dexamethasone suppression test, urinary catecholamines, and/or metanephrines) should be undertaken in those with symptoms or signs suggestive of functioning adrenal tumors or in those with tumors >1 cm. Adrenocortical carcinoma occurs in approximately 1% of MEN 1 patients but increases to >10% for adrenal tumors larger than 1 cm.

TREATMENT Adrenocortical Tumors

Consensus has not been reached about the management of MEN 1–associated nonfunctioning adrenal tumors, because the majority are benign. However, the risk of malignancy increases with size, particularly for tumors with a diameter >4 cm. Indications for surgery for adrenal tumors include: size >4 cm in diameter; atypical or suspicious radiologic features (e.g., increased Hounsfield unit on unenhanced CT scan) and size of 1–4 cm in diameter; or significant measurable growth over a 6-month period. The treatment of functioning (e.g., hormone-secreting) adrenal tumors is similar to that for tumors occurring in non–MEN 1 patients.

Meningioma

Central nervous system (CNS) tumors, including ependymomas, schwannomas, and meningiomas, have been reported in MEN 1 patients (Table 29-1). Meningiomas are found in <10% of patients with other clinical manifestations of MEN 1 (e.g., primary hyperparathyroidism) for >15 years. The majority of meningiomas are not associated with symptoms, and 60% do not enlarge. The treatment of MEN 1–associated meningiomas is similar to that in non–MEN 1 patients.

Lipomas

Subcutaneous lipomas occur in >33% of patients with MEN 1 (Table 29-1) and are frequently multiple. In addition, visceral, pleural, or retroperitoneal lipomas may occur in patients with MEN 1. Management is conservative. However, when surgically removed for cosmetic reasons, they typically do not recur.

Facial angiofibromas and collagenomas

The occurrence of multiple facial angiofibromas in patients with MEN 1 may range from >20 to >90%, and occurrence of collagenomas may range from 0 to >70% (Table 29-1). These cutaneous findings may allow presymptomatic diagnosis of MEN 1 in the relatives of a patient with MEN 1. Treatment for these cutaneous lesions is usually not required.

Thyroid tumors

Thyroid tumors, including adenomas, colloid goiters, and carcinomas, have been reported to occur in >25% of patients with MEN 1. However, the prevalence of thyroid disorders in the general population is high, and it has been suggested that the association of thyroid abnormalities in patients with MEN 1 may be incidental. The treatment of thyroid tumors in MEN 1 patients is similar to that for non–MEN 1 patients.

Genetics and screening

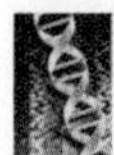

The *MEN1* gene is located on chromosome 11q13 and consists of 10 exons, which encode a 610–amino acid protein, menin, that regulates transcription, genome stability, cell division, and proliferation. The pathophysiology of MEN 1 follows the Knudson two-hit hypothesis with a tumor-suppressor role for menin. Inheritance of a germline *MEN1* mutation predisposes an individual to developing a tumor that arises following a somatic mutation, which may be a point mutation or more commonly a deletion, leading to loss of heterozygosity (LOH) in the tumor DNA. The germline mutations of the *MEN1* gene are scattered throughout the entire 1830-bp coding region and splice sites, and there is no apparent correlation between the location of *MEN1* mutations and clinical manifestations of the disorder, in contrast with the situation in patients with MEN 2 (Table 29-1). More than 10% of *MEN1* germline mutations arise de novo and may be transmitted to subsequent generations. Some families with MEN 1 mutations develop parathyroid tumors as the sole endocrinopathy, and this condition is referred to as familial isolated hyperparathyroidism (FIHP). However, between 5 and 25% of patients with MEN 1 do not harbor germline mutations or deletions of the *MEN1* gene. Such patients with MEN 1–associated tumors but without *MEN1* mutations may represent phenocopies or have mutations involving other genes. Other genes associated with MEN 1–like features include: *CDC73*, which encodes parafibromin, whose mutations result in the hyperparathyroid-jaw tumor syndrome; the calcium-sensing receptor gene (*CaSR*), whose mutations result in familial benign hypocalciuric hypercalcemia (FBHH); and the aryl hydrocarbon receptor interacting protein gene (*AIP*), a tumor suppressor located on chromosome 11q13 whose mutations are associated with familial isolated pituitary adenomas (FIPA). Genetic testing to determine the *MEN1* mutation status in symptomatic family members within a MEN 1 kindred, as well as to all index cases (e.g., patients) with two or more endocrine tumors, is advisable. If an *MEN1* mutation is not identified in the index case with two or more endocrine tumors, then clinical and genetic tests for other disorders such as hyperparathyroid-jaw tumor syndrome, FBHH, FIPA, MEN 2, or MEN 4 should be considered, because these patients may represent phenocopies for MEN 1.

The current guidelines recommend that *MEN1* mutational analysis should be undertaken in: (1) an index case with two or more MEN 1–associated endocrine tumors (e.g., parathyroid, pancreatic, or pituitary tumors); (2) asymptomatic first-degree relatives of a known *MEN1* mutation carrier; and (3) first-degree relatives of a *MEN1* mutation carrier with symptoms, signs, or biochemical or radiologic evidence for one or more MEN 1–associated tumors. In addition, *MEN1* mutational analysis should be considered in patients with suspicious or atypical MEN 1. This would include individuals with parathyroid adenomas before the age of 30 years or multigland parathyroid disease;

individuals with gastrinoma or multiple pancreatic NETs at any age; or individuals who have two or more MEN 1–associated tumors that are not part of the classical triad of parathyroid, pancreatic islet, and anterior pituitary tumors (e.g., parathyroid tumor plus adrenal tumor). Family members, including asymptomatic individuals who have been identified to harbor a *MEN1* mutation, will require biochemical and radiologic screening (Table 29-3). In contrast, relatives who do not harbor the *MEN1* mutation have a risk of developing MEN 1–associated endocrine tumors that is similar to that of the general population; thus, relatives without the *MEN1* mutation do not require repeated screening.

Mutational analysis in asymptomatic individuals should be undertaken at the earliest opportunity and, if possible, in the first decade of life because tumors have developed in some children by the age of 5 years. Appropriate biochemical and radiologic investigations (Table 29-3) aimed at detecting the development of tumors should then be undertaken in affected individuals. Mutant gene carriers should undergo biochemical screening at least once per annum and also have baseline pituitary and abdominal imaging (e.g., MRI or CT), which should then be repeated at 1- to 3-year intervals (Table 29-3). Screening should commence after 5 years of age and should continue for life because the disease may develop as late as the eighth decade. The screening history and physical examination elicit the symptoms and signs of hypercalcemia, nephrolithiasis, peptic ulcer disease, neuroglycopenia, hypopituitarism, galactorrhea and amenorrhea in women, acromegaly, Cushing's disease, and visual field loss and the presence of subcutaneous lipomas, angiofibromas, and collagenomas. Biochemical screening should include measurements of serum calcium, PTH, gastrointestinal hormones (e.g., gastrin, insulin with a fasting glucose, glucagon, VIP, PP), chromogranin A, prolactin, and IGF-I in all individuals. More specific endocrine function tests should be undertaken in individuals who have symptoms or signs suggestive of a specific clinical syndrome. Biochemical screening for the development of MEN 1 tumors in asymptomatic members of families with MEN 1 is of great importance to reduce morbidity and mortality from the associated tumors.

MULTIPLE ENDOCRINE NEOPLASIA TYPE 2 AND TYPE 3

Clinical manifestations

MEN type 2 (MEN 2), which is also called Sipple's syndrome, is characterized by the association of medullary thyroid carcinoma (MTC), pheochromocytomas, and parathyroid tumors (Table 29-1). Three clinical variants of MEN 2 are recognized: MEN 2A, MEN 2B, and MTC only. MEN 2A, which is often referred to as MEN 2, is the most common variant. In MEN 2A, MTC is associated with pheochromocytomas in 50% of patients (may be bilateral) and with parathyroid tumors in 20% of patients. MEN 2A may rarely occur in association with Hirschsprung's disease, caused by the absence of autonomic ganglion cells in the terminal hindgut, resulting in colonic dilatation, severe constipation, and obstruction. MEN 2A may also be associated with cutaneous lichen amyloidosis, which is a pruritic lichenoid lesion that is usually located on the upper back. MEN 2B, which is also referred to as MEN 3, represents 5% of all cases of MEN 2 and is characterized by the occurrence of MTC and pheochromocytoma in association with a Marfanoid habitus; mucosal neuromas of the lips, tongue, and eyelids; medullated corneal fibers; and intestinal autonomic ganglion dysfunction leading to multiple diverticulae and megacolon. Parathyroid tumors do not usually occur in MEN 2B. MTC only (FMTC) is a variant in which MTC is the sole manifestation of the syndrome. However, the distinction between FMTC and MEN 2A is difficult and should only be considered if there are at least four family members above the age of 50 years who are affected by MTC but not pheochromocytomas or primary hyperparathyroidism. All of the MEN 2 variants are due to mutations of the rearranged during transfection (*RET*) protooncogene, which encodes a TKR. Moreover, there is a correlation between the locations of *RET* mutations and MEN 2 variants. Thus, ~95% of MEN 2A patients have mutations involving the cysteine-rich extracellular domain, with mutations of codon 634 accounting for ~85% of MEN 2A mutations; FMTC patients also have mutations of the cysteine-rich extracellular domain, with most mutations occurring in codon 618. In contrast, ~95% of MEN 2B/MEN 3 patients have mutations of codon 918 of the intracellular tyrosine kinase domain (Table 29-1 and Table 29-4).

Medullary thyroid carcinoma

MTC is the most common feature of MEN 2A and MEN 2B and occurs in almost all affected individuals. MTC represents 5–10% of all thyroid gland carcinomas, and 20% of MTC patients have a family history of the disorder. The use of *RET* mutational analysis to identify family members at risk for hereditary forms of MTC has altered the presentation of MTC from that of symptomatic tumors to a preclinical disease for which prophylactic thyroidectomy (Table 29-4) is undertaken to improve the prognosis and ideally result in cure. However, in patients who do not have a known family history of MEN 2A, FMTC, or MEN 2B, and therefore have not had *RET* mutational analysis, MTC may present as a palpable mass in the neck, which may be asymptomatic or associated

TABLE 29-4

RECOMMENDATIONS FOR TESTS AND SURGERY IN MEN 2 AND MEN 3[a]

RET MUTATION, EXON (EX) LOCATION, AND CODON INVOLVED	RISK[b]	RECOMMENDED AGE (YEARS) FOR TEST/INTERVENTION				
		RET MUTATIONAL ANALYSIS	FIRST SERUM CALCITONIN AND NECK ULTRASOUND	PROPHYLACTIC THYROIDECTOMY	SCREENING FOR PHEOCHROMOCYTOMA	SCREENING FOR PHPT
Ex13 (768, 790)[c]; Ex14 (804)[c]; Ex15 (891)[c]	+	<3–5	<3–5	5[d]	20	20
Ex10 (609, 611, 618, 620)[c]; Ex11 (630)[c]	++	<3–5	<3–5	<5[e]	20	20
Ex11 (634)[c]	+++	<3–5	<3–5	<5	8	20
Ex15 (883)[f]; Ex16 (918)f	++++	ASAP and by <1	ASAP and by <0.5–1	ASAP and by <1	8	—[g]

[a]Adapted from American Thyroid Association Guidelines, RT Kloos et al: Thyroid 6:565, 2009.
[b]Risk for early development of metastasis and aggressive growth of medullary thyroid cancer: ++++, highest; +++, high; ++, intermediate; and +, lowest.
[c]Mutations associated with MEN 2A (or medullary thyroid carcinoma only).
[d]Consider surgery at 5 years or later if serum calcitonin is normal, neck ultrasound is normal, and there is a less aggressive family history and family preference.
[e]Consider surgery before 5 years or later if serum calcitonin is normal, neck ultrasound is normal, and there is a less aggressive family history and family preference.
[f]Mutations associated with MEN 2B (MEN 3).
[g]Not required because PHPT is not a feature of MEN 2B (MEN 3).
Abbreviations: ASAP, as soon as possible; MEN, multiple endocrine neoplasia; PHPT, primary hyperparathyroidism.

with symptoms of pressure or dysphagia in >15% of patients. Diarrhea occurs in 30% of patients and is associated either with elevated circulating concentrations of calcitonin or tumor-related secretion of serotonin and prostaglandins. Some patients may also experience flushing. In addition, ectopic ACTH production by MTC may cause Cushing's syndrome. The diagnosis of MTC relies on the demonstration of hypercalcitoninemia (>90 pg/mL in the basal state); stimulation tests using IV pentagastrin (0.5 mg/kg) and or calcium infusion (2 mg/kg) are rarely used now, reflecting improvements in the assay for calcitonin. Neck ultrasonography with fine-needle aspiration of the nodules can confirm the diagnosis. Radionucleotide thyroid scans may reveal MTC tumors as "cold" nodules. Radiography may reveal dense irregular calcification within the involved portions of the thyroid gland and in lymph nodes involved with metastases. Positron emission tomography (PET) may help to identify the MTC and metastases (Fig. 29-2). Metastases of MTC usually occur to the cervical lymph nodes in the early stages and to the mediastinal nodes, lung, liver, trachea, adrenal, esophagus, and bone in later stages. Elevations in serum calcitonin concentrations are often the first sign of recurrence or persistent disease, and the serum calcitonin doubling time is useful for determining prognosis. MTC can have an aggressive clinical course, with early metastases and death in approximately 10% of patients. A family history of aggressive MTC or MEN 2B may be elicited.

TREATMENT Medullary Thyroid Carcinoma

Individuals with *RET* mutations who do not have clinical manifestations of MTC should be offered prophylactic surgery between the ages of <1 and 5 years. The timing of surgery will depend on the type of *RET* mutation and its associated risk for early development, metastasis, and aggressive growth of MTC (Table 29-4). Such patients should have a total thyroidectomy with a systematic central neck dissection to remove occult nodal metastasis, although the value of undertaking a central neck dissection has been subject to debate. Prophylactic thyroidectomy, with life-long thyroxine replacement, has dramatically improved outcomes in patients with MEN 2 and MEN 3, such that ~90% of young patients with *RET* mutations who had a prophylactic thyroidectomy have no evidence of persistent or recurrent MTC at 7 years after surgery. In patients with clinically evident MTC, a total thyroidectomy with bilateral central resection is recommended, and an ipsilateral lateral neck dissection should be undertaken if the primary tumor is >1 cm in size or there is evidence of nodal metastasis in the central neck. Surgery is the only curative therapy for MTC. The 10-year survival in patients with metastatic MTC is ~20%. For inoperable MTC

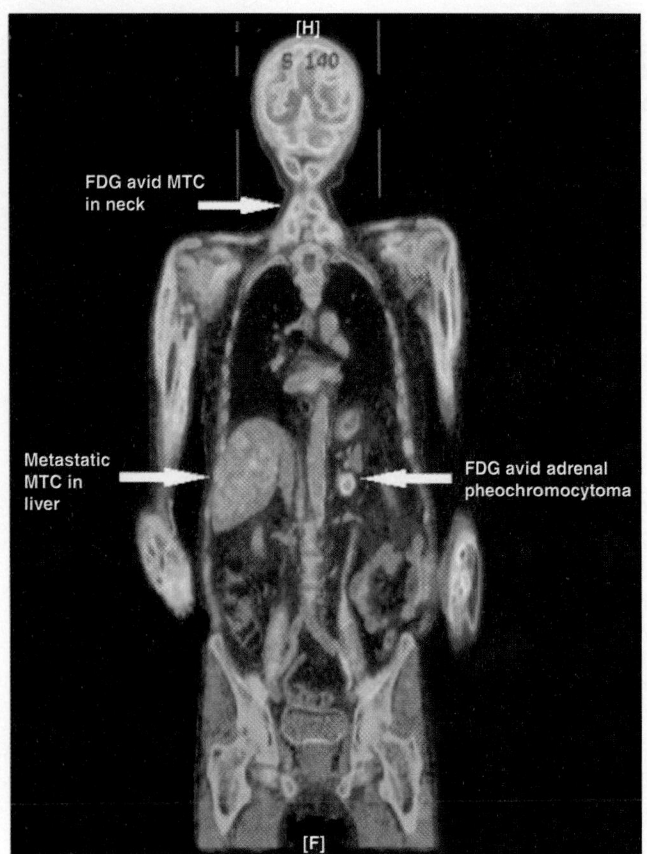

FIGURE 29-2
Fluorodeoxyglucose (FDG) positron emission tomography scan in a patient with multiple endocrine neoplasia type 2A, showing medullary thyroid cancer (MTC) with hepatic and skeletal (left arm) metastasis and a left adrenal pheochromocytoma. Note the presence of excreted FDG compound in the bladder. *(Reproduced with permission from A Naziat et al: Clin Endocrinol [Oxf] 78:966, 2013.)*

or metastatic disease, the tyrosine kinase inhibitors, vandetanib and cabozantinib, have improved the progression-free survival times. Other types of chemotherapy are of limited efficacy, but radiotherapy may help to palliate local disease.

Pheochromocytoma

(See also Chap. 9) These noradrenaline- and adrenaline-secreting tumors occur in >50% of patients with MEN 2A and MEN 2B and are a major cause of morbidity and mortality. Patients may have symptoms and signs of catecholamine secretion (e.g., headaches, palpitations, sweating, poorly controlled hypertension), or they may be asymptomatic with detection through biochemical screening based on a history of familial MEN 2A, MEN 2B, or MTC. Pheochromocytomas in patients with MEN 2A and MEN 2B differ significantly in distribution when compared with patients without MEN 2A and MEN 2B. Extra-adrenal pheochromocytomas, which occur in 10% of patients without MEN 2A and MEN 2B, are observed rarely in patients with MEN 2A and MEN 2B. Malignant pheochromocytomas are much less common in patients with MEN 2A and MEN 2B. The biochemical and radiologic investigation of pheochromocytoma in patients with MEN 2A and MEN 2B is similar to that in non–MEN 2 patients and includes the measurement of plasma (obtained from supine patients) and urinary free fractionated metanephrines (e.g., normetanephrine and metanephrines measured separately), CT or MRI scanning, radionuclide scanning with meta-iodo-(^{123}I or ^{131}I)-benzyl guanidine (MIBG), and PET using (^{18}F)-fluorodopamine or (^{18}F)-fluoro-2-dexoxy-d-glucose (Fig. 29-2).

TREATMENT **Pheochromocytoma**

Surgical removal of pheochromocytoma, using α and β adrenoreceptor blockade before and during the operation, is the recommended treatment. Endoscopic adrenal-sparing surgery, which decreases postoperative morbidity, hospital stay, and expense, as opposed to open surgery, has become the method of choice.

Parathyroid tumors

(See also Chap. 34) Parathyroid tumors occur in 10–25% of patients with MEN 2A. However, >50% of these patients do not have hypercalcemia. The presence of abnormally enlarged parathyroids, which are unusually hyperplastic, is often seen in the normocalcemic patient undergoing thyroidectomy for MTC. The biochemical investigation and treatment of hypercalcemic patients with MEN 2A is similar to that of patients with MEN 1.

Genetics and screening

To date, approximately 50 different *RET* mutations have been reported, and these are located in exons 5, 8, 10, 11, 13, 14, 15, and 16. *RET* germline mutations are detected in >95% of MEN 2A, FMTC, and MEN 2B families, with Cys634Arg being most common in MEN 2A, Cys618Arg being most common in FMTC, and Met918Thr being most common in MEN 2B (Tables 29-1 and 29-4). Between 5 and 10% of patients with MTC or MEN 2A–associated tumors have de novo *RET* germline mutations, and ~50% of patients with MEN 2B have de novo *RET* germline mutations. These de novo *RET* germline mutations always occur on the paternal allele. Approximately 5% of patients with sporadic pheochromocytoma have a germline *RET* mutation, but such germline *RET* mutations do not appear to be associated with sporadic primary hyperparathyroidism. Thus, *RET* mutational analysis should be performed in: (1) all patients with MTC who have a family history of tumors associated with MEN 2, FMTC, or MEN 3, such that the diagnosis can be confirmed and genetic testing offered to asymptomatic relatives; (2) all patients with MTC and pheochromocytoma without a known family history of MEN 2 or MEN 3; (3) all patients with MTC, but without a family history of MEN 2, FMTC, or MEN 3, because these patients may have a de novo germline *RET* mutations; (4) all patients with bilateral pheochromocytoma; and (5) patients with unilateral pheochromocytoma, particularly if this occurs with increased calcitonin levels.

Screening for MEN 2/MEN 3–associated tumors in patients with *RET* germline mutations should be undertaken annually and include serum calcitonin measurements, a neck ultrasound for MTC, plasma and 24-h urinary fractionated metanephrines for pheochromocytoma, and albumin-corrected serum calcium or ionized calcium with PTH for primary hyperparathyroidism. In patients with MEN 2–associated *RET* mutations, screening for MTC should begin by 3 to 5 years; for pheochromocytoma by 20 years; and for primary hyperparathyroidism by 20 years of age (Table 29-4).

MULTIPLE ENDOCRINE NEOPLASIA TYPE 4

Clinical manifestations

Patients with MEN 1–associated tumors, such as parathyroid adenomas, pituitary adenomas, and pancreatic NETs, occurring in association with gonadal, adrenal, renal, and thyroid tumors have been reported to have mutations of the gene encoding the 196–amino acid cyclin-dependent kinase inhibitor (CK1) p27 kip1 (*CDNKIB*). Such families with MEN 1–associated tumors and *CDNKIB* mutations are designated to have MEN 4 (Table 29-1). The investigations and treatments for the MEN 4–associated tumors are similar to those for MEN 1 and non–MEN 1 tumors.

Genetics and screening

To date, eight different MEN 4–associated mutations of *CDNKIB*, which is located on chromosome 12p13, have been reported, and all of these are associated with a loss of function. These MEN 4 patients may represent ~3% of the 5–10% of patients with MEN 1 who do not have mutations of the *MEN1* gene. Germline *CDNKIB* mutations may rarely be found in patients with sporadic (i.e., nonfamilial) forms of primary hyperparathyroidism.

HYPERPARATHYROIDISM-JAW TUMOR SYNDROME

Clinical manifestations

Hyperparathyroidism-jaw tumor (HPT-JT) syndrome is an autosomal dominant disorder characterized by the development of parathyroid tumors (15% are carcinomas) and fibro-osseous jaw tumors **(see also Chap. 34)**. In addition, some patients may also develop Wilms' tumors, renal cysts, renal hematomas, renal cortical adenomas, papillary renal cell carcinomas, pancreatic adenocarcinomas, uterine tumors, testicular mixed germ cell tumors with a major seminoma component, and Hürthle cell thyroid adenomas. The parathyroid tumors may occur in isolation and without any evidence of jaw tumors, and this may cause confusion with other hereditary hypercalcemic disorders, such as MEN 1. However, genetic testing to identify the causative mutation will help to establish the correct diagnosis. The investigation and treatment for HPT-JT-associated tumors are similar to those in non-HPT-JT patients, except that early parathyroidectomy is advisable because of the increased frequency of parathyroid carcinoma.

Genetics and screening

The gene that causes HPT-JT is located on chromosome 1q31.2 and encodes a 531–amino acid protein, parafibromin (Table 29-2). Parafibromin is also referred to as cell division cycle protein 73 (CDC73) and has a role in transcription. Genetic testing in families helps to identify mutation carriers who should be periodically screened for the development of tumors (Table 29-5).

TABLE 29-5

HPT-JT SCREENING GUIDELINES

TUMOR[a]	TEST	FREQUENCY[b]
Parathyroid	Serum Ca, PTH	6–12 months
Ossifying jaw fibroma	Panoramic jaw x-ray with neck shielding[c]	5 years
Renal	Abdominal MRI[c,d]	5 years
Uterine	Ultrasound (transvaginal or transabdominal) and additional imaging ± D&C if indicated[e]	Annual

[a]Screening for most common HPT-JT–associated tumors is considered. Assessment for other reported tumor types may be indicated (e.g., pancreatic, thyroid, testicular tumors).

[b]Frequency of repeating test after baseline tests performed.

[c]X-rays and imaging involving ionizing radiation should ideally be avoided to minimize risk of generating subsequent mutations.

[d]Ultrasound scan recommended if MRI unavailable.

[e]Such selective pelvic imaging should be considered after obtaining a detailed menstrual history.

Abbreviations: Ca, calcium; D&C, dilatation and curettage; HPT-JT, hyperparathyroidism-jaw tumor syndrome; MRI, magnetic resonance imaging; PTH, parathyroid hormone.

Source: Reproduced from PJ Newey et al: Hum Mutat 31:295, 2010.

VON HIPPEL-LINDAU DISEASE

Clinical manifestations

von Hippel-Lindau (VHL) disease is an autosomal dominant disorder characterized by hemangioblastomas of the retina and CNS; cysts involving the kidneys, pancreas, and epididymis; renal cell carcinomas; pheochromocytomas; and pancreatic islet cell tumors **(See also Chap. 9)**. The retinal and CNS hemangioblastomas are benign vascular tumors that may be multiple; those in the CNS may cause symptoms by compressing adjacent structures and/or increasing intracranial pressure. In the CNS, the cerebellum and spinal cord are the most frequently involved sites. The renal abnormalities consist of cysts and carcinomas, and the lifetime risk of a renal cell carcinoma (RCC) in VHL is 70%. The endocrine tumors in VHL consist of pheochromocytomas and pancreatic islet cell tumors. The clinical presentation of pheochromocytoma in VHL disease is similar to that in sporadic cases, except there is a higher frequency of bilateral or multiple tumors, which may involve extra-adrenal sites in VHL disease. The most frequent pancreatic lesions in VHL are multiple cyst-adenomas, which rarely cause clinical disease. However, nonsecreting pancreatic islet cell tumors occur in <10% of VHL patients, who are usually asymptomatic. The pancreatic tumors in these patients are often detected by regular screening using abdominal imaging. Pheochromocytomas should be investigated and treated as described earlier for MEN 2. The pancreatic islet cell tumors frequently become malignant, and early surgery is recommended.

Genetics and screening

The *VHL* gene, which is located on chromosome 3p26-p25, is widely expressed in human tissues and encodes a 213–amino acid protein (pVHL) (Table 29-2). A wide variety of germline *VHL* mutations have been identified. *VHL* acts as a tumor-suppressor gene. A correlation appears to exist between the type of mutation and the clinical phenotype; large deletions and protein-truncating mutations are associated with a low incidence of pheochromocytomas, whereas some missense mutations in VHL patients are associated with pheochromocytoma (referred to as VHL type 2C). Other missense mutations may be associated with hemangioblastomas and RCC but not pheochromocytoma (referred to as VHL type 1), whereas distinct missense mutations are associated with hemangioblastomas, RCC, and pheochromocytoma (VHL type 2B). VHL type 2A, which refers to the occurrence of hemangioblastomas and pheochromocytoma without RCC, is associated with rare missense mutations. The basis for these complex genotype-phenotype relationships remains to be elucidated. One major function of pVHL, which is also referred to as elongin, is to downregulate the expression of vascular endothelial growth factor (VEGF) and other hypoxia-inducible mRNAs. Thus, pVHL, in complex with other proteins, regulates the expression of hypoxia-inducible factors (HIF-1 and HIF-2) such that loss of functional pVHL leads to a stabilization of the HIF protein complexes, resulting in VEGF overexpression and tumor angiogenesis. Screening for the development of pheochromocytomas and pancreatic islet cell tumors is as described earlier for MEN 2 and MEN 1, respectively (Tables 29-3 and 29-4).

NEUROFIBROMATOSIS

Clinical manifestations

Neurofibromatosis type 1 (NF1), which is also referred to as von Recklinghausen's disease, is an autosomal dominant disorder characterized by the following manifestations: neurologic (e.g., peripheral and spinal neurofibromas); ophthalmologic (e.g., optic gliomas and iris hamartomas such as Lisch nodules); dermatologic (e.g., café au lait macules); skeletal (e.g., scoliosis, macrocephaly, short stature, and pseudoarthrosis); vascular (e.g., stenoses of renal and intracranial arteries); and endocrine (e.g., pheochromocytoma, carcinoid tumors, and precocious puberty). Neurofibromatosis type 2 (NF2) is also an autosomal dominant disorder but is characterized by the development of bilateral vestibular schwannomas (acoustic neuromas) that lead to deafness, tinnitus, or vertigo. Some patients with NF2 also develop meningiomas, spinal schwannomas, peripheral nerve neurofibromas, and café au lait macules. Endocrine abnormalities are not found in NF2 and are associated solely with NF1. Pheochromocytomas, carcinoid tumors, and precocious puberty occur in about 1% of patients with NF1, and growth hormone deficiency has been also reported. The features of pheochromocytomas in NF1 are similar to those in non-NF1 patients, with 90% of tumors being located within the adrenal medulla and the remaining 10% at an extra-adrenal location, which often involves the para-aortic region. Primary carcinoid tumors are often periampullary and may also occur in the ileum but rarely in the pancreas, thyroid, or lungs. Hepatic metastases are associated with symptoms of the carcinoid syndrome, which include flushing, diarrhea, bronchoconstriction, and tricuspid valve disease. Precocious puberty is usually associated with the extension of an optic glioma into the hypothalamus with resultant early activation of gonadotropin-releasing hormone secretion. Growth hormone deficiency has also been observed in some NF1 patients, who may or may not have optic chiasmal gliomas, but it is important to note that short stature is frequent in the absence of growth hormone deficiency in patients with NF1. The investigation and treatment for tumors are similar to those undertaken for each respective tumor type in non-NF1 patients.

Genetics and screening

The *NF1* gene, which is located on chromosome 17q11.2 and acts as a tumor suppressor, consists of 60 exons that span more than 350 kb of genomic DNA (Table 29-2). Mutations in *NF1* are of diverse types and are scattered throughout the exons. The NF1 gene product is the protein neurofibromin, which has homologies to the p120GAP (GTPase activating protein) and acts on p21ras by converting the active GTP bound form to its inactive GDP form. Mutations of *NF1* impair this downregulation of the p21ras signaling pathways, which in turn results in abnormal cell proliferation. Screening for the development of pheochromocytomas and carcinoid tumors is as described earlier for MEN 2 and MEN 1, respectively (Tables 29-3 and 29-4).

CARNEY COMPLEX

Clinical manifestations

Carney complex (CNC) is an autosomal dominant disorder characterized by spotty skin pigmentation (usually of the face, labia, and conjunctiva), myxomas (usually of the eyelids and heart, but also the tongue, palate, breast, and skin), psammomatous melanotic schwannomas (usually of the sympathetic nerve chain and upper gastrointestinal tract), and endocrine tumors that involve the adrenals, Sertoli cells, somatotropes, thyroid, and ovary. Cushing's syndrome, the result of primary pigmented nodular adrenal disease (PPNAD), is the most common endocrine manifestation of CNC and may occur in one-third of patients. Patients with CNC and Cushing's syndrome often have an atypical appearance by being thin (as opposed to having truncal obesity). In addition, they may have short stature, muscle and skin wasting, and osteoporosis. These patients often have levels of urinary free cortisol that are normal or increased only marginally. Cortisol production may fluctuate periodically with days or weeks of hypercortisolism; this pattern is referred to as "periodic Cushing's syndrome." Patients with Cushing's syndrome usually have loss of the circadian rhythm of cortisol production. Acromegaly, the result of a somatotrope tumor, affects ~10% of patients with CNC. Testicular tumors may also occur in one-third of patients with CNC. These may either be large-cell calcifying Sertoli cell tumors, adrenocortical rests, or Leydig cell tumors. The Sertoli cell tumors occasionally may be estrogen-secreting and lead to precocious puberty or gynecomastia. Some patients with CNC have been reported to develop thyroid follicular tumors, ovarian cysts, or breast duct adenomas.

Genetics and screening

CNC type 1 (CNC1) is due to mutations of the protein kinase A (PKA) regulatory subunit 1 α (R1α) (*PPKAR1A*), a tumor suppressor, whose gene is located on chromosome 17q.24.2 (Table 29-2). The gene causing CNC type 2 (CNC2) is located on chromosome 2p16 and has not yet been identified. It is interesting to note, however, that some tumors do not show LOH of 2p16 but instead show genomic instability, suggesting that this CNC gene may not be a tumor suppressor. Screening and treatment of these endocrine tumors are similar to those described earlier for patients with MEN 1 and MEN 2 (Tables 29-3 and 29-4).

COWDEN'S SYNDROME

Clinical manifestations

Multiple hamartomatous lesions, especially of the skin, mucous membranes (e.g., buccal, intestinal, and colonic), breast, and thyroid are characteristic of Cowden's (CWD) syndrome, which is an autosomal dominant disorder. Thyroid abnormalities occur in two-thirds of patients with CWD syndrome, and these usually consist of multinodular goiters or benign adenomas, although <10% of patients may have a follicular thyroid carcinoma. Breast abnormalities occur in >75% of patients and consist of either fibrocystic disease or adenocarcinomas. The investigation and treatment for CWD tumors are similar to those undertaken for non-CWD patients.

Genetics and screening

CWD syndrome is genetically heterogenous, and six types (CWD1–6) are recognized (Table 29-2). CWD is due to mutations of the phosphate and tensin homologue deleted on chromosome 10 (*PTEN*) gene, located on chromosome 10q23.31. CWD2 is caused by mutations of the succinate dehydrogenase subunit B (*SDHB*) gene, located on chromosome 1p36.13; and CWD3 is caused by mutations of the *SDHD* gene, located on chromosome 11q13.1. *SDHB* and *SDHD* mutations are also associated with pheochromocytoma. CWD4 is caused by hypermethylation of the Killin (*KLLN*) gene, the promoter of which shares the same transcription site as *PTEN* on chromosome 10q23.31. CWD5 is caused by mutations of the phosphatidylinositol 3-kinase catalytic alpha (*PIK3CA*) gene on chromosome 3q26.32, and CWD6 is caused by mutations of the V-Akt murine thymoma viral oncogene homolog 1 (*AKT1*) gene on chromosome 14q32.33. Screening for thyroid abnormalities entails neck ultrasonography and fine-needle aspiration with analysis of cell cytology.

MCCUNE-ALBRIGHT SYNDROME

Clinical manifestations

McCune-Albright syndrome (MAS) is characterized by the triad of polyostotic fibrous dysplasia, which may be associated with hypophosphatemic rickets; café au lait skin pigmentation; and peripheral precocious puberty; other endocrine abnormalities include thyrotoxicosis, which may be associated with a multinodular goiter, somatotrope tumors, and Cushing's syndrome (due to adrenal tumors) **(See also Chap. 36)**. Investigation and treatment for each endocrinopathy are similar to those used in patients without MAS.

Genetics and screening

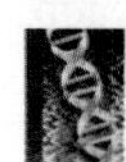

MAS is a disorder of mosaicism that results from postzygotic somatic cell mutations of the G protein α stimulating subunit (Gsα), encoded by the *GNAS1* gene, located on chromosome 20q13.32 (Table 29-2). The Gsα mutations, which include Arg-201Cys, Arg201His, Glu227Arg, or Glu227His, are activating and are found only in cells of the abnormal tissues. Screening for hyperfunction of relevant endocrine glands and development of hypophosphatemia, which may be associated with elevated serum fibroblast growth factor 23 (FGF23) concentrations, is undertaken in MAS patients.

ACKNOWLEDGMENTS

The author is grateful to the Medical Research Council (UK) for support and to Mrs. Tracey Walker for typing the manuscript.

CHAPTER 30

AUTOIMMUNE POLYENDOCRINE SYNDROMES

Peter A. Gottlieb

Polyglandular deficiency syndromes have been given many different names, reflecting the wide spectrum of disorders that have been associated with these syndromes and the heterogeneity of their clinical presentations. The name used in this chapter for this group of disorders is *autoimmune polyendocrine syndrome* (APS). In general, these disorders are divided into two major categories, APS type 1 (APS-1) and APS type 2 (APS-2). Some groups have further subdivided APS-2 into APS type 3 (APS-3) and APS type 4 (APS-4) depending on the type of autoimmunity involved. For the most part, this additional classification does not clarify our understanding of disease pathogenesis or prevention of complications in individual patients. Importantly, there are many nonendocrine disease associations included in these syndromes, suggesting that although the underlying autoimmune disorder predominantly involves endocrine targets, it does not exclude other tissues. The disease associations found in APS-1 and APS-2 are summarized in Table 30-1. Understanding these syndromes and their disease manifestations can lead to early diagnosis and treatment of additional disorders in patients and their family members.

APS-1

APS-1 (Online Mendelian Inheritance in Man [OMIM] 240300) has also been called autoimmune polyendocrinopathy–candidiasis–ectodermal dystrophy (APECED). Mucocutaneous candidiasis, hypoparathyroidism, and Addison's disease form the three major components of this disorder. However, as summarized in Table 30-1, many other organ systems can be involved over time. APS-1 is rare, with fewer than 500 cases reported in the literature. It is an autosomal recessive disorder caused by mutations in the *AIRE* gene (autoimmune regulator gene) found on chromosome 21. This gene is most highly expressed in thymic medullary epithelial cells (mTECs) where it appears to control the expression of tissue-specific self-antigens (e.g., insulin). Deletion of this regulator leads to decreased expression of tissue-specific self-antigens and is hypothesized to allow autoreactive T cells to avoid clonal deletion, which normally occurs during T cell maturation in the thymus. The *AIRE* gene is also expressed in epithelial cells found in peripheral lymphoid organs, but its role in these extrathymic cells remains controversial. A number of mutations have been described in this gene, and there is a higher frequency within certain ethnic groups including Iranian Jews, Sardinians, Finns, Norwegians, and Irish.

Clinical manifestations

APS-1 develops very early in life, often in infancy (Table 30-2). Chronic mucocutaneous candidiasis without signs of systemic disease is often the first manifestation. It affects the mouth and nails more frequently than the skin and esophagus. Chronic oral candidiasis can result in atrophic disease with areas suggestive of leukoplakia, which can pose a risk for future carcinoma. The etiology is associated with anticytokine autoantibodies (anti-IL-17A, -IL-17F, and -IL-22) related to T helper (T_H) 17 T cells and depressed production of these cytokines by peripheral blood mononuclear cells. Hypoparathyroidism usually develops next, followed by adrenal insufficiency. The time from development of one component of the disorder to the next can be many years, and the order of disease appearance is variable.

Chronic candidiasis is nearly always present and is not very responsive to treatment. Hypoparathyroidism is found in >85% of cases, and Addison's disease is found in nearly 80%. Gonadal failure appears to affect women more than men (70% vs 25%, respectively), and hypoplasia of the dental enamel also occurs frequently (77% of patients). Other endocrine disorders that occur less frequently include type 1 diabetes (23%) and autoimmune thyroid disease (18%). Nonendocrine

TABLE 30-1

DISEASE ASSOCIATIONS WITH AUTOIMMUNE POLYENDOCRINE SYNDROMES

AUTOIMMUNE POLYENDOCRINE SYNDROME TYPE 1	AUTOIMMUNE POLYENDOCRINE SYNDROME TYPE 2	OTHER AUTOIMMUNE POLYENDOCRINE DISORDERS
Endocrine	**Endocrine**	IPEX (immune dysfunction polyendocrinopathy X-linked)
Addison's disease	Addison's disease	Thymic tumors
Hypoparathyroidism	Type 1 diabetes	Anti-insulin receptor antibodies
Hypogonadism	*Graves' disease or autoimmune thyroiditis*	POEMS syndrome
Graves' disease or autoimmune thyroiditis	*Hypogonadism*	Insulin autoimmune syndrome (Hirata's syndrome)
Type 1 diabetes		Adult combined pituitary hormone deficiency (CPHD) with anti-Pit1 autoantibodies
		Kearns-Sayre syndrome
		DIDMOAD syndrome
Nonendocrine	**Nonendocrine**	Congenital rubella associated with thyroiditis and/or diabetes
Mucocutaneous candidiasis	Celiac disease, dermatitis herpetiformis	
Chronic active hepatitis	Pernicious anemia	
Pernicious anemia	Vitiligo	
Vitiligo	*Alopecia*	
Asplenism	*Myasthenia gravis*	
Ectodermal dysplasia	*IgA deficiency*	
Alopecia	*Parkinson's disease*	
Malabsorption syndromes	*Idiopathic thrombocytopenia*	
IgA deficiency		

Abbreviations: DIDMOAD, *d*iabetes *i*nsipidus, *d*iabetes *m*ellitus, progressive bilateral optic *a*trophy, and sensorineural *d*eafness; POEMS, *p*olyneuropathy, *o*rganomegaly, *e*ndocrinopathy, *M*-protein, and *s*kin changes.
Note: Italics denote less common disorders.

TABLE 30-2

COMPARISON OF APS-1 AND APS-2

APS-1	APS-2
Early onset: infancy	Later onset
Siblings often affected and at risk	Multigenerational
Equivalent sex distribution	Females > males affected
Monogenic: *AIRE* gene, chromosome 21, autosomal recessive	Polygenic: *HLA, MICA, PTNP22, CTLA4*
Not HLA associated for entire syndrome, some specific component risk	DR3/DR4 associated; other HLA class III gene associations noted
Autoantibodies to type 1 interferons and IL-17 and IL-22	No autoantibodies to cytokines
Autoantibodies to specific target organs	Autoantibodies to specific target organs
Asplenism	No defined immunodeficiency
Mucocutaneous candidiasis	Association with other nonendocrine immunologic disorders like myasthenia gravis and idiopathic thrombocytopenic purpura

Abbreviations: APS, autoimmune polyendocrine syndrome; IL, interleukin.

manifestations that present less frequently include alopecia (40%), vitiligo (26%), intestinal malabsorption (18%), pernicious anemia (31%), chronic active hepatitis (17%), and nail dystrophy. An unusual and debilitating manifestation of the disorder is the development of refractory diarrhea/obstipation that may be related to autoantibody-mediated destruction of enterochromaffin or enterochromaffin-like cells. The incidence rates for many of these disorders peak in the first or second decade of life, but the individual disease components continue to emerge over time. Therefore, prevalence rates may be higher than originally reported.

Diagnosis

The diagnosis of APS-1 is usually made clinically when two of the three major component disorders are found in an individual patient. Siblings of individuals with APS-1 should be considered affected even if only one component disorder has been detected due to the known inheritance of the syndrome. Genetic analysis of the *AIRE* gene should be undertaken to identify mutations. Initial sequencing may detect the common mutations, but rare mutations are continually being noted, and an initial negative genetic analysis should not dissuade one from the clinical diagnosis until more extensive DNA sequencing can be performed. Detection of anti–interferon α and anti–interferon o antibodies can identify nearly 100% of cases with APS-1. The autoantibody arises independent of the type of *AIRE* gene mutation and is not found in other autoimmune disorders.

Diagnosis of each underlying disorder should be done based on their typical clinical presentations (Table 30-3). Mucocutaneous candidiasis may present throughout the gastrointestinal tract, and it may be detected in the oral mucosa or from stool samples. Evaluation by a gastroenterologist to examine the esophagus for candidiasis or secondary stricture may be merited based on symptoms. Other gastrointestinal manifestations of APS-1, including malabsorption and obstipation, may also bring these young patients to the attention of gastroenterologists for first evaluation. Specific physical examination findings of

TABLE 30-3

CLINICAL FEATURES AND RECOMMENDED FOLLOW-UP FOR APS-1 AND APS-2

COMPONENT DISEASE	RECOMMENDED EVALUATION
APS-1	
Addison's disease	Sodium, potassium, ACTH, cortisol, 21- and 17-hydroxylase autoantibodies
Diarrhea	History
Ectodermal dysplasia	Physical examination
Hypoparathyroidism	Serum calcium, phosphate, PTH
Hepatitis	Liver function tests
Hypothyroidism/Graves' disease	TSH; thyroid peroxidase and/or thyroglobulin autoantibodies and anti-TSH receptor Ab
Male hypogonadism	FSH/LH, testosterone
Malabsorption	Physical examination, anti-IL-17 and anti-IL-22 autoantibodies
Mucocutaneous candidiasis	Physical examination, mucosal swab, stool samples
Obstipation	History
Ovarian failure	FSH/LH, estradiol
Pernicious anemia	CBC, vitamin B_{12} levels
Splenic atrophy	Blood smear for Howell-Jolly bodies; platelet count; ultrasound if positive
Type 1 diabetes	Glucose, hemoglobin A_{1c}, diabetes-associated autoantibodies (insulin, GAD65, IA-2, ZnT8)
APS-2	
Addison's disease	21-Hydroxylase autoantibodies, ACTH stimulation testing if positive
Alopecia	Physical examination
Autoimmune hyper- or hypothyroidism	TSH; thyroid peroxidase and/or thyroglobulin autoantibodies, anti-TSH receptor Ab
Celiac disease	Transglutaminase autoantibodies; small intestine biopsy if positive
Cerebellar ataxia	Dictated by signs and symptoms of disease
Chronic inflammatory demyelinating polyneuropathy	Dictated by signs and symptoms of disease
Hypophysitis	Dictated by signs and symptoms of disease, anti-Pit1 autoantibody
Idiopathic heart block	Dictated by signs and symptoms of disease
IgA deficiency	IgA level
Myasthenia gravis	Dictated by signs and symptoms of disease, antiacetylcholinesterase Ab
Myocarditis	Dictated by signs and symptoms of disease
Pernicious anemia	Anti–parietal cell autoantibodies
	CBC, vitamin B_{12} levels if positive
Serositis	Dictated by signs and symptoms of disease
Stiff man syndrome	Dictated by signs and symptoms of disease
Vitiligo	Physical examination, NALP-1 polymorphism

Abbreviations: Ab, antibody; ACTH, adrenocorticotropic hormone; APS, autoimmune polyendocrine syndrome; CBC, complete blood count; FSH, follicle-stimulating hormone; IL, interleukin; LH, luteinizing hormone; PTH, parathyroid hormone; TSH, thyroid-stimulating hormone.

hyperpigmentation, vitiligo, alopecia, tetany, and signs of hyper- or hypothyroidism should be considered as signs of development of component disorders.

The development of disease-specific autoantibody assays can help confirm disease and also detect risk for future disease. For example, where possible, detection of anticytokine antibodies to interleukin (IL) 17 and IL-22 would confirm the diagnosis of mucocutaneous candidiasis due to APS-1. The presence of anti-21-hydroxylase antibody or anti-17-hydroxylase antibody (which may be found more commonly in adrenal insufficiency associated with APS-1) would confirm the presence or risk for Addison's disease. Other autoantibodies found in type 1 diabetes (e.g., anti-GAD65), pernicious anemia, and other component conditions should be screened for on a regular basis (6- to 12-month intervals depending on the age of the subject).

Laboratory tests, including a complete metabolic panel, phosphorous and magnesium, thyroid-stimulating hormone (TSH), adrenocorticotropic hormone (ACTH; morning), hemoglobin A_{1c}, plasma vitamin B_{12} level, and complete blood count with peripheral smear looking for Howell-Jolly bodies (asplenism), should also be performed at these time points. Detection of abnormal physical findings or test results should prompt subsequent examinations of the relevant organ system (e.g., presence of Howell-Jolly bodies indicates need for ultrasound of spleen).

TREATMENT APS-1

Therapy of individual disease components is carried out as outlined in other relevant chapters. Replacement of deficient hormones (e.g., adrenal, pancreas, ovaries/testes) will treat most of the endocrinopathies noted. Several unique issues merit special emphasis. Adrenal insufficiency can be masked by primary hypothyroidism by prolonging the half-life of cortisol. The caveat therefore is that replacement therapy with thyroid hormone can precipitate an adrenal crisis in an undiagnosed individual. Hence, all patients with hypothyroidism and the possibility of APS should be screened for adrenal insufficiency to allow treatment with glucocorticoids prior to the initiation of thyroid hormone replacement. Treatment of mucocutaneous candidiasis with ketoconazole in an individual with subclinical adrenal insufficiency may also precipitate adrenal crisis. Furthermore, mucocutaneous candidiasis may be difficult to eradicate entirely. Severe cases of disease involvement may require systemic immunomodulatory therapy, but this is not commonly needed.

APS-2

APS-2 (OMIM 269200) is more common than APS-1 with a prevalence of 1 in 100,000. It has a gender bias and occurs more often in female patients with a ratio of at least 3:1 compared to male patients. In contrast to APS-1, APS-2 often has its onset in adulthood with a peak incidence between 20 and 60 years of age. It shows a familial, multigenerational heritage (Table 30-2). The presence of two or more of the following endocrine deficiencies in the same patient defines the presence of APS-2: primary adrenal insufficiency (Addison's disease; 50–70%), Graves' disease or autoimmune thyroiditis (15–69%), type 1 diabetes mellitus (T1D; 40–50%), and primary hypogonadism. Frequently associated autoimmune conditions include celiac disease (3–15%), myasthenia gravis, vitiligo, alopecia, serositis, and pernicious anemia. These conditions occur with increased frequency in affected patients but are also are found in their family members (Table 30-3).

Genetic considerations

The overwhelming risk factor for APS-2 has been localized to the genes in the human lymphocyte antigen complex on chromosome 6. Primary adrenal insufficiency in APS-2, but not APS-1, is strongly associated with both HLA-DR3 and HLA-DR4. Other class I and class II genes and alleles, such as HLA-B8, HLA-DQ2 and HLA-DQ8, and HLA-DR subtype such as DRB1*0404, appear to contribute to organ-specific disease susceptibility (Table 30-4). HLA-B8- and HLA-DR3-associated illnesses include selective IgA deficiency, juvenile dermatomyositis, dermatitis herpetiformis, alopecia, scleroderma, autoimmune thrombocytopenia purpura, hypophysitis, metaphyseal osteopenia, and serositis.

Several other immune genes have been proposed to be associated with Addison's disease and therefore with APS-2 (Table 30-3). The "5.1" allele of a major histocompatibility complex (MHC) gene is an atypical class I HLA molecule MIC-A. The MIC-A5.1 allele has a very strong association with Addison's disease that is not accounted for by linkage disequilibrium with DR3 or DR4. Its role is complicated because certain HLA class I genes can offset this effect. PTPN22 codes for a polymorphism in a protein tyrosine phosphatase, which acts on intracellular signaling pathways in both T and B lymphocytes. It has been implicated in T1D, Addison's disease, and other autoimmune conditions. CTLA4 is a receptor on the T cell surface that modulates the activation state of the cell as part of the signal 2 pathway. Polymorphisms of this gene appear to cause downregulation of the cell surface expression of the receptor, leading to decreased T cell activation and proliferation. This appears to contribute to disease in Addison's disease and potentially other components of APS-2. Allelic variants of the IL-2Rα are linked to development of T1D and autoimmune thyroid disease and could contribute to the phenotype of APS-2 in certain individuals.

TABLE 30-4

APS-2 AND OTHER POLYENDOCRINE DISORDER ASSOCIATIONS

DISEASE	HLA ASSOCIATION	INITIATING FACTOR	MECHANISM	AUTOANTIGEN
Graves' Disease	DR3	Iodine Anti-CD52	Antibody	TSH receptor
Myasthenia gravis	DR3, DR7	Thymoma Penicillamine	Antibody	Acetylcholine receptor
Anti-insulin receptor	?	SLE or other autoimmune disease	Antibody	Insulin receptor
Hypoparathyroidism	?	?	Antibody	Cell surface inhibitor
Insulin autoimmune syndrome	DR4, DRB1*0406	Methimazole Sulfhydryl-containing drugs	Antibody	Insulin
Celiac disease	DQ2/DQ8	Gluten diet	T cell	Transglutaminase
Type 1 diabetes	DR3/DR4 DQ2/DQ8	? Congenital rubella	T cell	Insulin, GAD65, IA-2, ZnT8, IGRP
Addison's disease	DR3/DR4 DRB1*0404	Unknown	T cell	21-Hydroxylase P450-5cc
Thyroiditis	DR3/DQB1*0201 DQA1*0301	Iodine Interferon α	T cell	Thyroglobulin Thyroid peroxidase
Pernicious anemia	?	?	T cell	Intrinsic factor H+/K+ ATPase
Vitiligo	?	Melanoma Antigen Immunization	?	Melanocyte
Chromosome dysgenesis–trisomy 21 and Turner's syndrome	DQA1*0301	?	?	Thyroid, islet, transglutaminase
Hypophysitis	?	Pit-1, TDRD6	?	Pituitary, Pit-1

Abbreviations: APS, autoimmune polyendocrine syndrome; SLE, systemic lupus erythematosus; TSH, thyroid-stimulating hormone.

Diagnosis

When one of the component disorders is present, a second associated disorder occurs more commonly than in the general population (Table 30-3). There is controversy as to which tests to use and how often to screen individuals for disease. A strong family history of autoimmunity should raise suspicion in an individual with an initial component diagnosis. The development of a rarer form of autoimmunity, such as Addison's disease, should prompt more extensive screening for other linked disorders compared to the diagnosis of autoimmune thyroid disease, which is relatively common.

Circulating autoantibodies, as previously discussed, can precede the development of disease by many years but would allow the clinician to follow the patient and identify the disease onset at its earliest time point (Tables 30-3 and 30-4). For each of the endocrine components of the disorder, appropriate autoantibody assays are listed and, if positive, should prompt physiologic testing to diagnose clinical or subclinical disease. For Addison's disease, antibodies to 21-hydroxylase antibodies are highly diagnostic for risk of adrenal insufficiency. However, individuals may take many years to develop overt hypoadrenalism. Screening of 21-hydroxylase antibody–positive patients can be performed measuring morning ACTH and cortisol on a yearly basis. Rising ACTH values over time or low morning cortisol in association with signs or symptoms of adrenal insufficiency should prompt testing via the cosyntropin stimulation test **(Chap. 8)**. T1D can be screened for by measuring autoantibodies including anti-insulin, anti-GAD65, anti-IA-2, and anti-ZnT8. Risk for progression to disease can be based on the number of antibodies, and in some cases the titer (insulin autoantibody), as well as other metabolic factors (impaired oral glucose tolerance test). National Institutes of Health–sponsored trial groups such as Type 1 Diabetes TrialNet are screening first- and second-degree family members for these autoantibodies and identifying prediabetic individuals who may qualify for intervention trials to change the course of the disease prior to onset.

Screening tests for thyroid disease can include anti–thyroid peroxidase (TPO) or anti-thyroglobulin autoantibodies or anti-TSH receptor antibodies for Graves' disease. Yearly measurements of TSH can then be used to follow these individuals. Celiac disease can be screened for using the anti–tissue transglutaminase (tTg) antibody test. For those <20 years of age, testing every 1–2 years should be performed, whereas less frequent testing is indicated after the age of 20 because the majority of individuals who develop celiac disease have the antibody earlier in life. Positive tTg antibody test results should be confirmed on repeat testing, followed by small-bowel biopsy to document pathologic changes of celiac disease. Many patients have asymptomatic celiac disease that is nevertheless associated with osteopenia and impaired growth. If left untreated, symptomatic celiac disease has been reported to be associated with an increased risk of gastrointestinal malignancy, especially lymphoma.

The knowledge of the particular disease associations should guide other autoantibody or laboratory testing. A complete history and physical examination should be performed every 1–3 years including CBC, metabolic panel, TSH, and vitamin B_{12} levels to screen for most of the possible abnormalities. More specific tests should be based on specific findings from the history and physical.

TREATMENT APS-2

With the exception of Graves' disease, the management of each of the endocrine components of APS-2 involves hormone replacement and is covered in detail in the chapters on adrenal **(Chap. 8)**, thyroid **(Chap. 7)**, gonadal **(Chaps. 11 and 13)**, and parathyroid disease **(Chap. 34)**. As noted for APS-1, adrenal insufficiency can be masked by primary hypothyroidism and should be considered and treated as discussed above. In patients with T1D, decreasing insulin requirements or hypoglycemia, without obvious secondary causes, may indicate the emergence of adrenal insufficiency. Hypocalcemia in APS-2 patients is more likely due to malabsorption than hypoparathyroidism.

Immunotherapy for autoimmune endocrine disease has been reserved for T1D, for the most part, reflecting the lifetime burden of the disease for the individual patient and society. Although several immunotherapies (e.g., modified anti-CD3, rituximab, abatacept) can prolong the honeymoon phase of T1D, none has achieved long-term success. Active research using new approaches and combination therapy may change the treatment of this disease or other autoimmune conditions that share similar pathways. Furthermore, treatment of subclinical disease diagnosed by the presence of autoantibodies may provide a mechanism to preempt the development of overt disease and is the subject of active basic and clinical research.

IPEX

*I*mmune dysregulation, *p*olyendocrinopathy, *e*nteropathy, and *X*-linked disease (IPEX; OMIM 304790) is a rare X-linked recessive disorder. The disease onset is in infancy and is characterized by severe enteropathy, T1D, and skin disease, as well as variable association with several other autoimmune disorders. Many infants die within the first days of life, but the course is variable, with some children surviving for 12–15 years. Early onset of T1D, often at birth, is highly suggestive of the diagnosis because nearly 80% of IPEX patients develop T1D. Although treatment of the individual disorders can temporarily improve the situation, treatment of the underlying immune deficiency is required and includes immunosuppressive therapy generally followed by hematopoietic stem cell transplantation. Transplantation is the only life-saving form of therapy and can be fully curative by normalizing the imbalanced immune system found in this disorder.

IPEX is caused by mutations in the *FOXP3* gene, which is also mutated in the Scurfy mouse, an animal model that shares much of the phenotype of IPEX patients. The FOXP3 transcription factor is expressed in regulatory T cells designated CD4+CD25+FOXP3+ (Treg). Lack of this factor causes a profound deficiency of this Treg population and results in rampant autoimmunity due to the lack of peripheral tolerance normally provided by these cells. Certain mutations may lead to varying forms of expression of the full syndrome, and there are rare cases where the *FOXP3* gene is intact but other genes involved in this pathway (e.g., CD25, IL-2Rα) may be causative.

THYMIC TUMORS

Thymomas and thymic hyperplasia are associated with several autoimmune diseases, with the most common being myasthenia gravis (44%) and red cell aplasia (20%). Graves' disease, T1D, and Addison's disease may also be associated with thymic tumors. Patients with myasthenia gravis and thymoma may have unique anti–acetylcholine receptor autoantibodies. Many thymomas lack AIRE expression within the thymoma, and this could be a potential factor in the development of autoimmunity. In support of this concept, thymoma is the one other disease with "frequent" development of anticytokine antibodies and mucocutaneous candidiasis in adults. The majority of tumors are malignant, and temporary remissions of the autoimmune condition can occur with resection of the tumor.

ANTI-INSULIN RECEPTOR ANTIBODIES

This is a very rare disorder where severe insulin resistance (type B) is caused by the presence of anti-insulin receptor antibodies. It is associated with acanthosis nigricans, which can also be associated with other forms of less severe insulin resistance. About one-third of patients have an associated autoimmune illness such as systemic lupus erythematosus or Sjögren's syndrome. Therefore, the presence of antinuclear antibodies, elevated erythrocyte sedimentation rate, hyperglobulinemia, leukopenia, and hypocomplementemia may accompany the presentation. The presence of anti-insulin receptor autoantibodies leads to marked insulin resistance, requiring more than 100,000 units of insulin to be given daily with only partial control of hyperglycemia. Patients can also have severe hypoglycemia due to partial activation of the insulin receptor by the antibody. The course of the disease is variable, and several patients have had spontaneous remissions. Therapy targeting B lymphocytes including rituximab, cyclophosphamide, and pulse steroids can induce remission of the disease.

INSULIN AUTOIMMUNE SYNDROME (HIRATA'S SYNDROME)

The insulin autoimmune syndrome, associated with Graves' disease and methimazole therapy (or other sulfhydryl-containing medications), is of particular interest due to a remarkably strong association with a specific HLA haplotype. Such patients with elevated titers of anti-insulin autoantibodies frequently present with hypoglycemia. In Japan, the disease is restricted to HLA-DR4-positive individuals with DRB1*0406. Curiously, a recent report demonstrated that five out of six Caucasian patients taking lipoic acid (sulfhydryl group) who developed insulin autoimmune syndrome were primarily DRB1*0403 (which is related to DRB1*0406); the sixth was DRB1*0406. In Hirata's syndrome the anti-insulin autoantibodies are often polyclonal. Discontinuation of the medication generally leads to resolution of the syndrome over time.

POEMS SYNDROME

POEMS (*p*olyneuropathy, *o*rganomegaly, *e*ndocrinopathy, *M*-protein, and *s*kin changes; also known as Crow-Fukase syndrome; OMIM 192240) patients usually present with a progressive sensorimotor polyneuropathy, diabetes mellitus (50%), primary gonadal failure (70%), and a plasma cell dyscrasia with sclerotic bony lesions. Associated findings can be hepatosplenomegaly, lymphadenopathy, and hyperpigmentation. Patients often present in the fifth to sixth decade of life and have a median survival after diagnosis of less than 3 years. The syndrome is assumed to be secondary to circulating immunoglobulins, but patients have excess vascular endothelial growth factor as well as elevated levels of other inflammatory cytokines such as IL1-β, IL-6, and tumor necrosis factor α. A small series of patients have been treated with thalidomide, leading to a decrease in vascular endothelial growth factor. Hyperglycemia responds to small, subcutaneous doses of insulin. The hypogonadism is due to primary gonadal disease with elevated plasma levels of follicle-stimulating hormone and luteinizing hormone. Temporary resolution of the features of POEMS, including normalization of blood glucose, may occur after radiotherapy for localized plasma cell lesions of bone or after chemotherapy, thalidomide, plasmapheresis, autologous stem cell transplantation, or treatment with all-*trans*-retinoic acid.

OTHER DISORDERS

Other diseases can exhibit polyendocrine deficiencies, including Kearns-Sayre syndrome, DIDMOAD syndrome (*d*iabetes *i*nsipidus, *d*iabetes *m*ellitus, progressive bilateral *o*ptic *a*trophy, and sensorineural *d*eafness; also termed Wolfram's syndrome), Down's syndrome or trisomy 21 (OMIM 190685), Turner's syndrome (monosomy X, 45,X), and congenital rubella.

Kearns-Sayre syndrome (OMIM 530000) is a rare mitochondrial DNA disorder characterized by myopathic abnormalities leading to ophthalmoplegia and progressive weakness in association with several endocrine abnormalities, including hypoparathyroidism, primary gonadal failure, diabetes mellitus, and hypopituitarism. Crystalline mitochondrial inclusions are found in muscle biopsy specimens, and such inclusions have also been observed in the cerebellum. Antiparathyroid antibodies have not been described; however, antibodies to the anterior pituitary gland and striated muscle have been identified, and the disease may have autoimmune components. These mitochondrial DNA mutations occur sporadically and do not appear to be associated with a familial syndrome.

Wolfram's syndrome (OMIM 222300, chromosome 4; OMIM 598500, mitochondrial) is a rare autosomal recessive disease that is also called DIDMOAD. Neurologic and psychiatric disturbances are prominent in most patients and can cause severe disability. The disease is caused by defects in wolframin, a 100-kDa transmembrane protein that has been localized to the endoplasmic reticulum and is found in neuronal and neuroendocrine tissue. Its expression induces ion channel activity with a resultant increase in intracellular calcium and may play an important role in intracellular calcium homeostasis. Wolfram's syndrome appears to be a slowly progressive neurodegenerative process, and there is nonautoimmune selective destruction of the pancreatic beta cells. Diabetes mellitus with an onset in childhood is usually the first manifestation. Diabetes mellitus and optic atrophy are present in all reported cases, but expression of the other features is variable.

Down's syndrome, or trisomy 21 (OMIM 190685), is associated with the development of T1D, thyroiditis, and celiac disease. Patients with Turner's syndrome also appear to be at increased risk for the development of thyroid disease and celiac disease. It is recommended to screen patients with trisomy 21 and Turner's syndrome for associated autoimmune diseases on a regular basis.

CHAPTER 31

PARANEOPLASTIC SYNDROMES: ENDOCRINOLOGIC/HEMATOLOGIC

J. Larry Jameson ■ Dan L. Longo

Neoplastic cells can produce a variety of products that can stimulate hormonal, hematologic, dermatologic, and neurologic responses. *Paraneoplastic syndromes* is the term used to refer to the disorders that accompany benign or malignant tumors but are not directly related to mass effects or invasion. Tumors of neuroendocrine origin, such as small-cell lung carcinoma (SCLC) and carcinoids, produce a wide array of peptide hormones and are common causes of paraneoplastic syndromes. However, almost every type of tumor has the potential to produce hormones or to induce cytokine and immunologic responses. Careful studies of the prevalence of paraneoplastic syndromes indicate that they are more common than is generally appreciated. The signs, symptoms, and metabolic alterations associated with paraneoplastic disorders may be overlooked in the context of a malignancy and its treatment. Consequently, atypical clinical manifestations in a patient with cancer should prompt consideration of a paraneoplastic syndrome. The most common endocrinologic and hematologic syndromes associated with underlying neoplasia will be discussed here.

ENDOCRINE PARANEOPLASTIC SYNDROMES

Etiology

Hormones can be produced from eutopic or ectopic sources. *Eutopic* refers to the expression of a hormone from its normal tissue of origin, whereas *ectopic* refers to hormone production from an atypical tissue source. For example, adrenocorticotropic hormone (ACTH) is expressed eutopically by the corticotrope cells of the anterior pituitary, but it can be expressed ectopically in SCLC. Many hormones are produced at low levels from a wide array of tissues in addition to the classic endocrine source. Thus, ectopic expression is often a quantitative change rather than an absolute change in tissue expression. Nevertheless, the term *ectopic expression* is firmly entrenched and conveys the abnormal physiology associated with hormone production by neoplastic cells. In addition to high levels of hormones, ectopic expression typically is characterized by abnormal regulation of hormone production (e.g., defective feedback control) and peptide processing (resulting in large, unprocessed precursors).

A diverse array of molecular mechanisms has been suggested to cause ectopic hormone production. In rare instances, genetic rearrangements explain aberrant hormone expression. For example, translocation of the parathyroid hormone (*PTH*) gene can result in high levels of PTH expression in tissues other than the parathyroid gland because the genetic rearrangement brings the *PTH* gene under the control of atypical regulatory elements. A related phenomenon is well documented in many forms of leukemia and lymphoma, in which somatic genetic rearrangements confer a growth advantage and alter cellular differentiation and function. Although genetic rearrangements cause selected cases of ectopic hormone production, this mechanism is rare, as many tumors are associated with excessive production of numerous peptides. Cellular dedifferentiation probably underlies most cases of ectopic hormone production. Many cancers are poorly differentiated, and certain tumor products, such as human chorionic gonadotropin (hCG), parathyroid hormone–related protein (PTHrP), and α fetoprotein, are characteristic of gene expression at earlier developmental stages. In contrast, the propensity of certain cancers to produce particular hormones (e.g., squamous cell carcinomas produce PTHrP) suggests that dedifferentiation is partial or that selective pathways are derepressed. These expression profiles probably reflect epigenetic modifications that alter transcriptional repression, microRNA expression, and other pathways that govern cell differentiation.

In SCLC, the pathway of differentiation has been relatively well defined. The neuroendocrine phenotype is dictated in part by the basic-helix-loop-helix (bHLH) transcription factor human achaete-scute homologue 1 (hASH-1), which is expressed at abnormally high levels in SCLC associated with ectopic ACTH. The activity of hASH-1 is inhibited by hairy enhancer of split 1 (HES-1) and by Notch proteins, which also are capable of inducing growth arrest. Thus, abnormal expression of these developmental transcription factors appears to provide a link between cell proliferation and differentiation.

Ectopic hormone production would be merely an epiphenomenon associated with cancer if it did not result in clinical manifestations. Excessive and unregulated production of hormones such as ACTH, PTHrP, and vasopressin can lead to substantial morbidity and complicate the cancer treatment plan. Moreover, the paraneoplastic endocrinopathies may be a presenting clinical feature of underlying malignancy and prompt the search for an unrecognized tumor.

A large number of paraneoplastic endocrine syndromes have been described, linking overproduction of particular hormones with specific types of tumors. However, certain recurring syndromes emerge from this group (Table 31-1). The most common paraneoplastic endocrine syndromes include hypercalcemia from overproduction of PTHrP and other factors, hyponatremia from excess vasopressin, and Cushing's syndrome from ectopic ACTH.

HYPERCALCEMIA CAUSED BY ECTOPIC PRODUCTION OF PTHRP

(See also Chap. 34)

Etiology

Humoral hypercalcemia of malignancy (HHM) occurs in up to 20% of patients with cancer. HHM is most common in cancers of the lung, head and neck, skin, esophagus, breast, and genitourinary tract and in multiple myeloma and lymphomas. There are several distinct humoral causes of HHM, but it is caused most commonly by overproduction of PTHrP. In addition to acting as a circulating humoral factor, bone metastases (e.g., breast, multiple myeloma) may produce PTHrP, leading to local osteolysis and hypercalcemia. PTHrP may also affect the initiation and progression of tumors by acting through pro-survival and chemokine pathways.

PTHrP is structurally related to PTH and binds to the PTH receptor, explaining the similar biochemical features of HHM and hyperparathyroidism. PTHrP plays a key role in skeletal development and regulates cellular proliferation and differentiation in other tissues, including skin, bone marrow, breast, and hair follicles. The mechanism of PTHrP induction in malignancy is incompletely understood; however, tumor-bearing tissues commonly associated with HHM normally produce PTHrP during development or cell renewal. PTHrP expression is stimulated by hedgehog pathways and Gli transcription factors that are active in many malignancies. Transforming growth factor β (TGF-β), which is produced by many tumors, also stimulates PTHrP, in part by activating the Gli pathway. Mutations in certain oncogenes, such as *Ras*, also can activate PTHrP expression. In adult T cell lymphoma, the transactivating Tax protein produced by human T cell lymphotropic virus 1 (HTLV-1) stimulates PTHrP promoter activity. Metastatic lesions to bone are more likely to produce PTHrP than are metastases in other tissues, suggesting that bone produces factors (e.g., TGF-β) that enhance PTHrP production or that PTHrP-producing metastases have a selective growth advantage in bone. PTHrP activates the pro-survival AKT pathway and the chemokine receptor CXCR4. Thus, PTHrP production can be stimulated by mutations in oncogenes, altered expression of viral or cellular transcription factors, and local growth factors. In addition to its role in HHM, the PTHrP pathway may also provide a potential target for therapeutic intervention to impede cancer growth.

Another relatively common cause of HHM is excess production of 1,25-dihydroxyvitamin D. Like granulomatous disorders associated with hypercalcemia, lymphomas can produce an enzyme that converts 25-hydroxyvitamin D to the more active 1,25-dihydroxyvitamin D, leading to enhanced gastrointestinal calcium absorption. Other causes of HHM include tumor-mediated production of osteolytic cytokines and inflammatory mediators.

Clinical manifestations

The typical presentation of HHM is a patient with a known malignancy who is found to be hypercalcemic on routine laboratory tests. Less often, hypercalcemia is the initial presenting feature of malignancy. Particularly when calcium levels are markedly increased (>3.5 mmol/L [>14 mg/dL]), patients may experience fatigue, mental status changes, dehydration, or symptoms of nephrolithiasis.

Diagnosis

Features that favor HHM, as opposed to primary hyperparathyroidism, include known malignancy, recent onset of hypercalcemia, and very high serum calcium levels.

TABLE 31-1

PARANEOPLASTIC SYNDROMES CAUSED BY ECTOPIC HORMONE PRODUCTION

PARANEOPLASTIC SYNDROME	ECTOPIC HORMONE	TYPICAL TUMOR TYPES[a]
Common		
Hypercalcemia of malignancy	Parathyroid hormone–related protein (PTHrP)	Squamous cell (head and neck, lung, skin), breast, genitourinary, gastrointestinal
	1,25-dihydroxyvitamin D	Lymphomas
	Parathyroid hormone (PTH) (rare)	Lung, ovary
	Prostaglandin E_2 (PGE_2) (rare)	Renal, lung
Syndrome of inappropriate antidiuretic hormone secretion (SIADH)	Vasopressin	Lung (squamous, small cell), gastrointestinal, genitourinary, ovary
Cushing's syndrome	Adrenocorticotropic hormone (ACTH)	Lung (small cell, bronchial carcinoid, adenocarcinoma, squamous), thymus, pancreatic islet, medullary thyroid carcinoma
	Corticotropin-releasing hormone (CRH) (rare)	Pancreatic islet, carcinoid, lung, prostate
	Ectopic expression of gastric inhibitory peptide (GIP), luteinizing hormone (LH)/human chorionic gonadotropin (hCG), other G protein–coupled receptors (rare)	Macronodular adrenal hyperplasia
Less Common		
Non–islet cell hypoglycemia	Insulin-like growth factor type II (IGF-II)	Mesenchymal tumors, sarcomas, adrenal, hepatic, gastrointestinal, kidney, prostate
	Insulin (rare)	Cervix (small-cell carcinoma)
Male feminization	hCG[b]	Testis (embryonal, seminomas), germinomas, choriocarcinoma, lung, hepatic, pancreatic islet
Diarrhea or intestinal hypermotility	Calcitonin[c]	Lung, colon, breast, medullary thyroid carcinoma
	Vasoactive intestinal peptide (VIP)	Pancreas, pheochromocytoma, esophagus
Rare		
Oncogenic osteomalacia	Phosphatonin (fibroblast growth factor 23 [FGF23])	Hemangiopericytomas, osteoblastomas, fibromas, sarcomas, giant cell tumors, prostate, lung
Acromegaly	Growth hormone–releasing hormone (GHRH)	Pancreatic islet, bronchial, and other carcinoids
	Growth hormone (GH)	Lung, pancreatic islet
Hyperthyroidism	Thyroid-stimulating hormone (TSH)	Hydatidiform mole, embryonal tumors, struma ovarii
Hypertension	Renin	Juxtaglomerular tumors, kidney, lung, pancreas, ovary

[a]Only the most common tumor types are listed. For most ectopic hormone syndromes, an extensive list of tumors has been reported to produce one or more hormones.

[b]hCG is produced eutopically by trophoblastic tumors. Certain tumors produce disproportionate amounts of the hCG α or hCG β subunit. High levels of hCG rarely cause hyperthyroidism because of weak binding to the TSH receptor.

[c]Calcitonin is produced eutopically by medullary thyroid carcinoma and is used as a tumor marker.

Like hyperparathyroidism, hypercalcemia caused by PTHrP is accompanied by hypercalciuria and hypophosphatemia. Patients with HHM typically have metabolic alkalosis rather than hyperchloremic acidosis, as is seen in hyperparathyroidism. Measurement of PTH is useful to exclude primary hyperparathyroidism; the PTH level should be suppressed in HHM. An elevated PTHrP level confirms the diagnosis, and it is increased in ~80% of hypercalcemic patients with cancer. 1,25-Dihydroxyvitamin D levels may be increased in patients with lymphoma.

TREATMENT Humoral Hypercalcemia of Malignancy

The management of HHM begins with removal of excess calcium in the diet, medications, or IV solutions. Saline rehydration (typically 200–500 mL/h) is used to dilute serum calcium and promote calciuresis; exercise caution in patients with cardiac, hepatic, or renal insufficiency. Forced diuresis with furosemide (20–80 mg IV in escalating doses) or other loop diuretics can enhance calcium excretion but provides relatively little value except in life-threatening hypercalcemia. When used, loop diuretics should be administered only after complete rehydration and with careful monitoring of fluid balance. Oral phosphorus (e.g., 250 mg Neutra-Phos 3–4 times daily) should be given until serum phosphorus is >1 mmol/L (>3 mg/dL). Bisphosphonates such as pamidronate (60–90 mg IV), zoledronate (4–8 mg IV), and etidronate (7.5 mg/kg per day PO for 3–7 consecutive days) can reduce serum calcium within 1–2 days and suppress calcium release for several weeks. Bisphosphonate infusions can be repeated, or oral bisphosphonates can be used for chronic treatment. Dialysis should be considered in severe hypercalcemia when saline hydration and bisphosphonate treatments are not possible or are too slow in onset. Previously used agents such as calcitonin and mithramycin have little utility now that bisphosphonates are available. Calcitonin (2–8 U/kg SC every 6–12 h) should be considered when rapid correction of severe hypercalcemia is needed. Hypercalcemia associated with lymphomas, multiple myeloma, or leukemia may respond to glucocorticoid treatment (e.g., prednisone 40–100 mg PO in four divided doses).

ECTOPIC VASOPRESSIN: TUMOR-ASSOCIATED SIADH

Etiology

Vasopressin is an antidiuretic hormone normally produced by the posterior pituitary gland. Ectopic vasopressin production by tumors is a common cause of the syndrome of inappropriate antidiuretic hormone (SIADH), occurring in at least half of patients with SCLC. SIADH also can be caused by a number of nonneoplastic conditions, including central nervous system (CNS) trauma, infections, and medications (**Chap. 6**). Compensatory responses to SIADH, such as decreased thirst, may mitigate the development of hyponatremia. However, with prolonged production of excessive vasopressin, the osmostat controlling thirst and hypothalamic vasopressin secretion may become reset. In addition, intake of free water, orally or intravenously, can quickly worsen hyponatremia because of reduced renal diuresis.

Tumors with neuroendocrine features, such as SCLC and carcinoids, are the most common sources of ectopic vasopressin production, but it also occurs in other forms of lung cancer and with CNS lesions, head and neck cancer, and genitourinary, gastrointestinal, and ovarian cancers. The mechanism of activation of the vasopressin gene in these tumors is unknown but often involves concomitant expression of the adjacent oxytocin gene, suggesting derepression of this locus.

Clinical manifestations

Most patients with ectopic vasopressin secretion are asymptomatic and are identified because of the presence of hyponatremia on routine chemistry testing. Symptoms may include weakness, lethargy, nausea, confusion, depressed mental status, and seizures. The severity of symptoms reflects the rapidity of onset as well as the severity of hyponatremia. Hyponatremia usually develops slowly but may be exacerbated by the administration of IV fluids or the institution of new medications.

Diagnosis

The diagnostic features of ectopic vasopressin production are the same as those of other causes of SIADH (**Chap. 6**). Hyponatremia and reduced serum osmolality occur in the setting of an inappropriately normal or increased urine osmolality. Urine sodium excretion is normal or increased unless volume depletion is present. Other causes of hyponatremia should be excluded, including renal, adrenal, or thyroid insufficiency. Physiologic sources of vasopressin stimulation (CNS lesions, pulmonary disease, nausea), adaptive circulatory mechanisms (hypotension, heart failure, hepatic cirrhosis), and medications, including many chemotherapeutic agents, also should be considered as possible causes of hyponatremia. Vasopressin measurements are not usually necessary to make the diagnosis.

TREATMENT Ectopic Vasopressin: Tumor-Associated SIADH

Most patients with ectopic vasopressin production develop hyponatremia over several weeks or months. The disorder should be corrected gradually unless mental status is altered or there is risk of seizures. Treatment of the underlying malignancy may reduce ectopic vasopressin production, but this response is slow if it occurs at all. Fluid restriction to less than urine output, plus insensible losses, is often sufficient to correct hyponatremia partially. However, strict monitoring of the amount and types of liquids consumed or administered intravenously is required for fluid restriction to be effective. Salt tablets and saline are not helpful unless volume depletion is also present. Demeclocycline (150–300 mg orally three to four times daily) can be used to inhibit vasopressin action on the renal distal tubule, but its onset of action is relatively slow (1–2 weeks). Conivaptan, a nonpeptide V_2-receptor antagonist, can be administered either PO (20–120 mg bid) or IV (10–40 mg) and is particularly effective when used in combination with fluid restriction in euvolemic hyponatremia. Tolvaptan (15 mg PO daily) is another vasopressin antagonist. The dose can be increased to 30–60 mg/d based on response. Severe hyponatremia (Na <115 meq/L) or mental status changes may require treatment with hypertonic (3%) or normal saline infusion together with furosemide to enhance free water clearance. The rate of sodium correction should be slow (0.5–1 meq/L per hour) to prevent rapid fluid shifts and the possible development of central pontine myelinolysis.

CUSHING'S SYNDROME CAUSED BY ECTOPIC ACTH PRODUCTION

(See also Chap. 8)

Etiology

Ectopic ACTH production accounts for 10–20% of cases of Cushing's syndrome. The syndrome is particularly common in neuroendocrine tumors. SCLC is the most common cause of ectopic ACTH, followed by bronchial and thymic carcinoids, islet cell tumors, other carcinoids, and pheochromocytomas. Ectopic ACTH production is caused by increased expression of the proopiomelanocortin (*POMC*) gene, which encodes ACTH, along with melanocyte-stimulating hormone (MSH), β lipotropin, and several other peptides. In many tumors, there is abundant but aberrant expression of the *POMC* gene from an internal promoter, proximal to the third exon, which encodes ACTH. However, because this product lacks the signal sequence necessary for protein processing, it is not secreted. Increased production of ACTH arises instead from less abundant, but unregulated, *POMC* expression from the same promoter site used in the pituitary. However, because the tumors lack many of the enzymes needed to process the POMC polypeptide, it is typically released as multiple large, biologically inactive fragments along with relatively small amounts of fully processed, active ACTH.

Rarely, corticotropin-releasing hormone (CRH) is produced by pancreatic islet cell tumors, SCLC, medullary thyroid cancer, carcinoids, or prostate cancer. When levels are high enough, CRH can cause pituitary corticotrope hyperplasia and Cushing's syndrome. Tumors that produce CRH sometimes also produce ACTH, raising the possibility of a paracrine mechanism for ACTH production.

A distinct mechanism for ACTH-independent Cushing's syndrome involves ectopic expression of various G protein–coupled receptors in the adrenal nodules. Ectopic expression of the gastric inhibitory peptide (GIP) receptor is the best-characterized example of this mechanism. In this case, meals induce GIP secretion, which inappropriately stimulates adrenal growth and glucocorticoid production.

Clinical manifestations

The clinical features of hypercortisolemia are detected in only a small fraction of patients with documented ectopic ACTH production. Patients with ectopic ACTH syndrome generally exhibit less marked weight gain and centripetal fat redistribution, probably because the exposure to excess glucocorticoids is relatively brief and because cachexia reduces the propensity for weight gain and fat deposition. The ectopic ACTH syndrome is associated with several clinical features that distinguish it from other causes of Cushing's syndrome (e.g., pituitary adenomas, adrenal adenomas, iatrogenic glucocorticoid excess). The metabolic manifestations of ectopic ACTH syndrome are dominated by fluid retention and hypertension, hypokalemia, metabolic alkalosis, glucose intolerance, and occasionally steroid psychosis. The very high ACTH levels often cause increased pigmentation, and melanotrope-stimulating hormone (MSH) activity derived from the POMC precursor peptide is also increased. The extraordinarily high glucocorticoid levels in patients with ectopic sources of ACTH can lead to marked skin fragility and easy bruising. In addition, the high cortisol levels often overwhelm the renal 11β-hydroxysteroid dehydrogenase type II enzyme, which normally inactivates cortisol and prevents it from binding to renal mineralocorticoid receptors. Consequently, in addition to the excess mineralocorticoids produced by ACTH stimulation of the adrenal gland, high levels of cortisol exert activity through the mineralocorticoid receptor, leading to severe hypokalemia.

Diagnosis

The diagnosis of ectopic ACTH syndrome is usually not difficult in the setting of a known malignancy. Urine free cortisol levels fluctuate but are typically greater than two to four times normal, and the plasma ACTH level is usually >22 pmol/L (>100 pg/mL). A suppressed ACTH level excludes this diagnosis and indicates an

ACTH-independent cause of Cushing's syndrome (e.g., adrenal or exogenous glucocorticoid). In contrast to pituitary sources of ACTH, most ectopic sources of ACTH do not respond to glucocorticoid suppression. Therefore, high-dose dexamethasone (8 mg PO) suppresses 8:00 A.M. serum cortisol (50% decrease from baseline) in ~80% of pituitary ACTH-producing adenomas but fails to suppress ectopic ACTH in ~90% of cases. Bronchial and other carcinoids are well-documented exceptions to these general guidelines, as these ectopic sources of ACTH may exhibit feedback regulation indistinguishable from pituitary adenomas, including suppression by high-dose dexamethasone, and ACTH responsiveness to adrenal blockade with metyrapone. If necessary, petrosal sinus catheterization can be used to evaluate a patient with ACTH-dependent Cushing's syndrome when the source of ACTH is unclear. After CRH stimulation, a 3:1 petrosal sinus:peripheral ACTH ratio strongly suggests a pituitary ACTH source. Imaging studies (computed tomography or magnetic resonance imaging) are also useful in the evaluation of suspected carcinoid lesions, allowing biopsy and characterization of hormone production using special stains. If available, positron emission tomography or octreotide scanning may identify some sources of ACTH production.

TREATMENT Cushing's Syndrome Caused by Ectopic ACTH Production

The morbidity associated with the ectopic ACTH syndrome can be substantial. Patients may experience depression or personality changes because of extreme cortisol excess. Metabolic derangements, including diabetes mellitus and hypokalemia, can worsen fatigue. Poor wound healing and predisposition to infections can complicate the surgical management of tumors, and opportunistic infections caused by organisms such as *Pneumocystis carinii* and mycoses are often the cause of death in patients with ectopic ACTH production. These patients likely have increased risk of venous thromboembolism reflecting the combination of malignancy and altered coagulation factor profiles. Depending on prognosis and treatment plans for the underlying malignancy, measures to reduce cortisol levels are often indicated. Treatment of the underlying malignancy may reduce ACTH levels but is rarely sufficient to reduce cortisol levels to normal. Adrenalectomy is not practical for most of these patients but should be considered during surgery for the malignancy or if the underlying tumor is not resectable and the prognosis is otherwise favorable (e.g., carcinoid). Medical therapy with ketoconazole (300–600 mg PO bid), metyrapone (250–500 mg PO every 6 h), mitotane (3–6 g PO in four divided doses, tapered to maintain low cortisol production), or other agents that block steroid synthesis or action is often the most practical strategy for managing the hypercortisolism associated with ectopic ACTH production. Glucocorticoid replacement should be provided to prevent adrenal insufficiency **(Chap. 8)**. Unfortunately, many patients eventually progress despite medical blockade.

TUMOR-INDUCED HYPOGLYCEMIA CAUSED BY EXCESS PRODUCTION OF IGF-II

(See also Chap. 26) Mesenchymal tumors, hemangiopericytomas, hepatocellular tumors, adrenal carcinomas, and a variety of other large tumors have been reported to produce excessive amounts of insulin-like growth factor type II (IGF-II) precursor, which binds weakly to insulin receptors and more strongly to IGF-I receptors, leading to insulin-like actions. The gene encoding IGF-II resides on a chromosome 11p15 locus that is normally imprinted (that is, expression is exclusively from a single parental allele). Biallelic expression of the IGF-II gene occurs in a subset of tumors, suggesting loss of methylation and loss of imprinting as a mechanism for gene induction. In addition to increased IGF-II production, IGF-II bioavailability is increased due to complex alterations in circulating binding proteins. Increased IGF-II suppresses growth hormone (GH) and insulin, resulting in reduced IGF binding protein 3 (IGFBP-3), IGF-I, and acid-labile subunit (ALS). The reduction in ALS and IGFBP-3, which normally sequester IGF-II, causes it to be displaced to a small circulating complex that has greater access to insulin target tissues. For this reason, circulating IGF-II levels may not be markedly increased despite causing hypoglycemia. In addition to IGF-II–mediated hypoglycemia, tumors may occupy enough of the liver to impair gluconeogenesis.

In most cases, a tumor causing hypoglycemia is clinically apparent (usually >10 cm in size) and hypoglycemia develops in association with fasting. The diagnosis is made by documenting low serum glucose and suppressed insulin levels in association with symptoms of hypoglycemia. Serum IGF-II levels may not be increased (IGF-II assays may not detect IGF-II precursors). Increased IGF-II mRNA expression is found in most of these tumors. Any medications associated with hypoglycemia should be eliminated. Treatment of the underlying malignancy, if possible, may reduce the predisposition to hypoglycemia. Frequent meals and IV glucose, especially during sleep or fasting, are often necessary to prevent hypoglycemia. Glucagon and glucocorticoids have also been used to enhance glucose production.

HUMAN CHORIONIC GONADOTROPIN

hCG is composed of α and β subunits and can be produced as intact hormone, which is biologically active, or as uncombined biologically inert subunits. Ectopic production of intact hCG occurs most often in association with testicular embryonal tumors, germ cell tumors, extragonadal germinomas, lung cancer, hepatoma, and pancreatic islet tumors. Eutopic production of hCG occurs with trophoblastic malignancies. hCG α subunit production is particularly common in lung cancer and pancreatic islet cancer. In men, high hCG levels stimulate steroidogenesis and aromatase activity in testicular Leydig cells, resulting in increased estrogen production and the development of gynecomastia. Precocious puberty in boys or gynecomastia in men should prompt measurement of hCG and consideration of a testicular tumor or another source of ectopic hCG production. Most women are asymptomatic. hCG is easily measured. Treatment should be directed at the underlying malignancy.

ONCOGENIC OSTEOMALACIA

Hypophosphatemic oncogenic osteomalacia, also called tumor-induced osteomalacia (TIO), is characterized by markedly reduced serum phosphorus and renal phosphate wasting, leading to muscle weakness, bone pain, and osteomalacia. Serum calcium and PTH levels are normal, and 1,25-dihydroxyvitamin D is low. Oncogenic osteomalacia is usually caused by benign mesenchymal tumors, such as hemangiopericytomas, fibromas, and giant cell tumors, often of the skeletal extremities or head. It has also been described in sarcomas and in patients with prostate and lung cancer. Resection of the tumor reverses the disorder, confirming its humoral basis. The circulating phosphaturic factor is called *phosphatonin*—a factor that inhibits renal tubular reabsorption of phosphate and renal conversion of 25-hydroxyvitamin D to 1,25-dihydroxyvitamin D. Phosphatonin has been identified as fibroblast growth factor 23 (FGF23). FGF23 levels are increased in some, but not all, patients with osteogenic osteomalacia. FGF23 forms a ternary complex with the klotho protein and renal FGF receptors to reduce renal phosphate reabsorption. Treatment involves removal of the tumor, if possible, and supplementation with phosphate and vitamin D. Octreotide treatment reduces phosphate wasting in some patients with tumors that express somatostatin receptor subtype 2. Octreotide scans may also be useful in detecting these tumors.

HEMATOLOGIC SYNDROMES

The elevation of granulocyte, platelet, and eosinophil counts in most patients with myeloproliferative disorders is caused by the proliferation of the myeloid elements due to the underlying disease rather than to a paraneoplastic syndrome. The paraneoplastic hematologic syndromes in patients with solid tumors are less well characterized than are the endocrine syndromes because the ectopic hormone(s) or cytokines responsible have not been identified in most of these tumors (Table 31-2). The extent of the paraneoplastic syndromes parallels the course of the cancer.

TABLE 31-2
PARANEOPLASTIC HEMATOLOGIC SYNDROMES

SYNDROME	PROTEINS	CANCERS TYPICALLY ASSOCIATED WITH SYNDROME
Erythrocytosis	Erythropoietin	Renal cancers, hepatocarcinoma, cerebellar hemangioblastomas
Granulocytosis	G-CSF, GM-CSF, IL-6	Lung cancer, gastrointestinal cancer, ovarian cancer, genitourinary cancer, Hodgkin's disease
Thrombocytosis	IL-6	Lung cancer, gastrointestinal cancer, breast cancer, ovarian cancer, lymphoma
Eosinophilia	IL-5	Lymphoma, leukemia, lung cancer
Thrombophlebitis	Unknown	Lung cancer, pancreatic cancer, gastrointestinal cancer, breast cancer, genitourinary cancer, ovarian cancer, prostate cancer, lymphoma

Abbreviations: G-CSF, granulocyte colony-stimulating factor; GM-CSF, granulocyte-macrophage colony-stimulating factor; IL, interleukin.

ERYTHROCYTOSIS

Ectopic production of erythropoietin by cancer cells causes most paraneoplastic erythrocytosis. The ectopically produced erythropoietin stimulates the production of red blood cells (RBCs) in the bone marrow and raises the hematocrit. Other lymphokines and hormones produced by cancer cells may stimulate erythropoietin release but have not been proved to cause erythrocytosis.

Most patients with erythrocytosis have an elevated hematocrit (>52% in men, >48% in women) that is detected on a routine blood count. Approximately 3% of patients with renal cell cancer, 10% of patients with hepatoma, and 15% of patients with cerebellar hemangioblastomas have erythrocytosis. In most cases, the erythrocytosis is asymptomatic.

Patients with erythrocytosis due to a renal cell cancer, hepatoma, or CNS cancer should have measurement of red cell mass. If the red cell mass is elevated, the serum erythropoietin level should be measured. Patients with an appropriate cancer, elevated erythropoietin levels, and no other explanation for erythrocytosis (e.g., hemoglobinopathy that causes increased O_2 affinity) have the paraneoplastic syndrome.

TREATMENT Erythrocytosis

Successful resection of the cancer usually resolves the erythrocytosis. If the tumor cannot be resected or treated effectively with radiation therapy or chemotherapy, phlebotomy may control any symptoms related to erythrocytosis.

GRANULOCYTOSIS

Approximately 30% of patients with solid tumors have granulocytosis (granulocyte count >8000/μL). In about half of patients with granulocytosis and cancer, the granulocytosis has an identifiable nonparaneoplastic etiology (infection, tumor necrosis, glucocorticoid administration, etc.). The other patients have proteins in urine and serum that stimulate the growth of bone marrow cells. Tumors and tumor cell lines from patients with lung, ovarian, and bladder cancers have been documented to produce granulocyte colony-stimulating factor (G-CSF), granulocyte-macrophage colony-stimulating factor (GM-CSF), and/or interleukin 6 (IL-6). However, the etiology of granulocytosis has not been characterized in most patients.

Patients with granulocytosis are nearly all asymptomatic, and the differential white blood cell count does not have a shift to immature forms of neutrophils. Granulocytosis occurs in 40% of patients with lung and gastrointestinal cancers, 20% of patients with breast cancer, 30% of patients with brain tumors and ovarian cancers, 20% of patients with Hodgkin's disease, and 10% of patients with renal cell carcinoma. Patients with advanced-stage disease are more likely to have granulocytosis than are those with early-stage disease.

Paraneoplastic granulocytosis does not require treatment. The granulocytosis resolves when the underlying cancer is treated.

THROMBOCYTOSIS

Some 35% of patients with thrombocytosis (platelet count >400,000/μL) have an underlying diagnosis of cancer. IL-6, a candidate molecule for the etiology of paraneoplastic thrombocytosis, stimulates the production of platelets in vitro and in vivo. Some patients with cancer and thrombocytosis have elevated levels of IL-6 in plasma. Another candidate molecule is thrombopoietin, a peptide hormone that stimulates megakaryocyte proliferation and platelet production. The etiology of thrombocytosis has not been established in most cases.

Patients with thrombocytosis are nearly all asymptomatic. Thrombocytosis is not clearly linked to thrombosis in patients with cancer. Thrombocytosis is present in 40% of patients with lung and gastrointestinal cancers; 20% of patients with breast, endometrial, and ovarian cancers; and 10% of patients with lymphoma. Patients with thrombocytosis are more likely to have advanced-stage disease and have a poorer prognosis than do patients without thrombocytosis. In ovarian cancer, IL-6 has been shown to directly promote tumor growth. Paraneoplastic thrombocytosis does not require treatment other than treatment of the underlying tumor.

EOSINOPHILIA

Eosinophilia is present in ~1% of patients with cancer. Tumors and tumor cell lines from patients with lymphomas or leukemia may produce IL-5, which stimulates eosinophil growth. Activation of IL-5 transcription in lymphomas and leukemias may involve translocation of the long arm of chromosome 5, to which the genes for IL-5 and other cytokines map.

Patients with eosinophilia are typically asymptomatic. Eosinophilia is present in 10% of patients with lymphoma, 3% of patients with lung cancer, and occasional patients with cervical, gastrointestinal, renal, and breast cancer. Patients with markedly elevated eosinophil counts (>5000/μL) can develop shortness of breath and wheezing. A chest radiograph may reveal diffuse pulmonary infiltrates from eosinophil infiltration and activation in the lungs.

TREATMENT Eosinophilia

Definitive treatment is directed at the underlying malignancy: Tumors should be resected or treated with radiation or chemotherapy. In most patients who develop shortness of breath related to eosinophilia, symptoms resolve with the use of oral or inhaled glucocorticoids. IL-5 antagonists exist but have not been evaluated in this clinical setting.

THROMBOPHLEBITIS

Deep venous thrombosis and pulmonary embolism are the most common thrombotic conditions in patients with cancer. Migratory or recurrent thrombophlebitis may be the initial manifestation of cancer. Nearly 15% of patients who develop deep venous thrombosis or pulmonary embolism have a diagnosis of cancer. The coexistence of peripheral venous thrombosis with visceral carcinoma, particularly pancreatic cancer, is called *Trousseau's syndrome*.

Pathogenesis

Patients with cancer are predisposed to thromboembolism because they are often at bed rest or immobilized, and tumors may obstruct or slow blood flow. Postoperative deep venous thrombosis is twice as common in cancer patients who undergo surgery. Chronic IV catheters also predispose to clotting. In addition, clotting may be promoted by release of procoagulants or cytokines from tumor cells or associated inflammatory cells or by platelet adhesion or aggregation. The specific molecules that promote thromboembolism have not been identified.

Chemotherapeutic agents, particularly those associated with endothelial damage, can induce venous thrombosis. The annual risk of venous thrombosis in patients with cancer receiving chemotherapy is about 11%, sixfold higher than the risk in the general population. Bleomycin, L-asparaginase, thalidomide analogues, cisplatin-based regimens, and high doses of busulfan and carmustine are all associated with an increased risk.

In addition to cancer and its treatment causing secondary thrombosis, primary thrombophilic diseases may be associated with cancer. For example, the antiphospholipid antibody syndrome is associated with a wide range of pathologic manifestations. About 20% of patients with this syndrome have cancers. Among patients with cancer and antiphospholipid antibodies, 35–45% develop thrombosis.

Clinical manifestations

Patients with cancer who develop deep venous thrombosis usually develop swelling or pain in the leg, and physical examination reveals tenderness, warmth, and redness. Patients who present with pulmonary embolism develop dyspnea, chest pain, and syncope, and physical examination shows tachycardia, cyanosis, and hypotension. Some 5% of patients with no history of cancer who have a diagnosis of deep venous thrombosis or pulmonary embolism will have a diagnosis of cancer within 1 year. The most common cancers associated with thromboembolic episodes include lung, pancreatic, gastrointestinal, breast, ovarian, and genitourinary cancers; lymphomas; and brain tumors. Patients with cancer who undergo surgical procedures requiring general anesthesia have a 20–30% risk of deep venous thrombosis.

Diagnosis

The diagnosis of deep venous thrombosis in patients with cancer is made by impedance plethysmography or bilateral compression ultrasonography of the leg veins. Patients with a noncompressible venous segment have deep venous thrombosis. If compression ultrasonography is normal and there is a high clinical suspicion for deep venous thrombosis, venography should be done to look for a luminal filling defect. Elevation of D-dimer is not as predictive of deep venous thrombosis in patients with cancer as it is in patients without cancer; elevations are seen in people over age 65 years without concomitant evidence of thrombosis, probably as a consequence of increased thrombin deposition and turnover in aging.

Patients with symptoms and signs suggesting a pulmonary embolism should be evaluated with a chest radiograph, electrocardiogram, arterial blood gas analysis, and ventilation-perfusion scan. Patients with mismatched segmental perfusion defects have a pulmonary embolus. Patients with equivocal ventilation-perfusion findings should be evaluated as described above for deep venous thrombosis in their legs. If deep venous thrombosis is detected, they should be anticoagulated. If deep venous thrombosis is not detected, they should be considered for a pulmonary angiogram.

Patients without a diagnosis of cancer who present with an initial episode of thrombophlebitis or pulmonary embolus need no additional tests for cancer other than a careful history and physical examination. In light of the many possible primary sites, diagnostic testing in asymptomatic patients is wasteful. However, if the clot is refractory to standard treatment or is in an unusual site or if the thrombophlebitis is migratory or recurrent, efforts to find an underlying cancer are indicated.

TREATMENT Thrombophlebitis

Patients with cancer and a diagnosis of deep venous thrombosis or pulmonary embolism should be treated initially with IV unfractionated heparin or low-molecular-weight heparin for at least 5 days, and warfarin should be started within 1 or 2 days. The warfarin dose should be adjusted so that the international normalized ratio (INR) is 2–3. Patients with proximal deep venous thrombosis and a relative contraindication to heparin anticoagulation (hemorrhagic brain metastases or pericardial effusion) should be considered for placement of a filter in the inferior vena cava (Greenfield filter) to prevent pulmonary embolism. Warfarin should be administered for 3–6 months. An alternative approach is to use low-molecular-weight heparin for 6 months. Patients with cancer who undergo a major surgical procedure should be considered for heparin prophylaxis or pneumatic boots. Breast cancer patients undergoing chemotherapy and patients with implanted catheters should be considered for prophylaxis. Guidelines recommend that hospitalized patients with cancer and patients receiving a thalidomide analogue receive prophylaxis with low-molecular-weight heparin or low-dose aspirin. Use of prophylaxis routinely during chemotherapy is controversial and not recommended by the American Society of Clinical Oncology.

ACKNOWLEDGMENT

The authors acknowledge the contributions of Bruce E. Johnson to prior versions of this chapter.

SECTION VI

DISORDERS OF BONE AND CALCIUM METABOLISM

CHAPTER 32

BONE AND MINERAL METABOLISM IN HEALTH AND DISEASE

F. Richard Bringhurst ■ Marie B. Demay ■ Stephen M. Krane ■ Henry M. Kronenberg

BONE STRUCTURE AND METABOLISM

Bone is a dynamic tissue that is remodeled constantly throughout life. The arrangement of compact and cancellous bone provides strength and density suitable for both mobility and protection. In addition, bone provides a reservoir for calcium, magnesium, phosphorus, sodium, and other ions necessary for homeostatic functions. Bone also hosts and regulates hematopoiesis by providing niches for hematopoietic cell proliferation and differentiation. The skeleton is highly vascular and receives about 10% of the cardiac output. Remodeling of bone is accomplished by two distinct cell types: osteoblasts produce bone matrix, and osteoclasts resorb the matrix.

The extracellular components of bone consist of a solid mineral phase in close association with an organic matrix, of which 90–95% is type I collagen. The noncollagenous portion of the organic matrix is heterogeneous and contains serum proteins such as albumin as well as many locally produced proteins, whose functions are incompletely understood. Those proteins include cell attachment/signaling proteins such as thrombospondin, osteopontin, and fibronectin; calcium-binding proteins such as matrix gla protein and osteocalcin; and proteoglycans such as biglycan and decorin. Some of the proteins organize collagen fibrils; others influence mineralization and binding of the mineral phase to the matrix.

The mineral phase is made up of calcium and phosphate and is best characterized as a poorly crystalline hydroxyapatite. The mineral phase of bone is deposited initially in intimate relation to the collagen fibrils and is found in specific locations in the "holes" between the collagen fibrils. This architectural arrangement of mineral and matrix results in a two-phase material well suited to withstand mechanical stresses. The organization of collagen influences the amount and type of mineral phase formed in bone. Although the primary structures of type I collagen in skin and bone tissues are similar, there are differences in posttranslational modifications and distribution of intermolecular cross-links. The holes in the packing structure of the collagen are larger in mineralized collagen of bone and dentin than in unmineralized collagens such as those in tendon. Single amino acid substitutions in the helical portion of either the α1 (*COL1A1*) or α2 (*COL1A2*) chains of type I collagen disrupt the organization of bone in osteogenesis imperfecta. The severe skeletal fragility associated with this group of disorders highlights the importance of the fibrillar matrix in the structure of bone.

Osteoblasts synthesize and secrete the organic matrix and regulate its mineralization. They are derived from cells of mesenchymal origin (Fig. 32-1A). Active osteoblasts are found on the surface of newly forming bone. As an osteoblast secretes matrix, which then is mineralized, the cell becomes an *osteocyte*, still connected with its blood supply through a series of canaliculi. Osteocytes account for the vast majority of the cells in bone. They are thought to be the mechanosensors in bone that communicate signals to surface osteoblasts and their progenitors through the canalicular network and thereby serve as master regulators of bone formation and resorption. Remarkably, osteocytes also secrete fibroblast growth factor 23 (FGF23), a major regulator of phosphate metabolism (see below). Mineralization of the matrix, both in trabecular bone and in osteones of compact cortical bone (*Haversian systems*), begins soon after the matrix is secreted (primary mineralization) but is not completed for several weeks or even longer (secondary mineralization). Although this mineralization

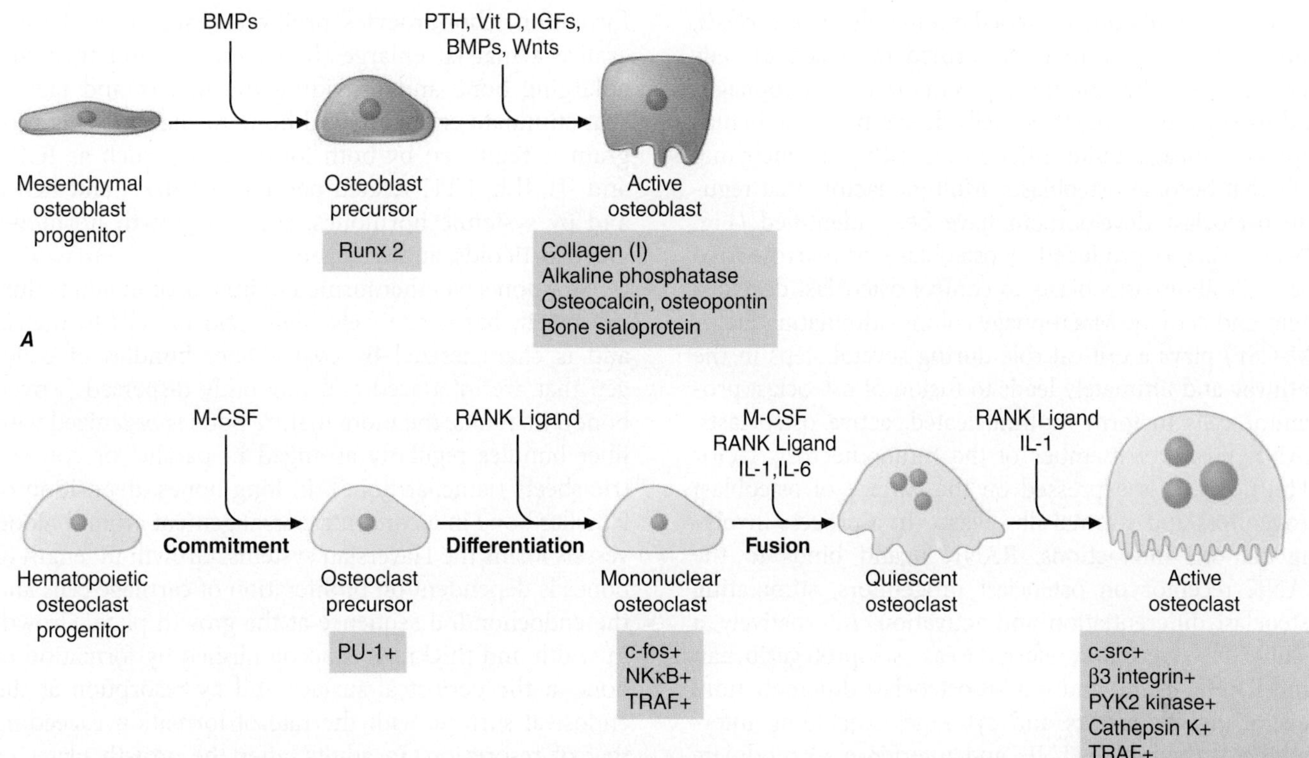

FIGURE 32-1

Pathways regulating development of (*A*) osteoblasts and (*B*) osteoclasts. Hormones, cytokines, and growth factors that control cell proliferation and differentiation are shown above the arrows. Transcription factors and other markers specific for various stages of development are depicted below the arrows. BMPs, bone morphogenic proteins; IGFs, insulin-like growth factors; IL-1, interleukin 1; IL-6, interleukin 6; M-CSF, macrophage colony-stimulating factor; NFκB, nuclear factor κB; PTH, parathyroid hormone; PU-1, a monocyte- and B lymphocyte–specific ets family transcription factor; RANK ligand, receptor activator of NFκB ligand; Runx2, Runt-related transcription factor 2; TRAF, tumor necrosis factor receptor–associated factors; Vit D, vitamin D; wnts, wingless-type mouse mammary tumor virus integration site. *(Modified from T Suda et al: Endocr Rev 20:345, 1999, with permission.)*

takes advantage of the high concentrations of calcium and phosphate, already near saturation in serum, mineralization is a carefully regulated process that is dependent on the activity of osteoblast-derived alkaline phosphatase, which probably works by hydrolyzing inhibitors of mineralization.

Genetic studies in humans and mice have identified several key genes that control osteoblast development. *Runx2* is a transcription factor expressed specifically in chondrocyte (cartilage cells) and osteoblast progenitors as well as in hypertrophic chondrocytes and mature osteoblasts. *Runx2* regulates the expression of several important osteoblast proteins, including osterix (another transcription factor needed for osteoblast maturation), osteopontin, bone sialoprotein, type I collagen, osteocalcin, and receptor-activator of NFκB (RANK) ligand. *Runx2* expression is regulated in part by bone morphogenic proteins (BMPs). *Runx2*-deficient mice are devoid of osteoblasts, whereas mice with a deletion of only one allele (*Runx2* +/−) exhibit a delay in formation of the clavicles and some cranial bones. The latter abnormalities are similar to those in the human disorder *cleidocranial dysplasia*, which is also caused by heterozygous inactivating mutations in *Runx2*.

The paracrine signaling molecule, Indian hedgehog (Ihh), also plays a critical role in osteoblast development, as evidenced by Ihh-deficient mice that lack osteoblasts in the type of bone formed on a cartilage mold (endochondral ossification). Signals originating from members of the wnt (wingless-type mouse mammary tumor virus integration site) family of paracrine factors are also important for osteoblast proliferation and differentiation. Numerous other growth-regulatory factors affect osteoblast function, including the three closely related transforming growth factor βs, fibroblast growth factors (FGFs) 2 and 18, platelet-derived growth factor, and insulin-like growth factors (IGFs) I and II. Hormones such as parathyroid hormone (PTH) and 1,25-dihydroxyvitamin D (1,25[OH]$_2$D) activate receptors expressed by osteoblasts to assure mineral homeostasis and influence a variety of bone cell functions.

Resorption of bone is carried out mainly by *osteoclasts*, multinucleated cells that are formed by fusion of cells derived from the common precursor of macrophages and osteoclasts. Thus, these cells derive from the hematopoietic lineage, quite different from the mesenchymal cells that become osteoblasts. Multiple factors that regulate osteoclast development have been identified (Fig. 32-1B). Factors produced by osteoblasts or marrow stromal cells allow osteoblasts to control osteoclast development and activity. Macrophage colony-stimulating factor (M-CSF) plays a critical role during several steps in the pathway and ultimately leads to fusion of osteoclast progenitor cells to form multinucleated, active osteoclasts. RANK ligand, a member of the tumor necrosis factor (TNF) family, is expressed on the surface of osteoblast progenitors and stromal fibroblasts. In a process involving cell-cell interactions, RANK ligand binds to the RANK receptor on osteoclast progenitors, stimulating osteoclast differentiation and activation. Alternatively, a soluble decoy receptor, referred to as osteoprotegerin, can bind RANK ligand and inhibit osteoclast differentiation. Several growth factors and cytokines (including interleukins 1, 6, and 11; TNF; and interferon γ) modulate osteoclast differentiation and function. Most hormones that influence osteoclast function do not target these cells directly but instead act on cells of the osteoblast lineage to increase production of M-CSF and RANK. Both PTH and $1,25(OH)_2D$ increase osteoclast number and activity by this indirect mechanism. Calcitonin, in contrast, binds to its receptor on the basal surface of osteoclasts and directly inhibits osteoclast function. Estradiol has multiple cellular targets in bone, including osteoclasts, immune cells, and osteoblasts; actions on all these cells serve to decrease osteoclast number and decrease bone resorption.

Osteoclast-mediated resorption of bone takes place in scalloped spaces (*Howship's lacunae*) where the osteoclasts are attached through a specific $\alpha_v\beta_3$ integrin to components of the bone matrix such as osteopontin. The osteoclast forms a tight seal to the underlying matrix and secretes protons, chloride, and proteinases into a confined space that has been likened to an extracellular lysosome. The active osteoclast surface forms a ruffled border that contains a specialized proton pump ATPase that secretes acid and solubilizes the mineral phase. Carbonic anhydrase (type II isoenzyme) within the osteoclast generates the needed protons. The bone matrix is resorbed in the acid environment adjacent to the ruffled border by proteases, such as cathepsin K, that act at low pH.

In the embryo and the growing child, bone develops mostly by remodeling and replacing previously calcified cartilage (endochondral bone formation) or, in a few bones, is formed without a cartilage matrix (intramembranous bone formation). During endochondral bone formation, chondrocytes proliferate, secrete and mineralize a matrix, enlarge (hypertrophy), and then die, enlarging bone and providing the matrix and factors that stimulate endochondral bone formation. This program is regulated by both local factors, such as IGF-I and -II, Ihh, PTH-related peptide (PTHrP), and FGFs, and by systemic hormones, such as growth hormone, glucocorticoids, and estrogen.

New bone, whether formed in infants or in adults during repair, has a relatively high ratio of cells to matrix and is characterized by coarse fiber bundles of collagen that are interlaced and randomly dispersed (woven bone). In adults, the more mature bone is organized with fiber bundles regularly arranged in parallel or concentric sheets (lamellar bone). In long bones, deposition of lamellar bone in a concentric arrangement around blood vessels forms the Haversian systems. Growth in length of bones is dependent on proliferation of cartilage cells and the endochondral sequence at the growth plate. Growth in width and thickness is accomplished by formation of bone at the periosteal surface and by resorption at the endosteal surface, with the rate of formation exceeding that of resorption. In adults, after the growth plates of cartilage close, growth in length and endochondral bone formation cease except for some activity in the cartilage cells beneath the articular surface. Even in adults, however, remodeling of bone (within Haversian systems as well as along the surfaces of trabecular bone) continues throughout life. In adults, ~4% of the surface of trabecular bone (such as iliac crest) is involved in active resorption, whereas 10–15% of trabecular surfaces are covered with osteoid, unmineralized new bone formed by osteoblasts. Radioisotope studies indicate that as much as 18% of the total skeletal calcium is deposited and removed each year. Thus, bone is an active metabolizing tissue that requires an intact blood supply. The cycle of bone resorption and formation is a highly orchestrated process carried out by the basic multicellular unit, which is composed of a group of osteoclasts and osteoblasts (Fig. 32-2).

The response of bone to fractures, infection, and interruption of blood supply and to expanding lesions is relatively limited. Dead bone must be resorbed, and new bone must be formed, a process carried out in association with growth of new blood vessels into the involved area. In injuries that disrupt the organization of the tissue such as a fracture in which apposition of fragments is poor or when motion exists at the fracture site, progenitor stromal cells recapitulate the endochondral bone formation of early development and form cartilage that is replaced by bone and, variably, fibrous tissue. When there is good apposition with fixation and little motion at the fracture site, repair occurs predominantly by formation of new bone without other mediating tissue.

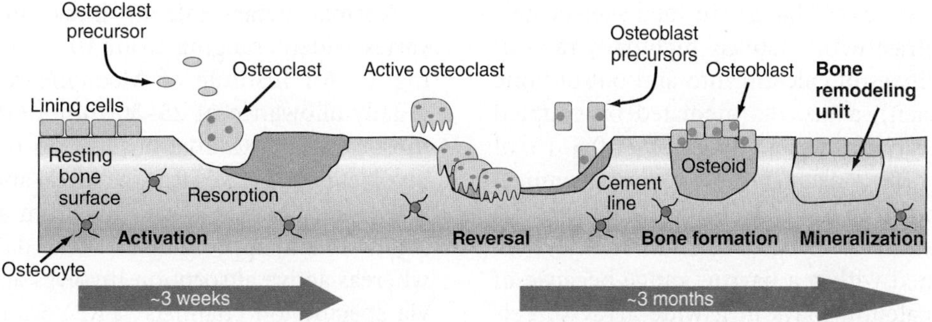

FIGURE 32-2

Schematic representation of bone remodeling. The cycle of bone remodeling is carried out by the basic multicellular unit (BMU), which consists of a group of osteoclasts and osteoblasts. In cortical bone, the BMUs tunnel through the tissue, whereas in cancellous bone, they move across the trabecular surface. The process of bone remodeling is initiated by contraction of the lining cells and the recruitment of osteoclast precursors. These precursors fuse to form multinucleated, active osteoclasts that mediate bone resorption. Osteoclasts adhere to bone and subsequently remove it by acidification and proteolytic digestion. As the BMU advances, osteoclasts leave the resorption site and osteoblasts move in to cover the excavated area and begin the process of new bone formation by secreting osteoid, which eventually is mineralized into new bone. After osteoid mineralization, osteoblasts flatten and form a layer of lining cells over new bone.

Remodeling of bone occurs along lines of force generated by mechanical stress. The signals from these mechanical stresses are sensed by osteocytes, which transmit signals to osteoclasts and osteoblasts or their precursors. One such signal made by osteocytes is sclerostin, an inhibitor of wnt signaling. Mechanical forces suppress sclerostin production and thus increase bone formation by osteoblasts. Expanding lesions in bone such as tumors induce resorption at the surface in contact with the tumor by producing ligands such as PTHrP that stimulate osteoclast differentiation and function. Even in a disorder as architecturally disruptive as Paget's disease, remodeling is dictated by mechanical forces. Thus, bone plasticity reflects the interaction of cells with each other and with the environment.

Measurement of the products of osteoblast and osteoclast activity can assist in the diagnosis and management of bone diseases. Osteoblast activity can be assessed by measuring serum bone-specific alkaline phosphatase. Similarly, osteocalcin, a protein secreted from osteoblasts, is made virtually only by osteoblasts. Osteoclast activity can be assessed by measurement of products of collagen degradation. Collagen molecules are covalently linked to each other in the extracellular matrix through the formation of hydroxypyridinium cross-links. After digestion by osteoclasts, these cross-linked peptides can be measured both in urine and in blood.

CALCIUM METABOLISM

Over 99% of the 1–2 kg of calcium present normally in the adult human body resides in the skeleton, where it provides mechanical stability and serves as a reservoir sometimes needed to maintain extracellular fluid (ECF) calcium concentration (Fig. 32-3). Skeletal calcium accretion first becomes significant during the third trimester of fetal life, accelerates throughout childhood and adolescence, reaches a peak in early adulthood, and gradually declines thereafter at rates that rarely exceed

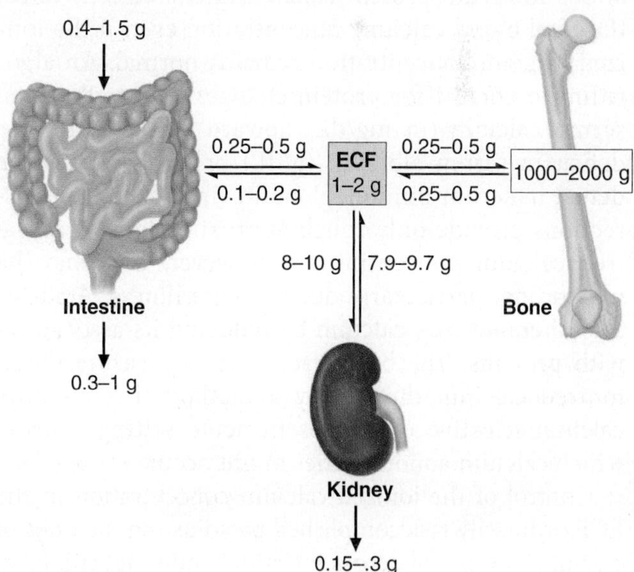

FIGURE 32-3

Calcium homeostasis. Schematic illustration of calcium content of extracellular fluid (ECF) and bone as well as of diet and feces; magnitude of calcium flux per day as calculated by various methods is shown at sites of transport in intestine, kidney, and bone. Ranges of values shown are approximate and were chosen to illustrate certain points discussed in the text. In conditions of calcium balance, rates of calcium release from and uptake into bone are equal.

1–2% per year. These slow changes in total skeletal calcium content contrast with relatively high daily rates of closely matched fluxes of calcium into and out of bone (~250–500 mg each), a process mediated by coupled osteoblastic and osteoclastic activity. Another 0.5–1% of skeletal calcium is freely exchangeable (e.g., in chemical equilibrium) with that in the ECF.

The concentration of ionized calcium in the ECF must be maintained within a narrow range because of the critical role calcium plays in a wide array of cellular functions, especially those involved in neuromuscular activity, secretion, and signal transduction. Intracellular cytosolic free calcium levels are ~100 nmol/L and are 10,000-fold lower than ionized calcium concentrations in the blood and ECF (1.1–1.3 mmol/L). Cytosolic calcium does not play the structural role played by extracellular calcium; instead, it serves a signaling function. The steep chemical gradient of calcium from outside to inside the cell promotes rapid calcium influx through various membrane calcium channels that can be activated by hormones, metabolites, or neurotransmitters, swiftly changing cellular function. In blood, total calcium concentration is normally 2.2–2.6 m*M* (8.5–10.5 mg/dL), of which ~50% is ionized. The remainder is bound ionically to negatively charged proteins (predominantly albumin and immunoglobulins) or loosely complexed with phosphate, citrate, sulfate, or other anions. Alterations in serum protein concentrations directly affect the total blood calcium concentration even if the ionized calcium concentration remains normal. An algorithm to correct for protein changes adjusts the total serum calcium (in mg/dL) upward by 0.8 times the deficit in serum albumin (g/dL) or by 0.5 times the deficit in serum immunoglobulin (in g/dL). Such corrections provide only rough approximations of actual free calcium concentrations, however, and may be misleading, particularly during acute illness. Acidosis also alters ionized calcium by reducing its association with proteins. The best practice is to measure blood ionized calcium directly by a method that employs calcium-selective electrodes in acute settings during which calcium abnormalities might occur.

Control of the ionized calcium concentration in the ECF ordinarily is accomplished by adjusting the rates of calcium movement across intestinal and renal epithelia. These adjustments are mediated mainly via changes in blood levels of the hormones, PTH and $1,25(OH)_2D$. Blood ionized calcium directly suppresses PTH secretion by activating calcium-sensing receptors (CaSRs) in parathyroid cells. Also, ionized calcium indirectly affects PTH secretion by lowering $1,25(OH)_2D$ production. This active vitamin D metabolite inhibits PTH production by an incompletely understood mechanism of negative feedback **(Chap. 34)**.

Normal dietary calcium intake in the United States varies widely, ranging from 10–37 mmol/d (400–1500 mg/d). An Institute of Medicine report recommends a daily allowance of 25–30 mmol (1000–1200 mg) for most adults. Intestinal absorption of ingested calcium involves both active (transcellular) and passive (paracellular) mechanisms. Passive calcium absorption is nonsaturable and approximates 5% of daily calcium intake, whereas active absorption involves apical calcium entry via specific ion channels (TRPV5 and TRPV6), whose expression is controlled principally by $1,25(OH)_2D$, and normally ranges from 20 to 70%. Active calcium transport occurs mainly in the proximal small bowel (duodenum and proximal jejunum), although some active calcium absorption occurs in most segments of the small intestine. Optimal rates of calcium absorption require gastric acid. This is especially true for weakly dissociable calcium supplements such as calcium carbonate. In fact, large boluses of calcium carbonate are poorly absorbed because of their neutralizing effect on gastric acid. In achlorhydric subjects and for those taking drugs that inhibit gastric acid secretion, supplements should be taken with meals to optimize their absorption. Use of calcium citrate may be preferable in these circumstances. Calcium absorption may also be blunted in disease states such as pancreatic or biliary insufficiency, in which ingested calcium remains bound to unabsorbed fatty acids or other food constituents. At high levels of calcium intake, synthesis of $1,25(OH)_2D$ is reduced; this decreases the rate of active intestinal calcium absorption. The opposite occurs with dietary calcium restriction. Some calcium, ~2.5–5 mmol/d (100–200 mg/d), is excreted as an obligate component of intestinal secretions and is not regulated by calciotropic hormones.

The feedback-controlled hormonal regulation of intestinal absorptive efficiency results in a relatively constant daily net calcium absorption of ~5–7.5 mmol/d (200–400 mg/d) despite large changes in daily dietary calcium intake. This daily load of absorbed calcium is excreted by the kidneys in a manner that is also tightly regulated by the concentration of ionized calcium in the blood. Approximately 8–10 g/d of calcium is filtered by the glomeruli, of which only 2–3% appears in the urine. Most filtered calcium (65%) is reabsorbed in the proximal tubules via a passive, paracellular route that is coupled to concomitant NaCl reabsorption and not specifically regulated. The cortical thick ascending limb of Henle's loop (cTAL) reabsorbs roughly another 20% of filtered calcium, also via a paracellular mechanism. Calcium reabsorption in the cTAL requires a tight-junctional protein called paracellin-1 and is inhibited by increased blood concentrations of calcium or magnesium, acting via the CaSR, which is highly expressed on basolateral membranes in this nephron segment. Operation of the renal CaSR provides a mechanism, independent of those engaged directly by PTH or 1,25(OH)$_2$D, by which serum ionized calcium can control renal calcium reabsorption. Finally, ~10% of filtered calcium is reabsorbed in the distal convoluted tubules (DCTs) by a transcellular mechanism. Calcium enters the luminal surface of the cell through specific apical calcium channels (TRPV5), whose number is regulated. It then moves across the cell in association with a specific calcium-binding protein (calbindin-D28k) that buffers cytosolic calcium concentrations from the large mass of transported calcium. Ca^{2+}-ATPases and Na^+/Ca^{2+} exchangers actively extrude calcium across the basolateral surface and thereby maintain the transcellular calcium gradient. All these processes are stimulated directly or indirectly by PTH. The DCT is also the site of action of thiazide diuretics, which lower urinary calcium excretion by inducing sodium depletion and thereby augmenting proximal calcium reabsorption. Conversely, dietary sodium loads, or increased distal sodium delivery caused by loop diuretics or saline infusion, induce calciuresis.

The homeostatic mechanisms that normally maintain a constant serum ionized calcium concentration may fail at extremes of calcium intake or when the hormonal systems or organs involved are compromised. Thus, even with maximal activity of the vitamin D–dependent intestinal active transport system, sustained calcium intakes <5 mmol/d (<200 mg/d) cannot provide enough net calcium absorption to replace obligate losses via the intestine, the kidney, sweat, and other secretions. In this case, increased blood levels of PTH and 1,25(OH)$_2$D activate osteoclastic bone resorption to obtain needed calcium from bone, which leads to progressive bone loss and negative calcium balance. Increased PTH and 1,25(OH)$_2$D also enhance renal calcium reabsorption, and 1,25(OH)$_2$D enhances calcium absorption in the gut. At very high calcium intakes (>100 mmol/d [>4 g/d]), passive intestinal absorption continues to deliver calcium into the ECF despite maximally downregulated intestinal active transport and renal tubular calcium reabsorption. This can cause severe hypercalciuria, nephrocalcinosis, progressive renal failure, and hypercalcemia (e.g., "milk-alkali syndrome"). Deficiency or excess of PTH or vitamin D, intestinal disease, and renal failure represent other commonly encountered challenges to normal calcium homeostasis **(Chap. 34)**.

PHOSPHORUS METABOLISM

Although 85% of the ~600 g of body phosphorus is present in bone mineral, phosphorus is also a major intracellular constituent both as the free anion(s) and as a component of numerous organophosphate compounds, including structural proteins, enzymes, transcription factors, carbohydrate and lipid intermediates, high-energy stores (adenosine triphosphate [ATP], creatine phosphate), and nucleic acids. Unlike calcium, phosphorus exists intracellularly at concentrations close to those present in ECF (e.g., 1–2 mmol/L). In cells and in the ECF, phosphorus exists in several forms, predominantly as $H_2PO_4^-$ or $NaHPO_4^-$, with perhaps 10% as HPO_4^{2-}. This mixture of anions will be referred to here as "phosphate." In serum, about 12% of phosphorus is bound to proteins. Concentrations of phosphates in blood and ECF generally are expressed in terms of elemental phosphorus, with the normal range in adults being 0.75–1.45 mmol/L (2.5–4.5 mg/dL). Because the volume of the intracellular fluid compartment is twice that of the ECF, measurements of ECF phosphate may not accurately reflect phosphate availability within cells that follows even modest shifts of phosphate from one compartment to the other.

Phosphate is widely available in foods and is absorbed efficiently (65%) by the small intestine even in the absence of vitamin D. However, phosphate absorptive efficiency may be enhanced (to 85–90%) via active transport mechanisms that are stimulated by 1,25(OH)$_2$D. These mechanisms involve activation of Na^+/PO_4^{2-} co-transporters that move phosphate into intestinal cells against an unfavorable electrochemical gradient. Daily net intestinal phosphate absorption varies widely with the composition of the diet but is generally in the range of 500–1000 mg/d. Phosphate absorption can be inhibited by large doses of calcium salts or by sevelamer hydrochloride (Renagel), strategies commonly used to control levels of serum phosphate in renal failure. Aluminum hydroxide antacids also reduce phosphate absorption but are used less commonly because of the potential for aluminum toxicity. Low serum phosphate stimulates renal proximal tubular synthesis of 1,25(OH)$_2$D, perhaps by suppressing blood levels of FGF23 (see below).

Serum phosphate levels vary by as much as 50% on a normal day. This reflects the effect of food intake but also an underlying circadian rhythm that produces a nadir between 7:00 and 10:00 A.M. Carbohydrate administration, especially as IV dextrose solutions in fasting subjects, can decrease serum phosphate by >0.7 mmol/L (2 mg/dL) due to rapid uptake into and utilization by cells. A similar response is observed in the treatment of diabetic ketoacidosis and during metabolic or respiratory alkalosis. Because of this wide variation in serum phosphate, it is best to perform measurements in the basal, fasting state.

Control of serum phosphate is determined mainly by the rate of renal tubular reabsorption of the filtered load, which is ~4–6 g/d. Because intestinal phosphate absorption is highly efficient, urinary excretion is not constant but varies directly with dietary intake. The fractional excretion of phosphate (ratio of phosphate to creatinine clearance) is generally in the range of 10–15%. The proximal tubule is the principal site at which renal phosphate reabsorption is regulated. This is accomplished by changes in the levels of apical expression and activity of specific Na^+/PO_4^{2-} co-transporters (NaPi-2a and NaPi-2c) in the proximal tubule. Levels of these transporters at the apical surface of these cells are reduced rapidly by PTH, a major hormonal regulator of renal phosphate excretion. FGF23 can impair phosphate reabsorption dramatically by a similar mechanism. Activating *FGF23* mutations cause the rare disorder autosomal dominant hypophosphatemic rickets. In contrast to PTH, FGF23 also leads to reduced synthesis of $1,25(OH)_2D$, which may worsen the resulting hypophosphatemia by lowering intestinal phosphate absorption. Renal reabsorption of phosphate is responsive to changes in dietary intake such that experimental dietary phosphate restriction leads to a dramatic lowering of urinary phosphate within hours, preceding any decline in serum phosphate (e.g., filtered load). This physiologic renal adaptation to changes in dietary phosphate availability occurs independently of PTH and may be mediated in part by changes in levels of serum FGF23. Findings in *FGF23*-knockout mice suggest that FGF23 normally acts to lower blood phosphate and $1,25(OH)_2D$ levels. In turn, elevation of blood phosphate increases blood levels of FGF23.

Renal phosphate reabsorption is impaired by hypocalcemia, hypomagnesemia, and severe hypophosphatemia. Phosphate clearance is enhanced by ECF volume expansion and impaired by dehydration. Phosphate retention is an important pathophysiologic feature of renal insufficiency.

HYPOPHOSPHATEMIA

Causes

Hypophosphatemia can occur by one or more of three primary mechanisms: (1) inadequate intestinal phosphate absorption, (2) excessive renal phosphate excretion, and (3) rapid redistribution of phosphate from the ECF into bone or soft tissue (Table 32-1). Because phosphate is so abundant in foods, inadequate intestinal absorption is almost never observed now that aluminum hydroxide antacids, which bind phosphate in the gut, are no longer widely used. Fasting or starvation, however, may result in depletion of body phosphate and predispose to subsequent hypophosphatemia during refeeding, especially if this is accomplished with IV glucose alone.

Chronic hypophosphatemia usually signifies a persistent renal tubular phosphate-wasting disorder.

TABLE 32-1

CAUSES OF HYPOPHOSPHATEMIA

- I. Reduced renal tubular phosphate reabsorption
  - A. PTH/PTHrP-dependent
    - 1. Primary hyperparathyroidism
    - 2. Secondary hyperparathyroidism
      - a. Vitamin D deficiency/resistance
      - b. Calcium starvation/malabsorption
      - c. Bartter's syndrome
      - d. Autosomal recessive renal hypercalciuria with hypomagnesemia
    - 3. PTHrP-dependent hypercalcemia of malignancy
    - 4. Familial hypocalciuric hypercalcemia
  - B. PTH/PTHrP-independent
    - 1. Excess FGF23 or other "phosphatonins"
      - a. X-linked hypophosphatemic rickets (XLH)
      - b. Autosomal recessive hypophosphatemia (ARHP)
      - c. Autosomal dominant hypophosphatemic rickets (ADHR) (DMP1, ENPP1 deficiency)
      - d. Tumor-induced osteomalacia syndrome (TIO)
      - e. McCune-Albright syndrome (fibrous dysplasia)
      - f. Epidermal nevus syndrome
    - 2. Intrinsic renal disease
      - a. Fanconi's syndrome(s)
      - b. Cystinosis
      - c. Wilson's disease
      - d. NaPi-2a or NaPi-2c mutations
    - 3. Other systemic disorders
      - a. Poorly controlled diabetes mellitus
      - b. Alcoholism
      - c. Hyperaldosteronism
      - d. Hypomagnesemia
      - e. Amyloidosis
      - f. Hemolytic-uremic syndrome
      - g. Renal transplantation or partial liver resection
      - h. Rewarming or induced hyperthermia
    - 4. Drugs or toxins
      - a. Ethanol
      - b. Acetazolamide, other diuretics
      - c. High-dose estrogens or glucocorticoids
      - d. Heavy metals (lead, cadmium, saccharated ferric oxide)
      - e. Toluene, *N*-methyl formamide
      - f. Cisplatin, ifosfamide, foscarnet, rapamycin
- II. Impaired intestinal phosphate absorption
  - A. Aluminum-containing antacids
  - B. Sevelamer

(continued)

TABLE 32-1

CAUSES OF HYPOPHOSPHATEMIA (CONTINUED)

- III. Shifts of extracellular phosphate into cells
  - A. Intravenous glucose
  - B. Insulin therapy for prolonged hyperglycemia or diabetic ketoacidosis
  - C. Catecholamines (epinephrine, dopamine, albuterol)
  - D. Acute respiratory alkalosis
  - E. Gram-negative sepsis, toxic shock syndrome
  - F. Recovery from starvation or acidosis
  - G. Rapid cellular proliferation
    1. Leukemic blast crisis
    2. Intensive erythropoietin, other growth factor therapy
- IV. Accelerated net bone formation
  - A. After parathyroidectomy
  - B. Treatment of vitamin D deficiency, Paget's disease
  - C. Osteoblastic metastases

Abbreviations: PTH, parathyroid hormone; PTHrP, parathyroid hormone–related peptide.

Excessive activation of PTH/PTHrP receptors in the proximal tubule as a result of primary or secondary hyperparathyroidism or because of the PTHrP-mediated hypercalcemia syndrome in malignancy **(Chap. 34)** is among the more common causes of renal hypophosphatemia, especially because of the high prevalence of vitamin D deficiency in older Americans. Familial hypocalciuric hypercalcemia and Jansen's chondrodystrophy are rare examples of genetic disorders in this category **(Chap. 34)**.

Several genetic and acquired diseases cause PTH/PTHrP-independent tubular phosphate wasting with associated rickets and osteomalacia. All these diseases manifest severe hypophosphatemia; renal phosphate wasting, sometimes accompanied by aminoaciduria; inappropriately low blood levels of 1,25$(OH)_2$D; low-normal serum levels of calcium; and evidence of impaired cartilage or bone mineralization. Analysis of these diseases led to the discovery of the hormone FGF23, which is an important physiologic regulator of phosphate metabolism. FGF23 decreases phosphate reabsorption in the proximal tubule and also suppresses the 1α-hydroxylase responsible for synthesis of 1,25$(OH)_2$D. FGF23 is synthesized by cells of the osteoblast lineage, primarily osteocytes. High-phosphate diets increase FGF23 levels, and low-phosphate diets decrease them. Autosomal dominant hypophosphatemic rickets (ADHR) was the first disease linked to abnormalities in FGF23. ADHR results from activating mutations in the gene that encodes FGF23. These mutations alter a cleavage site that ordinarily allows for inactivation of intact FGF23. Several other genetic disorders exhibit elevated FGF23 and hypophosphatemia. The most common of these is X-linked hypophosphatemic rickets (XLH), which results from inactivating mutations in an endopeptidase termed *PHEX* (*p*hosphate-regulating gene with *h*omologies to *e*ndopeptidases on the *X* chromosome) that is expressed most abundantly on the surface of osteocytes and mature osteoblasts. Patients with XLH usually have high FGF23 levels, and ablation of the *FGF23* gene reverses the hypophosphatemia found in the mouse version of XLH. How inactivation of *PHEX* leads to increased levels of FGF23 has not been determined. Two rare autosomal recessive hypophosphatemic syndromes associated with elevated FGF23 are due to inactivating mutations of dentin matrix protein-1 (*DMP1*) and ectonucleotide pyrophosphatase/phosphodiesterase 1 (*ENPP1*), both of which normally are highly expressed in bone and regulate FGF23 production. An unusual hypophosphatemic disorder, tumor-induced osteomalacia (TIO), is an acquired disorder in which tumors, usually of mesenchymal origin and generally histologically benign, secrete FGF23 and/or other molecules that induce renal phosphate wasting. The hypophosphatemic syndrome resolves completely within hours to days after successful resection of the responsible tumor. Such tumors typically express large amounts of FGF23 mRNA, and patients with TIO usually exhibit elevations of FGF23 in their blood.

Dent's disease is an X-linked recessive disorder caused by inactivating mutations in *CLCN5*, a chloride transporter expressed in endosomes of the proximal tubule; features include hypercalciuria, hypophosphatemia, and recurrent kidney stones. Renal phosphate wasting is common among poorly controlled diabetic patients and alcoholics, who therefore are at risk for iatrogenic hypophosphatemia when treated with insulin or IV glucose, respectively. Diuretics and certain other drugs and toxins can cause defective renal tubular phosphate reabsorption (Table 32-1).

In hospitalized patients, hypophosphatemia is often attributable to massive redistribution of phosphate from the ECF into cells. Insulin therapy for diabetic ketoacidosis is a paradigm for this phenomenon, in which the severity of the hypophosphatemia is related to the extent of antecedent depletion of phosphate and other electrolytes **(Chap. 23)**. The hypophosphatemia is usually greatest at a point many hours after initiation of insulin therapy and is difficult to predict from baseline measurements of serum phosphate at the time of presentation, when prerenal azotemia can obscure significant phosphate depletion. Other factors that may contribute to such acute redistributive hypophosphatemia include antecedent starvation or malnutrition, administration of IV glucose without other nutrients, elevated blood catecholamines (endogenous or exogenous), respiratory alkalosis, and recovery from metabolic acidosis.

Hypophosphatemia also can occur transiently (over weeks to months) during the phase of accelerated net bone formation that follows parathyroidectomy for severe primary hyperparathyroidism or during treatment of vitamin D deficiency or lytic Paget's disease. This is usually most prominent in patients who preoperatively have evidence of high bone turnover (e.g., high serum levels of alkaline phosphatase). Osteoblastic metastases can also lead to this syndrome.

Clinical and laboratory findings

The clinical manifestations of severe hypophosphatemia reflect a generalized defect in cellular energy metabolism because of ATP depletion, a shift from oxidative phosphorylation toward glycolysis, and associated tissue or organ dysfunction. Acute, severe hypophosphatemia occurs mainly or exclusively in hospitalized patients with underlying serious medical or surgical illness and preexisting phosphate depletion due to excessive urinary losses, severe malabsorption, or malnutrition. Chronic hypophosphatemia tends to be less severe, with a clinical presentation dominated by musculoskeletal complaints such as bone pain, osteomalacia, pseudofractures, and proximal muscle weakness or, in children, rickets and short stature.

Neuromuscular manifestations of severe hypophosphatemia are variable but may include muscle weakness, lethargy, confusion, disorientation, hallucinations, dysarthria, dysphagia, oculomotor palsies, anisocoria, nystagmus, ataxia, cerebellar tremor, ballismus, hyporeflexia, impaired sphincter control, distal sensory deficits, paresthesia, hyperesthesia, generalized or Guillain-Barré–like ascending paralysis, seizures, coma, and even death. Serious sequelae such as paralysis, confusion, and seizures are likely only at phosphate concentrations <0.25 mmol/L (<0.8 mg/dL). Rhabdomyolysis may develop during rapidly progressive hypophosphatemia. The diagnosis of hypophosphatemia-induced rhabdomyolysis may be overlooked, as up to 30% of patients with acute hypophosphatemia (<0.7 m*M*) have creatine phosphokinase elevations that peak 1–2 days after the nadir in serum phosphate, when the release of phosphate from injured myocytes may have led to a near normalization of circulating levels of phosphate.

Respiratory failure and cardiac dysfunction, which are reversible with phosphate treatment, may occur at serum phosphate levels of 0.5–0.8 mmol/L (1.5–2.5 mg/dL). Renal tubular defects, including tubular acidosis, glycosuria, and impaired reabsorption of sodium and calcium, may occur. Hematologic abnormalities correlate with reductions in intracellular ATP and 2,3-diphosphoglycerate and may include erythrocyte microspherocytosis and hemolysis; impaired oxyhemoglobin dissociation; defective leukocyte chemotaxis, phagocytosis, and bacterial killing; and platelet dysfunction with spontaneous gastrointestinal hemorrhage.

TREATMENT Hypophosphatemia

Severe hypophosphatemia (<0.75 mmol/L [<2 mg/dL]), particularly in the setting of underlying phosphate depletion, constitutes a dangerous electrolyte abnormality that should be corrected promptly. Unfortunately, the cumulative deficit in body phosphate cannot be predicted easily from knowledge of the circulating level of phosphate, and therapy must be approached empirically. The threshold for IV phosphate therapy and the dose administered should reflect consideration of renal function, the likely severity and duration of the underlying phosphate depletion, and the presence and

TABLE 32-2

INTRAVENOUS THERAPY FOR HYPOPHOSPHATEMIA

Consider

Likely severity of underlying phosphate depletion
Concurrent parenteral glucose administration
Presence of neuromuscular, cardiopulmonary, or hematologic complications of hypophosphatemia
Renal function (reduce dose by 50% if serum creatinine >220 μmol/L [>2.5 mg/dL])
Serum calcium level (correct hypocalcemia first; reduce dose by 50% in hypercalcemia)
Guidelines

Serum Phosphorus, m*M* (mg/dL)	Rate of Infusion, mmol/h	Duration, h	Total Administered, mmol
<0.8 (<2.5)	2	6	12
<0.5 (<1.5)	4	6	24
<0.3 (<1)	8	6	48

Note: Rates shown are calculated for a 70-kg person; levels of serum calcium and phosphorus must be measured every 6–12 h during therapy; infusions can be repeated to achieve stable serum phosphorus levels >0.8 mmol/L (>2.5 mg/dL); most formulations available in the United States provide 3 mmol/mL of sodium or potassium phosphate.

severity of symptoms consistent with those of hypophosphatemia. In adults, phosphate may be safely administered IV as neutral mixtures of sodium or potassium phosphate salts at initial doses of 0.2–0.8 mmol/kg of elemental phosphorus over 6 h (e.g., 10–50 mmol over 6 h), with doses >20 mmol/6 h reserved for those who have serum levels <0.5 mmol/L (1.5 mg/dL) and normal renal function. A suggested approach is presented in Table 32-2. Serum levels of phosphate and calcium must be monitored closely (every 6–12 h) throughout treatment. It is necessary to avoid a serum calcium-phosphorus product >50 to reduce the risk of heterotopic calcification. Hypocalcemia, if present, should be corrected before administering IV phosphate. Less severe hypophosphatemia, in the range of 0.5–0.8 mmol/L (1.5–2.5 mg/dL), usually can be treated with oral phosphate in divided doses of 750–2000 mg/d as elemental phosphorus; higher doses can cause bloating and diarrhea.

Management of chronic hypophosphatemia requires knowledge of the cause(s) of the disorder. Hypophosphatemia related to the secondary hyperparathyroidism of vitamin D deficiency usually responds to treatment with vitamin D and calcium alone. XLH, ADHR, TIO, and related renal tubular disorders usually are managed with divided oral doses of phosphate, often with calcium and $1,25(OH)_2D$ supplements to bypass the block in renal $1,25(OH)_2D$ synthesis and prevent secondary hyperparathyroidism caused by suppression of ECF calcium levels. Thiazide diuretics may be used to prevent nephrocalcinosis in patients who are managed this way. Complete normalization of hypophosphatemia is generally not possible in these conditions. Optimal therapy for TIO is extirpation of the responsible tumor, which may be localized by radiographic skeletal survey or bone scan (many are located in bone) or by radionuclide scanning using sestamibi or labeled octreotide. Successful treatment of TIO-induced hypophosphatemia with octreotide has been reported in a small number of patients.

HYPERPHOSPHATEMIA

Causes

When the filtered load of phosphate and glomerular filtration rate (GFR) are normal, control of serum phosphate levels is achieved by adjusting the rate at which phosphate is reabsorbed by the proximal tubular NaPi-2 co-transporters. The principal hormonal regulators of NaPi-2 activity are PTH and FGF23. Hyperphosphatemia, defined in adults as a fasting serum phosphate concentration >1.8 mmol/L (5.5 mg/dL), usually results from impaired glomerular filtration, hypoparathyroidism, excessive delivery of phosphate into the ECF (from bone, gut, or parenteral phosphate therapy), or a combination of these factors (Table 32-3). The upper limit of normal serum phosphate concentrations is higher in children and neonates (2.4 mmol/L [7 mg/dL]). It is useful to distinguish hyperphosphatemia caused by impaired renal phosphate excretion from that which results from excessive delivery of phosphate into the ECF (Table 32-3).

TABLE 32-3

CAUSES OF HYPERPHOSPHATEMIA

I. Impaired renal phosphate excretion
  A. Renal insufficiency
  B. Hypoparathyroidism
    1. Developmental
    2. Autoimmune
    3. After neck surgery or radiation
    4. Activating mutations of the calcium-sensing receptor
  C. Parathyroid suppression
    1. Parathyroid-independent hypercalcemia
      a. Vitamin D or vitamin A intoxication
      b. Sarcoidosis, other granulomatous diseases
      c. Immobilization, osteolytic metastases
      d. Milk-alkali syndrome
    2. Severe hypermagnesemia or hypomagnesemia
  D. Pseudohypoparathyroidism
  E. Acromegaly
  F. Tumoral calcinosis
  G. Heparin therapy
II. Massive extracellular fluid phosphate loads
  A. Rapid administration of exogenous phosphate (intravenous, oral, rectal)
  B. Extensive cellular injury or necrosis
    1. Crush injuries
    2. Rhabdomyolysis
    3. Hyperthermia
    4. Fulminant hepatitis
    5. Cytotoxic therapy
    6. Severe hemolytic anemia
  C. Transcellular phosphate shifts
    1. Metabolic acidosis
    2. Respiratory acidosis

In chronic renal insufficiency, reduced GFR leads to phosphate retention. Hyperphosphatemia in turn further impairs renal synthesis of $1,25(OH)_2D$, increases FGF23 levels, and stimulates PTH secretion and hypertrophy both directly and indirectly (by lowering blood ionized calcium levels). Thus, hyperphosphatemia is a major cause of the secondary hyperparathyroidism of renal failure and must be addressed early in the course of the disease **(Chap. 34)**.

Hypoparathyroidism leads to hyperphosphatemia via increased expression of NaPi-2 co-transporters in the proximal tubule. Hypoparathyroidism, or parathyroid suppression, has multiple potential causes, including autoimmune disease; developmental, surgical, or radiation-induced absence of functional parathyroid tissue; vitamin D intoxication or other causes of PTH-independent hypercalcemia; cellular PTH resistance (pseudohypoparathyroidism or hypomagnesemia); infiltrative disorders such as Wilson's disease and hemochromatosis; and impaired PTH secretion caused by hypermagnesemia, severe hypomagnesemia, or activating mutations in the CaSR. Hypocalcemia may also contribute directly to impaired phosphate clearance, as calcium infusion can induce phosphaturia in hypoparathyroid subjects. Increased tubular phosphate reabsorption also occurs in acromegaly, during heparin administration, and in tumoral calcinosis. Tumoral calcinosis is caused by a rare group of genetic disorders in which FGF23 is processed in a way that leads to low levels of active FGF23 in the bloodstream. This may result from mutations in the FGF23 sequence or via inactivating mutations in the *GALNT3* gene, which encodes a galactosaminyl transferase that normally adds sugar residues to FGF23 that slow its proteolysis. A similar syndrome results from FGF23 resistance due to inactivating mutations of the FGF23 co-receptor Klotho. These abnormalities cause elevated serum $1,25(OH)_2D$, parathyroid suppression, increased intestinal calcium absorption, and focal hyperostosis with large, lobulated periarticular heterotopic ossifications (especially at shoulders or hips) and are accompanied by hyperphosphatemia. In some forms of tumoral calcinosis, serum phosphorus levels are normal.

When large amounts of phosphate are delivered rapidly into the ECF, hyperphosphatemia can occur despite normal renal function. Examples include overzealous IV phosphate therapy, oral or rectal administration of large amounts of phosphate-containing laxatives or enemas (especially in children), extensive soft tissue injury or necrosis (crush injuries, rhabdomyolysis, hyperthermia, fulminant hepatitis, cytotoxic chemotherapy), extensive hemolytic anemia, and transcellular phosphate shifts induced by severe metabolic or respiratory acidosis.

Clinical findings

The clinical consequences of acute, severe hyperphosphatemia are due mainly to the formation of widespread calcium phosphate precipitates and resulting hypocalcemia. Thus, tetany, seizures, accelerated nephrocalcinosis (with renal failure, hyperkalemia, hyperuricemia, and metabolic acidosis), and pulmonary or cardiac calcifications (including development of acute heart block) may occur. The severity of these complications relates to the elevation of serum phosphate levels, which can reach concentrations as high as 7 mmol/L (20 mg/dL) in instances of massive soft tissue injury or tumor lysis syndrome.

TREATMENT Hyperphosphatemia

Therapeutic options for management of severe hyperphosphatemia are limited. Volume expansion may enhance renal phosphate clearance. Aluminum hydroxide antacids or sevelamer may be helpful in chelating and limiting absorption of offending phosphate salts present in the intestine. Hemodialysis is the most effective therapeutic strategy and should be considered early in the course of severe hyperphosphatemia, especially in the setting of renal failure and symptomatic hypocalcemia.

MAGNESIUM METABOLISM

Magnesium is the major intracellular divalent cation. Normal concentrations of extracellular magnesium and calcium are crucial for normal neuromuscular activity. Intracellular magnesium forms a key complex with ATP and is an important cofactor for a wide range of enzymes, transporters, and nucleic acids required for normal cellular function, replication, and energy metabolism. The concentration of magnesium in serum is closely regulated within the range of 0.7–1 mmol/L (1.5–2 meq/L; 1.7–2.4 mg/dL), of which 30% is protein-bound and another 15% is loosely complexed to phosphate and other anions. One-half of the 25 g (1000 mmol) of total body magnesium is located in bone, only one-half of which is insoluble in the mineral phase. Almost all extraskeletal magnesium is present within cells, where the total concentration is 5 m*M*, 95% of which is bound to proteins and other macromolecules. Because only 1% of body magnesium resides in the ECF, measurements of serum magnesium levels may not accurately reflect the level of total body magnesium stores.

Dietary magnesium content normally ranges from 6 to 15 mmol/d (140–360 mg/d), of which 30–40% is absorbed, mainly in the jejunum and ileum. Intestinal magnesium absorptive efficiency is stimulated by $1,25(OH)_2D$ and can reach 70% during magnesium deprivation. Urinary magnesium excretion normally matches net intestinal absorption and is ~4 mmol/d (100 mg/d). Regulation of serum magnesium concentrations is achieved mainly by control of renal magnesium reabsorption. Only 20% of filtered magnesium is reabsorbed in the proximal tubule, whereas 60% is reclaimed in the cTAL and another 5–10% in the DCT. Magnesium reabsorption in the cTAL occurs via a paracellular route that requires both a lumen-positive potential, created by NaCl reabsorption, and tight-junction proteins encoded by members of the Claudin gene family. Magnesium reabsorption in the cTAL is increased by PTH but inhibited by hypercalcemia or hypermagnesemia, both of which activate the CaSR in this nephron segment.

HYPOMAGNESEMIA

Causes

Hypomagnesemia usually signifies substantial depletion of body magnesium stores (0.5–1 mmol/kg). Hypomagnesemia can result from intestinal malabsorption;

protracted vomiting, diarrhea, or intestinal drainage; defective renal tubular magnesium reabsorption; or rapid shifts of magnesium from the ECF into cells, bone, or third spaces (Table 32-4). Dietary magnesium deficiency is unlikely except possibly in the setting of alcoholism. A rare genetic disorder that causes selective intestinal magnesium malabsorption has been described (primary infantile hypomagnesemia). Another rare inherited disorder (hypomagnesemia with secondary hypocalcemia) is caused by mutations in the gene encoding TRPM6, a protein that, along with TRPM7, forms a channel important for both intestinal and distal-tubular renal transcellular magnesium transport. Malabsorptive states, often compounded by vitamin D deficiency, can critically limit magnesium absorption and produce hypomagnesemia despite the compensatory effects of secondary hyperparathyroidism and of hypocalcemia and hypomagnesemia to enhance cTAL magnesium reabsorption. Diarrhea or surgical drainage fluid may contain ≥5 mmol/L of magnesium. Proton pump inhibitors (omeprazole and others) may produce hypomagnesemia by an unknown mechanism that does not involve renal wasting of magnesium.

TABLE 32-4

CAUSES OF HYPOMAGNESEMIA

I. Impaired intestinal absorption
  A. Hypomagnesemia with secondary hypocalcemia (TRPM6 mutations)
  B. Malabsorption syndromes
  C. Vitamin D deficiency
  D. Proton pump inhibitors
II. Increased intestinal losses
  A. Protracted vomiting/diarrhea
  B. Intestinal drainage, fistulas
III. Impaired renal tubular reabsorption
  A. Genetic magnesium-wasting syndromes
    1. Gitelman's syndrome
    2. Bartter's syndrome
    3. Claudin 16 or 19 mutations
    4. Potassium channel mutations (Kv1.1, Kir4.1)
    5. Na^+, K^+-ATPase γ-subunit mutations (FXYD2)
  B. Acquired renal disease
    1. Tubulointerstitial disease
    2. Postobstruction, ATN (diuretic phase)
    3. Renal transplantation
  C. Drugs and toxins
    1. Ethanol
    2. Diuretics (loop, thiazide, osmotic)
    3. Cisplatin
    4. Pentamidine, foscarnet
    5. Cyclosporine
    6. Aminoglycosides, amphotericin B
    7. Cetuximab
  D. Other
    1. Extracellular fluid volume expansion
    2. Hyperaldosteronism
    3. SIADH
    4. Diabetes mellitus
    5. Hypercalcemia
    6. Phosphate depletion
    7. Metabolic acidosis
    8. Hyperthyroidism
IV. Rapid shifts from extracellular fluid
  A. Intracellular redistribution
    1. Recovery from diabetic ketoacidosis
    2. Refeeding syndrome
    3. Correction of respiratory acidosis
    4. Catecholamines
  B. Accelerated bone formation
    1. Postparathyroidectomy
    2. Treatment of vitamin D deficiency
    3. Osteoblastic metastases
  C. Other
    1. Pancreatitis, burns, excessive sweating
    2. Pregnancy (third trimester) and lactation

Abbreviations: ATN, acute tubular necrosis; SIADH, syndrome of inappropriate antidiuretic hormone.

Several genetic magnesium-wasting syndromes have been described, including inactivating mutations of genes encoding the DCT NaCl co-transporter (Gitelman's syndrome), proteins required for cTAL Na-K-2Cl transport (Bartter's syndrome), claudin 16 or claudin 19 (autosomal recessive renal hypomagnesemia with hypercalciuria), a DCT Na^+, K^+-ATPase γ-subunit (autosomal dominant renal hypomagnesemia with hypocalciuria), DCT K^+ channels (Kv1.1, Kir4.1), and a mitochondrial gene encoding a tRNA. Activating mutations of the CaSR can cause hypomagnesemia as well as hypocalcemia. ECF expansion, hypercalcemia, and severe phosphate depletion may impair magnesium reabsorption, as can various forms of renal injury, including those caused by drugs such as cisplatin, cyclosporine, aminoglycosides, and pentamidine as well as the epidermal growth factor (EGF) receptor inhibitory antibody, cetuximab (EGF action is required for normal DCT apical expression of TRPM6) (Table 32-4). A rising blood concentration of ethanol directly impairs tubular magnesium reabsorption, and persistent glycosuria with osmotic diuresis leads to magnesium wasting and probably contributes to the high frequency of hypomagnesemia in poorly controlled diabetic patients. Magnesium depletion is aggravated by metabolic acidosis, which causes intracellular losses as well.

Hypomagnesemia due to rapid shifts of magnesium from ECF into the intracellular compartment can occur during recovery from diabetic ketoacidosis, starvation, or respiratory acidosis. Less acute shifts may be seen during rapid bone formation after parathyroidectomy, with treatment of vitamin D deficiency, or with osteoblastic metastases. Large amounts of magnesium may be lost with acute pancreatitis, extensive burns, or protracted and severe sweating and during pregnancy and lactation.

Clinical and laboratory findings

Hypomagnesemia may cause generalized alterations in neuromuscular function, including tetany, tremor, seizures, muscle weakness, ataxia, nystagmus, vertigo, apathy, depression, irritability, delirium, and psychosis. Patients are usually asymptomatic when serum magnesium concentrations are >0.5 mmol/L (1 meq/L; 1.2 mg/dL), although the severity of symptoms may not correlate with serum magnesium levels. Cardiac arrhythmias may occur, including sinus tachycardia, other supraventricular tachycardias, and ventricular arrhythmias. Electrocardiographic abnormalities may include prolonged PR or QT intervals, T-wave flattening or inversion, and ST straightening. Sensitivity to digitalis toxicity may be enhanced.

Other electrolyte abnormalities often seen with hypomagnesemia, including hypocalcemia (with hypocalciuria) and hypokalemia, may not be easily corrected unless magnesium is administered as well. The hypocalcemia may be a result of concurrent vitamin D deficiency, although hypomagnesemia can cause impaired synthesis of $1,25(OH)_2D$, cellular resistance to PTH, and, at very low serum magnesium (<0.4 mmol/L [0.8 meq/L; <1 mg/dL]), a defect in PTH secretion; these abnormalities are reversible with therapy.

TREATMENT Hypomagnesemia

Mild, asymptomatic hypomagnesemia may be treated with oral magnesium salts ($MgCl_2$, MgO, $Mg[OH]_2$) in divided doses totaling 20–30 mmol/d (40–60 meq/d). Diarrhea may occur with larger doses. More severe hypomagnesemia should be treated parenterally, preferably with IV $MgCl_2$, which can be administered safely as a continuous infusion of 50 mmol/d (100 meq Mg^{2+}/d) if renal function is normal. If GFR is reduced, the infusion rate should be lowered by 50–75%. Use of IM $MgSO_4$ is discouraged; the injections are painful and provide relatively little magnesium (2 mL of 50% $MgSO_4$ supplies only 4 mmol). $MgSO_4$ may be given IV instead of $MgCl_2$, although the sulfate anions may bind calcium in serum and urine and aggravate hypocalcemia. Serum magnesium should be monitored at intervals of 12–24 h during therapy, which may continue for several days because of impaired renal conservation of magnesium (only 50–70% of the daily IV magnesium dose is retained) and delayed repletion of intracellular deficits, which may be as high as 1–1.5 mmol/kg (2–3 meq/kg).

It is important to consider the need for calcium, potassium, and phosphate supplementation in patients with hypomagnesemia. Vitamin D deficiency frequently coexists and should be treated with oral or parenteral vitamin D or 25(OH)D (but not with $1,25[OH]_2D$, which may impair tubular magnesium reabsorption, possibly via PTH suppression). In severely hypomagnesemic patients with concomitant hypocalcemia and hypophosphatemia, administration of IV magnesium alone may worsen hypophosphatemia, provoking neuromuscular symptoms or rhabdomyolysis, due to rapid stimulation of PTH secretion. This is avoided by administering both calcium and magnesium.

HYPERMAGNESEMIA

Causes

Hypermagnesemia is rarely seen in the absence of renal insufficiency, as normal kidneys can excrete large amounts (250 mmol/d) of magnesium. Mild hypermagnesemia due to excessive reabsorption in the cTAL occurs with CaSR mutations in familial hypocalciuric hypercalcemia and has been described in some patients with adrenal insufficiency, hypothyroidism, or hypothermia. Massive exogenous magnesium exposures, usually via the gastrointestinal tract, can overwhelm renal excretory capacity and cause life-threatening hypermagnesemia (Table 32-5). A notable example of this is prolonged retention of even normal amounts of magnesium-containing cathartics in patients with intestinal ileus, obstruction, or perforation. Extensive soft tissue injury or necrosis can also deliver large amounts of magnesium into the ECF in patients who have suffered trauma, shock, sepsis, cardiac arrest, or severe burns.

Clinical and laboratory findings

The most prominent clinical manifestations of hypermagnesemia are vasodilation and neuromuscular blockade, which may appear at serum magnesium concentrations >2 mmol/L (>4 meq/L; >4.8 mg/dL). Hypotension that is refractory to vasopressors or volume expansion may be an early sign. Nausea, lethargy, and weakness may progress to respiratory failure, paralysis, and coma, with hypoactive tendon reflexes, at serum magnesium levels >4 mmol/L. Other findings may include gastrointestinal hypomotility or ileus;

TABLE 32-5

CAUSES OF HYPERMAGNESEMIA

I. Excessive magnesium intake
  A. Cathartics, urologic irrigants
  B. Parenteral magnesium administration
II. Rapid mobilization from soft tissues
  A. Trauma, shock, sepsis
  B. Cardiac arrest
  C. Burns
III. Impaired magnesium excretion
  A. Renal failure
  B. Familial hypocalciuric hypercalcemia
IV. Other
  A. Adrenal insufficiency
  B. Hypothyroidism
  C. Hypothermia

facial flushing; pupillary dilation; paradoxical bradycardia; prolongation of PR, QRS, and QT intervals; heart block; and, at serum magnesium levels approaching 10 mmol/L, asystole.

Hypermagnesemia, acting via the CaSR, causes hypocalcemia and hypercalciuria due to both parathyroid suppression and impaired cTAL calcium reabsorption.

TREATMENT Hypermagnesemia

Successful treatment of hypermagnesemia generally involves identifying and interrupting the source of magnesium and employing measures to increase magnesium clearance from the ECF. Use of magnesium-free cathartics or enemas may be helpful in clearing ingested magnesium from the gastrointestinal tract. Vigorous IV hydration should be attempted, if appropriate. Hemodialysis is effective and may be required in patients with significant renal insufficiency. Calcium, administered IV in doses of 100–200 mg over 1–2 h, has been reported to provide temporary improvement in signs and symptoms of hypermagnesemia.

VITAMIN D

SYNTHESIS AND METABOLISM

1,25-Dihydroxyvitamin D (1,25[OH]$_2$D) is the major steroid hormone involved in mineral ion homeostasis regulation. Vitamin D and its metabolites are hormones and hormone precursors rather than vitamins, since in the proper biologic setting, they can be synthesized endogenously (Fig. 32-4). In response to ultraviolet radiation of the skin, a photochemical cleavage results in the formation of vitamin D from 7-dehydrocholesterol. Cutaneous production of vitamin D is decreased by melanin and high solar protection factor sunblocks, which effectively impair skin penetration by ultraviolet light. The increased use of sunblocks in North America and Western Europe and a reduction in the magnitude of solar exposure of the general population over the last several decades has led to an increased reliance on dietary sources of vitamin D. In the United States and Canada, these sources largely consist of fortified cereals and dairy products, in addition to fish oils and egg yolks. Vitamin D from plant sources is in the form of vitamin D_2, whereas that from animal sources is vitamin D_3. These two forms have equivalent biologic activity and are activated equally well by the vitamin D hydroxylases in humans. Vitamin D enters the circulation, whether absorbed from the intestine or synthesized cutaneously, bound to vitamin D–binding protein, an α-globulin synthesized in the liver. Vitamin D is subsequently 25-hydroxylated in the liver by cytochrome P450–like enzymes in the mitochondria and microsomes. The activity of this hydroxylase is not tightly regulated, and the resultant metabolite, 25-hydroxyvitamin D (25[OH]D), is the major circulating and storage form of vitamin D. Approximately 88% of 25(OH)D circulates bound to the vitamin D–binding protein, 0.03% is free, and the rest circulates bound to albumin. The half-life of 25(OH)D is approximately 2–3 weeks; however, it is shortened dramatically when vitamin D–binding protein levels are reduced, as can occur with increased urinary losses in the nephrotic syndrome.

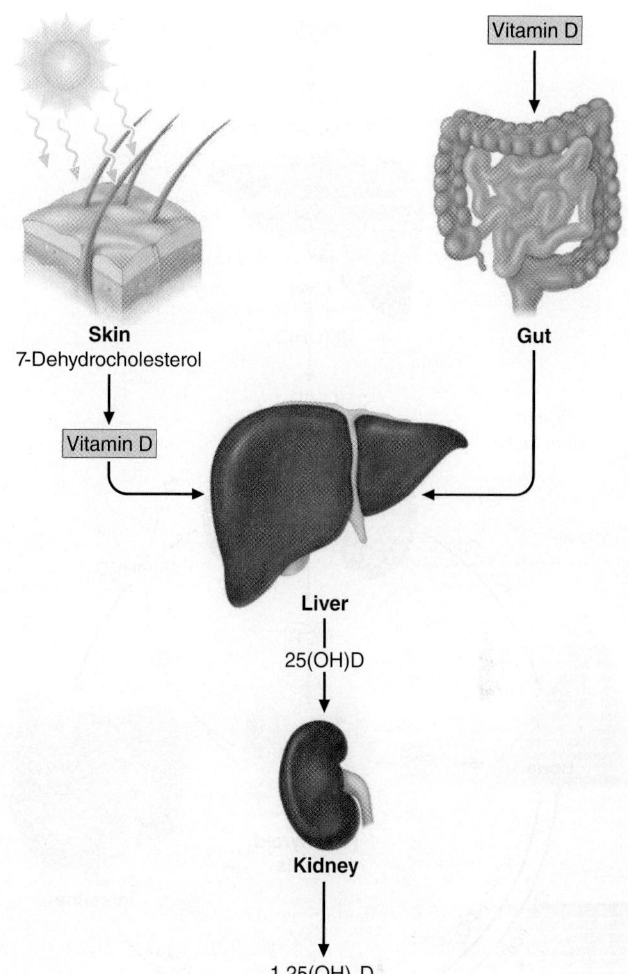

FIGURE 32-4

Vitamin D synthesis and activation. Vitamin D is synthesized in the skin in response to ultraviolet radiation and also is absorbed from the diet. It is then transported to the liver, where it undergoes 25-hydroxylation. This metabolite is the major circulating form of vitamin D. The final step in hormone activation, 1α-hydroxylation, occurs in the kidney.

The second hydroxylation, required for the formation of the mature hormone, occurs in the kidney (Fig. 32-5). The 25-hydroxyvitamin D-1α-hydroxylase is a tightly regulated cytochrome P450–like mixed-function oxidase expressed in the proximal convoluted tubule cells of the kidney. PTH and hypophosphatemia

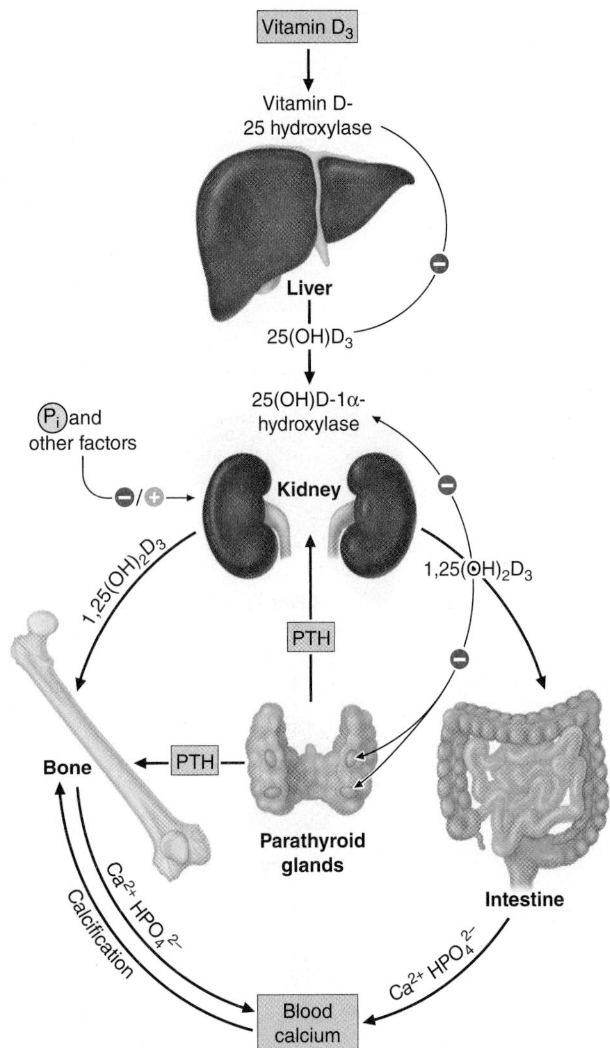

FIGURE 32-5

Schematic representation of the hormonal control loop for vitamin D metabolism and function. A reduction in the serum calcium below ~2.2 mmol/L (8.8 mg/dL) prompts a proportional increase in the secretion of parathyroid hormone (PTH) and so mobilizes additional calcium from the bone. PTH promotes the synthesis of $1,25(OH)_2D$ in the kidney, which in turn stimulates the mobilization of calcium from bone and intestine and regulates the synthesis of PTH by negative feedback.

are the major inducers of this microsomal enzyme, whereas calcium, FGF23, and the enzyme's product, $1,25(OH)_2D$, repress it. The 25-hydroxyvitamin D-1α-hydroxylase is also present in epidermal keratinocytes, but keratinocyte production of $1,25(OH)_2D$ is not thought to contribute to circulating levels of this hormone. In addition to being present in the trophoblastic layer of the placenta, the 1α-hydroxylase is produced by macrophages associated with granulomas and lymphomas. In these latter pathologic states, the activity of the enzyme is induced by interferon γ and TNF-α but is not regulated by calcium or $1,25(OH)_2D$; therefore, hypercalcemia, associated with elevated levels of $1,25(OH)_2D$, may be observed. Treatment of sarcoidosis-associated hypercalcemia with glucocorticoids, ketoconazole, or chloroquine reduces $1,25(OH)_2D$ production and effectively lowers serum calcium. In contrast, chloroquine has not been shown to lower the elevated serum $1,25(OH)_2D$ levels in patients with lymphoma.

The major pathway for inactivation of vitamin D metabolites is an additional hydroxylation step by the vitamin D 24-hydroxylase, an enzyme that is expressed in most tissues. $1,25(OH)_2D$ is the major inducer of this enzyme; therefore, this hormone promotes its own inactivation, thereby limiting its biologic effects. Mutations of the gene encoding this enzyme (CYP24A1) can lead to infantile hypercalcemia and, in those less severely affected, long-standing hypercalciuria, nephrocalcinosis, and nephrolithiasis.

Polar metabolites of $1,25(OH)_2D$ are secreted into the bile and reabsorbed via the enterohepatic circulation. Impairment of this recirculation, which is seen with diseases of the terminal ileum, leads to accelerated losses of vitamin D metabolites.

ACTIONS OF $1,25(OH)_2D$

$1,25(OH)_2D$ mediates its biologic effects by binding to a member of the nuclear receptor superfamily, the vitamin D receptor (VDR). This receptor belongs to the subfamily that includes the thyroid hormone receptors, the retinoid receptors, and the peroxisome proliferator–activated receptors; however, in contrast to the other members of this subfamily, only one VDR isoform has been isolated. The VDR binds to target DNA sequences as a heterodimer with the retinoid X receptor, recruiting a series of coactivators that modify chromatin and approximate the VDR to the basal transcriptional apparatus, resulting in the induction of target gene expression. The mechanism of transcriptional repression by the VDR varies with different target genes but has been shown to involve either interference with the action of activating transcription factors or the recruitment of novel proteins to the VDR complex, resulting in transcriptional repression.

The affinity of the VDR for $1,25(OH)_2D$ is approximately three orders of magnitude higher than that for other vitamin D metabolites. In normal physiologic circumstances, these other metabolites are not thought to stimulate receptor-dependent actions. However, in states of vitamin D toxicity, the markedly elevated levels of 25(OH)D may lead to hypercalcemia by interacting directly with the VDR and by displacing $1,25(OH)_2D$ from vitamin D–binding protein, resulting in increased bioavailability of the active hormone.

The VDR is expressed in a wide range of cells and tissues. The molecular actions of $1,25(OH)_2D$ have been studied most extensively in tissues involved in the regulation of mineral ion homeostasis. This hormone is a major inducer of calbindin 9K, a calcium-binding protein expressed in the intestine, which is thought to play an important role in the active transport of calcium across the enterocyte. The two major calcium transporters expressed by intestinal epithelia, TRPV5 and TRPV6 (transient receptor potential vanilloid), are also vitamin D responsive. By inducing the expression of these and other genes in the small intestine, $1,25(OH)_2D$ increases the efficiency of intestinal calcium absorption, and it also has been shown to have several important actions in the skeleton. The VDR is expressed in osteoblasts and regulates the expression of several genes in this cell. These genes include the bone matrix proteins osteocalcin and osteopontin, which are upregulated by $1,25(OH)_2D$, in addition to type I collagen, which is transcriptionally repressed by $1,25(OH)_2D$. Both $1,25(OH)_2D$ and PTH induce the expression of RANK ligand, which promotes osteoclast differentiation and increases osteoclast activity, by binding to RANK on osteoclast progenitors and mature osteoclasts. This is the mechanism by which $1,25(OH)_2D$ induces bone resorption. However, the skeletal features associated with VDR-knockout mice (rickets, osteomalacia) are largely corrected by increasing calcium and phosphorus intake, underscoring the importance of vitamin D action in the gut.

The VDR is expressed in the parathyroid gland, and $1,25(OH)_2D$ has been shown to have antiproliferative effects on parathyroid cells and to suppress the transcription of the PTH gene. These effects of $1,25(OH)_2D$ on the parathyroid gland are an important part of the rationale for current therapies directed at preventing and treating hyperparathyroidism associated with renal insufficiency.

The VDR is also expressed in tissues and organs that do not play a role in mineral ion homeostasis. Notable in this respect is the observation that $1,25(OH)_2D$ has an antiproliferative effect on several cell types, including keratinocytes, breast cancer cells, and prostate cancer cells. The effects of $1,25(OH)_2D$ and the VDR on keratinocytes are particularly intriguing. Alopecia is seen in humans and mice with mutant VDRs but is not a feature of vitamin D deficiency; thus, the effects of the VDR on the hair follicle are ligand-independent.

VITAMIN D DEFICIENCY

The mounting concern about the relationship between solar exposure and the development of skin cancer has led to increased reliance on dietary sources of vitamin D. Although the prevalence of vitamin D deficiency varies, the third National Health and Nutrition Examination Survey (NHANES III) revealed that vitamin D deficiency is prevalent throughout the United States. The clinical syndrome of vitamin D deficiency can be a result of deficient production of vitamin D in the skin, lack of dietary intake, accelerated losses of vitamin D, impaired vitamin D activation, or resistance to the biologic effects of $1,25(OH)_2D$ (Table 32-6). The elderly and nursing home residents are particularly at risk for vitamin D deficiency, since both the efficiency of vitamin D synthesis in the skin and the absorption of vitamin D from the intestine decline with age. Similarly, intestinal malabsorption of dietary fats and short bowel syndrome, including that associated with intestinal bypass surgery, can lead to vitamin D deficiency. This is further exacerbated in the presence of terminal ileal disease, which results in impaired enterohepatic circulation of vitamin D metabolites. In addition to intestinal diseases, accelerated inactivation of vitamin D metabolites can be seen with drugs that induce hepatic cytochrome P450 mixed-function oxidases such as barbiturates, phenytoin, and rifampin. Impaired 25-hydroxylation, associated with severe liver disease or isoniazid, is an uncommon cause of vitamin D deficiency. A mutation in the gene responsible for 25-hydroxylation has been identified in one kindred. Impaired 1α-hydroxylation is prevalent in the population with profound renal dysfunction due to an increase in circulating FGF23 levels and a decrease in functional renal mass. Thus, therapeutic interventions should be considered in patients whose creatinine clearance is <0.5 mL/s (30 mL/min). Mutations in the renal 1α-hydroxylase are the basis for the genetic disorder, pseudovitamin D–deficiency rickets. This autosomal recessive disorder presents with the syndrome of vitamin D deficiency in the first year of life. Patients present with growth retardation, rickets, and hypocalcemic seizures. Serum $1,25(OH)_2D$ levels are low

TABLE 32-6

CAUSES OF IMPAIRED VITAMIN D ACTION	
Vitamin D deficiency	Impaired 1α-hydroxylation
Impaired cutaneous production	Hypoparathyroidism
Dietary absence	Renal failure
Malabsorption	Ketoconazole
Accelerated loss of vitamin D	1α-hydroxylase mutation
Increased metabolism (barbiturates, phenytoin, rifampin)	Oncogenic osteomalacia X-linked hypophosphatemic rickets
Impaired enterohepatic circulation	Target organ resistance
Nephrotic syndrome	Vitamin D receptor mutation
Impaired 25-hydroxylation	Phenytoin
Liver disease, isoniazid	

despite normal 25(OH)D levels and elevated PTH levels. Treatment with vitamin D metabolites that do not require 1α-hydroxylation results in disease remission, although lifelong therapy is required. A second autosomal recessive disorder, hereditary vitamin D–resistant rickets, a consequence of vitamin D receptor mutations, is a greater therapeutic challenge. These patients present in a similar fashion during the first year of life, but alopecia often accompanies the disorder, demonstrating a functional role of the VDR in postnatal hair regeneration. Serum levels of 1,25$(OH)_2$D are dramatically elevated in these individuals both because of increased production due to stimulation of 1α-hydroxylase activity as a consequence of secondary hyperparathyroidism and because of impaired inactivation, since induction of the 24-hydroxylase by 1,25$(OH)_2$D requires an intact VDR. Because the receptor mutation results in hormone resistance, daily calcium and phosphorus infusions may be required to bypass the defect in intestinal mineral ion absorption.

Regardless of the cause, the clinical manifestations of vitamin D deficiency are largely a consequence of impaired intestinal calcium absorption. Mild to moderate vitamin D deficiency is asymptomatic, whereas long-standing vitamin D deficiency results in hypocalcemia accompanied by secondary hyperparathyroidism, impaired mineralization of the skeleton (osteopenia on x-ray or decreased bone mineral density), and proximal myopathy. Vitamin D deficiency also has been shown to be associated with an increase in overall mortality, including cardiovascular causes. In the absence of an intercurrent illness, the hypocalcemia associated with long-standing vitamin D deficiency rarely presents with acute symptoms of hypocalcemia such as numbness, tingling, and seizures. However, the concurrent development of hypomagnesemia, which impairs parathyroid function, or the administration of potent bisphosphonates, which impair bone resorption, can lead to acute symptomatic hypocalcemia in vitamin D–deficient individuals.

Rickets and osteomalacia

In children, before epiphyseal fusion, vitamin D deficiency results in growth retardation associated with an expansion of the growth plate known as *rickets*. Three layers of chondrocytes are present in the normal growth plate: the reserve zone, the proliferating zone, and the hypertrophic zone. Rickets associated with impaired vitamin D action is characterized by expansion of the hypertrophic chondrocyte layer. The proliferation and differentiation of the chondrocytes in the rachitic growth plate are normal, and the expansion of the growth plate is a consequence of impaired apoptosis of the late hypertrophic chondrocytes, an event that precedes replacement of these cells by osteoblasts during endochondral bone formation. Investigations in murine models demonstrate that hypophosphatemia, which in vitamin D deficiency is a consequence of secondary hyperparathyroidism, is a key etiologic factor in the development of the rachitic growth plate.

The hypocalcemia and hypophosphatemia that accompany vitamin D deficiency result in impaired mineralization of bone matrix proteins, a condition known as *osteomalacia*. Osteomalacia is also a feature of long-standing hypophosphatemia, which may be a consequence of renal phosphate wasting or chronic use of etidronate or phosphate-binding antacids. This hypomineralized matrix is biomechanically inferior to normal bone; as a result, patients with vitamin D deficiency are prone to bowing of weight-bearing extremities and skeletal fractures. Vitamin D and calcium supplementation have been shown to decrease the incidence of hip fracture among ambulatory nursing home residents in France, suggesting that undermineralization of bone contributes significantly to morbidity in the elderly. Proximal myopathy is a striking feature of severe vitamin D deficiency both in children and in adults. Rapid resolution of the myopathy is observed upon vitamin D treatment.

Although vitamin D deficiency is the most common cause of rickets and osteomalacia, many disorders lead to inadequate mineralization of the growth plate and bone. Calcium deficiency without vitamin D deficiency, the disorders of vitamin D metabolism previously discussed, and hypophosphatemia can all lead to inefficient mineralization. Even in the presence of normal calcium and phosphate levels, chronic acidosis and drugs such as bisphosphonates can lead to osteomalacia. The inorganic calcium/phosphate mineral phase of bone cannot form at low pH, and bisphosphonates bind to and prevent mineral crystal growth. Because alkaline phosphatase is necessary for normal mineral deposition, probably because the enzyme can hydrolyze inhibitors of mineralization such as inorganic pyrophosphate, genetic inactivation of the alkaline phosphatase gene (hereditary hypophosphatasia) also can lead to osteomalacia in the setting of normal calcium and phosphate levels.

Diagnosis of vitamin D deficiency, rickets, and osteomalacia

The most specific screening test for vitamin D deficiency in otherwise healthy individuals is a serum 25(OH)D level. Although the normal ranges vary, levels of 25(OH)D <37 nmol/L (<15 ng/mL) are associated with increasing PTH levels and lower bone density. The Institute of Medicine has defined vitamin D sufficiency as a vitamin D level >50 nmol/L (>20 ng/mL), although higher levels may be required to optimize intestinal calcium absorption in the elderly and those with underlying disease states. Vitamin D deficiency leads to impaired intestinal absorption of calcium, resulting in decreased serum total and ionized calcium values. This hypocalcemia results in secondary hyperparathyroidism, a homeostatic response that initially maintains serum calcium levels at the expense of the skeleton. Due to the PTH-induced increase in bone turnover, alkaline phosphatase levels are often increased. In addition to increasing bone resorption, PTH decreases urinary calcium excretion while promoting phosphaturia. This results in hypophosphatemia, which exacerbates the mineralization defect in the skeleton. With prolonged vitamin D deficiency resulting in osteomalacia, calcium stores in the skeleton become relatively inaccessible, since osteoclasts cannot resorb unmineralized osteoid, and frank hypocalcemia ensues. Because PTH is a major stimulus for the renal 25(OH) D 1α-hydroxylase, there is increased synthesis of the active hormone, $1,25(OH)_2D$. Paradoxically, levels of this hormone are often normal in severe vitamin D deficiency. Therefore, measurements of $1,25(OH)_2D$ are not accurate reflections of vitamin D stores and should not be used to diagnose vitamin D deficiency in patients with normal renal function.

Radiologic features of vitamin D deficiency in children include a widened, expanded growth plate that is characteristic of rickets. These findings not only are apparent in the long bones but also are present at the costochondral junction, where the expansion of the growth plate leads to swellings known as the "rachitic rosary." Impairment of intramembranous bone mineralization leads to delayed fusion of the calvarial sutures and a decrease in the radiopacity of cortical bone in the long bones. If vitamin D deficiency occurs after epiphyseal fusion, the main radiologic finding is a decrease in cortical thickness and relative radiolucency of the skeleton. A specific radiologic feature of osteomalacia, whether associated with phosphate wasting or vitamin D deficiency, is pseudofractures, or Looser's zones. These are radiolucent lines that occur where large arteries are in contact with the underlying skeletal elements; it is thought that the arterial pulsations lead to the radiolucencies. As a result, these pseudofractures are usually a few millimeters wide, are several centimeters long, and are seen particularly in the scapula, the pelvis, and the femoral neck.

TREATMENT Vitamin D Deficiency

Based on the Institute of Medicine 2010 report, the recommended daily intake of vitamin D is 600 IU from 1 to 70 years of age, and 800 IU for those over 70. Based on the observation that 800 IU of vitamin D, with calcium supplementation, decreases the risk of hip fractures in elderly women, this higher dose is thought to be an appropriate daily intake for prevention of vitamin D deficiency in adults. The safety margin for vitamin D is large, and vitamin D toxicity usually is observed only in patients taking doses in the range of 40,000 IU daily. Treatment of vitamin D deficiency should be directed at the underlying disorder, if possible, and also should be tailored to the severity of the condition. Vitamin D should always be repleted in conjunction with calcium supplementation because most of the consequences of vitamin D deficiency are a result of impaired mineral ion homeostasis. In patients in whom 1α-hydroxylation is impaired, metabolites that do not require this activation step are the treatment of choice. They include $1,25(OH)_2D_3$ (calcitriol [Rocaltrol], 0.25–0.5 μg/d) and 1α-hydroxyvitamin D_2 (Hectorol, 2.5–5 μg/d). If the pathway required for activation of vitamin D is intact, severe vitamin D deficiency can be treated with pharmacologic repletion initially (50,000 IU weekly for 3–12 weeks), followed by maintenance therapy (800 IU daily). Pharmacologic doses may be required for maintenance therapy in patients who are taking medications, such as barbiturates or phenytoin, that accelerate metabolism of or cause resistance to $1,25(OH)_2D$. Calcium supplementation should include 1.5–2 g/d of elemental calcium. Normocalcemia is usually observed within 1 week of the institution of therapy, although increases in PTH and alkaline phosphatase levels may persist for 3–6 months. The most efficacious methods to monitor treatment and resolution of vitamin D deficiency are serum and urinary calcium measurements. In patients who are vitamin D replete and are taking adequate calcium supplementation, the 24-h urinary calcium excretion should be in the range of 100–250 mg/24 h. Lower levels suggest problems with adherence to the treatment regimen or with absorption of calcium or vitamin D supplements. Levels >250 mg/24 h predispose to nephrolithiasis and should lead to a reduction in vitamin D dosage and/or calcium supplementation.

CHAPTER 33
HYPERCALCEMIA AND HYPOCALCEMIA

Sundeep Khosla

The calcium ion plays a critical role in normal cellular function and signaling, regulating diverse physiologic processes such as neuromuscular signaling, cardiac contractility, hormone secretion, and blood coagulation. Thus, extracellular calcium concentrations are maintained within an exquisitely narrow range through a series of feedback mechanisms that involve parathyroid hormone (PTH) and the active vitamin D metabolite 1,25-dihydroxyvitmin D [$1,25(OH)_2D$]. These feedback mechanisms are orchestrated by integrating signals between the parathyroid glands, kidney, intestine, and bone (Fig. 33-1; **Chap. 32**). Disorders of serum calcium concentration are relatively common and often serve as a harbinger of underlying disease. This chapter provides a brief summary of the approach to patients with altered serum calcium levels. **See Chap. 34 for a detailed discussion of this topic.**

HYPERCALCEMIA

ETIOLOGY

The causes of hypercalcemia can be understood and classified based on derangements in the normal feedback mechanisms that regulate serum calcium (Table 33-1). Excess PTH production, which is not appropriately suppressed by increased serum calcium concentrations, occurs in primary neoplastic disorders of the parathyroid glands (parathyroid adenomas; hyperplasia; or, rarely, carcinoma) that are associated with increased parathyroid cell mass and impaired feedback inhibition by calcium. Inappropriate PTH secretion for the ambient level of serum calcium also occurs with heterozygous inactivating calcium sensor receptor (CaSR) or G protein mutations, which impair extracellular calcium sensing by the parathyroid glands and the kidneys, resulting in familial hypocalciuric hypercalcemia (FHH). Although PTH secretion by tumors is extremely rare, many solid tumors produce PTH-related peptide (PTHrP), which shares homology with PTH in the first 13 amino acids and binds the PTH receptor, thus mimicking effects of PTH on bone and the kidney. In PTHrP-mediated hypercalcemia of malignancy, PTH levels are suppressed by the high serum calcium levels. Hypercalcemia associated with granulomatous disease (e.g., sarcoidosis) or lymphomas is caused by enhanced conversion of 25(OH)D to the potent $1,25(OH)_2D$. In these disorders, $1,25(OH)_2D$ enhances intestinal calcium absorption, resulting in hypercalcemia and suppressed PTH. Disorders that directly increase calcium mobilization from bone, such as hyperthyroidism or osteolytic metastases, also lead to hypercalcemia with suppressed PTH secretion as does exogenous calcium overload, as in milk-alkali syndrome, or total parenteral nutrition with excessive calcium supplementation.

CLINICAL MANIFESTATIONS

Mild hypercalcemia (up to 11–11.5 mg/dL) is usually asymptomatic and recognized only on routine calcium measurements. Some patients may complain of vague neuropsychiatric symptoms, including trouble concentrating, personality changes, or depression. Other presenting symptoms may include peptic ulcer disease or nephrolithiasis, and fracture risk may be increased. More severe hypercalcemia (>12–13 mg/dL), particularly if it develops acutely, may result in lethargy, stupor, or coma, as well as gastrointestinal symptoms (nausea, anorexia, constipation, or pancreatitis). Hypercalcemia decreases renal concentrating ability, which may cause polyuria and polydipsia. With long-standing hyperparathyroidism, patients may present with bone pain or pathologic fractures. Finally, hypercalcemia can result in significant electrocardiographic changes, including bradycardia, AV block, and short QT interval; changes in serum calcium can be monitored by following the QT interval.

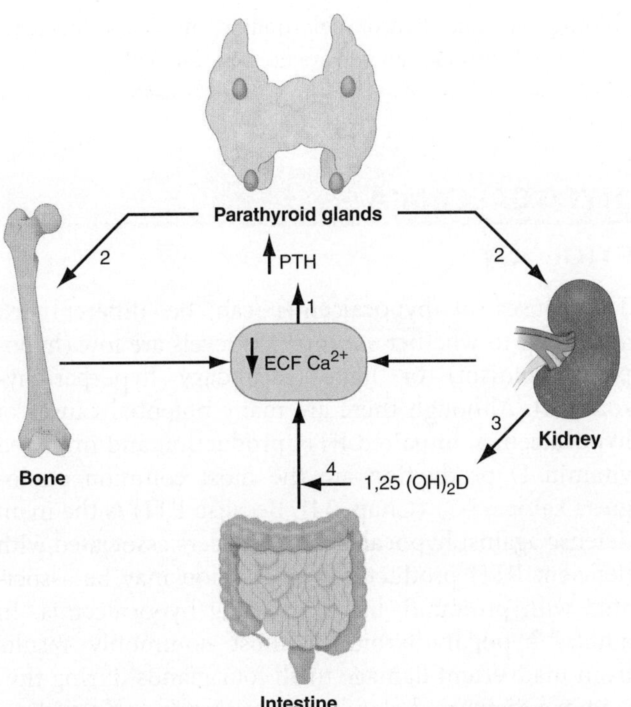

FIGURE 33-1

Feedback mechanisms maintaining extracellular calcium concentrations within a narrow, physiologic range (8.9–10.1 mg/dL [2.2–2.5 m*M*]). A decrease in extracellular (ECF) calcium (Ca^{2+}) triggers an increase in parathyroid hormone (PTH) secretion (1) via the calcium sensor receptor on parathyroid cells. PTH, in turn, results in increased tubular reabsorption of calcium by the kidney (2) and resorption of calcium from bone (2) and also stimulates renal $1,25(OH)_2D$ production (3). $1,25(OH)_2D$, in turn, acts principally on the intestine to increase calcium absorption (4). Collectively, these homeostatic mechanisms serve to restore serum calcium levels to normal.

DIAGNOSTIC APPROACH

The first step in the diagnostic evaluation of hyper- or hypocalcemia is to ensure that the alteration in serum calcium levels is not due to abnormal albumin concentrations. About 50% of total calcium is ionized, and the rest is bound principally to albumin. Although direct measurements of ionized calcium are possible, they are easily influenced by collection methods and other artifacts; thus, it is generally preferable to measure total calcium and albumin to "correct" the serum calcium. When serum albumin concentrations are reduced, a corrected calcium concentration is calculated by adding 0.2 m*M* (0.8 mg/dL) to the total calcium level for every decrement in serum albumin of 1.0 g/dL below the reference value of 4.1 g/dL for albumin, and, conversely, for elevations in serum albumin.

A detailed history may provide important clues regarding the etiology of the hypercalcemia (Table 33-1). Chronic hypercalcemia is most commonly caused by primary hyperparathyroidism, as opposed to the second most common etiology of hypercalcemia, an underlying malignancy. The history should include medication use, previous neck surgery, and systemic symptoms suggestive of sarcoidosis or lymphoma.

TABLE 33-1

CAUSES OF HYPERCALCEMIA

Excessive PTH production
Primary hyperparathyroidism (adenoma, hyperplasia, rarely carcinoma)
Tertiary hyperparathyroidism (long-term stimulation of PTH secretion in renal insufficiency)
Ectopic PTH secretion (very rare)
Inactivating mutations in the CaSR or in G proteins (FHH)
Alterations in CaSR function (lithium therapy)
Hypercalcemia of malignancy
Overproduction of PTHrP (many solid tumors)
Lytic skeletal metastases (breast, myeloma)
Excessive $1,25(OH)_2D$ production
Granulomatous diseases (sarcoidosis, tuberculosis, silicosis)
Lymphomas
Vitamin D intoxication
Primary increase in bone resorption
Hyperthyroidism
Immobilization
Excessive calcium intake
Milk-alkali syndrome
Total parenteral nutrition
Other causes
Endocrine disorders (adrenal insufficiency, pheochromocytoma, VIPoma)
Medications (thiazides, vitamin A, antiestrogens)

Abbreviations: CaSR, calcium sensor receptor; FHH, familial hypocalciuric hypercalcemia; PTH, parathyroid hormone; PTHrP, PTH-related peptide.

Once true hypercalcemia is established, the second most important laboratory test in the diagnostic evaluation is a PTH level using a two-site assay for the intact hormone. Increases in PTH are often accompanied by hypophosphatemia. In addition, serum creatinine should be measured to assess renal function; hypercalcemia may impair renal function, and renal clearance of PTH may be altered depending on the fragments detected by the assay. If the PTH level is increased (or "inappropriately normal") in the setting of elevated calcium and low phosphorus, the diagnosis is almost always primary hyperparathyroidism. Because individuals with FHH may also present with mildly elevated PTH levels and hypercalcemia, this diagnosis should be considered and excluded because parathyroid surgery is ineffective in this condition. A calcium/creatinine clearance ratio (calculated as urine calcium/serum calcium divided by urine creatinine/serum creatinine) of <0.01

is suggestive of FHH, particularly when there is a family history of mild, asymptomatic hypercalcemia. In addition, sequence analysis of the CaSR gene is now commonly performed for the definitive diagnosis of FHH, although in some families, FHH may be caused by mutations in G proteins that mediate signaling by the CaSR. Ectopic PTH secretion is extremely rare.

A suppressed PTH level in the face of hypercalcemia is consistent with non-parathyroid-mediated hypercalcemia, most often due to underlying malignancy. Although a tumor that causes hypercalcemia is generally overt, a PTHrP level may be needed to establish the diagnosis of hypercalcemia of malignancy. Serum 1,25$(OH)_2$D levels are increased in granulomatous disorders, and clinical evaluation in combination with laboratory testing will generally provide a diagnosis for the various disorders listed in Table 33-1.

TREATMENT Hypercalcemia

Mild, asymptomatic hypercalcemia does not require immediate therapy, and management should be dictated by the underlying diagnosis. By contrast, significant, symptomatic hypercalcemia usually requires therapeutic intervention independent of the etiology of hypercalcemia. Initial therapy of significant hypercalcemia begins with volume expansion because hypercalcemia invariably leads to dehydration; 4–6 L of intravenous saline may be required over the first 24 h, keeping in mind that underlying comorbidities (e.g., congestive heart failure) may require the use of loop diuretics to enhance sodium and calcium excretion. However, loop diuretics should not be initiated until the volume status has been restored to normal. If there is increased calcium mobilization from bone (as in malignancy or severe hyperparathyroidism), drugs that inhibit bone resorption should be considered. Zoledronic acid (e.g., 4 mg intravenously over ~30 min), pamidronate (e.g., 60–90 mg intravenously over 2–4 h), and ibandronate (2 mg intravenously over 2 h) are bisphosphonates that are commonly used for the treatment of hypercalcemia of malignancy in adults. Onset of action is within 1–3 days, with normalization of serum calcium levels occurring in 60–90% of patients. Bisphosphonate infusions may need to be repeated if hypercalcemia relapses. An alternative to the bisphosphonates is gallium nitrate (200 mg/m^2 intravenously daily for 5 days), which is also effective, but has potential nephrotoxicity. In rare instances, dialysis may be necessary. Finally, although intravenous phosphate chelates calcium and decreases serum calcium levels, this therapy can be toxic because calcium-phosphate complexes may deposit in tissues and cause extensive organ damage.

In patients with 1,25$(OH)_2$D-mediated hypercalcemia, glucocorticoids are the preferred therapy, as they decrease 1,25$(OH)_2$D production. Intravenous hydrocortisone (100–300 mg daily) or oral prednisone (40–60 mg daily) for 3–7 days is used most often. Other drugs, such as ketoconazole, chloroquine, and hydroxychloroquine, may also decrease 1,25$(OH)_2$D production and are used occasionally.

HYPOCALCEMIA

ETIOLOGY

The causes of hypocalcemia can be differentiated according to whether serum PTH levels are low (hypoparathyroidism) or high (secondary hyperparathyroidism). Although there are many potential causes of hypocalcemia, impaired PTH production and impaired vitamin D production are the most common etiologies (Table 33-2) **(Chap. 34)**. Because PTH is the main defense against hypocalcemia, disorders associated with deficient PTH production or secretion may be associated with profound, life-threatening hypocalcemia. In adults, hypoparathyroidism most commonly results from inadvertent damage to all four glands during thyroid or parathyroid gland surgery. Hypoparathyroidism is a cardinal feature of autoimmune endocrinopathies **(Chap. 29)**; rarely, it may be associated with infiltrative diseases such as sarcoidosis. Impaired PTH secretion may be secondary to magnesium deficiency or to activating mutations in the CaSR or in the G proteins that mediate CaSR signaling, which suppress PTH, leading to effects that are opposite to those that occur in FHH.

Vitamin D deficiency, impaired 1,25$(OH)_2$D production (primarily secondary to renal insufficiency), or vitamin D resistance also cause hypocalcemia. However, the degree of hypocalcemia in these disorders is generally not as severe as that seen with hypoparathyroidism because the parathyroids are capable of mounting a compensatory increase in PTH secretion. Hypocalcemia may also occur in conditions associated with severe tissue injury such as burns, rhabdomyolysis, tumor lysis, or pancreatitis. The cause of hypocalcemia in these settings may include a combination of low albumin, hyperphosphatemia, tissue deposition of calcium, and impaired PTH secretion.

CLINICAL MANIFESTATIONS

Patients with hypocalcemia may be asymptomatic if the decreases in serum calcium are relatively mild and chronic, or they may present with life-threatening complications. Moderate to severe hypocalcemia is associated with paresthesias, usually of the fingers, toes, and circumoral regions, and is caused by increased neuromuscular irritability. On physical examination, a Chvostek's sign (twitching of the circumoral muscles in response to gentle tapping of the facial nerve just anterior to the ear) may be elicited, although it is also present in ~10% of normal individuals. Carpal spasm

TABLE 33-2

CAUSES OF HYPOCALCEMIA

Low Parathyroid Hormone Levels (Hypoparathyroidism)
Parathyroid agenesis
Isolated
DiGeorge's syndrome
Parathyroid destruction
Surgical
Radiation
Infiltration by metastases or systemic diseases
Autoimmune
Reduced parathyroid function
Hypomagnesemia
Activating CaSR or G protein mutations
High Parathyroid Hormone Levels (Secondary Hyperparathyroidism)
Vitamin D deficiency or impaired $1,25(OH)_2D$ production/action
Nutritional vitamin D deficiency (poor intake or absorption)
Renal insufficiency with impaired $1,25(OH)_2D$ production
Vitamin D resistance, including receptor defects
Parathyroid hormone resistance syndromes
PTH receptor mutations
Pseudohypoparathyroidism (G protein mutations)
Drugs
Calcium chelators
Inhibitors of bone resorption (bisphosphonates, plicamycin)
Altered vitamin D metabolism (phenytoin, ketoconazole)
Miscellaneous causes
Acute pancreatitis
Acute rhabdomyolysis
Hungry bone syndrome after parathyroidectomy
Osteoblastic metastases with marked stimulation of bone formation (prostate cancer)

Abbreviations: CaSR, calcium sensor receptor; PTH, parathyroid hormone.

may be induced by inflation of a blood pressure cuff to 20 mmHg above the patient's systolic blood pressure for 3 min (Trousseau's sign). Severe hypocalcemia can induce seizures, carpopedal spasm, bronchospasm, laryngospasm, and prolongation of the QT interval.

DIAGNOSTIC APPROACH

In addition to measuring serum calcium, it is useful to determine albumin, phosphorus, and magnesium levels. As for the evaluation of hypercalcemia, determining the PTH level is central to the evaluation of hypocalcemia. A suppressed (or "inappropriately low") PTH level in the setting of hypocalcemia establishes absent or reduced PTH secretion (hypoparathyroidism) as the cause of the hypocalcemia. Further history will often elicit the underlying cause (i.e., parathyroid agenesis vs. destruction). By contrast, an elevated PTH level (secondary hyperparathyroidism) should direct attention to the vitamin D axis as the cause of the hypocalcemia. Nutritional vitamin D deficiency is best assessed by obtaining serum 25-hydroxyvitamin D levels, which reflect vitamin D stores. In the setting of renal insufficiency or suspected vitamin D resistance, serum $1,25(OH)_2D$ levels are informative.

TREATMENT Hypocalcemia

The approach to treatment depends on the severity of the hypocalcemia, the rapidity with which it develops, and the accompanying complications (e.g., seizures, laryngospasm). Acute, symptomatic hypocalcemia is initially managed with calcium gluconate, 10 mL 10% wt/vol (90 mg or 2.2 mmol) intravenously, diluted in 50 mL of 5% dextrose or 0.9% sodium chloride, given intravenously over 5 min. Continuing hypocalcemia often requires a constant intravenous infusion (typically 10 ampules of calcium gluconate or 900 mg of calcium in 1 L of 5% dextrose or 0.9% sodium chloride administered over 24 h). Accompanying hypomagnesemia, if present, should be treated with appropriate magnesium supplementation.

Chronic hypocalcemia due to hypoparathyroidism is treated with calcium supplements (1000–1500 mg/d elemental calcium in divided doses) and either vitamin D_2 or D_3 (25,000–100,000 U daily) or calcitriol [$1,25(OH)_2D$, 0.25–2 μg/d]. Other vitamin D metabolites (dihydrotachysterol, alfacalcidiol) are now used less frequently. Vitamin D deficiency, however, is best treated using vitamin D supplementation, with the dose depending on the severity of the deficit and the underlying cause. Thus, nutritional vitamin D deficiency generally responds to relatively low doses of vitamin D (50,000 U, 2–3 times per week for several months), whereas vitamin D deficiency due to malabsorption may require much higher doses (100,000 U/d or more). The treatment goal is to bring serum calcium into the low normal range and to avoid hypercalciuria, which may lead to nephrolithiasis.

GLOBAL CONSIDERATIONS

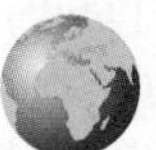

In countries with more limited access to health care or screening laboratory testing of serum calcium levels, primary hyperparathyroidism often presents in its severe form with skeletal complications (osteitis fibrosa cystica) in contrast to the asymptomatic form that is common in developed countries. In addition, vitamin D deficiency is paradoxically common in some countries despite extensive sunlight (e.g., India) due to avoidance of sun exposure and poor dietary vitamin D intake.

CHAPTER 34

DISORDERS OF THE PARATHYROID GLAND AND CALCIUM HOMEOSTASIS

John T. Potts, Jr. ■ Harald Jüppner

The four parathyroid glands are located posterior to the thyroid gland. They produce parathyroid hormone (PTH), which is the primary regulator of calcium physiology. PTH acts directly on bone, where it induces calcium release; on the kidney, where it enhances calcium reabsorption in the distal tubules; and in the proximal renal tubules, where it synthesizes 1,25-dihydroxyvitamin D (1,25[OH]$_2$D), a hormone that increases gastrointestinal calcium absorption. Serum PTH levels are tightly regulated by a negative feedback loop. Calcium, acting through the calcium-sensing receptor, and vitamin D, acting through its nuclear receptor, reduce PTH release and synthesis. Additional evidence indicates that fibroblast growth factor 23 (FGF23), a phosphaturic hormone, can suppress PTH secretion. Understanding the hormonal pathways that regulate calcium levels and bone metabolism is essential for effective diagnosis and management of a wide array of hyper- and hypocalcemic disorders.

Hyperparathyroidism, characterized by excess production of PTH, is a common cause of hypercalcemia and is usually the result of autonomously functioning adenomas or hyperplasia. Surgery for this disorder is highly effective and has been shown to reverse some of the deleterious effects of long-standing PTH excess on bone density. Humoral hypercalcemia of malignancy is also common and is usually due to the overproduction of parathyroid hormone–related peptide (PTHrP) by cancer cells. The similarities in the biochemical characteristics of hyperparathyroidism and humoral hypercalcemia of malignancy, first noted by Albright in 1941, are now known to reflect the actions of PTH and PTHrP through the same G protein–coupled PTH/PTHrP receptor.

The genetic basis of multiple endocrine neoplasia (MEN) types 1 and 2, familial hypocalciuric hypercalcemia (FHH), different forms of pseudohypoparathyroidism, Jansen's syndrome, disorders of vitamin D synthesis and action, and the molecular events associated with parathyroid gland neoplasia have provided new insights into the regulation of calcium homeostasis. PTH and *possibly some* of its analogues are promising therapeutic agents for the treatment of postmenopausal or senile osteoporosis, and calcimimetic agents, which activate the calcium-sensing receptor, have provided new approaches for PTH suppression.

PARATHYROID HORMONE

PHYSIOLOGY

The primary function of PTH is to maintain the extracellular fluid (ECF) calcium concentration within a narrow normal range. The hormone acts directly on bone and kidney and indirectly on the intestine through its effects on synthesis of 1,25(OH)$_2$D to increase serum calcium concentrations; in turn, PTH production is closely regulated by the concentration of serum ionized calcium. This feedback system is the critical homeostatic mechanism for maintenance of ECF calcium. Any tendency toward hypocalcemia, as might be induced by calcium- or vitamin D–deficient diets, is counteracted by an increased secretion of PTH. This in turn (1) increases the rate of dissolution of bone mineral, thereby increasing the flow of calcium from bone into blood; (2) reduces the renal clearance of calcium, returning more of the calcium and phosphate filtered at the glomerulus into ECF; and (3) increases the efficiency of calcium absorption in the intestine by stimulating the production of 1,25(OH)$_2$D. Immediate control of blood calcium is due to PTH effects on bone and, to a lesser extent, on renal calcium clearance. Maintenance of steady-state calcium balance, on the other hand, probably results from the effects of $1,25(OH)_2D$ on calcium absorption **(Chap. 32)**. The renal actions of the hormone are exerted at multiple sites and include inhibition of phosphate transport (proximal tubule), augmentation of calcium reabsorption (distal tubule), and stimulation of the renal 25(OH)D-1α-hydroxylase. As much as 12 mmol (500 mg) of calcium is transferred between the ECF and bone each day (a large amount in relation to the total ECF calcium pool), and PTH has a major effect on this transfer. The homeostatic role of the hormone can preserve calcium concentration in blood at the cost of bone demineralization.

PTH has multiple actions on bone, some direct and some indirect. PTH-mediated changes in bone calcium release can be seen within minutes. The chronic effects of PTH are to increase the number of bone cells, both osteoblasts and osteoclasts, and to increase the remodeling of bone; these effects are apparent within hours after the hormone is given and persist for hours after PTH is withdrawn. Continuous exposure to elevated PTH (as in hyperparathyroidism or long-term infusions in animals) leads to increased osteoclast-mediated bone resorption. However, the intermittent administration of PTH, elevating hormone levels for 1–2 h each day, leads to a net stimulation of bone formation rather than bone breakdown. Striking increases, especially in trabecular bone in the spine and hip, have been reported with the use of PTH in combination with estrogen. PTH (1–34) as monotherapy caused a highly significant reduction in fracture incidence in a worldwide placebo-controlled trial.

Osteoblasts (or stromal cell precursors), which have PTH/PTHrP receptors, are crucial to this bone-forming effect of PTH; osteoclasts, which mediate bone breakdown, lack such receptors. PTH-mediated stimulation of osteoclasts is indirect, acting in part through cytokines released from osteoblasts to activate osteoclasts; in experimental studies of bone resorption in vitro, osteoblasts must be present for PTH to activate osteoclasts to resorb bone **(Chap. 32)**.

STRUCTURE

PTH is an 84-amino-acid single-chain peptide. The amino-terminal portion, PTH (1–34), is highly conserved and is critical for the biologic actions of the molecule. Modified synthetic fragments of the amino-terminal sequence as small as PTH (1–11) are sufficient to activate the PTH/PTHrP receptor (see below). The carboxyl-terminal region of the full-length PTH (1–84) molecule also can bind to a separate binding protein/receptor (cPTH-R), but this receptor has been incompletely characterized. Fragments shortened at the amino-terminus possibly by binding to cPTH-R can reduce, directly or indirectly, some of the biologic actions of full-length PTH (1–84) and of PTH (1–34).

BIOSYNTHESIS, SECRETION, AND METABOLISM

Synthesis

Parathyroid cells have multiple methods of adapting to increased needs for PTH production. Most rapid (within minutes) is secretion of preformed hormone in response to hypocalcemia. Second, within hours, PTH mRNA expression is induced by sustained hypocalcemia. Finally, protracted challenge leads within days to cellular replication to increase parathyroid gland mass.

PTH is initially synthesized as a larger molecule (preproparathyroid hormone, consisting of 115 amino acids). After a first cleavage step to remove the "pre" sequence of 25 amino acid residues, a second cleavage step removes the "pro" sequence of 6 amino acid residues before secretion of the mature peptide comprising 84 residues. Mutations in the preprotein region of the gene can cause hypoparathyroidism by interfering with hormone synthesis, transport, or secretion.

Transcriptional suppression of the PTH gene by calcium is nearly maximal at physiologic calcium concentrations. Hypocalcemia increases transcriptional activity within hours. $1,25(OH)_2D$ strongly suppresses PTH gene transcription. In patients with renal failure, IV administration of supraphysiologic levels of $1,25(OH)_2D$ or analogues of this active metabolite can dramatically suppress PTH overproduction, which is sometimes difficult to control due to severe secondary hyperparathyroidism. Regulation of proteolytic destruction of preformed hormone (posttranslational regulation of hormone production) is an important mechanism for mediating rapid (within minutes) changes in hormone availability. High calcium increases and low calcium inhibit the proteolytic destruction of stored hormone.

Regulation of PTH secretion

PTH secretion increases steeply to a maximum value of about five times the basal rate of secretion as the calcium concentration falls from normal to the range of 1.9–2.0 mmol/L (7.6–8.0 mg/dL; measured as total calcium). However, the ionized fraction of blood calcium is the important determinant of hormone secretion. Severe intracellular magnesium deficiency impairs PTH secretion (see below).

ECF calcium controls PTH secretion by interaction with a calcium-sensing receptor (CaSR), a G protein–coupled receptor (GPCR) for which Ca^{2+} ions act as the primary ligand (see below). This receptor is a member of a distinctive subgroup of the GPCR superfamily that mediates its actions through the alpha-subunits of two related signaling G proteins, namely Gq and G11, and is characterized by a large extracellular domain suitable for "clamping" the small-molecule ligand. Stimulation of the CaSR by high calcium levels suppresses PTH secretion. The CaSR is present in parathyroid glands and the calcitonin-secreting cells of the thyroid (C cells), as well as in multiple other sites, including brain and kidney. Genetic evidence has revealed a key biologic role for the CaSR in parathyroid gland responsiveness to calcium and in renal calcium clearance. Heterozygous loss-of-function mutations in CaSR cause the syndrome of FHH, in which the blood calcium abnormality resembles that observed in hyperparathyroidism but with hypocalciuria; two more recently defined variants of FHH, FHH2 and FHH3, are caused either by heterozygous mutations in G11, one of the signaling proteins downstream of the CaSR, or by heterozygous mutations in *AP2S1*. Homozygous loss-of-function mutations in the CaSR are the cause of severe neonatal hyperparathyroidism, a disorder that can be lethal if not treated within the first days of life. On the other hand, heterozygous gain-of-function mutations cause a form of hypocalcemia resembling hypoparathyroidism (see below).

Metabolism

The secreted form of PTH is indistinguishable by immunologic criteria and by molecular size from the 84-amino-acid peptide (PTH[1–84]) extracted from glands. However, much of the immunoreactive material found in the circulation is smaller than the extracted or secreted hormone. The principal circulating fragments of immunoreactive hormone lack a portion of the critical amino-terminal sequence required for biologic activity and, hence, are biologically inactive fragments (so-called middle and carboxyl-terminal fragments). Much of the proteolysis of the hormone occurs in the liver and kidney. Peripheral metabolism of PTH does not appear to be regulated by physiologic states (high versus low calcium, etc.); hence, peripheral metabolism of hormone, although responsible for rapid clearance of secreted hormone, appears to be a high-capacity, metabolically invariant catabolic process.

The rate of clearance of the secreted 84-amino-acid peptide from blood is more rapid than the rate of clearance of the biologically inactive fragment(s) corresponding to the middle and carboxyl-terminal regions of PTH. Consequently, the interpretation of results obtained with earlier PTH radioimmunoassays was influenced by the nature of the peptide fragments detected by the antibodies.

Although the problems inherent in PTH measurements have been largely circumvented by use of double-antibody immunometric assays, it is now known that some of these assays detect, besides the intact molecule, large amino-terminally truncated forms of PTH, which are present in normal and uremic individuals in addition to PTH(1–84). The concentration of these fragments relative to that of intact PTH(1–84) is higher with induced hypercalcemia than in eucalcemic or hypocalcemic conditions and is higher in patients with impaired renal function. PTH(7–84) has been identified as a major component of these amino-terminally truncated fragments. Growing evidence suggests that the PTH(7–84) (and probably related amino-terminally truncated fragments) can act, through yet undefined mechanisms, as an inhibitor of PTH action and may be of clinical significance, particularly in patients with chronic kidney disease. In this group of patients, efforts to prevent secondary hyperparathyroidism by a variety of measures (vitamin D analogues, higher calcium intake, higher dialysate calcium, phosphate-lowering strategies, and calcimetic drugs) can lead to oversuppression of the parathyroid glands since some amino-terminally truncated PTH fragments, such as PTH(7–84), react in many immunometric PTH assays (now termed second-generation assays; see below under "Diagnosis"), thus overestimating the levels of biologically active, intact PTH. Such excessive parathyroid gland suppression in chronic kidney disease can lead to adynamic bone disease (see below), which has been associated with further impaired growth in children and increased bone fracture rates in adults, and can furthermore lead to significant hypercalcemia. The measurement of PTH with newer third-generation immunoassays, which use detection antibodies directed against extreme amino-terminal PTH epitopes and thus detect only full-length PTH(1–84), may provide some advantage to prevent bone disease in chronic kidney disease.

PARATHYROID HORMONE–RELATED PROTEIN (PTHrP)

PTHrP is responsible for most instances of humoral hypercalcemia of malignancy **(Chap. 31)**, a syndrome that resembles primary hyperparathyroidism but without elevated PTH levels. Most cell types normally produce PTHrP, including brain, pancreas, heart, lung, mammary tissue, placenta, endothelial cells, and smooth muscle. In fetal animals, PTHrP directs transplacental calcium transfer, and high concentrations of PTHrP are produced in mammary tissue and secreted into milk, but the biologic significance of the very high concentrations of this hormone in breast milk is unknown. PTHrP also plays an essential role in endochondral bone formation and in branching morphogenesis of the breast, and possibly in uterine contraction and other biologic functions.

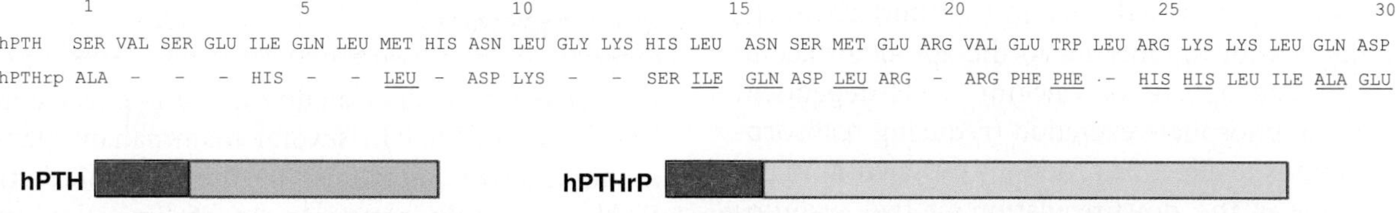

FIGURE 34-1

Schematic diagram to illustrate similarities and differences in structure of human parathyroid hormone (PTH) and human PTH-related peptide (PTHrP). Close structural (and functional) homology exists between the first 30 amino acids of hPTH and hPTHrP. The PTHrP sequence may be ≥144 amino acid residues in length. PTH is only 84 residues long; after residue 30, there is little structural homology between the two. *Dashed lines* in the PTHrP sequence indicate identity; *underlined residues*, although different from those of PTH, still represent conservative changes (charge or polarity preserved). Ten amino acids are identical, and a total of 20 of 30 are homologues.

PTH and PTHrP, although products of different genes, exhibit considerable functional and structural homology (Fig. 34-1) and have evolved from a shared ancestral gene. The structure of the gene encoding human PTHrP, however, is more complex than that of PTH, containing multiple additional exons, which can undergo alternate splicing patterns during formation of the mature mRNA. Protein products of 139, 141, and 173 amino acids are produced, and other molecular forms may result from tissue-specific degradation at accessible internal cleavage sites. The biologic roles of these various molecular species and the nature of the circulating forms of PTHrP are unclear. In fact, it is uncertain whether PTHrP circulates at any significant level in adults. As a paracrine factor, PTHrP may be produced, act, and be destroyed locally within tissues. In adults, PTHrP appears to have little influence on calcium homeostasis, except in disease states, when large tumors, especially of the squamous cell type as well as renal cell carcinomas, lead to massive overproduction of the hormone and hypercalcemia.

PTH AND PTHrP HORMONE ACTION

Both PTH and PTHrP bind to and activate the PTH/PTHrP receptor. The PTH/PTHrP receptor (also known as the PTH-1 receptor, PTH1R) belongs to a subfamily of GPCRs that includes the receptors for calcitonin, glucagon, secretin, vasoactive intestinal peptide, and other peptides. Although both ligands activate the PTH1R, the two peptides induce distinct responses in the receptor, which explains how a single receptor without isoforms can serve two biologic roles. The extracellular regions of the receptor are involved in hormone binding, and the intracellular domains, after hormone activation, bind G protein subunits to transduce hormone signaling into cellular responses through the stimulation of second messenger formation. A second receptor that binds PTH, originally termed the *PTH-2 receptor* (PTH2R), is primarily expressed in brain, pancreas, and testis. Different mammalian PTH1Rs respond equivalently to PTH and PTHrP, at least when tested with traditional assays, whereas only the human PTH2R responds efficiently to PTH (but not to PTHrP). PTH2Rs from other species show little or no stimulation of second-messenger formation in response to PTH or PTHrP. The endogenous ligand of the PTH2R was shown to be a hypothalamic peptide referred to as tubular infundibular peptide of 39 residues, TIP39, that is distantly related to PTH and PTHrP. The PTH1R and the PTH2R can be traced backward in evolutionary time to fish; in fact, the zebrafish genome contains, in addition to the PTH1R and the PTH2R orthologs, a third receptor, the PTH3R, that is more closely related to the fish PTH1R than to the fish PTH2R. The evolutionary conservation of structure and function suggests important biologic roles for these receptors, even in fish, which lack discrete parathyroid glands but produce two molecules that are closely related to mammalian PTH.

Studies using the cloned PTH1R confirm that it can be coupled to more than one G protein and second-messenger pathway, apparently explaining the multiplicity of pathways stimulated by PTH. Activation of protein kinases (A and C) and calcium transport channels is associated with a variety of hormone-specific tissue responses. These responses include inhibition of phosphate and bicarbonate transport, stimulation of calcium transport, and activation of renal 1α-hydroxylase in the kidney. The responses in bone include effects on collagen synthesis, alkaline phosphatase, ornithine decarboxylase, citrate decarboxylase, and glucose-6-phosphate dehydrogenase activities; phospholipid synthesis; and calcium and phosphate transport. Ultimately, these biochemical events lead to an integrated hormonal response in bone turnover and calcium homeostasis. PTH also activates Na^+/Ca^{2+} exchangers at renal distal tubular sites and stimulates translocation of preformed calcium transport channels, moving them from the interior to the apical surface to increase tubular uptake of calcium. PTH-dependent stimulation of phosphate excretion (reducing reabsorption—the opposite effect from actions on calcium in the kidney) involves the downregulation of two sodium-dependent phosphate co-transporters, NPT2a and NPT2c, and their expression at the apical membrane, thereby reducing phosphate reabsorption in the proximal renal tubules. Similar mechanisms may be involved in other renal tubular transporters that are influenced by PTH. Recent studies reaffirm the critical linkage of blood phosphate lowering to net calcium entry into blood by PTH action and emphasize the participation of bone cells other than osteoclasts in the rapid calcium-elevating actions of PTH.

PTHrP exerts important developmental influences on fetal bone development and in adult physiology. A homozygous ablation of the gene encoding PTHrP (or disruption of the PTH1R gene) in mice causes a lethal phenotype in which animals are born with pronounced acceleration of chondrocyte maturation that resembles a lethal form of chondrodysplasia in humans that is caused by homozygous or compound heterozygous, inactivating PTH1R mutations (Fig. 34-2). Heterozygous PTH1R mutations in humans furthermore can be a cause of delayed tooth eruption, and mice that are heterozygous for ablation of the PTHrP gene display reduced mineral density consistent with osteoporosis. Experiments with these mouse models point to a hitherto unappreciated role of PTHrP as a paracrine/autocrine factor that modulates bone metabolism in adults as well as during bone development.

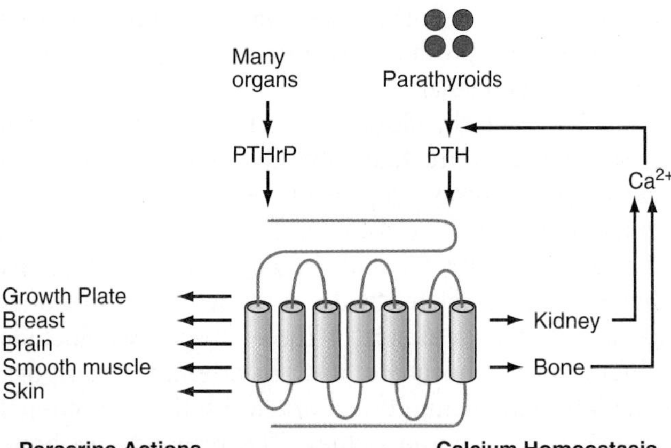

FIGURE 34-2

Dual role for the actions of the PTH/PTHrP receptor (PTH1R). Parathyroid hormone (PTH; endocrine-calcium homeostasis) and PTH-related peptide (PTHrP; paracrine–multiple tissue actions including growth plate cartilage in developing bone) use the single receptor for their disparate functions mediated by the amino-terminal 34 residues of either peptide. Other regions of both ligands interact with other receptors (not shown).

CALCITONIN

(See also Chap. 29) Calcitonin is a hypocalcemic peptide hormone that in several mammalian species acts as an indirect antagonist to the calcemic actions of PTH. Calcitonin seems to be of limited physiologic significance in humans, at least with regard to calcium homeostasis. It is of medical significance because of its role as a tumor marker in sporadic and hereditary cases of medullary carcinoma and its medical use as an adjunctive treatment in severe hypercalcemia and in Paget's disease of bone.

The hypocalcemic activity of calcitonin is accounted for primarily by inhibition of osteoclast-mediated bone resorption and secondarily by stimulation of renal calcium clearance. These effects are mediated by receptors on osteoclasts and renal tubular cells. Calcitonin exerts additional effects through receptors present in the brain, the gastrointestinal tract, and the immune system. The hormone, for example, exerts analgesic effects directly on cells in the hypothalamus and related structures, possibly by interacting with receptors for related peptide hormones such as calcitonin gene–related peptide (CGRP) or amylin. Both of these ligands have specific high-affinity receptors that share considerable structural similarity with the PTH1R and can also bind to and activate calcitonin receptors. The calcitonin receptor shares considerable structural similarity with the PTH1R.

The thyroid is the major source of the hormone, and the cells involved in calcitonin synthesis arise from neural crest tissue. During embryogenesis, these cells migrate into the ultimobranchial body, derived from the last branchial pouch. In submammalian vertebrates, the ultimobranchial body constitutes a discrete organ, anatomically separate from the thyroid gland; in mammals, the ultimobranchial gland fuses with and is incorporated into the thyroid gland.

The naturally occurring calcitonins consist of a peptide chain of 32 amino acids. There is considerable sequence variability among species. Calcitonin from salmon, which is used therapeutically, is 10–100 times more potent than mammalian forms in lowering serum calcium.

There are two calcitonin genes, α and β; the transcriptional control of these genes is complex. Two different mRNA molecules are transcribed from the α gene; one is translated into the precursor for calcitonin, and the other message is translated into an alternative product, CGRP. CGRP is synthesized wherever the calcitonin mRNA is expressed (e.g., in medullary carcinoma of the thyroid). The β, or CGRP-2, gene is transcribed into the mRNA for CGRP in the central nervous system (CNS); this gene does not produce calcitonin, however. CGRP has cardiovascular actions and may serve as a neurotransmitter or play a developmental role in the CNS.

The circulating level of calcitonin in humans is lower than that in many other species. In humans, even extreme variations in calcitonin production do not change calcium and phosphate metabolism; no definite effects are attributable to calcitonin deficiency (totally thyroidectomized patients receiving only replacement thyroxine) or excess (patients with medullary carcinoma of the thyroid, a calcitonin-secreting tumor) **(Chap. 29)**. Calcitonin has been a useful pharmacologic agent to suppress bone resorption in Paget's disease **(Chap. 36)** and osteoporosis **(Chap. 35)** and in the treatment of hypercalcemia of malignancy (see below). However, bisphosphonates are usually more effective, and the physiologic role, if any, of calcitonin in humans is uncertain. On the other hand, ablation of the calcitonin gene (combined because of the close proximity with ablation of the CGRP gene) in mice leads to reduced bone mineral density, suggesting that its biologic role in mammals is still not fully understood.

HYPERCALCEMIA

(See also Chap. 33) Hypercalcemia can be a manifestation of a serious illness such as malignancy or can be detected coincidentally by laboratory testing in a patient with no obvious illness. The number of patients recognized with asymptomatic hypercalcemia, usually hyperparathyroidism, increased in the late twentieth century.

Whenever hypercalcemia is confirmed, a definitive diagnosis must be established. Although hyperparathyroidism, a frequent cause of asymptomatic hypercalcemia, is a chronic disorder in which manifestations, if any, may be expressed only after months or years, hypercalcemia can also be the earliest manifestation of malignancy, the second most common cause of hypercalcemia in the adult. The causes of hypercalcemia are numerous (Table 34-1), but hyperparathyroidism and cancer account for 90% of all cases.

Before undertaking a diagnostic workup, it is essential to be sure that true hypercalcemia, not a false-positive laboratory test, is present. A false-positive diagnosis of hypercalcemia is usually the result of inadvertent hemoconcentration during blood collection or elevation in serum proteins such as albumin. Hypercalcemia is a chronic problem, and it is cost-effective to obtain several serum calcium measurements; these tests need not be in the fasting state.

Clinical features are helpful in differential diagnosis. Hypercalcemia in an adult who is asymptomatic is usually due to primary hyperparathyroidism. In malignancy-associated hypercalcemia, the disease is usually not occult; rather, symptoms of malignancy bring the patient to the physician, and hypercalcemia is discovered during the evaluation. In such patients, the interval between detection of hypercalcemia and death, especially without vigorous treatment, is often <6 months. Accordingly, if an asymptomatic individual has had hypercalcemia or some manifestation of hypercalcemia such as kidney stones for more than 1 or 2 years, it is unlikely that malignancy is the cause. Nevertheless, differentiating primary hyperparathyroidism from occult malignancy can occasionally be difficult, and careful evaluation is required, particularly when the duration of the hypercalcemia is unknown. Hypercalcemia not due to hyperparathyroidism or malignancy can result from excessive vitamin D action, impaired metabolism of 1,25(OH)2D, high bone turnover from any of several causes, or renal failure (Table 34-1). Dietary history and a history of ingestion of vitamins or drugs are often helpful in diagnosing some of the less frequent causes. Immunometric PTH assays serve as the principal laboratory test in establishing the diagnosis.

Hypercalcemia from any cause can result in fatigue, depression, mental confusion, anorexia, nausea, vomiting, constipation, reversible renal tubular defects, increased urine output, a short QT interval in the electrocardiogram, and, in some patients, cardiac arrhythmias. There

TABLE 34-1

CLASSIFICATION OF CAUSES OF HYPERCALCEMIA

I. Parathyroid-Related
   A. Primary hyperparathyroidism
      1. Adenoma(s)
      2. Multiple endocrine neoplasia
      3. Carcinoma
   B. Lithium therapy
   C. Familial hypocalciuric hypercalcemia
II. Malignancy-Related
   A. Solid tumor with metastases (breast)
   B. Solid tumor with humoral mediation of hypercalcemia (lung, kidney)
   C. Hematologic malignancies (multiple myeloma, lymphoma, leukemia)
III. Vitamin D–Related
   A. Vitamin D intoxication
   B. ↑ $1,25(OH)_2D$; sarcoidosis and other granulomatous diseases
   C. ↑ $1,25(OH)_2D$; impaired $1,25(OH)_2D$ metabolism due to 24-hydroxylase deficiency
IV. Associated with High Bone Turnover
   A. Hyperthyroidism
   B. Immobilization
   C. Thiazides
   D. Vitamin A intoxication
   E. Fat necrosis
V. Associated with Renal Failure
   A. Severe secondary hyperparathyroidism
   B. Aluminum intoxication
   C. Milk-alkali syndrome

is a variable relation from one patient to the next between the severity of hypercalcemia and the symptoms. Generally, symptoms are more common at calcium levels >2.9–3.0 mmol/L (11.6–12.0 mg/dL), but some patients, even at this level, are asymptomatic. When the calcium level is >3.2 mmol/L (12.8 mg/dL), calcification in kidneys, skin, vessels, lungs, heart, and stomach occurs and renal insufficiency may develop, particularly if blood phosphate levels are normal or elevated due to impaired renal excretion. Severe hypercalcemia, usually defined as ≥3.7–4.5 mmol/L (14.8–18.0 mg/dL), can be a medical emergency; coma and cardiac arrest can occur.

Acute management of the hypercalcemia is usually successful. The type of treatment is based on the severity of the hypercalcemia and the nature of associated symptoms, as outlined below.

PRIMARY HYPERPARATHYROIDISM

Natural history and incidence

Primary hyperparathyroidism is a generalized disorder of calcium, phosphate, and bone metabolism due to an increased secretion of PTH. The elevation of circulating hormone usually leads to hypercalcemia and hypophosphatemia. There is great variation in the manifestations. Patients may present with multiple signs and symptoms, including recurrent nephrolithiasis, peptic ulcers, mental changes, and, less frequently, extensive bone resorption. However, with greater awareness of the disease and wider use of multiphasic screening tests, including measurements of blood calcium, the diagnosis is frequently made in patients who have no symptoms and minimal, if any, signs of the disease other than hypercalcemia and elevated levels of PTH. The manifestations may be subtle, and the disease may have a benign course for many years or a lifetime. This milder form of the disease is usually termed *asymptomatic hyperparathyroidism*. Rarely, hyperparathyroidism develops or worsens abruptly and causes severe complications such as marked dehydration and coma, so-called hypercalcemic parathyroid crisis.

The annual incidence of the disease is calculated to be as high as 0.2% in patients >60, with an estimated prevalence, including undiscovered asymptomatic patients, of ≥1%; some reports suggest the incidence may be declining. If confirmed, these changing estimates may reflect less frequent routine testing of serum calcium in recent years, earlier overestimates in incidence, or unknown factors. The disease has a peak incidence between the third and fifth decades but occurs in young children and in the elderly.

Etiology

Parathyroid tumors are most often encountered as isolated adenomas without other endocrinopathy. They may also arise in hereditary syndromes such as MEN syndromes. Parathyroid tumors may also arise as secondary to underlying disease (excessive stimulation in secondary hyperparathyroidism, especially chronic renal failure) or after other forms of excessive stimulation such as lithium therapy. These etiologies are discussed below.

Solitary adenomas

A single abnormal gland is the cause in ~80% of patients; the abnormality in the gland is usually a benign neoplasm or adenoma and rarely a parathyroid carcinoma. Some surgeons and pathologists report that the enlargement of multiple glands is common; double adenomas are reported. In ~15% of patients, all glands are hyperfunctioning; *chief cell parathyroid hyperplasia* is usually hereditary and frequently associated with other endocrine abnormalities.

Hereditary syndromes and multiple parathyroid tumors

Hereditary hyperparathyroidism can occur without other endocrine abnormalities but is usually part of a *multiple endocrine neoplasia* (MEN) syndrome **(Chap. 29)**. MEN 1 (Wermer's syndrome) consists of hyperparathyroidism and tumors of the pituitary and pancreas, often associated with gastric hypersecretion and peptic ulcer disease (Zollinger-Ellison syndrome). MEN 2A is characterized by pheochromocytoma and medullary carcinoma of the thyroid, as well as hyperparathyroidism; MEN 2B has additional associated features such as multiple neuromas but usually lacks hyperparathyroidism. Each of these MEN syndromes is transmitted in an apparent autosomal dominant manner, although, as noted below, the genetic basis of MEN 1 involves biallelic loss of a tumor suppressor.

The *hyperparathyroidism jaw tumor* (HPT-JT) syndrome occurs in families with parathyroid tumors (sometimes carcinomas) in association with benign jaw tumors. This disorder is caused by mutations in *CDC73* (*HRPT2*), and mutations in this gene are also observed in parathyroid cancers. Some kindreds exhibit hereditary hyperparathyroidism without other endocrinopathies. This disorder is often termed *nonsyndromic familial isolated hyperparathyroidism* (FIHP). There is speculation that these families may be examples of variable expression of the other syndromes such as MEN 1, MEN 2, or the HPT-JT syndrome, but they may also have distinctive, still unidentified genetic causes.

Pathology

Adenomas are most often located in the inferior parathyroid glands, but in 6–10% of patients, parathyroid adenomas may be located in the thymus, the thyroid, the pericardium, or behind the esophagus. Adenomas are usually 0.5–5 g in size but may be as large as

10–20 g (normal glands weigh 25 mg on average). Chief cells are predominant in both hyperplasia and adenoma. With chief cell hyperplasia, the enlargement may be so asymmetric that some involved glands appear grossly normal. If generalized hyperplasia is present, however, histologic examination reveals a uniform pattern of chief cells and disappearance of fat even in the absence of an increase in gland weight. Thus, microscopic examination of biopsy specimens of several glands is essential to interpret findings at surgery.

Parathyroid carcinoma is often not aggressive. Long-term survival without recurrence is common if at initial surgery the entire gland is removed without rupture of the capsule. Recurrent parathyroid carcinoma is usually slow-growing with local spread in the neck, and surgical correction of recurrent disease may be feasible. Occasionally, however, parathyroid carcinoma is more aggressive, with distant metastases (lung, liver, and bone) found at the time of initial operation. It may be difficult to appreciate initially that a primary tumor is carcinoma; increased numbers of mitotic figures and increased fibrosis of the gland stroma may precede invasion. The diagnosis of carcinoma is often made in retrospect. Hyperparathyroidism from a parathyroid carcinoma may be indistinguishable from other forms of primary hyperparathyroidism but is usually more severe clinically. A potential clue to the diagnosis is offered by the degree of calcium elevation. Calcium values of 3.5–3.7 mmol/L (14–15 mg/dL) are frequent with carcinoma and may alert the surgeon to remove the abnormal gland with care to avoid capsular rupture. Recent findings concerning the genetic basis of parathyroid carcinoma (distinct from that of benign adenomas) indicate the need, in these kindreds, for family screening (see below).

GENETIC DEFECTS ASSOCIATED WITH HYPERPARATHYROIDISM

As in many other types of neoplasia, two fundamental types of genetic defects have been identified in parathyroid gland tumors: (1) overactivity of protooncogenes and (2) loss of function of tumor-suppressor genes. The former, by definition, can lead to uncontrolled cellular growth and function by activation (gain-of-function mutation) of a single allele of the responsible gene, whereas the latter requires loss of function of both allelic copies. Biallelic loss of function of a tumor-suppressor gene is usually characterized by a germline defect (all cells) and an additional somatic deletion/mutation in the tumor (Fig. 34-3).

Mutations in the *MEN1* gene locus, encoding the protein MENIN, on chromosome 11q13 are responsible for causing MEN 1; the normal allele of this gene fits the definition of a tumor-suppressor gene. Inheritance of one mutated allele in this hereditary syndrome, followed by loss of the other allele via somatic cell mutation, leads to monoclonal expansion and tumor development. Also, in ~15–20% of sporadic parathyroid adenomas, both alleles of the *MEN1* locus on chromosome 11 are somatically deleted, implying that the same defect responsible for MEN 1 can also cause the sporadic disease (Fig. 34-3A). Consistent with the Knudson hypothesis for two-step neoplasia in certain inherited cancer syndromes, the earlier onset of hyperparathyroidism in the hereditary syndromes reflects the need for only one mutational event to trigger the monoclonal outgrowth. In sporadic adenomas, typically occurring later in life, two different somatic events must occur before the *MEN1* gene is silenced.

Other presumptive anti-oncogenes involved in hyperparathyroidism include a still unidentified gene mapped to chromosome 1p seen in 40% of sporadic parathyroid adenomas and a gene mapped to chromosome Xp11 in patients with secondary hyperparathyroidism and renal failure, who progressed to "tertiary" hyperparathyroidism, now known to reflect monoclonal outgrowths within previously hyperplastic glands.

A more complex pattern, still incompletely resolved, arises with genetic defects and carcinoma of the parathyroids. This appears to be due to biallelic loss of a functioning copy of a gene, *HRPT2* (or CDC73), originally identified as the cause of the HPT-JT syndrome. Several inactivating mutations have been identified in *HRPT2* (located on chromosome 1q21-31), which encodes a 531-amino-acid protein called parafibromin. The responsible genetic mutations in *HRPT2* appear to be necessary, but not sufficient, for parathyroid cancer.

In general, the detection of additional genetic defects in these parathyroid tumor–related syndromes and the variations seen in phenotypic expression/penetrance indicate the multiplicity of the genetic factors responsible. Nonetheless, the ability to detect the presence of the major genetic contributors has greatly aided a more informed management of family members of patients identified in the hereditary syndromes such as MEN 1, MEN 2, and HPT-JT.

An important contribution from studies on the genetic origin of parathyroid carcinoma has been the realization that the mutations involve a different pathway than that involved with the benign gland enlargements. Unlike the pathogenesis of genetic alterations seen in colon cancer, where lesions evolve from benign adenomas to malignant disease by progressive genetic changes, the alterations commonly seen in most parathyroid cancers (*HRPT2* mutations) are infrequently seen in sporadic parathyroid adenomas.

Abnormalities at the *Rb* gene were the first to be noted in parathyroid cancer. The *Rb* gene, a tumor-suppressor gene located on chromosome 13q14, was

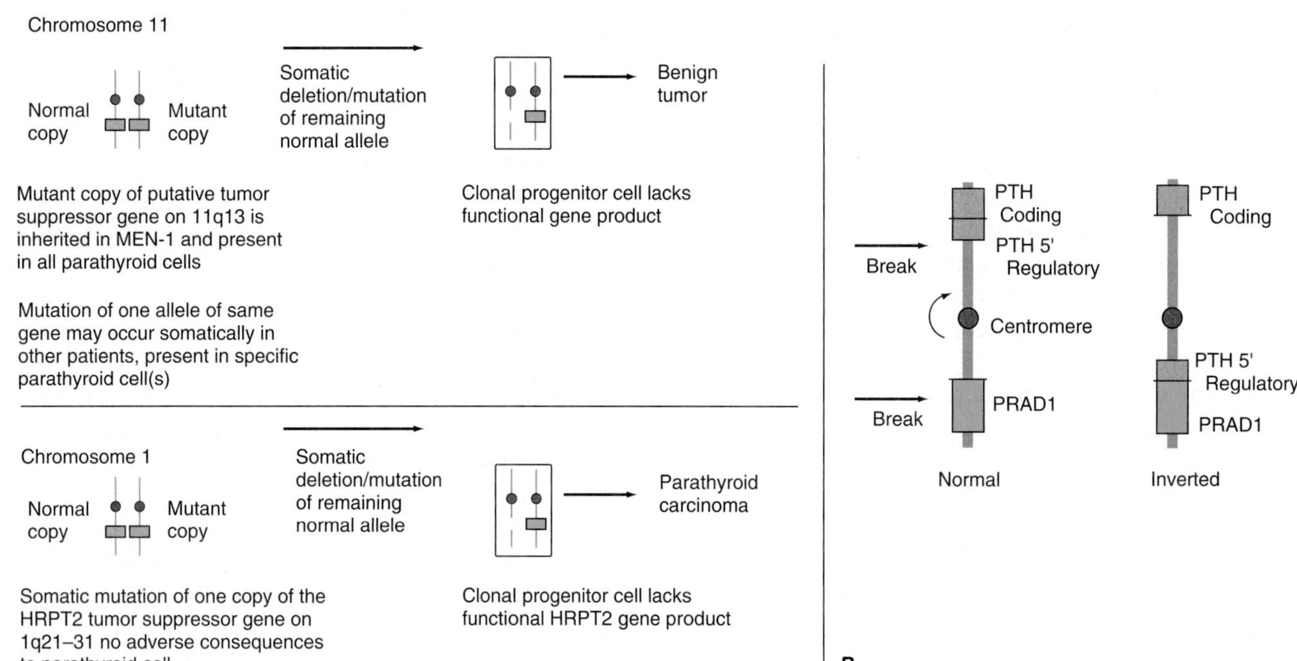

FIGURE 34-3

A. Schematic diagram indicating molecular events in tumor susceptibility. The patient with the hereditary abnormality (multiple endocrine neoplasia [MEN]) is envisioned as having one defective gene inherited from the affected parent on chromosome 11, but one copy of the normal gene is present from the other parent. In the monoclonal tumor (benign tumor), a somatic event, here partial chromosomal deletion, removes the remaining normal gene from a cell. In nonhereditary tumors, two successive somatic mutations must occur, a process that takes a longer time. By either pathway, the cell, deprived of growth-regulating influence from this gene, has unregulated growth and becomes a tumor. A different genetic locus also involving loss of a tumor-suppressor gene termed HRPT2 is involved in the pathogenesis of parathyroid carcinoma. *(From A Arnold: J Clin Endocrine Metab 77:1108, 1993. Copyright 1993, The Endocrine Society.)* ***B.*** Schematic illustration of the mechanism and consequences of gene rearrangement and overexpression of the *PRAD1* protooncogene (pericentromeric inversion of chromosome 11) in parathyroid adenomas. The excessive expression of PRAD1 (a cell cycle control protein, cyclin D_1) by the highly active parathyroid hormone (PTH) gene promoter in the parathyroid cell contributes to excess cellular proliferation. *(From J Habener et al, in L DeGroot, JL Jameson [eds]: Endocrinology, 4th ed. Philadelphia, Saunders, 2001; with permission.)*

initially associated with retinoblastoma but has since been implicated in other neoplasias, including parathyroid carcinoma. Early studies implicated allelic deletions of the *Rb* gene in many parathyroid carcinomas and decreased or absent expression of the Rb protein. However, because there are often large deletions in chromosome 13 that include many genes in addition to the *Rb* locus (with similar findings in some pituitary carcinomas), it remains possible that other tumor-suppressor genes on chromosome 13 may be playing a role in parathyroid carcinoma.

Study of the parathyroid cancers found in some patients with the HPT-JT syndrome has led to identification of a much larger role for mutations in the *HRPT2* gene in most parathyroid carcinomas, including those that arise sporadically, without apparent association with the HPT-JT syndrome. Mutations in the coding region have been identified in 75–80% of all parathyroid cancers analyzed, leading to the conclusion that, with addition of presumed mutations in the noncoding regions, this genetic defect may be seen in essentially all parathyroid carcinomas. Of special importance was the discovery that, in some sporadic parathyroid cancers, germline mutations have been found; this, in turn, has led to careful investigation of the families of these patients and a new clinical indication for genetic testing in this setting.

Hypercalcemia occurring in family members (who are also found to have the germline mutations) can lead to the finding, at parathyroid surgery, of premalignant parathyroid tumors.

Overall, it seems there are multiple factors in parathyroid cancer, in addition to the *HRPT2* and *Rb* gene, although the *HRPT2* gene mutation is the most invariant abnormality. *RET* encodes a tyrosine kinase type receptor; specific inherited germline mutations lead to a constitutive activation of the receptor, thereby explaining the autosomal dominant mode of transmission and the relatively early onset of neoplasia. In the MEN 2 syndrome, the *RET* protooncogene may be responsible for the earliest disorder detected, the polyclonal disorder (C cell hyperplasia, which then is transformed into a clonal outgrowth—a medullary carcinoma with the participation of other, still uncharacterized genetic defects).

In some parathyroid adenomas, activation of a protooncogene has been identified (Fig. 34-3B). A reciprocal translocation involving chromosome 11 has been identified that juxtaposes the *PTH* gene promoter upstream of a gene product termed *PRAD-1*, encoding a cyclin D protein that plays a key role in normal cell division. This translocation plus other mechanisms that cause an equivalent overexpression of cyclin D1 are found in 20–40% of parathyroid adenomas.

Mouse models have confirmed the role of several of the major identified genetic defects in parathyroid disease and the MEN syndromes. Loss of the *MEN1* gene locus or overexpression of the *PRAD-1* protooncogene or the mutated *RET* protooncogene have been analyzed by genetic manipulation in mice, with the expected onset of parathyroid tumors or medullary carcinoma, respectively.

Signs and symptoms

Many patients with hyperparathyroidism are asymptomatic. Manifestations of hyperparathyroidism involve primarily the kidneys and the skeletal system. Kidney involvement, due either to deposition of calcium in the renal parenchyma or to recurrent nephrolithiasis, was present in 60–70% of patients prior to 1970. With earlier detection, renal complications occur in <20% of patients in many large series. Renal stones are usually composed of either calcium oxalate or calcium phosphate. In occasional patients, repeated episodes of nephrolithiasis or the formation of large calculi may lead to urinary tract obstruction, infection, and loss of renal function. Nephrocalcinosis may also cause decreased renal function and phosphate retention.

The distinctive bone manifestation of hyperparathyroidism is *osteitis fibrosa cystica*, which occurred in 10–25% of patients in series reported 50 years ago. Histologically, the pathognomonic features are an increase in the giant multinucleated osteoclasts in scalloped areas on the surface of the bone (Howship's lacunae) and a replacement of the normal cellular and marrow elements by fibrous tissue. X-ray changes include resorption of the phalangeal tufts and replacement of the usually sharp cortical outline of the bone in the digits by an irregular outline (subperiosteal resorption). In recent years, osteitis fibrosa cystica is very rare in primary hyperparathyroidism, probably due to the earlier detection of the disease.

Dual-energy x-ray absorptiometry (DEXA) of the spine provides reproducible quantitative estimates (within a few percent) of spinal bone density. Similarly, bone density in the extremities can be quantified by densitometry of the hip or of the distal radius at a site chosen to be primarily cortical. Computed tomography (CT) is a very sensitive technique for estimating spinal bone density, but reproducibility of standard CT is no better than 5%. Newer CT techniques (spiral, "extreme" CT) are more reproducible but are currently available in a limited number of medical centers. Cortical bone density is reduced while cancellous bone density, especially in the spine, is relatively preserved. In symptomatic patients, dysfunctions of the CNS, peripheral nerve and muscle, gastrointestinal tract, and joints also occur. It has been reported that severe neuropsychiatric manifestations may be reversed by parathyroidectomy. When present in symptomatic patients, neuromuscular manifestations may include proximal muscle weakness, easy fatigability, and atrophy of muscles and may be so striking as to suggest a primary neuromuscular disorder. The distinguishing feature is the complete regression of neuromuscular disease after surgical correction of the hyperparathyroidism.

Gastrointestinal manifestations are sometimes subtle and include vague abdominal complaints and disorders of the stomach and pancreas. Again, cause and effect are unclear. In MEN 1 patients with hyperparathyroidism, duodenal ulcer may be the result of associated pancreatic tumors that secrete excessive quantities of gastrin (Zollinger-Ellison syndrome). Pancreatitis has been reported in association with hyperparathyroidism, but the incidence and the mechanism are not established.

Much attention has been paid in recent years to the manifestations of and optimum management strategies for asymptomatic hyperparathyroidism. This is now the most prevalent form of the disease. *Asymptomatic primary hyperparathyroidism* is defined as biochemically confirmed hyperparathyroidism (elevated or inappropriately normal PTH levels despite hypercalcemia) with the absence of signs and symptoms typically associated with more severe hyperparathyroidism such as features of renal or bone disease.

Three conferences on the topic have been held in the United States over the past two decades, with the most recent in 2008. The published proceedings include discussion of more subtle manifestations of disease, its natural history (without parathyroidectomy), and guidelines both for indications for surgery and medical monitoring in nonoperated patients.

Issues of concern include the potential for cardiovascular deterioration, the presence of subtle neuropsychiatric symptoms, and the longer-term status of skeletal integrity in patients not treated surgically. The current consensus is that medical monitoring rather than surgical correction of hyperparathyroidism may be justified in certain patients. The current recommendation is that patients who show mild disease, as defined by specific

TABLE 34-2

GUIDELINES FOR SURGERY IN ASYMPTOMATIC PRIMARY HYPERPARATHYROIDISM[a]

PARAMETER	GUIDELINE
Serum calcium (above normal)	>1 mg/dL
24-h urinary calcium	No indication
Creatinine clearance (calculated)[b]	If <60 mL/min
Bone density	T score <–2.5 at any of 3 sites[c]
Age	<50

[a]JP Bilezikian et al: Guidelines for the management of asymptomatic primary hyperparathyroidism: Summary statement from the third international workshop. J Clin Endocrinol Metab 94:335, 2009.
[b]Creatinine clearance calculated by Cockcroft-Gault equation or Modification of Diet in Renal Disease (MDRD) equation.
[c]Spine, distal radius, hip.

criteria (Table 34-2), can be safely followed under management guidelines (Table 34-3). There is, however, growing uncertainty about subtle disease manifestations and whether surgery is therefore indicated in most patients. Among the issues is the evidence of eventual (>8 years) deterioration in bone mineral density after a decade of relative stability. There is concern that this late-onset deterioration in bone density in nonoperated patients could contribute significantly to the well-known age-dependent fracture risk (osteoporosis). One study reported significant and sustained improvements in bone mineral density after successful parathyroidectomy, again raising the issue regarding benefits of surgery. Other randomized studies, however, did not report major gains after surgery.

Cardiovascular disease including left ventricular hypertrophy, cardiac functional defects, and endothelial dysfunction have been reported as reversible in European patients with more severe symptomatic disease after surgery, leading to numerous studies of these

TABLE 34-3

GUIDELINES FOR MONITORING IN ASYMPTOMATIC PRIMARY HYPERPARATHYROIDISM[a]

PARAMETER	GUIDELINE
Serum calcium	Annually
24-h urinary calcium	Recommended
Creatinine clearance	Recommended
Serum creatinine[b]	Annually
Bone density	Annually (3 sites)[a]

[a]Updates guidelines (JP Bilezikian et al: J Clin Endocrinol Metab 2014; epub ahead of print).
[b]Creatinine clearance calculated by Cockcroft-Gault equation or Modification of Diet in Renal Disease (MDRD) equation.

cardiovascular features in those with milder disease. There are reports of endothelial dysfunction in patients with mild asymptomatic hyperparathyroidism, but the expert panels concluded that more observation is needed, especially regarding whether there is reversibility with surgery.

A topic of considerable interest and some debate is assessment of neuropsychiatric status and health-related quality of life (QOL) status in hyperparathyroid patients both before surgery and in response to parathyroidectomy. Several observational studies suggest considerable improvements in symptom score after surgery. Randomized studies of surgery versus observation, however, have yielded inconclusive results, especially regarding benefits of surgery. Most studies report that hyperparathyroidism is associated with increased neuropsychiatric symptoms, so the issue remains a significant factor in decisions regarding the impact of surgery in this disease.

DIAGNOSIS

The diagnosis is typically made by detecting an elevated immunoreactive PTH level in a patient with asymptomatic hypercalcemia (see "Differential Diagnosis: Special Tests," below). Serum phosphate is usually low but may be normal, especially if renal failure has developed.

Several modifications in PTH assays have been introduced in efforts to improve their utility in light of information about metabolism of PTH (as discussed above). First-generation assays were based on displacement of radiolabeled PTH from antibodies that reacted with PTH (often also PTH fragments). Double-antibody or immunometric assays (one antibody that is usually directed against the carboxyl-terminal portion of intact PTH to capture the hormone and a second radio- or enzyme-labeled antibody that is usually directed against the amino-terminal portion of intact PTH) greatly improved the diagnostic discrimination of the tests by eliminating interference from circulating biologically inactive fragments, detected by the original first-generation assays. Double-antibody assays are now referred to as second-generation. Such PTH assays have in some centers and testing laboratories been replaced by third-generation assays after it was discovered that large PTH fragments, devoid of only the extreme amino-terminal portion of the PTH molecule, are also present in blood and are detected, incorrectly, as intact PTH. These amino-terminally truncated PTH fragments were prevented from registering in the newer third-generation assays by use of a detection antibody directed against the extreme amino-terminal epitope. These assays may be useful for clinical research studies as in management of chronic renal disease, but the consensus is that either second- or third-generation assays are useful in the diagnosis of

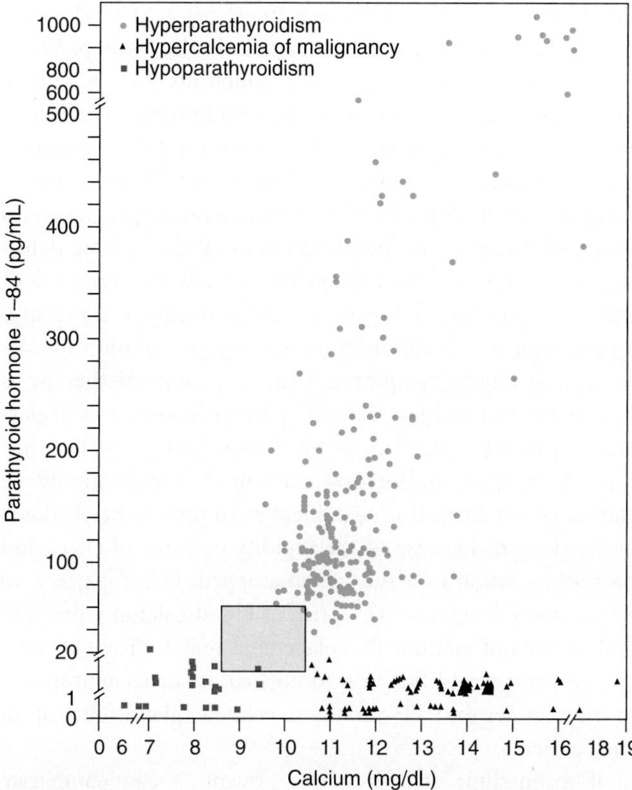

FIGURE 34-4

Levels of immunoreactive parathyroid hormone (PTH) detected in patients with primary hyperparathyroidism, hypercalcemia of malignancy, and hypoparathyroidism. *Boxed area* represents the upper and normal limits of blood calcium and/or immunoreactive PTH. *(From SR Nussbaum, JT Potts, Jr, in L DeGroot, JL Jameson [eds]: Endocrinology, 4th ed. Philadelphia, Saunders, 2001; with permission.)*

primary hyperparathyroidism and for the diagnosis of high-turnover bone disease in chronic kidney disease.

Many tests based on renal responses to excess PTH (renal calcium and phosphate clearance; blood phosphate, chloride, magnesium; urinary or nephrogenous cyclic AMP [cAMP]) were used in earlier decades. These tests have low specificity for hyperparathyroidism and are therefore not cost-effective; they have been replaced by PTH immunometric assays combined with simultaneous blood calcium measurements (Fig. 34-4).

TREATMENT Hyperparathyroidism

Surgical excision of the abnormal parathyroid tissue is the definitive therapy for this disease. As noted above, medical surveillance without operation for patients with mild, asymptomatic disease is, however, still preferred by some physicians and patients, particularly when the patients are more elderly. Evidence favoring surgery, if medically feasible, is growing because of concerns about skeletal, cardiovascular, and neuropsychiatric disease, even in mild hyperparathyroidism.

Two surgical approaches are generally practiced. The conventional parathyroidectomy procedure was neck exploration with general anesthesia; this procedure is being replaced in many centers, whenever feasible, by an outpatient procedure with local anesthesia, termed *minimally invasive parathyroidectomy.*

Parathyroid exploration is challenging and should be undertaken by an experienced surgeon. Certain features help in predicting the pathology (e.g., multiple abnormal glands in familial cases). However, some critical decisions regarding management can be made only during the operation.

With conventional surgery, one approach is still based on the view that typically only one gland (the adenoma) is abnormal. If an enlarged gland is found, a normal gland should be sought. In this view, if a biopsy of a normal-sized second gland confirms its histologic (and presumed functional) normality, no further exploration, biopsy, or excision is needed. At the other extreme is the minority viewpoint that all four glands be sought and that most of the total parathyroid tissue mass be removed. The concern with the former approach is that the recurrence rate of hyperparathyroidism may be high if a second abnormal gland is missed; the latter approach could involve unnecessary surgery and an unacceptable rate of hypoparathyroidism. When normal glands are found in association with one enlarged gland, excision of the single adenoma usually leads to cure or at least years free of symptoms. Long-term follow-up studies to establish true rates of recurrence are limited.

Recently, there has been growing experience with new surgical strategies that feature a minimally invasive approach guided by improved preoperative localization and intraoperative monitoring by PTH assays. Preoperative ^{99m}Tc sestamibi scans with single-photon emission CT (SPECT) are used to predict the location of an abnormal gland and intraoperative sampling of PTH before and at 5-min intervals after removal of a suspected adenoma to confirm a rapid fall (>50%) to normal levels of PTH. In several centers, a combination of preoperative sestamibi imaging, cervical block anesthesia, minimal surgical incision, and intraoperative PTH measurements has allowed successful outpatient surgical management with a clear-cut cost benefit compared to general anesthesia and more extensive neck surgery. The use of these minimally invasive approaches requires clinical judgment to select patients unlikely to have multiple gland disease (e.g., MEN or secondary hyperparathyroidism). The growing acceptance of the technique and its relative ease for the patient has lowered the threshold for surgery.

Severe hypercalcemia may provide a preoperative clue to the presence of parathyroid carcinoma. In such cases, when neck exploration is undertaken, the tissue should be widely excised; care is taken to avoid rupture of the capsule to prevent local seeding of tumor cells.

Multiple-gland hyperplasia, as predicted in familial cases, poses more difficult questions of surgical management. Once a diagnosis of hyperplasia is established, all the glands must be identified. Two schemes have been proposed for surgical management. One is to totally remove three glands with partial excision of the fourth gland; care is taken to leave a good blood supply for the remaining gland. Other surgeons advocate total parathyroidectomy with immediate transplantation of a portion of a removed, minced parathyroid gland into the muscles of the forearm, with the view that surgical excision is easier from the ectopic site in the arm if there is recurrent hyperfunction.

In a minority of cases, if no abnormal parathyroid glands are found in the neck, the issue of further exploration must be decided. There are documented cases of five or six parathyroid glands and of unusual locations for adenomas such as in the mediastinum.

When a second parathyroid exploration is indicated, the minimally invasive techniques for preoperative localization such as ultrasound, CT scan, and isotope scanning are combined with venous sampling and/or selective digital arteriography in one of the centers specializing in these procedures. Intraoperative monitoring of PTH levels by rapid PTH immunoassays may be useful in guiding the surgery. At one center, long-term cures have been achieved with selective embolization or injection of large amounts of contrast material into the end-arterial circulation feeding the parathyroid tumor.

A decline in serum calcium occurs within 24 h after successful surgery; usually blood calcium falls to low-normal values for 3–5 days until the remaining parathyroid tissue resumes full hormone secretion. Acute postoperative hypocalcemia is likely only if severe bone mineral deficits are present or if injury to all the normal parathyroid glands occurs during surgery. In general, there are few problems encountered in patients with uncomplicated disease such as a single adenoma (the clear majority), who do not have symptomatic bone disease or a large deficit in bone mineral, who are vitamin D and magnesium sufficient, and who have good renal and gastrointestinal function. The extent of postoperative hypocalcemia varies with the surgical approach. If all glands are biopsied, hypocalcemia may be transiently symptomatic and more prolonged. Hypocalcemia is more likely to be symptomatic after second parathyroid explorations, particularly when normal parathyroid tissue was removed at the initial operation and when the manipulation and/or biopsy of the remaining normal glands are more extensive in the search for the missing adenoma.

Patients with hyperparathyroidism have efficient intestinal calcium absorption due to the increased levels of $1,25(OH)_2D$ stimulated by PTH excess. Once hypocalcemia signifies successful surgery, patients can be put on a high-calcium intake or be given oral calcium supplements. Despite mild hypocalcemia, most patients do not require parenteral therapy. If the serum calcium falls to <2 mmol/L (8 mg/dL), *and if the phosphate level rises simultaneously,* the possibility that surgery has caused hypoparathyroidism must be considered. With unexpected hypocalcemia, coexistent hypomagnesemia should be considered, because it interferes with PTH secretion and causes functional hypoparathyroidism **(Chap. 32)**.

Signs of hypocalcemia include symptoms such as muscle twitching, a general sense of anxiety, and positive Chvostek's and Trousseau's signs coupled with serum calcium consistently <2 mmol/L (8 mg/dL). Parenteral calcium replacement at a low level should be instituted when hypocalcemia is symptomatic. The rate and duration of IV therapy are determined by the severity of the symptoms and the response of the serum calcium to treatment. An infusion of 0.5–2 mg/kg per hour or 30–100 mL/h of a 1-mg/mL solution usually suffices to relieve symptoms. Usually, parenteral therapy is required for only a few days. If symptoms worsen or if parenteral calcium is needed for >2–3 days, therapy with a vitamin D analogue and/or oral calcium (2–4 g/d) should be started (see below). It is cost-effective to use calcitriol (doses of 0.5–1 μg/d) because of the rapidity of onset of effect and prompt cessation of action when stopped, in comparison to other forms of vitamin D. A rise in blood calcium after several months of vitamin D replacement may indicate restoration of parathyroid function to normal. It is also appropriate to monitor serum PTH serially to estimate gland function in such patients.

If magnesium deficiency was present, it can complicate the postoperative course since magnesium deficiency impairs the secretion of PTH. Hypomagnesemia should be corrected whenever detected. Magnesium replacement can be effective orally (e.g., $MgCl_2$, $MgOH_2$), but parenteral repletion is usual to ensure postoperative recovery, if magnesium deficiency is suspected due to low blood magnesium levels. Because the depressant effect of magnesium on central and peripheral nerve functions does not occur at levels <2 mmol/L (normal range 0.8–1.2 mmol/L), parenteral replacement can be given rapidly. A cumulative dose as great as 0.5–1 mmol/kg of body weight can be administered if severe hypomagnesemia is present; often, however, total doses of 20–40 mmol are sufficient.

MEDICAL MANAGEMENT The guidelines for recommending surgical intervention, if feasible (Table 34-2), as well as for monitoring patients with asymptomatic hyperparathyroidism who elect not to undergo parathyroidectomy (Table 34-3), reflect the changes over time since the first conference on the topic in 1990. Medical monitoring rather than corrective surgery is still acceptable, but it is clear that surgical intervention is the more frequently recommended option for the reasons noted above. Tightened guidelines favoring surgery include lowering the recommended level of serum calcium elevation, more careful attention to skeletal integrity through reference to peak skeletal mass at baseline (T scores) rather than age-adjusted bone density (Z scores), as well as the presence of any fragility fracture. The other changes noted in the two guidelines (Tables 34-2 and 34-3) reflect accumulated experience and practical consideration, such as a difficulty in quantity of urine collections. Despite the usefulness of the guidelines, the importance of individual patient and physician judgment and preference is clear in all recommendations.

When surgery is not selected, or not medically feasible, there is interest in the potential value of specific medical therapies. There is no long-term experience regarding specific clinical outcomes such as fracture prevention, but it has been established that bisphosphonates increase bone mineral density significantly without changing serum calcium (as does estrogen, but the latter is not favored because of reported adverse effects in other organ systems). Calcimimetics that lower PTH secretion lower calcium but do not affect bone mineral density.

OTHER PARATHYROID-RELATED CAUSES OF HYPERCALCEMIA

Lithium therapy

Lithium, used in the management of bipolar depression and other psychiatric disorders, causes hypercalcemia in ~10% of treated patients. The hypercalcemia is dependent on continued lithium treatment, remitting and recurring when lithium is stopped and restarted. The parathyroid adenomas reported in some hypercalcemic patients with lithium therapy may reflect the presence of an independently occurring parathyroid tumor; a permanent effect of lithium on parathyroid gland growth need not be implicated as most patients have complete reversal of hypercalcemia when lithium is stopped. However, long-standing stimulation of parathyroid cell replication by lithium may predispose to development of adenomas (as is documented in secondary hyperparathyroidism and renal failure).

At the levels achieved in blood in treated patients, lithium can be shown in vitro to shift the PTH secretion curve to the right in response to calcium; i.e., higher calcium levels are required to lower PTH secretion, probably acting at the calcium sensor (see below). This effect can cause elevated PTH levels and consequent hypercalcemia in otherwise normal individuals. Fortunately, there are usually alternative medications for the underlying psychiatric illness. Parathyroid surgery should not be recommended unless hypercalcemia and elevated PTH levels persist after lithium is discontinued.

GENETIC DISORDERS CAUSING HYPERPARATHYROID-LIKE SYNDROMES

Familial hypocalciuric hypercalcemia

FHH (also called *familial benign hypercalcemia*) is inherited as an autosomal dominant trait. Affected individuals are discovered because of asymptomatic hypercalcemia. Most cases of FHH (FHH1) are caused by an inactivating mutation in a single allele of the CaSR (see below), leading to inappropriately normal or even increased secretion of PTH, whereas another hypercalcemic disorder, namely the exceedingly rare Jansen's disease, is caused by a constitutively active PTH/PTHrP receptor in target tissues. Neither FHH1 nor Jansen's disease, however, is a growth disorder of the parathyroids. Other forms of FHH are caused either by heterozygous mutations in *GNA11* (encoding G11), one of the signaling proteins downstream of the CaSR (FHH2), or by mutations in *AP2S1* (FHH3).

The pathophysiology of FHH1 is now understood. The primary defect is abnormal sensing of the blood calcium by the parathyroid gland and renal tubule, causing inappropriate secretion of PTH and excessive reabsorption of calcium in the distal renal tubules. The CaSR is a member of the third family of GPCRs (type C or type III). The receptor responds to increased ECF calcium concentration by suppressing PTH secretion through second-messenger signaling involving the G protein alpha-subunits G11 and Gq, thereby providing negative-feedback regulation of PTH secretion. Many different inactivating CaSR mutations have been identified in patients with FHH1. These mutations lower the capacity of the sensor to bind calcium, and the mutant receptors function as though blood calcium levels were low; excessive secretion of PTH occurs from an otherwise normal gland. Approximately two-thirds of patients with FHH have mutations within the protein-coding region of the CaSR gene. The remaining one-third of kindreds may have mutations in the promoter of the CaSR gene or are caused by mutations in other genes.

Even before elucidation of the pathophysiology of FHH, abundant clinical evidence served to separate the disorder from primary hyperparathyroidism; these clinical features are still useful in differential diagnosis. Patients with primary hyperparathyroidism have <99% renal calcium reabsorption, whereas most patients with FHH have >99% reabsorption. The hypercalcemia in FHH is often detectable in affected members of the kindreds in the first decade of life, whereas hypercalcemia rarely occurs in patients with primary hyperparathyroidism or the MEN syndromes who are age <10 years. PTH may be elevated in the different forms of FHH, but the values are usually normal or lower for the same degree of calcium elevation than is observed in patients with primary hyperparathyroidism. Parathyroid surgery performed in a few patients with FHH before the nature of the syndrome was understood led to permanent hypoparathyroidism; nevertheless, hypocalciuria persisted, establishing that hypocalciuria is not PTH-dependent (now known to be due to the abnormal CaSR in the kidney).

Few clinical signs or symptoms are present in patients with FHH, whereas other endocrine abnormalities are not. Most patients are detected as a result of family screening after hypercalcemia is detected in a proband. In those patients inadvertently operated upon for primary hyperparathyroidism, the parathyroids appeared normal or moderately hyperplastic. Parathyroid surgery is not appropriate, nor, in view of the lack of symptoms, does medical treatment seem needed to lower the calcium. One striking exception to the rule against parathyroid surgery in this syndrome is the occurrence, usually in consanguineous marriages (due to the rarity of the gene mutation), of a homozygous or compound heterozygote state, resulting in severe impairment of CaSR function. In this condition, neonatal severe hypercalcemia, total parathyroidectomy is mandatory, but calcimetics have been used as a temporary measure. Rare but well-documented cases of acquired hypocalciuric hypercalcemia are reported due to antibodies against the CaSR. They appear to be a complication of an underlying autoimmune disorder and respond to therapies directed against the underlying disorder.

Jansen's disease

Activating mutations in the PTH/PTHrP receptor (PTH1R) have been identified as the cause of this rare autosomal dominant syndrome. Because the mutations lead to constitutive activation of receptor function, one abnormal copy of the mutant receptor is sufficient to cause the disease, thereby accounting for its dominant mode of transmission. The disorder leads to short-limbed dwarfism due to abnormal regulation of chondrocyte maturation in the growth plates of the bone that are formed through the endochondral process. In adult life, there are numerous abnormalities in bone, including multiple cystic resorptive areas resembling those seen in severe hyperparathyroidism. Hypercalcemia and hypophosphatemia with undetectable or low PTH levels are typically observed. The pathogenesis of the growth plate abnormalities in Jansen's disease has been confirmed by transgenic experiments in which targeted expression of the mutant PTH/PTHrP receptor to the proliferating chondrocyte layer of growth plate emulated several features of the human disorder. Some of these genetic mutations in the parathyroid gland or PTH target cells that affect Ca^{2+} metabolism are illustrated in Fig. 34-5.

MALIGNANCY-RELATED HYPERCALCEMIA

Clinical syndromes and mechanisms of hypercalcemia

Hypercalcemia due to malignancy is common (occurring in as many as 20% of cancer patients, especially with certain types of tumor such as lung carcinoma), often severe and difficult to manage, and, on rare occasions, difficult to distinguish from primary hyperparathyroidism. Although malignancy is often clinically obvious or readily detectable by medical history, hypercalcemia can occasionally be due to an occult tumor. Previously, hypercalcemia associated with malignancy was thought to be due to local invasion and destruction of bone by tumor cells; many cases are now known to result from the elaboration by the malignant cells of humoral mediators of hypercalcemia. PTHrP is the responsible humoral agent in most solid tumors that cause hypercalcemia.

The histologic character of the tumor is more important than the extent of skeletal metastases in predicting hypercalcemia. Small-cell carcinoma (oat cell) and adenocarcinoma of the lung, although the most common lung tumors associated with skeletal metastases, rarely cause hypercalcemia. By contrast, many patients with squamous cell carcinoma of the lung develop hypercalcemia. Histologic studies of bone in patients with squamous cell or epidermoid carcinoma of the lung, in sites invaded by tumor as well as areas remote from tumor invasion, reveal increased bone resorption.

Two main mechanisms of hypercalcemia are operative in cancer hypercalcemia. Many solid tumors associated with hypercalcemia, particularly squamous cell and renal tumors, produce and secrete PTHrP that causes increased bone resorption and mediate the hypercalcemia through systemic actions on the skeleton. Alternatively, direct bone marrow invasion occurs with hematologic malignancies such as leukemia, lymphoma, and multiple myeloma. Lymphokines and cytokines (including PTHrP) produced by cells involved in the marrow response to the tumors promote resorption of bone through local destruction. Several hormones, hormone analogues, cytokines, and growth factors have been implicated as the result of clinical assays, in vitro tests, or chemical isolation. The etiologic factor produced by activated normal lymphocytes and by myeloma and lymphoma cells, originally termed *osteoclast activation factor*, now appears to represent the biologic action of several different cytokines, probably interleukin 1 and lymphotoxin or tumor necrosis factor (TNF). In some lymphomas, there is a third mechanism, caused by an increased blood level of $1,25(OH)_2D$, produced by the abnormal lymphocytes.

In the more common mechanism, usually termed *humoral hypercalcemia of malignancy*, solid tumors (cancers of the lung and kidney, in particular), in which bone metastases are absent, minimal, or not detectable clinically, secrete PTHrP measurable by immunoassay. Secretion by the tumors of the PTH-like factor, PTHrP, activates the PTH1R, resulting in a pathophysiology closely resembling hyperparathyroidism, but with normal or suppressed PTH levels. The clinical picture resembles primary hyperparathyroidism

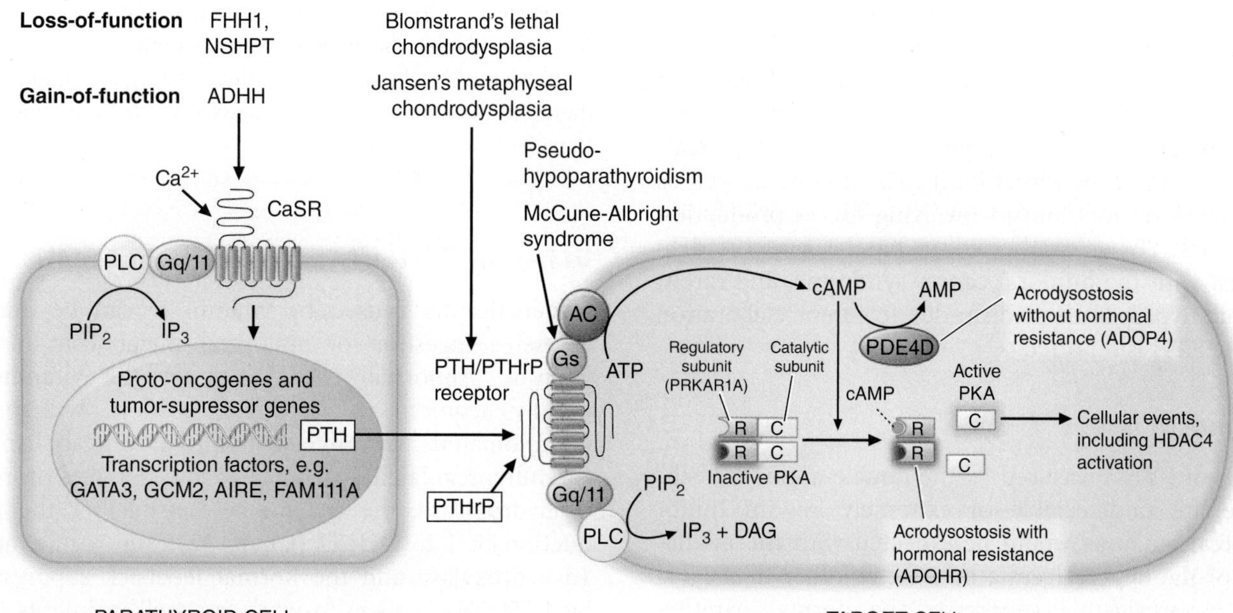

FIGURE 34-5

Illustration of some genetic mutations that alter calcium metabolism by effects on the parathyroid cell or target cells of parathyroid hormone (PTH) action. Alterations in PTH production by the parathyroid cell can be caused by changes in the response to extracellular fluid calcium (Ca^{2+}) that are detected by the calcium-sensing receptor (CaSR). Furthermore, PTH (or PTH-related peptide [PTHrP]) can show altered efficacy in target cells such as in proximal tubular cells, by altered function of its receptor (PTH/PTHrP receptor) or the signal transduction proteins, G proteins such as $G_s\alpha$, which is linked to adenylate cyclase (AC), the enzyme responsible for producing cyclic AMP (cAMP) (also illustrated are Gq/11, which activate an alternate pathway of receptor signal transmission involving the generation of inositol triphosphate [IP_3] or diacylglycerol [DAG]). Heterozygous loss-of-function mutations in the CaSR cause familial benign hypocalciuric hypercalcemia (FBHH), homozygous mutations (both alleles mutated), and severe neonatal hyperparathyroidism (NSHPT); heterozygous gain-of-function causes autosomal dominant hypercalciuric hypocalcemia (ADHH). Other defects in parathyroid cell function that occur at the level of gene regulation (oncogenes or tumor-suppressor genes) or transcription factors are discussed in the text. Blomstrand's lethal chondrodysplasia is due to homozygous or compound heterozygous loss-of-function mutations in the PTH/PTHrP receptor, a neonatally lethal disorder, while pseudohypoparathyroidism involves inactivation at the level of the G proteins, specifically mutations that eliminate or reduce $G_s\alpha$ activity in the kidney (see text for details). Acrodysostosis can occur with (acrodysostosis with hormonal resistance [ADOHR]; mutant regulatory subunit of PKA) or without hormonal resistance (ADOP4; mutant PDE4D). Jansen's metaphyseal chondrodysplasia and McCune-Albright syndrome represent gain-of-function mutations in the PTH/PTHrP receptor and $G_s\alpha$ protein, respectively.

(hypophosphatemia accompanies hypercalcemia), and elimination or regression of the primary tumor leads to disappearance of the hypercalcemia.

As in hyperparathyroidism, patients with the humoral hypercalcemia of malignancy have elevated urinary nephrogenous cAMP excretion, hypophosphatemia, and increased urinary phosphate clearance. However, in humoral hypercalcemia of malignancy, immunoreactive PTH is undetectable or suppressed, making the differential diagnosis easier. Other features of the disorder differ from those of true hyperparathyroidism. Although the biologic actions of PTH and PTHrP are exerted through the same receptor, subtle differences in receptor activation by the two ligands must account for some of the discordance in pathophysiology, when an excess of one or the other peptide occurs. Other cytokines elaborated by the malignancy may contribute to the variations from hyperparathyroidism in these patients as well. Patients with humoral hypercalcemia of malignancy may have low to normal levels of $1{,}25(OH)_2D$ instead of elevated levels as in true hyperparathyroidism. In some patients with the humoral hypercalcemia of malignancy, osteoclastic resorption is unaccompanied by an osteoblastic or bone-forming response, implying inhibition of the normal coupling of bone formation and resorption.

Several different assays (single- or double-antibody, different epitopes) have been developed to detect PTHrP. Most data indicate that circulating PTHrP levels are undetectable (or low) in normal individuals except perhaps in pregnancy (high in human milk) and elevated in most cancer patients with the humoral syndrome. The etiologic mechanisms in cancer hypercalcemia may be multiple in the same patient. For example, in breast carcinoma (metastatic to bone) and in a distinctive type of T cell lymphoma/leukemia initiated by human T cell lymphotropic virus I, hypercalcemia is caused by direct local lysis of bone as well as by a humoral mechanism involving excess production of PTHrP. Hyperparathyroidism has been reported to coexist with the humoral cancer syndrome, and rarely, ectopic hyperparathyroidism due to tumor elaboration of true PTH is reported.

Diagnostic issues

Levels of PTH measured by the double-antibody technique are undetectable or extremely low in tumor hypercalcemia, as would be expected with the mediation of the hypercalcemia by a factor other than PTH (the hypercalcemia suppresses the normal parathyroid glands). In a patient with minimal symptoms referred for hypercalcemia, low or undetectable PTH levels would focus attention on a possible occult malignancy (except for very rare cases of ectopic hyperparathyroidism).

Ordinarily, the diagnosis of cancer hypercalcemia is not difficult because tumor symptoms are prominent when hypercalcemia is detected. Indeed, hypercalcemia may be noted incidentally during the workup of a patient with known or suspected malignancy. Clinical suspicion that malignancy is the cause of the hypercalcemia is heightened when there are other signs or symptoms of a paraneoplastic process such as weight loss, fatigue, muscle weakness, or unexplained skin rash, or when symptoms specific for a particular tumor are present. Squamous cell tumors are most frequently associated with hypercalcemia, particularly tumors of the lung, kidney, head and neck, and urogenital tract. Radiologic examinations can focus on these areas when clinical evidence is unclear. Bone scans with technetium-labeled bisphosphonate are useful for detection of osteolytic metastases; the sensitivity is high, but specificity is low; results must be confirmed by conventional x-rays to be certain that areas of increased uptake are due to osteolytic metastases per se. Bone marrow biopsies are helpful in patients with anemia or abnormal peripheral blood smears.

TREATMENT Malignancy-Related Hypercalcemia

Treatment of the hypercalcemia of malignancy is first directed to control of tumor; reduction of tumor mass usually corrects hypercalcemia. If a patient has severe hypercalcemia yet has a good chance for effective tumor therapy, treatment of the hypercalcemia should be vigorous while awaiting the results of definitive therapy. If hypercalcemia occurs in the late stages of a tumor that is resistant to antitumor therapy, the treatment of the hypercalcemia should be judicious as high calcium levels can have a mild sedating effect. Standard therapies for hypercalcemia (discussed below) are applicable to patients with malignancy.

VITAMIN D–RELATED HYPERCALCEMIA

Hypercalcemia caused by vitamin D can be due to excessive ingestion or abnormal metabolism of the vitamin. Abnormal metabolism of the vitamin is usually acquired in association with a widespread granulomatous disorder. Vitamin D metabolism is carefully regulated, particularly the activity of renal 1α-hydroxylase, the enzyme responsible for the production of $1,25(OH)_2D$ **(Chap. 32)**. The regulation of 1α-hydroxylase and the normal feedback suppression by $1,25(OH)_2D$ seem to work less well in infants than in adults and to operate poorly, if at all, in sites other than the renal tubule; these phenomena may explain the occurrence of hypercalcemia secondary to excessive $1,25(OH)_2D$ production in infants with Williams' syndrome (see below) and in adults with sarcoidosis or lymphoma.

Vitamin D intoxication

Chronic ingestion of 40–100 times the normal physiologic requirement of vitamin D (amounts >40,000–100,000 U/d) is usually required to produce significant hypercalcemia in otherwise healthy individuals. The stated upper limit of safe dietary intake is 2000 U/d (50 μg/d) in adults because of concerns about potential toxic effects of cumulative supraphysiologic doses. These recommendations are now regarded as too restrictive, because some estimates are that in elderly individuals in northern latitudes, 2000 U/d or more may be necessary to avoid vitamin D insufficiency.

Hypercalcemia in vitamin D intoxication is due to an excessive biologic action of the vitamin, perhaps the consequence of increased levels of 25(OH)D rather than merely increased levels of the active metabolite $1,25(OH)_2D$ (the latter may not be elevated in vitamin D intoxication). 25(OH)D has definite, if low, biologic activity in the intestine and bone. The production of 25(OH)D is less tightly regulated than is the production of $1,25(OH)_2D$. Hence concentrations of 25(OH)D are elevated several-fold in patients with excess vitamin D intake.

The diagnosis is substantiated by documenting elevated levels of 25(OH)D >100 mg/mL. Hypercalcemia is usually controlled by restriction of dietary calcium intake and appropriate attention to hydration. These measures, plus discontinuation of vitamin D, usually lead to resolution of hypercalcemia. However, vitamin

D stores in fat may be substantial, and vitamin D intoxication may persist for weeks after vitamin D ingestion is terminated. Such patients are responsive to glucocorticoids, which in doses of 100 mg/d of hydrocortisone or its equivalent usually return serum calcium levels to normal over several days; severe intoxication may require intensive therapy.

Sarcoidosis and other granulomatous diseases

In patients with sarcoidosis and other granulomatous diseases, such as tuberculosis and fungal infections, excess $1,25(OH)_2D$ is synthesized in macrophages or other cells in the granulomas. Indeed, increased $1,25(OH)_2D$ levels have been reported in anephric patients with sarcoidosis and hypercalcemia. Macrophages obtained from granulomatous tissue convert 25(OH)D to $1,25(OH)_2D$ at an increased rate. There is a positive correlation in patients with sarcoidosis between 25(OH)D levels (reflecting vitamin D intake) and the circulating concentrations of $1,25(OH)_2D$, whereas normally there is no increase in $1,25(OH)_2D$ with increasing 25(OH)D levels due to multiple feedback controls on renal 1α-hydroxylase **(Chap. 32)**. The usual regulation of active metabolite production by calcium and phosphate or by PTH does not operate in these patients. Clearance of $1,25(OH)_2D$ from blood may be decreased in sarcoidosis as well. PTH levels are usually low and $1,25(OH)_2D$ levels are elevated, but primary hyperparathyroidism and sarcoidosis may coexist in some patients.

Management of the hypercalcemia can often be accomplished by avoiding excessive sunlight exposure and limiting vitamin D and calcium intake. Presumably, however, the abnormal sensitivity to vitamin D and abnormal regulation of $1,25(OH)_2D$ synthesis will persist as long as the disease is active. Alternatively, glucocorticoids in the equivalent of 100 mg/d of hydrocortisone or equivalent doses of glucocorticoids may help control hypercalcemia. Glucocorticoids appear to act by blocking excessive production of $1,25(OH)_2D$, as well as the response to it in target organs.

Idiopathic hypercalcemia of infancy

This rare disorder, usually referred to as *Williams' syndrome,* is an autosomal dominant disorder characterized by multiple congenital development defects, including supravalvular aortic stenosis, mental retardation, and an elfin facies, in association with hypercalcemia due to abnormal sensitivity to vitamin D. The hypercalcemia associated with the syndrome was first recognized in England after fortification of milk with vitamin D. The cardiac and developmental abnormalities were independently described, but the connection between these defects and hypercalcemia were not described until later. Levels of $1,25(OH)_2D$ can be elevated, ranging from 46 to 120 nmol/L (150–500 pg/mL). The mechanism of the abnormal sensitivity to vitamin D and of the increased circulating levels of $1,25(OH)_2D$ is still unclear. Studies suggest that genetic mutations involving microdeletions at the elastin locus and perhaps other genes on chromosome 7 may play a role in the pathogenesis. Another cause of hypercalcemia in infants and young children is a 24-hydroxylase deficiency that impairs metabolism of $1,25(OH)_2D$.

HYPERCALCEMIA ASSOCIATED WITH HIGH BONE TURNOVER

Hyperthyroidism

As many as 20% of hyperthyroid patients have high-normal or mildly elevated serum calcium concentrations; hypercalciuria is even more common. The hypercalcemia is due to increased bone turnover, with bone resorption exceeding bone formation. Severe calcium elevations are not typical, and the presence of such suggests a concomitant disease such as hyperparathyroidism. Usually, the diagnosis is obvious, but signs of hyperthyroidism may occasionally be occult, particularly in the elderly **(Chap. 7)**. Hypercalcemia is managed by treatment of the hyperthyroidism. Reports that thyroid-stimulating hormone (TSH) itself normally has a bone-protective effect suggest that suppressed TSH levels also play a role in hypercalcemia.

Immobilization

Immobilization is a rare cause of hypercalcemia in adults in the absence of an associated disease but may cause hypercalcemia in children and adolescents, particularly after spinal cord injury and paraplegia or quadriplegia. With resumption of ambulation, the hypercalcemia in children usually returns to normal.

The mechanism appears to involve a disproportion between bone formation and bone resorption; the former decreased and the latter increased. Hypercalciuria and increased mobilization of skeletal calcium can develop in normal volunteers subjected to extensive bed rest, although hypercalcemia is unusual. Immobilization of an adult with a disease associated with high bone turnover, however, such as Paget's disease, may cause hypercalcemia.

Thiazides

Administration of benzothiadiazines (thiazides) can cause hypercalcemia in patients with high rates of bone turnover. Traditionally, thiazides are associated with aggravation of hypercalcemia in primary hyperparathyroidism, but this effect can be seen in other high-bone-turnover states as well. The mechanism of thiazide action is complex. Chronic thiazide administration leads to reduction in urinary calcium; the hypocalciuric effect appears to reflect the enhancement of proximal tubular resorption of sodium and calcium in response to sodium depletion. Some of this renal effect is due to augmentation of PTH action and is more pronounced in individuals with intact PTH secretion. However, thiazides cause hypocalciuria in hypoparathyroid patients on high-dose vitamin D and oral calcium replacement if sodium intake is restricted. This finding is the rationale for the use of thiazides as an adjunct to therapy in hypoparathyroid patients, as discussed below. Thiazide administration to normal individuals causes a transient increase in blood calcium (usually within the high-normal range) that reverts to preexisting levels after a week or more of continued administration. If hormonal function and calcium and bone metabolism are normal, homeostatic controls are reset to counteract the calcium-elevating effect of the thiazides. In the presence of hyperparathyroidism or increased bone turnover from another cause, homeostatic mechanisms are ineffective. The abnormal effects of the thiazide on calcium metabolism disappear within days of cessation of the drug.

Vitamin A intoxication

Vitamin A intoxication is a rare cause of hypercalcemia and is most commonly a side effect of dietary faddism. Calcium levels can be elevated into the 3–3.5-mmol/L (12–14 mg/dL) range after the ingestion of 50,000–100,000 units of vitamin A daily (10–20 times the minimum daily requirement). Typical features of severe hypercalcemia include fatigue, anorexia, and, in some, severe muscle and bone pain. Excess vitamin A intake is presumed to increase bone resorption.

The diagnosis can be established by history and by measurement of vitamin A levels in serum. Occasionally, skeletal x-rays reveal periosteal calcifications, particularly in the hands. Withdrawal of the vitamin is usually associated with prompt disappearance of the hypercalcemia and reversal of the skeletal changes. As in vitamin D intoxication, administration of 100 mg/d of hydrocortisone or its equivalent leads to a rapid return of the serum calcium to normal.

HYPERCALCEMIA ASSOCIATED WITH RENAL FAILURE

Severe secondary hyperparathyroidism

The pathogenesis of secondary hyperparathyroidism in chronic kidney disease is incompletely understood. Resistance to the normal level of PTH is a major factor contributing to the development of hypocalcemia, which, in turn, is a stimulus to parathyroid gland enlargement. However, recent findings have indicated that an increase of FGF23 production by osteocytes (and possibly osteoblasts) in bone occurs well before an elevation in PTH is detected. FGF23 is a potent inhibitor of the renal 1-alpha hydroxylase, and the FGF23-dependent reduction in 1,25(OH)$_2$ vitamin D seems to be an important stimulus for the development of secondary hyperparathyroidism.

Secondary hyperparathyroidism occurs not only in patients with renal failure but also in those with osteomalacia due to multiple causes **(Chap. 32)**, including deficiency of vitamin D action and pseudohypoparathyroidism (deficient response to PTH downstream of PTHR1). For both disorders, hypocalcemia seems to be the common denominator in initiating the development of secondary hyperparathyroidism. Primary (1°) and secondary (2°) hyperparathyroidism can be distinguished conceptually by the autonomous growth of the parathyroid glands in primary hyperparathyroidism (presumably irreversible) and the adaptive response of the parathyroids in secondary hyperparathyroidism (typically reversible). In fact, reversal over weeks from an abnormal pattern of secretion, presumably accompanied by involution of parathyroid gland mass to normal, occurs in patients with osteomalacia who have been treated effectively with calcium and vitamin D. However, it is now recognized that a true clonal outgrowth (irreversible) can arise in long-standing, inadequately treated chronic kidney disease (e.g., tertiary [3°] hyperparathyroidism; see below).

Patients with secondary hyperparathyroidism may develop bone pain, ectopic calcification, and pruritus. The bone disease seen in patients with secondary hyperparathyroidism and chronic kidney disease is termed *renal osteodystrophy* and affects primarily bone turnover. However, osteomalacia is frequently encountered as well and may be related to the circulating levels of FGF23.

Two other skeletal disorders have been frequently associated in the past with chronic kidney disease (CKD) patients treated by long-term dialysis, who received aluminum-containing phosphate binders. Aluminum deposition in bone (see below) leads to an osteomalacia-like picture. The other entity is a low-turnover bone disease termed "aplastic" or "adynamic" bone disease; PTH levels are lower than typically observed in CKD patients with secondary hyperparathyroidism. It is believed that the condition is caused, at least in part, by excessive PTH suppression, which may be even greater than previously appreciated in light of evidence that some of the immunoreactive PTH detected by most commercially available PTH assays is not the full-length biologically active molecule (as discussed above) but may consist of amino-terminally truncated fragments that do not activate the PTH1R.

TREATMENT Secondary Hyperparathyroidism

Medical therapy to reverse secondary hyperparathyroidism in CKD includes reduction of excessive blood phosphate by restriction of dietary phosphate, the use of nonabsorbable phosphate binders, and careful, selective addition of calcitriol (0.25–2 μg/d) or related analogues. Calcium carbonate became preferred over aluminum-containing antacids to prevent aluminum-induced bone disease. However, synthetic gels that also bind phosphate (such as sevelamer) are now widely used, with the advantage of avoiding not only aluminum retention, but also excess calcium loading, which may contribute to cardiovascular calcifications. Intravenous calcitriol (or related analogues), administered as several pulses each week, helps control secondary hyperparathyroidism. Aggressive but carefully administered medical therapy can often, but not always, reverse hyperparathyroidism and its symptoms and manifestations.

Occasional patients develop severe manifestations of secondary hyperparathyroidism, including hypercalcemia, pruritus, extraskeletal calcifications, and painful bones, despite aggressive medical efforts to suppress the hyperparathyroidism. PTH hypersecretion no longer responsive to medical therapy, a state of severe hyperparathyroidism in patients with CKD that requires surgery, has been referred to as *tertiary hyperparathyroidism*. Parathyroid surgery is necessary to control this condition. Based on genetic evidence from examination of tumor samples in these patients, the emergence of autonomous parathyroid function is due to a monoclonal outgrowth of one or more previously hyperplastic parathyroid glands. The adaptive response has become an independent contributor to disease; this finding seems to emphasize the importance of optimal medical management to reduce the proliferative response of the parathyroid cells that enables the irreversible genetic change.

Aluminum intoxication

Aluminum intoxication (and often hypercalcemia as a complication of medical treatment) in the past occurred in patients on chronic dialysis; manifestations included acute dementia and unresponsive and severe osteomalacia. Bone pain, multiple nonhealing fractures, particularly of the ribs and pelvis, and a proximal myopathy occur. Hypercalcemia develops when these patients are treated with vitamin D or calcitriol because of impaired skeletal responsiveness. Aluminum is present at the site of osteoid mineralization, osteoblastic activity is minimal, and calcium incorporation into the skeleton is impaired. The disorder is now rare because of the avoidance of aluminum-containing antacids or aluminum excess in the dialysis regimen.

Milk-alkali syndrome

The milk-alkali syndrome is due to excessive ingestion of calcium and absorbable antacids such as milk or calcium carbonate. It is much less frequent since proton pump inhibitors and other treatments became available for peptic ulcer disease. For a time, the increased use of calcium carbonate in the management of secondary hyperparathyroidism led to reappearance of the syndrome. Several clinical presentations—acute, subacute, and chronic—have been described, all of which feature hypercalcemia, alkalosis, and renal failure. The chronic form of the disease, termed *Burnett's syndrome*, is associated with irreversible renal damage. The acute syndromes reverse if the excess calcium and absorbable alkali are stopped.

Individual susceptibility is important in the pathogenesis, because some patients are treated with calcium carbonate and alkali regimens without developing the syndrome. One variable is the fractional calcium absorption as a function of calcium intake. Some individuals absorb a high fraction of calcium, even with intakes ≥2 g of elemental calcium per day, instead of reducing calcium absorption with high intake, as occurs in most normal individuals. Resultant mild hypercalcemia after meals in such patients is postulated to contribute to the generation of alkalosis. Development of hypercalcemia causes increased sodium excretion and some depletion of total-body water. These phenomena and perhaps some suppression of endogenous PTH secretion due to mild hypercalcemia lead to increased bicarbonate resorption and to alkalosis in the face of continued calcium carbonate ingestion. Alkalosis per se selectively enhances calcium resorption in the distal nephron, thus aggravating the hypercalcemia. The cycle of mild hypercalcemia → bicarbonate retention → alkalosis → renal calcium retention → severe hypercalcemia perpetuates and aggravates hypercalcemia and alkalosis as long as calcium and absorbable alkali are ingested.

DIFFERENTIAL DIAGNOSIS: SPECIAL TESTS

Differential diagnosis of hypercalcemia is best achieved by using clinical criteria, but immunometric assays to measure PTH are especially useful in distinguishing among major causes (Fig. 34-6). The clinical features that deserve emphasis are the presence or absence of symptoms or signs of disease and evidence of chronicity. If one discounts fatigue or depression, >90% of patients with primary hyperparathyroidism have *asymptomatic hypercalcemia*; symptoms of malignancy are usually present in cancer-associated hypercalcemia.

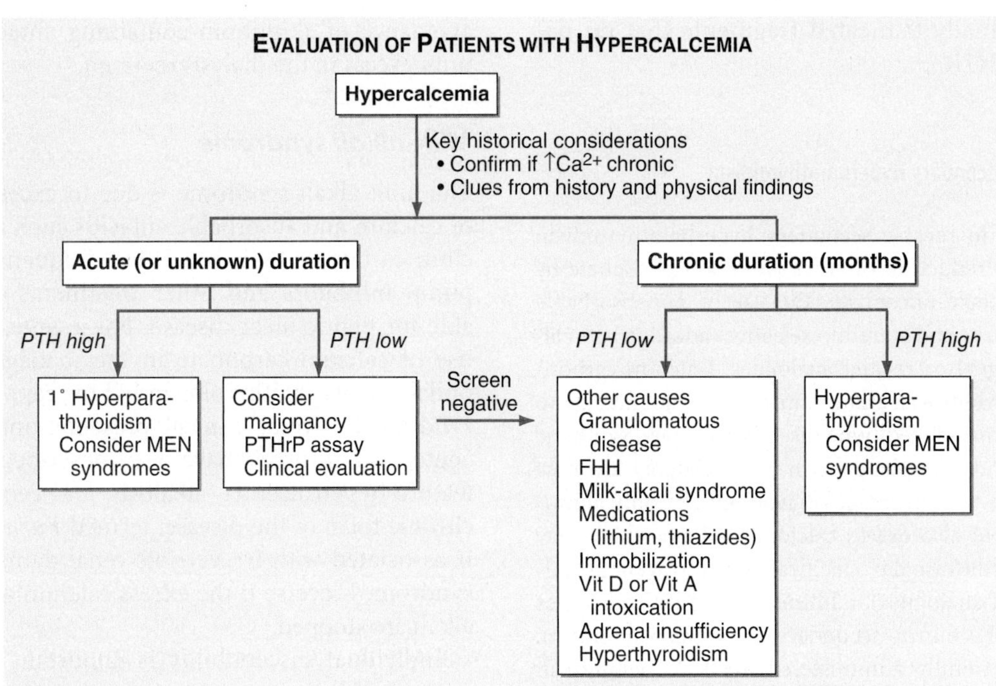

FIGURE 34-6

Algorithm for the evaluation of patients with hypercalcemia. See text for details. FHH, familial hypocalciuric hypercalcemia; MEN, multiple endocrine neoplasia; PTH, parathyroid hormone; PTHrP, parathyroid hormone–related peptide.

Disorders other than hyperparathyroidism and malignancy cause <10% of cases of hypercalcemia, and some of the nonparathyroid causes are associated with clear-cut manifestations such as renal failure.

Hyperparathyroidism is the likely diagnosis in patients with *chronic hypercalcemia*. If hypercalcemia has been manifest for >1 year, malignancy can usually be excluded as the cause. A striking feature of malignancy-associated hypercalcemia is the rapidity of the course, whereby signs and symptoms of the underlying malignancy are evident within months of the detection of hypercalcemia. Although clinical considerations are helpful in arriving at the correct diagnosis of the cause of hypercalcemia, appropriate laboratory testing is essential for definitive diagnosis. The immunoassay for PTH usually separates hyperparathyroidism from all other causes of hypercalcemia (exceptions are very rare reports of ectopic production of excess PTH by nonparathyroid tumors). Patients with hyperparathyroidism have elevated PTH levels despite hypercalcemia, whereas patients with malignancy and the other causes of hypercalcemia (except for disorders mediated by PTH such as lithium-induced hypercalcemia) have levels of hormone below normal or undetectable levels. Assays based on the double-antibody method for PTH exhibit very high sensitivity (especially if serum calcium is simultaneously evaluated) and specificity for the diagnosis of primary hyperparathyroidism (Fig. 34-4).

In summary, PTH values are elevated in >90% of parathyroid-related causes of hypercalcemia, undetectable or low in malignancy-related hypercalcemia, and undetectable or normal in vitamin D–related and high-bone-turnover causes of hypercalcemia. In view of the specificity of the PTH immunoassay and the high frequency of hyperparathyroidism in hypercalcemic patients, it is cost-effective to measure the PTH level in all hypercalcemic patients unless malignancy or a specific nonparathyroid disease is obvious. False-positive PTH assay results are rare. Immunoassays for PTHrP are helpful in diagnosing certain types of malignancy-associated hypercalcemia. Although FHH is parathyroid-related, the disease should be managed distinctively from hyperparathyroidism. Clinical features and the low urinary calcium excretion can help make the distinction. Because the incidence of malignancy and hyperparathyroidism both increase with age, they can coexist as two independent causes of hypercalcemia.

$1,25(OH)_2D$ levels are elevated in many (but not all) patients with primary hyperparathyroidism. In other disorders associated with hypercalcemia, concentrations of $1,25(OH)_2D$ are low or, at the most, normal. However, this test is of low specificity and is not cost-effective, as not all patients with hyperparathyroidism have elevated $1,25(OH)_2D$ levels and not all nonparathyroid hypercalcemic patients have suppressed $1,25(OH)_2D$. Measurement of $1,25(OH)_2D$ is, however, critically valuable in establishing the cause of hypercalcemia in sarcoidosis and certain lymphomas.

A useful general approach is outlined in Fig. 34-6. If the patient is *asymptomatic* and there is evidence of *chronicity* to the hypercalcemia, hyperparathyroidism is almost certainly the cause. If PTH levels (usually measured at least twice) are elevated, the clinical impression is confirmed and little additional evaluation is necessary. If there is only a short history or no data as to the duration of the hypercalcemia, *occult malignancy* must be considered; if the PTH levels are not elevated, then a thorough workup must be undertaken for malignancy, including chest x-ray, CT of chest and abdomen, and bone scan. Immunoassays for PTHrP may be especially useful in such situations. Attention should also be paid to clues for underlying hematologic disorders such as anemia, increased plasma globulin, and abnormal serum immunoelectrophoresis; bone scans can be negative in some patients with metastases such as in multiple myeloma. Finally, if a patient with chronic hypercalcemia is asymptomatic and malignancy therefore seems unlikely on clinical grounds, but PTH values are not elevated, it is useful to search for other chronic causes of hypercalcemia such as occult sarcoidosis. A careful history of dietary supplements and drug use may suggest intoxication with vitamin D or vitamin A or the use of thiazides.

TREATMENT Hypercalcemic States

The approach to medical treatment of hypercalcemia varies with its severity (Table 34-4). Mild hypercalcemia, <3 mmol/L (12 mg/dL), can be managed by hydration. More severe hypercalcemia (levels of 3.2–3.7 mmol/L [13–15 mg/dL]) must be managed aggressively; above that level, hypercalcemia can be life-threatening and requires emergency measures. By using a combination of approaches in severe hypercalcemia, the serum calcium concentration can be decreased by 0.7–2.2 mmol/L (3–9 mg/dL) within 24–48 h in most patients, enough to relieve acute symptoms, prevent death from hypercalcemic crisis, and permit diagnostic evaluation. Therapy can then be directed at the underlying disorder—the second priority.

Hypercalcemia develops because of excessive skeletal calcium release, increased intestinal calcium absorption, or inadequate renal calcium excretion. Understanding the particular pathogenesis helps guide therapy. For example, hypercalcemia in patients with malignancy is primarily due to excessive skeletal calcium release and is, therefore, minimally improved by restriction of dietary calcium. On the other hand, patients with vitamin D hypersensitivity or vitamin D intoxication have excessive intestinal calcium absorption, and restriction of dietary calcium is beneficial. Decreased renal function or ECF depletion decreases urinary calcium excretion. In such situations, rehydration may rapidly reduce or reverse the hypercalcemia, even though increased bone resorption persists. As outlined below, the more severe the hypercalcemia, the greater the number of combined therapies that should be used. Rapid-acting (hours) approaches—rehydration, forced diuresis, and calcitonin—can be used with the most effective antiresorptive agents such as bisphosphonates (since severe hypercalcemia usually involves excessive bone resorption).

HYDRATION, INCREASED SALT INTAKE, MILD AND FORCED DIURESIS The first principle of treatment is to restore normal hydration. Many hypercalcemic patients are dehydrated because of vomiting, inanition, and/or hypercalcemia-induced defects in urinary concentrating ability. The resultant drop in glomerular filtration rate is accompanied by an additional decrease in renal tubular sodium and calcium clearance. Restoring a normal ECF volume corrects these abnormalities and increases urine calcium excretion by 2.5–7.5 mmol/d (100–300 mg/d). Increasing urinary sodium excretion to 400–500 mmol/d increases urinary calcium excretion even further than simple rehydration. After rehydration has been achieved, saline can be administered, or furosemide or ethacrynic acid can be given twice daily to depress the tubular reabsorptive mechanism for calcium (care must be taken to prevent dehydration). The combined use of these therapies can increase urinary calcium excretion to ≥12.5 mmol/d (500 mg/d) in most hypercalcemic patients. Because this is a substantial percentage of the exchangeable calcium pool, the serum calcium concentration usually falls 0.25–0.75 mmol/L (1–3 mg/dL) within 24 h. Precautions should be taken to prevent potassium and magnesium depletion; calcium-containing renal calculi are a potential complication.

Under life-threatening circumstances, the preceding approach can be pursued more aggressively, but the availability of effective agents to block bone resorption (such as bisphosphonates) has reduced the need for extreme diuresis regimens (Table 34-4). Depletion of potassium and magnesium is inevitable unless replacements are given; pulmonary edema can be precipitated. The potential complications can be reduced by careful monitoring of central venous pressure and plasma or urine electrolytes; catheterization of the bladder may be necessary. Dialysis treatment may be needed when renal function is compromised.

BISPHOSPHONATES The bisphosphonates are analogues of pyrophosphate, with high affinity for bone, especially in areas of increased bone turnover, where they are powerful inhibitors of bone resorption. These bone-seeking compounds are stable in vivo because phosphatase enzymes cannot hydrolyze the central carbon-phosphorus-carbon bond. The bisphosphonates are concentrated in areas of high bone turnover and are taken up by and inhibit osteoclast action; the mechanism of action is complex. The bisphosphonate molecules that contain amino groups in the side chain structure (see below) interfere with prenylation of proteins and can lead to cellular apoptosis. The highly active nonamino group–containing bisphosphonates are also metabolized to cytotoxic products.

TABLE 34-4

THERAPIES FOR SEVERE HYPERCALCEMIA

TREATMENT	ONSET OF ACTION	DURATION OF ACTION	ADVANTAGES	DISADVANTAGES
Most Useful Therapies				
Hydration with saline	Hours	During infusion	Rehydration invariably needed	Volume overload
Forced diuresis; saline plus loop diuretic	Hours	During treatment	Rapid action	Volume overload, cardiac decompensation, intensive monitoring, electrolyte disturbance, inconvenience
Pamidronate	1–2 days	10–14 days to weeks	High potency; intermediate onset of action	Fever in 20%, hypophosphatemia, hypocalcemia, hypomagnesemia, rarely jaw necrosis
Zoledronate	1–2 days	>3 weeks	Same as for pamidronate (may last longer)	Same as pamidronate above
Calcitonin	Hours	1–2 days	Rapid onset of action; useful as adjunct in severe hypercalcemia	Rapid tachyphylaxis
Special Use Therapies				
Phosphate oral	24 h	During use	Chronic management (with hypophosphatemia); low toxicity if phosphate <4 mg/dL	Limited use except as adjuvant or chronic therapy
Glucocorticoids	Days	Days, weeks	Oral therapy, antitumor agent	Active only in certain malignancies, vitamin D excess and sarcoidosis; glucocorticoid side effects
Dialysis	Hours	During use and 24–48 h afterward	Useful in renal failure; onset of effect in hours; can immediately reverse life-threatening hypercalcemia	Complex procedure, reserved for extreme or special circumstances

The initial bisphosphonate widely used in clinical practice, etidronate, was effective but had several disadvantages, including the capacity to inhibit bone formation as well as blocking resorption. Subsequently, a number of second- or third-generation compounds have become the mainstays of antiresorptive therapy for treatment of hypercalcemia and osteoporosis. The newer bisphosphonates have a highly favorable ratio of blocking resorption versus inhibiting bone formation; they inhibit osteoclast-mediated skeletal resorption yet do not cause mineralization defects at ordinary doses. Although the bisphosphonates have similar structures, the routes of administration, efficacy, toxicity, and side effects vary. The potency of the compounds for inhibition of bone resorption varies more than 10,000-fold, increasing in the order of etidronate, tiludronate, pamidronate, alendronate, risedronate, and zoledronate. The IV use of pamidronate and zoledronate is approved for the treatment of hypercalcemia; between 30 and 90 mg pamidronate, given as a single IV dose over a few hours, returns serum calcium to normal within 24–48 h with an effect that lasts for weeks in 80–100% of patients. Zoledronate given in doses of 4 or 8 mg/5-min infusion has a more rapid and more sustained effect than pamidronate in direct comparison.

These drugs are used extensively in cancer patients. Absolute survival improvements are noted with pamidronate and zoledronate in multiple myeloma, for example. However, although still rare, there are increasing reports of jaw necrosis, especially after dental surgery, mainly in cancer patients treated with multiple doses of the more potent bisphosphonates.

CALCITONIN Calcitonin acts within a few hours of its administration, principally through receptors on osteoclasts, to block bone resorption. Calcitonin, after 24 h of use, is no longer effective in lowering calcium. Tachyphylaxis, a known phenomenon with this drug, seems to explain the results, since the drug is often effective in the first 24 h of use. Therefore, in life-threatening hypercalcemia, calcitonin can be used effectively within the first 24 h in combination with rehydration and saline diuresis while waiting for more sustained effects from a simultaneously administered bisphosphonate such as pamidronate. Usual doses of calcitonin are 2–8 U/kg of body weight IV, SC, or IM every 6–12 h.

OTHER THERAPIES *Denosumab*, an antibody that blocks the RANK ligand (RANKL) and dramatically reduces osteoclast number and function, is approved for therapy of osteoporosis. It also appears to be an effective treatment to reverse hypercalcemia of malignancy, but is not yet approved for this indication. *Plicamycin* (formerly mithramycin), which inhibits bone resorption, and *gallium nitrate,* which exerts a hypocalcemic action also by inhibiting bone resorption, are no longer used because of superior alternatives such as bisphosphonates.

Glucocorticoids have utility, especially in hypercalcemia complicating certain malignancies. They increase urinary calcium excretion and decrease intestinal calcium absorption when given in pharmacologic doses, but they also cause negative skeletal calcium balance. In normal individuals and in patients with primary hyperparathyroidism, glucocorticoids neither increase nor decrease the serum calcium concentration. In patients with hypercalcemia due to certain osteolytic malignancies, however, glucocorticoids may be effective as a result of antitumor effects. The malignancies in which hypercalcemia responds to glucocorticoids include multiple myeloma, leukemia, Hodgkin's disease, other lymphomas, and carcinoma of the breast, at least early in the course of the disease. Glucocorticoids are also effective in treating hypercalcemia due to vitamin D intoxication and sarcoidosis. Glucocorticoids are also useful in the rare form of hypercalcemia, now recognized in certain autoimmune disorders in which inactivating antibodies against the receptor imitate FHH. Elevated PTH and calcium levels are effectively lowered by the glucocorticoids. In all the preceding situations, the hypocalcemic effect develops over several days, and the usual glucocorticoid dosage is 40–100 mg prednisone (or its equivalent) daily in four divided doses. The side effects of chronic glucocorticoid therapy may be acceptable in some circumstances.

Dialysis is often the treatment of choice for severe hypercalcemia complicated by renal failure, which is difficult to manage medically. Peritoneal dialysis with calcium-free dialysis fluid can remove 5–12.5 mmol (200–500 mg) of calcium in 24–48 h and lower the serum calcium concentration by 0.7–3 mmol/L (3–12 mg/dL). Large quantities of phosphate are lost during dialysis, and serum inorganic phosphate concentration usually falls, potentially aggravating hypercalcemia. Therefore, the serum inorganic phosphate concentration should be measured after dialysis, and phosphate supplements should be added to the diet or to dialysis fluids if necessary.

Phosphate therapy, PO or IV, has a limited role in certain circumstances **(Chap. 32)**. Correcting hypophosphatemia lowers the serum calcium concentration by several mechanisms, including bone/calcium exchange. The usual oral treatment is 1–1.5 g of phosphorus per day for several days, given in divided doses. It is generally believed, but not established, that toxicity does not occur if therapy is limited to restoring serum inorganic phosphate concentrations to normal.

Raising the serum inorganic phosphate concentration above normal decreases serum calcium levels, sometimes strikingly. Intravenous phosphate is one of the most dramatically effective treatments available for severe hypercalcemia but is toxic and even dangerous (fatal hypocalcemia). For these reasons, it is used rarely and only in severely hypercalcemic patients with cardiac or renal failure where dialysis, the preferable alternative, is not feasible or is unavailable.

SUMMARY The various therapies for hypercalcemia are listed in Table 34-4. The choice depends on the underlying disease, the severity of the hypercalcemia, the serum inorganic phosphate level, and the renal, hepatic, and bone marrow function. Mild hypercalcemia (≤3 mmol/L [12 mg/dL]) can usually be managed by hydration. Severe hypercalcemia (≥3.7 mmol/L [15 mg/dL]) requires rapid correction. Calcitonin should be given for its rapid, albeit short-lived, blockade of bone resorption, and IV pamidronate or zoledronate should be administered, although its onset of action is delayed for 1–2 days. In addition, for the first 24–48 h, aggressive sodium-calcium diuresis with IV saline should be given and, following rehydration, large doses of furosemide or ethacrynic acid, but only if appropriate monitoring is available and cardiac and renal function are adequate. Intermediate degrees of hypercalcemia between 3 and 3.7 mmol/L (12 and 15 mg/dL) should be approached with vigorous hydration and then the most appropriate selection for the patient of the combinations used with severe hypercalcemia.

HYPOCALCEMIA

(See also Chap. 33)

PATHOPHYSIOLOGY OF HYPOCALCEMIA: CLASSIFICATION BASED ON MECHANISM

Chronic hypocalcemia is less common than hypercalcemia; causes include chronic renal failure, hereditary and acquired hypoparathyroidism, vitamin D deficiency, pseudohypoparathyroidism, and hypomagnesemia (Table 34-5).

Acute rather than chronic hypocalcemia is seen in critically ill patients or as a consequence of certain medications and often does not require specific

TABLE 34-5

FUNCTIONAL CLASSIFICATION OF HYPOCALCEMIA (EXCLUDING NEONATAL CONDITIONS)

PTH Absent	
Hereditary hypoparathyroidism	Hypomagnesemia
Acquired hypoparathyroidism	
PTH Ineffective	
Chronic kidney disease	Active vitamin D ineffective
Active vitamin D lacking	Intestinal malabsorption
↓ Dietary intake or sunlight	Vitamin D–dependent rickets type II
Defective metabolism:	Pseudohypoparathyroidism
Anticonvulsant therapy	
Vitamin D–dependent rickets type I	
PTH Overwhelmed	
Severe, acute hyperphosphatemia	Osteitis fibrosa after parathyroidectomy
Tumor lysis	
Acute kidney injury	
Rhabdomyolysis	

Abbreviation: PTH, parathyroid hormone.

treatment. Transient hypocalcemia is seen with severe sepsis, burns, acute kidney injury, and extensive transfusions with citrated blood. Although as many as one-half of patients in an intensive care setting are reported to have calcium concentrations of <2.1 mmol/L (8.5 mg/dL), most do not have a reduction in ionized calcium. Patients with severe sepsis may have a decrease in ionized calcium (true hypocalcemia), but in other severely ill individuals, hypoalbuminemia is the primary cause of the reduced total calcium concentration. Alkalosis increases calcium binding to proteins, and in this setting, direct measurements of ionized calcium should be made.

Medications such as protamine, heparin, and glucagon may cause transient hypocalcemia. These forms of hypocalcemia are usually not associated with tetany and resolve with improvement in the overall medical condition. The hypocalcemia after repeated transfusions of citrated blood usually resolves quickly.

Patients with *acute pancreatitis* have hypocalcemia that persists during the acute inflammation and varies in degree with disease severity. The cause of hypocalcemia remains unclear. PTH values are reported to be low, normal, or elevated, and both resistance to PTH and impaired PTH secretion have been postulated. Occasionally, a chronic low total calcium and low ionized calcium concentration are detected in an elderly patient without obvious cause and with a paucity of symptoms; the pathogenesis is unclear.

Chronic hypocalcemia, however, is usually symptomatic and requires treatment. Neuromuscular and neurologic manifestations of chronic hypocalcemia include muscle spasms, carpopedal spasm, facial grimacing, and, in extreme cases, laryngeal spasm and convulsions. Respiratory arrest may occur. Increased intracranial pressure occurs in some patients with long-standing hypocalcemia, often in association with papilledema. Mental changes include irritability, depression, and psychosis. The QT interval on the electrocardiogram is prolonged, in contrast to its shortening with hypercalcemia. Arrhythmias occur, and digitalis effectiveness may be reduced. Intestinal cramps and chronic malabsorption may occur. Chvostek's or Trousseau's sign can be used to confirm latent tetany.

The classification of hypocalcemia shown in Table 34-5 is based on an organizationally useful premise that PTH is responsible for minute-to-minute regulation of plasma calcium concentration and, therefore, that the occurrence of hypocalcemia must mean a failure of the homeostatic action of PTH. Failure of the PTH response can occur if there is hereditary or acquired parathyroid gland failure, if PTH is ineffective in target organs, or if the action of the hormone is overwhelmed by the loss of calcium from the ECF at a rate faster than it can be replaced.

PTH ABSENT

Whether hereditary or acquired, hypoparathyroidism has a number of common components. Symptoms of untreated hypocalcemia are shared by both types of hypoparathyroidism, although the onset of hereditary hypoparathyroidism can be more gradual and associated with other developmental defects. Basal ganglia calcification and extrapyramidal syndromes are more common and earlier in onset in hereditary hypoparathyroidism. In previous decades, acquired hypoparathyroidism secondary to surgery in the neck was more common than hereditary hypoparathyroidism, but the frequency of surgically induced parathyroid failure has diminished as a result of improved surgical techniques that spare the parathyroid glands and increased use of nonsurgical therapy for hyperthyroidism. Pseudohypoparathyroidism, an example of ineffective PTH action rather than a failure of parathyroid gland production, may share several features with hypoparathyroidism, including extraosseous calcification and extrapyramidal manifestations such as choreoathetotic movements and dystonia.

Papilledema and raised intracranial pressure may occur in both hereditary and acquired hypoparathyroidism, as do chronic changes in fingernails and hair and lenticular cataracts, the latter usually reversible with treatment of hypocalcemia. Certain skin manifestations, including alopecia and candidiasis, are characteristic of hereditary hypoparathyroidism associated with autoimmune polyglandular failure **(Chap. 29)**.

Hypocalcemia associated with hypomagnesemia is associated with both deficient PTH release and impaired responsiveness to the hormone. Patients with hypocalcemia secondary to hypomagnesemia have absent or low levels of circulating PTH, indicative of diminished hormone release despite a maximum physiologic stimulus by hypocalcemia. Plasma PTH levels return to normal with correction of the hypomagnesemia. Thus hypoparathyroidism with low levels of PTH in blood can be due to hereditary gland failure, acquired gland failure, or acute but reversible gland dysfunction (hypomagnesemia).

Genetic abnormalities and hereditary hypoparathyroidism

Hereditary hypoparathyroidism can occur as an isolated entity without other endocrine or dermatologic manifestations. More typically, it occurs in association with other abnormalities such as defective development of the thymus or failure of other endocrine organs such as the adrenal, thyroid, or ovary **(Chap. 29)**. Hereditary hypoparathyroidism is often manifest within the first decade but may appear later.

Genetic defects associated with hypoparathyroidism serve to illuminate the complexity of organ development, hormonal biosynthesis and secretion, and tissue-specific patterns of endocrine effector function (Fig. 34-5). Often, hypoparathyroidism is isolated, signifying a highly specific functional disturbance. When hypoparathyroidism is associated with other developmental or organ defects, treatment of the hypocalcemia can still be effective.

A form of hypoparathyroidism associated with defective development of both the thymus and the parathyroid glands is termed the *DiGeorge syndrome*, or the *velocardiofacial syndrome*. Congenital cardiovascular, facial, and other developmental defects are present, and patients may die in early childhood with severe infections, hypocalcemia and seizures, or cardiovascular complications. Patients can survive into adulthood, and milder, incomplete forms occur. Most cases are sporadic, but an autosomal dominant form involving microdeletions of chromosome 22q11.2 has been described. Smaller deletions in chromosome 22 are seen in incomplete forms of the DiGeorge syndrome, appearing in childhood or adolescence, that are manifest primarily by parathyroid gland failure. The chromosome 22 defect is now termed *DSG1*; more recently, a defect in chromosome 10p is also recognized—now called *DSG2*. The phenotypes seem similar. Studies on the chromosome 22 defect have pinpointed a transcription factor, TBX1. Deletions of the orthologous mouse gene show a phenotype similar to the human syndrome.

Another autosomal dominant developmental defect, featuring hypoparathyroidism, deafness, and renal dysplasia (HDR), has been studied at the genetic level. Cytogenetic abnormalities in some, but not all kindreds, point to translocation defects on chromosome 10, as in DiGeorge syndrome. However, the lack of immunodeficiency and heart defects distinguishes the two syndromes. Mouse models, as well as deletional analysis in some HDR patients, has identified the transcription factor GATA3, which is important in embryonic development and is expressed in developing kidney, ear structures, and the parathyroids.

Another pair of linked developmental disorders involving the parathyroids is recognized. *Kenney-Caffey syndrome type I* features hypoparathyroidism, short stature, osteosclerosis, and thick cortical bones. A defect seen in Middle Eastern patients, particularly in Saudi Arabia, termed *Sanjad-Sakati syndrome*, also exhibits growth failure and other dysmorphic features. This syndrome, which is clearly autosomal recessive, involves a gene on chromosome 1q42-q43. Both syndromes apparently involve a chaperone protein, called *TBCE*, relevant to tubulin function. Recently, a defect in FAM111A was identified as the cause of *Kenney-Caffey syndrome type 2*.

Hypoparathyroidism can occur in association with a complex hereditary autoimmune syndrome involving failure of the adrenals, the ovaries, the immune system, and the parathyroids in association with recurrent mucocutaneous candidiasis, alopecia, vitiligo, and pernicious anemia **(Chap. 29)**. The responsible gene on chromosome 21q22.3 has been identified. The protein product, which resembles a transcription factor, has been termed the *autoimmune regulator*, or AIRE. A stop codon mutation occurs in many Finnish families with the disorder, commonly referred to as *polyglandular autoimmune type 1 deficiency*, whereas another AIRE mutation (Y85C) is typically observed in Jews of Iraqi and Iranian descent.

Hypoparathyroidism is seen in two disorders associated with mitochondrial dysfunction and myopathy, one termed the *Kearns-Sayre syndrome* (KSS), with ophthalmoplegia and pigmentary retinopathy, and the other termed the *MELAS syndrome* (*m*itochondrial *e*ncephalopathy, *l*actic *a*cidosis, and *s*troke-like episodes). Mutations or deletions in mitochondrial genes have been identified.

Several forms of hypoparathyroidism, each rare in frequency, are seen as isolated defects; the genetic mechanisms are varied. The inheritance includes autosomal dominant, autosomal recessive, and X-linked modes. Three separate autosomal defects involving the parathyroid gene have been recognized: one is dominant and the other two are recessive. The dominant form has a point mutation in the signal sequence, a critical region involved in intracellular transport of the hormone precursor. An Arg for Cys mutation interferes with processing of the precursor and is believed to trigger an apoptotic cellular response, hence acting as a dominant negative. The other two forms are recessive. One point mutation also blocks cleavage of the PTH precursor but requires both alleles to cause hypoparathyroidism. The third involves a single-nucleotide base change that results in an exon splicing defect; the lost exon contains the promoter—hence, the gene is silenced. An X-linked recessive form of hypoparathyroidism has been described in males, and the defect has been localized to chromosome Xq26-q27, perhaps involving the *SOX3* gene.

Abnormalities in the CaSR are detected in three distinctive hypocalcemic disorders. All are rare, but more than 10 different gain-of-function mutations have been found in one form of hypocalcemia termed *autosomal dominant hypocalcemic hypercalciuria (ADHH)*. The receptor senses the ambient calcium level as excessive and suppresses PTH secretion, leading to hypocalcemia. The hypocalcemia is aggravated by constitutive receptor activity in the renal tubule causing excretion of inappropriate amounts of calcium. Recognition of the syndrome is important because efforts to treat the hypocalcemia with vitamin D analogues and increased oral calcium exacerbate the already excessive urinary calcium excretion (several grams or more per 24 h), leading to irreversible renal damage from stones and ectopic calcification.

Other causes of isolated hypoparathyroidism include homozygous, inactivating mutations in the parathyroid-specific transcription factor GCM2, which lead to an autosomal recessive form of the disease, or heterozygous point mutations in GCM2, which have a dominant negative effect on the wild-type protein and thus lead to an autosomal dominant form of hypoparathyroidism. Furthermore, heterozygous mutations in G11, one of the two signaling proteins downstream of the CaSR, have been identified as a cause of autosomal dominant hypoparathyroidism.

Bartter's syndrome is a group of disorders associated with disturbances in electrolyte and acid/base balance, sometimes with nephrocalcinosis and other features. Several types of ion channels or transporters are involved. Curiously, *Bartter's syndrome type V* has the electrolyte and pH disturbances seen in the other syndromes but appears to be due to a gain of function in the CaSR. The defect may be more severe than in ADHH and explains the additional features seen beyond hypocalcemia and hypercalciuria.

As with autoimmune disorders that block the CaSR (discussed above under hypercalcemic conditions), there are autoantibodies that at least transiently activate the CaSR, leading to suppressed PTH secretion and hypocalcemia. This disorder may wax and wane.

Acquired hypoparathyroidism

Acquired chronic hypoparathyroidism is usually the result of inadvertent surgical removal of all the parathyroid glands; in some instances, not all the tissue is removed, but the remainder undergoes vascular supply compromise secondary to fibrotic changes in the neck after surgery. In the past, the most frequent cause of acquired hypoparathyroidism was surgery for hyperthyroidism. Hypoparathyroidism now usually occurs after surgery for hyperparathyroidism when the surgeon, facing the dilemma of removing too little tissue and thus not curing the hyperparathyroidism, removes too much. Parathyroid function may not be totally absent in all patients with postoperative hypoparathyroidism.

Rare causes of acquired chronic hypoparathyroidism include radiation-induced damage subsequent to radioiodine therapy of hyperthyroidism and glandular damage in patients with hemochromatosis or hemosiderosis after repeated blood transfusions. Infection may involve one or more of the parathyroids but usually does not cause hypoparathyroidism because all four glands are rarely involved.

Transient hypoparathyroidism is frequent following surgery for hyperparathyroidism. After a variable period of hypoparathyroidism, normal parathyroid function may return due to hyperplasia or recovery of remaining tissue. Occasionally, recovery occurs months after surgery.

TREATMENT Acquired and Hereditary Hypoparathyroidism

Treatment involves replacement with vitamin D or $1,25(OH)_2D$ (calcitriol) combined with a high oral calcium intake. In most patients, blood calcium and phosphate levels are satisfactorily regulated, but some patients show resistance and a brittleness, with a tendency to alternate between hypocalcemia and hypercalcemia. For many patients, vitamin D in doses of 40,000–120,000 U/d (1–3 mg/d) combined with ≥1 g elemental calcium is satisfactory. The wide dosage range reflects the variation encountered from patient to patient; precise regulation of each patient is required. Compared to typical daily requirements in euparathyroid patients of 200 U/d (or in older patients as high as 800 U/d), the high dose of vitamin D (as much as 100-fold higher) reflects the reduced conversion of vitamin D to $1,25(OH)_2D$. Many physicians now use 0.5–1 μg of calcitriol in management of such patients, especially if they are difficult to control. Because of its storage in fat, when vitamin D is withdrawn, weeks are required for the disappearance of the biologic effects, compared with a few days for calcitriol, which has a rapid turnover.

Oral calcium and vitamin D restore the overall calcium-phosphate balance but do not reverse the lowered urinary calcium reabsorption typical of hypoparathyroidism. Therefore, care must be taken to avoid excessive urinary calcium excretion after vitamin D and calcium replacement therapy; otherwise, nephrocalcinosis and kidney stones can develop, and the risk of CKD is increased. Thiazide diuretics lower urine calcium by as much as 100 mg/d in hypoparathyroid patients on vitamin D, provided they are maintained on a low-sodium diet. Use of thiazides seems to be of benefit in mitigating hypercalciuria and easing the daily management of these patients.

There are now trials of parenterally administered PTH (either PTH[1–34] or PTH[1–84]) in patients with hypoparathyroidism providing greater ease of maintaining serum calcium and reducing urinary calcium excretion (desirable to protect any renal damage). However, PTH therapy for the treatment of hypoparathyroidism is not approved as of yet.

Hypomagnesemia

Severe hypomagnesemia (<0.4 mmol/L; <0.8 meq/L) is associated with hypocalcemia **(Chap. 32)**. Restoration of the total-body magnesium deficit leads to rapid reversal of hypocalcemia. There are at least two causes of the hypocalcemia—impaired PTH secretion and reduced responsiveness to PTH. **For further discussion of causes and treatment of hypomagnesemia, see Chap. 32.**

The effects of magnesium on PTH secretion are similar to those of calcium; hypermagnesemia suppresses and hypomagnesemia stimulates PTH secretion. The effects of magnesium on PTH secretion are normally of little significance, however, because the calcium effects dominate. Greater change in magnesium than in calcium is needed to influence hormone secretion. Nonetheless, hypomagnesemia might be expected to increase hormone secretion. It is therefore surprising to find that severe hypomagnesemia is associated with blunted secretion of PTH. The explanation for the paradox is that severe, chronic hypomagnesemia leads to intracellular magnesium deficiency, which interferes with secretion and peripheral responses to PTH. The mechanism of the cellular abnormalities caused by hypomagnesemia is unknown, although effects on adenylate cyclase (for which magnesium is a cofactor) have been proposed.

PTH levels are undetectable or inappropriately low in severe hypomagnesemia despite the stimulus of severe hypocalcemia, and acute repletion of magnesium leads to a rapid increase in PTH level. Serum phosphate levels are often not elevated, in contrast to the situation with acquired or idiopathic hypoparathyroidism, probably because phosphate deficiency is often seen in hypomagnesemia.

Diminished peripheral responsiveness to PTH also occurs in some patients, as documented by subnormal response in urinary phosphorus and urinary cAMP excretion after administration of exogenous PTH to patients who are hypocalcemic and hypomagnesemic. Both blunted PTH secretion and lack of renal response to administered PTH can occur in the same patient. When acute magnesium repletion is undertaken, the restoration of PTH levels to normal or supranormal may precede restoration of normal serum calcium by several days.

TREATMENT Hypomagnesemia

Repletion of magnesium cures the condition. Repletion should be parenteral. Attention must be given to restoring the intracellular deficit, which may be considerable. After IV magnesium administration, serum magnesium may return transiently to the normal range, but unless replacement therapy is adequate, serum magnesium will again fall. If the cause of the hypomagnesemia is renal magnesium wasting, magnesium may have to be given long-term to prevent recurrence **(Chap. 32)**.

PTH INEFFECTIVE

PTH is not sufficiently active to fully prevent hypocalcemia (although retaining phosphaturic activity, for example). This problem occurs when the PTH1R–signaling protein complex is defective (as in the different forms of pseudohypoparathyroidism [PHP], discussed below); when PTH action to promote calcium absorption from the diet via the synthesis of 1,25(OH)2D is insufficient because of vitamin D deficiency or because vitamin D is ineffective (defects in vitamin D receptor or vitamin D synthesis); or in CKD in which the calcium-elevating action of PTH is impaired.

Typically, hypophosphatemia is more severe than hypocalcemia in vitamin D deficiency states because of the increased secretion of PTH, which, although only partly effective in elevating blood calcium, is readily capable of promoting urinary phosphate excretion.

PHP, on the other hand, has a pathophysiology that is different from the other disorders of ineffective PTH action. PHP resembles hypoparathyroidism (in which PTH synthesis is deficient) and is manifested by hypocalcemia and hyperphosphatemia, yet elevated PTH levels. The cause of the disorder is defective

PTH-dependent activation of the stimulatory G protein complex or the downstream effector protein kinase A, resulting in failure of PTH to increase intracellular cAMP or to respond to elevated cAMP levels (see below).

Chronic kidney disease

Improved medical management of CKD now allows many patients to survive for decades and hence allows time enough to develop features of renal osteodystrophy, which must be controlled to avoid additional morbidity. Impaired production of $1,25(OH)_2D$ is now thought to be the principal factor that causes calcium deficiency, secondary hyperparathyroidism, and bone disease; hyperphosphatemia typically occurs only in the later stages of the disease. Low levels of $1,25(OH)_2D$ due to increased FGF23 production in bone are critical in the development of hypocalcemia. The uremic state also causes impairment of intestinal absorption by mechanisms other than defects in vitamin D metabolism. Nonetheless, treatment with supraphysiologic amounts of vitamin D or calcitriol can correct the impaired calcium absorption. Because increased FGF23 levels are seen even in early stages of CKD and have been reported to correlate with increased mortality and left ventricular hypertrophy, there is current interest in approaches to lower intestinal phosphate absorption early during the course of kidney disease and to thereby lower FGF23 levels. However, there is concern as to whether vitamin D supplementation increases the circulating FGF23 levels in CKD patients. Although vitamin D analogs improve survival in this patient population, it is notable that there are often dramatic elevations of FGF23.

Hyperphosphatemia in CKD lowers blood calcium levels by several mechanisms, including extraosseous deposition of calcium and phosphate, impairment of the bone-resorbing action of PTH, and reduction in $1,25(OH)_2D$ production by remaining renal tissue.

TREATMENT Chronic Kidney Disease

Therapy of CKD involves appropriate management of patients prior to dialysis and adjustment of regimens once dialysis is initiated. Attention should be paid to restriction of phosphate in the diet; avoidance of aluminum-containing phosphate-binding antacids to prevent the problem of aluminum intoxication; provision of an adequate calcium intake by mouth, usually 1–2 g/d; and supplementation with 0.25–1 μg/d calcitriol or other activated forms of vitamin D. Each patient must be monitored closely. The aim of therapy is to restore normal calcium balance to prevent osteomalacia and severe secondary hyperparathyroidism (it is usually recommended to maintain PTH levels between 100 and 300 pg/mL) and, in light of evidence of genetic changes and monoclonal outgrowths of parathyroid glands in CKD patients, to prevent secondary hyperparathyroidism from becoming autonomous hyperparathyroidism. Reduction of hyperphosphatemia and restoration of normal intestinal calcium absorption by calcitriol can improve blood calcium levels and reduce the manifestations of secondary hyperparathyroidism. Because adynamic bone disease can occur in association with low PTH levels, it is important to avoid excessive suppression of the parathyroid glands while recognizing the beneficial effects of controlling the secondary hyperparathyroidism. These patients should probably be closely monitored with PTH assays that detect only the full-length PTH(1–84) to ensure that biologically active PTH and not inactive, inhibitory PTH fragments are measured. Use of phosphate-binding agents such as sevelamer is approved only in end-stage renal disease, but it may be necessary to initiate such treatment much earlier during the course of kidney disease to prevent the increase in FGF23 and its "off-target" effects.

Vitamin D deficiency due to inadequate diet and/or sunlight

Vitamin D deficiency due to inadequate intake of dairy products enriched with vitamin D, lack of vitamin supplementation, and reduced sunlight exposure in the elderly, particularly during winter in northern latitudes, is more common in the United States than previously recognized. Biopsies of bone in elderly patients with hip fracture (documenting osteomalacia) and abnormal levels of vitamin D metabolites, PTH, calcium, and phosphate indicate that vitamin D deficiency may occur in as many as 25% of elderly patients, particularly in northern latitudes in the United States. Concentrations of 25(OH)D are low or low-normal in these patients. Quantitative histomorphometric analysis of bone biopsy specimens from such individuals reveals widened osteoid seams consistent with osteomalacia **(Chap. 32)**. PTH hypersecretion compensates for the tendency for the blood calcium to fall but also increases renal phosphate excretion and thus causes osteomalacia.

Treatment involves adequate replacement with vitamin D and calcium until the deficiencies are corrected. Severe hypocalcemia rarely occurs in moderately severe vitamin D deficiency of the elderly, but vitamin D deficiency must be considered in the differential diagnosis of mild hypocalcemia.

Mild hypocalcemia, secondary hyperparathyroidism, severe hypophosphatemia, and a variety of nutritional deficiencies occur with gastrointestinal diseases. Hepatocellular dysfunction can lead to reduction in 25(OH)D levels, as in portal or biliary cirrhosis of the liver, and malabsorption of vitamin D and its metabolites, including $1,25(OH)_2D$, may occur in a variety of bowel diseases, hereditary or acquired. Hypocalcemia itself can lead to steatorrhea, due to deficient production of pancreatic enzymes and bile salts. Depending on the disorder, vitamin D or its metabolites can be given parenterally, guaranteeing adequate blood levels of active metabolites.

Defective vitamin D metabolism

Anticonvulsant therapy

Anti-convulsant therapy with any of several agents induces acquired vitamin D deficiency by increasing the conversion of vitamin D to inactive compounds and/or causing resistance to its action. The more marginal the vitamin D intake in the diet, the more likely that anti-convulsant therapy will lead to abnormal mineral and bone metabolism.

Vitamin D–dependent rickets type I

Vitamin D–dependent rickets type I, previously termed *pseudo-vitamin D–resistant rickets*, differs from true vitamin D–resistant rickets (vitamin D–dependent rickets type II, see below) in that it is typically less severe and the biochemical and radiographic abnormalities can be reversed with appropriate doses of the vitamin's active metabolite, $1,25(OH)_2D$. Physiologic amounts of calcitriol cure the disease **(Chap. 32)**. This finding fits with the pathophysiology of the disorder, which is autosomal recessive, and is now known to be caused by mutations in the gene encoding 25(OH)D-1α-hydroxylase. Both alleles are inactivated in affected patients, and compound heterozygotes, harboring distinct mutations, are common.

Clinical features include hypocalcemia, often with tetany or convulsions, hypophosphatemia, secondary hyperparathyroidism, and osteomalacia, often associated with skeletal deformities and increased alkaline phosphatase. Treatment involves physiologic replacement doses of $1,25(OH)_2D$ **(Chap. 32)**.

Vitamin D–dependent rickets type II

Vitamin D–dependent rickets type II results from end-organ resistance to the active metabolite $1,25(OH)_2D$. The clinical features resemble those of the type I disorder and include hypocalcemia, hypophosphatemia, secondary hyperparathyroidism, and rickets but also partial or total alopecia. Plasma levels of $1,25(OH)_2D$ are elevated, in keeping with the refractoriness of the end organs. This disorder is caused by mutations in the gene encoding the vitamin D receptor; treatment is difficult and requires regular, usually nocturnal calcium infusions, which dramatically improve growth but do not restore hair growth **(Chap. 32)**.

Pseudohypoparathyroidism

PHP refers to a group of distinct inherited disorders. Patients affected by PHP type Ia (PHP-Ia) are characterized by symptoms and signs of hypocalcemia in association with distinctive skeletal and developmental defects. The hypocalcemia is due to a deficient response to PTH, which is probably restricted to the proximal renal tubules. Hyperplasia of the parathyroids, a response to hormone-resistant hypocalcemia, causes elevation of PTH levels. Studies, both clinical and basic, have clarified some aspects of these disorders, including the variable clinical spectrum, the pathophysiology, the genetic defects, and their mode of inheritance.

A working classification of the various forms of PHP is given in Table 34-6. The classification scheme is based on the signs of ineffective PTH action (low calcium and high phosphate), low or normal urinary cAMP response to exogenous PTH, the presence or absence of *Albright's hereditary osteodystrophy* (AHO), and assays to measure the concentration of the $G_s\alpha$ subunit of the adenylate cyclase enzyme. Using these criteria, there are four types:

TABLE 34-6

CLASSIFICATION OF PSEUDOHYPOPARATHYROIDISM (PHP) AND PSEUDOPSEUDOHYPOPARATHYROIDISM (PPHP)

TYPE	HYPOCALCEMIA, HYPERPHOSPHATEMIA	RESPONSE OF URINARY cAMP TO PTH	SERUM PTH	$G_s\alpha$ SUBUNIT DEFICIENCY	AHO	RESISTANCE TO HORMONES OTHER THAN PTH
PHP-Ia	Yes	↓	↑	Yes	Yes	Yes
PPHP	No	Normal	Normal	Yes	Yes	No
PHP-Ib	Yes	↓	↑	No	No	Yes (in some patients)
PHP-II	Yes	Normal	↑	No	No	No
Acrodysostosis with hormonal resistance	Yes	Normal (but ↓ phosphaturic response)	↑	No	Yes	Yes

Abbreviations: ↓, decreased; ↑, increased; AHO, Albright's hereditary osteodystrophy; PTH, parathyroid hormone.

PHP types Ia and Ib; pseudopseudohypoparathyroidism (PPHP), and PHP-II.

PHP-IA and PHP-IB

Individuals with PHP-I, the most common of the disorders, show a deficient urinary cAMP response to administration of exogenous PTH. Patients with PHP-I are divided into type Ia and type Ib. Patients with PHP-Ia show evidence for AHO and reduced amounts of $G_s\alpha$ protein/activity, as determined in readily accessible tissues such as erythrocytes, lymphocytes, and fibroblasts. Patients with PHP-Ib typically lack evidence for AHO and they have normal $G_s\alpha$ activity. PHP-Ic, sometimes listed as a third form of PHP-I, is really a variant of PHP-Ia, although the mutant $G_s\alpha$ shows normal activity in certain in vitro assays.

Most patients who have PHP-Ia reveal characteristic features of AHO, which consist of short stature, round face, obesity, skeletal anomalies (brachydactyly), intellectual impairment, and/or heterotopic calcifications. Patients have low calcium and high phosphate levels, as with true hypoparathyroidism. PTH levels, however, are elevated, reflecting resistance to hormone action.

Amorphous deposits of calcium and phosphate are found in the basal ganglia in about one-half of patients. The defects in metacarpal and metatarsal bones are sometimes accompanied by short phalanges as well, possibly reflecting premature closing of the epiphyses. The typical findings are short fourth and fifth metacarpals and metatarsals. The defects are usually bilateral. Exostoses and radius curvus are frequent.

Inheritance and genetic defects

Multiple defects at the *GNAS* locus have now been identified in PHP-Ia, PHP-Ib, and PPHP patients. This gene, which is located on chromosome 20q13.3, encodes the α-subunit of the stimulatory G protein ($G_s\alpha$), among other products (see below). Mutations include abnormalities in splice junctions associated with deficient mRNA production, point mutations, insertions, and/or deletion that all result in a protein with defective function resulting in a 50% reduction of $G_s\alpha$ activity in erythrocytes or other cells.

Detailed analyses of disease transmission in affected kindreds have clarified many features of PHP-Ia, PPHP, and PHP-Ib (Fig. 34-7). The former two entities, often traced through multiple generations, have an inheritance pattern consistent with genetic imprinting. The phenomenon of gene imprinting, involving methylation of genetic loci, independent of any mutation, impairs transcription from either the maternal or the paternal allele. The $G_s\alpha$ transcript is biallelically expressed in most tissues; expression from paternal allele is silenced through as-of-yet unknown mechanisms in some tissues including the proximal renal tubules and the thyroid; consequently, inheritance of a defective paternal allele has no implications with regard to hormonal function. Thus, females affected by either PHP-Ia or PPHP will have offspring with PHP-Ia, if these children inherit the allele carrying the *GNAS* mutation; in contrast, if the mutant allele is inherited from a male affected by either disorder, the offspring will exhibit PPHP. Consistent with these data in humans, gene-ablation studies in mice have shown that inheritance of the mutant $G_s\alpha$ allele from the female causes much reduced $G_s\alpha$ protein in renal cortex, hypocalcemia, and resistance to PTH. Offspring inheriting the mutant allele from the male showed no evidence of PTH resistance or hypocalcemia.

Imprinting is tissue selective. Paternal $G_s\alpha$ expression is not silenced in most tissues. It seems likely, therefore, that the AHO phenotype recognized in PPHP as well as PHP-Ia reflects $G_s\alpha$ haploinsufficiency during embryonic or postnatal development.

The complex mechanisms that control the *GNAS* gene contribute to challenges involved in unraveling the pathogenesis of these disorders, especially that of PHP-Ib. Much intensive work with families in which

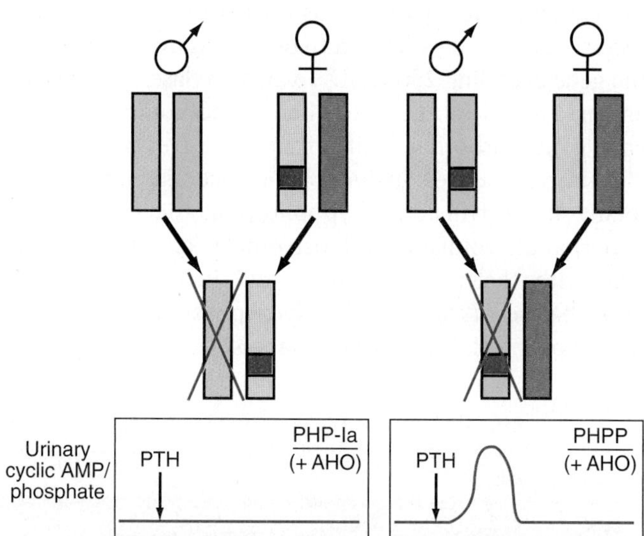

FIGURE 34-7

Paternal imprinting of renal parathyroid hormone (PTH) resistance. An impaired excretion of urinary cyclic AMP and phosphate is observed in patients with pseudohypoparathyroidism type Ia (PHP-Ia). In the renal cortex, there is selective silencing of paternal $G_s\alpha$ expression. The disease becomes manifest only in patients who inherit the defective gene from an obligate female carrier (*left*). If the genetic defect is inherited from an obligate male gene carrier, there is no biochemical abnormality; administration of PTH causes an appropriate increase in the urinary cyclic AMP and phosphate concentration (pseudo-PHP [PPHP]; *right*). Both patterns of inheritance lead to Albright's hereditary osteodystrophy (AHO), perhaps because of haplotype insufficiency—i.e., both copies of $G_s\alpha$ must be active for normal bone development.

multiple members are affected by PHP-Ib, as well as studies of the complex regulation of the *GNAS* gene locus, have now shown that PHP-Ib is caused by microdeletions within or upstream of the *GNAS* locus, which are associated with a loss of DNA methylation at one or several loci of the maternal allele (Table 34-6). These abnormalities in methylation silence the expression of the gene. This leads in the proximal renal tubules—where $G_s\alpha$ appears to be expressed exclusively from the maternal allele—to PTH resistance.

PHP-Ib, lacking the AHO phenotype in most instances, shares with PHP-Ia the hypocalcemia and hyperphosphatemia caused by PTH resistance, and thus the blunted urinary cAMP response to administered PTH, a standard test to assess the presence or absence of hormone resistance (Table 34-6). Furthermore, these endocrine abnormalities become apparent only if the disease-causing mutation is inherited maternally. Bone responsiveness may be excessive rather than blunted in PHP-Ib (and in PHP-Ia) patients, based on case reports that have emphasized an osteitis fibrosa–like pattern in several PHP-Ib patients.

PHP-II refers to patients with hypocalcemia and hyperphosphatemia, who have a normal urinary cAMP but an impaired urinary phosphaturic response to PTH. In a PHP-II variant, referred to as acrodysostosis with hormonal resistance (ADOHR), patients have a defect in the regulatory subunit of PKA (PRKAR1A) that mediates the response to PTH distal to cAMP production. Acrodysostosis without hormonal resistance is caused by mutations in the cAMP-selective phosphodiesterase 4 (ADOP4). It remains unclear why the PTH-resistance in some patients, labeled as PHP-II without bony abnormalities, resolves upon treatment with vitamin D supplements.

The diagnosis of these hormone-resistant states can usually be made without difficulty when there is a positive family history for features of AHO, in association with the signs and symptoms of hypocalcemia. In both categories—PHP-Ia and PHP-Ib—serum PTH levels are elevated, particularly when patients are hypocalcemic. However, patients with PHP-Ib or PHP-II without acrodysostosis present only with hypocalcemia and high PTH levels, as evidence for hormone resistance. In PHP-Ia and PHP-Ib, the response of urinary cAMP to the administration of exogenous PTH is blunted. The diagnosis of PHP-II, in the absence of acrodysostosis, is more complex, and vitamin D deficiency must be excluded before such a diagnosis can be entertained.

TREATMENT Pseudohypoparathyroidism

Treatment of PHP is similar to that of hypoparathyroidism, except that calcium and vitamin D doses are usually higher. Patients with PHP show no PTH-resistance in the distal tubules—hence, urinary calcium clearance is typically reduced, and they are not at risk of developing nephrocalcinosis as are patients with true hypoparathyroidism, unless overtreatment occurs, for example, after the completion of pubertal development and skeletal mutation, when calcium and $1,25(OH)_2D$ treatment should be reduced. Variability in response makes it necessary to establish the optimal regimen for each patient, based on maintaining appropriate blood calcium level and urinary calcium excretion and keeping the PTH level within or slightly above the normal range.

PTH OVERWHELMED

Occasionally, loss of calcium from the ECF is so severe that PTH cannot compensate. Such situations include acute pancreatitis and severe, acute hyperphosphatemia, often in association with renal failure, conditions in which there is rapid efflux of calcium from the ECF. Severe hypocalcemia can occur quickly; PTH rises in response to hypocalcemia but does not return blood calcium to normal.

Severe, acute hyperphosphatemia

Severe hyperphosphatemia is associated with extensive tissue damage or cell destruction **(Chap. 32)**. The combination of increased release of phosphate from muscle and impaired ability to excrete phosphorus because of renal failure causes moderate to severe hyperphosphatemia, the latter causing calcium loss from the blood and mild to moderate hypocalcemia. Hypocalcemia is usually reversed with tissue repair and restoration of renal function as phosphorus and creatinine values return to normal. There may even be a mild hypercalcemic period in the oliguric phase of renal function recovery. This sequence, severe hypocalcemia followed by mild hypercalcemia, reflects widespread deposition of calcium in muscle and subsequent redistribution of some of the calcium to the ECF after phosphate levels return to normal.

Other causes of hyperphosphatemia include hypothermia, massive hepatic failure, and hematologic malignancies, either because of high cell turnover of malignancy or because of cell destruction by chemotherapy.

TREATMENT Severe, Acute Hyperphosphatemia

Treatment is directed toward lowering of blood phosphate by the administration of phosphate-binding antacids or dialysis, often needed for the management of CKD. Although calcium replacement may be necessary if hypocalcemia is severe and symptomatic, calcium administration during the hyperphosphatemic period tends to increase extraosseous calcium deposition and aggravate tissue damage. The levels of 1,25$(OH)_2$D may be low during the hyperphosphatemic phase and return to normal during the oliguric phase of recovery.

Osteitis fibrosa after parathyroidectomy

Severe hypocalcemia after parathyroid surgery is rare now that osteitis fibrosa cystica is an infrequent manifestation of hyperparathyroidism. When osteitis fibrosa cystica is severe, however, bone mineral deficits can be large. After parathyroidectomy, hypocalcemia can persist for days if calcium replacement is inadequate. Treatment may require parenteral administration of calcium; addition of calcitriol and oral calcium supplementation is sometimes needed for weeks to a month or two until bone defects are filled (which, of course, is of therapeutic benefit in the skeleton), making it possible to discontinue parenteral calcium and/or reduce the amount.

DIFFERENTIAL DIAGNOSIS OF HYPOCALCEMIA

Care must be taken to ensure that true hypocalcemia is present; in addition, acute transient hypocalcemia can be a manifestation of a variety of severe, acute illnesses, as discussed above. *Chronic hypocalcemia*, however, can usually be ascribed to a few disorders associated with absent or ineffective PTH. Important clinical criteria include the duration of the illness, signs or symptoms of associated disorders, and the presence of features that suggest a hereditary abnormality. A nutritional history can be helpful in recognizing a low intake of vitamin D and calcium in the elderly, and a history of excessive alcohol intake may suggest magnesium deficiency.

Hypoparathyroidism and PHP are typically lifelong illnesses, usually (but not always) appearing by adolescence; hence, a recent onset of hypocalcemia in an adult is more likely due to nutritional deficiencies, renal failure, or intestinal disorders that result in deficient or ineffective vitamin D. Neck surgery, even long past, however, can be associated with a delayed onset of postoperative hypoparathyroidism. A history of seizure disorder raises the issue of anticonvulsive medication. Developmental defects may point to the diagnosis of PHP. Rickets and a variety of neuromuscular syndromes and deformities may indicate ineffective vitamin D action, either due to defects in vitamin D metabolism or to vitamin D deficiency.

A pattern of *low calcium with high phosphorus* in the absence of renal failure or massive tissue destruction almost invariably means hypoparathyroidism or PHP. A *low calcium and low phosphorus* pattern points to absent or ineffective vitamin D, thereby impairing the action of PTH on calcium metabolism (but not phosphate clearance). The relative ineffectiveness of PTH in calcium homeostasis in vitamin D deficiency, anticonvulsant therapy, gastrointestinal disorders, and hereditary defects in vitamin D metabolism leads to secondary hyperparathyroidism as a compensation. The excess PTH on renal tubule phosphate transport accounts for renal phosphate wasting and hypophosphatemia.

Exceptions to these patterns may occur. Most forms of hypomagnesemia are due to long-standing nutritional deficiency as seen in chronic alcoholics. Despite the fact that the hypocalcemia is principally due to an acute absence of PTH, phosphate levels are usually low, rather than elevated, as in hypoparathyroidism. Chronic renal failure is often associated with hypocalcemia and hyperphosphatemia, despite secondary hyperparathyroidism.

Diagnosis is usually established by application of the PTH immunoassay, tests for vitamin D metabolites, and measurements of the urinary cAMP response to exogenous PTH. In hereditary and acquired hypoparathyroidism and in severe hypomagnesemia, PTH is either undetectable or inappropriately in the normal range (Fig. 34-4). This finding in a hypocalcemic patient is supportive of hypoparathyroidism, as distinct from ineffective PTH action, in which even mild hypocalcemia is associated with elevated PTH levels. Hence a failure to detect elevated PTH levels establishes the diagnosis of hypoparathyroidism; elevated levels suggest the presence of secondary hyperparathyroidism, as found in many of the situations in which the hormone is ineffective due to associated abnormalities in vitamin D action. Assays for 25(OH)D can be helpful. Low or low-normal 25(OH)D indicates vitamin D deficiency due to lack of sunlight, inadequate vitamin D intake, or intestinal malabsorption. Recognition that mild hypocalcemia, rickets, and hypophosphatemia are due to anticonvulsant therapy is made by history.

TREATMENT Hypocalcemic States

The management of hypoparathyroidism, PHP, chronic renal failure, and hereditary defects in vitamin D metabolism involves the use of vitamin D or vitamin D metabolites and calcium supplementation. Vitamin D itself is the least expensive form of vitamin D replacement and is frequently used in the management of uncomplicated hypoparathyroidism and some disorders associated with ineffective vitamin D action. When vitamin D is used prophylactically, as in the elderly or in those with chronic anticonvulsant therapy, there is a wider margin of safety than with the more potent metabolites. However, most of the conditions in which vitamin D is administered chronically for hypocalcemia require amounts

50–100 times the daily replacement dose because the formation of 1,25$(OH)_2$D is deficient. In such situations, vitamin D is no safer than the active metabolite because intoxication can occur with high-dose therapy (because of storage in fat). Calcitriol is more rapid in onset of action and also has a short biologic half-life.

Vitamin D (at least 1000 U/d [2–3 μg/d] [higher levels required in older persons]) or calcitriol (0.25–1 μg/d) is required to prevent rickets in normal individuals. In contrast, 40,000–120,000 U (1–3 mg) of vitamin D_2 or D_3 is typically required in hypoparathyroidism. The dose of calcitriol is unchanged in hypoparathyroidism, because the defect is in hydroxylation by the 25(OH)D-1α-hydroxylase. Calcitriol is also used in disorders of 25(OH)D-1α-hydroxylase; vitamin D receptor defects are much more difficult to treat.

Patients with hypoparathyroidism should be given 2–3 g of elemental calcium PO each day. The two agents, vitamin D or calcitriol and oral calcium, can be varied independently. Urinary calcium excretion needs to be monitored carefully. If hypocalcemia alternates with episodes of hypercalcemia in high-brittleness patients with hypoparathyroidism, administration of calcitriol and use of thiazides, as discussed above, may make management easier. Clinical trials with PTH(1–34) or PTH(1–84) are promising, but these alternative treatments have not yet been approved.

CHAPTER 35
OSTEOPOROSIS

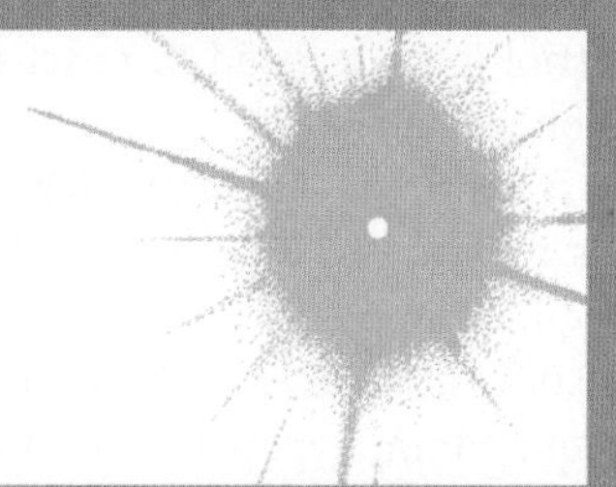

Robert Lindsay ■ Felicia Cosman

Osteoporosis, a condition characterized by decreased bone strength, is prevalent among postmenopausal women but also occurs in men and women with underlying conditions or major risk factors associated with bone demineralization. Its chief clinical manifestations are vertebral and hip fractures, although fractures can occur at almost any skeletal site. Osteoporosis affects almost 10 million individuals in the United States, but only a small proportion are diagnosed and treated.

DEFINITION

Osteoporosis is defined as a reduction in the strength of bone that leads to an increased risk of fractures. Loss of bone tissue is associated with deterioration in skeletal microarchitecture. The World Health Organization (WHO) operationally defines osteoporosis as a bone density that falls 2.5 standard deviations (SD) below the mean for young healthy adults of the same sex—also referred to as a *T-score* of –2.5. Postmenopausal women who fall at the lower end of the young normal range (a T-score <–1.0) are defined as having low bone density and are also at increased risk of osteoporosis. Although risk is lower in this group, more than 50% of fractures among postmenopausal women, including hip fractures, occur in this group with low bone density, because the number of individuals in this category is so much larger than that in the osteoporosis range. As a result, there are ongoing attempts to identify individuals within the low bone density range who are at high risk of fracture and might benefit from pharmacologic intervention. Furthermore, some have advocated using fracture risk as the "diagnostic" criterion for osteoporosis.

EPIDEMIOLOGY

In the United States, as many as 9 million adults have osteoporosis (T-score <–2.5 in either spine or hip), and an additional 48 million individuals have bone mass levels that put them at increased risk of developing osteoporosis (e.g., bone mass T-score <–1.0). Osteoporosis occurs more frequently with increasing age as bone tissue is lost progressively. In women, the loss of ovarian function at menopause (typically about age 50) precipitates rapid bone loss so that most women meet the diagnostic criterion for osteoporosis by age 70–80. As the population continues to age, the number of individuals with osteoporosis and fractures will also continue to increase, despite a recognized reduction in age-specific risk. It is estimated that about 2 million fractures occur each year in the United States as a consequence of osteoporosis, and that number is expected to increase as the population continues to age.

The epidemiology of fractures follows the trend for loss of bone density, with exponential increases in both hip and vertebral fractures with age. Fractures of the distal radius have a somewhat different epidemiology, increasing in frequency before age 50 and plateauing by age 60, with only a modest age-related increase thereafter. In contrast, incidence rates for hip fractures double every 5 years after age 70 (Fig. 35-1). This distinct epidemiology may be related to the way the elderly fall as they age, with fewer falls on an outstretched hand and more falls directly on the hip. About 300,000 hip fractures occur each year in the United States, most of which require hospital admission and surgical intervention. The probability that a 50-year-old white individual will have a hip fracture during his or her lifetime is 14% for women and 5% for men; the risk for African Americans is lower (about one-half those rates), and the risk for Asians is roughly equal to that for whites. Hip fractures are associated with a high incidence of deep vein thrombosis and pulmonary embolism (20–50%) and a mortality rate between 5 and 20% during the year after surgery. There is also significant morbidity, with about 20–40% of survivors requiring long-term care, and

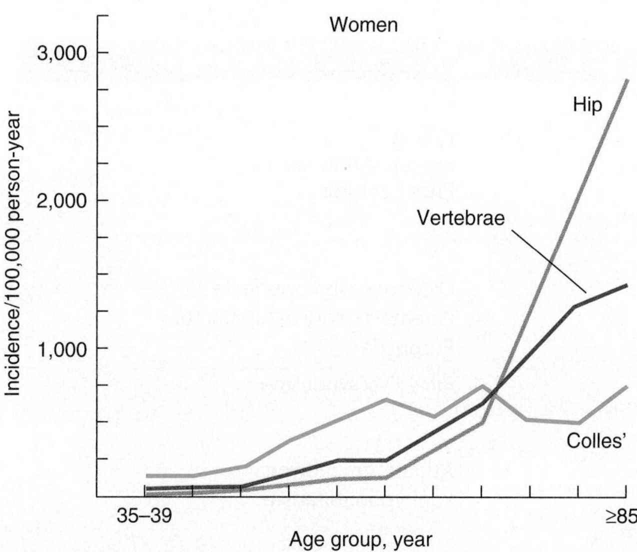

FIGURE 35-1
Epidemiology of vertebral, hip, and Colles' fractures with age. *(Adapted from C Cooper, LJ Melton III: Trends Endocrinol Metab 3:224, 1992; with permission.)*

many who are unable to function as they did before the fracture.

There are about 550,000 vertebral crush fractures per year in the United States. Only a fraction (estimated to be one-third) of them are recognized clinically, because many are relatively asymptomatic and are identified incidentally during radiography for other purposes (Fig. 35-2). Vertebral fractures rarely require hospitalization but are associated with long-term morbidity and a slight increase in mortality rates, primarily related to pulmonary disease. Multiple vertebral fractures lead to height loss (often of several inches), kyphosis, and secondary pain and discomfort related to altered biomechanics of the back. Thoracic fractures can be associated with restrictive lung disease, whereas lumbar fractures are associated with abdominal symptoms that include distention, early satiety, and constipation.

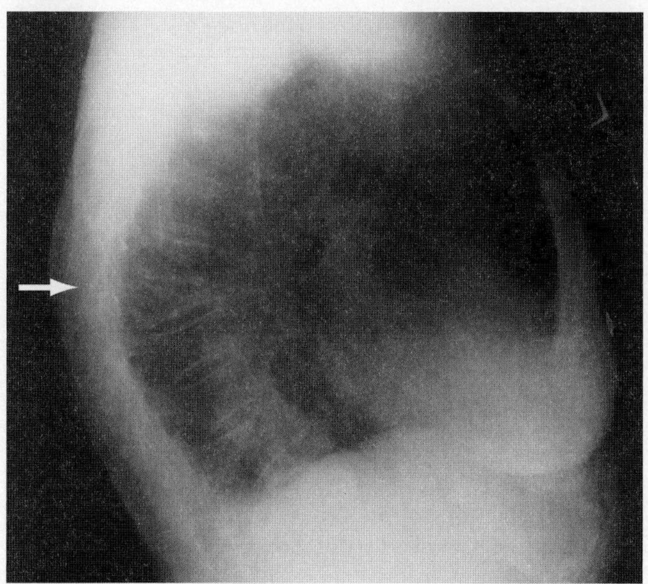

FIGURE 35-2
Lateral spine x-ray showing severe osteopenia and a severe wedge-type deformity (severe anterior compression).

Approximately 400,000 wrist fractures and 135,000 pelvic fractures occur in the United States each year. Fractures of the humerus and other bones (estimated to be about 675,000 per year) also occur with osteoporosis; this is not surprising in light of the fact that bone loss is a systemic phenomenon. Although some fractures result from major trauma, the threshold for fracture is reduced for an osteoporotic bone (Fig. 35-3). In addition to bone density, there are a number of risk factors for fracture; the common ones are summarized in Table 35-1 Age, prior fractures (especially recent fractures), a family history of osteoporosis-related fractures, low body weight, smoking, and excessive alcohol use are all independent predictors of fracture. Chronic diseases with inflammatory components that increase skeletal remodeling such as rheumatoid arthritis, increase the risk of osteoporosis, as do diseases associated with malabsorption. Chronic diseases that increase the risk of falling or frailty, including dementia, Parkinson's disease, and multiple sclerosis, also increase fracture risk.

In the United States and Europe, osteoporosis-related fractures are more common among women than men, presumably due to a lower peak bone mass as well as postmenopausal bone loss in women. However, this sex difference in bone density and age-related increase in hip fractures is not as apparent in some other cultures, possibly due to genetics, physical activity level, or diet.

Fractures are themselves risk factors for future fractures (Table 35-1). Vertebral fractures increase the risk of other vertebral fractures as well as fractures of the peripheral skeleton such as the hip and wrist. Wrist fractures also increase the risk of vertebral and hip fractures. The risk for subsequent fractures is particularly high in the first several years after the first fracture, and the risk

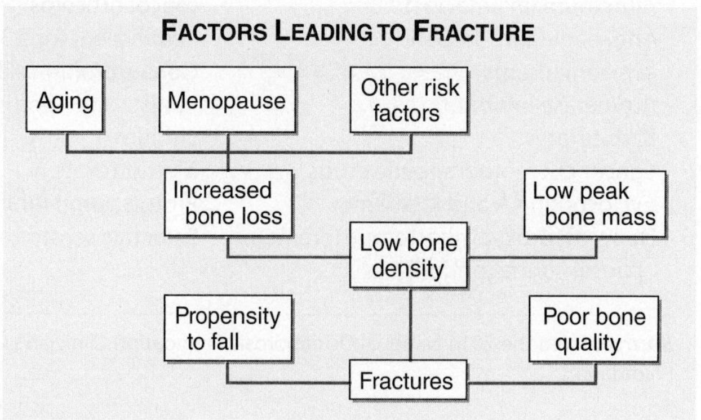

FIGURE 35-3
Factors leading to osteoporotic fractures.

TABLE 35-1

CONDITIONS, DISEASES, AND MEDICATIONS THAT CONTRIBUTE TO OSTEOPOROSIS AND FRACTURES

Lifestyle factors		
Alcohol abuse Low calcium intake Vitamin D insufficiency Excess vitamin A	High salt intake Inadequate physical activity Immobilization Smoking (active or passive)	Falling Excessive thinness Prior fractures
Genetic factors		
Cystic fibrosis Ehlers-Danlos syndrome Gaucher's disease Glycogen storage diseases Hemochromatosis	Homocystinuria Hypophosphatasia Idiopathic hypercalciuria Marfan's syndrome Menkes' steely hair syndrome	Osteogenesis imperfecta Parental history of hip fracture Porphyria Riley-Day syndrome
Hypogonadal states		
Androgen insensitivity Anorexia nervosa and bulimia Turner's & Klinefelter's syndromes	Hyperprolactinemia Premature menopause Premature ovarian failure	Athletic amenorrhea Panhypopituitarism
Endocrine disorders		
Adrenal insufficiency Diabetes mellitus (types 1 and 2)	Cushing's syndrome Hyperparathyroidism	Central adiposity Thyrotoxicosis
Gastrointestinal disorders		
Celiac disease Gastric bypass Gastrointestinal surgery	Inflammatory bowel disease Malabsorption Pancreatic disease	Primary biliary cirrhosis
Hematologic disorders		
Multiple myeloma Hemophilia Thalassemia	Monoclonal gammopathies Leukemia and lymphomas	Sickle cell disease Systemic mastocytosis
Rheumatologic and autoimmune diseases		
Ankylosing spondylitis Other rheumatic and autoimmune diseases	Lupus	Rheumatoid arthritis
Central nervous system disorders		
Epilepsy Multiple sclerosis	Parkinson's disease Spinal cord injury	Stroke
Miscellaneous conditions and diseases		
AIDS/HIV Alcoholism Amyloidosis Chronic metabolic acidosis Chronic obstructive lung disease	Congestive heart failure Depression End-stage renal disease Hypercalciuria Idiopathic scoliosis Muscular dystrophy	Posttransplant bone disease Sarcoidosis Weight loss
Medications		
Aluminum (in antacids) Anticoagulants (heparin) Anticonvulsants Aromatase inhibitors Barbiturates Cancer chemotherapeutic drugs Cyclosporine A and tacrolimus Depo-medroxyprogesterone (premenopausal contraception)	Glucocorticoids (≥5 mg/d prednisone or equivalent for ≥3 months) Gonadotropin-releasing hormone antagonists and agonists Lithium Methotrexate Proton pump inhibitors Selective serotonin reuptake inhibitors	Tamoxifen (premenopausal use) Thiazolidinediones (such as pioglitazone and rosiglitazone) Thyroid hormones (in excess) Parenteral nutrition

Source: From the 2014 National Osteoporosis Foundation Clinician's Guide to the Prevention and Treatment of Osteoporosis.

wanes considerably thereafter. Consequently, among individuals over age 50, any fracture should be considered as potentially related to osteoporosis regardless of the circumstances of the fracture. Osteoporotic bone is more likely to fracture than normal bone at any level of trauma, and a fracture in a person over 50 should trigger evaluation for osteoporosis. This often does not occur because postfracture care is not always well coordinated.

PATHOPHYSIOLOGY

BONE REMODELING

Osteoporosis results from bone loss due to age-related changes in bone remodeling as well as extrinsic and intrinsic factors that exaggerate this process. These changes may be superimposed on a low peak bone mass. Consequently, understanding the bone remodeling process is fundamental to understanding the pathophysiology of osteoporosis **(Chap. 32)**. During growth, the skeleton increases in size by linear growth and by apposition of new bone tissue on the outer surfaces of the cortex (Fig. 35-4). The latter process is called *modeling*, a process that also allows the long bones to adapt in shape to the stresses placed on them. Increased sex hormone production at puberty is required for skeletal maturation, which reaches maximum mass and density in early adulthood. It is around puberty that the sexual dimorphism in skeletal size becomes obvious, although true bone density remains similar between the sexes. Nutrition and lifestyle also play an important role in growth, although genetic factors primarily determine peak skeletal mass and density. Numerous genes control skeletal growth, peak bone mass, and body size, as well as skeletal structure and density. Heritability estimates of 50–80% for bone density and size have been derived on the basis of twin studies. Although peak bone mass is often lower among individuals with a family history of osteoporosis, association studies of candidate genes (vitamin D receptor; type I collagen, the estrogen receptor [ER], and interleukin 6 [IL-6]; and insulin-like growth factor I [IGF-I]) and bone mass, bone turnover, and fracture prevalence have been inconsistent. Linkage studies suggest that a genetic locus on chromosome 11 is associated with high bone mass. Families with high bone mass and without much apparent age-related bone loss have been shown to have a point mutation in *LRP5*, a low-density lipoprotein receptor–related protein. The role of this gene in the general population is not clear, although a nonfunctional mutation results in osteoporosis-pseudoglioma syndrome, and *LRP5* signaling appears to be important in controlling bone formation. *LRP5* acts through the Wnt signaling pathway. With *LRP5* and Wnt activation, beta-catenin is translocated to the nucleus, allowing stimulation of osteoblast formation, activation, and life span as well as suppression of osteoclast activity, thereby increasing bone formation. The osteocyte product, sclerostin, is a negative inhibitor of Wnt signaling.

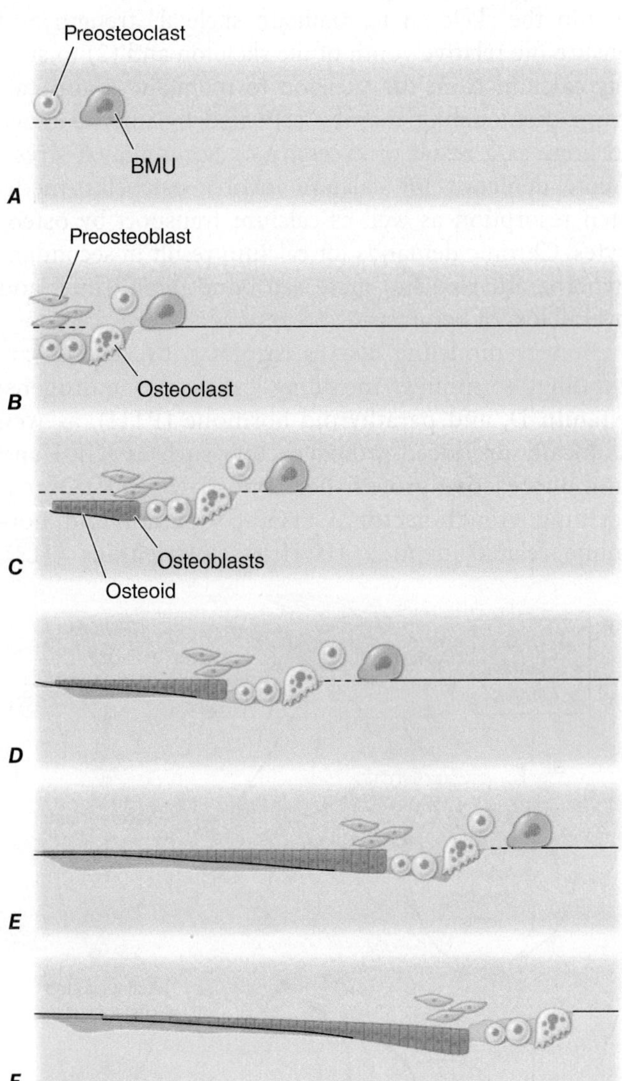

FIGURE 35-4

Mechanism of bone remodeling. The basic molecular unit (BMU) moves along the trabecular surface at a rate of about 10 μm/d. The figure depicts remodeling over ~120 days. ***A.*** Origination of BMU-lining cells contracts to expose collagen and attract preosteoclasts. ***B.*** Osteoclasts fuse into multinucleated cells that resorb a cavity. Mononuclear cells continue resorption, and preosteoblasts are stimulated to proliferate. ***C.*** Osteoblasts align at bottom of cavity and start forming osteoid (*black*). ***D.*** Osteoblasts continue formation and mineralization. Previous osteoid starts to mineralize (*horizontal lines*). ***E.*** Osteoblasts begin to flatten. ***F.*** Osteoblasts turn into lining cells; bone remodeling at initial surface (*left of drawing*) is now complete, but BMU is still advancing (*to the right*). *(Adapted from SM Ott, in JP Bilezikian et al [eds]: Principles of Bone Biology, vol. 18. San Diego, Academic Press, 1996, pp 231–241.)*

Genome-wide scans for low bone mass suggest multiple genes are involved, many of which are also implicated in control of body size.

In adults, bone remodeling, not modeling, is the principal metabolic skeletal process. Bone remodeling has two primary functions: (1) to repair microdamage within the skeleton to maintain skeletal strength and ensure the relative youth of the skeleton and (2) to supply calcium from the skeleton to maintain serum calcium. Remodeling may be activated by microdamage to bone as a result of excessive or accumulated stress. Acute demands for calcium involve osteoclast-mediated resorption as well as calcium transport by osteocytes. Chronic demands for calcium result in secondary hyperparathyroidism, increased bone remodeling, and overall loss of bone tissue.

Bone remodeling also is regulated by several circulating hormones, including estrogens, androgens, vitamin D, and parathyroid hormone (PTH), as well as locally produced growth factors such as IGF-I and immunoreactive growth hormone II (IGH-II), transforming growth factor β (TGF-β), parathyroid hormone–related peptide (PTHrP), interleukins (ILs), prostaglandins, and members of the tumor necrosis factor (TNF) superfamily. These factors primarily modulate the rate at which new remodeling sites are activated, a process that results initially in bone resorption by osteoclasts, followed by a period of repair during which new bone tissue is synthesized by osteoblasts. The cytokine responsible for communication between the osteoblasts, other marrow cells, and osteoclasts is RANK ligand (RANKL; receptor activator of nuclear factor-κB [NF-κB]). RANKL, a member of the TNF family, is secreted by osteoblasts and certain cells of the immune system **(Chap. 32)**. The osteoclast receptor for this protein is referred to as *RANK*. Activation of RANK by RANKL is a final common path in osteoclast development, activation, and life span. A humoral decoy for RANKL, also secreted by osteoblasts, is *osteoprotegerin* (Fig. 35-5). Modulation of osteoclast recruitment and activity appears to be related to the interplay among these three factors. It appears that estrogens are pivotal in modulating secretion of osteoprotegerin (OPG) and perhaps also RANKL. Additional influences include nutrition (particularly calcium intake) and physical activity level.

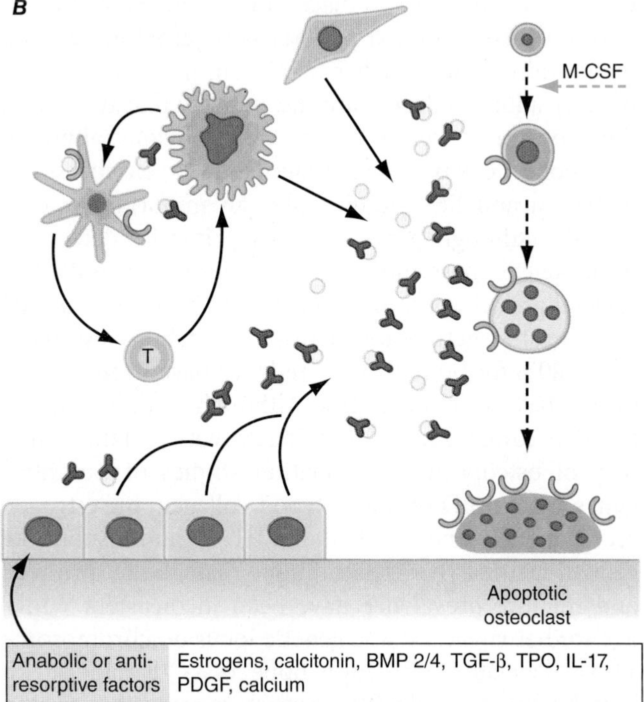

FIGURE 35-5

Hormonal control of bone resorption. *A.* Proresorptive and calciotropic factors. ***B.*** Anabolic and antiosteoclastic factors. RANK ligand (RANKL) expression is induced in osteoblasts, activated T cells, synovial fibroblasts, and bone marrow stromal cells. It binds to membrane-bound receptor RANK to promote osteoclast differentiation, activation, and survival. Conversely, osteoprotegerin (OPG) expression is induced by factors that block bone catabolism and promote anabolic effects. OPG binds and neutralizes RANKL, leading to a block in osteoclastogenesis and decreased survival of preexisting osteoclasts. CFU-GM, colony-forming units, granulocyte macrophage; IL, interleukin; LIF, leukemia inhibitory factor; M-CSF, macrophage colony-stimulating factor; OPG-L, osteoprotegerin-ligand; PDGF, platelet-derived growth factor; PGE_2, prostaglandin E_2; PTH, parathyroid hormone; RANKL, receptor activator of nuclear factor nuclear factor-κB; TGF-β, transforming growth factor β; TNF, tumor necrosis factor; TPO, thrombospondin. *(From WJ Boyle et al: Nature 423: 337, 2003.)*

In young adults, resorbed bone is replaced by an equal amount of new bone tissue. Thus, the mass of the skeleton remains constant after peak bone mass is achieved in adulthood. After age 30–45, however, the resorption and formation processes become imbalanced, and resorption exceeds formation. This imbalance may begin at different ages and varies at different skeletal sites; it becomes exaggerated in women after menopause. Excessive bone loss can be due to an increase in osteoclastic activity and/or a decrease in osteoblastic activity. In addition, an increase in remodeling activation frequency, and thus the number of remodeling sites, can magnify the small imbalance seen at each remodeling unit. Increased recruitment of bone remodeling sites produces a reversible reduction in bone tissue but also can result in permanent loss of tissue and disrupted skeletal architecture. In trabecular bone, if the osteoclasts penetrate trabeculae, they leave no template for new bone formation to occur, and, consequently, rapid bone loss ensues and cancellous connectivity becomes impaired. A higher number of remodeling sites increases the likelihood of this event. In cortical bone, increased activation of remodeling creates more porous bone. The effect of this increased porosity on cortical bone strength may be modest if the overall diameter of the bone is not changed. However, decreased apposition of new bone on the periosteal surface coupled with increased endocortical resorption of bone decreases the biomechanical strength of long bones. Even a slight exaggeration in normal bone loss increases the risk of osteoporosis-related fractures because of the architectural changes that occur, and osteoporosis is primarily a disease of disordered skeletal architecture. The main clinically available tool (dual-energy x-ray absorptiometry) measures mass not architecture. Emerging data from high-resolution peripheral quantitative computed tomography (CT) scans suggest that aging is associated with changes in microstructure of bone tissue, including increased cortical porosity and reduced cortical thickness.

CALCIUM NUTRITION

Peak bone mass may be impaired by inadequate calcium intake during growth among other nutritional factors (calories, protein, and other minerals), leading to increased risk of osteoporosis later in life. During the adult phase of life, insufficient calcium intake contributes to relative secondary hyperparathyroidism and an increase in the rate of bone remodeling to maintain normal serum calcium levels. PTH stimulates the hydroxylation of vitamin D in the kidney, leading to increased levels of 1,25-dihydroxyvitamin D [$1,25(OH)_2D$] and enhanced gastrointestinal calcium absorption. PTH also reduces renal calcium loss. Although these are all appropriate compensatory homeostatic responses for adjusting calcium economy, the long-term effects are detrimental to the skeleton because the increased remodeling rates and the ongoing imbalance between resorption and formation at remodeling sites combine to accelerate loss of bone tissue.

Total daily calcium intakes <400 mg are detrimental to the skeleton, and intakes in the range of 600–800 mg, which is about the average intake among adults in the United States, are also probably suboptimal. The recommended daily required intake of 1000–1200 mg for adults accommodates population heterogeneity in controlling calcium balance. Such intakes should preferentially come from dietary sources, and supplements should be used only when dietary intakes fall short. The supplement should contain enough calcium to bring total intake to about 1200 mg/d.

VITAMIN D

(See also Chap. 32) Severe vitamin D deficiency causes rickets in children and osteomalacia in adults. However, there is accumulating evidence that vitamin D insufficiency may be more prevalent than previously thought, particularly among individuals at increased risk such as the elderly; those living in northern latitudes; and individuals with poor nutrition, malabsorption, or chronic liver or renal disease. Dark-skinned individuals are also at high risk of vitamin D deficiency. There is controversy regarding optimal levels of serum 25-hydroxy-vitamin D [25(OH)D], with some advocating levels >20 ng/mL and others advocating optimal targets >75 nmol/L (30 ng/mL). To achieve this level for most adults requires an intake of 800–1000 units/d, particularly in individuals who avoid sunlight or routinely use ultra-violet-blocking lotions. Vitamin D insufficiency leads to compensatory secondary hyperparathyroidism and is an important risk factor for osteoporosis and fractures. Some studies have shown that >50% of inpatients on a general medical service exhibit biochemical features of vitamin D deficiency, including increased levels of PTH and alkaline phosphatase and lower levels of ionized calcium. In women living in northern latitudes, vitamin D levels decline during the winter months. This is associated with seasonal bone loss, reflecting increased bone turnover. Even among healthy ambulatory individuals, mild vitamin D deficiency is increasing in prevalence, in part due to decreased exposure to sunlight coupled with increased use of potent sunscreens. Treatment with vitamin D can return levels to normal and prevent the associated increase in bone remodeling, bone loss, and fractures. Improved muscle function and gait associated with reduced falls and fracture rates also have been documented among individuals in northern latitudes who have greater vitamin D intake and higher 25(OH)D levels (see below). Vitamin

D adequacy also may affect risk and/or severity of other diseases, including cancers (colorectal, prostate, and breast), autoimmune diseases, and diabetes; however, many observational studies suggesting these potential extraskeletal benefits have not been confirmed with randomized controlled trials.

ESTROGEN STATUS

Estrogen deficiency probably causes bone loss by two distinct but interrelated mechanisms: (1) activation of new bone remodeling sites and (2) exaggeration of the imbalance between bone formation and resorption. The change in activation frequency causes a transient bone loss until a new steady state between resorption and formation is achieved. The remodeling imbalance, however, results in a permanent decrement in mass. In addition, the very presence of more remodeling sites in the skeleton increases the probability that trabeculae will be penetrated, eliminating the template on which new bone can be formed and accelerating the loss of bony tissue.

The most common estrogen-deficient state is the cessation of ovarian function at the time of menopause, which occurs on average at age 51 **(Chap. 16)**. Thus, with current life expectancy, an average woman will spend about 30 years without an ovarian supply of estrogen. The mechanism by which estrogen deficiency causes bone loss is summarized in Fig. 35-5. Marrow cells (macrophages, monocytes, osteoclast precursors, mast cells) as well as bone cells (osteoblasts, osteocytes, osteoclasts) express ERs α and β. Loss of estrogen increases production of RANKL and may reduce production of OPG, increasing osteoclast recruitment. Estrogen also may play an important role in determining the life span of bone cells by controlling the rate of apoptosis. Thus, in situations of estrogen deprivation, the life span of osteoblasts may be decreased, whereas the longevity and activity of osteoclasts are increased. The rate and duration of bone loss after menopause are heterogeneous and unpredictable. Once surfaces are lost in cancellous bone, the rate of bone loss must decline. In cortical bone, loss is slower but continues for a longer time period.

Because remodeling is initiated at the surface of bone, it follows that trabecular bone—which has a considerably larger surface area (80% of the total) than cortical bone—will be affected preferentially by estrogen deficiency. Fractures occur earliest at sites where trabecular bone contributes most to bone strength; consequently, vertebral fractures are the most common early consequence of estrogen deficiency.

PHYSICAL ACTIVITY

Inactivity, such as prolonged bed rest or paralysis, results in significant bone loss. Concordantly, athletes have higher bone mass than does the general population. These changes in skeletal mass are most marked when the stimulus begins during growth and before the age of puberty. Adults are less capable than children of increasing bone mass after restoration of physical activity. Epidemiologic data support the beneficial effects on the skeleton of chronic high levels of physical activity. Fracture risk is lower in rural communities and in countries where physical activity is maintained into old age. However, when exercise is initiated during adult life, the effects of moderate exercise on the skeleton are modest, with a bone mass increase of 1–2% in short-term studies of <2 years in duration. It is argued that more active individuals are less likely to fall and are more capable of protecting themselves upon falling, thereby reducing fracture risk.

CHRONIC DISEASE

Various genetic and acquired diseases are associated with an increase in the risk of osteoporosis (Table 35-1). Mechanisms that contribute to bone loss are unique for each disease and typically result from multiple factors, including nutrition, reduced physical activity levels, and factors that affect rates of bone remodeling. In most, but not all, circumstances the primary diagnosis is made before osteoporosis presents clinically.

MEDICATIONS

A large number of medications used in clinical practice have potentially detrimental effects on the skeleton (Table 35-1). *Glucocorticoids* are the most common cause of medication-induced osteoporosis. It is often not possible to determine the extent to which osteoporosis is related to glucocorticoids or to other factors, because treatment is superimposed on the effects of the primary disease, which in itself may be associated with bone loss (e.g., rheumatoid arthritis). Excessive doses of thyroid hormone can accelerate bone remodeling and result in bone loss.

Other medications have less detrimental effects on the skeleton than pharmacologic doses of glucocorticoids. *Anticonvulsants* are thought to increase the risk of osteoporosis, although many affected individuals have concomitant insufficiency of 1,25(OH)2D, as some anticonvulsants induce the cytochrome P450 system and vitamin D metabolism. Patients undergoing transplantation are at high risk for rapid bone loss and fracture not only from glucocorticoids but also from treatment with other *immunosuppressants* such as cyclosporine and tacrolimus (FK506). In addition, these patients often have underlying metabolic abnormalities, such as hepatic or renal failure, that predispose to bone loss.

Aromatase inhibitors, which potently block the aromatase enzyme that converts androgens and other adrenal precursors to estrogen, reduce circulating postmenopausal estrogen levels dramatically. These agents, which are used in various stages for breast cancer treatment, also have been shown to have a detrimental effect on bone density and risk of fracture. More recently a variety of agents have been implicated in increased bone loss and fractures. These include selective serotonin reuptake inhibitors, proton pump inhibitors, and thiazolidinediones. It is difficult in some cases to separate the risk accrued by the underlying disease from that attributable to the medication. For example, both depression and diabetes are risk factors for fracture by themselves.

CIGARETTE CONSUMPTION

The use of cigarettes over a long period has detrimental effects on bone mass. These effects may be mediated directly by toxic effects on osteoblasts or indirectly by modifying estrogen metabolism. On average, cigarette smokers reach menopause 1–2 years earlier than the general population. Cigarette smoking also produces secondary effects that can modulate skeletal status, including intercurrent respiratory and other illnesses, frailty, decreased exercise, poor nutrition, and the need for additional medications (e.g., glucocorticoids for lung disease).

MEASUREMENT OF BONE MASS

Several noninvasive techniques are available for estimating skeletal mass or density. They include dual-energy x-ray absorptiometry (DXA), single-energy x-ray absorptiometry (SXA), quantitative CT, and ultrasound (US). DXA is a highly accurate x-ray technique that has become the standard for measuring bone density. Although it can be used for measurement in any skeletal site, clinical determinations usually are made of the lumbar spine and hip. DXA also can be used to measure body composition. In the DXA technique, two x-ray energies are used to estimate the area of mineralized tissue, and the mineral content is divided by the area, which partially corrects for body size. However, this correction is only partial because DXA is a two-dimensional scanning technique and cannot estimate the depth or posteroanterior length of the bone. Thus, small slim people tend to have lower than average bone mineral density (BMD), a feature that is important in interpreting BMD measurements when performed in young adults, and something that must be taken into account at any age. Bone spurs, which are common in osteoarthritis, tend to falsely increase bone density of the spine and are a particular problem in measuring the spine in older individuals. Because DXA instrumentation is provided by several different manufacturers, the output varies in absolute terms. Consequently, it has become standard practice to relate the results to "normal" values by using T-scores (a T-score of 1 equals 1 SD), which compare individual results to those in a young population that is matched for race and sex. Z-scores (also measured in SD) compare individual results to those of an age-matched population that also is matched for race and sex. Thus, a 60-year-old woman with a Z-score of −1 (1 SD below mean for age) has a T-score of −2.5 (2.5 SD below mean for a young control group) (Fig. 35-6). A T-score below −2.5 in the lumbar spine, femoral neck, or total hip has been defined as a diagnosis of osteoporosis. As noted above, because more than 50% of fractures occur in individuals with low bone mass rather than BMD osteoporosis, attempts are ongoing to redefine the disease as a fracture risk rather than a specific BMD. Consistent with this concept, fractures of the spine and hip that occur in the absence of major trauma would be considered to be sufficient to diagnose osteoporosis, regardless of BMD. Fractures of other sites, such as pelvis, proximal humerus, and wrist, would be tantamount to an osteoporosis diagnosis in the presence of low BMD. CT can also be used to measure the spine and the hip, but is rarely used clinically, in part because of higher radiation exposure and cost, in addition to a lesser body of data confirming its ability to predict fracture risk, compared with BMD by DXA. High-resolution peripheral CT is used to measure bone in the forearm or tibia as a research tool to noninvasively provide some measure of skeletal architecture. Magnetic resonance imaging (MRI) can also be used in research settings to obtain some architectural information on the forearm and perhaps the hip.

DXA equipment can also be used to obtain lateral images of the spine, from T4 through L4, a technique called vertebral fracture assessment (VFA). Although

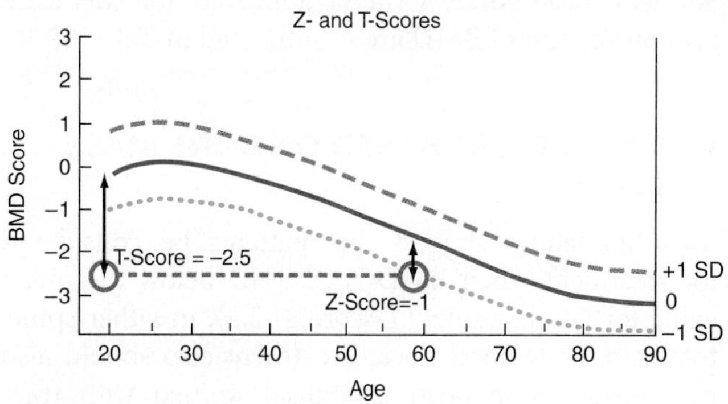

FIGURE 35-6
Relationship between Z-scores and T-scores in a 60-year-old woman. BMD, bone mineral density; SD, standard deviation.

not as definitive as radiography, it is a useful screening tool when height loss, back pain, or postural change suggests the presence of an undiagnosed vertebral fracture. Furthermore, because vertebral fractures are so prevalent with advancing age, screening vertebral imaging is recommended in women and men with low bone mass (T-score <1) by age 70 and 80, respectively.

US is used to measure bone mass by calculating the attenuation of the signal as it passes through bone or the speed with which it traverses the bone. It is unclear whether US assesses properties of bone other than mass (e.g., quality), but this is a potential advantage of the technique. Because of its relatively low cost and mobility, US is amenable for use as a screening procedure in stores or at health fairs.

All of these techniques for measuring BMD have been approved by the U.S. Food and Drug Administration (FDA) on the basis of their capacity to predict fracture risk. The hip is the preferred site of measurement in most individuals, because it predicts the risk of hip fracture, the most important consequence of osteoporosis, better than any other bone density measurement site. When hip measurements are performed by DXA, the spine can be measured at the same time. In younger individuals such as perimenopausal or early postmenopausal women, spine measurements may be the most sensitive indicator of bone loss. A risk assessment tool (FRAX) incorporates femoral neck BMD to assess 10-year fracture risk (see below).

WHEN TO MEASURE BONE MASS

Clinical guidelines have been developed for the use of bone densitometry in clinical practice. The original National Osteoporosis Foundation guidelines recommend bone mass measurements in postmenopausal women, assuming they have one or more risk factors for osteoporosis in addition to age, sex, and estrogen deficiency. The guidelines further recommend that bone mass measurement be considered in *all* women by age 65, a position ratified by the U.S. Preventive Health Services Task Force. Criteria approved for Medicare reimbursement of BMD are summarized in Table 35-2.

WHEN TO TREAT BASED ON BONE MASS RESULTS

Most guidelines suggest that patients be considered for treatment when BMD is >2.5 SD below the mean value for young adults (T-score ≤–2.5), in either spine, total hip, or femoral neck. Treatment also should also be considered in postmenopausal women with fracture risk factors even if BMD is not in the osteoporosis range. Risk factors (age, prior fracture, family history of hip fracture, low body weight, cigarette consumption, excessive alcohol use, steroid use, and rheumatoid arthritis) can be combined with BMD to assess the likelihood of a fracture over a 5- or 10-year period. Treatment threshold depends on cost-effectiveness analyses but probably is ~1% per year of risk in the United States.

TABLE 35-2

INDICATIONS FOR BONE DENSITY TESTING

Consider BMD testing in the following individuals:

- Women age 65 and older and men age 70 and older, regardless of clinical risk factors
- Younger postmenopausal women, women in the menopausal transition and men age 50–69 with clinical risk factors for fracture
- Adults who have a fracture after age 50
- Adults with a condition (e.g., rheumatoid arthritis) or taking a medication (e.g., glucocorticoids in a daily dose ≥5 mg prednisone or equivalent for ≥3 months) associated with low bone mass or bone loss

Source: From the 2014 National Osteoporosis Foundation Clinician's Guide to the Prevention and Treatment of Osteoporosis. © National Osteoporosis Foundation.

APPROACH TO THE PATIENT: Osteoporosis

The perimenopausal transition is a good opportunity to initiate a discussion about risk factors for osteoporosis and consideration of indications for a BMD test. A careful history and physical examination should be performed to identify risk factors for osteoporosis. A low Z-score increases the suspicion of a secondary disease. Height loss >2.5–3.8 cm (>1–1.5 in.) is an indication for VFA by DXA or radiography to rule out asymptomatic vertebral fractures, as is the presence of significant kyphosis or back pain, particularly if it began after menopause. In appropriate individuals, screening BMD and screening vertebral imaging should be recommended as above, even in the absence of any specific risk factors (Table 35-3). For patients who present with fractures, it is important to ensure that the fractures are not caused by an underlying malignancy. Usually this is clear on routine radiography, but on occasion, CT, MRI, or radionuclide scans may be necessary.

ROUTINE LABORATORY EVALUATION There is no established algorithm for the evaluation of women who present with osteoporosis. A general evaluation that includes complete blood count, serum and 24-h urine calcium, renal and hepatic function tests, and a 25(OH)D level is useful for identifying selected secondary causes of low bone mass, particularly for women with fractures or very low Z-scores. An elevated serum calcium level

TABLE 35-3

INDICATIONS FOR VERTEBRAL IMAGING

Consider vertebral imaging tests in the following individuals:

- In all women age 70 and older and all men age 80 and older if bone mineral density (BMD) T-score is −1.0 or below
- In women age 65–69 and men age 75–79 if BMD T-score is −1.5 or below
- In postmenopausal women age 50–64 and men age 50–69 with specific risk factors:
  - Low-trauma fracture
  - Historical height loss of 1.5 in. or more (4 cm)
  - Prospective height loss of 0.8 in. or more (2 cm)
  - Recent or ongoing long-term glucocorticoid treatment

Source: From the 2014 National Osteoporosis Foundation Clinician's Guide to the Prevention and Treatment of Osteoporosis. © National Osteoporosis Foundation.

suggests hyperparathyroidism or malignancy, whereas a reduced serum calcium level may reflect malnutrition and osteomalacia. In the presence of hypercalcemia, a serum PTH level differentiates between hyperparathyroidism (PTH↑) and malignancy (PTH↓), and a high PTHrP level can help document the presence of humoral hypercalcemia of malignancy **(Chap. 34)**. A low urine calcium (<50 mg/24 h) suggests osteomalacia, malnutrition, or malabsorption; a high urine calcium (>300 mg/24 h) is indicative of hypercalciuria and must be investigated further. Hypercalciuria occurs primarily in three situations: (1) a renal calcium leak, which is more common in males with osteoporosis; (2) absorptive hypercalciuria, which can be idiopathic or associated with increased 1,25(OH)$_2$D in granulomatous disease; or (3) hematologic malignancies or conditions associated with excessive bone turnover such as Paget's disease, hyperparathyroidism, and hyperthyroidism. Renal hypercalciuria is treated with thiazide diuretics, which lower urine calcium and help improve calcium economy.

Individuals who have osteoporosis-related fractures or bone density in the osteoporotic range should have a measurement of serum 25(OH)D level, because the intake of vitamin D required to achieve a target level >20–30 ng/mL is highly variable. Vitamin D levels should be optimized in all individuals being treated for osteoporosis. Hyperthyroidism should be evaluated by measuring thyroid-stimulating hormone (TSH).

When there is clinical suspicion of Cushing's syndrome, urinary free cortisol levels or a fasting serum cortisol should be measured after overnight dexamethasone. When bowel disease, malabsorption, or malnutrition is suspected, serum albumin, cholesterol, and a complete blood count should be checked. Asymptomatic malabsorption may be heralded by anemia (macrocytic—vitamin B$_{12}$ or folate deficiency; microcytic—iron deficiency) or low serum cholesterol or urinary calcium levels. If these or other features suggest malabsorption, further evaluation is required. Asymptomatic celiac disease with selective malabsorption is being found with increasing frequency; the diagnosis can be made by testing for antigliadin, anti-endomysial, or transglutaminase antibodies but may require endoscopic biopsy. A trial of a gluten-free diet can be confirmatory. When osteoporosis is found associated with symptoms of rash, multiple allergies, diarrhea, or flushing, mastocytosis should be excluded by using 24-h urine histamine collection or serum tryptase.

Myeloma can masquerade as generalized osteoporosis, although it more commonly presents with bone pain and characteristic "punched-out" lesions on radiography. Serum and urine electrophoresis and or serum free light chains are required to exclude this diagnosis. More commonly, a monoclonal gammopathy of unclear significance (MGUS) is found, and the patient is subsequently monitored to ensure that this is not an incipient myeloma. Approximately 1% of patients with MGUS progress to myeloma each year. A bone marrow biopsy may be required to rule out myeloma (in patients with equivocal electrophoretic results) and also can be used to exclude mastocytosis, leukemia, and other marrow infiltrative disorders such as Gaucher's disease. MGUS syndromes, although benign, may also be associated with reduced bone mass and elevated bone turnover.

BONE BIOPSY Tetracycline labeling of the skeleton allows determination of the rate of remodeling as well as evaluation for other metabolic bone diseases. The current use of BMD tests, in combination with hormonal evaluation and biochemical markers of bone remodeling, has largely replaced the clinical use of bone biopsy, although it remains an important tool in clinical research and assessment of mechanism of action of medication for osteoporosis.

BIOCHEMICAL MARKERS Several biochemical tests are available that provide an index of the overall rate of bone remodeling (Table 35-4). Biochemical markers usually are characterized as those related primarily to *bone formation* or *bone resorption*. These tests measure the overall state of bone remodeling at a single point in time. Clinical use of these tests has been hampered by biologic variability (in part related to circadian rhythm) as well as analytic variability, although the latter is improving.

Biochemical markers of bone resorption may help in the prediction of fracture risk, independently of bone density, particularly in older individuals. In women ≥65 years, when bone density results are greater than the usual treatment thresholds noted above, a high level of bone resorption should prompt consideration

TABLE 35-4

INDICATIONS FOR BIOCHEMICAL MARKERS

Biochemical markers of bone turnover may:

- Predict risk of fracture independently of bone density.
- Predict extent of fracture risk reduction when repeated after 3–6 months of treatment with FDA-approved therapies.
- Predict magnitude of BMD increases with FDA-approved therapies.
- Predict rapidity of bone loss.
- Help determine adequacy of patient compliance and persistence with osteoporosis therapy.
- Help determine duration of "drug holiday" (data are quite limited to support this use, but studies are under way).

Abbreviations: BMD, bone mineral density; FDA, U.S. Food and Drug Administration.

Source: Adapted from the 2014 National Osteoporosis Foundation Clinician's Guide to the Prevention and Treatment of Osteoporosis. © National Osteoporosis Foundation.

of treatment. The primary use of biochemical markers is for monitoring the response to treatment. With the introduction of antiresorptive therapeutic agents, bone remodeling declines rapidly, with the fall in resorption occurring earlier than the fall in formation. Inhibition of bone resorption is maximal within 3 months or so. Thus, measurement of bone resorption (C-telopeptide [CTX] is the preferred marker) before initiating therapy and 3–6 months after starting therapy provides an earlier estimate of patient response than does bone densitometry. A decline in resorptive markers can be ascertained after treatment with potent antiresorptive agents such as bisphosphonates, denosumab, or standard-dose estrogen; this effect is less marked after treatment with weaker agents such as raloxifene or intranasal calcitonin. A biochemical marker response to therapy is particularly useful for asymptomatic patients and may help ensure long-term adherence to treatment. Bone turnover markers are also useful in monitoring the effects of osteoanabolic agents such as 1-34hPTH, or teriparatide, which rapidly increases bone formation (P1NP is preferred, but osteocalcin is a reasonable alternative) and later bone resorption. The recent suggestion of "drug holidays" (see below) has created another use for biochemical markers, allowing evaluation of the off effect of drugs such as bisphosphonates.

TREATMENT Osteoporosis

MANAGEMENT OF PATIENTS WITH FRACTURES Treatment of a patient with osteoporosis frequently involves management of acute fractures as well as treatment of the underlying disease. Hip fractures almost always require surgical repair if the patient is to become ambulatory again. Depending on the location and severity of the fracture, condition of the neighboring joint, and general status of the patient, procedures may include open reduction and internal fixation with pins and plates, hemiarthroplasties, and total arthroplasties. These surgical procedures are followed by intense rehabilitation in an attempt to return patients to their prefracture functional level. Long bone fractures (e.g., wrist) often require either external or internal fixation. Other fractures (e.g., vertebral, rib, and pelvic fractures) usually are managed with supportive care, requiring no specific orthopedic treatment.

Only ~25–30% of vertebral compression fractures present with sudden-onset back pain. For acutely symptomatic fractures, treatment with analgesics is required, including nonsteroidal anti-inflammatory agents and/or acetaminophen, sometimes with the addition of a narcotic agent (codeine or oxycodone). A few small, randomized clinical trials suggest that calcitonin may reduce pain related to acute vertebral compression fracture. Percutaneous injection of artificial cement (polymethylmethacrylate) into the vertebral body (vertebroplasty or kyphoplasty) may offer significant immediate pain relief in patients with severe pain from acute or subacute vertebral fractures. Safety concerns include extravasation of cement with neurologic sequelae and increased risk of fracture in neighboring vertebrae due to mechanical rigidity of the treated bone. Exactly which patients are the optimal candidates for this procedure remains unknown. Short periods of bed rest may be helpful for pain management, but in general, early mobilization is recommended because it helps prevent further bone loss associated with immobilization. Occasionally, use of a soft elastic-style brace may facilitate earlier mobilization. Muscle spasms often occur with acute compression fractures and can be treated with muscle relaxants and heat treatments.

Severe pain usually resolves within 6–10 weeks. More chronic severe pain might suggest the possibility of multiple myeloma or underlying metastatic disease. Chronic pain following vertebral fracture is probably not bony in origin; instead, it is related to abnormal strain on muscles, ligaments, and tendons and to secondary facet-joint arthritis associated with alterations in thoracic and/or abdominal shape. Chronic pain is difficult to treat effectively and may require analgesics, sometimes including narcotic analgesics. Frequent intermittent rest in a supine or semireclining position is often required to allow the soft tissues, which are under tension, to relax. Back-strengthening exercises (paraspinal) may be beneficial. Heat treatments help relax muscles and reduce the muscular component of discomfort. Various physical modalities, such as US and transcutaneous nerve stimulation, may be beneficial in some patients. Pain also occurs in the neck region, not as a result of compression fractures (which almost never occur in the cervical spine as a result of osteoporosis) but because of chronic strain associated with trying to elevate the head in a person with a significant thoracic kyphosis.

Multiple vertebral fractures often are associated with psychological symptoms; this is not always appreciated. The changes in body configuration and back pain can lead to marked loss of self-image and a secondary depression. Altered balance, precipitated by the kyphosis and the anterior movement of the body's center of gravity, leads to a fear of falling, a consequent tendency to remain indoors, and the onset of social isolation. These symptoms sometimes can be alleviated by family support and/or psychotherapy. Medication may be necessary when depressive features are present. Multiple thoracic vertebral fractures may be associated with restrictive lung disease symptoms and increased pulmonary infections. Multiple lumbar vertebral fractures are often associated with abdominal pain, constipation, protuberance, and early satiety. Multiple vertebral fractures are associated with greater age-specific mortality.

Multiple studies show that the majority of patients presenting in adulthood with fractures are not evaluated or treated for osteoporosis. Estimates suggest only about 20% of fracture patients receive follow-up care. Patients who sustain acute fractures are at dramatically elevated risk for more fractures, particularly within the first several years, and pharmacologic intervention can reduce that risk substantially. Recently, several studies have demonstrated the effectiveness of a relatively simple and inexpensive program that reduces the risk of subsequent fractures. In the Kaiser system, it is estimated that a 20% decline in hip fracture occurrence was seen with the introduction of what is called a fracture liaison service. This typically involves a health care professional (usually a nurse) whose job is to coordinate follow-up care and education of fracture patients. If the Kaiser experience can be repeated, there would be significant savings of health care dollars, as well as a dramatic drop in hip fracture incidence and a marked improvement in morbidity and mortality among the aging population.

MANAGEMENT OF THE UNDERLYING DISEASE Patients presenting with typical osteoporosis-related fractures (certainly hip and spine) can be assumed to have osteoporosis and can be treated appropriately. Patients with osteoporosis by BMD are handled in a similar fashion. Other fracture patients and those with reduced bone mass can be classified according to their future risk of fracture and treated if that risk is sufficiently high. It must be emphasized, however, that risk assessment is an inexact science when applied to individual patients. Fractures are chance occurrences that can happen to anyone. Patients often do not understand the relative benefits of medications, compared to the perceived risks of the medications themselves.

Risk Factor Reduction Several tools exist for risk assessment. The most commonly available is the FRAX tool, developed by a working party for the WHO, and available as part of the report from many DXA machines. It is also available online *(http://www.shef.ac.uk/FRAX/tool.jsp?locationValue=9)* (Fig. 35-7). In the United States, it has been estimated that it is cost-effective to treat a patient if the 10-year major fracture risk (including hip, clinical spine, proximal humerus, and tibia) from FRAX is ≥20% and/or the 10-year risk of hip fracture is ≥3%. FRAX is an imperfect tool because it does not include any assessment of fall risk and secondary causes are excluded when BMD is entered. Moreover, it does not include any term for multiple fractures or recent versus remote fracture. Nonetheless, it is useful as an educational tool for patients.

After risk assessment, patients should be thoroughly educated to reduce the impact of modifiable risk factors associated with bone loss and falling. All medications that increase risk of falls, bone loss, or fractures should be reviewed to ensure that they are necessary and being used at the lowest required dose. For those on thyroid hormone replacement, TSH testing should be performed to confirm that an excessive dose is not being used, because biochemical and symptomatic thyrotoxicosis can be associated with increased bone loss. In patients who smoke, efforts should be made to facilitate smoking cessation. Reducing risk factors for falling also include alcohol abuse treatment and a review of the medical regimen for any drugs that might be associated with orthostatic hypotension and/or sedation, including hypnotics and anxiolytics. If nocturia occurs, the frequency should be reduced, if possible (e.g., by decreasing or modifying diuretic use), because arising in the middle of sleep is a common precipitant of a fall. Patients should be instructed about environmental safety with regard to eliminating exposed wires, curtain strings, slippery rugs, and mobile tables. Avoiding stocking feet on wood floors, checking carpet condition (particularly on stairs), and providing good light in paths to bathrooms and outside the home are important preventive measures. Treatment for impaired vision is recommended, particularly a problem with depth perception, which is specifically associated with increased falling risk. Elderly patients with neurologic impairment (e.g., stroke, Parkinson's disease, Alzheimer's disease) are particularly at risk of falling and require specialized supervision and care.

Nutritional Recommendations

Calcium A large body of data indicates that optimal calcium intake reduces bone loss and suppresses bone turnover. Recommended intakes from an Institute of Medicine report are shown in Table 35-5.

The National Health and Nutrition Examination Surveys (NHANES) have consistently documented that average calcium intakes fall considerably short of these recommendations. Food sources of calcium are dairy products (milk, yogurt, and cheese) and fortified foods such as certain cereals, waffles, snacks, juices, and crackers. Some of these fortified foods contain as much calcium per serving as milk. Green leafy vegetables and nuts, particularly almonds, are also sources of calcium, although their bioavailability may be lower than with dairy products. Calcium intake from the diet can also be assessed (Table 35-6) and calculators are available at *NOF.org* or *NYSOPEP.org*.

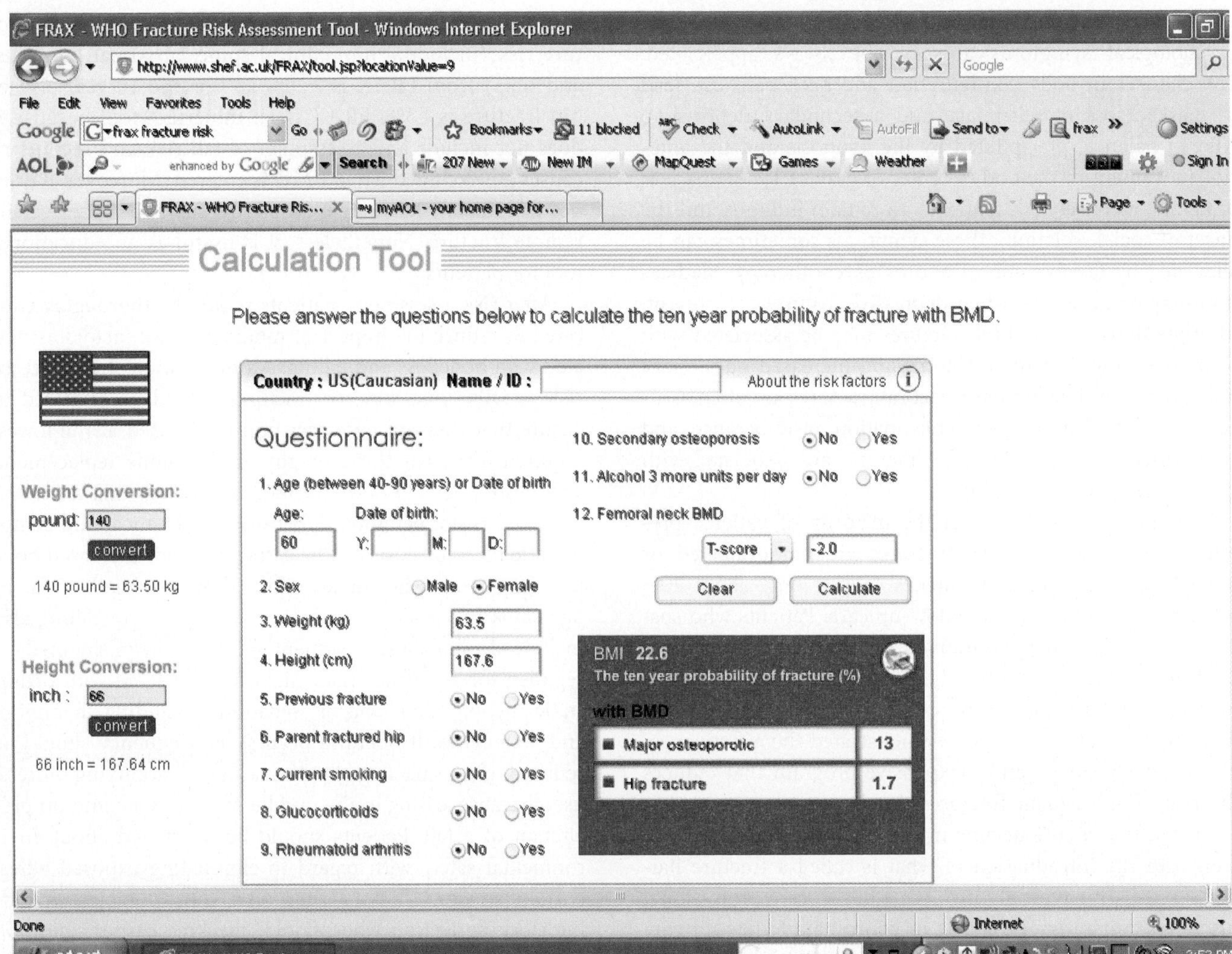

FIGURE 35-7
FRAX calculation tool. When the answers to the indicated questions are filled in, the calculator can be used to assess the 10-year probability of fracture. The calculator (available online at *http://www.shef.ac.uk/FRAX/tool.jsp?locationValue=9*) also can risk adjust for various ethnic groups.

TABLE 35-5
ADEQUATE CALCIUM INTAKE

LIFE STAGE GROUP	ESTIMATED ADEQUATE DAILY CALCIUM INTAKE, MG/D
Young children (1–3 years)	500
Older children (4–8 years)	800
Adolescents and young adults (9–18 years)	1300
Men and women (19–50 years)	1000
Men and women (51 and older)	1200

Note: Pregnancy and lactation needs are the same as for nonpregnant women (e.g., 1300 mg/d for adolescents/young adults and 1000 mg/d for ≥19 years).
Source: Adapted from the Standing Committee on the Scientific Evaluation of Dietary Reference Intakes. Food and Nutrition Board. Institute of Medicine. Washington, DC, 1997, National Academy Press.

If a calcium supplement is required, it should be taken in doses sufficient to supplement dietary intake to bring total intake to the required level (1000–1200 mg/d). Doses of supplements should be ≤600 mg at a time, because the calcium absorption fraction decreases at higher doses. Calcium supplements should be calculated on the basis of the elemental calcium content of the supplement, not the weight of the calcium salt. Calcium supplements containing carbonate are best taken with food because they require acid for solubility. Calcium citrate supplements can be taken at any time. To confirm bioavailability, calcium supplements can be placed in distilled vinegar. They should dissolve within 30 min.

Several controlled clinical trials of calcium, mostly plus vitamin D, have confirmed reductions in clinical fractures, including fractures of the hip (~20–30% risk reduction). All recent studies of pharmacologic agents have been conducted in the context of calcium replacement (± vitamin D). Thus, it is standard practice to ensure an adequate calcium and

TABLE 35-6

SIMPLE METHOD FOR CALCULATING DIETARY CALCIUM INTAKE

STEP 1: Estimate calcium intake from calcium-rich foods

Product	# of Servings/d	Estimated calcium/ serving, in mg	Calcium in mg
Milk (8 oz.)	________	× 300	= ________
Yogurt (6 oz.)	________	× 300	= ________
Cheese (1 oz. or 1 cubic in.)	________	× 200	= ________
Fortified foods or juices	________	× 80 to 1000	= ________
	Subtotal = ________		

STEP 2: Total from above + 250 mg for nondairy sources

= total dietary calcium TOTAL Calcium, in mg = ________

Source: Adapted from SM Krane, MF Holick, Chap. 355, in *Harrison's Principles of Internal Medicine*, 14th ed. New York, McGraw-Hill, 1998.

vitamin D intake in patients with osteoporosis whether they are receiving additional pharmacologic therapy or not. A systematic review confirmed a greater BMD response to antiresorptive therapy when calcium intake was adequate.

Although side effects from supplemental calcium are minimal (eructation and constipation mostly with carbonate salts), individuals with a history of kidney stones should have a 24-h urine calcium determination before starting increased calcium to avoid significant hypercalciuria. Many studies confirm a small but significant increase in the risk of renal stones with calcium supplements, but not dietary calcium. A recent analysis of published data has suggested that high intakes of calcium from supplements are associated with an increase in the risk of heart disease. This is an evolving story with additional studies that confirm or refute this finding. Because high calcium supplement intakes increase the risk of renal stones and confer no extra benefit to the skeleton, the recommendation that total intakes should be between 1000 and 1200 mg/d is reasonable.

Vitamin D Vitamin D is synthesized in skin under the influence of heat and ultraviolet light **(Chap. 32)**. However, large segments of the population do not obtain sufficient vitamin D to maintain what is now considered an adequate supply [serum 25(OH)D consistently >75 μmol/L (30 ng/mL)]. Because vitamin D supplementation at doses that would achieve these serum levels is safe and inexpensive, the Institute of Medicine (based on obtaining a serum level of 20 ng/mL) recommends daily intakes of 200 IU for adults <50 years of age, 400 IU for those 50–70 years, and 600 IU for those >70 years. Multivitamin tablets usually contain 400 IU, and many calcium supplements also contain vitamin D. Some data suggest that higher doses (≥1000 IU) may be required in the elderly and chronically ill. The Institute of Medicine report suggests that it is safe to take up to 4000 IU/d. For those with osteoporosis or those at risk of osteoporosis, 1000–2000 IU/d can usually maintain serum 25(OH)D above 30 ng/mL.

Other Nutrients Other nutrients such as salt, high animal protein intakes, and caffeine may have modest effects on calcium excretion or absorption. Adequate vitamin K status is required for optimal carboxylation of osteocalcin. States in which vitamin K nutrition or metabolism is impaired, such as with long-term warfarin therapy, have been associated with reduced bone mass. Research concerning cola intake is controversial but suggests a possible link to reduced bone mass through factors that are independent of caffeine. Although dark green leafy vegetables such as spinach and kale contain a fair amount of calcium, the high oxalate content reduces absorption of this calcium (but does not inhibit absorption of calcium from other food eaten simultaneously).

Magnesium is abundant in foods, and magnesium deficiency is quite rare in the absence of a serious chronic disease. Magnesium supplementation may be warranted in patients with inflammatory bowel disease, celiac disease, chemotherapy, severe diarrhea, malnutrition, or alcoholism. Dietary phytoestrogens, which are derived primarily from soy products and legumes (e.g., garbanzo beans [chickpeas] and lentils), exert some estrogenic activity but are insufficiently potent to justify their use in place of a pharmacologic agent in the treatment of osteoporosis.

Patients with hip fractures are often frail and relatively malnourished. Some data suggest an improved outcome in such patients when they are provided calorie and protein supplementation. Excessive protein intake can increase renal calcium excretion, but this can be corrected by an adequate calcium intake.

Exercise Exercise in young individuals increases the likelihood that they will attain the maximal genetically determined peak bone mass. Meta-analyses of studies performed in postmenopausal women indicate that weight-bearing exercise helps prevent bone loss but does not appear to result in substantial gain of bone mass. This beneficial effect wanes if exercise is discontinued. Most of the studies are short term, and a more substantial effect on bone mass is likely if exercise is continued over a long period. Exercise also has beneficial effects on neuromuscular function, and it improves coordination, balance, and strength, thereby reducing the risk of falling. A walking program is a practical way to start. Other activities, such as dancing, racquet sports, cross-country skiing, and use of gym equipment, are also recommended, depending on the patient's personal preference and general condition. Even women who cannot walk benefit from swimming or water exercises, not so much for the effects on bone, which are quite minimal, but because of effects on muscle. Exercise habits should be consistent, optimally at least three times a week.

PHARMACOLOGIC THERAPIES Before the mid-1990s, estrogen treatment, either by itself or in concert with a progestin, was the primary therapeutic agent for prevention or treatment of osteoporosis. There are now a number of new medications approved for osteoporosis and more under development. Some are agents that specifically treat osteoporosis (bisphosphonates, calcitonin, denosumab, and teriparatide [1-34hPTH]); others, such as selective estrogen response modulators (SERMs) and, most recently, an estrogen/SERM combination medication, have broader effects. The availability of these drugs allows therapy to be tailored to the needs of an individual patient.

Estrogens A large body of clinical trial data indicates that various types of estrogens (conjugated equine estrogens, estradiol, estrone, esterified estrogens, ethinyl estradiol, and mestranol) reduce bone turnover, prevent bone loss, and induce small increases in bone mass of the spine, hip, and total body. The effects of estrogen are seen in women with natural or surgical menopause and in late postmenopausal women with or without established osteoporosis. Estrogens are efficacious when administered orally or transdermally. For both oral and transdermal routes of administration, combined estrogen/progestin preparations are now available in many countries, obviating the problem of taking two tablets or using a patch and oral progestin.

Dose of Estrogen For oral estrogens, the standard recommended doses have been 0.3 mg/d for esterified estrogens, 0.625 mg/d for conjugated equine estrogens, and 5 μg/d for ethinyl estradiol. For transdermal estrogen, the commonly used dose supplies 50 μg estradiol per day, but a lower dose may be appropriate for some individuals. Dose-response data for conjugated equine estrogens indicate that lower doses (0.3 and 0.45 mg/d) are effective. Doses even lower have been associated with bone mass protection.

Fracture Data Epidemiologic databases indicate that women who take estrogen replacement have a 50% reduction, on average, of osteoporotic fractures, including hip fractures. The beneficial effect of estrogen is greatest among those who start replacement early and continue the treatment; the benefit declines after discontinuation to the extent that there is no residual protective effect against fracture by 10 years after discontinuation. The first clinical trial evaluating fractures as secondary outcomes, the Heart and Estrogen-Progestin Replacement Study (HERS) trial, showed no effect of hormone therapy on hip or other clinical fractures in women with established coronary artery disease. These data made the results of the Women's Health Initiative (WHI) exceedingly important **(Chap. 16)**. The estrogen-progestin arm of the WHI in >16,000 postmenopausal healthy women indicated that hormone therapy reduces the risk of hip and clinical spine fracture by 34% and reduces the risk of all clinical fractures by 24%. There was similar antifracture efficacy seen with estrogen alone in women who had had a hysterectomy.

A few smaller clinical trials have evaluated spine fracture occurrence as an outcome with estrogen therapy. They have consistently shown that estrogen treatment reduces the incidence of vertebral compression fracture.

The WHI has provided a vast amount of data on the multisystemic effects of hormone therapy. Although earlier observational studies suggested that estrogen replacement might reduce heart disease, the WHI showed that combined estrogen-progestin treatment increased risk of fatal and nonfatal myocardial infarction by ~29%, confirming data from the HERS study. Other important relative risks included a 40% increase in stroke, a 100% increase in venous thromboembolic disease, and a 26% increase in risk of breast cancer. Subsequent analyses have confirmed the increased risk of stroke and, in a substudy, showed a twofold increase in dementia. Benefits other than the fracture reductions noted above included a 37% reduction in the risk of colon cancer. These relative risks have to be interpreted in light of absolute risk (Fig. 35-8). For example, out of 10,000 women treated with estrogen-progestin for 1 year, there will be 8 excess heart attacks, 8 excess breast cancers, 18 excess venous thromboembolic events, 5 fewer hip fractures, 44 fewer clinical fractures, and 6 fewer colorectal cancers. These numbers must be multiplied by years of hormone treatment. There was no effect of hormone treatment on the risk of uterine cancer or total mortality.

It is important to note that these WHI findings apply specifically to hormone treatment in the form of conjugated equine estrogen plus medroxyprogesterone acetate. The relative benefits and risks of unopposed estrogen in women who had hysterectomies vary somewhat. They still show benefits against fracture occurrence and increased risk of venous thrombosis and stroke, similar in magnitude to the risks for combined hormone therapy. In contrast, though, the estrogen-only arm of WHI indicated no increased risk of heart attack or breast cancer. The data suggest that at least some of the detrimental effects of combined therapy are related to the progestin component. In addition, there is the possibility, suggested by primate data, that the risk accrues mainly to women who have some years of estrogen deficiency before initiating treatment. (The average woman in the WHI was

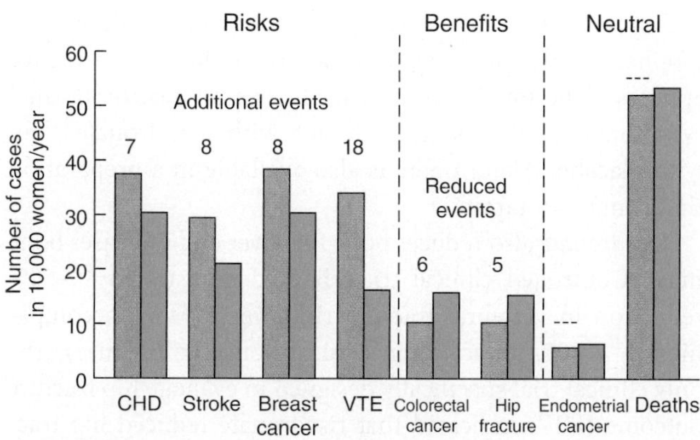

FIGURE 35-8

Effects of hormone therapy on event rates: green, placebo; purple, estrogen and progestin. CHD, coronary heart disease; VTE, venous thromboembolic events. *(Adapted from Women's Health Initiative. WHI HRT Update. Available at http://www.nhlbi.nih.gov/health/women/upd2002.htm.)*

more than 10 years from the last menstrual period). Nonetheless, there is reluctance among women to use estrogen/hormone therapy, and the U.S. Preventive Services Task Force has specifically suggested that estrogen/hormone therapy not be used for disease prevention.

Mode of Action Two subtypes of ERs, α and β, have been identified in bone and other tissues. Cells of monocyte lineage express both ERα and ERβ, as do osteoblasts. Estrogen-mediated effects vary with the receptor type. Using ER knock-out mouse models, elimination of ERα produces a modest reduction in bone mass, whereas mutation of ERβ has less of an effect on bone. A male patient with a homozygous mutation of ERα had markedly decreased bone density as well as abnormalities in epiphyseal closure, confirming the important role of ERα in bone biology. The mechanism of estrogen action in bone is an area of active investigation **(Fig. 35-5)**. Although data are conflicting, estrogens may inhibit osteoclasts directly. However, the majority of estrogen (and androgen) effects on bone resorption are mediated through paracrine factors produced by osteoblasts and osteocytes. These actions include decreasing RANKL production and increasing OPG production by osteoblasts.

Progestins In women with a uterus, daily progestin or cyclical progestins at least 12 days per month are prescribed in combination with estrogens to reduce the risk of uterine cancer. Medroxyprogesterone acetate and norethindrone acetate blunt the high-density lipoprotein response to estrogen, but micronized progesterone does not. Neither medroxyprogesterone acetate nor micronized progesterone appears to have an independent effect on bone; at lower doses of estrogen, norethindrone acetate may have an additive benefit. On breast tissue, progestins may increase the risk of breast cancer.

SERMs Two SERMs are used currently in postmenopausal women: raloxifene, which is approved for the prevention and treatment of osteoporosis as well as the prevention of breast cancer, and tamoxifen, which is approved for the prevention and treatment of breast cancer. A third SERM, bazedoxifene, has been complexed with conjugated estrogen, creating a tissue selective estrogen complex (TSEC). This agent has been approved for prevention of osteoporosis.

Tamoxifen reduces bone turnover and bone loss in postmenopausal women compared with placebo groups. These findings support the concept that tamoxifen acts as an estrogenic agent in bone. There are limited data on the effect of tamoxifen on fracture risk, but the Breast Cancer Prevention Study indicated a possible reduction in clinical vertebral, hip, and Colles' fractures. The major benefit of tamoxifen is on breast cancer occurrence. The breast cancer prevention trial indicated that tamoxifen administration over 4–5 years reduced the incidence of new invasive and noninvasive breast cancer by ~45% in women at increased risk of breast cancer. The incidence of ER-positive breast cancers was reduced by 65%. Tamoxifen increases the risk of uterine cancer and increases risk of venous thrombosis, cataracts, and possibly stroke in postmenopausal women, limiting its use for breast cancer prevention in women at low or moderate risk.

Raloxifene (60 mg/d) has effects on bone turnover and bone mass that are very similar to those of tamoxifen, indicating that this agent is also estrogenic on the skeleton. The effect of raloxifene on bone density (+1.4–2.8% vs placebo in the spine, hip, and total body) is somewhat less than that seen with standard doses of estrogens. Raloxifene reduces the occurrence of vertebral fracture by 30–50%, depending on the population; however, there are no data confirming that raloxifene can reduce the risk of nonvertebral fractures over 8 years of observation.

Raloxifene, like tamoxifen and estrogen, has effects in other organ systems. The most beneficial effect appears to be a reduction in invasive breast cancer (mainly decreased ER-positive) occurrence of ~65% in women who take raloxifene compared to placebo. In a head-to-head study, raloxifene was as effective as tamoxifen in preventing breast cancer in high-risk women, and raloxifene is now FDA approved for this indication. In a further study, raloxifene had no effect on heart disease in women with increased risk for this outcome. In contrast to tamoxifen, raloxifene is not associated with an increase in the risk of uterine cancer or benign uterine disease. Raloxifene increases the occurrence of hot flashes but reduces serum total and low-density lipoprotein cholesterol, lipoprotein(a), and fibrinogen. Raloxifene, with positive effects on breast cancer and vertebral fractures, has become a useful agent for the treatment of the younger asymptomatic postmenopausal woman. In some women, a recurrence of menopausal hot flashes may occur. Usually this is evanescent, but occasionally, it is sufficiently impactful on daily life and sleep that the drug must be withdrawn. Raloxifene increases the risk of deep vein thrombosis and may increase the risk of death from stroke among older women. Consequently, it is not usually recommended for women over 70 years of age.

The main advantage of the *bazedoxifene/conjugated estrogen* compound is that the bazedoxifene protects uterine tissue from the effects of estrogen and makes it possible to avoid taking a progestin, while using an estrogen primarily for control of menopausal symptoms. The TSEC prevents bone loss somewhat more potently than raloxifene alone and appears safe for the breast.

Mode of Action of Serms All SERMs bind to the ER, but each agent produces a unique receptor-drug conformation. As a result, specific co-activator or co-repressor proteins are bound to the receptor **(Chap. 2)**, resulting in differential effects on gene transcription that vary depending on other transcription factors present in the cell. Another aspect of selectivity is the affinity of each SERM for the different ERα and ERβ subtypes, which are expressed differentially in various tissues. These tissue-selective effects of SERMs offer the possibility of tailoring estrogen therapy to best meet the needs and risk factor profile of an individual patient.

Bisphosphonates Alendronate, risedronate, ibandronate, and zoledronic acid are approved for the prevention and treatment of postmenopausal osteoporosis. Alendronate, risedronate, and zoledronic acid are also approved for the treatment of steroid-induced osteoporosis, and risedronate and zoledronic acid are approved for prevention of steroid-induced osteoporosis. Alendronate, risedronate, and zoledronic acid are approved for treatment of osteoporosis in men.

Alendronate has been shown to decrease bone turnover and increase bone mass in the spine by up to 8% versus placebo and by 6% versus placebo in the hip. Multiple trials have evaluated its effect on fracture occurrence. The Fracture Intervention Trial provided evidence in >2000 women with prevalent vertebral fractures that daily alendronate treatment (5 mg/d for 2 years and 10 mg/d for 9 months afterward) reduces vertebral fracture risk by about 50%, multiple vertebral fractures by up to 90%, and hip fractures by up to 50%. Several subsequent trials have confirmed these findings (Fig. 35-9). For example, in a study of >1900 women with low bone mass treated with alendronate (10 mg/d) versus placebo, the incidence of all nonvertebral fractures was reduced by ~47% after only 1 year. In the United States, the 10-mg dose is approved for treatment of osteoporosis and 5 mg/d is used for prevention.

Trials comparing once-weekly alendronate, 70 mg, with daily 10-mg dosing have shown equivalence with regard to bone mass and bone turnover responses. Consequently, once-weekly therapy generally is preferred because of the low incidence of gastrointestinal side effects and ease of administration. Alendronate should be given with a full glass of water before breakfast, because bisphosphonates are poorly absorbed. Because of the potential for esophageal irritation, alendronate is contraindicated in patients who have stricture or inadequate emptying of the esophagus. It is recommended that patients remain upright for at least 30 min after taking the medication to avoid esophageal irritation. Cases of esophagitis, esophageal ulcer, and esophageal stricture have been described, but the incidence appears to be low. In clinical trials, overall gastrointestinal symptomatology was no different with alendronate than with placebo. Alendronate is also available in a preparation that contains vitamin D.

Risedronate also reduces bone turnover and increases bone mass. Controlled clinical trials have demonstrated 40–50% reduction in vertebral fracture risk over 3 years, accompanied by a 40% reduction in clinical nonspine fractures. The only clinical trial specifically designed to evaluate hip fracture outcome (HIP) indicated that risedronate reduced hip fracture risk in women in their seventies with confirmed osteoporosis by 40%. In contrast, risedronate was not effective at reducing hip fracture occurrence in older women (80+ years) without proven osteoporosis. Studies have shown that 35 mg of risedronate administered once weekly is therapeutically equivalent to 5 mg/d and that 150 mg once monthly is therapeutically equivalent to 35 mg once weekly. Patients should take risedronate with a full glass of plain water to facilitate delivery to the stomach and should not lie down for 30 min after taking the drug. The incidence of gastrointestinal side effects in trials with risedronate was similar to that of placebo. A new preparation, which allows risedronate to be taken with food, was recently approved.

Etidronate was the first bisphosphonate to be approved, initially for use in Paget's disease and hypercalcemia. This agent has also been used in osteoporosis trials of smaller magnitude than those performed for alendronate and risedronate but is not approved by the FDA for treatment of osteoporosis. Etidronate probably has some efficacy against vertebral fracture when given as an intermittent cyclical regimen (2 weeks on, 2.5 months off). Its effectiveness against nonvertebral fractures has not been studied.

Ibandronate is the third amino-bisphosphonate approved in the United States. Ibandronate (2.5 mg/d) has been shown in clinical trials to reduce vertebral fracture risk by ~40% but with no overall effect on nonvertebral fractures. In a post hoc analysis of subjects with a femoral neck T-score of –3 or below, ibandronate reduced the risk of nonvertebral fractures by ~60%. In clinical trials, ibandronate doses of 150 mg/month PO or 3 mg every 3 months IV had greater effects on turnover and bone mass than did 2.5 mg/d. Patients should take oral ibandronate in the same way as other bisphosphonates, but with 1 h elapsing before other food or drink (other than plain water).

Zoledronic acid is a potent bisphosphonate with a unique administration regimen (5 mg by slow IV infusion annually). The data confirm that it is highly effective in fracture risk reduction. In a study of >7000 women followed for 3 years, zoledronic acid (three annual infusions) reduced the risk of vertebral fractures by 70%, nonvertebral fractures by 25%, and hip fractures by 40%. These results were associated with less height loss and disability. In the treated population, there was an increased risk of transient postdose symptoms

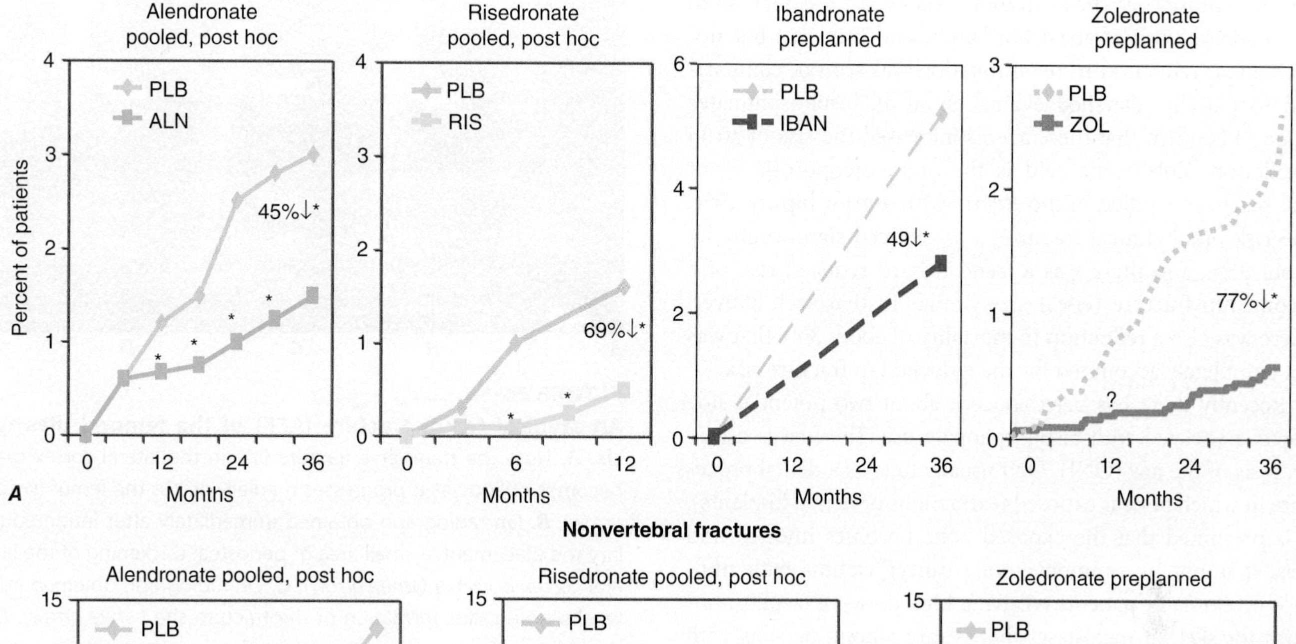

Nonvertebral fractures

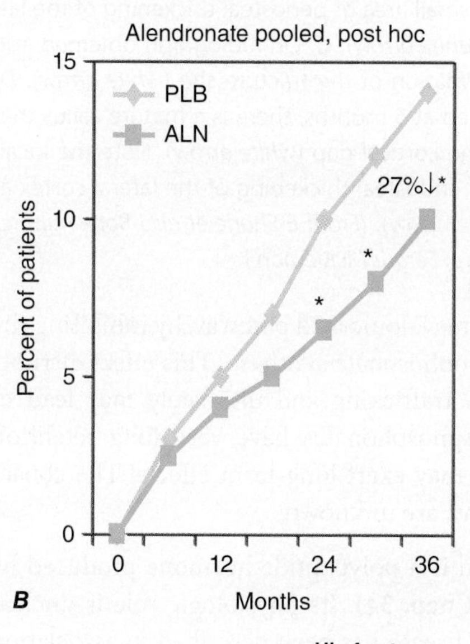

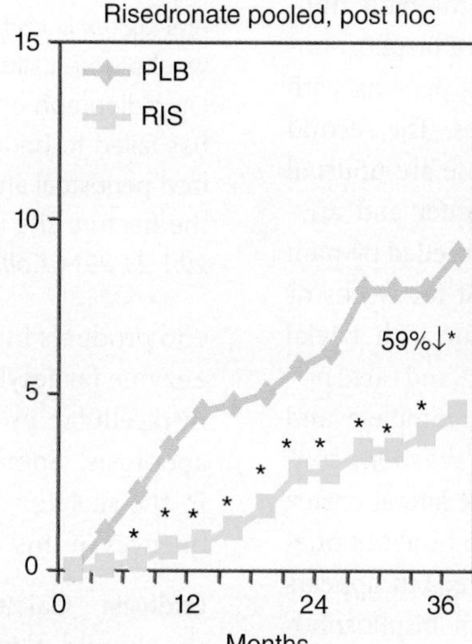

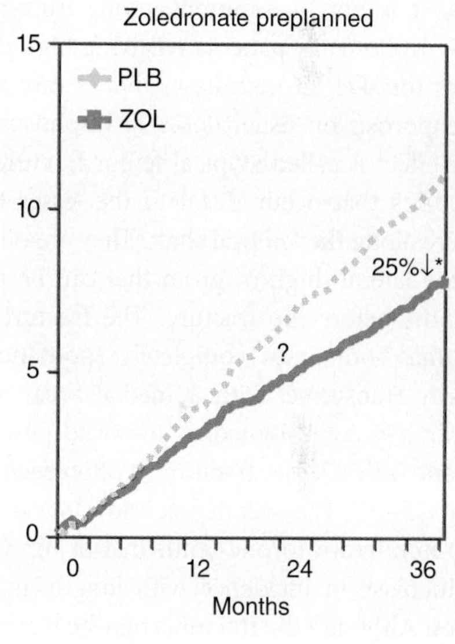

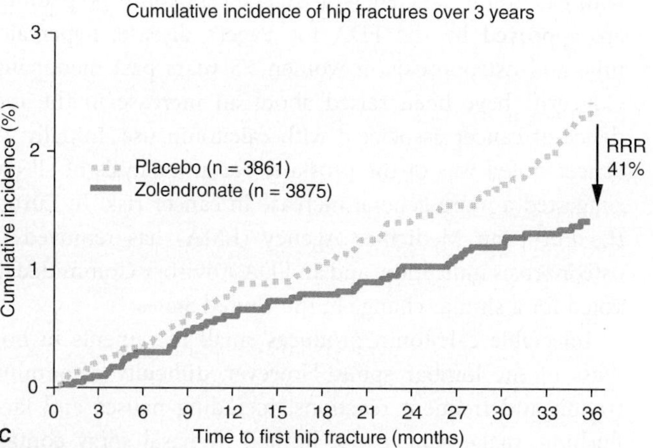

FIGURE 35-9

Effects of various bisphosphonates on clinical vertebral fractures **A.** nonvertebral fractures **B.** and hip fractures **C.** PLB, placebo; RRR, relative risk reduction. *(After DM Black et al: J Clin Endocrinol Metab 85:4118, 2000; C Roux et al: Curr Med Res Opin 4:433, 2004; CH Chesnut et al: J Bone Miner Res 19:1241, 2004; DM Black et al: N Engl J Med 356:1809, 2007; JT Harrington et al: Calcif Tissue Int 74:129, 2003.)*

(acute-phase reaction) manifested by fever, arthralgia, myalgias, and headache. The symptoms usually last less than 48 h. An increased risk of atrial fibrillation and transient but not permanent reduction in renal function was seen in comparison to placebo. Detailed evaluation of all bisphosphonates failed to confirm that these agents increased the risk of atrial fibrillation. Zoledronic acid is the only osteoporosis agent that has been studied in the elderly with a prior hip fracture. The risk of all clinical fractures was reduced significantly by about 35%, and there was a trend toward reduced risk of a second hip fracture (effect size similar to that seen above). There was also a reduction in mortality of about 30% that was not completely accounted for the reduced hip fracture risk.

Recently there has been concern about two potential side effects associated with bisphosphonate use. The first is osteonecrosis of the jaw (ONJ). ONJ usually follows a dental procedure in which bone is exposed (extractions or dental implants). It is presumed that the exposed bone becomes infected and dies. It is not uncommon among cancer victims with multiple myeloma or patients receiving high doses of bisphosphonates for skeletal metastases, but is rare among persons with osteoporosis on usual doses of bisphosphonates. The second side effect is called atypical femur fracture. These are unusual fractures that occur distal to the lesser trochanter and anywhere along the femoral shaft. They are often preceded by pain in the lateral thigh or groin that can be present for weeks or months before the fracture. The fractures occur with trivial trauma, sometimes completely spontaneously, and are primarily transverse, with a medial break when complete and minimally comminuted. A localized periosteal reaction, consistent with a stress fracture, is often seen in the lateral cortex (Fig. 35-10). The overall risk is low (suggested to be about one-one hundredth to one-tenth that of hip fracture) but appears to increase in incidence with long-term use of bisphosphonates. Although the fractures may be bisphosphonate related in many individuals, they clearly occur in patients with no prior bisphosphonate exposure. When complete, they require surgical fixation and may be difficult to heal. Anabolic medication may accelerate healing of these fractures in some patients, and surgery can sometimes be avoided. Patients initiating bisphosphonates need to be warned that if they develop thigh or groin pain they must notify their physician. Routine x-rays will sometimes pick up cortical thickening or even a stress fracture, but more commonly MRI or technetium bone scan is required. The presence of an abnormality requires at minimum a period of modified weight bearing and may need prophylactic rodding of the femur. It is important to realize that these fractures may be bilateral, and when an abnormality is found, the other femur should be investigated.

Mode of Action Bisphosphonates are structurally related to pyrophosphates, compounds that are incorporated into bone matrix. Bisphosphonates specifically impair osteoclast function and reduce osteoclast number, in part by inducing apoptosis. Recent evidence suggests that the nitrogen-containing bisphosphonates also inhibit protein prenylation, one of the end products in the mevalonic acid pathway, by inhibiting the enzyme farnesyl pyrophosphate synthase. This effect disrupts intracellular protein trafficking and ultimately may lead to apoptosis. Some bisphosphonates have very long retention in the skeleton and may exert long-term effects. The consequences of this, if any, are unknown.

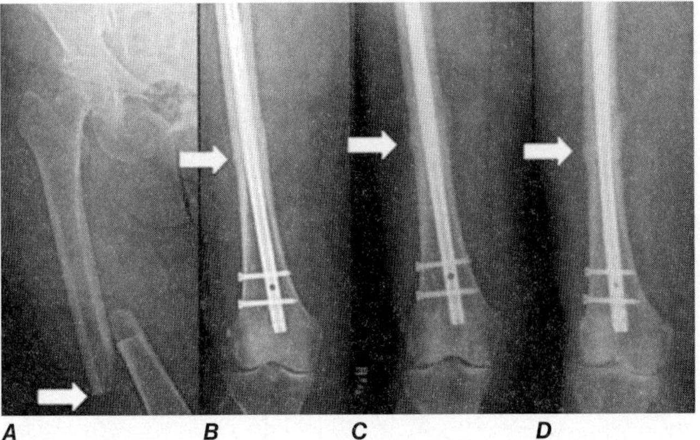

FIGURE 35-10

An atypical femur fracture (AFF) of the femoral diaphysis. *A.* Note the transverse fracture line in the lateral cortex that becomes oblique as it progresses medially across the femur (*white arrow*). ***B.*** On radiograph obtained immediately after intramedullary rod placement, a small area of periosteal thickening of the lateral cortex is visible (*white arrow*). ***C.*** On radiograph obtained at 6 weeks, note callus formation of the fracture site (*white arrow*). ***D.*** On radiograph obtained at 3 months, there is a mature callus that has failed to bridge the cortical gap (*white arrow*). Note the localized periosteal and/or endosteal thickening of the lateral cortex at the fracture site (*white arrow*). *(From E Shane et al: J Bone Min Res 29:1-23, 2014. Courtesy of Fergus McKiernan.)*

Calcitonin Calcitonin is a polypeptide hormone produced by the thyroid gland **(Chap. 34)**. Its physiologic role is unclear because no skeletal disease has been described in association with calcitonin deficiency or excess. Calcitonin preparations are approved by the FDA for Paget's disease, hypercalcemia, and osteoporosis in women >5 years past menopause. Concerns have been raised about an increase in the incidence of cancer associated with calcitonin use. Initially, the cancer noted was of the prostate, but an analysis of all data suggested a more general increase in cancer risk. In Europe, the European Medicines Agency (EMA) has removed the osteoporosis indication, and an FDA Advisory Committee has voted for a similar change in the United States.

Injectable calcitonin produces small increments in bone mass of the lumbar spine. However, difficulty of administration and frequent reactions, including nausea and facial flushing, make general use limited. A nasal spray containing calcitonin (200 IU/d) is available for treatment of osteoporosis in postmenopausal women. One study suggests that nasal calcitonin produces small increments in bone mass and a small reduction in new vertebral fractures in calcitonin-treated patients versus those on calcium alone. There has been no proven effectiveness against nonvertebral fractures.

Calcitonin is not indicated for prevention of osteoporosis and is not sufficiently potent to prevent bone loss in early postmenopausal women. Calcitonin might have an analgesic effect on bone pain, both in the subcutaneous and possibly the nasal form.

Mode of Action Calcitonin suppresses osteoclast activity by direct action on the osteoclast calcitonin receptor. Osteoclasts exposed to calcitonin cannot maintain their active ruffled border, which normally maintains close contact with underlying bone.

Denosumab A novel agent that was given twice yearly by SC administration in a randomized controlled trial in postmenopausal women with osteoporosis has been shown to increase BMD in the spine, hip, and forearm and reduce vertebral, hip, and nonvertebral fractures over a 3-year period by 70, 40, and 20%, respectively (Fig. 35-11). Other clinical trials indicate ability to increase bone mass in postmenopausal women with low bone mass (above osteoporosis range) and in postmenopausal women with breast cancer treated with hormonal agents. Furthermore, a study of men with prostate cancer treated with gonadotropin-releasing hormone (GnRH) agonist therapy indicated the ability of denosumab to improve bone mass and reduce vertebral fracture occurrence. Denosumab was approved by the FDA in 2010 for the treatment of postmenopausal women who have a high risk for osteoporotic fractures, including those with a history of fracture or multiple risk factors for fracture, and those who have failed or are intolerant to other osteoporosis therapy. Denosumab is also approved for the treatment of osteoporosis in men at high risk, men with prostate cancer on GnRH agonist therapy, and women with breast cancer on aromatase inhibitor therapy.

Mode of Action Denosumab is a fully human monoclonal antibody to RANKL, the final common effector of osteoclast formation, activity, and survival. Denosumab binds to RANKL, inhibiting its ability to initiate formation of mature osteoclasts from osteoclast precursors and to bring mature osteoclasts to the bone surface and initiate bone resorption. Denosumab also plays a role in reducing the survival of the osteoclast. Through these actions on the osteoclast, denosumab induces potent antiresorptive action, as assessed biochemically and histomorphometrically, and may contribute to the occurrence of ONJ. Atypical femur fractures have also been noted. Serious adverse reactions include hypocalcemia, skin infections (usually cellulitis of the lower extremity), and dermatologic reactions such as dermatitis, rashes, and eczema. The effects of denosumab are rapidly reversible. If denosumab is stopped, bone will be lost rapidly if another agent is not used.

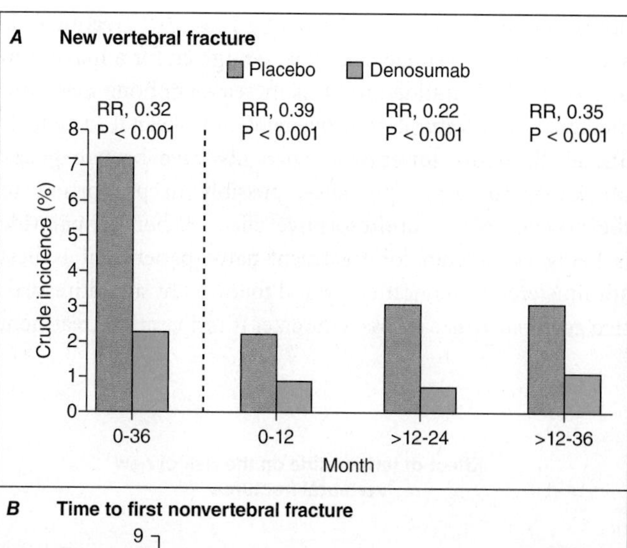

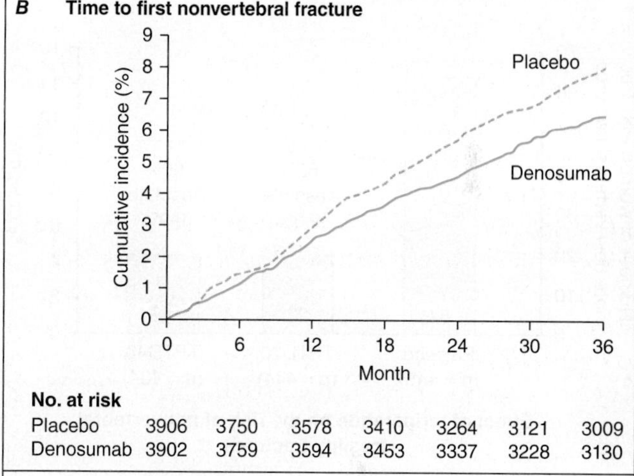

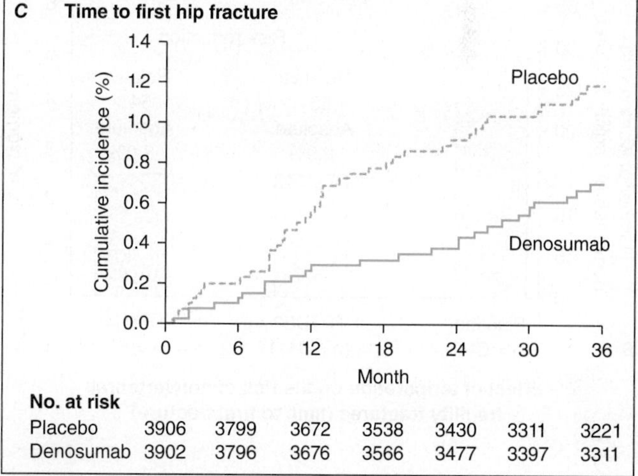

FIGURE 35-11

Effects of denosumab on new vertebral fractures ***A.*** and times to nonvertebral and hip fracture ***B.*** and ***C.*** RR, relative risk. *(After SR Cummings et al: N Engl J Med 361:756, 2009.)*

Parathyroid Hormone Endogenous PTH is an 84-amino-acid peptide that is largely responsible for calcium homeostasis **(Chap. 34)**. Although chronic elevation of PTH, as occurs in hyperparathyroidism, is associated with bone loss (particularly cortical bone), PTH when given exogenously as a daily injection exerts anabolic effects on bone. Teriparatide (1-34hPTH) is approved for the treatment of osteoporosis in both men and women at high risk for fracture. In a pivotal study (median time of treatment, 19 months' duration), 20 μg of teriparatide daily by SC injection reduced vertebral fractures by 65% and nonvertebral fractures by 45% (Fig. 35-12). Treatment is administered as a single daily injection given for a maximum of 2 years. Teriparatide produces increases in bone mass and mediates architectural improvements in skeletal structure. These effects are lower when patients have been exposed previously to bisphosphonates, possibly in proportion to the potency of the antiresorptive effect. When teriparatide is being considered for treatment-naive patients, it is best administered as monotherapy and followed by an antiresorptive agent such as a bisphosphonate. If teriparatide treatment is not followed by an antiresorptive agent, the bone gained is rapidly lost.

Side effects of teriparatide are generally mild and can include leg cramps, muscle pain, weakness, dizziness, headache, and nausea. Rodents given prolonged treatment with PTH in relatively high doses developed osteogenic sarcomas. Long-term surveillance studies suggest no association between 2 years of teriparatide administration and osteosarcoma risk in humans.

PTH use may be limited by its mode of administration; alternative modes of delivery are being investigated. The optimal frequency of administration also remains to be established, and it is possible that PTH might be effective when used intermittently. Cost also may be a limiting factor. In some settings, the effect of PTH might be enhanced by combination with an antiresorptive agent. This might be particularly important in patients who have been treated previously with bisphosphonate medications.

Mode of Action Exogenously administered PTH appears to have direct actions on osteoblast activity, with biochemical and histomorphometric evidence of de novo bone formation early in response to PTH, before activation of bone resorption. Subsequently, PTH activates bone remodeling but still appears to favor bone formation over bone resorption. PTH stimulates Wnt signaling, IGF-I, and collagen production and appears to increase osteoblast number by stimulating replication, enhancing osteoblast recruitment, and inhibiting apoptosis. Unlike all other treatments, PTH produces a true increase in bone tissue and an apparent restoration of bone microarchitecture (Fig. 35-13).

Fluoride Fluoride has been available for many years and is a potent stimulator of osteoprogenitor cells when studied in vitro. It has been used in multiple osteoporosis studies with conflicting results, in part because of the use of varying doses and preparations. Despite increments in bone mass of up to 10%, there are no consistent effects of fluoride on vertebral or nonvertebral fracture; the latter may actually increase when high doses of fluoride are used. Fluoride

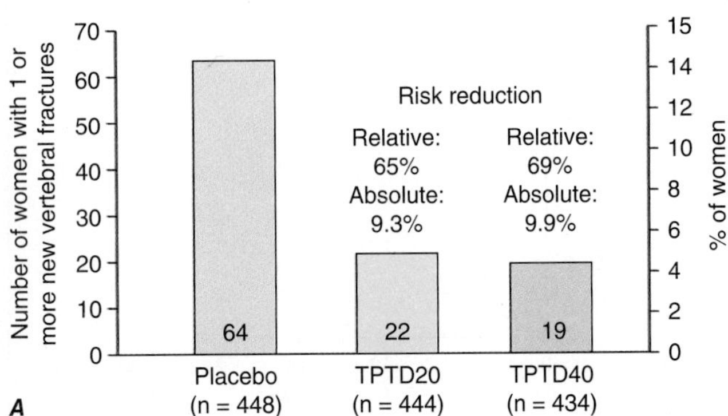

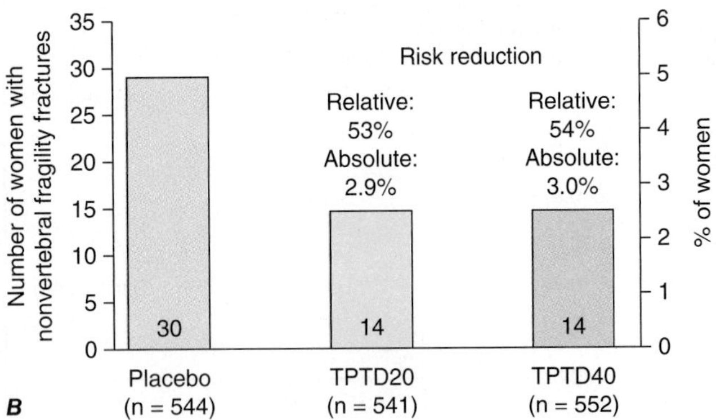

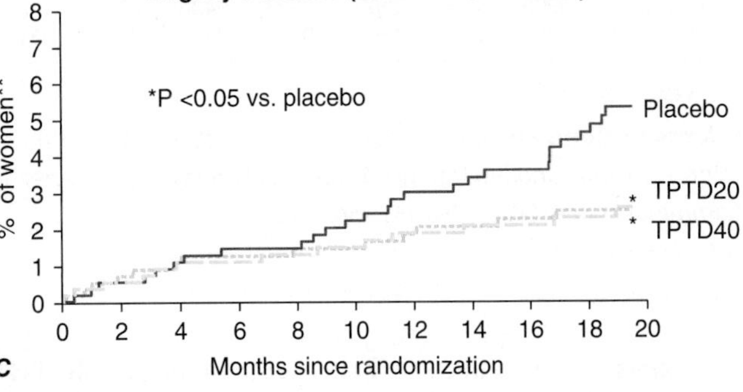

FIGURE 35-12

Effects of teriparatide (TPTD) on new vertebral fractures ***A.*** and nonvertebral fragility fractures ***B.*** and ***C.*** *(After RM Neer et al: N Engl J Med 344:1434, 2001.)*

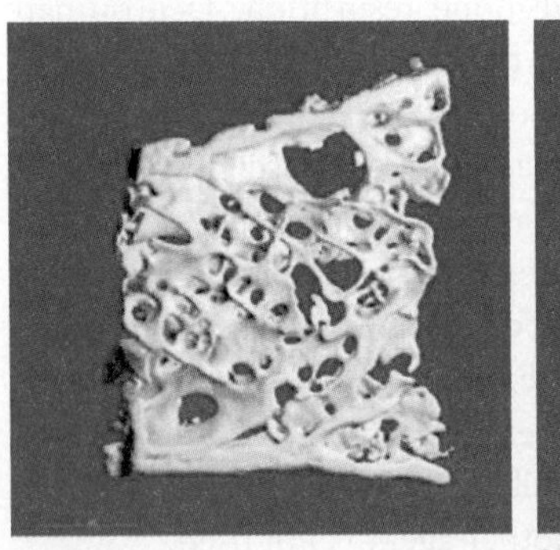

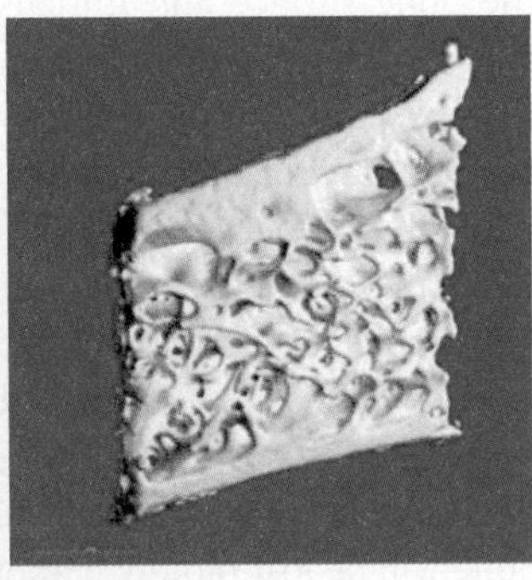

FIGURE 35-13

Effect of parathyroid hormone (PTH) treatment on bone microarchitecture. Paired biopsy specimens from a 64-year-old woman before ***A.*** and after ***B.*** treatment with PTH. *(From DW Dempster et al: J Bone Miner Res 16:1846, 2001.)*

remains an experimental agent despite its long history and multiple studies.

Strontium Ranelate Strontium ranelate is approved in several European countries for the treatment of osteoporosis. It increases bone mass throughout the skeleton; in clinical trials, the drug reduced the risk of vertebral fractures by 37% and that of nonvertebral fractures by 14%. It appears to be modestly antiresorptive while at the same time not causing as much of a decrease in bone formation (measured biochemically). Strontium is incorporated into hydroxyapatite, replacing calcium, a feature that might explain some of its fracture benefits. Small increased risks of venous thrombosis, sometimes severe dermatologic reactions, seizures, and abnormal cognition have been seen and require further study. An increase in risk of cardiovascular disease has also been associated with use of strontium, such that the EMA has restricted its use at present.

Other Potential Anabolic Agents Several small studies of growth hormone (GH), alone or in combination with other agents, have not shown consistent or substantial positive effects on skeletal mass. Many of these studies have been relatively short term, and the effects of GH, growth hormone–releasing hormone, and the IGFs are still under investigation. Anabolic steroids, mostly derivatives of testosterone, act primarily as antiresorptive agents to reduce bone turnover but also may stimulate osteoblastic activity. Effects on bone mass remain unclear but appear weak in general, and use is limited by masculinizing side effects. Several observational studies suggested that the statin drugs, used to treat hypercholesterolemia, may be associated with increased bone mass and reduced fractures, but conclusions from clinical trials have been largely negative. Early studies with sclerostin antibodies, which inhibit sclerostin, activate Wnt, and might be highly anabolic to bone, are under development. Odanacatib is a mixed antiresorptive, partial bone formation stimulator that is currently in the late stages of development.

NONPHARMACOLOGIC APPROACHES In some early studies, protective pads worn around the outer thigh, which cover the trochanteric region of the hip, were able to prevent hip fractures in elderly residents in nursing homes. Randomized controlled trials of hip protectors have been unable to confirm these early findings. Therefore, the efficacy of hip protectors remains controversial at this time.

Kyphoplasty and *vertebroplasty* are also useful nonpharmacologic approaches for the treatment of painful vertebral fractures. However, no long-term data are available.

TREATMENT MONITORING There are currently no well-accepted guidelines for monitoring treatment of osteoporosis. Because most osteoporosis treatments produce small or moderate bone mass increments on average, it is reasonable to consider BMD as a monitoring tool. Changes must exceed ~4% in the spine and 6% in the hip to be considered significant in any individual. The hip is the preferred site due to larger surface area and greater reproducibility. Medication-induced increments may require several years to produce changes of this magnitude (if they do at all). Consequently, it can be argued that BMD should be repeated at intervals >2 years. Only significant BMD reductions should prompt a change in medical regimen, because it is expected that many individuals will not show responses greater than the detection limits of the current measurement techniques.

Biochemical markers of bone turnover may prove useful for treatment monitoring, but little hard evidence currently supports this concept; it remains unclear which endpoint is most useful. If bone turnover markers are used, a determination should be made before therapy is started and repeated ≥4 months after therapy is initiated. In general, a change in bone turnover markers must be 30–40% lower than the baseline to be significant because of the biologic and technical variability in these tests. A positive change in biochemical markers and/or bone density can be useful to help patients adhere to treatment regimens.

GLUCOCORTICOID-INDUCED OSTEOPOROSIS

Osteoporotic fractures are a well-characterized consequence of the hypercortisolism associated with Cushing's syndrome. However, the therapeutic use of glucocorticoids is by far the most common form of glucocorticoid-induced osteoporosis. Glucocorticoids are used widely in the treatment of a variety of disorders, including chronic lung disorders, rheumatoid arthritis and other connective tissue diseases, inflammatory bowel disease, and after transplantation. Osteoporosis and related fractures are serious side effects of chronic glucocorticoid therapy. Because the effects of glucocorticoids on the skeleton are often superimposed on the consequences of aging and menopause, it is not surprising that women and the elderly are most frequently affected. The skeletal response to steroids is remarkably heterogeneous, however, and even young, growing individuals treated with glucocorticoids can present with fractures.

The risk of fractures depends on the dose and duration of glucocorticoid therapy, although recent data suggest that there may be no completely safe dose. Bone loss is more rapid during the early months of treatment, and trabecular bone is affected more severely than cortical bone. As a result, fractures have been shown to increase within 3 months of steroid treatment. There is an increase in fracture risk in both the axial skeleton and the appendicular skeleton, including risk of hip fracture. Bone loss can occur with any route of steroid administration, including high-dose inhaled glucocorticoids and intraarticular injections. Alternate-day delivery does not appear to ameliorate the skeletal effects of glucocorticoids.

PATHOPHYSIOLOGY

Glucocorticoids increase bone loss by multiple mechanisms, including (1) inhibition of osteoblast function and an increase in osteoblast apoptosis, resulting in impaired synthesis of new bone; (2) stimulation of bone resorption, probably as a secondary effect; (3) impairment of the absorption of calcium across the intestine, probably by a vitamin D–independent effect; (4) increase of urinary calcium loss and perhaps induction of some degree of secondary hyperparathyroidism; (5) reduction of adrenal androgens and suppression of ovarian and testicular secretion of estrogens and androgens; and (6) induction of glucocorticoid myopathy, which may exacerbate effects on skeletal and calcium homeostasis as well as increase the risk of falls.

EVALUATION OF THE PATIENT

Because of the prevalence of glucocorticoid-induced bone loss, it is important to evaluate the status of the skeleton in all patients starting or already receiving long-term glucocorticoid therapy. Modifiable risk factors should be identified, including those for falls. Examination should include testing of height and muscle strength. Laboratory evaluation should include an assessment of 24-h urinary calcium. All patients on long-term (>3 months) glucocorticoids should have measurement of bone mass at both the spine and the hip using DXA. If only one skeletal site can be measured, it is best to assess the spine in individuals <60 years and the hip in those >60 years.

PREVENTION

Bone loss caused by glucocorticoids can be prevented and the risk of fractures significantly reduced. Strategies must include using the lowest dose of glucocorticoid for disease management. Topical and inhaled routes of administration are preferred, where appropriate. Risk factor reduction is important, including smoking cessation, limitation of alcohol consumption, and participation in weight-bearing exercise, when appropriate. All patients should receive an adequate calcium and vitamin D intake from the diet or from supplements.

TREATMENT Glucocorticoid-Induced Osteoporosis

Several bisphosphonates (alendronate, risedronate, and zoledronic acid) have been demonstrated in large clinical trials to reduce the risk of vertebral fractures in patients being treated with glucocorticoids, as well as improve bone mass in spine and hip. Teriparatide also improves bone mass and reduces fracture risk in glucocorticoid-treated osteoporosis compared to an active comparator (alendronate).

CHAPTER 36

PAGET'S DISEASE AND OTHER DYSPLASIAS OF BONE

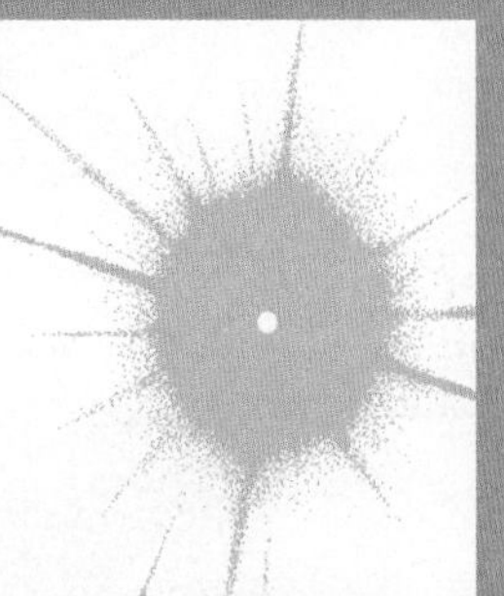

Murray J. Favus ■ Tamara J. Vokes

PAGET'S DISEASE OF BONE

Paget's disease is a localized bone-remodeling disorder that affects widespread, noncontiguous areas of the skeleton. The pathologic process is initiated by overactive osteoclastic bone resorption followed by a compensatory increase in osteoblastic new bone formation, resulting in a structurally disorganized mosaic of woven and lamellar bone. Pagetic bone is expanded, less compact, and more vascular; thus, it is more susceptible to deformities and fractures. Although most patients are asymptomatic, symptoms resulting directly from bony involvement (bone pain, secondary arthritis, fractures) or secondarily from the expansion of bone causing compression of surrounding neural tissue are not uncommon.

Epidemiology

There is a marked geographic variation in the frequency of Paget's disease, with high prevalence in Western Europe (Great Britain, France, and Germany, but not Switzerland or Scandinavia) and among those who have immigrated to Australia, New Zealand, South Africa, and North and South America. The disease is rare in native populations of the Americas, Africa, Asia, and the Middle East; when it does occur, the affected subjects usually have evidence of European ancestry, supporting the migration theory. For unclear reasons, the prevalence and severity of Paget's disease are decreasing, and the age of diagnosis is increasing.

The prevalence is greater in males and increases with age. Autopsy series reveal Paget's disease in about 3% of those over age 40. Prevalence of positive skeletal radiographs in patients over age 55 is 2.5% for men and 1.6% for women. Elevated alkaline phosphatase (ALP) levels in asymptomatic patients have an age-adjusted incidence of 12.7 and 7 per 100,000 person-years in men and women, respectively.

Etiology

The etiology of Paget's disease of bone remains unknown, but evidence supports both genetic and viral etiologies. A positive family history is found in 15–25% of patients and, when present, raises the prevalence of the disease seven- to tenfold among first-degree relatives.

A clear genetic basis has been established for several rare familial bone disorders that clinically and radiographically resemble Paget's disease but have more severe presentation and earlier onset. A homozygous deletion of the *TNFRSF11B* gene, which encodes osteoprotegrin (Fig. 36-1), causes *juvenile Paget's disease,* also known as *familial idiopathic hyperphosphatasia*, a disorder characterized by uncontrolled osteoclastic differentiation and resorption. Familial patterns of disease in several large kindred are consistent with an autosomal dominant pattern of inheritance with variable penetrance. *Familial expansile osteolysis, expansile skeletal hyperphosphatasia, and early-onset Paget's disease* are associated with mutations in *TNFRSF11A* gene, which encodes RANK (receptor activator of nuclear factor-κB), a member of the tumor necrosis factor superfamily critical for osteoclast differentiation (Fig. 36-1). Finally, mutations in the gene for valosin-containing protein cause a rare syndrome with autosomal dominant inheritance and variable penetrance known as *inclusion body myopathy with Paget's disease and frontotemporal dementia (IBMPFD)*. The role of genetic factors is less clear in the more common form of late-onset Paget's disease. Although a few families with mutations in the gene encoding RANK have been reported, the most common mutations identified in

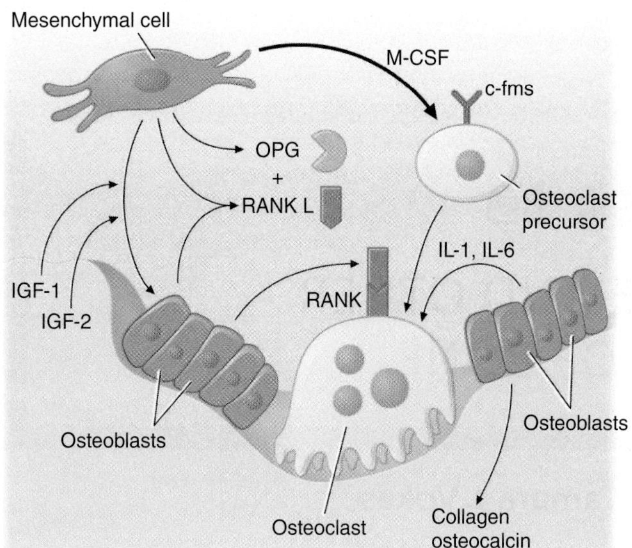

FIGURE 36-1
Diagram illustrating factors that promote differentiation and function of osteoclasts and osteoblasts and the role of the RANK pathway. Stromal bone marrow (mesenchymal) cells and differentiated osteoblasts produce multiple growth factors and cytokines, including macrophage colony-stimulating factor (M-CSF), to modulate osteoclastogenesis. RANKL (receptor activator of nuclear factor-κB ligand) is produced by osteoblast progenitors and mature osteoblasts and can bind to a soluble decoy receptor known as OPG (osteoprotegerin) to inhibit RANKL action. Alternatively, a cell-cell interaction between osteoblast and osteoclast progenitors allows RANKL to bind to its membrane-bound receptor, RANK, thereby stimulating osteoclast differentiation and function. RANK binds intracellular proteins called TRAFs (tumor necrosis factor receptor–associated factors) that mediate receptor signaling through transcription factors such as NF-κB. M-CSF binds to its receptor, c-fms, which is the cellular homologue of the *fms* oncogene. See text for the potential role of these pathways in disorders of osteoclast function such as Paget's disease and osteopetrosis. IL, interleukin; IGF, insulin-like growth factor.

familial and sporadic cases of Paget's disease have been in the *SQSTM1* gene (sequestasome-1 or p62 protein) in the C-terminal ubiquitin-binding domain. The p62 protein is involved in nuclear factor κB (NF-κB) signaling and regulates osteoclastic differentiation. The phenotypic variability in patients with *SQSTM1* mutations suggests that additional factors, such as other genetic influences or viral infection, may influence clinical expression of the disease.

Several lines of evidence suggest that a viral infection may contribute to the clinical manifestations of Paget's disease, including (1) the presence of cytoplasmic and nuclear inclusions resembling paramyxoviruses (measles and respiratory syncytial virus) in pagetic osteoclasts and (2) viral mRNA in precursor and mature osteoclasts. The viral etiology is further supported by conversion of osteoclast precursors to pagetic-like osteoclasts by vectors containing the measles virus nucleocapsid or matrix genes. However, the viral etiology has been questioned by the inability to culture a live virus from pagetic bone and by failure to clone the full-length viral genes from material obtained from patients with Paget's disease.

Pathophysiology

The principal abnormality in Paget's disease is the increased number and activity of osteoclasts. Pagetic osteoclasts are large, increased 10- to 100-fold in number, and have a greater number of nuclei (as many as 100 compared to 3–5 nuclei in the normal osteoclast). The overactive osteoclasts may create a sevenfold increase in resorptive surfaces and an erosion rate of 9 μg/d (normal is 1 μg/d). Several causes for the increased number and activity of pagetic osteoclasts have been identified: (1) osteoclastic precursors are hypersensitive to $1,25(OH)_2D_3$; (2) osteoclasts are hyperresponsive to RANK ligand (RANKL), the osteoclast stimulatory factor that mediates the effects of most osteotropic factors on osteoclast formation; (3) marrow stromal cells from pagetic lesions have increased RANKL expression; (4) osteoclast precursor recruitment is increased by interleukin (IL) 6, which is increased in the blood of patients with active Paget's disease and is overexpressed in pagetic osteoclasts; (5) expression of the protooncogene *c-fos*, which increases osteoclastic activity, is increased; and (6) the antiapoptotic oncogene *Bcl*-2 in pagetic bone is overexpressed. Numerous osteoblasts are recruited to active resorption sites and produce large amounts of new bone matrix. As a result, bone turnover is high, and bone mass is normal or increased, not reduced, unless there is concomitant deficiency of calcium and/or vitamin D.

The characteristic feature of Paget's disease is increased bone resorption accompanied by accelerated bone formation. An initial osteolytic phase involves prominent bone resorption and marked hypervascularization. Radiographically, this manifests as an advancing lytic wedge, or "blade of grass" lesion. The second phase is a period of very active bone formation and resorption that replaces normal lamellar bone with haphazard (woven) bone. Fibrous connective tissue may replace normal bone marrow. In the final sclerotic phase, bone resorption declines progressively and leads to a hard, dense, less vascular pagetic or mosaic bone, which represents the so-called burned-out phase of Paget's disease. All three phases may be present at the same time at different skeletal sites.

Clinical manifestations

Diagnosis is often made in asymptomatic patients because they have elevated ALP levels on routine blood chemistry testing or an abnormality on a skeletal radiograph obtained for another indication. The skeletal sites most commonly involved are the pelvis, vertebral bodies, skull, femur, and tibia. Familial cases with an early presentation often have numerous active sites of skeletal involvement.

The most common presenting symptom is pain, which may result from increased bony vascularity, expanding lytic lesions, fractures, bowing, or other deformities. Bowing of the femur or tibia causes gait abnormalities and abnormal mechanical stresses with secondary osteoarthritis of the hip or knee joints. Long bone bowing also causes extremity pain by stretching the muscles attached to the bone softened by the pagetic process. Back pain results from enlarged pagetic vertebrae, vertebral compression fractures, spinal stenosis, degenerative changes of the joints, and altered body mechanics with kyphosis and forward tilt of the upper back. Rarely, spinal cord compression may result from bone enlargement or from the vascular steal syndrome. Skull involvement may cause headaches, symmetric or asymmetric enlargement of the parietal or frontal bones (frontal bossing), and increased head size. Cranial expansion may narrow cranial foramens and cause neurologic complications including hearing loss from cochlear nerve damage from temporal bone involvement, cranial nerve palsies, and softening of the base of the skull (*platybasia*) with the risk of brainstem compression. Pagetic involvement of the facial bones may cause facial deformity; loss of teeth and other dental conditions; and, rarely, airway compression.

Fractures are serious complications of Paget's disease and usually occur in long bones at areas of active or advancing lytic lesions. Common fracture sites are the femoral shaft and subtrochanteric regions. Neoplasms arising from pagetic bone are rare (<0.5%). The incidence of sarcoma appears to be decreasing, possibly because of earlier, more effective treatment with potent antiresorptive agents. The majority of tumors are osteosarcomas, which usually present with new pain in a long-standing pagetic lesion. Osteoclast-rich benign giant cell tumors may arise in areas adjacent to pagetic bone, and they respond to glucocorticoid therapy.

Cardiovascular complications may occur in patients with involvement of large (15–35%) portions of the skeleton and a high degree of disease activity (ALP four times above normal). The extensive arteriovenous shunting and marked increases in blood flow through the vascular pagetic bone lead to a high-output state and cardiac enlargement. However, high-output heart failure is relatively rare and usually develops in patients with concomitant cardiac pathology. In addition, calcific aortic stenosis and diffuse vascular calcifications have been associated with Paget's disease.

Diagnosis

The diagnosis may be suggested on clinical examination by the presence of an enlarged skull with frontal bossing, bowing of an extremity, or short stature with simian posturing. An extremity with an area of warmth and tenderness to palpation may suggest an underlying pagetic lesion. Other findings include bony deformity of the pelvis, skull, spine, and extremities; arthritic involvement of the joints adjacent to lesions; and leg-length discrepancy resulting from deformities of the long bones.

Paget's disease is usually diagnosed from radiologic and biochemical abnormalities. Radiographic findings typical of Paget's disease include enlargement or expansion of an entire bone or area of a long bone, cortical thickening, coarsening of trabecular markings, and typical lytic and sclerotic changes. Skull radiographs (Fig. 36-2) reveal regions of "cotton wool," or

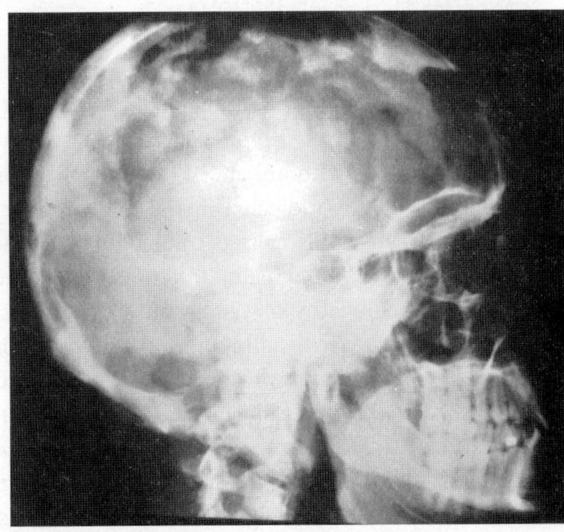

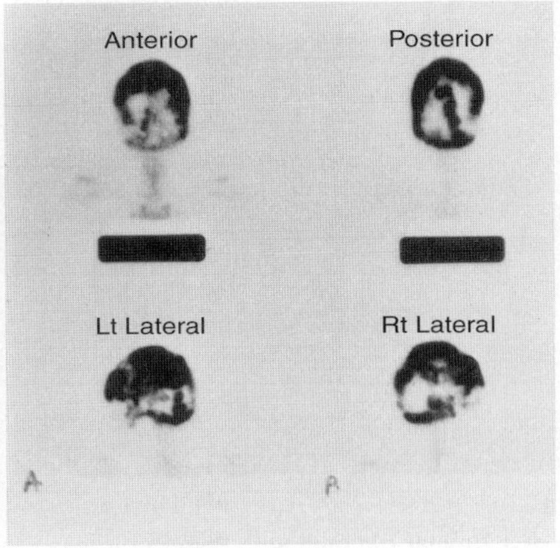

FIGURE 36-2
A 48-year-old woman with Paget's disease of the skull. ***Left*.** Lateral radiograph showing areas of both bone resorption and sclerosis. ***Right*.** ^{99m}Tc HDP bone scan with anterior, posterior, and lateral views of the skull showing diffuse isotope uptake by the frontal, parietal, occipital, and petrous bones.

osteoporosis circumscripta, thickening of diploic areas, and enlargement and sclerosis of a portion or all of one or more skull bones. Vertebral cortical thickening of the superior and inferior end plates creates a "picture frame" vertebra. Diffuse radiodense enlargement of a vertebra is referred to as "ivory vertebra." Pelvic radiographs may demonstrate disruption or fusion of the sacroiliac joints; porotic and radiodense lesions of the ilium with whorls of coarse trabeculation; thickened and sclerotic iliopectineal line (brim sign); and softening with protrusio acetabuli, with axial migration of the hips and functional flexion contracture. Radiographs of long bones reveal bowing deformity and typical pagetic changes of cortical thickening and expansion and areas of lucency and sclerosis (Fig. 36-3). Radionuclide ^{99m}Tc bone scans are less specific but are more sensitive than standard radiographs for identifying sites of active skeletal lesions. Although computed tomography (CT) and magnetic resonance imaging (MRI) studies are not necessary in most cases, CT may be useful for the assessment of possible fracture, and MRI is necessary to assess the possibility of sarcoma, giant cell tumor, or metastatic disease in pagetic bone. Definitive diagnosis of malignancy often requires bone biopsy.

Biochemical evaluation is useful in the diagnosis and management of Paget's disease. The marked increase in bone turnover can be monitored using biochemical markers of bone formation and resorption. The parallel rise in markers of bone formation and resorption confirms the coupling of bone formation and resorption in Paget's disease. The degree of bone marker elevation reflects the extent and severity of the disease. Patients with the highest elevation of ALP (10 × the upper limit of normal) typically have involvement of the skull and at least one other skeletal site. Lower values suggest less extensive involvement or a quiescent phase of the disease. For most patients, serum total ALP remains the test of choice both for diagnosis and assessing response to therapy. Occasionally, a symptomatic patient with evidence of progression at a single site may have a normal total ALP level but increased bone-specific ALP. For unclear reasons, serum osteocalcin, another marker of bone formation, is not always elevated and is not recommended for use in diagnosis or management of Paget's disease. Bone resorption markers (serum or urine N-telopeptide or C-telopeptide measured in the blood or urine) are also elevated in active Paget's disease and decrease more rapidly in response to therapy than does ALP.

Serum calcium and phosphate levels are normal in Paget's disease. Immobilization of a patient with active Paget's disease may rarely cause hypercalcemia and hypercalciuria and increase the risk for nephrolithiasis. However, the discovery of hypercalcemia, even in the presence of immobilization, should prompt a search for another cause of hypercalcemia. In contrast, hypocalcemia or mild secondary hyperparathyroidism may develop in Paget's patients with very active bone formation and insufficient calcium and vitamin D intake, particularly during bisphosphonate therapy when bone resorption is rapidly suppressed and active bone formation continues. Therefore, adequate calcium and vitamin D intake should be instituted prior to administration of bisphosphonates.

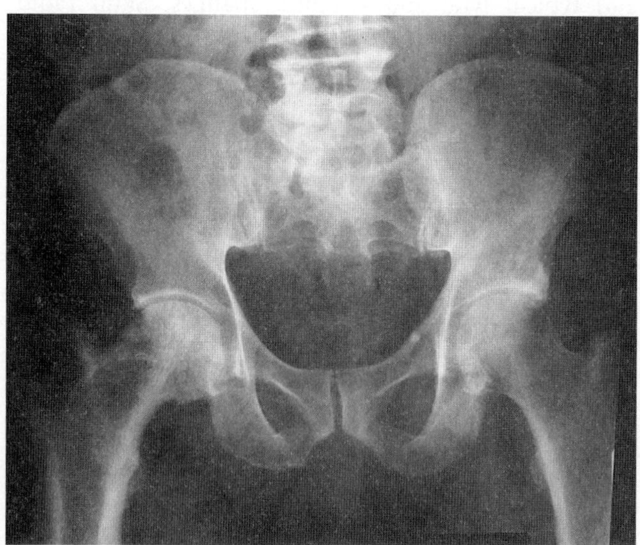

FIGURE 36-3

Radiograph of a 73-year-old man with Paget's disease of the right proximal femur. Note the coarsening of the trabecular pattern with marked cortical thickening and narrowing of the joint space consistent with osteoarthritis secondary to pagetic deformity of the right femur.

TREATMENT Paget's Disease of Bone

The development of effective and potent pharmacologic agents (Table 36-1) has changed the treatment philosophy from treating only symptomatic patients to treating asymptomatic patients who are at risk for complications. Pharmacologic therapy is indicated in the following circumstances: to control symptoms caused by metabolically active Paget's disease such as bone pain, fracture, headache, pain from pagetic radiculopathy or arthropathy, or neurologic complications; to decrease local blood flow and minimize operative blood loss in patients who need surgery at an active pagetic site; to reduce hypercalciuria that may occur during immobilization; and to decrease the risk of complications when disease activity is high (elevated ALP) and when the site of involvement involves weight-bearing bones, areas adjacent to major joints, vertebral bodies, and the skull. Whether or not early therapy prevents late complications remains to be determined. A randomized study of over 1200 patients from the United Kingdom showed no difference in bone pain, fracture

TABLE 36-1

PHARMACOLOGIC AGENTS APPROVED FOR TREATMENT OF PAGET'S DISEASE

NAME	DOSE AND MODE OF DELIVERY	NORMALIZATION OF ALP
Zoledronic acid	5 mg IV over 15 min	90% of patients at 6 mo
Pamidronate	30 mg IV/d over 4 h on 3 days	~50% of patients
Risedronate	30 mg PO/d for 2 mo	73% of patients
Alendronate	40 mg PO/d for 6 mo	63% of patients
Tiludronate	800 mg PO daily for 3 mo	35% of patients
Etidronate	200–400 mg PO/d × 6 mo	15% of patients
Calcitonin (Miacalcin)	100 U SC daily for 6–18 mo (may reduce to 50 U 3 × per wk)	(Reduction of ALP by up to 50%)

rates, quality of life, and hearing loss between patients who received pharmacologic therapy to control symptoms (bone pain) and those receiving bisphosphonates to normalize serum ALP. However, the most potent agent (zoledronic acid) was not used, and the duration of observation (mean of 3 years with a range of 2 to 5 years) may not be long enough to assess the impact of treatment on long-term outcomes. It seems likely that the restoration of normal bone architecture following suppression of pagetic activity will prevent further deformities and complications.

Agents approved for treatment of Paget's disease suppress the very high rates of bone resorption and secondarily decrease the high rates of bone formation (Table 36-1). As a result of decreasing bone turnover, pagetic structural patterns, including areas of poorly mineralized woven bone, are replaced by more normal cancellous or lamellar bone. Reduced bone turnover can be documented by a decline in serum ALP and urine or serum resorption markers (N-telopeptide, C-telopeptide).

The first clinically useful agent, etidronate, is now rarely used because the doses required to suppress bone resorption may impair mineralization, necessitating that the drug be given for a maximum of 6 months followed by a 6-month drug-free period. The second-generation oral bisphosphonates—tiludronate, alendronate, and risedronate—are more potent than etidronate in controlling bone turnover and, thus, induce a longer remission at a lower dose. The lower doses reduce the risks of impaired mineralization and osteomalacia. Oral bisphosphonates should be taken first thing in the morning on an empty stomach, followed by maintenance of upright posture with no food, drink, or other medications for 30–60 min. The efficacy of different agents, based on their ability to normalize or decrease ALP levels, is summarized in Table 36-1, although the response rates are not comparable because they are obtained from different studies.

Intravenous bisphosphonates approved for Paget's disease include pamidronate and zoledronic acid. Although the recommended dose for pamidronate is 30 mg dissolved in 500 mL of normal saline or dextrose IV over 4 h on 3 consecutive days, a more commonly used simpler regimen is a single infusion of 60–90 mg in patients with mild elevation of serum ALP and multiple 90-mg infusions in those with higher levels of ALP. In many patients, particularly those who have severe disease or need rapid normalization of bone turnover (neurologic symptoms, severe bone pain due to a lytic lesion, risk of an impending fracture, or pretreatment prior to elective surgery in an area of active disease), treatment with zoledronic acid is the first choice. It normalizes ALP in about 90% of patients by 6 months, and the therapeutic effect persists for at least 6 more months in most patients. About 10–20% of patients experience a flulike syndrome after the first infusion, which can be partly ameliorated by pretreatment with acetaminophen or nonsteroidal anti-inflammatory drugs (NSAIDs). In patients with high bone turnover, vitamin D and calcium should be provided to prevent hypocalcemia and secondary hyperparathyroidism. Remission following treatment with IV bisphosphonates, particularly zoledronic acid, may persist for well over 1 year. Bisphosphonates should not be used in patients with renal insufficiency (glomerular filtration rate <35 mL/min).

The subcutaneous injectable form of salmon calcitonin is approved for the treatment of Paget's disease. The common side effects of calcitonin therapy are nausea and facial flushing. Secondary resistance after prolonged use may be due to either the formation of anticalcitonin antibodies or downregulation of osteoclastic cell–surface calcitonin receptors. The lower potency and injectable mode of delivery make this agent a less attractive treatment option that should be reserved for patients who either do not tolerate bisphosphonates or have a contraindication to their use. In early reports, denosumab, an antibody to RANKL, has shown promise but has not been approved for this indication.

SCLEROSING BONE DISORDERS

OSTEOPETROSIS

Osteopetrosis refers to a group of disorders caused by severe impairment of osteoclast-mediated bone resorption. Other terms that are often used include marble bone disease, which captures the solid x-ray appearance of the involved skeleton, and Albers-Schonberg disease, which refers to the milder, adult form of osteopetrosis also known as autosomal dominant osteopetrosis type II. The major types of osteopetrosis include malignant (severe, infantile, autosomal recessive) osteopetrosis and benign (adult, autosomal dominant) osteopetrosis types I and II. A rare autosomal recessive intermediate form has a more benign prognosis. Autosomal recessive carbonic anhydrase (CA) II deficiency produces osteopetrosis of intermediate severity associated with renal tubular acidosis and cerebral calcification.

Etiology and genetics

Naturally occurring and gene-knockout animal models with phenotypes similar to those of the human disorders have been used to explore the genetic basis of osteopetrosis. The primary defect in osteopetrosis is the loss of osteoclastic bone resorption and preservation of normal osteoblastic bone formation. Osteoprotegerin (OPG) is a soluble decoy receptor that binds osteoblast-derived RANK ligand, which mediates osteoclast differentiation and activation (Fig. 36-1). Transgenic mice that overexpress OPG develop osteopetrosis, presumably by blocking RANK ligand. Mice deficient in RANK lack osteoclasts and develop severe osteopetrosis.

Recessive mutations of CA II prevent osteoclasts from generating an acid environment in the clear zone between its ruffled border and the adjacent mineral surface. Absence of CA II, therefore, impairs osteoclastic bone resorption. Other forms of human disease have less clear genetic defects. About one-half of the patients with malignant infantile osteopetrosis have a mutation in the *TCIRG1* gene encoding the osteoclast-specific subunit of the vacuolar proton pump, which mediates the acidification of the interface between bone mineral and the osteoclast ruffled border. Mutations in the *CICN7* chloride channel gene cause autosomal dominant osteopetrosis type II.

Clinical presentation

The incidence of autosomal recessive severe (malignant) osteopetrosis ranges from 1 in 200,000 to 1 in 500,000 live births. As bone and cartilage fail to undergo modeling, paralysis of one or more cranial nerves may occur due to narrowing of the cranial foramens. Failure of skeletal modeling also results in inadequate marrow space, leading to extramedullary hematopoiesis with hypersplenism and pancytopenia. Hypocalcemia due to lack of osteoclastic bone resorption may occur in infants and young children. The untreated infantile disease is fatal, often before age 5.

Adult (benign) osteopetrosis is an autosomal dominant disease that is usually diagnosed by the discovery of typical skeletal changes in young adults who undergo radiologic evaluation of a fracture. The prevalence is 1 in 100,000 to 1 in 500,000 adults. The course is not always benign, because fractures may be accompanied by loss of vision, deafness, psychomotor delay, mandibular osteomyelitis, and other complications usually associated with the juvenile form. In some kindred, nonpenetrance results in skip generations, while in other families, severely affected children are born into families with benign disease. The milder form of the disease does not usually require treatment.

Radiography

Typically, there are generalized symmetric increases in bone mass with thickening of both cortical and trabecular bone. Diaphyses and metaphyses are broadened, and alternating sclerotic and lucent bands may be seen in the iliac crests, at the ends of long bones, and in vertebral bodies. The cranium is usually thickened, particularly at the base of the skull, and the paranasal and mastoid sinuses are underpneumatized.

Laboratory findings

The only significant laboratory findings are elevated serum levels of osteoclast-derived tartrate-resistant acid phosphatase (TRAP) and the brain isoenzyme of creatine kinase. Serum calcium may be low in severe disease, and parathyroid hormone and 1,25-dihydroxyvitamin D levels may be elevated in response to hypocalcemia.

TREATMENT Osteopetrosis

Allogeneic HLA-identical bone marrow transplantation has been successful in some children. Following transplantation, the marrow contains progenitor cells and normally functioning osteoclasts. A cure is most likely when children are transplanted before age 4. Marrow transplantation from nonidentical HLA-matched donors has a much higher failure rate. Limited studies in small numbers of patients have suggested variable benefits following treatment with interferon γ-1β, 1,25-dihydroxyvitamin D (which stimulates osteoclasts directly), methylprednisolone, and a low-calcium/high-phosphate diet.

Surgical intervention is indicated to decompress optic or auditory nerve compression. Orthopedic management is required for the surgical treatment of fractures and their complications including malunion and postfracture deformity.

PYKNODYSOSTOSIS

This is an autosomal recessive form of osteosclerosis that is believed to have affected the French impressionist painter Henri de Toulouse-Lautrec. The molecular basis involves mutations in the gene that encodes cathepsin K, a lysosomal metalloproteinase highly expressed in osteoclasts and important for bone-matrix degradation. Osteoclasts are present but do not function normally. Pyknodysostosis is a form of short-limb dwarfism that presents with frequent fractures but usually a normal life span. Clinical features include short stature; kyphoscoliosis and deformities of the chest; high arched palate; proptosis; blue sclerae; dysmorphic features including small face and chin, frontooccipital prominence, pointed beaked nose, large cranium, and obtuse mandibular angle; and small, square hands with hypoplastic nails. Radiographs demonstrate a generalized increase in bone density, but in contrast to osteopetrosis, the long bones are normally shaped. Separated cranial sutures, including the persistent patency of the anterior fontanel, are characteristic of the disorder. There may also be hypoplasia of the sinuses, mandible, distal clavicles, and terminal phalanges. Persistence of deciduous teeth and sclerosis of the calvarium and base of the skull are also common. Histologic evaluation shows normal cortical bone architecture with decreased osteoblastic and osteoclastic activities. Serum chemistries are normal, and unlike osteopetrosis, there is no anemia. There is no known treatment for this condition, and there are no reports of attempted bone marrow transplant.

PROGRESSIVE DIAPHYSEAL DYSPLASIA

Also known as *Camurati-Engelmann disease*, progressive diaphyseal dysplasia is an autosomal dominant disorder that is characterized radiographically by diaphyseal hyperostosis and a symmetric thickening and increased diameter of the endosteal and periosteal surfaces of the diaphyses of the long bones, particularly the femur and tibia, and, less often, the fibula, radius, and ulna. The genetic defect responsible for the disease has been localized to the area of chromosome 19q13.2 encoding tumor growth factor (TGF) β1. The mutation promotes activation of TGF-β1. The clinical severity is variable. The most common presenting symptoms are pain and tenderness of the involved areas, fatigue, muscle wasting, and gait disturbance. The weakness may be mistaken for muscular dystrophy. Characteristic body habitus includes thin limbs with little muscle mass yet prominent and palpable bones and, when the skull is involved, large head with prominent forehead and proptosis. Patients may also display signs of cranial nerve palsies, hydrocephalus, central hypogonadism, and Raynaud's phenomenon. Radiographically, patchy progressive endosteal and periosteal new bone formation is observed along the diaphyses of the long bones. Bone scintigraphy shows increased radiotracer uptake in involved areas.

Treatment with low-dose glucocorticoids relieves bone pain and may reverse the abnormal bone formation. Intermittent bisphosphonate therapy has produced clinical improvement in a limited number of patients.

HYPEROSTOSIS CORTICALIS GENERALISATA

This is also known as *van Buchem's disease*; it is an autosomal recessive disorder characterized by endosteal hyperostosis in which osteosclerosis involves the skull, mandible, clavicles, and ribs. The major manifestations are due to narrowed cranial foramens with neural compressions that may result in optic atrophy, facial paralysis, and deafness. Adults may have an enlarged mandible. Serum ALP levels may be elevated, which reflect the uncoupled bone remodeling with high osteoblastic formation rates and low osteoclastic resorption. As a result, there is increased accumulation of normal bone. Endosteal hyperostosis with syndactyly, known as *sclerosteosis*, is a more severe form. The genetic defects for both sclerosteosis and van Buchem's disease have been assigned to the same region of the chromosome 17q12-q21. It is possible that both conditions may have deactivating mutations in the *BEER* (bone-expressed equilibrium regulator) gene.

MELORHEOSTOSIS

Melorheostosis (Greek, "flowing hyperostosis") may occur sporadically or follow a pattern consistent with an autosomal recessive disorder. The major manifestation is progressive linear hyperostosis in one or more bones of one limb, usually a lower extremity. The name comes from the radiographic appearance of the involved bone, which resembles melted wax that has dripped down a candle. Symptoms appear during childhood as pain or stiffness in the area of sclerotic bone. There may be associated ectopic soft tissue masses, composed of cartilage or osseous tissue, and skin changes overlying the involved bone, consisting of scleroderma-like areas and hypertrichosis. The disease does not progress in adults, but pain and stiffness may persist. Laboratory tests are unremarkable. No specific etiology is known. There is no specific treatment. Surgical interventions to correct contractures are often unsuccessful.

OSTEOPOIKILOSIS

The literal translation of osteopoikilosis is "spotted bones"; it is a benign autosomal dominant condition in which numerous small, variably shaped (usually round or oval) foci of bony sclerosis are seen in the epiphyses and adjacent metaphyses. The lesions may involve any bone except the skull, ribs, and vertebrae. They may be misidentified as metastatic lesions. The main differentiating points are that bony lesions of osteopoikilosis are stable over time and do not accumulate radionucleotide on bone scanning. In some kindred, osteopoikilosis is associated with connective tissue nevi known as *dermatofibrosis lenticularis disseminata*, also known as *Buschke-Ollendorff syndrome*. Histologic inspection reveals thickened but otherwise normal trabeculae and islands of normal cortical bone. No treatment is indicated.

HEPATITIS C–ASSOCIATED OSTEOSCLEROSIS

Hepatitis C–associated osteosclerosis (HCAO) is a rare acquired diffuse osteosclerosis in adults with prior hepatitis C infection. After a latent period of several years, patients develop diffuse appendicular bone pain and a generalized increase in bone mass with elevated serum ALP. Bone biopsy and histomorphometry reveal increased rates of bone formation, decreased bone resorption with a marked decrease in osteoclasts, and dense lamellar bone. One patient had increased serum OPG levels, and bone biopsy showed large numbers of osteoblasts positive for OPG and reduced osteoclast number. Empirical therapy includes pain control, and there may be beneficial response to bisphosphonate. Long-term antiviral therapy may reverse the bone disease.

DISORDERS ASSOCIATED WITH DEFECTIVE MINERALIZATION

HYPOPHOSPHATASIA

This is a rare inherited disorder that presents as rickets in infants and children or osteomalacia in adults with paradoxically low serum levels of ALP. The frequency of the severe neonatal and infantile forms is about 1 in 100,000 live births in Canada, where the disease is most common because of its high prevalence among Mennonites and Hutterites. It is rare in African Americans. The severity of the disease is remarkably variable, ranging from intrauterine death associated with profound skeletal hypomineralization at one extreme to premature tooth loss as the only manifestation in some adults. Severe cases are inherited in an autosomal recessive manner, but the genetic patterns are less clear for the milder forms. The disease is caused by a deficiency of tissue nonspecific (bone/liver/kidney) ALP (TNSALP), which, although ubiquitous, results only in bone abnormalities. Protein levels and functions of the other ALP isozymes (germ cell, intestinal, placental) are normal. Defective ALP permits accumulation of its major naturally occurring substrates including phosphoethanolamine (PEA), inorganic pyrophosphate (PPi), and pyridoxal 5′-phosphate (PLP). The accumulation of PPi interferes with mineralization through its action as a potent inhibitor of hydroxyapatite crystal growth.

Perinatal hypophosphatasia becomes manifest during pregnancy and is often complicated by polyhydramnios and intrauterine death. The infantile form becomes clinically apparent before the age of 6 months with failure to thrive, rachitic deformities, functional craniosynostosis despite widely open fontanels (which are actually hypomineralized areas of the calvarium), raised intracranial pressure, and flail chest with predisposition to pneumonia. Hypercalcemia and hypercalciuria are common. This form has a mortality rate of about 50%. Prognosis seems to improve for the children who survive infancy. Childhood hypophosphatasia has variable clinical presentation. Premature loss of deciduous teeth (before age 5) is the hallmark of the disease. Rickets causes delayed walking with waddling gait, short stature, and dolichocephalic skull with frontal bossing. The disease often improves during puberty but may recur in adult life. Adult hypophosphatasia presents during middle age with painful, poorly healing metatarsal stress fractures or thigh pain due to femoral pseudofractures.

Laboratory investigation reveals low ALP levels and normal or elevated levels of serum calcium and phosphorus despite clinical and radiologic evidence of rickets or osteomalacia. Serum parathyroid hormone, 25-hydroxyvitamin D, and 1,25-dihydroxyvitamin D levels are normal. The elevation of PLP is specific for the disease and may even be present in asymptomatic parents of severely affected children. Because vitamin B_6 increases PLP levels, vitamin B_6 supplements should be discontinued 1 week before testing. Clinical testing is available to detect loss-of-function mutation(s) within the *ALPL* gene that encodes TNSALP.

There is no established medical therapy. In contrast to other forms of rickets and osteomalacia, calcium and vitamin D supplementation should be avoided because they may aggravate hypercalcemia and hypercalciuria. A low-calcium diet, glucocorticoids, and calcitonin have been used in a small number of patients with variable responses. Because fracture healing is poor, placement of intramedullary rods is best for acute fracture repair and for prophylactic prevention of fractures.

AXIAL OSTEOMALACIA

This is a rare disorder characterized by defective skeletal mineralization despite normal serum calcium and phosphate levels. Clinically, the disorder presents in middle-aged or elderly men with chronic axial skeletal discomfort. Cervical spine pain may also be present. Radiographic findings are mainly osteosclerosis due to coarsened trabecular patterns typical of osteomalacia. Spine, pelvis, and ribs are most commonly affected.

Histologic changes show defective mineralization and flat, inactive osteoblasts. The primary defect appears to be an acquired defect in osteoblast function. The course is benign, and there is no established treatment. Calcium and vitamin D therapies are not effective.

FIBROGENESIS IMPERFECTA OSSIUM

This is a rare condition of unknown etiology. It presents in both sexes; in middle age or later; and with progressive, intractable skeletal pain and fractures; worsening immobilization; and a debilitating course. Radiographic evaluation reveals generalized osteomalacia, osteopenia, and occasional pseudofractures. Histologic features include a tangled pattern of collagen fibrils with abundant osteoblasts and osteoclasts. There is no effective treatment. Spontaneous remission has been reported in a small number of patients. Calcium and vitamin D have not been beneficial.

FIBROUS DYSPLASIA AND MCCUNE-ALBRIGHT SYNDROME

Fibrous dysplasia is a sporadic disorder characterized by the presence of one (monostotic) or more (polyostotic) expanding fibrous skeletal lesions composed of bone-forming mesenchyme. The association of the polyostotic form with café au lait spots and hyperfunction of an endocrine system such as pseudoprecocious puberty of ovarian origin is known as *McCune-Albright syndrome* (MAS). A spectrum of the phenotypes is caused by activating mutations in the *GNAS1* gene, which encodes the α subunit of the stimulatory G protein ($G_s\alpha$). As the postzygotic mutations occur at different stages of early development, the extent and type of tissue affected are variable and explain the mosaic pattern of skin and bone changes. GTP binding activates the $G_s\alpha$ regulatory protein and mutations in regions of $G_s\alpha$ that selectively inhibit GTPase activity, which results in constitutive stimulation of the cyclic AMP–protein kinase A signal transduction pathway. Such mutations of the $G_s\alpha$ protein–coupled receptor may cause autonomous function in bone (parathyroid hormone receptor); skin (melanocyte-stimulating hormone receptor); and various endocrine glands including ovary (follicle-stimulating hormone receptor), thyroid (thyroid-stimulating hormone receptor), adrenal (adrenocorticotropic hormone receptor), and pituitary (growth hormone–releasing hormone receptor). The skeletal lesions are composed largely of mesenchymal cells that do not differentiate into osteoblasts, resulting in the formation of imperfect bone. In some areas of bone, fibroblast-like cells develop features of osteoblasts in that they produce extracellular matrix that organizes into woven bone. Calcification may occur in some areas. In other areas, cells have features of chondrocytes and produce cartilage-like extracellular matrix.

CLINICAL PRESENTATION

Fibrous dysplasia occurs with equal frequency in both sexes, whereas MAS with precocious puberty is more common (10:1) in girls. The monostotic form is the most common and is usually diagnosed in patients between 20 and 30 years of age without associated skin lesions. The polyostotic form typically manifests in children <10 years old and may progress with age. Early-onset disease is generally more severe. Lesions may become quiescent in puberty and progress during pregnancy or with estrogen therapy. In polyostotic fibrous dysplasia, the lesions most commonly involve the maxilla and other craniofacial bones, ribs, and metaphyseal or diaphyseal portions of the proximal femur or tibia. Expanding bone lesions may cause pain, deformity, fractures, and nerve entrapment. Sarcomatous degeneration involving the facial bones or femur is infrequent (<1%). The risk of malignant transformation is increased by radiation, which has proven to be ineffective treatment. In rare patients with widespread lesions, renal phosphate wasting and hypophosphatemia may cause rickets or osteomalacia. Hypophosphatemia may be due to production of a phosphaturic factor by the abnormal fibrous tissue.

MAS patients may have café au lait spots, which are flat, hyperpigmented skin lesions that have rough borders ("coast of Maine") in contrast to the café au lait lesions of neurofibromatosis that have smooth borders ("coast of California"). The most common endocrinopathy is isosexual pseudoprecocious puberty in girls. Other less common endocrine disorders include thyrotoxicosis, Cushing's syndrome, acromegaly, hyperparathyroidism, hyperprolactinemia, and pseudoprecocious puberty in boys.

RADIOGRAPHIC FINDINGS

In long bones, the fibrous dysplastic lesions are typically well-defined, radiolucent areas with thin cortices and a ground-glass appearance. Lesions may be lobulated with trabeculated areas of radiolucency (Fig. 36-4). Involvement of facial bones usually presents as radiodense lesions, which may create a leonine appearance (leontiasis osea). Expansile cranial lesions may narrow foramens and cause optic lesions, reduce hearing, and create other manifestations of cranial nerve compression.

LABORATORY RESULTS

Serum ALP is occasionally elevated but calcium, parathyroid hormone, 25-hydroxyvitamin D, and

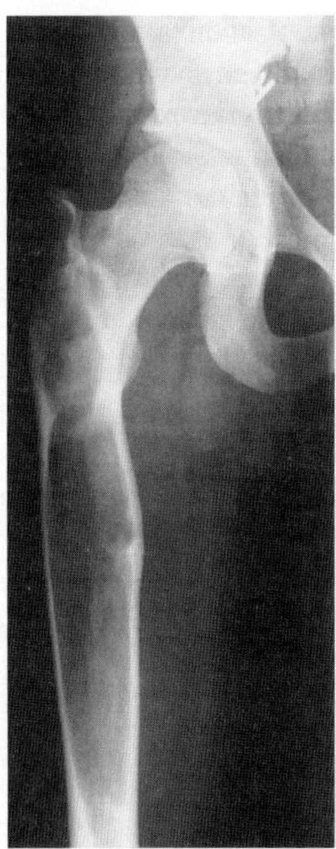

FIGURE 36-4
Radiograph of a 16-year-old male with fibrous dysplasia of the right proximal femur. Note the multiple cystic lesions, including the large lucent lesion in the proximal midshaft with scalloping of the interior surface. The femoral neck contains two lucent cystic lesions.

1,25-dihydroxy-vitamin D levels are normal. Patients with extensive polyostotic lesions may have hypophosphatemia, hyperphosphaturia, and osteomalacia. The hypophosphatemia and phosphaturia are directly related to the levels of fibroblast growth factor 23 (FGF23). Biochemical markers of bone turnover may be elevated.

TREATMENT Fibrous Dysplasia and McCune-Albright Syndrome

Spontaneous healing of the lesions does not occur, and there is no established effective treatment. Improvement in bone pain and partial or complete resolution of radiographic lesions have been reported after IV bisphosphonate therapy. Surgical stabilization is used to prevent pathologic fracture or destruction of a major joint space and to relieve nerve root or cranial nerve compression or sinus obstruction.

OTHER DYSPLASIAS OF BONE AND CARTILAGE

PACHYDERMOPERIOSTOSIS

Pachydermoperiostosis, or hypertrophic osteoarthropathy (primary or idiopathic), is an autosomal dominant disorder characterized by periosteal new bone formation that involves the distal extremities. The lesions present as clubbing of the digits and hyperhidrosis and thickening of the skin, primarily of the face and forehead. The changes usually appear during adolescence, progress over the next decade, and then become quiescent. During the active phase, progressive enlargement of the hands and feet produces a paw-like appearance, which may be mistaken for acromegaly. Arthralgias, pseudogout, and limited mobility may also occur. The disorder must be differentiated from secondary hypertrophic osteopathy that develops during the course of serious pulmonary disorders. The two conditions can be differentiated by standard radiography of the digits in which secondary pachydermoperiostosis has exuberant periosteal new bone formation and a smooth and undulating surface. In contrast, primary hypertrophic osteopathy has an irregular periosteal surface.

There are no diagnostic blood or urine tests. Synovial fluid does not have an inflammatory profile. There is no specific therapy, although a limited experience with colchicine suggests some benefit in controlling the arthralgias.

OSTEOCHONDRODYSPLASIAS

These include several hundred heritable disorders of connective tissue. These primary abnormalities of cartilage manifest as disturbances in cartilage and bone growth. Selected growth-plate chondrodysplasias are described here.

Achondrodysplasia

This is a relatively common form of short-limb dwarfism that occurs in 1 in 15,000 to 1 in 40,000 live births. The disease is caused by a mutation of the fibroblast growth factor receptor 3 (*FGFR3*) gene that results in a gain-of-function state. Most cases are sporadic mutations. However, when the disorder appears in families, the inheritance pattern is consistent with an autosomal dominant disorder. The primary defect is abnormal chondrocyte proliferation at the growth plate that causes development of short, but proportionately thick, long bones. Other regions of the long bones may be relatively unaffected. The disorder is manifest by the presence of short limbs (particularly the proximal portions), normal trunk, large head, saddle nose, and an exaggerated lumbar lordosis. Severe spinal deformity may lead to cord compression. The homozygous disorder is more serious than the sporadic form and may cause neonatal death. Pseudoachondroplasia clinically resembles achondrodysplasia but has no skull abnormalities.

Enchondromatosis

This is also called *dyschondroplasia* or *Ollier's disease*; it is also a disorder of the growth plate in which the primary cartilage is not resorbed. Cartilage ossification proceeds normally, but it is not resorbed normally, leading to cartilage accumulation. The changes are most marked at the ends of long bones, where the highest growth rates occur. Chondrosarcoma develops infrequently. The association of enchondromatosis and cavernous hemangiomas of the skin and soft tissues is known as *Maffucci's syndrome*. Both Ollier's disease and Maffucci's syndrome are associated with various malignancies, including granulosa cell tumor of the ovary and cerebral glioma.

Multiple exostoses

This is also called *diaphyseal aclasis* or *osteochondromatosis*; it is a genetic disorder that follows an autosomal dominant pattern of inheritance. In this condition, areas of growth plates become displaced, presumably by growing through a defect in the perichondrium. The lesion begins with vascular invasion of the growth-plate cartilage, resulting in a characteristic radiographic finding of a mass that is in direct communication with the marrow cavity of the parent bone. The underlying cortex is resorbed. The disease is caused by inactivating mutations of the *EXT1* and *EXT2* genes, whose products normally regulate processing of chondrocyte cytoskeletal proteins. The products of the *EXT* gene likely function as tumor suppressors, with the loss-of-function mutation resulting in abnormal proliferation of growth-plate cartilage. Solitary or multiple lesions are located in the metaphyses of long bones. Although usually asymptomatic, the lesions may interfere with joint or tendon function or compress peripheral nerves. The lesions stop growing when growth ceases but may recur during pregnancy. There is a small risk for malignant transformation into chondrosarcoma.

EXTRASKELETAL (ECTOPIC) CALCIFICATION AND OSSIFICATION

Deposition of calcium phosphate crystals (*calcification*) or formation of true bone (*ossification*) in nonosseous soft tissue may occur by one of three mechanisms: (1) metastatic calcification due to a supranormal calcium × phosphate concentration product in extracellular fluid; (2) dystrophic calcification due to mineral deposition into metabolically impaired or dead tissue despite normal serum levels of calcium and phosphate; and (3) ectopic ossification, or true bone formation. Disorders that may cause extraskeletal calcification or ossification are listed in Table 36-2.

METASTATIC CALCIFICATION

Soft tissue calcification may complicate diseases associated with significant hypercalcemia, hyperphosphatemia, or both. In addition, vitamin D and phosphate treatments or calcium administration in the presence of mild hyperphosphatemia, such as during hemodialysis, may induce ectopic calcification. Calcium phosphate precipitation may complicate any disorder when the serum calcium × phosphate concentration product is >75. The initial calcium phosphate deposition is in the form of small, poorly organized crystals, which subsequently organize into hydroxyapatite crystals. Calcifications that occur in hypercalcemic states with normal or low phosphate have a predilection for kidney, lungs, and gastric mucosa. Hyperphosphatemia with normal or low serum calcium may promote soft tissue calcification with predilection for the kidney and arteries. The disturbances of calcium and phosphate in renal failure and hemodialysis are common causes of soft tissue (metastatic) calcification.

TABLE 36-2

DISEASES AND CONDITIONS ASSOCIATED WITH ECTOPIC CALCIFICATION AND OSSIFICATION

Metastatic calcification	Dystrophic calcification
Hypercalcemic states	Inflammatory disorders
Primary hyperparathyroidism	Scleroderma
Sarcoidosis	Dermatomyositis
Vitamin D intoxication	Systemic lupus erythematosus
Milk-alkali syndrome	Trauma-induced
Renal failure	Ectopic ossification
Hyperphosphatemia	Myositis ossificans
Tumoral calcinosis	Postsurgery
Secondary hyperparathyroidism	Burns
Pseudohypoparathyroidism	Neurologic injury
Renal failure	Other trauma
Hemodialysis	Fibrodysplasia ossificans progressiva
Cell lysis following chemotherapy	
Therapy with vitamin D and phosphate	

TUMORAL CALCINOSIS

This is a rare genetic disorder characterized by masses of metastatic calcifications in soft tissues around major joints, most often shoulders, hips, and ankles. Tumoral calcinosis differs from other disorders in that the periarticular masses contain hydroxyapatite crystals or amorphous calcium phosphate complexes, while in fibrodysplasia ossificans progressiva (below), true bone is formed in soft tissues. About one-third of tumoral calcinosis cases are familial, with both autosomal recessive and autosomal dominant modes of inheritance reported. The disease is also associated with a variably expressed abnormality of dentition marked by short bulbous roots, pulp calcification, and radicular dentin deposited in swirls. The primary defect responsible for the metastatic calcification appears to be hyperphosphatemia resulting from the increased capacity of the renal tubule to reabsorb filtered phosphate. Spontaneous soft tissue calcification is related to the elevated serum phosphate, which, along with normal serum calcium, exceeds the concentration product of 75.

All of the North American patients reported have been African American. The disease usually presents in childhood and continues throughout the patient's life. The calcific masses are typically painless and grow at variable rates, sometimes becoming large and bulky. The masses are often located near major joints but remain extracapsular. Joint range of motion is not usually restricted unless the tumors are very large. Complications include compression of neural structures and ulceration of the overlying skin with drainage of chalky fluid and risk of secondary infection. Small deposits not detected by standard radiographs may be detected by ^{99m}Tc bone scanning. The most common laboratory findings are hyperphosphatemia and elevated serum 1,25-dihydroxyvitamin D levels. Serum calcium, parathyroid hormone, and ALP levels are usually normal. Renal function is also usually normal. Urine calcium and phosphate excretions are low, and calcium and phosphate balances are positive.

An acquired form of the disease may occur with other causes of hyperphosphatemia, such as secondary hyperparathyroidism associated with hemodialysis, hypoparathyroidism, pseudohypoparathyroidism, and massive cell lysis following chemotherapy for leukemia. Tissue trauma from joint movement may contribute to the periarticular calcifications. Metastatic calcifications are also seen in conditions associated with hypercalcemia, such as in sarcoidosis, vitamin D intoxication, milk-alkali syndrome, and primary hyperparathyroidism. In these conditions, however, mineral deposits are more likely to occur in proton-transporting organs such as kidney, lungs, and gastric mucosa in which an alkaline milieu is generated by the proton pumps.

TREATMENT Tumoral Calcinosis

Therapeutic successes have been achieved with surgical removal of subcutaneous calcified masses, which tend not to recur if all calcification is removed from the site. Reduction of serum phosphate by chronic phosphorus restriction may be accomplished using low dietary phosphorus intake alone or in combination with oral phosphate binders. The addition of the phosphaturic agent acetazolamide may be useful. Limited experience using the phosphaturic action of calcitonin deserves further testing.

DYSTROPHIC CALCIFICATION

Posttraumatic calcification may occur with normal serum calcium and phosphate levels and normal ion-solubility product. The deposited mineral is either in the form of amorphous calcium phosphate or hydroxyapatite crystals. Soft tissue calcification complicating connective tissue disorders such as scleroderma, dermatomyositis, and systemic lupus erythematosus may involve localized areas of the skin or deeper subcutaneous tissue and is referred to as *calcinosis circumscripta*. Mineral deposition at sites of deeper tissue injury including periarticular sites is called *calcinosis universalis*.

ECTOPIC OSSIFICATION

True extraskeletal bone formation that begins in areas of fasciitis following surgery, trauma, burns, or neurologic injury is referred to as *myositis ossificans*. The bone formed is organized as lamellar or trabecular, with normal osteoblasts and osteoclasts conducting active remodeling. Well-developed haversian systems and marrow elements may be present. A second cause of ectopic bone formation occurs in an inherited disorder, *fibrodysplasia ossificans progressiva*.

FIBRODYSPLASIA OSSIFICANS PROGRESSIVA

This is also called *myositis ossificans progressiva*; it is a rare autosomal dominant disorder characterized by congenital deformities of the hands and feet and episodic soft tissue swellings that ossify. Ectopic bone formation occurs in fascia, tendons, ligaments, and connective tissue within voluntary muscles. Tender, rubbery induration, sometimes precipitated by trauma, develops in the soft tissue and gradually calcifies. Eventually, heterotopic bone forms at these sites of soft tissue trauma. Morbidity results from heterotopic bone interfering with normal movement and function of muscle and other soft tissues. Mortality is usually related to restrictive lung disease caused by an inability of the chest to expand. Laboratory tests are unremarkable.

There is no effective medical therapy. Bisphosphonates, glucocorticoids, and a low-calcium diet have largely been ineffective in halting progression of the ossification. Surgical removal of ectopic bone is not recommended, because the trauma of surgery may precipitate formation of new areas of heterotopic bone. Dental complications including frozen jaw may occur following injection of local anesthetics. Thus, CT imaging of the mandible should be undertaken to detect early sites of soft tissue ossification before they are appreciated by standard radiography.

APPENDIX

LABORATORY VALUES OF CLINICAL IMPORTANCE

Alexander Kratz ■ Michael A. Pesce ■ Robert C. Basner ■ Andrew J. Einstein

This Appendix contains tables of reference values for common laboratory tests. A variety of factors can influence reference values. Such variables include the population studied, the duration and means of specimen transport, laboratory methods and instrumentation, and even the type of container used for the collection of the specimen. The reference or "normal" ranges given in this appendix may therefore not be appropriate for all laboratories, and these values should only be used as general guidelines. Whenever possible, reference values provided by the laboratory performing the testing should be used in the interpretation of laboratory data. Values supplied in this Appendix reflect typical reference ranges in nonpregnant adults. Pediatric reference ranges and values in pregnant patients may vary significantly from the data presented in the Appendix.

In preparing the Appendix, the authors have taken into account the fact that the system of international units (SI, système international d'unités) is used in most countries and in some medical journals. However, clinical laboratories may continue to report values in "traditional" or conventional units. Therefore, both systems are provided in the Appendix. The dual system is also used in the text except for those instances in which the numbers remain the same and only the terminology is changed (mmol/L for meq/L or IU/L for mIU/mL), when only the SI units are given.

TABLE 1

HEMATOLOGY AND COAGULATION

ANALYTE	SPECIMEN	SI UNITS	CONVENTIONAL UNITS
Activated clotting time	WB	70–180 s	70–180 s
Activated protein C resistance (factor V Leiden)	P	Not applicable	Ratio >2.1
ADAMTS13 activity	P	≥0.67	≥67%
ADAMTS13 inhibitor activity	P	Not applicable	≤0.4 U
ADAMTS13 antibody	P	Not applicable	≤18 U
Alpha$_2$ antiplasmin	P	0.87–1.55	87–155%
Antiphospholipid antibody panel			
PTT-LA (lupus anticoagulant screen)	P	Negative	Negative
Platelet neutralization procedure	P	Negative	Negative
Dilute viper venom screen	P	Negative	Negative
Anticardiolipin antibody	S		
IgG		0–15 arbitrary units	0–15 GPL
IgM		0–15 arbitrary units	0–15 MPL

(continued)

TABLE 1

HEMATOLOGY AND COAGULATION (CONTINUED)

ANALYTE	SPECIMEN	SI UNITS	CONVENTIONAL UNITS
Beta-2 glycoprotein 1 antibodies	S		
IgG		0–20 arbitrary units	0–20 SGU
IgM		0–20 arbitrary units	0–20 SMU
Antithrombin III	P		
Antigenic		220–390 mg/L	22–39 mg/dL
Functional		0.7–1.30 U/L	70–130 %
Anti-Xa assay (heparin assay)	P		
Unfractionated heparin		0.3–0.7 kIU/L	0.3–0.7 IU/mL
Low-molecular-weight heparin		0.5–1.0 kIU/L	0.5–1.0 IU/mL
Danaparoid (Orgaran)		0.5–0.8 kIU/L	0.5–0.8 IU/mL
Autohemolysis test	WB	0.004–0.045	0.4–4.50%
Autohemolysis test with glucose	WB	0.003–0.007	0.3–0.7%
Bleeding time (adult)		<7.1 min	<7.1 min
C4 binding protein	P	305–695 mg/L	30.5–69.5 mg/dL
	S	275–604 mg/L	27.5–60.4 mg/dL
Clot retraction	WB	0.50–1.00/2 h	50–100%/2 h
Cryofibrinogen	P	Negative	Negative
D-dimer	P	220–740 ng/mL FEU	220–740 ng/mL FEU
Differential blood count	WB		
Relative counts:			
Neutrophils		0.40–0.70	40–70%
Bands		0.0–0.05	0–5%
Lymphocytes		0.20–0.50	20–50%
Monocytes		0.04–0.08	4–8%
Eosinophils		0.0–0.6	0–6%
Basophils		0.0–0.02	0–2%
Absolute counts:			
Neutrophils		$1.42–6.34 \times 10^9$/L	1420–6340/mm^3
Bands		$0–0.45 \times 10^9$/L	0–450/mm^3
Lymphocytes		$0.71–4.53 \times 10^9$/L	710–4530/mm^3
Monocytes		$0.14–0.72 \times 10^9$/L	140–720/mm^3
Eosinophils		$0–0.54 \times 10^9$/L	0–540/mm^3
Basophils		$0–0.18 \times 10^9$/L	0–180/mm^3
Erythrocyte count	WB		
Adult males		$4.30–5.60 \times 10^{12}$/L	$4.30–5.60 \times 10^6$/mm^3
Adult females		$4.00–5.20 \times 10^{12}$/L	$4.00–5.20 \times 10^6$/mm^3
Erythrocyte life span	WB		
Normal survival		120 days	120 days
Chromium labeled, half-life ($t_{1/2}$)		25–35 days	25–35 days
Erythrocyte sedimentation rate	WB		
Females		0–20 mm/h	0–20 mm/h
Males		0–15 mm/h	0–15 mm/h

(*continued*)

TABLE 1

HEMATOLOGY AND COAGULATION (CONTINUED)

ANALYTE	SPECIMEN	SI UNITS	CONVENTIONAL UNITS
Euglobulin lysis time	P	7200–14400 s	120–240 min
Factor II, prothrombin	P	0.50–1.50	50–150%
Factor V	P	0.50–1.50	50–150%
Factor VII	P	0.50–1.50	50–150%
Factor VIII	P	0.50–1.50	50–150%
Factor IX	P	0.50–1.50	50–150%
Factor X	P	0.50–1.50	50–150%
Factor XI	P	0.50–1.50	50–150%
Factor XII	P	0.50–1.50	50–150%
Factor XIII screen	P	Not applicable	Present
Factor inhibitor assay	P	<0.5 Bethesda Units	<0.5 Bethesda Units
Fibrin(ogen) degradation products	P	0–1 mg/L	0–1 μg/mL
Fibrinogen	P	2.33–4.96 g/L	233–496 mg/dL
Glucose-6-phosphate dehydrogenase (erythrocyte)	WB	<2400 s	<40 min
Ham's test (acid serum)	WB	Negative	Negative
Hematocrit	WB		
Adult males		0.388–0.464	38.8–46.4
Adult females		0.354–0.444	35.4–44.4
Hemoglobin			
Plasma	P	6–50 mg/L	0.6–5.0 mg/dL
Whole blood:	WB		
Adult males		133–162 g/L	13.3–16.2 g/dL
Adult females		120–158 g/L	12.0–15.8 g/dL
Hemoglobin electrophoresis	WB		
Hemoglobin A		0.95–0.98	95–98%
Hemoglobin A_2		0.015–0.031	1.5–3.1%
Hemoglobin F		0–0.02	0–2.0%
Hemoglobins other than A, A_2, or F		Absent	Absent
Heparin-induced thrombocytopenia antibody	P	Negative	Negative
Immature platelet fraction (IPF)	WB	0.011–0.061	1.1–6.1%
Joint fluid crystal	JF	Not applicable	No crystals seen
Joint fluid mucin	JF	Not applicable	Only type I mucin present
Leukocytes			
Alkaline phosphatase (LAP)	WB	0.2–1.6 μkat/L	13–100 μ/L
Count (WBC)	WB	$3.54–9.06 \times 10^9$/L	$3.54–9.06 \times 10^3/mm^3$
Mean corpuscular hemoglobin (MCH)	WB	26.7–31.9 pg/cell	26.7–31.9 pg/cell
Mean corpuscular hemoglobin concentration (MCHC)	WB	323–359 g/L	32.3–35.9 g/dL
Mean corpuscular hemoglobin of reticulocytes (CH)	WB	24–36 pg	24–36 pg
Mean corpuscular volume (MCV)	WB	79–93.3 fL	79–93.3 μm^3
Mean platelet volume (MPV)	WB	9.00–12.95 fL	9.00–12.95

(continued)

TABLE 1

HEMATOLOGY AND COAGULATION (CONTINUED)

ANALYTE	SPECIMEN	SI UNITS	CONVENTIONAL UNITS
Osmotic fragility of erythrocytes	WB		
Direct		0.0035–0.0045	0.35–0.45%
Indirect		0.0030–0.0065	0.30–0.65%
Partial thromboplastin time, activated	P	26.3–39.4 s	26.3–39.4 s
Plasminogen	P		
Antigen		84–140 mg/L	8.4–14.0 mg/dL
Functional		0.70–1.30	70–130%
Plasminogen activator inhibitor 1	P	4–43 μg/L	4–43 ng/mL
Platelet aggregation	PRP	Not applicable	>65% aggregation in response to adenosine diphosphate, epinephrine, collagen, ristocetin, and arachidonic acid
Platelet count	WB	165–415 × 10^9/L	165–415 × 10^3/mm^3
Platelet, mean volume	WB	6.4–11 fL	6.4–11.0 μm^3
Prekallikrein assay	P	0.50–1.5	50–150%
Prekallikrein screen	P		No deficiency detected
Protein C	P		
Total antigen		0.70–1.40	70–140%
Functional		0.70–1.30	70–130%
Protein S	P		
Total antigen		0.70–1.40	70–140%
Functional		0.65–1.40	65–140%
Free antigen		0.70–1.40	70–140%
Prothrombin gene mutation G20210A	WB	Not applicable	Not present
Prothrombin time	P	12.7–15.4 s	12.7–15.4 s
Protoporphyrin, free erythrocyte	WB	0.28–0.64 μmol/L of red blood cells	16–36 μg/dL of red blood cells
Red cell distribution width	WB	<0.145	<14.5%
Reptilase time	P	16–23.6 s	16–23.6 s
Reticulocyte count	WB		
Adult males		0.008–0.023 red cells	0.8–2.3% red cells
Adult females		0.008–0.020 red cells	0.8–2.0% red cells
Reticulocyte hemoglobin content	WB	>26 pg/cell	>26 pg/cell
Ristocetin cofactor (functional von Willebrand factor)	P		
Blood group O		0.75 mean of normal	75% mean of normal
Blood group A		1.05 mean of normal	105% mean of normal
Blood group B		1.15 mean of normal	115% mean of normal
Blood group AB		1.25 mean of normal	125% mean of normal
Serotonin release assay	S	<0.2 release	<20% release
Sickle cell test	WB	Negative	Negative
Sucrose hemolysis	WB	<0.1	<10% hemolysis
Thrombin time	P	15.3–18.5 s	15.3–18.5 s
Thrombin-antithrombin (TAT) complex	P	<4 μg/L	<4 ng/mL

(*continued*)

TABLE 1

HEMATOLOGY AND COAGULATION (CONTINUED)

ANALYTE	SPECIMEN	SI UNITS	CONVENTIONAL UNITS
Total eosinophils	WB	150–300 × 10^6/L	150–300/mm^3
Transferrin receptor	S, P	9.6–29.6 nmol/L	9.6–29.6 nmol/L
Viscosity			
Plasma	P	1.7–2.1	1.7–2.1
Serum	S	1.4–1.8	1.4–1.8
von Willebrand factor (VWF) antigen (factor VIII:R antigen)	P		
Blood group O		0.75 mean of normal	75% mean of normal
Blood group A		1.05 mean of normal	105% mean of normal
Blood group B		1.15 mean of normal	115% mean of normal
Blood group AB		1.25 mean of normal	125% mean of normal
von Willebrand factor collagen binding	P	590–2490 units/L	59–249 units/dL
von Willebrand factor multimers	P	Normal distribution	Normal distribution
White blood cells: see "Leukocytes"			

Abbreviations: JF, joint fluid; P, plasma; PRP, platelet-rich plasma; S, serum; WB, whole blood.

TABLE 2

CLINICAL CHEMISTRY AND IMMUNOLOGY

ANALYTE	SPECIMEN	SI UNITS	CONVENTIONAL UNITS
Acetoacetate	P	49–294 μmol/L	0.5–3.0 mg/dL
Adrenocorticotropin (ACTH)	P	1.3–16.7 pmol/L	6.0–76.0 pg/mL
Alanine aminotransferase (ALT, SGPT)	S	0.12–0.70 μkat/L	7–41 U/L
Albumin	S	40–50 g/L	4.0–5.0 mg/dL
Aldolase	S	26–138 nkat/L	1.5–8.1 U/L
Aldosterone (adult)			
Supine, normal sodium diet	S, P	<443 pmol/L	<16 ng/dL
Upright, normal.	S, P	111–858 pmol/L	4–31 ng/dL
Alpha fetoprotein (adult)	S	0–8.5 μg/L	0–8.5 ng/mL
Alpha-1-acid glycoprotein	S	0.50–1.2 g/L	50–120 mg/dL
Alpha$_1$ antitrypsin	S	1.0–2.0 g/L	100–200 mg/dL
Ammonia, as NH_3	P	11–35 μmol/L	19–60 μg/dL
Amylase (method dependent)	S	0.34–1.6 μkat/L	20–96 U/L
Androstenedione (adult)	S		
Males		0.81–3.1 nmol/L	23–89 ng/dL
Females			
Premenopausal		0.91–7.5 nmol/L	26–214 ng/dL
Postmenopausal		0.46–2.9 nmol/L	13–82 ng/dL
Angiotensin-converting enzyme (ACE)	S	0.15–1.1 μkat/L	9–67 U/L
Anion gap	S	7–16 mmol/L	7–16 mmol/L
Apolipoprotein A-1	S		
Male		0.94–1.78 g/L	94–178 mg/dL
Female		1.01–1.99 g/L	101–199 mg/dL

(*continued*)

TABLE 2

CLINICAL CHEMISTRY AND IMMUNOLOGY (CONTINUED)

ANALYTE	SPECIMEN	SI UNITS	CONVENTIONAL UNITS
Apolipoprotein B	S		
Male		0.55–1.40 g/L	55–140 mg/dL
Female		0.55–1.25 g/L	55–125 mg/dL
Arterial blood gases	WB		
(HCO_3^-)		22–30 mmol/L	22–30 meq/L
P_{CO_2} (Sea Level, F_{IO_2} 0.21)		4.7–6.0 kPa	35–45 mmHg
pH		7.35–7.45	7.35–7.45
P_{O_2} (Sea Level, F_{IO_2} 0.21, age related)		8.9–13.8 kPa	67–104 mmHg
Carboxyhemoglobin and methemoglobin at pH 7.40 and 37°C		≤0.01	≤1%
Aspartate aminotransferase (AST, SGOT)	S	0.20–0.65 μkat/L	12–38 U/L
Autoantibodies	S		
Anti-centromere antibody IgG		≤29 AU/mL	≤29 AU/mL
Anti-double-strand (native) DNA		<25 IU/L	<25 IU/L
Anti-glomerular basement membrane antibodies			
Qualitative IgG, IgA		Negative	Negative
Quantitative IgG antibody		≤19 AU/mL	≤19 AU/mL
Anti-histone antibodies		<1.0 U	<1.0 U
Anti-Jo-1 antibody		≤29 AU/mL	≤29 AU/mL
Anti-mitochondrial antibody		Not applicable	<20 Units
Anti-neutrophil cytoplasmic autoantibodies		Not applicable	<1:20
Serine proteinase 3 antibodies		≤19 AU/mL	≤19 AU/mL
Myeloperoxidase antibodies		≤19 AU/mL	≤19 AU/mL
Antinuclear antibody		Not applicable	Negative at 1:40
Anti-parietal cell antibody		Not applicable	None detected
Anti-RNP antibody		Not applicable	<1.0 U
Anti-Scl 70 antibody		Not applicable	<1.0 U
Anti-Smith antibody		Not applicable	<1.0 U
Anti-smooth muscle antibody		Not applicable	<1.0 U
Anti-SSA antibody		Not applicable	<1.0 U
Anti-SSB antibody		Not applicable	Negative
Anti-thyroglobulin antibody		<40 KIU/mL	<40 IU/mL
Anti-thyroid peroxidase antibody		<35 KIU/L	<35 IU/L
B-type natriuretic peptide (BNP)	P	Age and gender specific: <100 ng/L	Age and gender specific: <100 pg/mL
Bence Jones protein, serum qualitative	S	Not applicable	None detected
Bence Jones protein, serum quantitative	S		
Free kappa		3.3–19.4 mg/L	0.33–1.94 mg/dL
Free lambda		5.7–26.3 mg/L	0.57–2.63 mg/dL
K/L ratio		0.26–1.65	0.26–1.65
Beta-2-microglobulin	S	1.1–2.4 mg/L	1.1–2.4 mg/L

(*continued*)

TABLE 2

CLINICAL CHEMISTRY AND IMMUNOLOGY (CONTINUED)

ANALYTE	SPECIMEN	SI UNITS	CONVENTIONAL UNITS
Bile acids	S		
Cholic acid		0–1.9 µmol/L	0–1.9 µmol/L
Chenodeoxycholic acid		0–3.4 µmol/L	0–3.4 µmol/L
Deoxycholic acid		0–2.5 µmol/L	0–2.5 µmol/L
Ursodeoxycholic acid		0–1.0 µmol/L	0–1.0 µmol/L
Total		0–7.0 µmol/L	0–7.0 µmol/L
Bilirubin	S		
Total		5.1–22 µmol/L	0.3–1.3 mg/dL
Direct		1.7–6.8 µmol/L	0.1–0.4 mg/dL
Indirect		3.4–15.2 µmol/L	0.2–0.9 mg/dL
C peptide	S	0.27–1.19 nmol/L	0.8–3.5 ng/mL
C1-esterase-inhibitor protein	S	210–390 mg/L	21–39 mg/dL
CA 125	S	<35 kU/L	<35 U/mL
CA 19-9	S	<37 kU/L	<37 U/mL
CA 15-3	S	<33 kU/L	<33 U/mL
CA 27-29	S	0–40 kU/L	0–40 U/mL
Calcitonin	S		
Male		0–7.5 ng/L	0–7.5 pg/mL
Female		0–5.1 ng/L	0–5.1 pg/mL
Calcium	S	2.2–2.6 mmol/L	8.7–10.2 mg/dL
Calcium, ionized	WB	1.12–1.32 mmol/L	4.5–5.3 mg/dL
Carbon dioxide content (TCO_2)	P (sea level)	22–30 mmol/L	22–30 meq/L
Carboxyhemoglobin (carbon monoxide content)	WB		
Nonsmokers (in a nonsmoking environment)		0.0–0.025	0–2.5% of total hemoglobin (Hgb) value
Smokers		0.04–0.09	4–9% of total Hgb value
Loss of consciousness and death		>0.50	>50% of total Hgb value
Carcinoembryonic antigen (CEA)	S		
Nonsmokers		0.0–3.0 µg/L	0.0–3.0 ng/mL
Smokers		0.0–5.0 µg/L	0.0–5.0 ng/mL
Ceruloplasmin	S	250–630 mg/L	25–63 mg/dL
Chloride	S	102–109 mmol/L	102–109 meq/L
Cholesterol (LCL, Total, HDL): Ranges depend on individual patient factors; see 2013 ACC/AHA Guideline on the Treatment of Blood Cholesterol			
Cholinesterase	S	5–12 kU/L	5–12 U/mL
Chromogranin A	S	0–95 µg/L	0–95 ng/mL
Complement	S		
C3		0.83–1.77 g/L	83–177 mg/dL
C4		0.16–0.47 g/L	16–47 mg/dL
Complement total		60–144 CAE units	60–144 CAE units
Cortisol			
Fasting, 8 A.M.–12 noon	S	138–690 nmol/L	5–25 µg/dL
12 noon–8 P.M.		138–414 nmol/L	5–15 µg/dL
8 P.M.–8 A.M.		0–276 nmol/L	0–10 µg/dL
C-reactive protein	S	<10 mg/L	<10 mg/L

(continued)

TABLE 2

CLINICAL CHEMISTRY AND IMMUNOLOGY (CONTINUED)

ANALYTE	SPECIMEN	SI UNITS	CONVENTIONAL UNITS
C-reactive protein, high sensitivity	S	Cardiac risk Low: <1.0 mg/L Average: 1.0–3.0 mg/L High: >3.0 mg/L	Cardiac risk Low: <1.0 mg/L Average: 1.0–3.0 mg/L High: >3.0 mg/L
Creatine kinase (total)	S		
Females		0.66–4.0 µkat/L	39–238 U/L
Males		0.87–5.0 µkat/L	51–294 U/L
Creatine kinase-MB	S		
Mass		0.0–5.5 µg/L	0.0–5.5 ng/mL
Fraction of total activity (by electrophoresis)		0–0.04	0–4.0%
Creatinine	S		
Female		44–80 µmol/L	0.5–0.9 mg/dL
Male		53–106 µmol/L	0.6–1.2 mg/dL
Cryoglobulins	S	Not applicable	None detected
Cyclic citrullinated peptide (CCP) antibody (IgG)	S	Negative: <20 Units Weak positive: 20–39 Units Moderate positive: 40–59 Units Strong positive: ≥60 Units	Negative: <20 Units Weak positive: 20–39 Units Moderate positive: 40–59 Units Strong positive: ≥60 Units
Cystatin C	S	0.5–1.0 mg/L	0.5–1.0 mg/L
Deamidated gliadin peptide (DGP) antibody, IgA	S		
Negative Weak positive Positive		≤19 Units 20–30 Units ≥31 Units	≤19 Units 20–30 Units ≥31 Units
Deamidated gliadin peptide (DGP) antibody, IgG	S		
Negative Weak positive Positive		≤19 Units 20–30 Units ≥31 Units	≤19 Units 20–30 Units ≥31 Units
Dehydroepiandrosterone (DHEA) (adult)			
Male	S	6.2–43.4 nmol/L	180–1250 ng/dL
Female		4.5–34.0 nmol/L	130–980 ng/dL
Dehydroepiandrosterone (DHEA) sulfate	S		
Male (adult)		100–6190 µg/L	10–619 µg/dL
Female (adult, premenopausal)		120–5350 µg/L	12–535 µg/dL
Female (adult, postmenopausal)		300–2600 µg/L	30–260 µg/dL
11-Deoxycortisol (adult) (compound S)	S	0.34–4.56 nmol/L	12–158 ng/dL
Dihydrotestosterone			
Male	S, P	1.03–2.92 nmol/L	30–85 ng/dL
Female		0.14–0.76 nmol/L	4–22 ng/dL
Dopamine	P	0–130 pmol/L	0–20 pg/mL
Endomysial antibody, IgA	S	<1:10	<1:10
Endomysial antibody, IgG	S	<1:10	<1:10

(continued)

TABLE 2

CLINICAL CHEMISTRY AND IMMUNOLOGY (CONTINUED)

ANALYTE	SPECIMEN	SI UNITS	CONVENTIONAL UNITS
Epinephrine	P		
Supine (30 min)		<273 pmol/L	<50 pg/mL
Sitting		<328 pmol/L	<60 pg/mL
Standing (30 min)		<491pmol/L	<90 pg/mL
Erythropoietin	S	4–27 U/L	4–27 U/L
Estradiol	S, P		
Female			
Menstruating:			
Follicular phase		74–532 pmol/L	<20–145 pg/mL
Midcycle peak		411–1626 pmol/L	112–443 pg/mL
Luteal phase		74–885 pmol/L	<20–241 pg/mL
Postmenopausal		217 pmol/L	<59 pg/mL
Male		74 pmol/L	<20 pg/mL
Estrone	S, P		
Female			
Menstruating:			
Follicular phase		<555 pmol/L	<150 pg/mL
Luteal phase		<740 pmol/L	<200 pg/mL
Postmenopausal		11–118 pmol/L	3–32 pg/mL
Male		33–133 pmol/L	9–36 pg/mL
Fatty acids, free (nonesterified)	P	0.1–0.6 mmol/L	2.8–16.8 mg/dL
Ferritin	S		
Female		10–150 µg/L	10–150 ng/mL
Male		29–248 µg/L	29–248 ng/mL
Follicle-stimulating hormone (FSH)	S, P		
Female			
Menstruating			
Follicular phase		3.0–20.0 IU/L	3.0–20.0 mIU/mL
Ovulatory phase		9.0–26.0 IU/L	9.0–26.0 mIU/mL
Luteal phase		1.0–12.0 IU/L	1.0–12.0 mIU/mL
Postmenopausal		18.0–153.0 IU/L	18.0–153.0 mIU/mL
Male		1.0–12.0 IU/L	1.0–12.0 mIU/mL
Fructosamine	S	<285 µmol/L	<285 µmol/L
Galectin-3	S		
Low risk Intermediate risk Higher risk		≤17.8 µg/L 17.9–25.9 µg/L >25.9 µg/L	≤17.8 ng/mL 17.9–25.9 ng/mL >25.9 ng/mL
Gamma glutamyltransferase	S	0.15–0.99 µkat/L	9–58 U/L
Gastrin	S	<100 ng/L	<100 pg/mL
Glucagon	P	40–130 ng/L	40–130 pg/mL
Glucose	WB	3.6–5.3 mmol/L	65–95 mg/dL
Glucose (fasting)	P		
Normal		4.2–5.6 mmol/L	75–100 mg/dL
Increased risk for diabetes		5.6–6.9 mmol/L	100–125 mg/dL

(*continued*)

TABLE 2

CLINICAL CHEMISTRY AND IMMUNOLOGY (CONTINUED)

ANALYTE	SPECIMEN	SI UNITS	CONVENTIONAL UNITS
Diabetes mellitus		Fasting ≥7.0 mmol/L	Fasting ≥126 mg/dL
		A 2-h level of ≥11.1 mmol/L during an oral glucose tolerance test	A 2-h level of ≥200 mg/dL during an oral glucose tolerance test
		A random glucose level of ≥11.1 mmol/L in patients with symptoms of hyperglycemia	A random glucose level of ≥200 mg/dL in patients with symptoms of hyperglycemia
Growth hormone	S	0–5 μg/L	0–5 ng/mL
Hemoglobin A_{lc}	WB	0.04–0.06 Hgb fraction	4.0–5.6%
Prediabetes		0.057–0.064 Hgb fraction	5.7–6.4%
Diabetes mellitus		A hemoglobin A_{1c} level of ≥0.065 Hgb fraction as suggested by the American Diabetes Association	A hemoglobin A_{1c} level of ≥6.5% as suggested by the American Diabetes Association
Hemoglobin A_{1c} with estimated average glucose (eAG)	WB	eAg mmoL/L = 1.59 × HbA_{1c} – 2.59	eAg (mg/dL) = 28.7 × HbA_{1c} – 46.7
Homocysteine	P	4.4–10.8 μmol/L	4.4–10.8 μmol/L
Human chorionic gonadotropin (HCG)	S		
Nonpregnant female		<5 IU/L	<5 mIU/mL
1–2 weeks postconception		9–130 IU/L	9–130 mIU/mL
2–3 weeks postconception		75–2600 IU/L	75–2600 mIU/mL
3–4 weeks postconception		850–20,800 IU/L	850–20,800 mIU/mL
4–5 weeks postconception		4000–100,200 IU/L	4000–100,200 mIU/mL
5–10 weeks postconception		11,500–289,000 IU/L	11,500–289,000 mIU/mL
10–14 weeks postconception		18,300–137,000 IU/L	18,300–137,000 mIU/mL
Second trimester		1400–53,000 IU/L	1400–53,000 mIU/mL
Third trimester		940–60,000 IU/L	940–60,000 mIU/mL
Human epididymis protein 4 (HE-4)	S	0–150 pmol/L	0–150 pmol/L
β-Hydroxybutyrate	P	60–170 μmol/L	0.6–1.8 mg/dL
17-Hydroxyprogesterone (adult)	S		
Male		<4.17 nmol/L	<139 ng/dL
Female			
Follicular phase		0.45–2.1 nmol/L	15–70 ng/dL
Luteal phase		1.05–8.7 nmol/L	35–290 ng/dL
Immunofixation	S	Not applicable	No bands detected
Immunoglobulin, quantitation (adult)			
IgA	S	0.70–3.50 g/L	70–350 mg/dL
IgD	S	0–140 mg/L	0–14 mg/dL
IgE	S	1–87 KIU/L	1–87 IU/mL
IgG	S	7.0–17.0 g/L	700–1700 mg/dL
IgG_1	S	2.7–17.4 g/L	270–1740 mg/dL
IgG_2	S	0.3–6.3 g/L	30–630 mg/dL
IgG_3	S	0.13–3.2 g/L	13–320 mg/dL
IgG_4	S	0.11–6.2 g/L	11–620 mg/dL
IgM	S	0.50–3.0 g/L	50–300 mg/dL

(*continued*)

TABLE 2

CLINICAL CHEMISTRY AND IMMUNOLOGY (CONTINUED)

ANALYTE	SPECIMEN	SI UNITS	CONVENTIONAL UNITS
Inhibin A	S		
Males		≤2.0 ng/L	≤2.0 pg/mL
Females			
Early follicular phase		1.8–17.3 ng/L	1.8–17.3 pg/mL
Mid follicular phase		3.5–31.7 ng/L	3.5–17.3 pg/mL
Late follicular phase		9.8–90.3 ng/L	9.8–90.3 pg/mL
Midcycle		16.9–91.8 ng/L	16.9–91.8 pg/mL
Early luteal phase		16.1–97.5 ng/L	16.1–97.5 pg/mL
Mid luteal phase		3.9–87.7 ng/L	3.9–87.7 pg/mL
Late luteal phase		2.7–47.1 ng/L	2.7–47.1 pg/mL
Postmenopausal		<1.0–2.1 ng/L	<1.0–2.1 pg/mL
Insulin	S, P	14.35–143.5 pmol/L	2–20 μU/mL
Iron	S	7–25 μmol/L	41–141 μg/dL
Iron-binding capacity	S	45–73 μmol/L	251–406 μg/dL
Iron-binding capacity saturation	S	0.16–0.35	16–35%
Ischemia modified albumin	S	<85 KU/L	<85 U/mL
Joint fluid crystal	JF	Not applicable	No crystals seen
Joint fluid mucin	JF	Not applicable	Only type I mucin present
Ketone (acetone)	S	Negative	Negative
Lactate	P, arterial	0.5–1.6 mmol/L	4.5–14.4 mg/dL
	P, venous	0.5–2.2 mmol/L	4.5–19.8 mg/dL
Lactate dehydrogenase	S	2.0–3.8 μkat/L	115–221 U/L
Lamellar body count	AMF		
Immature		<15,000/μL	<15,000/μL
Indeterminate		15,000–50,000/μL	15,000-50,000/μL
Mature		>50,000/μL	>50,000/μL
Lecithin/sphingomyelin (L/S) ratio	AMF		
Immature		≤1.5	≤1.5
Transitional		1.5–1.9	1.5–1.9
Mature		2.0–2.5 or greater	2.0–2.5 or greater
Lipase	S	0.51–0.73 μkat/L	3–43 U/L
Lipoprotein (a)	S	0–300 mg/L	0–30 mg/dL
Lipoprotein associated phospholipase A2	S, P	0–234 μg/L	0–234 ng/mL
Luteinizing hormone (LH)	S, P		
Female			
Menstruating			
Follicular phase		2.0–15.0 U/L	2.0–15.0 mIU/mL
Ovulatory phase		22.0–105.0 U/L	22.0–105.0 mIU/mL
Luteal phase		0.6–19.0 U/L	0.6–19.0 mIU/mL
Postmenopausal		16.0–64.0 U/L	16.0–64.0 mIU/mL
Male		2.0–12.0 U/L	2.0–12.0 mIU/mL
Magnesium	S	0.62–0.95 mmol/L	1.5–2.3 mg/dL
Metanephrine	P	<0.5 nmol/L	<100 pg/mL
Methemoglobin	WB	0.0–0.01	0–1% of total Hgb value
Myoglobin	S		
Male		20–71 μg/L	20–71 μg/L
Female		25–58 μg/L	25–58 μg/L

(*continued*)

TABLE 2

CLINICAL CHEMISTRY AND IMMUNOLOGY (CONTINUED)

ANALYTE	SPECIMEN	SI UNITS	CONVENTIONAL UNITS
Norepinephrine	P		
Supine (30 min)		650–2423 pmol/L	110–410 pg/mL
Sitting		709–4019 pmol/L	120–680 pg/mL
Standing (30 min)		739–4137 pmol/L	125–700 pg/mL
N-telopeptide (cross-linked), NTx	S		
Female, premenopausal		6.2–19.0 nmol BCE	6.2–19.0 nmol BCE
Male		5.4–24.2 nmol BCE	5.4–24.2 nmol BCE
BCE = bone collagen equivalent			
NT-proBNP	S, P	<125 ng/L up to 75 years	<125 pg/mL up to 75 years
		<450 ng/L >75 years	<450 pg/mL >75 years
5' Nucleotidase	S	0.00–0.19 µkat/L	0–11 U/L
Osmolality	P	275–295 mOsmol/kg serum water	275–295 mOsmol/kg serum water
Osteocalcin	S	11–50 µg/L	11–50 ng/mL
Oxygen content (age and gender related)	WB		
Arterial (sea level)		17–21 mL/dL	17–21 vol%
Venous (sea level)		10–16 mL/dL	10–16 vol%
Oxygen saturation (sea level)	WB	Fraction:	Percent:
Arterial		0.91–1.0	91–100%
Venous, arm		0.60–0.85	60–85%
Parathyroid hormone (intact)	S	8–51 ng/L	8–51 pg/mL
Phosphatase, alkaline	S	0.56–1.63 µkat/L	33–96 U/L
Phosphatase, alkaline bone	S		
Male		≤20 µg/L	≤20 ng/mL
Female			
Premenopausal		≤14 µg/L	≤14 ng/mL
Postmenopausal		≤22 µg/L	≤22 ng/mL
Phosphorus, inorganic	S	0.81–1.4 mmol/L	2.5–4.3 mg/dL
Potassium	S	3.5–5.0 mmol/L	3.5–5.0 meq/L
Prealbumin (transthyretin)	S	170–340 mg/L	17–34 mg/dL
Procalcitonin	S	<0.1 µg/L	<0.1 ng/mL
Progesterone	S, P		
Female: Follicular		<3.18 nmol/L	<1.0 ng/mL
Midluteal		9.54–63.6 nmol/L	3–20 ng/mL
Male		<3.18 nmol/L	<1.0 ng/mL
Prolactin	S		
Male		53–360 mg/L	2.5–17 ng/mL
Female		40–530 mg/L	1.9–25 ng/mL
Prostate-specific antigen (PSA)	S	0.0–4.0 µg/L	0.0–4.0 ng/mL

(*continued*)

TABLE 2

CLINICAL CHEMISTRY AND IMMUNOLOGY (CONTINUED)

ANALYTE	SPECIMEN	SI UNITS	CONVENTIONAL UNITS
Prostate-specific antigen, free	S	With total PSA between 4 and 10 µg/L and when the free PSA is:	With total PSA between 4 and 10 ng/mL and when the free PSA is:
		>0.25 decreased risk of prostate cancer	>25% decreased risk of prostate cancer
		<0.10 increased risk of prostate cancer	<10% increased risk of prostate cancer
Protein fractions:	S		
Albumin		35–55 g/L	3.5–5.5 g/dL (50–60%)
Globulin		20–35 g/L	2.0–3.5 g/dL (40–50%)
$Alpha_1$		2–4 g/L	0.2–0.4 g/dL (4.2–7.2%)
$Alpha_2$		5–9 g/L	0.5–0.9 g/dL (6.8–12%)
Beta		6–11 g/L	0.6–1.1 g/dL (9.3–15%)
Gamma		7–17 g/L	0.7–1.7 g/dL (13–23%)
Protein, total	S	67–86 g/L	6.7–8.6 g/dL
Pyruvate	P	40–130 µmol/L	0.35–1.14 mg/dL
Retinol-binding protein	S	0.71–2.9 µmol/L	1.5–6.0 mg/dL
Rheumatoid factor	S	<15 kIU/L	<15 IU/mL
Serotonin	WB	0.28–1.14 µmol/L	50–200 ng/mL
Serum protein electrophoresis	S	Not applicable	Normal pattern
Sex hormone–binding globulin (adult)	S		
Male		11–80 nmol/L	11–80 nmol/L
Female		30–135 nmol/L	30–135 nmol/L
Sodium	S	136–146 mmol/L	136–146 meq/L
Somatomedin-C (IGF-1) (adult)	S		
16 years		226–903 µg/L	226–903 ng/mL
17 years		193–731 µg/L	193–731 ng/mL
18 years		163–584 µg/L	163–584 ng/mL
19 years		141–483 µg/L	141–483 ng/mL
20 years		127–424 µg/L	127–424 ng/mL
21–25 years		116–358 µg/L	116–358 ng/mL
26–30 years		117–329 µg/L	117–329 ng/mL
31–35 years		115–307 µg/L	115–307 ng/mL
36–40 years		119–204 µg/L	119–204 ng/mL
41–45 years		101–267 µg/L	101–267 ng/mL
46–50 years		94–252 µg/L	94–252 ng/mL
51–55 years		87–238 µg/L	87–238 ng/mL
56–60 years		81–225 µg/L	81–225 ng/mL
61–65 years		75–212 µg/L	75–212 ng/mL
66–70 years		69–200 µg/L	69–200 ng/mL
71–75 years		64–188 µg/L	64–188 ng/mL
76–80 years		59–177 µg/L	59–177 ng/mL
81–85 years		55–166 µg/L	55–166 ng/mL

(*continued*)

TABLE 2

CLINICAL CHEMISTRY AND IMMUNOLOGY (CONTINUED)

ANALYTE	SPECIMEN	SI UNITS	CONVENTIONAL UNITS
Somatostatin	P	<25 ng/L	<25 pg/mL
Testosterone, free			
Female, adult	S	10.4–65.9 pmol/L	3–19 pg/mL
Male, adult		312–1041 pmol/L	90–300 pg/mL
Testosterone, total,	S		
Female		0.21–2.98 nmol/L	6–86 ng/dL
Male		9.36–37.10 nmol/L	270–1070 ng/dL
Thyroglobulin	S	13–318 µg/L	1.3–31.8 ng/mL
Thyroid-binding globulin	S	13–30 mg/L	1.3–3.0 mg/dL
Thyroid-stimulating hormone (thyrotropin)	S	0.34–4.25 mIU/L	0.34–4.25 µIU/mL
Thyrotropin receptor antibody	S	≤1.75 IU/L	≤1.75 mIU/mL
Thyroxine, free (fT_4)	S	9.0–16 pmol/L	0.7–1.24 ng/dL
Thyroxine, total (T_4)	S	70–151 nmol/L	5.4–11.7 µg/dL
Thyroxine index (free)	S	6.7–10.9	6.7–10.9
Tissue transglutaminase (tTG) Antibody, IgA	S		
Negative		<4.0 Units/mL	<4.0 Units/mL
Weak positive		4.0–10.0 Units/mL	4.0–10.0 Units/mL
Positive		>10.0 Units/mL	>10.0 Units/mL
Tissue transglutaminase (tTG) antibody, IgG	S		
Negative		<6.0 Units/mL	<6.0 Units/mL
Weak positive		6.0–9.0 Units/mL	6.0–9.0 Units/mL
Positive		>9.0 Units/mL	>9.0 Units/mL
Transferrin	S	2.0–4.0 g/L	200–400 mg/dL
Transferrin, carbohydrate deficient, for alcohol use	S	0.017	1.7%
Triglycerides	S	0.34–2.26 mmol/L	30–200 mg/dL
Triiodothyronine, free (fT_3)	S	3.7–6.5 pmol/L	2.4–4.2 pg/mL
Triiodothyronine, total (T_3)	S	1.2–2.1 nmol/L	77–135 ng/dL
Troponin I	S, P		
99th percentile of a healthy population		Method-dependent	Method-dependent
Troponin T	S, P		
99th percentile of a healthy population		0–14 ng/L	0–14 ng/L
Urea nitrogen	S	2.5–7.1 mmol/L	7–20 mg/dL
Uric acid	S		
Females		0.15–0.33 mmol/L	2.5–5.6 mg/dL
Males		0.18–0.41 mmol/L	3.1–7.0 mg/dL
Vasoactive intestinal polypeptide	P	0–60 ng/L	0–60 pg/mL
Zinc protoporphyrin	WB	0–400 µg/L	0–40 µg/dL
Zinc protoporphyrin (ZPP)-to-heme ratio	WB	0–69 µmol ZPP/mol heme	0–69 µmol ZPP/mol heme

Abbreviations: AMF, amniotic fluid; P, plasma; S, serum; WB, whole blood.
Source: NJ Stone et al: J Am Coll Cardiol 63:2889–2934, 2014.

TABLE 3

VITAMINS AND SELECTED TRACE MINERALS

SPECIMEN	ANALYTE	REFERENCE RANGE	
		SI UNITS	CONVENTIONAL UNITS
Aluminum	S	<0.2 μmol/L	<5.41 μg/L
Arsenic	WB	0.0–0.17 μmol/L	0–13 μg/L
Cadmium	WB	<44.5 nmol/L	<5.0 μg/L
Coenzyme Q10 (ubiquinone)	P	433–1532 μg/L	433–1532 μg/L
β-Carotene	S	0.07–1.43 μmol/L	4–77 μg/dL
Copper	S	11–22 μmol/L	70–140 μg/dL
Folic acid	RC	340–1020 nmol/L cells	150–450 ng/mL cells
Folic acid	S	12.2–40.8 nmol/L	5.4–18.0 ng/mL
Lead	S		
Adult		<0.5 μmol/L	<10 μg/dL
Children		<0.25 μmol/L	<5 μg/dL
Mercury	WB	0–50 μmol/L	0–10 μg/L
Selenium	S	0.8–2.0 μmol/L	63–160 μg/L
Vitamin A	S	0.7–3.5 μmol/L	20–100 μg/dL
Vitamin B_1 (thiamine)	S	0–75 nmol/L	0–2 μg/dL
Vitamin B_2 (riboflavin)	S	106–638 nmol/L	4–24 μg/dL
Vitamin B_6	P	20–121 nmol/L	5–30 ng/mL
Vitamin B_{12}	S	206–735 pmol/L	279–996 pg/mL
Vitamin C (ascorbic acid)	S	23–57 μmol/L	0.4–1.0 mg/dL
Vitamin D 1,25-dihydroxy, total	S, P	36–180 pmol/L	15–75 pg/mL
Vitamin D 25-hydroxy, total	P	75–250 nmol/L	30–100 ng/mL
Vitamin E	S	12–42 μmol/L	5–18 μg/mL
Vitamin K	S	0.29–2.64 nmol/L	0.13–1.19 ng/mL
Zinc	S	11.5–18.4 μmol/L	75–120 μg/dL

Abbreviations: P, plasma; RC, red cells; S, serum; WB, whole blood.

TABLE 4

URINE ANALYSIS AND RENAL FUNCTION TESTS

	REFERENCE RANGE	
	SI UNITS	**CONVENTIONAL UNITS**
Acidity, titratable	20–40 mmol/d	20–40 meq/d
Aldosterone	Normal diet: 6–25 µg/d	Normal diet: 6–25 µg/d
	Low-salt diet: 17–44 µg/d	Low-salt diet: 17–44 µg/d
	High-salt diet: 0–6 µg/d	High-salt diet: 0–6 µg/d
Aluminum	0.19–1.11 µmol/L	5–30 µg/L
Ammonia	30–50 mmol/d	30–50 meq/d
Amylase		4–400 U/L
Amylase/creatinine clearance ratio ($[Cl_{am}/Cl_{cr}] \times 100$)	1–5	1–5
Arsenic	0.07–0.67 µmol/d	5–50 µg/d
Bence Jones protein, urine, qualitative	Not applicable	None detected
Bence Jones protein, urine, quantitative		
Free kappa	1.4–24.2 mg/L	0.14–2.42 mg/dL
Free lambda	0.2–6.7 mg/L	0.02–0.67 mg/dL
K/L ratio	2.04–10.37	2.04–10.37
Calcium (10 meq/d or 200 mg/d dietary calcium)	<7.5 mmol/d	<300 mg/d
Chloride	140–250 mmol/d	140–250 mmol/d
Citrate	320–1240 mg/d	320–1240 mg/d
Copper	<0.95 µmol/d	<60 µg/d
Coproporphyrins (types I and III)	0–20 µmol/mol creatinine	0–20 µmol/mol creatinine
Cortisol, free	55–193 nmol/d	20–70 µg/d
Creatine, as creatinine		
Female	<760 µmol/d	<100 mg/d
Male	<380 µmol/d	<50 mg/d
Creatinine	8.8–14 mmol/d	1.0–1.6 g/d
Dopamine	392–2876 nmol/d	60–440 µg/d
Eosinophils	<100 eosinophils/mL	<100 eosinophils/mL
Epinephrine	0–109 nmol/d	0–20 µg/d
Glomerular filtration rate	>60 mL/min/1.73 m^2	>60 mL/min/1.73 m^2
	For African Americans, multiply the result by 1.21	For African Americans, multiply the result by 1.21
Glucose (glucose oxidase method)	0.3–1.7 mmol/d	50–300 mg/d
5-Hydroindoleacetic acid (5-HIAA)	0–78.8 µmol/d	0–15 mg/d
Hydroxyproline	53–328 µmol/d	53–328 µmol/d
Iodine, spot urine		
WHO classification of iodine deficiency:		
Not iodine deficient	>100 µg/L	>100 µg/L
Mild iodine deficiency	50–100 µg/L	50–100 µg/L
Moderate iodine deficiency	20–49 µg/L	20–49 µg/L
Severe iodine deficiency	<20 µg/L	<20 µg/L
Ketone (acetone)	Negative	Negative
17 Ketosteroids	3–12 mg/d	3–12 mg/d

(continued)

TABLE 4

URINE ANALYSIS AND RENAL FUNCTION TESTS (CONTINUED)

	REFERENCE RANGE	
	SI UNITS	**CONVENTIONAL UNITS**
Metanephrines		
Metanephrine	30–350 µg/d	30–350 µg/d
Normetanephrine	50–650 µg/d	50–650 µg/d
Microalbumin		
Normal	0.0–0.03 g/d	0–30 mg/d
Microalbuminuria	0.03–0.30 g/d	30–300 mg/d
Clinical albuminuria	>0.3 g/d	>300 mg/d
Microalbumin/creatinine ratio		
Normal	0–3.4 g/mol creatinine	0–30 µg/mg creatinine
Microalbuminuria	3.4–34 g/mol creatinine	30–300 µg/mg creatinine
Clinical albuminuria	>34 g/mol creatinine	>300 µg/mg creatinine
β_2-Microglobulin	0–160 µg/L	0–160 µg/L
Norepinephrine	89–473 nmol/d	15–80 µg/d
N-telopeptide (cross-linked), NTx		
Female, premenopausal	17–94 nmol BCE/mmol creatinine	17–94 nmol BCE/mmol creatinine
Female, postmenopausal	26–124 nmol BCE/mmol creatinine	26–124 nmol BCE/mmol creatinine
Male	21–83 nmol BCE/mmol creatinine	21–83 nmol BCE/mmol creatinine
Osmolality	100–800 mosm/kg	100–800 mosm/kg
Oxalate		
Male	80–500 µmol/d	7–44 mg/d
Female	45–350 µmol/d	4–31 mg/d
pH	5.0–9.0	5.0–9.0
Phosphate (phosphorus) (varies with intake)	12.9–42.0 mmol/d	400–1300 mg/d
Porphobilinogen	None	None
Potassium (varies with intake)	25–100 mmol/d	25–100 meq/d
Protein	<0.15 g/d	<150 mg/d
Protein/creatinine ratio	Male: 15–68 mg/g Female: 10–107 mg/g	Male: 15–68 mg/g Female: 10–107 mg/g
Sediment		
Red blood cells	0–2/high-power field	
White blood cells	0–2/high-power field	
Bacteria	None	
Crystals	None	
Bladder cells	None	
Squamous cells	None	
Tubular cells	None	
Broad casts	None	
Epithelial cell casts	None	
Granular casts	None	

(*continued*)

TABLE 4

URINE ANALYSIS AND RENAL FUNCTION TESTS (CONTINUED)

	REFERENCE RANGE	
	SI UNITS	**CONVENTIONAL UNITS**
Hyaline casts	0–5/low-power field	
Red blood cell casts	None	
Waxy casts	None	
White cell casts	None	
Sodium (varies with intake)	100–260 mmol/d	100–260 meq/d
Specific gravity:		
After 12-h fluid restriction	>1.025	>1.025
After 12-h deliberate water intake	≤1.003	≤1.003
Tubular reabsorption, phosphorus	0.79–0.94 of filtered load	79–94% of filtered load
Urea nitrogen	214–607 mmol/d	6–17 g/d
Uric acid (normal diet)	1.49–4.76 mmol/d	250–800 mg/d
Vanillylmandelic acid (VMA)	<30 μmol/d	<6 mg/d

Abbreviation: BCE = bone collagen equivalent.

ACKNOWLEDGMENT

The contributions of Drs. Daniel J. Fink, Patrick M. Sluss, James L. Januzzi, Kent B. Lewandrowski, Amudha Palanisamy, and Scott Fink to this chapter in previous editions are gratefully acknowledged. We also express our gratitude to Drs. Alex Rai and Jeffrey Jhang for helpful suggestions.

REVIEW AND SELF-ASSESSMENT*

Charles M. Wiener ■ Cynthia D. Brown ■ Brian Houston

QUESTIONS

DIRECTIONS: Choose the **one best** response to each question.

1. All of the following hormones are produced by the anterior pituitary EXCEPT:

A. Adrenocorticotropic hormone
B. Growth hormone
C. Oxytocin
D. Prolactin
E. Thyroid stimulating hormone

2. A 45-year-old man reports to his primary care physician that his wife has noted coarsening of his facial features over several years. In addition, he reports low libido and decreased energy. Physical examination shows frontal bossing and enlarged hands. An MRI confirms that he has a pituitary mass. Which of the following screening tests should be ordered to diagnose the cause of the mass?

A. 24-hour urinary free cortisol
B. ACTH assay
C. Growth hormone level
D. Serum IGF-1 level
E. Serum prolactin level

3. Which of the following statements regarding the anatomy of the pituitary gland is TRUE?

A. Growth hormone is derived from the precursor POMC.
B. Prolactin-secreting cells form the majority of cells in the anterior pituitary.
C. The anterior pituitary secretes hormones directly synthesized in neuroendocrine cells in the hypothalamus.
D. The pituitary gland forms from Rathke's pouch embryonically.
E. The posterior pituitary has dual arterial blood supply.

4. A 58-year-old man undergoes severe head trauma and develops pituitary insufficiency. After recovery, he is placed on thyroid hormone, testosterone, glucocorticoids, and vasopressin. On a routine visit he questions his primary care physician regarding potential growth hormone deficiency. All of the following are potential signs or symptoms of growth hormone deficiency EXCEPT:

A. Abnormal lipid profile
B. Atherosclerosis
C. Increased bone mineral density
D. Increased waist:hip ratio
E. Left ventricular dysfunction

5. A 75-year-old man presents with development of abdominal obesity, proximal myopathy, and skin hyperpigmentation. His laboratory evaluation shows a hypokalemic metabolic alkalosis. Cushing's syndrome is suspected. Which of the following statements regarding this syndrome is TRUE?

A. Basal ACTH level is likely to be low
B. Circulating corticotropin releasing hormone is likely to be elevated
C. Pituitary MRI will visualize all ACTH-secreting tumors
D. Referral for urgent performance of inferior petrosal venous sampling is indicated
E. Serum potassium level $\leq$3.3 mmol/L is suggestive of ectopic ACTH production

6. Which of the following is common in patients with Kallmann's syndrome?

A. Anosmia
B. A white forelock
C. Precocious (early) puberty in females
D. Syndactyly in males
E. Hyperphagia-obesity

*Questions and answers were taken from Wiener C et al. (eds). *Harrison's Principles of Internal Medicine Self-Assessment and Board Review.* 19th ed. New York: McGraw-Hill; 2017.

7. A 22-year-old woman who is otherwise healthy undergoes an uneventful vaginal delivery of a full term infant. One day postpartum she complains of visual changes and severe headache. Two hours after these complaints, she is found unresponsive and profoundly hypotensive. She is intubated and placed on mechanical ventilation. Her blood pressure is 68/28 mmHg, regular heart rate of 148 beats/min, her oxygen saturation is 95% on FiO_2 0.40. Physical examination is unremarkable. Her laboratories are notable for glucose of 49 mg/dL, normal hematocrit and white blood cell count. Which of the following is most likely to reverse her hypotension?

   A. Activated drotrecogin alfa
   B. Hydrocortisone
   C. Piperacillin/tazobactam
   D. T_4
   E. Transfusion of packed red blood cells

8. You are caring for Mr. Gelston, a 19-year-old man who had a brain tumor when young and underwent cranial radiation. You note that he has short stature, and has not yet gone through puberty. You suspect that he has pituitary insufficiency due to radiation. You remember that which of the following is TRUE regarding acquired hypopituitarism due to radiation:

   A. At a dose of 50 Gy of radiation, only 5% of patients will manifest hypopituitarism.
   B. The majority of patients, who develop hypopituitarism after cranial radiation, do so within a year of treatment.
   C. Growth hormone is the most common hormonal deficiency.
   D. There is no correlation between radiation dose and likelihood of developing hypopituitarism.
   E. Older adults are at highest risk of radiation-induced hypopituitarism.

9. A 23-year-old college student is followed in the student health center for medical management of panhypopituitarism after resection of craniopharyngioma as a child. She reports moderate compliance with her medications but feels generally well. A TSH is checked and is below the limits of detection of the assay. Which of the following is the next most appropriate action?

   A. Decrease levothyroxine dose to half of current dose
   B. Do nothing
   C. Order free T_4 level
   D. Order MRI of her brain
   E. Thyroid uptake scan

10. A patient visited a local emergency room 1 week ago with a headache. She received a head MRI, which did not reveal a cause for her symptoms, but the final report states "an empty sella is noted. Advise clinical correlation." The patient was discharged from the emergency room with instructions to follow-up with her primary care physician as soon as possible. Her headache has resolved, and the patient has no complaints; however, she comes to your office 1 day later very concerned about this unexpected MRI finding. What should be the next step in her management?

    A. Diagnose her with subclinical panhypopituitarism, and initiate low-dose hormone replacement.
    B. Reassure her and follow laboratory results closely.
    C. Reassure her and repeat MRI in 6 months.
    D. This may represent early endocrine malignancy—whole-body positron-emission tomography/CT is indicated.
    E. This MRI finding likely represents the presence of a benign adenoma—refer to neurosurgery for resection.

11. Pituitary adenomas typically expand in which direction?

    A. Anteriorly
    B. Inferiorly
    C. Laterally
    D. Posteriorly
    E. Superiorly

12. On MRI of the pituitary, which of the following findings is abnormal in an adult?

    A. A slightly concave upper aspect of the pituitary
    B. Brighter T1 intensity of the posterior pituitary
    C. Heterogeneous anterior pituitary tissue
    D. Pituitary height of 8–12 mm
    E. Tissue which is lower intensity than the nearby brain tissue on T1 images and enhances on T2 images

13. Mr. Jones has a pituitary adenoma on imaging which has extended directly superiorly and is compressing his optic chiasm. Which of the below visual field deficits is most likely manifest?

    A. Bilateral inferior visual field deficits
    B. Bilateral superior visual field deficits
    C. Bitemporal hemianopia
    D. Central scotomas bilaterally
    E. Right homonymous hemianopia

14. All of the following features are in Carney's syndrome EXCEPT:

A. Acromegaly
B. Adrenal adenomas
C. Atrial myxomas
D. Hypertrophic cardiomyopathy
E. Spotty skin pigmentation

15. Which of the following is the most common cause of preventable mental deficiency in the world?

A. Beriberi disease
B. Cretinism
C. Folate deficiency
D. Scurvy
E. Vitamin A deficiency

16. All of the following are associated with increased levels of total T_4 in the plasma with a normal free T_4 EXCEPT:

A. Cirrhosis
B. Pregnancy
C. Sick-euthyroid syndrome
D. Familial dysalbuminemic hyperthyroxinemia
E. Familial excess thyroid binding globulin

17. Which of the following is the most common cause of hypothyroidism worldwide?

A. Graves' disease
B. Hashimoto's thyroiditis
C. Iatrogenic hypothyroidism
D. Iodine deficiency
E. Radiation exposure

18. A 75-year-old woman is diagnosed with hypothyroidism. She has longstanding coronary artery disease and is wondering about the potential consequences for her cardiovascular system. Which of the following statements is TRUE regarding the interaction of hypothyroidism and the cardiovascular system?

A. A reduced stroke volume is found with hypothyroidism.
B. Blood flow is diverted toward the skin in hypothyroidism.
C. Myocardial contractility is increased with hypothyroidism.
D. Pericardial effusions are a rare manifestation of hypothyroidism.
E. Reduced peripheral resistance is found in hypothyroidism and may be accompanied by hypotension.

19. A 38-year-old mother of three presents to her primary care office with complaints of fatigue. She feels that her energy level has been low for the past 3 months. She was previously healthy and taking no medications. She does report that she has gained about 10 lb and has severe constipation for which she has been taking a number of laxatives. A TSH is elevated at 25 mU/L. Free T_4 is low. She is wondering why she has hypothyroidism. Which of the following tests is most likely to diagnose the etiology?

A. Antithyroid peroxidase antibody
B. Antithyroglobulin antibody
C. Radioiodine uptake scan
D. Serum thyroglobulin level
E. Thyroid ultrasound

20. A 54-year-old woman with longstanding hypothyroidism is seen in her primary care physician's office for a routine evaluation. She reports feeling fatigued and somewhat constipated. Since her last visit, her other medical conditions, which include hypercholesterolemia and systemic hypertension are stable. She was diagnosed with uterine fibroids and started on iron recently. Her other medications include levothyroxine, atorvastatin, and hydrochlorothiazide. A TSH is checked and it is elevated to 15 mU/L. Which of the following is the most likely reason for her elevated TSH?

A. Celiac disease
B. Colon cancer
C. Medication noncompliance
D. Poor absorption of levothyroxine due to ferrous sulfate
E. TSH secreting pituitary adenoma

21. An 87-year-old woman is admitted to the intensive care unit with depressed level of consciousness, hypothermia, sinus bradycardia, hypotension, and hypoglycemia. She was previously healthy with the exception of hypothyroidism and systemic hypertension. Her family recently checked in on her and found that she was not taking any of her medications because of financial difficulties. There is no evidence of infection on examination, urine microscopy or chest radiograph. Her serum chemistries are notable for mild hyponatremia and a glucose of 48 mg/dL. A TSH is >100 mU/L. All of the following statements regarding this condition are true EXCEPT:

A. External warming is a critical feature of therapy in patients with a temperature <34°C
B. Hypotonic intravenous solutions should be avoided.

21. (*Continued*)

C. IV levothyroxine should be administered with IV glucocorticoids.
D. Sedation should be avoided if possible.
E. This condition occurs almost exclusively in the elderly and often is precipitated by an unrelated medical illness.

22. A 29-year-old woman is evaluated for anxiety, palpitations, and diarrhea and found to have Graves' disease. Before she begins therapy for her thyroid condition, she has an episode of acute chest pain and presents to the emergency department. Although a CT angiogram is ordered, the radiologist calls to notify the treating physician that this is potentially dangerous. Which of the following best explains the radiologist's recommendation?

A. Iodinated contrast exposure in patients with Graves' disease may exacerbate hyperthyroidism
B. Pulmonary embolism is exceedingly rare in Graves' disease
C. Radiation exposure in patients with hyperthyroidism is associated with increased risk of subsequent malignancy
D. Tachycardia with Graves' disease limits the image quality of CT angiography and will not allow accurate assessment of pulmonary embolism
E. The radiologist was mistaken, CT angiography is safe in Graves' disease

23. A patient has neurosurgery for a pituitary tumor that requires resection of the gland. Which of the following functions of the adrenal gland will be preserved in this patient immediately postoperatively?

A. Morning peak of plasma cortisol level
B. Release of cortisol in response to stress
C. Sodium retention in response to hypovolemia
D. None of the above

24. Which of the following is the most common cause of Cushing's syndrome?

A. ACTH-producing pituitary adenoma
B. Adrenocortical adenoma
C. Adrenocortical carcinoma
D. Ectopic ACTH secretion
E. McCune-Albright syndrome

25. All of the following are features of Conn's syndrome EXCEPT:

A. Alkalosis
B. Hyperkalemia
C. Muscle cramps
D. Normal serum sodium
E. Severe systemic hypertension

26. All of the following statements regarding asymptomatic adrenal masses (incidentalomas) are true EXCEPT:

A. All patients with incidentalomas should be screened for pheochromocytoma.
B. Fine-needle aspiration may distinguish between benign and malignant primary adrenal tumors.
C. In patients with a history of malignancy, the likelihood that the adrenal mass is a metastasis is ~50%.
D. The majority of adrenal incidentalomas are nonsecretory.
E. The vast majority of adrenal incidentalomas are benign.

27. You are designing an experiment to determine the effect of psychosocial stress exposure on peak daily cortisol secretion. When should you measure cortisol to ensure that you are most likely assessing peak cortisol levels?

A. Midnight (12:00 AM)
B. 4:00 AM
C. 8:30 AM
D. Noon (12:00 PM)
E. 8:30 PM

28. Mr. McTrap is admitted after a car accident. His medical history is unknown, and on presentation, he is obtunded and can provide no history. CT scan reveals a splenic laceration, and he is emergently taken to the operating room for splenectomy, which proceeds without complication. At the completion of the operation, bleeding has stopped, and he returns to the ICU. However, he remains deeply hypotensive with a BP of 70/50 mmHg with an increase only to 82/52 mmHg after a bolus of 2 L of normal saline intravenously. He is afebrile with a normal WBC count. Repeat CT scan of the chest, abdomen, and pelvis shows no hemorrhage. JVP is not visible above the clavicle. He has a round face and is obese, and you note the following on physical examination (see figures A–D below).

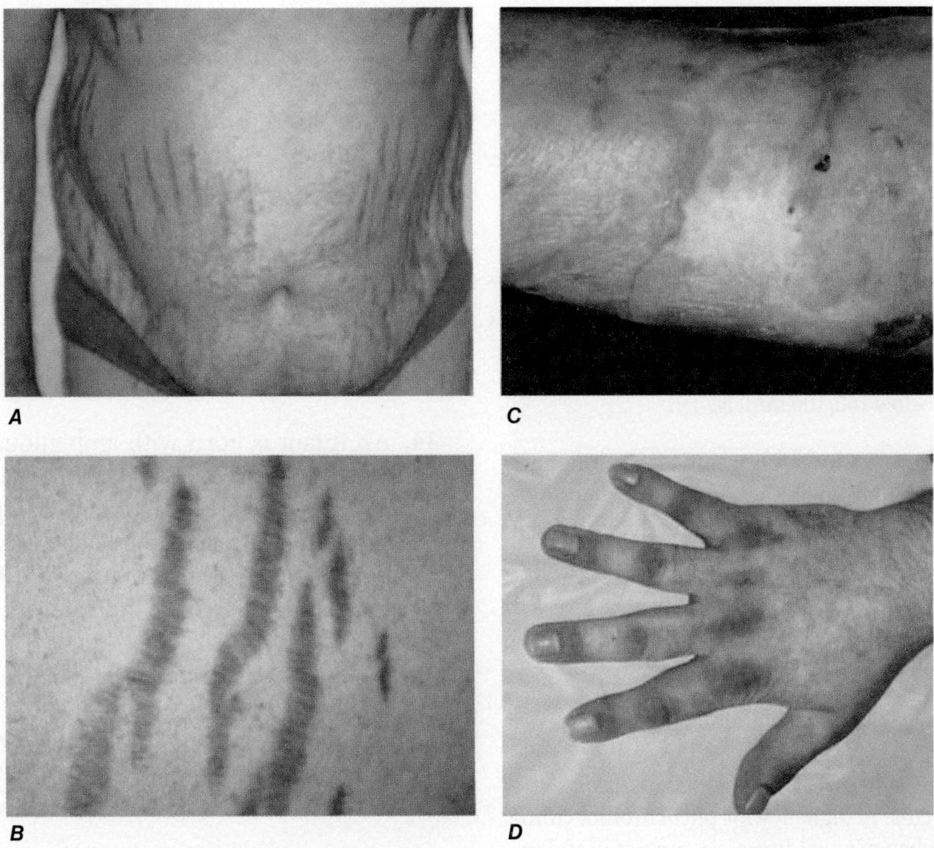

28. *(Continued)*
He has no hand hyperpigmentation. What is the next most appropriate step?

A. Return to the OR for exploratory laparotomy
B. Administer intravenous hydrocortisone, 100 mg IV
C. Administer vancomycin and piperacillin/tazobactam
D. Insert intra-aortic balloon pump for counterpulsation
E. Perform MRI of the spine

29. A 43-year-old man with episodic, severe hypertension is referred for evaluation of possible secondary causes of hypertension. He reports feeling well generally, except for episodes of anxiety, palpitations, and tachycardia with elevation in his blood pressure during these episodes. Exercise often brings on these events. The patient also has mild depression and is presently taking sertraline, labetalol, amlodipine, and lisinopril to control his blood pressure. Urine 24-hour total metanephrines are ordered and show an elevation of 1.5 times the upper limit of normal. Which of the following is the next most appropriate step?

A. Hold labetalol for 1 week and repeat testing
B. Hold sertraline for 1 week and repeat testing
C. Immediate referral for surgical evaluation

29. *(Continued)*
D. Measure 24-hour urine vanillylmandelic acid level
E. Obtain MRI of the abdomen

30. A 45-year-old man is diagnosed with pheochromocytoma after presentation with confusion, marked hypertension to 250/140 mmHg, tachycardia, headaches, and flushing. His fractionated plasma metanephrines show a normetanephrine level of 560 pg/mL and a metanephrine level of 198 pg/mL (normal values: normetanephrine: 18–111 pg/mL; metanephrine: 12–60 pg/mL). CT scanning of the abdomen with IV contrast demonstrates a 3-cm mass in the right adrenal gland. A brain MRI with gadolinium shows edema of the white matter near the parietooccipital junction consistent with reversible posterior leukoencephalopathy. You are asked to consult regarding management. Which of the following statements is TRUE regarding management of pheochromocytoma in this individual?

A. Beta-blockade is absolutely contraindicated for tachycardia even after adequate alpha-blockade has been attained.
B. Immediate surgical removal of the mass is indicated, because the patient presented with hypertensive crisis with encephalopathy.

30. (*Continued*)

C. Salt and fluid intake should be restricted to prevent further exacerbation of the patient's hypertension.
D. Treatment with phenoxybenzamine should be started at a high dose (20–30 mg three times daily) to rapidly control blood pressure, and surgery can be undertaken within 24–48 hours.
E. Treatment with IV phentolamine is indicated for treatment of the hypertensive crisis. Phenoxybenzamine should be started at a low dose and titrated to the maximum tolerated dose over 2–3 weeks. Surgery should not be planned until the blood pressure is consistently below 160/100 mmHg.

31. Mr. Robinson returns for a follow-up after a long hospital course for hypertension where he was diagnosed with a pheochromocytoma and ultimately underwent a left adrenalectomy. He reports feeling well since then, and his hypertension is well controlled. He is curious about whether his pheochromocytoma was considered malignant. You should tell him?

A. Approximately 50% of pheochromocytomas are malignant
B. Cellular atypia and invasion of blood vessels on pathology define malignancy for pheochromocytoma
C. ^{23}I-metaiodobenzylguanidine scans are not useful in locating distant metastases
D. The absence of distant metastases rules out malignant disease

32. A 37-year-old man is evaluated for infertility. He and his wife have been attempting to conceive a child for the past 2 years without success. He initially saw an infertility specialist, but was referred to endocrinology after sperm analysis showed no sperm. He is otherwise healthy and only takes a multivitamin. On physical examination his vital signs are normal. He is tall, has small testes, gynecomastia, minimal facial and axillary hair. Chromosomal analysis confirms Klinefelter's syndrome. Which of the following statements is TRUE?

A. Androgen supplementation is of little use in this condition
B. He is not at increased risk for breast tumors
C. Increased plasma concentrations of estrogen are present
D. Most cases are diagnosed prepubertally
E. Plasma concentrations of FSH and LH are decreased in this condition

33. A 17-year-old woman is evaluated in your office for primary amenorrhea. She does not feel as if she has entered puberty in that she has never had a menstrual period and has sparse axillary and pubic hair growth. On examination, she is noted to be 150 cm tall. She has a low hairline and slight webbing of her neck. Her follicle-stimulating hormone (FSH) level is 75 mIU/mL, luteinizing hormone is 20 mIU/mL, and estradiol level 2 pg/mL. You suspect Turner's syndrome. All of the following tests are indicated in this individual EXCEPT:

A. Buccal smear for nuclear heterochromatin (Barr body)
B. Echocardiogram
C. Karyotype analysis
D. Renal ultrasound
E. Thyroid-stimulating hormone (TSH)

34. An infant is born with ambiguous genitalia. While amniocentesis analysis during pregnancy showed a 46,XX genotype, this infant has phallic appearing genitalia and partially fused labia. You cannot palpate testes. Aside from standard blood test, which biochemical screen is indicated?

A. Flow cytometry of the peripheral blood
B. Serum cortisol levels
C. Serum 17-hydroxyprogesterone levels
D. Serum thyroid–stimulating hormone
E. Serum prolactin levels

35. A 58-year-old man is seen in his primary care physician's office for evaluation of bilateral breast enlargement. This has been present for several months and is accompanied by mild pain in both breasts. He reports no other symptoms. His other medical conditions include coronary artery disease with a history of congestive heart failure, atrial fibrillation, obesity, and type 2 diabetes mellitus. His current medications include lisinopril, spironolactone, furosemide, insulin, and digoxin. He denies illicit drug use and has fathered three children. Examination confirms bilateral breast enlargement with palpable glandular tissue that measures 2 cm bilaterally. Which of the following statements regarding his gynecomastia is TRUE?

A. He should be referred for mammography to rule out breast cancer.
B. His gynecomastia is most likely due to obesity with adipose tissue present in the breast.
C. Serum testosterone, LH, and FSH should be measured to evaluate for androgen insensitivity.
D. Spironolactone should be discontinued and examination followed for regression
E. Liver function testing should be performed to screen for cirrhosis.

36. All the following drugs may interfere with testicular function EXCEPT:

36. (*Continued*)
A. Cyclophosphamide
B. Ketoconazole
C. Metoprolol
D. Prednisone
E. Spironolactone

37. A 26-year-old man presents with pain and swelling of his right testicle that has persisted after an empiric treatment for epididymitis. Ultrasound confirms a 1.5 × 2 cm solid mass, suspicious for testicular cancer. Radical inguinal orchiectomy confirms the mass as a seminoma with disease limited to the testis (tumor stage pT1). Chest, abdomen, and pelvis CT show no evidence of metastatic disease or lymphadenopathy. Results of serum tumor markers demonstrate the following: AFP 5 ng/mL (<10 ng/mL), β-hCG 182 U/L (0.2–0.8 U/L), and LDH 432 U/L (100–190 U/L). Following resection, all tumor markers become undetectable after an appropriate interval. Which is the next best step in this patient's treatment?

A. Immediate retroperitoneal radiation therapy.
B. Nerve-sparing retroperitoneal lymph node dissection.
C. Single dose therapy with cisplatin.
D. Surveillance alone with treatment only if relapse detected.
E. Either A or D are associated with a near 100% cure rate.

38. Which of the following statements describes the relationship between testicular tumors and serum markers?

A. Beta-human chorionic gonadotropin (β-hCG) and α-fetoprotein (AFP) should be measured in following the progress of a tumor.
B. β-hCG is limited in its usefulness as a marker because it is identical to human luteinizing hormone.
C. Measurement of tumor markers the day after surgery for localized disease is useful in determining completeness of the resection.
D. More than 40% of nonseminomatous germ cell tumors produce no cell markers.
E. Pure seminomas produce AFP or β-hCG in more than 90% of cases.

39. Clinical signs and findings of the presence of ovulation include all of the following EXCEPT:

A. Detection of urinary LH surge
B. Estrogen peak during secretory phase of menstrual cycle
C. Increase in basal body temperature >0.5°F in second half of menstrual cycle
D. Presence of *mittelschmerz*
E. Progesterone level >5 ng/mL 7 days before expected menses

40. In the developmental progression from childhood through puberty to menopause, all of the following statements regarding levels of follicle-stimulating hormone (FSH) and luteinizing hormone (LH) are true EXCEPT:

A. FSH is suppressed from birth to 20 months of age.
B. LH is increased during neonatal year (birth to 20 months).
C. LH and FSH levels are reduced during childhood before puberty.
D. At the onset of puberty, pulsatile gonadotropin-releasing hormone (GnRH) drives pituitary FSH and LH levels.
E. LH and FSH levels rise sharply after menopause.

41. Which of the following occurs first in the majority of normal pubertal development for girls?

A. Achieving peak height velocity
B. Menarche
C. Breast development begins
D. The development of pubic hair
E. The development of axillary hair

42. A couple has been married for 5 years and have attempted to conceive a child for the last 12 months. Despite regular intercourse they have not achieved pregnancy. They are both 32 years of age and have no medical problems. Neither partner is taking medications. Which of the following is the most common cause of their infertility?

A. Endometriosis
B. Male causes
C. Ovulatory dysfunction
D. Tubal defect
E. Unexplained

43. A couple seeks advice regarding infertility. The female partner is 35 years old. She has never been pregnant and was taking oral contraceptive pills from age 20 until age 34. It is now 16 months since she discontinued her oral contraceptives. She is having menstrual cycles approximately once every 35 days, but occasionally will go as long as 60 days between cycles. Most months, she develops breast tenderness about 2–3 weeks after the start of her menstrual cycle. When she was in college, she was treated for Neisseria gonorrhoeae that was diagnosed when she presented to the student health center with a fever and pelvic pain. She otherwise has no medical history. She works about 60 hours weekly as a corporate attorney and exercises daily. She drinks coffee daily and alcohol at social occasions only. Her body mass index (BMI) is 19.8 kg/m^2. Her husband, who is 39 years old, accompanies her to the evaluation.

43. *(Continued)*
He also has never had children. He was married previously from the ages of 24–28. He and his prior wife attempted to conceive for about 15 months, but were unsuccessful. At that time, he was smoking marijuana on a daily basis and attributed their lack of success to his drug use. He has now been completely free of drugs for 9 years. He suffers from hypertension and is treated with lisinopril, 10 mg daily. He is not obese (BMI, 23.7 kg/m^2). They request evaluation for their infertility and request help with conception. Which of the following statements is TRUE in regards to their infertility and likelihood of success in conception?

A. Determination of ovulation is not necessary in the female partner as most of her cycles occur regularly, and she develops breast tenderness mid-cycle indicative of ovulation.
B. Lisinopril should be discontinued immediately because of the risk of birth defects associated with its use.
C. The female partner should be assessed for tubal patency by a hysterosalpingogram. If significant scarring is found, in vitro fertilization should be strongly considered to decrease the risk of ectopic pregnancy.
D. The prolonged use of oral contraceptives for >10 years has increased the risk of anovulation and infertility.
E. The use of marijuana by the male partner is directly toxic to sperm motility, and this is the likely cause of their infertility.

44. Which of the following forms of contraception have theoretical efficacy of >90%?

A. Condoms
B. Intrauterine devices
C. Oral contraceptives
D. Spermicides
E. All of the above

45. A 30-year-old male, the father of three children, has had progressive breast enlargement during the last 6 months. He does not use any drugs. Laboratory evaluation reveals that both LH and testosterone are low. Further evaluation of this patient should include which of the following?

A. 24-hour urine collection for the measurement of 17 ketosteroids
B. Blood sampling for serum glutamic-oxaloacetic transaminase (SGOT) and serum alkaline phosphatase and bilirubin levels
C. Breast biopsy
D. Karyotype analysis to exclude Klinefelter's syndrome
E. Measurement of estradiol and human chorionic gonadotropin (hCG) levels

46. You are seeing a 36-year-old woman in clinic as her family practitioner. In her history, she reports no illness and is taking no medications. She does mention that she and her husband have been trying to conceive a child unsuccessfully for the past 7 months. Which of the following would an appropriate response?

A. "You have likely entered menopause and cannot have a child."
B. "We do not recommend evaluation by a fertility specialist until you and her husband have tried for at least 12 months."
C. "I will refer you to an expert in fertility issues."
D. "Most causes of infertility are related to the male—I suggest you have him be evaluated."
E. "Advancing age does not reduce a woman's chance of becoming pregnant until she reaches menopause."

47. All of the following statements regarding menstrual function and dysfunction are true EXCEPT:

A. Pregnancy is the most common cause of secondary amenorrhea.
B. Primary amenorrhea is defined as the absence of ever having a first menstrual flow.
C. Secondary amenorrhea is defined as absence of a menstrual flow for >3–6 months in a woman that previously menstruated.
D. The absence of menarche at age 17 years old in a normally developing woman warrants evaluation for primary amenorrhea.
E. There is no evidence that race or ethnicity affect the prevalence of amenorrhea.

48. A 28-year-old woman seeks evaluation for secondary amenorrhea. She had a normal menarche at age 14 with regular monthly periods lasting 5–6 days for the last 13 years. Over the last year she's noticed greater irregularity and has had no menses for the last 6 months. She takes no medications and is sexually active with one partner using condoms as prophylaxis. Her physical examination is notable for normal vital signs, a BMI of 29 kg/m^2, normal breast development, and normal pelvic examination. Laboratory testing reveals a negative β-hCG, normal testosterone, normal DHEAS, elevated prolactin, and reduced FSH. Based on this information, the most likely diagnosis is:

A. Androgen insensitivity syndrome
B. Neuroendocrine tumor
C. Polycystic ovary syndrome
D. Pregnancy
E. Premature menopause

49. You are evaluating a 23-year-old woman with heavy uterine bleeding. She reports menarche at age 13 with regular monthly 5–6 day menses until the age of 19. Starting at age 20 she began having 3–4 menses/year only lasting 3 days. For the last year she has had four episodes of heavy uterine bleeding lasting 6–8 days. She has not had any menstruation for 9 months and is not sexually active. She has been diagnosed with type 2 diabetes and takes metformin. On examination she is mildly hirsute, her blood pressure is 130/85 with heart rate 85 beats/min and respiratory rate 14/min. Her BMI is 25 kg/m^2 and her SaO_2 on room air is 98%. Her β-hCG is negative, testosterone is elevated, and vaginal ultrasound reveals polycystic ovaries. Which of the following is the most effective treatment for her uterine bleeding?

A. Clomiphene
B. Letrozole
C. Prednisone
D. Progesterone
E. Testosterone

50. The Women's Health Initiative study investigated hormonal therapy in postmenopausal women. The study was stopped early due to increased risk of which of the following diseases in the estrogen only arm?

A. Deep venous thrombosis
B. Endometrial cancer
C. Myocardial infarction
D. Osteoporosis
E. Stroke

51. All of the following are traditional contraindications for oral hormone replacement therapy in postmenopausal women EXCEPT:

A. Active liver disease
B. Blood clotting disorder
C. Breast cancer
D. Coronary heart disease risk over ensuing 10 years of 5–10%
E. Unexplained vaginal bleeding

52. Ms. Chacco, a 19-year-old white woman, complains of worsening excess hairiness and is worried that she will be mocked as she starts college. She notes increasingly noticeable hair on her upper lip, chin, and arms. She takes no medications and reports a history of irregular menses. On examination she has normal vital signs and you note small to medium tufts of dark hair in the areas she mentioned plus in the midline above and below the umbilicus, along the inner thigh, and in the upper and lower back. All

52. *(Continued)* of the statements regarding her condition are true EXCEPT:

A. Further hormonal evaluation is likely necessary
B. She likely has elevated androgen levels
C. She meets the diagnostic criteria for hirsutism
D. The most common cause of her condition is congenital adrenal hyperplasia
E. This condition affects approximately 10% of women

53. For the patient described above, additional initial evaluation should include which of the following:

A. Abdominal/pelvic CT scan
B. ACTH stimulation test
C. Dexamethasone suppression test
D. Measurement of serum prolactin
E. Measurement of serum testosterone

54. All of the following statements regarding the risk of ovarian cancer are true EXCEPT:

A. Ten percent of women with ovarian cancer have a germline mutation in either *BRCA1 or BRCA2*
B. Early prophylactic oophorectomy in women with *BRCA1 or BRCA2* mutations reduces the risk of developing subsequent breast cancer
C. Individuals with a single copy of a *BRCA1 or BRCA2* mutant allele have an increased risk of breast and ovarian cancer
D. Women with a mutation in *BRCA1* have a higher risk of ovarian cancer than woman with a mutation in *BRCA2*
E. Women with *BRCA1*, *BRCA2*, or other at risk germ line mutations should be screened with serial measurement of the CA-125 tumor marker

55. A 42-year-old woman seeks evaluation for over 6 months of post-coital bleeding without dyspareunia. She also notes some recent spotting between her regular menses. She has no past medical history, is unmarried with multiple sexual partners and unprotected sex, and works as an accountant. She has not sought gynecologic evaluation for over 10 years. Pelvic examination reveals an abnormal appearance of the cervix with an abnormal Pap smear, positive HPV test, and negative HIV, chlamydia, gonorrhea, and syphilis studies. A cervical biopsy shows squamous cell carcinoma confined to the cervix. All of the following statements regarding this woman's condition are true EXCEPT:

A. Cervical cancer is an uncommon cancer worldwide
B. Her cancer is related to HPV infection

55. *(Continued)*

C. HPV vaccination before initiation of sexual activity can decrease the risk of developing an abnormal Pap smear
D. She has stage 1 cervical cancer
E. With surgical therapy her 5-year survival is >80%

56. All of the following statements regarding male sexual function are true EXCEPT:

A. Detumescence is mediated by the parasympathetic nervous system
B. Ejaculation is stimulated by the sympathetic nervous system
C. Nitric oxide enhances erection
D. Sildenafil maintains erection by inhibiting the breakdown of cGMP
E. Testosterone enhances libido

57. A 62-year-old man comes to clinic with his spouse complaining of erectile dysfunction. He has a 10-year history of moderately controlled diabetes mellitus and uses insulin. Over the last year, despite intact libido, he has been unable to attain or sustain an erection when attempting sexual intercourse with his wife. He reports that over this time he no longer awakes with an erection as he did previously. Serum chemistries are normal, Hgb A1c is 5.8%, and serum testosterone normal for his age. Which class of drug is most likely to improve his ability to achieve and maintain erection?

A. 5α-reductase inhibitor
B. Androgen
C. Corticosteroid
D. Phosphodiesterase-5 inhibitor
E. Selective serotonin reuptake inhibitor

58. A 54-year-old woman complains of difficulty having sex because of pain during intercourse. This symptom began about 8 years ago, but has worsened over the last year. She has one sexual partner and is on no medications. Which of the following is most likely to improve her symptoms?

A. Anastrozole
B. Estrogen cream
C. Paroxetine
D. Sildenafil
E. Tamoxifen

59. Metabolic syndrome was defined initially as a clinical entity by the World Health Organization in 1998 as a constellation of findings including central obesity, hypertriglyceridemia, low HDL, hyperglycemia,

59. *(Continued)*
and hypertension. Which of the following statements regarding the epidemiology of metabolic syndrome is TRUE?

A. After the age of 60, men are more likely to have metabolic syndrome than women.
B. Among patients with diabetes mellitus, presence of metabolic syndrome confers a higher risk of cardiovascular disease.
C. Body mass index is the strongest predictor of insulin resistance and diabetes risk in metabolic syndrome.
D. The highest recorded prevalence of metabolic syndrome in the United States is among Mexican-American women.
E. The nationality at the lowest risk of metabolic syndrome is the Japanese population.

60. A 47-year-old Chinese man is seen for an annual examination. He generally has no complaints, but lives a sedentary lifestyle. He works as an accountant and spends of his work days at a computer screen. He does not maintain a regular exercise routine. He admits his diet is poor. He is divorced and lives alone. He eats out or gets take out about four nights weekly. On other days, he prefers quick meals that he can heat up in the microwave. His past medical history is significant for hypertension and obesity. He is being treated with hydrochlorothiazide 25 mg daily. He has no allergies. His blood pressure today is 148/92. His waist circumference is 93 cm (36.6 in). He is 177.8 cm (70 in) and weighs 105 kg (225 lb). His BMI is 32.3 kg/m^2. On his annual fasting labs, his total cholesterol is 220 mg/dL, HDL is 28 mg/dL, triglycerides are 178 mg/dL, and LDL is 103 mg/dL. Fasting plasma glucose is 98 mg/dL. Which of the following is TRUE regarding a diagnosis of metabolic syndrome in this patient?

A. He cannot have metabolic syndrome because his fasting plasma glucose level is normal.
B. He has metabolic syndrome because he meets 3 out of 5 diagnostic criteria: high triglyceride levels, low HDL levels, and hypertension.
C. He has metabolic syndrome because he meets 4 out of 5 diagnostic criteria: body mass index, high triglyceride levels, low HDL level, and hypertension.
D. He has metabolic syndrome because he meets 4 out of 5 diagnostic criteria: waist circumference, high triglyceride levels, low HDL level, and hypertension.
E. Metabolic syndrome cannot be diagnosed on a single evaluation. Repeat testing is indicated in 3–6 months.

61. Which of the following ethnic populations in the United States has the highest risk of diabetes mellitus?

61. *(Continued)*

A. Ashkenazi Jews
B. Asian American
C. Hispanic
D. non-Hispanic black
E. non-Hispanic white

62. Which of the following defines **normal** glucose tolerance?

A. Fasting plasma glucose <100 mg/dL
B. Fasting plasma glucose <126 mg/dL following an oral glucose challenge
C. Fasting plasma glucose <100 mg/dL, plasma glucose <140 mg/dL following an oral glucose challenge and hemoglobin A1C <5.6%
D. Hemoglobin A1C <5.6% and fasting plasma glucose <140 mg/dL
E. Hemoglobin A1C <6.0%

63. A 37-year-old woman with obesity presents to clinic for routine health evaluation. She reports that over the last year she has had two yeast infections treated with over the counter remedies and frequently feels thirsty. She does report waking up at night to urinate. Which of the following studies is the most appropriate first test in evaluating the patient for diabetes mellitus?

A. Hemoglobin A1C
B. Oral glucose tolerance test
C. Plasma C peptide level
D. Plasma insulin level
E. Random plasma glucose level

64. A 27-year-old woman with mild obesity is seen by her primary care office for increased thirst and polyuria. Diabetes mellitus is suspected and a random plasma glucose of 211 mg/d confirms this diagnosis. Which of the following tests will strongly indicate that she has type 1 diabetes mellitus?

A. Anti-GAD-65 antibody
B. Peroxisom proliferator-activated receptor gamma-2 polymorphism testing
C. Plasma insulin level
D. Testing for HLA DR3
E. There is no laboratory test indicating type 1 diabetes mellitus

65. You have admitted an 18-year-old patient to the adult medical intensive care unit for diabetic ketoacidosis (DKA). The patient was not known previously to be diabetic, but her mother notes that she had been "going to bathroom a lot" recently, and "she had been really thirsty." The patient's BMI is 44 kg/m^2. There is no family history of diabetes. You successfully treat the patient for her DKA and note that serum anti-GAD antibodies and anti-ICA (islet cell antibodies) sent on admission are not detected. The patient and her mother want to know what "type" of diabetes she has. You should tell them which of the following?

A. "Due to the young age of onset, you likely have type 1 diabetes."
B. "Due to your presentation with diabetic ketoacidosis, you likely have type 1 diabetes."
C. "I suspect you have maturity-onset diabetes of the young (MODY)."
D. "You likely have type 2 diabetes mellitus."
E. "I suspect your diabetes was triggered by a virus."

66. A patient is evaluated in the emergency department for complications of diabetes mellitus due to an episode of life stressors. All of the following laboratory tests are consistent with the diagnosis of diabetic ketoacidosis EXCEPT:

A. Arterial pH = 7.1
B. Glucose = 550 mg/dL
C. Markedly positive plasma ketones
D. Normal serum potassium
E. Plasma osmolality 380 mOsm/mL

67. Pick the correct combination of onset of action and duration of action for the following insulins:

	Onset (h)	**Duration (h)**
A. Aspart	1	6
B. Detemir	2	12
C. Lispro	0.5	2
D. NPH	2	14
E. Regular	0.25	8

68. A 54-year-old woman is diagnosed with type 2 diabetes mellitus after a routine follow-up for impaired fasting glucose showed that her hemoglobin A1C is now 7.6%. She has attempted to lose weight and exercise with no improvement in her hemoglobin A1C, and drug therapy is now recommended. She has mild systemic hypertension that is well controlled and no other medical conditions. Which of the following is the most appropriate first line therapy?

A. Acarbose
B. Exenatide
C. Glyburide
D. Metformin
E. Sitagliptin

69. A 21-year-old female with a history of type 1 diabetes mellitus is brought to the emergency room with nausea, vomiting, lethargy, and dehydration. Her mother notes that she stopped taking insulin 1 day before presentation. She is lethargic, has dry mucous membranes, and is obtunded. Blood pressure is 80/40 mmHg, and heart rate is 112 beats/min. Heart sounds are normal. Lungs are clear. The abdomen is soft, and there is no organomegaly. She is responsive and oriented ×3 but diffusely weak. Serum sodium is 126 mEq/L, potassium is 4.3 mEq/L, magnesium is 1.2 mEq/L, blood urea nitrogen is 76 mg/ dL, creatinine is 2.2 mg/dL, bicarbonate is 10 mEq/L, and chloride is 88 mEq/L. Serum glucose is 720 mg/dL. All the following are appropriate management steps EXCEPT:

A. Three percent sodium solution
B. Arterial blood gas
C. Intravenous insulin
D. Intravenous potassium
E. Intravenous fluids

70. You are seeing a 28-year-old woman with long-standing type-1 diabetes on insulin. She tells you that she and her husband have decided to try to conceive. Which of the following is TRUE regarding reproductive issues and diabetes?

A. Women with diabetes have a reduced reproductive capacity.
B. Insulin crosses the placenta and may affect the fetus adversely.
C. The patient should expect her insulin requirements to increase during pregnancy.
D. High maternal serum glucose increases the risk of fetal abnormalities.
E. The most crucial period of glycemic control is in the third trimester to avoid fetal malformations.

71. Which of the following regarding care of the hospitalized diabetic patient is TRUE?

A. General anesthesia leads to insulin sensitization and higher risk for hypoglycemia.
B. A greater degree of hyperglycemia during hospitalization has NOT been associated with worse infectious outcomes.
C. In clinical trials, very strict glycemic control (goal 81–108 mg/dL) is superior to moderate glycemic control (target 140 mg/dL).
D. The initiation of total parenteral nutrition (TPN) is associated with increased insulin requirements.
E. In critically ill patients, subcutaneous insulin is invariably preferred over intravenous insulin.

72. In the following figure, what is the primary finding of this patient's fundus?

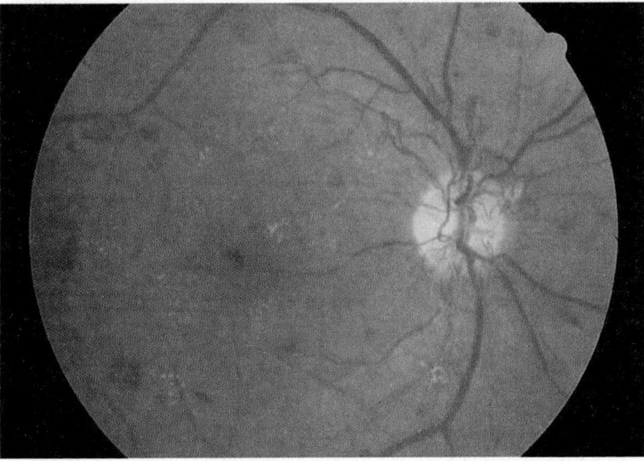

A. Arteriovenous nicking
B. Microaneurysms
C. Neovascularization
D. Papilledema

73. Which of the following patients should be treated with either an ACE inhibitor or angiotensin receptor blocker?

A. A 24-year-old woman with type 1 diabetes mellitus with two positive spot microalbuminuria tests 1 week apart
B. A 32-year-old woman with type 1 diabetes mellitus with a most blood glucose of 328 mg/dL and a positive spot microalbuminuria
C. A 48-year-old man with type 2 diabetes mellitus with a positive spot microalbuminuria test 1 week after starting a new exercise program
D. A 56-year-old man with type 2 diabetes mellitus with two positive spot microalbuminuria tests 3 months apart
E. A 62-year-old man with type 2 diabetes mellitus and hypertension with positive spot microalbuminuria. BP on day of testing was 190/118

74. A 58-year-old woman with type 2 diabetes mellitus is evaluated by her primary care provider for a tingling sensation in her hands and feet. She has had type 2 diabetes mellitus for 15 years with intermittently poor control. Her most recent hemoglobin A1C is 7.9%. She is currently managed with insulin detemir 40 units daily and metformin 1000 mg daily. On neurologic examination, there is loss of deep tendon reflexes at the ankles bilaterally. DTRs are 2+ at the knees, biceps, and triceps. Sensation is decreased to pinprick and light touch bilaterally to the ankle and wrists. She also has difficulty ascertaining if the great toe is being held in the up or down position when

74. *(Continued)*
her eyes are closed. She finds it difficult to sleep at night sometimes due to the pain in her legs. She is diagnosed with distal sensory polyneuropathy due to her diabetes. Which of the following medications have been approved by the U.S. Food and Drug Administration for the treatment of pain associated with diabetic neuropathy?

A. Duloxetine
B. Gabapentin
C. Pregabalin
D. A and C only
E. All of the above

75. Plasma glucose is normally tightly regulated in the body with fasting levels between 70–110 mg/dL. When the blood glucose falls below 80–85 mg/dL, which of the following physiologic changes is the first to occur?

A. Decrease in growth hormone
B. Decrease in insulin secretion
C. Increase in cortisol
D. Increase in epinephrine
E. Increase in glucagon

76. A 25-year-old health care worker is seen for evaluation of recurrent hypoglycemia. She has had several episodes at work over the past year in which she feels shaky, anxious, and sweaty. She measures her finger stick glucose and it is 40–55 mg/dL. This has been confirmed with plasma glucose during one episode of 50 mg/dL. She then drinks orange juice and feels better. These have not happened outside the work environment. Aside from oral contraceptives, she takes no medications and is otherwise healthy. Which of the following tests is most likely to demonstrate the underlying cause of her hypoglycemia?

A. Measurement of insulin-like growth factor 1
B. Measurement of fasting insulin and glucose levels
C. Measurement of fasting insulin, glucose, and C-peptide levels
D. Measurement of insulin, glucose, and C-peptide levels during an symptomatic episode
E. Measurement of plasma cortisol

77. All of the following statements regarding hypoglycemia in diabetes mellitus are true EXCEPT:

A. Individuals with type 2 diabetes mellitus experience less hypoglycemia than those with type 1 diabetes mellitus.
B. From 2–4% of deaths in type 1 diabetes mellitus are directly attributable to hypoglycemia.

77. *(Continued)*
C. Recurrent episodes of hypoglycemia predispose to the development of autonomic failure with defective glucose counterregulation and hypoglycemia unawareness.
D. The average person with type 1 diabetes mellitus has two episodes of symptomatic hypoglycemia weekly.
E. Thiazolidinediones and metformin cause hypoglycemia more frequently than sulfonylureas.

78. An 18-year-old man presents with severe mid-abdominal pain radiating to his back. Physical examination reveals a temperature of 38°C, blood pressure of 95/55, heart rate 110 beats/min, and respiratory rate 18/min with room air oxygen saturation 96%. His abdomen is diffusely tender with voluntary guarding and no rebound tenderness. There is enlargement of the liver and spleen. He also has eruptive xanthomas on his hands, feet, and legs. His lipase is 2300 U/L and he has a fasting triglyceride level of 1019 mg/dL. After appropriate evaluation, he is determined presumed to have pancreatitis and lipoprotein lipase deficiency. He stabilizes without complication and is ready for discharge after 4 days. What do you recommend for treatment?

A. Dietary fat restriction 15 g/d
B. Fish oil supplementation
C. Gemfibrozil 600 mg bid
D. Nicotinic acid sustained release 250 mg bid
E. Simvastatin 20 mg daily

79. A 32-year-old man is evaluated at a routine clinic visit for coronary risk factors. He report no tobacco use, his systemic blood pressure is normal and he does not have diabetes. He is otherwise healthy. His family history is notable for high cholesterol in his mother and maternal grandfather and grandmother. Physical examination shows tendon xanthomas. A fasting cholesterol is notable for an LDL-C of 387 mg/dL. Which of the following is the most likely genetic disorder affecting this individual?

A. ApoA-V deficiency
B. Familial defective apoB-100
C. Familial hepatic lipase deficiency
D. Familial hypercholesterolemia
E. Lipoprotein lipase deficiency

80. All of the following are potential causes of elevated LDL EXCEPT:

A. Anorexia nervosa
B. Cirrhosis
C. Hypothyroidism

80. *(Continued)*
D. Nephrotic syndrome
E. Thiazide diuretics

81. Your 60-year-old patient with a monoclonal gammopathy of unclear significance presents for a follow-up visit and to review recent laboratory data. His creatinine is newly elevated to 2.0 mg/dL, potassium is 3.7 mg/dL, calcium is 12.2 mg/dL, low-density lipoprotein (LDL) is 202 mg/dL, and triglycerides are 209 mg/dL. On further questioning he reports 3 months of swelling around the eyes and "foamy" urine. On examination, he has anasarca. Concerned for multiple myeloma and nephrotic syndrome, you order a urine protein/creatinine ratio, which returns at 14:1. Which treatment option would be most appropriate to treat his lipid abnormalities?

A. Cholesterol ester transfer protein inhibitor
B. Dietary management
C. HMG-CoA reductase inhibitors
D. Lipid apheresis
E. Niacin and fibrates

82. An 18-year-old girl is evaluated at her primary care physician's office for a routine physical. She is presently healthy. Her family history is notable for a father and two aunts with multiple endocrine neoplasia type 1 (MEN1) and the patient has undergone genetic testing and carries the MEN1 gene. Which of the following is the first and most common presentation for individuals with this genetic mutation?

A. Amenorrhea
B. Hypercalcemia
C. Hypoglycemia
D. Peptic ulcer disease
E. Uncontrolled systemic hypertension

83. You are seeing Mr. Avendaw in clinic today. He is a 35-year-old man, who last year had a partial thyroidectomy for medullary thyroid carcinoma. You noted that he was recently in the hospital and diagnosed with a pheochromocytoma, and after 2 weeks of intensive medical therapy, underwent unilateral adrenalectomy. He is recovering nicely. You are reviewing his chart before the visit, when you note that on the pathology from his thyroid surgery last year, a single parathyroid gland was removed which was shown to be a parathyroid tumor. When you meet with Mr. Avendaw, you will tell him which of the following?

A. "Family and genetic screening for similar cancers is not useful as the mutations causing these cancers are certainly unrelated and spontaneously arose."

83. *(Continued)*
B. "I suspect you have a syndrome called multiple endocrine neoplasia type 1."
C. "I suspect you have a syndrome called multiple endocrine neoplasia type 2."
D. "The partial thyroidectomy was an appropriate treatment for this condition."
E. "These tumors were likely caused by a mutation in the Menin gene."

84. Johnny Stewart, a 4-year-old boy, presents to the hospital with hypotension, lethargy, and hyponatremia. You also note that his potassium is elevated to 5.7 mEq/dL. He is afebrile and has a normal complete blood count. However, you note extensive oral thrush. On review of his chart you note that he has had multiple treatment courses for thrush and cutaneous candidal infections. HIV antibody tests have been negative. Also, you note that at 1 year of age, he had an episode of tetany prompting an emergent presentation to the hospital where he was found to be hypocalcemic. Ultimately, he was diagnosed with hypoparathyroidism. Given his current presentation, which of the following is the most appropriate course of treatment?

A. Calcium intravenously
B. Hydrocortisone intravenously
C. Kayexalate, IV insulin, and albuterol to treat presumed hyperkalemic periodic paralysis
D. Ketoconazole
E. Urgent echocardiogram for suspected cardiac tamponade

85. Mr. David presents to the emergency department with numbness and weakness in his legs and feet. On examination, you find that he is numb to the knees, and has marked weakness in ankle dorsiflexion and plantar flexion. Two years ago, he developed diabetes, and last year he was admitted when found to be profoundly hypothyroid. On examination, he has hepatosplenomegaly and appears dark tan despite having no sun exposure recently. Which of the following tests will likely help make his diagnosis?

A. Antinuclear antibody titer measurement
B. Antithymoglobulin antibody titer measurement
C. Blood cultures
D. Serum protein electrophoresis
E. Skin biopsy searching for intravascular clonal T-cells

86. A 63-year-old woman is brought to the emergency room by her nephew because of severe confusion and obtundation. Her vital signs are normal and there are no focal physical findings. She is found to have

86. *(Continued)*
hypercalcemia with a serum level of 14.8 mg/dL along with minimal elevation of BUN and creatinine. Initial evaluation reveals a chest radiograph with multiple nodules suggestive of metastatic disease. Unfortunately the nephew does not know anything about his aunt's medical history. He reports that she was in town attending a healing yoga conference. Subsequent laboratory testing reveals a normal parathyroid hormone level and an elevated parathyroid hormone-related protein level. All of the following are a likely primary malignancy in this woman EXCEPT:

A. Adenocarcinoma of the breast
B. Mantle cell lymphoma
C. Squamous cell of the lung
D. Squamous cell of the piriform sinus
E. Transitional cell of the bladder

87. In the patient described above, she should receive treatment with all of the following for her hypercalcemia EXCEPT:

A. Calcitonin
B. Furosemide
C. Normal saline
D. Pamidronate
E. Prednisone

88. A 55-year-old man is admitted to the intensive care unit with 1 week of fever and cough. He was well until 1 week before admission, when he noted progressive shortness of breath, cough, and productive sputum. On the day of admission the patient was noted by his wife to be lethargic. Emergency response found the patient unresponsive. He was intubated in the field and brought to the emergency department. His only medications are insulin glargine 20 units daily and insulin aspart with meals. The past medical history is notable for alcohol abuse and diabetes mellitus. His recent alcohol use has been at least 12 beers daily. Upon arrival to the hospital, the temperature is 38.9°C (102°F), blood pressure is 76/40 mmHg, and oxygen saturation 86% on ventilator setting of AC with a tidal volume of 420 mL, respiratory rate of 22/min, PEEP 5, and FiO_2 1.0. On examination, the patient is intubated on mechanical ventilation. Jugular venous pressure is normal. There are decreased breath sounds at the right lung base with egophony. Heart sounds are normal. The abdomen is soft. There is no peripheral edema. Chest radiography shows a right lower lobe infiltrate with a moderate pleural effusion. An electrocardiogram is normal. Sputum Gram stain shows gram-positive

88. *(Continued)*
diplococci. White blood cell count is 23 × 10^3/μL, with 70% polymorphonuclear cells and 6% bands. Blood urea nitrogen is 80 mg/dL, and creatinine is 3.1 mg/dL. Plasma glucose is 425 mg/dL. He is started on broad-spectrum antibiotics, intravenous fluids, omeprazole, and an insulin drip. A nasogastric tube is inserted, and tube feedings are started. On hospital day 2, his creatinine has improved to 1.6 mg/dL. However, plasma phosphate is 1.0 mg/dL (0.3 mmol/L) and calcium is 8.8 mg/dL. All of following are causes of hypophosphatemia in this patient EXCEPT:

A. Acute kidney injury
B. Alcoholism
C. Insulin
D. Malnutrition
E. Sepsis

89. In the patient above, what is the most appropriate approach to correcting the hypophosphatemia?

A. Administer intravenous calcium gluconate 1 g followed by infusion of intravenous phosphate at a rate of 8 mmol/h for 6 hours
B. Administer intravenous phosphate alone at a rate of 2 mmol/h for 6 hours
C. Administer intravenous phosphate alone at a rate of 8 mmol/h for 6 hours
D. Continued close observation as redistribution of phosphate is expected to normalize levels over the course of the next 24–48 hours
E. Initiate oral phosphate replacement at a dose of 1500 mg/d

90. You are caring for a 72-year-old man who has been living in a nursing home for the past 3 years. He has severe chronic obstructive pulmonary disease and requires continuous oxygen at 3 L/min. He also previously had a stroke which has left him with a right hemiparesis. His current medications include aspirin, losartan, hydrochlorothiazide, fluticasone/salmeterol, tiotropium, and albuterol. His body mass index is 18.5 kg/m^2. You are concerned that he may have vitamin D deficiency. Which of the following is the best test to determine if vitamin D deficiency is present?

A. 1,25-hydroxy vitamin D
B. 25-hydroxy vitamin D
C. Alkaline phosphatase
D. Parathyroid hormone
E. Serum total and ionized calcium levels

91. A 72-year-old woman has hospitalized with a right hip fracture. After initial surgical repair, she is transferred to rehabilitation for further care. While there,

91. *(Continued)*
she has a 25-hydroxy-vitamin D level checked, and it returns at 18.3 ng/L. What do you recommend for the treatment of this patient?

A. Vitamin D3 800 units daily
B. Vitamin D3 800 units daily plus calcium carbonate 1500 mg daily
C. Vitamin D3 2000 units daily
D. Vitamin D3 2000 units daily plus calcium carbonate 1500 mg daily
E. Vitamin D3 50,000 units weekly for 4 weeks then 800 units weekly, plus calcium 1500 mg daily

92. A 66-year-old man presents to the urgent care center with vague complaints of nausea and decreased appetite over the last 4–6 weeks. Physical examination reveals normal vital signs and no abnormality other than a thin man with mild diffuse abdominal tenderness without guarding or rebound. The patient is found to have reduced serum calcium of 7.8 mg/dL. He denies any musculoskeletal symptoms. Additional laboratory studies are presented below:

Sodium	139 mEq/dL
Bicarbonate	26 mEq/dL
Creatinine	1.2 mg/dL
Glucose	109 mg/dL
Total protein	6.2 g/dL
Albumin	2.0 g/dL
Bilirubin	1.2 mg/dL
Potassium	3.8 mg/dL

For the patient's hypocalcemia, what of the following is the most appropriate response?

A. Administer calcium gluconate 1 g intravenously
B. Check magnesium levels and replete if deficient
C. Check vitamin D levels and replete if deficient
D. No further response necessary
E. Prescribe oral calcium bicarbonate daily

93. Mr. Wassim is a 45-year-old man with metastatic nonsmall cell lung cancer undergoing chemotherapy. He presents to the hospital after his family noted that he was confused. Serum calcium is 11.5 mg/dL with a serum albumin of 2.5 g/dL. Vital signs are: HR 132 beats/min, blood pressure 90/55 mmHg, respiratory rate 18/min, temperature 37.2°C. What is the first appropriate therapeutic response for his hypercalcemia?

A. Furosemide 80 mg intravenously
B. Aggressive hydration with intravenous saline
C. Hydrocortisone 100 mg daily

93. *(Continued)*
D. No therapy is needed—the corrected serum calcium is normal
E. Zoledronic acid 4 mg intravenously

94. A 60-year-old woman is referred to your office for evaluation of hypercalcemia. A serum calcium level of 12.9 mg/dL was found incidentally on a chemistry panel that was drawn during a hospitalization for cholecystectomy. Despite fluid administration in the hospital, her serum calcium at discharge was 11.8 mg/dL. The patient is asymptomatic, and her parathyroid hormone level is 95 ng/L (reference value 10–65 ng/L). She is otherwise in good health and has had her recommended age-appropriate cancer screening. She denies constipation or bone pain and is now 8 weeks out from her surgical procedure. Today, her serum calcium level is 12.6 mg/dL, and phosphate is 2.3 mg/dL. Her hematocrit and all other chemistries including creatinine were normal. Which of the following would be an indication for surgery in this patient to definitively treat her underlying diagnosis?

A. Age >50
B. Elevated 24-hour urine calcium
C. Nephrolithiasis
D. Osteopenia on bone density testing
E. Serum calcium >1 mg/dL above normal

95. A 42-year-old man presents to the emergency department with acute onset right-sided flank pain. He describes the pain as 10 out of 10 in severity radiating to the groin. He has had one episode of hematuria. A noncontrast CT scan confirms the presence of a right sided renal stone that is currently located in the distal ureter. He has a past medical history of pulmonary sarcoidosis that is not currently treated. This was diagnosed by bronchoscopic biopsy showing noncaseating granulomas. His chest radiograph shows bilateral hilar adenopathy. His serum calcium level is 12.6 mg/dL. What is the mechanism of hypercalcemia in this patient?

A. Increased activation of 25-hydroxy vitamin D to 1,25-hydroxy vitamin D by macrophages within granulomas
B. Increased activation of 25-hydroxy vitamin D to 1,25-hydroxy vitamin D by the kidney
C. Increased activation of vitamin D to 25-hydroxy vitamin D by macrophages within granulomas
D. Missed diagnosis of lymphoma with subsequent bone marrow invasion and resorption of bone through local destruction
E. Production of parathyroid hormone-related peptide by macrophages within granulomas

96. A 52-year-old man has end stage kidney disease from long-standing hypertension and diabetes mellitus. He has been managed with hemodialysis for the past 8 years. Throughout this time, he has been poorly compliant with his medications and hemodialysis schedule, frequently missing one session weekly. He is now complaining of bone pain and dyspnea. His oxygen saturation is noted to be 92% on room air, and his chest radiograph shows hazy bilateral infiltrates. Chest CT shows ground glass infiltrates bilaterally. His laboratory data include a calcium of 12.3 mg/dL, phosphate of 8.1 mg/dL, and parathyroid hormone is 110 pg/mL. Which of the following would be the best approach to the treatment of the patient's current clinical condition?

A. Calcitriol 0.5 μg intravenously with hemodialysis with sevelamer three times daily
B. Calcitriol 0.5 μg orally daily with sevelamer 1600 mg three times daily
C. More aggressive hemodialysis to achieve optimal fluid and electrolyte balance
D. Parathyroidectomy
E. Sevelamer 1600 mg three times daily

97. A 54-year-old woman undergoes total thyroidectomy for follicular carcinoma of the thyroid. About 6 hours after surgery, the patient complains of tingling around her mouth. She subsequently develops a pins-and-needles sensation in the fingers and toes. The nurse calls the physician to the bedside to evaluate the patient after she has severe hand cramps when her blood pressure is taken. Upon evaluation, the patient is still complaining of intermittent cramping of her hands. Since surgery, she has received morphine sulfate for pain and metoclopramide for nausea. She has had no change in her vital signs and is afebrile. Tapping on the inferior portion of the zygomatic arch 2 cm anterior to the ear produces twitching at the corner of the mouth. An electrocardiogram (ECG) shows a QT interval of 575 ms. What is the next step in evaluation and treatment of this patient?

A. Administration of benztropine
B. Administration of calcium gluconate
C. Administration of magnesium sulphate
D. Measurement of calcium, magnesium, phosphate, and potassium levels
E. Measurement of forced vital capacity

98. A 68-year-old woman with stage IIIB squamous cell carcinoma of the lung is admitted to the hospital because of altered mental status and dehydration. Upon admission, she is found to have a calcium level of 19.6 mg/dL and phosphate of 1.8 mg/dL. Concomitant measurement of parathyroid hormone was 0.1 pg/mL (normal 10–65 pg/mL), and a screen for parathyroid hormone-related peptide was positive. Over the first 24 hours, the patient receives 4 L of normal saline with furosemide diuresis. The next morning, the patient's calcium is 17.6 mg/dL and phosphate is 2.2 mg/dL. She continues to have delirium. What is the best approach for ongoing treatment of this patient's hypercalcemia?

A. Continue therapy with large-volume fluid administration and forced diuresis with furosemide.
B. Continue therapy with large-volume fluid administration, but stop furosemide and treat with hydrochlorothiazide.
C. Initiate therapy with calcitonin alone.
D. Initiate therapy with pamidronate alone.
E. Initiate therapy with calcitonin and pamidronate.

99. Which of the following statements regarding the epidemiology of osteoporosis and bone fractures is correct?

A. For every 5-year period after age 70, the incidence of hip fractures increases by 25%.
B. Fractures of the distal radius increase in frequency before age 50 and plateau by age 60 with only a modest age-related increase.
C. Most women meet the diagnostic criteria for osteoporosis between the ages of 60–70.
D. The risk of hip fracture is equal when white women are compared to black women.
E. Women outnumber men with osteoporosis at a ratio of about 10 to 1.

100. A 50-year-old woman presents to your office to inquire about her risk of fracture related to osteoporosis. She has a positive family history of osteoporosis in her mother, but her mother never experienced any hip or vertebral fractures. The patient herself has also not experienced any fractures. She is Caucasian and has a 20 pack-year history of tobacco, quitting 10 years prior. At the age of 37, she had a total hysterectomy with bilateral salpingo-oophorectomy for endometriosis. She is lactose intolerant and does not consume dairy products. She currently takes calcium carbonate 500 mg daily. Her weight is 115 lb and her height is 66 in (BMI 18.6 kg/m^2). All of the following are risk factors for an osteoporotic fracture in this woman EXCEPT:

A. Early menopause
B. Female sex

100. *(Continued)*

C. History of cigarette smoking
D. Low body weight
E. Low calcium intake

101. A 54-year-old woman is referred to endocrinology clinic for evaluation of osteoporosis after a recent examination for back pain revealed a compression fracture of the T_4 vertebral body. She is perimenopausal with irregular menstrual periods and frequent hot flashes. She does not smoke. She otherwise is well and healthy. Her weight is 70 kg, and height is 168 cm. She has lost 5 cm from her maximum height. A bone mineral density scan shows a T-score of −3.5 SD and a Z-score of −2.5 SD. All of the following tests are indicated for the evaluation of osteoporosis in this patient EXCEPT:

A. 24-hour urine calcium
B. Follicle-stimulating hormone and luteinizing hormone levels
C. Serum calcium
D. Thyroid stimulating hormone
E. Vitamin D levels (25-hydroxyvitamin D)

102. A 45-year-old Caucasian woman seeks advice from her primary care physician regarding her risk for osteoporosis and the need for bone density screening. She is a lifelong nonsmoker and drinks alcohol only socially. She has a history of moderate-persistent asthma since adolescence. She is currently on fluticasone, 44 mg/puff twice daily, with good control currently. She last required oral prednisone therapy about 6 months ago when she had influenza that was complicated by an asthma flare. She took prednisone for a total of 14 days. She has had three pregnancies and two live births at ages 39 and 41. She currently has irregular periods occurring approximately every 42 days. Her follicle-stimulating hormone level is 25 mIU/L and 17β-estradiol level is 115 pg/mL on day 12 of her menstrual cycle. Her mother and maternal aunt both have been diagnosed with osteoporosis. Her mother also has rheumatoid arthritis and requires prednisone therapy, 5 mg daily. Her mother developed a compression fracture of the lumbar spine at age 68. On physical examination, the patient appears well and healthy. Her height is 168 cm. Her weight is 66.4 kg. The chest, cardiac, abdominal, muscular, and neurologic examinations are normal. What do you tell the patient about the need for bone density screening?

102. *(Continued)*

A. As she is currently perimenopausal, she should have a bone density screen every other year until she completes menopause and then have bone densitometry measured yearly thereafter.
B. Because of her family history, she should initiate bone density screening yearly beginning now.
C. Bone densitometry screening is not recommended until after completion of menopause.
D. Delayed childbearing until the fourth and fifth decade decreases her risk of developing osteoporosis so bone densitometry is not recommended.
E. Her use of low-dose inhaled glucocorticoids increases her risk of osteoporosis threefold, and she should undergo yearly bone density screening.

103–107. Match the following medications used for osteoporosis to the mechanism of action:

103. Calcitonin
104. Denosumab
105. Raloxifene
106. Teriparatide
107. Zoledronic acid

A. Recombinant parathyroid hormone (1-34hPTH) with direct stimulation of osteoblast activity
B. Polypeptide hormone that suppresses osteoclast activity through a specific receptor for the hormone
C. Bisphosphonate drug given on an annual basis that impairs osteoclast function and reduces osteoclast number
D. Selective estrogen receptor modulator
E. Human monoclonal antibody to RANKL, a protein necessary for osteoclast maturation

108. A 38-year-old woman with cystic fibrosis and vitamin D deficiency has a T-score of −2.8 in the lumbar spine and hip. She is initiated on treatment with alendronate 70 mg weekly, cholecalciferol 5000 units daily, and calcium carbonate 1500 mg daily. When should the bone densitometry testing be repeated to assess the response to therapy?

A. One year
B. Three years
C. Five years
D. Ten years
E. It does not need to be repeated. MRI imaging should be performed instead

ANSWERS

1. **The answer is C.**
(Chap. 3) Hormones produced by the anterior pituitary include adrenocorticotropic hormone, thyroid stimulating hormone, luteinizing hormone, follicle stimulating hormone, prolactin and growth hormone. The posterior pituitary produces vasopressin and oxytocin. The anterior and posterior pituitary have separate vascular supply and the posterior pituitary is directly innervated by the hypothalamic neurons via the pituitary stalk, thus making it susceptible to shear stress associated dysfunction. Hypothalamic control of anterior pituitary function is through secreted hormones, thus it is less susceptible to traumatic injury.

2. **The answer is D.**
(Chap. 3) Functional pituitary adenoma presentations include acromegaly, as in this patient, prolactinomas or Cushing's syndrome. Hypersecretion of growth hormone underlies this syndrome in patients with pituitary masses, though ectopic production of growth hormone, particularly by tumors, has been reported. Because growth hormone is secreted in a highly pulsatile fashion, obtaining random serum levels are not reliable. Thus, the downstream mediator of systemic effects of growth hormone, IGF-1, is measured to screen for growth hormone excess. IGF-1 is made by the liver in response to growth hormone stimulation. An oral glucose tolerance test with growth hormone obtained at 0, 30, and 60 minutes may also be used to screen for acromegaly as normal persons should suppress growth hormone to this challenge. Serum prolactin level is useful to screen for prolactinomas, 24-hour urinary free cortisol and ACTH assay are useful screens for Cushing's disease.

3. **The answer is D.**
(Chap. 3) The pituitary gland does form from Rathke's pouch embryonically. As shown below, blood supply of the pituitary gland comes from the superior and inferior hypophyseal arteries. The hypothalamic pituitary portal plexus provides the major blood source for the anterior pituitary, allowing reliable transmission of hypothalamic peptide pulses without significant systemic dilution; consequently, pituitary cells are exposed to releasing or inhibiting factors and in turn release their hormones as discrete pulses into the systemic circulation. The posterior pituitary is supplied by the inferior hypophyseal arteries. In contrast to the anterior pituitary, the posterior lobe is directly innervated by hypothalamic neurons (supraopticohypophyseal and tuberohypophyseal nerve tracts) via the pituitary stalk. Thus, posterior pituitary production of vasopressin (antidiuretic hormone [ADH]) and oxytocin is particularly sensitive to neuronal damage by lesions that affect the pituitary stalk or hypothalamus. ACTH is derived from POMC, and prolactin is secreted in the posterior pituitary (see **Figure 3-2**).

4. **The answer is C.**
(Chap. 3) Adult growth hormone deficiency is usually caused by hypothalamic or pituitary damage. Because growth hormone is no longer important for achieving stature, the presentation is different from childhood growth hormone deficiency. Although growth hormone has direct tissue effects, it primarily acts through increasing secretion of IGF-1 which in turn stimulate lipolysis, increase circulating fatty acids, reduced omental fat mass and enhanced lean body mass. Thus, deficiency of growth hormone causes the opposite effects. In addition, hypertension, left ventricular dysfunction, and increased plasma fibrinogen levels may also be present with deficient growth hormone. Reduced, not increased, bone mineral density may also occur in adults with growth hormone deficiency.

5. **The answer is E.**
(Chap. 3) The patient has a clinical presentation consistent with Cushing's syndrome. Although many cases of inappropriate elevation of ACTH are due to pituitary tumors, a substantial proportion is due to ectopic ACTH secretion. Clues to this diagnosis include a rapid onset of hypercortisolism features associated with skin hyperpigmentation and severe myopathy. Additionally, hypertension, hypokalemic metabolic alkalosis, glucose intolerance, and edema are more prominent in ectopic ACTH secretion than in pituitary tumors. Serum potassium <3.3 mmol/L is present in 70% of ectopic ACTH cases, but <10% of pituitary-dependent Cushing's syndrome. ACTH levels will be high, as this is the underlying cause of both types of Cushing's syndrome. Corticotropin releasing hormone is rarely the cause of Cushing's syndrome. Unfortunately, MRI of the pituitary gland will not visualize lesions <2 mm, thus occasionally sampling of the inferior petrosal veins is required, but this is not yet indicated in the case presented at this time in the evaluation.

6. **The answer is A.**
(Chap. 4) Kallmann's syndrome results from defective hypothalamic gonadotropin-releasing hormone

(GnRH) synthesis and is associated with anosmia or hyposmia due to olfactory bulb agenesis or hypoplasia. Classically, the syndrome may also be associated with color blindness, optic atrophy, nerve deafness, cleft palate, renal abnormalities, cryptorchidism, and neurologic abnormalities such as mirror movements. Associated clinical features, in addition to GnRH deficiency, vary depending on the genetic cause. GnRH deficiency prevents progression through puberty. Males present with delayed puberty and pronounced hypogonadal features, including micropenis, probably the result of low testosterone levels during infancy. Females present with primary amenorrhea and failure of secondary sexual development. A white forelock is typical of Waardenburg's syndrome, while hyperphagia obesity is common in Prader-Willi syndrome.

7. **The answer is B.**
   (Chap. 4) The patient has evidence of Sheehan's syndrome postpartum. In this syndrome, the hyperplastic pituitary postpartum is at increased risk for hemorrhage and/or infarction. This leads to bilateral visual changes, headache, and meningeal signs. Ophthalmoplegia may be observed. In severe cases, cardiovascular collapse and altered levels of consciousness may be observed. Laboratory evaluation commonly shows hypoglycemia. Pituitary CT or MRI may show signs of sellar hemorrhage if present. Involvement of all pituitary hormones may be seen, though the most acute finding is often hypoglycemia and hypotension from failure of adrenocorticotropic hormone. The hypoglycemia and hypotension present in this case suggest failure of glucocorticoid system, thus treatment with a corticosteroid is indicated. There is no evidence of sepsis, thus antibiotics and drotrecogin alfa are not indicated. With a normal hematocrit and no reported evidence of massive hemorrhage, packed red cell transfusion is unlikely to be helpful. Although thyroid stimulating hormone production is undoubtedly low in this patient, the most immediate concern is replacement of glucocorticoid.

8. **The answer is C.**
   (Chap. 4) Cranial irradiation may result in long-term hypothalamic and pituitary dysfunction, especially in children and adolescents, as they are more susceptible to damage after whole-brain or head and neck therapeutic irradiation. The development of hormonal abnormalities correlates strongly with irradiation dosage and the time interval after completion of radiotherapy. Up to two-thirds of patients ultimately develop hormone insufficiency after a median dose of 50 Gy (5000 rad) directed at the skull base. The development of hypopituitarism occurs over 5–15 years and usually reflects hypothalamic damage rather than primary destruction of pituitary cells. Although the pattern of hormone loss is variable, growth hormone deficiency is most common, followed by gonadotropin and ACTH deficiency. When deficiency of one or more hormones is documented, the possibility of diminished reserve of other hormones is likely. Accordingly, anterior pituitary function should be continually evaluated over the long term in previously irradiated patients, and replacement therapy instituted when appropriate.

9. **The answer is C.**
   (Chap. 4) The patient has panhypopituitarism and is unable to make TSH; thus her plasma TSH level will always be low, regardless of the adequacy of her T_4 replacement. A free T_4 level will allow determination of whether her plasma level is in the normal range of thyroid hormone. This, coupled with her symptoms, will aid in determination of proper levothyroxine dosing. There is no evidence of recurrent disease clinically, thus MRI is not useful. She is unlikely to have primary thyroid disease, and T_4 level is unknown presently, so thyroid uptake scan is not indicated at this time.

10. **The answer is B.**
   (Chap. 4) The identification of an empty sella is often the result of an incidental MRI finding. Typically these patients will have normal pituitary function and should be reassured. It is likely that the surrounding rim of pituitary tissue is functioning normally. An empty sella may signal the insidious onset of hypopituitarism, and laboratory results should be followed closely. Unless her clinical situation changes, repeat MRI is not indicated. Endocrine malignancy is unlikely, and surgery is not part of the management of an empty sella.

11. **The answer is E.**
   (Chap. 5) The dorsal sellar diaphragm presents the least resistance to soft tissue expansion from the sella; consequently, pituitary adenomas frequently extend in a suprasellar direction. Bony invasion may occur as well.

12. **The answer is E.**
   (Chap. 5) Pituitary gland height ranges from 6 mm in children to 8 mm in adults; during pregnancy and puberty, the height may reach 10–12 mm. The upper aspect of the adult pituitary is flat or slightly concave, but in adolescent and pregnant individuals,

this surface may be convex, reflecting physiologic pituitary enlargement. The stalk should be midline and vertical. Anterior pituitary gland soft tissue consistency is slightly heterogeneous on MRI, and signal intensity resembles that of brain matter on T1-weighted imaging. Adenoma density is usually lower than that of surrounding normal tissue on T1-weighted imaging, and the signal intensity increases with T2-weighted images. The high phospholipid content of the posterior pituitary results in a "pituitary bright spot."

13. **The answer is C.**
(Chap. 5) Because optic tracts may be contiguous to an expanding pituitary mass, reproducible visual field assessment using perimetry techniques should be performed on all patients with sellar mass lesions that impinge the optic chiasm. Bitemporal hemianopia, often more pronounced superiorly, is observed classically. It occurs because nasal ganglion cell fibers, which cross in the optic chiasm, are especially vulnerable to compression of the ventral optic chiasm. Occasionally, homonymous hemianopia occurs from postchiasmal compression or monocular temporal field loss from prechiasmal compression.

14. **The answer is D.**
(Chap. 5) Carney's syndrome is characterized by spotty skin pigmentation, myxomas, and endocrine tumors, including testicular, adrenal, and pituitary adenomas. Acromegaly occurs in about 20% of these patients. A subset of patients have mutations in the R1α regulatory subunit of protein kinase A (PRKAR1A).

15. **The answer is B.**
(Chap. 7) Nutritional and maternal iodine deficiencies are common in many parts of the developing world and, when severe, can result in cretinism. Cretinism is characterized by mental and growth retardation, but is preventable by administration of iodine and/or thyroid hormone early in life. Concomitant selenium deficiency can contribute to the neurologic manifestations. Iodine supplementation of bread, salt, and other foods has markedly decreased the rates of this disease. Beriberi disease is a nervous system ailment caused by a thiamine deficiency in the diet. Scurvy is due to vitamin C deficiency. Folate deficiency in pregnant women is associated with increased risk preterm labor and a number of congenital malformations, most notably involving the neural tube. Folate supplementation can lower the risk of spina bifida, anencephaly, congenital heart disease, cleft lips, and limb deformities. Vitamin A deficiency is a common cause of blindness in the developing world.

16. **The answer is C.**
(Chap. 7) There are a number of conditions associated with normal thyroid function, but hyperthyroxinemia. Although some of these are associated with clinical hyperthyroidism, many have simply elevated levels of total T_4 and normal conversion to T_3 and thus are clinically normal. Anything that increases liver production of thyroid binding globulin will produce elevated total T_4 levels and normal free T_4 and T_3 levels. In this category are pregnancy, estrogen containing oral contraceptives, cirrhosis, and familial excess thyroid binding globulin production. Familial dysalbuminemic hyperthyroxinemia results in an albumin mutation and increased T_4 with normal free T_4 and T_3 levels. Sick euthyroid syndrome occurs during acute medical and psychiatric illness. In this syndrome, there is transiently increased unbound T_4 and decreased TSH. Total T_4 and T_3 may be decreased particularly later in the course of disease.

17. **The answer is D.**
(Chap. 7) Iodine deficiency remains the most common cause of hypothyroidism worldwide. It is present at relatively high levels even in the developed world including Europe. In areas of iodine sufficiency, autoimmune disease (Hashimoto's thyroiditis) and iatrogenic hypothyroidism (treatment of hyperthyroidism) are the most common causes.

18. **The answer is A.**
(Chap. 7) There are a number of important effects of thyroid hormone (or its absence) on the cardiovascular system. Importantly, hypothyroidism is associated with bradycardia, reduced myocardial contractility and thereby reduced stroke volume. Increased peripheral resistance may be accompanied by systemic hypertension, particularly diastolic in hypothyroidism. Pericardial effusions are found in up to 30% of patients with hypothyroidism, though they rarely cause decreased cardiac function. Finally, in hypothyroid patients, blood flow is directed away from the skin and thus produces cool extremities.

19. **The answer is A.**
(Chap. 7) The most common cause of hypothyroidism in the United States is autoimmune thyroiditis, as it is an iodine-replete area. Although earlier in the disease, a radioiodine uptake scan may have shown diffusely increased uptake from lymphocytic infiltration, at this point in the disease when the infiltrate is "burned out" there is likely to be little found on the

scan. Likewise, a thyroid ultrasound would only be useful for presumed multinodular goiter. Antithyroid peroxidase antibodies are commonly found in patients with autoimmune thyroiditis, while antithyroglobulin antibodies are found less commonly. Antithyroglobulin antibodies are also found in other thyroid disorders (Graves' disease, thyrotoxicosis) as well as systemic autoimmune diseases (SLE; SLE refers to systemic lupus erythematosus). Thyroglobulin is released from the thyroid in all types of thyrotoxicosis with the exception of factitious disease. This patient, however, was hypothyroid and thus serum thyroglobulin levels are unlikely to be helpful.

20. The answer is D.
(Chap. 7) An increase in TSH in a patient with hypothyroidism that was previously stable in dosing for many years suggests either a failure of taking the medication, difficulty with absorption from bowel disease or medication interaction or drug-drug interaction affecting clearance. Patients with normal body weight taking >200 μg of levothyroxine per day with elevated TSH strongly suggest noncompliance. Such patients should be encouraged to take two tablets at one time on the day they remember to attempt to reach the weekly target dose; the long drug half-life makes this practice safe. Other causes of increased thyroxine requirements include malabsorption, such as with celiac disease or small bowel surgery, estrogen therapy, and drugs that interfere with T_4 absorption (e.g., ferrous sulfate and cholestyramine) or clearance, such as lovastatin, amiodarone, carbamazepine, and phenytoin.

21. The answer is A.
(Chap. 7) The patient has myxedema coma. This condition of profound hypothyroidism most commonly occurs in the elderly and often a precipitating condition may be identified such as myocardial infarction or infection. Clinical manifestations include altered level of consciousness, bradycardia, and hypothermia. Management includes repletion of thyroid hormone through IV levothyroxine, but also supplementation of glucocorticoids because there is impaired adrenal reserve in severe hypothyroidism. Care must be taken with rewarming as it may precipitate cardiovascular collapse. Therefore, external warming is indicated only if the temperature is <30°C. Hypertonic saline and glucose may be used if hyponatremia or hypoglycemia is severe; however, hypotonic solutions should be avoided as they may worsen fluid retention. Because metabolism of many substances is markedly reduced, sedation should be avoided or minimized. Similarly, blood levels of drugs should be monitored when available.

22. The answer is A.
(Chap. 7) Patients with Graves' disease produce thyroid stimulating immunoglobulins. They subsequently produce higher levels of T_4 compared with the normal population. As a result, many patients with Graves' disease are mildly iodine deficient and T_4 production is somewhat limited by the availability of iodine. Exposure to iodinated contrast thus reverses iodine deficiency and may precipitate worsening hyperthyroidism. Additionally, the reversal of mild iodine deficiency may make I-125 therapy for Graves' disease less successful because thyroid iodine uptake is lessened in the iodine-replete state.

23. The answer is C.
(Chap. 8) The adrenal gland has three major functions: (1) glucocorticoid synthesis, (2) aldosterone synthesis, and (3) androgen precursor synthesis. Glucocorticoid synthesis is controlled by the pituitary secretion of ACTH. The primary stimulus for aldosterone synthesis is the renin-angiotensin-aldosterone system, which is independent of the pituitary. Thus, morning cortisol secretion, release of cortisol in response to stress are regulated by the pituitary gland, while regulation of sodium retention and potassium excretion by aldosterone is independent of the pituitary and would be preserved in this patient.

24. The answer is A.
(Chap. 8) Cushing's syndrome is a constellation of features that result from chronic exposure to elevated levels of cortisol from any etiology. Although the most common etiology is ACTH-producing pituitary adenoma which accounts for 75% of Cushing's syndrome, 15% is due to ectopic ACTH syndromes such as bronchial or pancreatic tumors, small cell lung cancer and others. ACTH-independent Cushing's syndrome is much rarer. Adrenocortical adenoma underlies 5–10% of cases and adrenocortical carcinoma is present in 1% of Cushing's cases. McCune-Albright syndrome is a genetic cause of bone abnormalities, skin lesions (cafe au lait), and premature puberty particularly in girls. Interestingly, it is caused by a sporadic in utero mutation, not an inherited disorder, and thus will not be passed onto progeny.

25. The answer is B.
(Chap. 8) Conn's syndrome refers to an aldosterone producing adrenal adenoma. Although it accounts for 40% of hyperaldosterone states, bilateral micronodular adrenal hyperplasia is more common. Other causes of hyperaldosteronism are substantially more rare, accounting for <1% of disease. The hallmark of Conn's syndrome is hypertension

with hypokalemia. Because aldosterone stimulates sodium retention and potassium excretion, all patients should be hypokalemic at presentation. Serum sodium is usually normal because of concurrent fluid retention. Hypokalemia may be associated with muscle weakness, proximal myopathy or even paralysis. Hypokalemia may be exacerbated by thiazide diuretics. Additional features include metabolic alkalosis that may contribute to muscle cramps and tetany.

26. The answer is B.
(Chap. 8) Incidental adrenal masses are often discovered during radiographic testing for another condition and are found in ~6% of adult subjects at autopsy. Fifty percent of patients with a history of malignancy and a newly discovered adrenal mass will actually have an adrenal metastasis. Fine-needle aspiration of a suspected metastatic malignancy will often be diagnostic. In the absence of a suspected nonadrenal malignancy, most adrenal incidentalomas are benign. Primary adrenal malignancies are uncommon (<0.01%), and fine-needle aspiration is not useful to distinguish between benign and malignant primary adrenal tumors. Although 90% of these masses are nonsecretory, patients with an incidentaloma should be screened for pheochromocytoma and hypercortisolism with plasma-free metanephrines and an overnight dexamethasone suppression test, respectively. When radiographic features suggest a benign neoplasm (<3 cm), scanning should be repeated in 3–6 months. When masses are >6 cm, surgical removal (if more likely primary adrenal malignancy) or fine-needle aspiration (if more likely metastatic malignancy) is preferred.

27. The answer is C.
(Chap. 8) The release of CRH, and subsequently ACTH, occurs in a pulsatile fashion that follows a circadian rhythm under the control of the hypothalamus, specifically its suprachiasmatic nucleus (SCN), with additional regulation by a complex network of cell-specific clock genes. Reflecting the pattern of ACTH secretion, adrenal cortisol secretion exhibits a distinct circadian rhythm, starting to rise in the early morning hours prior to awakening, with peak levels in the morning and low levels in the evening (see **Figure 8-3**).

28. The answer is B.
(Chap. 8) This patient has obesity, abdominal stria, and a round (or moon) facies—all signs of glucocorticoid excess. Often, this is due to exogenous (corticosteroid) administration, though it could also be due to endogenous production (Cushing's syndrome). A physiologic stressor, such as trauma or infection, may trigger adrenal crisis. Importantly (though not present in this case), hyperthyroidism can also trigger adrenal crisis via increased glucocorticoid inactivation. Thus, glucocorticoids must always be provided first in the setting of concomitant thyroid and adrenal insufficiency. Acute adrenal insufficiency requires immediate initiation of rehydration, usually carried out by saline infusion at initial rates of 1 L/h with continuous cardiac monitoring. Glucocorticoid replacement should be initiated by bolus injection of 100 mg hydrocortisone, followed by the administration of 100–200 mg hydrocortisone over 24 hours, either by continuous infusion or by bolus IV or IM injections. Mineralocorticoid replacement can be initiated once the daily hydrocortisone dose has been reduced to <50 mg because at higher doses hydrocortisone provides sufficient stimulation of mineralocorticoid receptors.

29. The answer is A.
(Chap. 9) When the diagnosis of pheochromocytoma is entertained the first step is measurement of catecholamines and/or metanephrines. This can be achieved by urinary tests for vanillylmandelic acid, catecholamines, fractionated metanephrines or total metanephrines. Total metanephrines has a high sensitivity and therefore is frequently used. A value of three times the upper limit of normal is highly suggestive of pheochromocytoma. Borderline elevations, as this patient had, are likely to be false positives. The next most appropriate step is to remove potentially confounding dietary or drug exposures, if possible, and repeat the test. Likely culprit drugs include levodopa, sympathomimetics, diuretics, tricyclic antidepressants, and alpha and beta blockers (labetalol in this case). Sertraline is an SSRI antidepressant, not a tricyclic. Alternatively, a clonidine suppression test may be ordered.

30. The answer is E.
(Chap. 9) Complete removal of the pheochromocytoma is the only therapy that leads to a long-term cure, although 90% of tumors are benign. However, preoperative control of hypertension is necessary to prevent surgical complications and lower mortality. This patient is presenting with encephalopathy in a hypertensive crisis. The hypertension should be managed initially with IV medications to lower the mean arterial pressure by ~20% over the initial 24-hour period. Medications that can be used for hypertensive crisis in pheochromocytoma include nitroprusside, nicardipine, and phentolamine. Once

the acute hypertensive crisis has resolved, transition to oral α-adrenergic blockers is indicated. Phenoxybenzamine is the most commonly used drug and is started at low doses (5–10 mg three times daily) and titrated to the maximum tolerated dose (usually 20–30 mg daily). Once alpha blockers have been initiated, beta blockade can safely be utilized and is particularly indicated for ongoing tachycardia. Liberal salt and fluid intake helps expand plasma volume and treat orthostatic hypotension. Once blood pressure is maintained below 160/100 mmHg with moderate orthostasis, it is safe to proceed to surgery. If blood pressure remains elevated despite treatment with alpha blockade, addition of calcium channel blockers, angiotensin receptor blockers, or angiotensin-converting enzyme inhibitors should be considered. Diuretics should be avoided as they will exacerbate orthostasis.

31. The answer is D.
(Chap. 9) The diagnosis of malignant pheochromocytoma is problematic. The typical histologic criteria of cellular atypia, presence of mitoses, and invasion of vessels or adjacent tissues are insufficient for the diagnosis of malignancy in pheochromocytoma. Thus, the term malignant pheochromocytoma is restricted to tumors with distant metastases, most commonly found by nuclear medicine imaging in lungs, bone, or liver—locations suggesting a vascular pathway of spread.

32. The answer is C.
(Chap. 10) Klinefelter's syndrome is a chromosomal disorder with 47,XXY. Because the primary feature of this disorder is gonadal failure, low testosterone is present and thus increased LH and FSH are produced in an attempt to increase testosterone production in the feedback loop of sex hormones. Increased estrogen is often produced because of chronic Leydig cell stimulation by LH and because of aromatization of androstenedione by adipose tissue. The lower testosterone:estrogen ratio results in mild feminization with gynecomastia. Features of low testosterone are small testes and "eunuchoid" proportions with long legs and incomplete virilization. Biopsy of the testes, though rarely performed, shows hyalinization of the seminiferous tubules and azoospermia. Although severe cases are diagnosed prepubertally with small testes and impaired androgenization, approximately 75% of cases are not diagnosed and the frequency in the general population is 1/1000. Patients with Klinefelter's syndrome are at increased risk of breast tumors, thromboembolic disease, learning difficulties, obesity, diabetes mellitus (DM), and varicose veins.

33. The answer is A.
(Chap. 10) Turner's syndrome most frequently results from a 45,X karyotype, but mosaicism (45,X/46,XX) also can result in this disorder. Clinically, Turner's syndrome manifests as short stature and primary amenorrhea if presenting in young adulthood. In addition, chronic lymphedema of the hands and feet, nuchal folds, a low hairline, and high arched palate are also common features. To diagnose Turner's syndrome, karyotype analysis should be performed. A Barr body results from inactivation of one of the X chromosomes in women and is not seen in males. In Turner's syndrome, the Barr body should be absent, but only 50% of individuals with Turner's syndrome have the 45,X karyotype. Thus, the diagnosis could be missed in those with mosaicism or other structural abnormalities of the X chromosome. Multiple comorbid conditions are found in individuals with Turner's syndrome, and appropriate screening is recommended. Congenital heart defects affect 30% of women with Turner's syndrome, including bicuspid aortic valve, coarctation of the aorta, and aortic root dilatation. An echocardiogram should be performed, and the individual should be assessed with blood pressures in the arms and legs. Hypertension can also be associated with structural abnormalities of the kidney and urinary tract, most commonly horseshoe kidney. A renal ultrasound is also recommended. Autoimmune thyroid disease affects 15–30% of women with Turner's syndrome and should be assessed by screening TSH. Other comorbidities that may occur include sensorineural hearing loss, elevated liver function enzymes, osteoporosis, and celiac disease.

34. The answer is C.
(Chap. 10) This infant likely has congenital adrenal hyperplasia. The classic form of 21-hydroxylase deficiency (21-OHD) is the most common cause of CAH. It has an incidence between 1 in 10,000 and 1 in 15,000 and is the most common cause of androgenization in chromosomal 46,XX females. Affected individuals are homozygous or compound heterozygous for severe mutations in the enzyme 21-hydroxylase (CYP21A2). This mutation causes a block in adrenal glucocorticoid and mineralocorticoid synthesis, increasing 17-hydroxyprogesterone and shunting steroid precursors into the androgen synthesis pathway. Glucocorticoid insufficiency causes a compensatory elevation of adrenocorticotropin (ACTH), resulting in adrenal hyperplasia and additional synthesis of

steroid precursors proximal to the enzymatic block. Increased androgen synthesis in utero causes androgenization of the 46,XX fetus in the first trimester. Ambiguous genitalia are seen at birth, with varying degrees of clitoral enlargement and labial fusion. The salt-wasting form of 21-OHD results from severe combined glucocorticoid and mineralocorticoid deficiency. A salt-wasting crisis usually manifests between 5 and 21 days of life and is a potentially life threatening event that requires urgent fluid resuscitation and steroid treatment. Thus, a diagnosis of 21-OHD should be considered in any baby with atypical genitalia with bilateral nonpalpable gonads.

35. The answer is D.
(Chap. 11) Gynecomastia is a relatively common complaint in men and may be caused by either obesity with adipose tissue expansion in the breast or by an increased estrogen/androgen ratio in which there is true glandular enlargement, as in this case. If the breast is unilaterally enlarged or if it is hard or fixed to underlying tissue, mammography is indicated. Alternatively, if cirrhosis or a causative drug is present, these may be adequate explanations, particularly when gynecomastia develops later in life in previously fertile men. If the breast tissue is >4 cm or there is evidence of very small testes and no causative drugs or liver disease, a search for alterations in serum testosterone, LH, FSH estradiol, and hCG levels should be undertaken. An androgen deficiency or resistance syndrome may be present or an hCG secreting tumor may be found. In this case, spironolactone is the likely culprit and it may be stopped or switched to eplerenone and gynecomastia reassessed.

36. The answer is C.
(Chap. 11) Many drugs may interfere with testicular function through a variety of mechanisms. Cyclophosphamide damages the seminiferous tubules in a dose- and time-dependent fashion and causes azoospermia within a few weeks of initiation. This effect is reversible in approximately half these patients. Ketoconazole inhibits testosterone synthesis. Spironolactone causes a blockade of androgen action which may also cause gynecomastia. Glucocorticoids lead to hypogonadism predominantly through inhibition of hypothalamic-pituitary function. Sexual dysfunction has been described as a side effect of therapy with beta blockers. However, there is no evidence of an effect on testicular function. Most reports of sexual dysfunction were in patients receiving older beta blockers such as propranolol and timolol.

37. The answer is E.
(Chap. 12) Pure seminomas have the best survival of all forms of testicular cancer and represents approximately 50% of all germ cell tumors (GCTs). The median age of presentation is the fourth decade of life, and ~80% of individuals present with stage I disease, indicating any disease limited to the testis no matter the size at initial presentation. All men presenting with a testicular mass should be referred for radical inguinal orchiectomy as this approach mirrors the embryonic development of the testis and does not breach anatomic barriers to allow for other pathways of spread. In the staging work up of testicular cancers, men should undergo CT imaging of the chest, abdomen, and pelvis as well as measurement of the serum tumor markers alpha fetoprotein (AFP) and β-human chorionic gonadotropin hormone (β-hCG) in addition to LDH levels. These tumor markers assist with both diagnosis and prognosis in testicular cancer and help with determining the appropriate post-orchiectomy treatment. In pure seminomas, AFP levels should not be elevated. If the AFP level were to be elevated, this would indicate an occult nonseminomatous component, which may require more aggressive initial treatment with either retroperitoneal lymph node dissection or adjuvant chemotherapy depending upon local surgical expertise and preference of the patient and treating physician. β-hCG levels may be elevated in pure seminomas although this too is infrequent in men without advanced disease. LDH levels are less specific, but are increased in up to 80% of patients with advanced seminoma. After resection, the tumor markers should return to normal values within their expected half-lives following first order kinetics. The half-life of β-hCG is 24–36 hours, and AFP is 5–7 days. In stage I seminoma, survival is near 100% with either immediate post-orchiectomy radiation or with surveillance alone (option E). Given the concern about secondary malignancy due to radiation exposure, many providers chose watchful waiting with surveillance alone in men who are compliant with follow-ups. However, approximately 15% of patients will have relapse, and 5% of relapses occur after 5 years. So, extended follow-up is required. A single dose of carboplatin has been investigated as an alternative to radiation therapy, but long-term outcomes are as yet unknown.

38. The answer is A.
(Chap. 12) Ninety percent of persons with nonseminomatous germ cell tumors produce either AFP or β-hCG; in contrast, persons with pure seminomas usually produce neither. These tumor markers are present for some time after surgery; if the

presurgical levels are high, 30 days or more may be required before meaningful postsurgical levels can be obtained. The half-lives of AFP and β-hCG are 6 days and 1 day, respectively. After treatment, unequal reduction of β-hCG and AFP may occur, suggesting that the two markers are synthesized by heterogeneous clones of cells within the tumor; thus, both markers should be followed. β-hCG is similar to luteinizing hormone except for its distinctive beta subunit.

39. The answer is B.
(Chap. 13) Women who have regular monthly bleeding cycles that do not vary >4 days generally have ovulatory cycles, but several other indicators suggest that ovulation is likely. These include the presence of *mittelschmerz*, which is described as midcycle pelvic discomfort that is thought to be caused by rapid expansion of the dominant follicle at the time of ovulation or premenstrual symptoms such as breast tenderness, bloating, and food cravings. Additional objective parameters suggest the presence of ovulation including a progesterone level >5 ng/mL 7 days before expected menses, an increase in basal body temperature >0.5°F in second half of menstrual cycle and detection of urinary LH surge. Estrogen levels are elevated at the time of ovulation and during the secretory phase of the menstrual cycle, but are not useful in detection of ovulation.

40. The answer is A.
(Chap. 13) After birth and the loss of placenta-derived steroids, gonadotropin levels rise. FSH levels are much higher in girls than in boys. This rise in FSH results in ovarian activation (evident on ultrasound) and increased inhibin B and estradiol levels. Studies that have identified mutations in TAC3, which encodes neurokinin B, and its receptor, TAC3R, in patients with GnRH deficiency indicate that both are involved in control of GnRH secretion and may be particularly important at this early stage of development. By 12–20 months of age, the reproductive axis is again suppressed, and a period of relative quiescence persists until puberty. At the onset of puberty pulsatile GnRH secretion induces pituitary gonadotropin production. In the early stages of puberty, LH and FSH secretion are apparent only during sleep, but as puberty develops, pulsatile gonadotropin secretion occurs throughout the day and night. Gonadotropin levels are cyclic during the reproductive years and increase dramatically with the loss of negative feedback that accompanies menopause (see **Figure 13-5**).

41. The answer is C.
(Chap. 13) The first menstrual period (menarche) occurs relatively late in the series of developmental milestones that characterize normal pubertal development. Menarche is preceded by the appearance of pubic and then axillary hair (adrenarche) as a result of maturation of the zona reticularis in the adrenal gland and increased adrenal androgen secretion, particularly dehydroepiandrosterone (DHEA). The triggers for adrenarche remain unknown but may involve increases in body mass index, as well as in utero and neonatal factors. Menarche is also preceded by breast development (thelarche). The breast is exquisitely sensitive to the very low levels of estrogen that result from peripheral conversion of adrenal androgens and the low levels of estrogen secreted from the ovary early in pubertal maturation. Breast development precedes the appearance of pubic and axillary hair in ~60% of girls. The interval between the onset of breast development and menarche is ~2 years. There has been a gradual decline in the age of menarche over the past century, attributed in large part to improvement in nutrition, and there is a relationship between adiposity and earlier sexual maturation in girls.

42. The answer is C.
(Chap. 14) Infertility, defined as the inability to conceive after 12 months of unprotected intercourse is a common problem in the United States with estimates of 15% of couples affected. Initial evaluation should include an evaluation of current menstrual history, counseling regarding the appropriate timing of intercourse, and education regarding modifiable risk factors such as drug use, alcohol intake, smoking, caffeine, and obesity. Male factors are at root of approximately 25% of cases of infertility, unexplained infertility is found in 17% of cases, and female causes underlie 58% of infertility. Among the female causes, the most common is amenorrhea/ovulatory dysfunction that is present in 46% of cases. This is most frequently due to hypothalamic or pituitary cases or polycystic ovary syndrome. Tubal defects and endometriosis are less common.

43. The answer is C.
(Chap. 14) Evaluation of infertility should include evaluation of common male and female factors that could be contributing. Abnormalities of menstrual function are the most common cause of female infertility, and initial evaluation of infertility should include evaluation of ovulation and assessment of tubal and uterine patency. The female partner reports an episode of gonococcal infection with symptoms

of pelvic inflammatory disease, which would increase her risk of infertility due to tubal scarring and occlusion. A hysterosalpingogram is indicated. If there is evidence of tubal abnormalities, many experts recommend in vitro fertilization for conception as these women are at increased risk of ectopic pregnancy if conception occurs. The female partner reports some irregularity of her menses, suggesting anovulatory cycles, and thus, evidence of ovulation should be determined by assessing hormonal levels. There is no evidence that prolonged use of oral contraceptives affects fertility adversely (Farrow A et al. *Hum Reprod* 2002;17:2754). Angiotensin-converting enzyme inhibitors, including lisinopril, are known teratogens when taken by women, but have no effects on chromosomal abnormalities in men. Recent marijuana use may be associated with increased risk of infertility, and in vitro studies of human sperm exposed to a cannabinoid derivative showed decreased motility (Whan LB et al. *Fertil Steril* 2006;85:653). However, no studies have shown long-term decreased fertility in men who previously used marijuana.

44. The answer is E.
(Chap. 14) All of the choices have a theoretical efficacy in preventing pregnancy of >90%. However, the actual effectiveness can vary widely. Spermicides have the greatest failure rate of 21%. Barrier methods (condoms, cervical cap, diaphragm) have an actual efficacy between 82 and 88%. Oral contraceptives and intrauterine devices perform similarly, with 97% efficacy in preventing pregnancy in clinical practice.

45. The answer is E.
(Chap. 14) Pathologic gynecomastia develops when the effective ratio of testosterone to estrogen ratio is decreased owing to diminished testosterone production (as in primary testicular failure) or increased estrogen production. The latter may arise from direct estradiol secretion by a testis stimulated by LH or hCG or from an increase in peripheral aromatization of precursor steroids, most notably androstenedione. Elevated androstenedione levels may result from increased secretion by an adrenal tumor (leading to an elevated level of urinary 17-ketosteroids) or decreased hepatic clearance in patients with chronic liver disease. A variety of drugs, including diethylstilbestrol, heroin, digitalis, spironolactone, cimetidine, isoniazid, and tricyclic antidepressants, also can cause gynecomastia. In this patient, the history of paternity and the otherwise normal physical examination indicate that a karyotype is unnecessary, and the bilateral breast enlargement essentially excludes the presence of carcinoma and thus the need for biopsy. The presence of a low LH and testosterone suggests either estrogen or hCG production. Because of the normal testicular examination, a primary testicular tumor is not suspected. Carcinoma of the lung and germ cell tumors both can produce hCG, causing gynecomastia.

46. The answer is C.
(Chap. 14) The spectrum of infertility ranges from reduced conception rates or the need for medical intervention to irreversible causes of infertility. Infertility can be attributed primarily to male factors in 25% of couples and female factors in 58% of couples and is unexplained in about 17% of couples. Not uncommonly, both male and female factors contribute to infertility. Decreases in the ability to conceive as a function of age in women have led to recommendations that women >34 years old who are not at increased risk of infertility seek attention after 6 months, rather than 12 months as suggested for younger women, and receive an expedited work-up and approach to treatment.

47. The answer is D.
(Chap. 15) Amenorrhea refers to the absence of menstrual periods. Amenorrhea is classified as primary if menstrual bleeding has never occurred in the absence of hormonal treatment or secondary if menstrual periods cease for 3–6 months. Primary amenorrhea is a rare disorder that occurs in <1% of the female population. However, between 3 and 5% of women experience at least 3 months of secondary amenorrhea in any specific year. There is no evidence that race or ethnicity influences the prevalence of amenorrhea. However, because of the importance of adequate nutrition for normal reproductive function, both the age at menarche and the prevalence of secondary amenorrhea vary significantly in different parts of the world. The absence of menses by age 16 has been used traditionally to define primary amenorrhea. However, other factors, such as growth, secondary sexual characteristics, the presence of cyclic pelvic pain, and the secular trend toward an earlier age of menarche, particularly in African-American girls, also influence the age at which primary amenorrhea should be investigated. Thus, an evaluation for amenorrhea should be initiated by age 15 or 16 in the presence of normal growth and secondary sexual characteristics; age 13 in the absence of secondary sexual characteristics or if height is less than the third percentile; age 12 or 13 in the presence of breast development and cyclic

pelvic pain; or within 2 years of breast development if menarche, defined by the first menstrual period, has not occurred. Anovulation and irregular cycles are relatively common for up to 2 years after menarche and for 1–2 years before the final menstrual period. In the intervening years, menstrual cycle length is ~28 days, with an intermenstrual interval normally ranging between 25 and 35 days. Cycle-to-cycle variability in an individual woman who is ovulating consistently is generally +/– 2 days. Pregnancy is the most common cause of amenorrhea and should be excluded early in any evaluation of menstrual irregularity. However, many women occasionally miss a single period. Three or more months of secondary amenorrhea should prompt an evaluation, as should a history of intermenstrual intervals >35 or <21 days or bleeding that persists for >7 days.

48. The answer is B.

(Chap. 15) The first step in the evaluation of amenorrhea is assessment of the uterus and outflow tract. If normal, subsequent evaluation should include ruling out pregnancy followed by measurement of androgens (testosterone and DHEAS), FSH, and prolactin. As shown in **Figure 15-2**, this patient has findings consistent with a neuroendocrine tumor and should receive an MRI. Androgen resistance syndrome requires gonadectomy because there is risk of gonadoblastoma in the dysgenetic gonads. Whether this should be performed in early childhood or after completion of breast development is controversial.

49. The answer is D.

(Chap. 15) Polycystic ovarian syndrome (PCOS) is diagnosed based on a combination of clinical or biochemical evidence of hyperandrogenism, amenorrhea or oligomenorrhea, and the ultrasound appearance of polycystic ovaries. Approximately half of patients with PCOS are obese, and abnormalities in insulin dynamics are common, as is metabolic syndrome. Symptoms generally begin shortly after menarche and are slowly progressive. Patients may develop dysfunctional uterine bleeding as defined by frequent or heavy uterine bleeding. A major abnormality in patients with PCOS is the failure of regular predictable ovulation. Thus, these patients are at risk for the development of dysfunctional bleeding and endometrial hyperplasia associated with unopposed estrogen exposure. Endometrial protection can be achieved with the use of oral contraceptives or progestins (medroxyprogesterone acetate, 5–10 mg, or Prometrium, 200 mg daily for 10–14 days of each month). Oral contraceptives are also useful for management of hyperandrogenic symptoms, as is spironolactone which functions as weak androgen receptor blocker. Clomiphene and letrozole are used in PCOS patients that are interested in fertility. Corticosteroids will worsen her obesity and hyperglycemia. Testosterone will worsen the PCOS as the disorder is driven by androgen excess.

50. The answer is E.

(Chap. 16) The Women's Health Initiative was the largest study of hormone therapy to date including 27,000 postmenopausal women age 50–79 for an average of 5–7 years. It was presumed that hormone replacement in this group of women would decrease cardiovascular risk. However, the trial was stopped early because of an unfavorable risk-benefit ratio in the estrogen-progestin arm and an increased risk of stroke that was not offset by lower coronary heart disease in the estrogen-only arm. Endometrial cancer risk was higher in patients with estrogen only and an intact uterus. Use of progesterone eliminates this risk. Unopposed estrogen was associated with increased risk of stroke that far outweighed the decreased risk of coronary heart disease. Estrogen-progestin together was associated with an increased risk of coronary heart disease. Osteoporosis risk was decreased in both estrogen and estrogen-progestin groups. Venous thromboembolism risk was higher in both treatment groups as well. These therapies do reduce important menopausal symptoms such as hot flashes and vaginal drying. This seminal study caused a dramatic reevaluation of the use of estrogen/progesterone in postmenopausal women to reduce cardiovascular risk. Plus, it reiterated the importance of well-designed clinical studies to test accepted dogma.

51. The answer is D.

(Chap. 16) Traditional contraindications for oral hormone replacement therapy are unexplained vaginal bleeding; active liver disease; history of venous thromboembolism due to pregnancy, oral contraceptive use, or an unknown etiology; blood-clotting disorder; history of breast or endometrial cancer; and diabetes. Ten-year risk of CHD, based on Framingham Coronary Heart Disease Risk Score indicating a risk of 5–10% is not a traditional contraindication for OHT.

52. The answer is D.

(Chap. 17) Hirsutism, which is defined as androgen-dependent excessive male pattern hair growth, affects approximately 10% of women. Hirsutism is most often idiopathic or the consequence of androgen excess associated with the polycystic ovarian syndrome (PCOS). Less frequently, it may result from

adrenal androgen overproduction as occurs in nonclassic congenital adrenal hyperplasia (CAH). Historic elements relevant to the assessment of hirsutism include the age at onset and rate of progression of hair growth and associated symptoms or signs (e.g., acne). Depending on the cause, excess hair growth typically is first noted during the second and third decades of life. The growth is usually slow but progressive. Sudden development and rapid progression of hirsutism suggest the possibility of an androgen secreting neoplasm, in which case virilization also may be present. Physical examination should include measurement of height and weight and calculation of body mass index (BMI). A BMI >30 kg/m^2 is often seen in association with hirsutism, probably the result of increased conversion of androgen precursors to testosterone. Notation should be made of blood pressure, as adrenal causes may be associated with hypertension. Cutaneous signs sometimes associated with androgen excess and insulin resistance include acanthosis nigricans and skin tags. An objective clinical assessment of hair distribution and quantity is central to the evaluation in any woman presenting with hirsutism. This assessment permits the distinction between hirsutism and hypertrichosis and provides a baseline reference point to gauge the response to treatment. A simple and commonly used method to grade hair growth is the modified scale of Ferriman and Gallwey (as shown in **Figure 17-1**), in which each of nine androgen-sensitive sites is graded from 0 to 4. Approximately 95% of white women have a score below 8 on this scale; thus, it is normal for most women to have some hair growth in androgen sensitive sites. Scores above 8 suggest excess androgen-mediated hair growth, a finding that should be assessed further by means of hormonal evaluation. In racial/ethnic groups that are less likely to manifest hirsutism (e.g., Asian women), additional cutaneous evidence of androgen excess should be sought, including pustular acne and thinning scalp hair (see Figure 17-1).

53. The answer is E.

(Chap. 17) Androgens are secreted by the ovaries and adrenal glands in response to their respective tropic hormones: luteinizing hormone (LH) and adrenocorticotropic hormone (ACTH). The principal circulating steroids involved in the etiology of hirsutism are testosterone, androstenedione, dehydroepiandrosterone (DHEA), and its sulfated form (DHEAS). The ovaries and adrenal glands normally contribute about equally to testosterone production. The initial evaluation of hirsutism includes measurement of serum testosterone, free testosterone, and DHEAS. High levels of testosterone suggest a virilizing tumor and high levels of DHEAS suggest an adrenal source or polycystic ovarian syndrome. A suggested diagnostic algorithm is shown in **Figure 17-2**.

54. The answer is E.

(Chap. 18) A variety of genetic syndromes substantially increase a woman's risk of developing ovarian cancer. Approximately 10% of women with ovarian cancer have a germline mutation in one of two DNA repair genes: *BRCA1* (chromosome 17q12-21) or *BRCA2* (chromosome 13q12-13). Individuals inheriting a single copy of a mutant allele have a very high incidence of breast and ovarian cancer. Most of these women have a family history that is notable for multiple cases of breast and/or ovarian cancer, although inheritance through male members of the family can camouflage this genotype through several generations. The most common malignancy in these women is breast carcinoma, although women harboring germline *BRCA1* mutations have a marked increased risk of developing ovarian malignancies in their forties and fifties with a 30–50% lifetime risk of developing ovarian cancer. Women harboring a mutation in *BRCA2* have a lower penetrance of ovarian cancer with perhaps a 20–40% chance of developing this malignancy, with onset typically in their fifties or sixties. Women with a *BRCA2* mutation also are at slightly increased risk of pancreatic cancer. Likewise women with mutations in the DNA mismatch repair genes associated with Lynch syndrome, type 2 (*MSH2, MLH1, MLH6, PMS1, PMS2*) may have a risk of ovarian cancer as high as 1% per year in their forties and fifties. Finally, a small group of women with familial ovarian cancer may have mutations in other *BRCA*-associated genes such as *RAD51, CHK2,* and others. Screening studies in this select population suggest that current screening techniques, including serial evaluation of the CA-125 tumor marker and ultrasound, are insufficient at detecting early stage and curable disease, so women with these germline mutations are advised to undergo prophylactic removal of ovaries and fallopian tubes typically after completing childbearing and ideally before age 35–40 years. Early prophylactic oophorectomy also protects these women from subsequent breast cancer with a reduction of breast cancer risk of approximately 50%.

55. The answer is A.

(Chap. 18) Cervical cancer is the second most common and most lethal malignancy in women worldwide likely due to the widespread infection with high-risk strains of human papillomavirus (HPV) and limited

utilization of or access to Pap smear screening in many nations throughout the world. Nearly 500,000 cases of cervical cancer are expected worldwide, with approximately 240,000 deaths annually. Cancer incidence is particularly high in women residing in Central and South America, the Caribbean, and southern and eastern Africa. Mortality rate is disproportionately high in Africa. In the United States, 12,360 women were diagnosed with cervical cancer and 4020 women died in 2014. HPV is the primary neoplastic-initiating event in the vast majority of women with invasive cervical cancer. This double-strand DNA virus infects epithelium near the transformation zone of the cervix. More than 60 types of HPV are known, with approximately 20 types having the ability to generate high-grade dysplasia and malignancy. HPV-16 and -18 are the types most frequently associated with high-grade dysplasia and targeted by both U.S. Food and Drug Administration-approved vaccines. The large majority of sexually active adults are exposed to HPV, and most women clear the infection without specific intervention. Risk factors for HPV infection and, in particular, dysplasia include a high number of sexual partners, early age of first intercourse, and history of venereal disease. Smoking is a cofactor; heavy smokers have a higher risk of dysplasia with HPV infection. HIV infection, especially when associated with low CD4+ T cell counts, is associated with a higher rate of high-grade dysplasia and likely a shorter latency period between infection and invasive disease. The administration of highly active antiretroviral therapy reduces the risk of high-grade dysplasia associated with HPV infection. Currently approved vaccines include the recombinant proteins to the late proteins, L1 and L2, of HPV-16 and -18. Vaccination of women before the initiation of sexual activity dramatically reduces the rate of HPV-16 and -18 infection and subsequent dysplasia. Stage 1 disease, which accounts for almost half of staging at presentation, is defined by carcinoma confined to the cervix and has a >80% 5-year survival (see **Figure 18-1**).

56. The answer is A.
(Chap. 19) Normal male sexual function requires: (1) an intact libido, (2) the ability to achieve and maintain penile erection, (3) ejaculation, and (4) detumescence. Libido refers to sexual desire and is influenced by a variety of visual, olfactory, tactile, auditory, imaginative, and hormonal stimuli. Sex steroids, particularly testosterone, act to increase libido. Libido can be diminished by hormonal or psychiatric disorders and by medications. Nitric oxide, which induces vascular relaxation, promotes erection. Nitric oxide increases the production of cyclic GMP, which induces relaxation of smooth muscle. Cyclic GMP is gradually broken down by phosphodiesterase type 5 (PDE-5). Inhibitors of PDE-5, such as the oral medications sildenafil, vardenafil, and tadalafil, maintain erections by reducing the breakdown of cyclic GMP. Ejaculation is stimulated by the sympathetic nervous system; this results in contraction of the epididymis, vas deferens, seminal vesicles, and prostate, causing seminal fluid to enter the urethra. Seminal fluid emission is followed by rhythmic contractions of the bulbocavernosus and ischiocavernosus muscles, leading to ejaculation. Detumescence is mediated by norepinephrine from the sympathetic nerves, endothelin from the vascular surface, and smooth-muscle contraction induced by postsynaptic α-adrenergic receptors and activation of Rho kinase. These events increase venous outflow and restore the flaccid state.

57. The answer is D.
(Chap. 19) The phosphodiesterase-5 inhibitors including sildenafil, tadalafil, vardenafil, and avanafil are the only approved and effective oral agents for the treatment of erectile dysfunction (ED). They are effective for the treatment of a broad range of causes, including psychogenic, diabetic, vasculogenic, post-radical prostatectomy (nerve-sparing procedures), and spinal cord injury. Androgen therapy with testosterone may be effective to improve libido and erectile function in patients with low serum testosterone, but this patient has a normal serum testosterone for age. 5α-Reductase inhibitors, such as finasteride, are used to treat prostatic hypertrophy and act as antiandrogens, thus may cause ED. Corticosteroids and SSRI medications are associated with causing ED.

58. The answer is B.
(Chap. 19) In postmenopausal women, estrogen replacement therapy may be helpful in treating vaginal atrophy, decreasing coital pain, and improving clitoral sensitivity. Estrogen replacement in the form of local cream is the preferred method, as it avoids systemic side effects. There is no proven efficacy of phosphodiesterase-5 inhibitors, such as sildenafil, in female sexual dysfunction despite similar sexual response physiology in women as men. Selective serotonin reuptake inhibitors used for depression, such as paroxetine, may cause sexual dysfunction in women. Tamoxifen and anastrozole are antiestrogens used to treat breast cancer and may cause vaginal atrophy and female sexual dysfunction.

59. The answer is B.
(Chap. 22) Metabolic syndrome is a common disorder that features central obesity, hypertriglyceridemia,

low levels of HDL cholesterol, hyperglycemia, and hypertension. The prevalence of the disease varies around the world, reflecting the age, ethnicity, and varying diagnostic criteria applied. The highest prevalence of metabolic syndrome worldwide occurs in the Native American populations in the United States, with nearly 60% of women ages 45–49 and 45% of men ages 45–49 being affected. In the United States, African American men are less commonly affected while Mexican American women are more commonly affected. In France, the disease prevalence is generally the lowest in the world with <10% of individuals between 30 and 60 years of age affected although after age 60 the prevalence rises to 17.5%. Risk factors that confer increasing likelihood of developing metabolic syndrome included overweight/obesity, aging, sedentary lifestyle, DM, cardiovascular disease, and lipodystrophy. Central obesity is both a risk factor and a feature central to defining the presence of the disease. Central obesity as measured by waist circumference, not body mass index, is most strongly associated with insulin resistance and risk of DM and cardiovascular disease. The precise waist circumference at which the risk increases may vary between men and women and across different ethnicities. For instance, in Japanese women, the waist circumference that is used for diagnosis of metabolic syndrome is 90 cm compared to 85 cm for men. However, in individuals of Europoid descent, women are diagnosed with metabolic syndrome at a waist circumference ≥80 cm while men are diagnosed at a waist circumference ≥94 cm. Aging is also associated with increased risk of metabolic syndrome. Metabolic syndrome affects about half of the population older than 50, and after 60 women are more affected than men. Physical inactivity is a predictor of cardiovascular events and death in individuals with metabolic syndrome. Spending more than 4 hours daily watching television or videos or using a computer confers a twofold greater risk of metabolic syndrome. Insulin resistance is felt to be the pathophysiologic hallmark of the metabolic syndrome, and about 75% of individuals with type 2 DM or impaired glucose tolerance have metabolic syndrome. When these diseases coexist in an individual, there is a higher prevalence of cardiovascular disease than with T2DM or glucose tolerance alone.

60. The answer is D.

(Chap. 22) The most recent criteria for the diagnosis of metabolic syndrome is called the Harmonizing Definition and was published in 2009. This definition brought together multiple international medical societies to create a unifying definition including the International Diabetes Federation; the National Heart, Lung, and Blood Institute; the American Heart Association; the World Heart Federation; the International Atherosclerosis Society; and the International Association for the Study of Obesity. When compared to prior guidelines, the most important change was to recognize that the waist circumference that confers the risk of metabolic syndrome is different across ethnic groups. The harmonizing definition creates three different waist circumference groupings by gender and ethnic group (see **Table 22-1**). Furthermore, when compared with the NCEP:ATPIII 2001 classification, the waist circumference that is considered abnormal is lower by at least 8 cm in both men and women. The remaining diagnostic criteria for metabolic syndrome remain the same when compared to prior guidelines:

- Fasting triglycerides >150 mg/dL or specific medication
- HDL cholesterol <40 mg/dL in men or <50 mg/dL in women or specific medication
- Blood pressure >130 mmHg systolic or >85 mmHg diastolic or specific medication or previous diagnosis
- Fasting plasma glucose >100 mg/dL or drug treatment of elevated glucose level</BL>

This individual meets diagnostic criteria with elevated waist circumference (>90 cm in Chinese man), elevated triglyceride level, low HDL level, and hypertension.

61. The answer is D.

(Chap. 23) The risk of both type 1 and type 2 DM is rising in all populations, but the risk of type 2 diabetes is rising at a substantially faster rate. In the United States, the age-adjusted prevalence of DM is 7.1% in non-Hispanic whites, 7.5% in Asian Americans, 11.8% in Hispanics and 12.6% in non-Hispanic blacks. Comparable data is not available for individuals belonging to American-Indian, Alaska Native or Pacific Islander populations, but is thought to be even higher than the non-Hispanic black population.

62. The answer is C.

(Chap. 23) Glucose tolerance is classified into three categories: (1) normal glucose tolerance, (2) impaired glucose homeostasis, and (3) DM. Normal glucose tolerance is defined by the following: fasting plasma glucose <100 mg/dL, plasma glucose <140 mg/dL following an oral glucose challenge and hemoglobin A1C <5.6%. Abnormal glucose homeostasis is defined as fasting plasma glucose 100–125 mmol/dL

or plasma glucose 140–199 following oral glucose tolerance test or hemoglobin A1C of 5.7–6.4%. Actual DM is defined by either fasting plasma glucose >126 mg/dL, glucose of 200 mg/dL after oral glucose tolerance test or hemoglobin A1C ≥6.5%.

63. The answer is E.

(Chap. 23) Because the patient has symptoms, she is not being screened for DM. For screening, the fasting plasma glucose or hemoglobin A1C is recommended. Because the patient has symptoms, a random plasma glucose of >200 mg/dL is adequate to diagnose DM. Other criteria include fasting plasma glucose >126 mg/dL or hemoglobin A1C >6.4% or 2-hour plasma glucose >200 during an oral glucose tolerance test. C-peptide is a useful tool to determine if the normal cleavage of insulin from its precursor is occurring. A normal C-peptide level with hypoglycemia suggests surreptitious insulin use and a low C-peptide with hyperglycemia suggests pancreatic failure.

64. The answer is A.

(Chap. 23) Type 1 DM often has a more severe presentation with diabetic ketoacidosis and often presents in younger individuals compared with type 2 diabetes; however, there are some cases where the distinction of type 1 from type 2 is not straightforward. There is HLA DR3 localization preferences for type 1 diabetes; several haplotypes are present in 40% of children with type 1 DM, but it is still the minority. Immunologic destruction of the beta cell is the primary cause of disease in type 1 diabetes, and islet cell antibodies are commonly present. GAD, insulin, IA/ICA-512, and ZnT-8 are the most common targets. Commercially available assays for GAD-65 autoantibodies are widely available and can demonstrate antibodies in >85% of individuals with recent onset type 1 diabetes. These autoantibodies are infrequently present in type 2 DM at 5–10%. There may be some residual insulin in the plasma in early type 1 diabetes, thus this will not distinguish the two conditions reliably. Polymorphisms of the peroxisom proliferator-activated receptor gamma-2 have been described in type 2 DM, but cannot distinguish the two conditions.

65. The answer is D.

(Chap. 23) Individuals with type 2 DM often exhibit the following features: (1) develop diabetes after the age of 30 years; (2) are usually obese (80% are obese, but elderly individuals may be lean); (3) may not require insulin therapy initially; and (4) may have associated conditions such as insulin resistance, hypertension, cardiovascular disease, dyslipidemia, or PCOS. In type 2 DM, insulin resistance is often associated with abdominal obesity (as opposed to hip and thigh obesity) and hypertriglyceridemia. Although most individuals diagnosed with type 2 DM are older, the age of diagnosis is declining, and there is a marked increase among overweight children and adolescents. The age of the patient should not be the sole basis for determining the type of diabetes present. Some individuals with phenotypic type 2 DM present with diabetic ketoacidosis but lack autoimmune markers and may be later treated with oral glucose-lowering agents rather than insulin (this clinical picture is sometimes referred to as ketosis-prone type 2 DM). Monogenic forms of diabetes (MODY) should be considered in those with diabetes onset at <30 years of age, an autosomal pattern of diabetes inheritance (which this patient lacks), and the lack of nearly complete insulin deficiency.

66. The answer is E.

(Chap. 24) Diabetic ketoacidosis and hyperglycemic hyperosmolar state exist on a spectrum with diabetic ketoacidosis more common in patients with type 1 DM, but does occur with some frequency in patients with type 2 DM. Both conditions include hyperglycemia, dehydration, absolute or relative insulin deficiency and acid-base abnormalities. Ketosis is more common in diabetic ketoacidosis. In diabetic ketoacidosis, glucose normally ranges from 250 to 600 mg/dL, while it is frequently 600–1200 mg/dL in hyperglycemic hyperosmolar state. Sodium is often mildly depressed in ketoacidosis and is preserved in hyperosmolar state. Potassium is normal to elevated in diabetic ketoacidosis and normal in hyperglycemic hyperosmolar patients. Magnesium, chloride and phosphate are normal in both conditions. Creatinine may be slightly elevated in diabetic ketoacidosis, but is often moderately elevated in hyperglycemic hyperosmolar state. Plasma ketones may be slightly positive in hyperosmolar patients, but are always strongly positive in diabetic ketoacidosis. Because hyperosmolarity is the hallmark of hyperglycemic hyperosmolar patients, they have an osmolarity of 330–380 mOsm/mL, while patients with diabetic ketoacidosis typically have a slightly elevated plasma osmolarity ranging from 300 to 320 mOsm/mL. Serum bicarbonate is markedly depressed in diabetic ketoacidosis and normal or slightly depressed in hyperosmolar state. Arterial pH is depressed at <7.3 in ketoacidosis and >7.3 in hyperosmolar state. Finally, the anion gap is wide in diabetic ketoacidosis and normal to slightly elevated in hyperglycemic hyperosmolar state.

67. The answer is D.
(Chap. 24) Insulin preparations can be divided into short acting and long acting insulins. The short acting insulins include regular and new preparations including aspart, glulisine, and lispro. Regular insulin has an onset of action of 0.5–1 hour and is effective for 4–6 hours. The other three short acting insulins have an onset of action of <0.25 hours and are effective for 3–4 hours. Long-acting insulins include detemir, glargine, and NPH. Detemir and glargine have an onset of action of 1–4 hours and last up to 24 hours, while NPH has an onset of action of 1–4 hours and is effective for 10–16 hours. These insulins have a number of combination preparations that take advantage of the different durations of onset and action to provide optimal efficacy and compliance.

68. The answer is D.
(Chap. 24) First line oral therapy for patients with type 2 DM is metformin. It is contraindicated in patients with GFR <60 mL/min, any form of acidosis, congestive heart failure, liver disease, or severe hypoxemia, but is well tolerated in most individuals. Insulin secretagogues, biguanides, alpha-glucosidase inhibitors, thiazolidinediones, GLP-1 agonists, DPP-IV inhibitors, and insulin have all been approved as monotherapy for type 2 diabetes. Because of extensive clinical experience with metformin, favorable side effect profile and relatively low cost, it is the recommended first line agent. It has additional benefits of promotion of mild weight loss, lower insulin levels, and mild improvements in lipid profile. Sulfonylureas such as glyburide, GLP-1 agonists such as exenatide, insulin dipeptidyl peptidase-4 inhibitors such as sitagliptin may be appropriate as combination therapy, but are not considered first line therapy for most patients.

69. The answer is A.
(Chap. 24) Diabetic ketoacidosis is an acute complication of DM. It results from a relative or absolute deficiency of insulin combined with a counterregulatory hormone excess. In particular, a decrease in the ratio of insulin to glucagons promotes gluconeogenesis, glycogenolysis, and the formation of ketone bodies in the liver. Ketosis results from an increase in the release of free fatty acids from adipocytes, with a resultant shift toward ketone body synthesis in the liver. This is mediated by the relationship between insulin and the enzyme carnitine palmitoyltransferase I. At physiologic pH, ketone bodies exist as ketoacids, which are neutralized by bicarbonate. As bicarbonate stores are depleted, acidosis develops. Clinically, these patients have nausea, vomiting, and abdominal pain. They are dehydrated and may be hypotensive. Lethargy and severe central nervous system depression may occur. The treatment centers on replacement of the body's insulin, which will result in cessation of the formation of ketoacids and improvement of the acidotic state. Assessment of the level of acidosis may be done with an arterial blood gas. These patients have an anion gap acidosis and often a concomitant metabolic alkalosis resulting from volume depletion. Volume resuscitation with intravenous fluids is critical. Many electrolyte abnormalities may occur. Patients are total body sodium-, potassium-, and magnesium-depleted. As a result of the acidosis, intracellular potassium may shift out of cells and cause a normal or even elevated potassium level. However, with improvement in the acidosis, the serum potassium rapidly falls. Therefore, potassium repletion is critical despite the presence of a "normal" level. Because of the osmolar effects of glucose, fluid is drawn into the intravascular space. This results in a drop in the measured serum sodium. There is a drop of 1.6 mEq/L in serum sodium for each rise of 100 mg/dL in serum glucose. In this case, the serum sodium will improve with hydration alone. The use of 3% saline is not indicated because the patient has no neurologic deficits, and the expectation is for rapid resolution with intravenous fluids alone.

70. The answer is D.
(Chap. 24) Reproductive capacity in either men or women with DM appears to be normal. Menstrual cycles may be associated with alterations in glycemic control in women with DM. Pregnancy is associated with marked insulin resistance; the increased insulin requirements often precipitate DM and lead to the diagnosis of gestational DM (GDM). Glucose, which at high levels is a teratogen to the developing fetus, readily crosses the placenta, but insulin does not. Thus, hyperglycemia from the maternal circulation may stimulate insulin secretion in the fetus. The anabolic and growth effects of insulin may result in macrosomia. Pregnancy in individuals with known DM requires meticulous planning and adherence to strict treatment regimens. Intensive diabetes management and normalization of the HbA1c are essential for individuals with existing DM who are planning pregnancy. The most crucial period of glycemic control is soon after fertilization. The risk of fetal malformations is increased 4–10 times in individuals with uncontrolled DM at the time of conception, and normal plasma glucose during the

preconception period and throughout the periods of organ development in the fetus should be the goal.

71. The answer is D.

(Chap. 24) Virtually all medical and surgical subspecialties are involved in the care of hospitalized patients with diabetes. Hyperglycemia, whether in a patient with known diabetes or in someone without known diabetes, appears to be a predictor of poor outcome in hospitalized patients. General anesthesia, surgery, infection, or concurrent illness raises the levels of counterregulatory hormones (cortisol, growth hormone, catecholamines, and glucagon) and cytokines that may lead to transient insulin resistance and hyperglycemia. In a number of cross-sectional studies of patients with diabetes, a greater degree of hyperglycemia was associated with worse cardiac, neurologic, and infectious outcomes. In some studies, patients who do not have preexisting diabetes but who develop modest blood glucose elevations during their hospitalization appear to benefit from achieving near-normoglycemia using insulin treatment. However, a large randomized clinical trial (Normoglycemia in Intensive Care Evaluation Survival Using Glucose Algorithm Regulation [NICESUGAR]) of individuals in the ICU (most of whom were receiving mechanical ventilation) found an increased mortality rate and a greater number of episodes of severe hypoglycemia with very strict glycemic control (target blood glucose of 4.5–6 mmol/L or 81–108 mg/dL) compared to individuals with a more moderate glycemic goal (mean blood glucose of 8 mmol/L or 144 mg/dL). Total parenteral nutrition (TPN) greatly increases insulin requirements. In addition, individuals not previously known to have DM may become hyperglycemic during TPN and require insulin treatment. Insulin infusions are preferred in the ICU or in a clinically unstable setting. The absorption of SC insulin may be variable in such situations. Insulin infusions can also effectively control plasma glucose in the perioperative period and when the patient is unable to take anything by mouth.

72. The answer is C.

(Chap. 25) Diabetic retinopathy is the leading cause blindness in individuals between the ages of 20 and 74 in the United States. Individuals with DM are 25 times more likely to go legally blind than individuals without those with DM. Diabetic retinopathy is classified into two stages: (1) nonproliferative and (2) proliferative. Nonproliferative retinopathy typically appears late in the first decade or early in the second decade of the disease. Characteristic findings include cotton wool spots, blot hemorrhages, and retinal vascular microaneurysms. Mild proliferative retinopathy may progress to more extensive disease, characterized by changes in venous vessel caliber, intraretinal microvascular abnormalities, and more numerous microaneurysms and hemorrhages. Pathophysiologically, there is loss of retinal pericytes, increased retinal vascular permeability, alterations in retinal blood flow, and abnormal retinal microvasculature. Severe nonproliferative diabetic retinopathy creates retinal hypoxemia and establishes the environment for development the proliferative retinopathy. Neovascularization, as shown in this patient's fundus, is the hallmark of proliferative retinopathy. Neovascular vessels appear at the optic disc. The most effective therapy for the treatment of diabetic retinopathy is prevention with intensive glycemic and blood pressure control. However, in established diabetic retinopathy, improved glycemic control leads to transient worsening of the disease. When proliferative retinopathy and neovascularization is present retinal laser photocoagulation is required.

73. The answer is D.

(Chap. 25) Diabetes mellitus is the most common cause of chronic kidney disease, end stage renal disease, and chronic kidney disease requiring renal replacement therapy. In the first 5 years after diabetes onset, glomerular hyperfiltration and increased glomerular filtration rate are seen. The glomerular basement membrane subsequently thickens with concomitant mesangial volume and glomerular hypertrophy. Typically within 5–10 years, many individuals will begin to excrete small amounts of albumin in their urine. It is recommended to screen for albumin excretion annually with a 24-hour collection or spot albumin to creatinine ratio. Microalbuminuria is defined as >30–299 g/d in a 24-hour collection or 30–299 g/mg creatinine in a spot collection. However, interpretation may be clouded by conditions known to transiently increase albumin excretion including urinary tract infection, hematuria, heart failure, febrile illness, severe hyperglycemia (option B), severe hypertension (option E), pregnancy, and vigorous exercise (option C). If testing is positive, it should be repeated within 3–6 months, and treatment began at that time. This makes option A too soon for repeat testing and option D the most appropriate answer to the question. While direct comparisons have not been done, experts believe that ACE inhibitors and angiotensin receptor blockers are equivalent in the treatment of albuminuria and diabetic nephropathy.

74. The answer is D.

(Chap. 25) Diabetic neuropathy occurs in as much as 50% of individuals with long-standing type 1 and

type 2 DM and can manifests as polyneuropathy, mononeuropathy, and/or autonomic neuropathy. Like other complications of DM, the likelihood of developing neuropathy depends upon the duration of the disease and the degree of glycemic control. The most common form of neuropathy is distal symmetric polyneuropathy, which typically presents as distal sensory loss and pain. However, as many as 50% of individuals will have no symptoms at all. Alternatively, hyperesthesia, paresthesia, and dysesthesia may also occur. Clinically, patients often complain of a pins-and-needles sensation in the distal extremities. Other symptoms include burning, numbness, or a sharp pain. Both the hands and feet may be affected, but usually starts in the lower extremities. Pain is worse at rest and at night. An acute form of diabetic neuropathy may worsen in the setting of improved glycemic control. As the neuropathy progresses, the pain may subside with worsening numbness and sensory deficit. Physical examination shows sensory loss to light touch and pinprick with loss of ankle deep-tendon reflexes and abnormal position sense. Treatment of diabetic neuropathy is difficult. Improved glycemic control may improve nerve conduction velocity but symptoms of neuropathy may not improve. Avoidance of other neurotoxins, such as alcohol, smoking, and vitamin deficiencies, that could worsen neuropathy should be avoided. Multiple agents have been used to attempt treatment of painful neuropathy although the results of treatment are less than ideal. Of these, only two agents—duloxetine and pregabalin—have been approved by the FDA for the treatment of diabetic neuropathy. Other agents that are sometimes used off label include amitriptyline, gabapentin, valproate, and opioids.

75. The answer is B.

(Chap. 26) Maintenance of euglycemia involves a number of systems to lower elevated blood glucose, but also to restore normal levels when hypoglycemia is present or impending. This is particularly important for neurologic functioning as the brain cannot synthesize glucose and has only a few minutes' supply stored as glycogen. In a nondiabetic individual, the normal fasting plasma glucose level is normally tightly controlled between 70 and 110 mg/dL. When the plasma glucose begins to fall below about 80–85 mg/dL, the first line of defense to protect against development of hypoglycemia is to decrease insulin secretion. When this occurs, hepatic glycogenolysis and gluconeogenesis increase. In addition, lowered insulin levels lead to decreased peripheral glucose utilization. If the glucose continues to fall to about 65–70 mg/dL, other protective mechanisms are employed. The second line of defense against hypoglycemia is glucagon secretion, which further stimulates hepatic gluconeogenesis. Epinephrine may also be secreted although it is not normally critical unless glucagon is deficient. Cortisol and growth hormone are secreted later in the pathway when hypoglycemia is prolonged greater than 4 hours. These hormones have no role in acute hypoglycemia.

76. The answer is D.

(Chap. 26) The patient presents with recurrent episodes of hypoglycemia that meet Whipple's triad of symptoms: (1) symptoms of hypoglycemia; (2) low plasma glucose concentration measured with a precise method (not a glucose monitor); and (3) relief of symptoms with raising the plasma glucose level. The differential starts with measuring insulin levels during hypoglycemia. The levels must be obtained during an episode to be interpretable. If insulin is elevated, it suggests either endogenous hyperproduction from an insulin-secreting tumor or exogenous administration causing factitious hypoglycemia. Because C-peptide is cleaved from native proinsulin to make the secreted product, it will be high in the case of endogenous hyperinsulinemia and will be low during an episode of factitious hypoglycemia. Surreptitious ingestion of sulfonylurea could cause hypoglycemia along with high insulin and C-peptide levels since the drugs stimulate pancreatic insulin secretion. In this case, a sulfonylurea drug screen would be indicated. Red flags in this case that point to surreptitious insulin use include the patient being a health care worker and the presence of symptoms only at work. Other groups in which this is common is relatives of patients with diabetes and patients with a history of other factitious disorders. It is possible that she has an insulin-secreting beta cell tumor, but this is much less likely and symptoms would be present during times other than work. Evaluation is aimed at demonstrating that pancreatic insulin secretion is suppressed during the episode of hypoglycemia. Although a failure of counterregulatory hormones can produce hypoglycemia, this is a very rare cause of hypoglycemia and evaluation should be aimed at this only after surreptitious use is ruled out.

77. The answer is E.

(Chap. 26) The most common cause of hypoglycemia is related to the treatment of diabetes mellitus. Individuals with type 1 diabetes mellitus (T1DM) have more symptomatic hypoglycemia than individuals with type 2 diabetes mellitus (T2DM). On average,

those with T1DM experience two episodes of symptomatic hypoglycemia weekly; and at least once yearly, individuals with T1DM will have a severe episode of hypoglycemia that is at least temporarily disabling. It is estimated that 6–10% of individuals with T1DM will die from hypoglycemia. In addition, recurrent episodes of hypoglycemia in T1DM contribute to the development of hypoglycemia-associated autonomic failure. Clinically, this is manifested as hypoglycemia unawareness and defective glucose counterregulation, with lack of glucagon and epinephrine secretion as glucose levels fall. Individuals with T2DM are less likely to develop hypoglycemia. However, once an individual with T2DM becomes insulin requiring, the likelihood of symptomatic hypoglycemia increases, and while the incidence of hypoglycemia is overall lower in T2DM, the absolute number of individuals with T2DM with hypoglycemia episodes far outnumber those with T1DM given the higher prevalence of T2DM. Medications that are associated with hypoglycemia in T2DM are insulin and insulin secretagogues, such as sulfonylureas. Metformin, thiazolidinediones, α-glucosidase inhibitors, glucagon-like peptide-1 receptor agonists, and dipeptidyl peptidase-IV inhibitors should not cause hypoglycemia. However, when these medications are combined with another class of medications known to cause hypoglycemia, they do increase the risk of hypoglycemic episodes.

78. The answer is A.

(Chap. 27) Lipoprotein lipase (LPL) deficiency is a very rare autosomal recessive disorder that results in elevated fasting triglyceride levels as the absence of lipoprotein lipase results in the inability for chylomicrons to undergo hydrolysis of triglycerides. Thus, circulating levels of chylomicrons, VLDL, and triglycerides are high. Fasting triglyceride levels are typically >1000 mg/dL. LPL deficiency has an incidence of 1 in ~1,000,000 in the population. The disease typically presents in childhood or young adulthood with recurrent episodes of pancreatitis. Ophthalmologic examination may show lipemia retinalis with an opalescent appearance to the retinal blood vessels. Eruptive xanthomas are small, yellowish-white papules and may appear on the back, buttocks, and extensor surfaces of the arms and legs. Hepatosplenomegaly occurs because of uptake of the circulating chylomicrons by the reticuloendothelial system. Primary treatment of the disorder is to restrict dietary fat to 15 g/d or less. If dietary fat restriction alone is not sufficient to control the triglyceride level, fish oil has been useful in some patients.

79. The answer is D.

(Chap. 27) Familial hypercholesterolemia (FH) is the most common inherited cause of hypercholesterolemia and may be one of the most common single-gene disorders in humans. The incidence of the mutation that causes FH is estimated to be as common as 1 in 250 to 1 in 500 individuals in the population. FH is also known as autosomal dominant hypercholesterolemia, type 1, and is caused by a loss of function mutations in the gene encoding the LDL receptor. More than 1600 mutations in the gene have been reported. In the presence of a single mutation (heterozygous FH), there is a decrease of LDL receptors in the liver with a resulting decrease in clearance of LDL from the circulation, and plasma levels of LDL-C typically range from 200 to 400 mg/dL. In the presence of two mutations (homozygous FH), LDL receptors are markedly reduced or absent. In these patients, the LDL-C levels are markedly elevated to 400 to >1000 mg/dL. Many individuals with homozygous FH present in childhood with cutaneous xanthomas and early cardiovascular disease in late childhood or young adulthood. While heterozygous patients have hypercholesterolemia from birth, disease recognition is usually not until adulthood when patients are found to have tendon xanthomas or coronary artery disease. In patients with heterozygous disease, there is generally a family history on at least one side of the family. Familial defective apoB-100 has a similar presentation, but is less common (1/1000). ApoA-V deficiency presents with xanthomas, but also has pancreatitis and hepatosplenomegaly with elevated chylomicrons and VLDL. Familial hepatic lipase deficiency and lipoprotein lipase deficiency are associated with increased chylomicrons, not LDL-C, and present with eruptive xanthomas, hepatosplenomegaly, and pancreatitis. These conditions occur rarely (<1/1,000,000).

80. The answer is B.

(Chap. 27) There are many secondary forms of elevated LDL that warrant consideration in a patient found to have abnormal LDL. These include hypothyroidism, nephrotic syndrome, cholestasis, acute intermittent porphyria, anorexia nervosa, hepatoma, and drugs such as thiazides, cyclosporine, and tegretol. Cirrhosis is associated with reduced LDL because of inadequate production. Malabsorption, malnutrition, Gaucher's disease, chronic infectious disease, hyperthyroidism, and niacin toxicity are all similarly associated with reduced LDL.

81. The answer is C.

(Chap. 27) This patient has nephrotic syndrome, which is likely a result of multiple myeloma. The

hyperlipidemia of nephrotic syndrome appears to be due to a combination of increased hepatic production and decreased clearance of very low density lipoproteins, with increased LDL production. It is usually mixed but can manifest as hypercholesterolemia or hypertriglyceridemia. Effective treatment of the underlying renal disease normalizes the lipid profile. Of the choices presented, HMG-CoA reductase inhibitors would be the most effective to reduce this patient's LDL. Dietary management is an important component of lifestyle modification but seldom results in a >10% fall in LDL. Niacin and fibrates would be indicated if the triglycerides were higher, but the LDL is the more important lipid abnormality to address at this time. Lipid apheresis is reserved for patients who cannot tolerate the lipid-lowering drugs or who have a genetic lipid disorder refractory to medication. Cholesterol ester transfer protein inhibitors have been shown to raise high-density lipoprotein levels and their role in the treatment of lipoproteinemias is still under investigation.

82. The answer is B.
(Chap. 29) Multiple endocrine neoplasia (MEN) syndrome is defined as a disorder with neoplasms affecting two or more hormonal tissues in several members of the family. The most common of these is MEN type 1 (MEN1), which is caused by the gene coding the nuclear protein called Menin. MEN1 is associated with tumors or hyperplasia of the parathyroid, pancreas, pituitary, adrenal cortex, and foregut and/or subcutaneous or visceral lipomas. The most common and earliest manifestation is hyperparathyroidism with symptomatic hypercalcemia. This most commonly occurs in the late teenage years and 93–100% of mutation carriers develop this complication. Gastrinomas, insulinomas, and prolactinomas are less common and tend to occur in the 20s, 30s, and 40s. Pheochromocytoma may occur in MEN1, but is more commonly found in MEN2A or von Hippel-Lindau syndrome.

83. The answer is C.
(Chap. 29) Multiple endocrine neoplasia type 2 (MEN2), also called Sipple's syndrome, is characterized by the association of medullary thyroid carcinoma (MTC), pheochromocytomas, and parathyroid tumors. In MEN2A (the most common variant), MTC is associated with pheochromocytomas in 50% of patients (may be bilateral) and with parathyroid tumors in 20% of patients. MEN1, which is also referred to as Wermer's syndrome, is characterized by the triad of tumors involving the parathyroids, pancreatic islets, and anterior pituitary. MEN1 syndrome is caused by a mutation in the menin (or MEN1) gene. MEN2 is caused by a mutation in the RET gene. Family and genetic screening both have high value in this syndrome (MEN2) as prophylactic thyroidectomy, with life-long thyroxine replacement, has dramatically improved outcomes in patients with MEN2 and MEN3, such that ~90% of young patients with RET mutations who had a prophylactic thyroidectomy have no evidence of persistent or recurrent MTC at 7 years after surgery. Partial thyroidectomy was inappropriate for this patient; in patients with clinically evident MTC, a total thyroidectomy with bilateral central resection is recommended.

84. The answer is B.
(Chap. 30) This patient almost certainly is hypotensive, hyponatremic, and hyperkalemic from primary adrenal insufficiency. Given the concomitant presence of hypoparathyroidism and mucocutaneous candidiasis, he likely suffers from autoimmune polyendocrine syndrome type 1. Mucocutaneous candidiasis, hypoparathyroidism, and Addison's disease form the three major components of this disorder. It is an autosomal recessive disorder caused by mutations in the AIRE gene (autoimmune regulator gene) found on chromosome 21. APS-1 develops very early in life, often in infancy. Chronic mucocutaneous candidiasis without signs of systemic disease is often the first manifestation. Hypoparathyroidism usually develops next, followed by adrenal insufficiency. Regarding the treatment of adrenal crisis, several issues merit mention. Adrenal insufficiency can be masked by primary hypothyroidism by prolonging the half-life of cortisol. The caveat therefore is that replacement therapy with thyroid hormone can precipitate an adrenal crisis in an undiagnosed individual. Hence, all patients with hypothyroidism and the possibility of APS should be screened for adrenal insufficiency to allow treatment with glucocorticoids prior to the initiation of thyroid hormone replacement. Treatment of mucocutaneous candidiasis with ketoconazole in an individual with subclinical adrenal insufficiency may also precipitate adrenal crisis. This patient may have concurrent hypocalcemia that merits treatment in conjunction with the adrenal insufficiency.

85. The answer is D.
(Chap. 30) This patient likely has POEMS (polyneuropathy, organomegaly, endocrinopathy, M-protein, and skin changes). Patients usually present with a progressive sensorimotor polyneuropathy, DM (50%), primary

gonadal failure (70%), and a plasma cell dyscrasia with sclerotic bony lesions. Associated findings can be hepatosplenomegaly, lymphadenopathy, and hyperpigmentation. Patients often present in the fifth to sixth decade of life and have a median survival after diagnosis of <3 years. The detection of an M-protein on serum electrophoresis would make POEMS the most likely diagnosis.

86. The answer is B.

(Chap. 31) Humoral hypercalcemia of malignancy (HHM) occurs in up to 20% of patients with cancer. HHM is most common in cancers of the lung, head and neck, skin, esophagus, breast, and genitourinary tract and in multiple myeloma and lymphomas. There are several distinct humoral causes of HHM, but it is caused most commonly by overproduction of parathyroid hormone related-protein (PTHrP). In addition to acting as a circulating humoral factor, bone metastases (e.g., breast, multiple myeloma) may produce PTHrP, leading to local osteolysis and hypercalcemia. PTHrP is structurally related to parathyroid hormone (PTH) and binds to the PTH receptor, explaining the similar biochemical features of HHM and hyperparathyroidism. Metastatic lesions to bone are more likely to produce PTHrP than are metastases in other tissues. Another relatively common cause of HHM is excess production of 1,25-dihydroxyvitamin D. Like granulomatous disorders associated with hypercalcemia, lymphomas can produce an enzyme that converts 25-hydroxyvitamin D to the more active 1,25-dihydroxyvitamin D, leading to enhanced gastrointestinal calcium absorption. Other causes of HHM include tumor-mediated production of osteolytic cytokines and inflammatory mediators. In this case, the multiple metastatic nodules and elevated PTHrP make lymphoma the least likely malignancy.

87. The answer is E.

(Chap. 31) The management of severe symptomatic humoral hypercalcemia of malignancy (HHM) begins saline rehydration (typically 200–500 mL/h) to dilute serum calcium and promote calciuresis. Forced diuresis with furosemide or other loop diuretics can enhance calcium excretion but provides relatively little value except in life-threatening hypercalcemia. When used, loop diuretics should be administered only after complete rehydration and with careful monitoring of fluid balance. Oral phosphorus should be given until serum phosphorus is >1 mmol/L (>3 mg/dL). Bisphosphonates, such as pamidronate, zoledronate, and etidronate, can reduce serum calcium within 1–2 days and suppress calcium release for several weeks. Bisphosphonate infusions can be repeated, or oral bisphosphonates can be used for chronic treatment. Dialysis should be considered in severe hypercalcemia when saline hydration and bisphosphonate treatments are not possible or are too slow in onset. Previously used agents such as calcitonin and mithramycin have little utility now that bisphosphonates are available. Calcitonin should be considered when rapid correction of severe hypercalcemia is needed. Hypercalcemia associated with lymphomas, multiple myeloma, or leukemia may respond to glucocorticoid treatment. This patient most likely does not have lymphoma so initial treatment should not include corticosteroids.

88. and 89. The answers are A and C, respectively.

(Chap. 32) Hypophosphatemia results from one of three mechanisms: (1) inadequate intestinal phosphate absorption, (2) excessive renal phosphate excretion, and (3) rapid redistribution of phosphate from the extracellular space into bone or soft tissue. Inadequate intestinal absorption is rare since antacids containing aluminum hydroxide are no longer commonly prescribed. Malnutrition from fasting or starvation may result in depletion of phosphate. This is also commonly seen in alcoholism. In hospitalized patients, redistribution is the main cause. Insulin promotes phosphate entry into cells along with glucose. When nutrition is initiated, refeeding further increases redistribution of phosphate into cells and is more pronounced when IV glucose is used alone. Sepsis may cause destruction of cells and metabolic acidosis, resulting in a net shift of phosphate from the extracellular space into cells. Renal failure is associated with hyperphosphatemia, not hypophosphatemia, and initial prerenal azotemia, such as in this presentation can obscure underlying phosphate depletion. The approach to treating hypophosphatemia should take into account several factors, including the likelihood (and magnitude) of underlying phosphate depletion, renal function, serum calcium levels, and the concurrent administration of parenteral glucose. In addition, the treating physician should assess the patient for complications of hypophosphatemia that can include neuromuscular weakness, cardiac dysfunction, hemolysis, and platelet dysfunction. Severe hypophosphatemia generally occurs when the serum concentration falls below 2 mg/dL (<0.75 mmol/L). This becomes particularly dangerous when there is underlying chronic phosphate depletion. However, there is no simple formula to determine the body's phosphate needs from measurement of the serum phosphate levels because most phosphate is intracellular. It is generally

recommended to use oral phosphate repletion when the serum phosphate levels are greater than 1.5–2.5 mg/dL (0.5–0.8 mmol/L). The dose of oral phosphate is 750–2000 mg daily of elemental phosphate given in divided doses. More severe hypophosphatemia, as in the case presented, requires intravenous repletion. Intravenous phosphate repletion is given as neutral mixtures of sodium and potassium phosphate salts at doses of 0.2–0.8 mmol/kg given over 6 hours. **Table 32-2** outlines the total dose and recommended infusion rates for a range of phosphate levels. In this patient with a level of 1.0 mg/dL, the recommended infusion rate is 8 mmol/h over 6 hours for a total dose of 48 mmol. Until the underlying hypophosphatemia is corrected, one should measure phosphate and calcium levels every 6 hours. The infusion should be stopped if the calcium phosphate product rises to higher than 50 to decrease the risk of heterotopic calcification. Alternatively, if hypocalcemia is present coincident with the hypophosphatemia, it is important to correct the calcium prior to administering phosphate.

90. The answer is B.

(Chap. 32) Vitamin D deficiency is highly prevalent in the United States and is most common in older individuals who are hospitalized or institutionalized. Vitamin D deficiency can occur as a result of inadequate dietary intake, decreased production in the skin, decreased intestinal absorption, accelerated losses, or impaired vitamin D activation in the liver or kidney. Clinically, vitamin D deficiency in older individuals is most often silent. Often practitioners fail to consider vitamin D deficiency until a patient has been diagnosed with osteoporosis or suffered a fracture. However, some individuals can experience diffuse muscle and bone pain. When assessing vitamin D levels, the appropriate test is 25-hydroxy vitamin D [25(OH)D] levels. The Institute of Medicine has defined vitamin D sufficiency as a level of 25(OH)D >50 nmol/L (>20 ng/L). However, in the elderly and in some disease states, higher levels may be required to maximize intestinal calcium absorption. Levels <37 nmol/L (15 ng/mL) are associated with a rise in parathyroid hormone levels and a fall in bone density. Vitamin D deficiency may also lead to decreased intestinal absorption of calcium with resultant hypocalcemia and secondary hyperparathyroidism. In response to this, there is higher bone turnover and can be associated with an increase in alkaline phosphatase levels. In addition, elevated PTH stimulates renal conversion of 25-hydroxy vitamin D to 1,25-hydroxy vitamin D, the activated form of vitamin D. Thus, even in the face of severe vitamin D deficiency, the activated 1,25(OH)D levels may be normal and do not accurately reflect vitamin D stores. Thus, 1,25(OH)D should not be used to make a diagnosis of vitamin D deficiency. While vitamin D deficiency may be associated with abnormalities in PTH, alkaline phosphatase, and calcium levels, these biochemical abnormalities are seen in many other disease and are neither sensitive nor specific for the diagnosis of vitamin D deficiency.

91. The answer is D.

(Chap. 32) Vitamin D deficiency is common in all areas of the United States and has resulted from decreased solar exposure with deficient production of vitamin D in the skin, lack of dietary intake accelerated losses of vitamin D, impaired vitamin D activation, or resistance to the biologic effects of $1,25(OH)_2D$, the activated form of vitamin D. Vitamin D stores are best assessed by measuring 25-hydroxyvitamin D, 25(OH)D. Levels <20 ng/L (<50 nmol/L) should be repleted. The recommended daily intake in the absence of vitamin D deficiency is 800 IU of vitamin D, typically administered as vitamin D3, or cholecalciferol, daily. However, higher doses of vitamin D are required when vitamin D deficiency is present to return vitamin D levels to normal. In most individuals, supplementation with vitamin D3 at 2000 IU daily along with calcium supplementation would be recommended. In severe cases of vitamin D deficiency, high dose repletion may be required. This is given as ergocalciferol (vitamin D) 50,000 IU weekly for 3–12 weeks before dropping to maintenance daily dose of 800 IU of cholecalciferol daily.

92. The answer is D.

(Chap. 33) The first step in the diagnostic evaluation of hyper- or hypocalcemia is to ensure that the alteration in serum calcium levels is not due to abnormal albumin concentrations. About 50% of total calcium is ionized, and the rest is bound principally to albumin. Although direct measurements of ionized calcium are possible, they are easily influenced by collection methods and other artifacts; thus, it is generally preferable to measure total calcium and albumin to "correct" the serum calcium. When serum albumin concentrations are reduced, a corrected calcium concentration is calculated by adding 0.2 mM (0.8 mg/dL) to the total calcium level for every decrement in serum albumin of 1.0 g/dL below the reference value of 4.1 g/dL for albumin, and, conversely, for elevations in serum albumin. For this patient, their albumin is 2.5, or ~1.5 below the reference value. Thus, we would add 1.6

(or 0.8 × 1.5) to the measured calcium level, arriving at a corrected value of 9.4 mg/dL—a value requiring no treatment for the hypocalcemia. Additional evaluation may be in order for the symptoms and reduced serum albumin.

93. The answer is B.

(Chap. 33) When serum albumin concentrations are reduced, a corrected calcium concentration is calculated by adding 0.2 mM (0.8 mg/dL) to the total calcium level for every decrement in serum albumin of 1.0 g/dL below the reference value of 4.1 g/dL for albumin, and, conversely, for elevations in serum albumin. For this patient, the corrected serum calcium is elevated at 12.7 (11.5 + [4 − 2.5] × 0.8). Significant symptomatic hypercalcemia usually requires therapeutic intervention independent of the etiology of hypercalcemia. Initial therapy of significant hypercalcemia begins with volume expansion because hypercalcemia invariably leads to dehydration; 4–6 L of intravenous saline may be required over the first 24 hours, keeping in mind that underlying comorbidities (e.g., congestive heart failure) may require the use of loop diuretics to enhance sodium and calcium excretion. However, loop diuretics should not be initiated until the volume status has been restored to normal. If there is increased calcium mobilization from bone (as in malignancy or severe hyperparathyroidism), drugs that inhibit bone resorption should be considered. Zoledronic acid (e.g., 4 mg intravenously over ~30 min), pamidronate (e.g., 60–90 mg intravenously over 2–4 hours), and ibandronate (2 mg intravenously over 2 hours) are bisphosphonates that are commonly used for the treatment of hypercalcemia of malignancy in adults. In patients with 1,25(OH)2D-mediated hypercalcemia, glucocorticoids are the preferred therapy, as they decrease 1,25(OH)2D production. Intravenous hydrocortisone (100–300 mg daily) or oral prednisone (40–60 mg daily) for 3–7 days is used most often.

94. The answer is E.

(Chap. 34) Primary hyperparathyroidism is the most common cause of hypercalcemia and is the most likely cause in an adult who is asymptomatic. Primary hyperparathyroidism results from autonomous secretion of parathyroid hormone (PTH) that is no longer regulated by serum calcium levels, usually related to development of parathyroid adenomas. Most patients are asymptomatic or have minimal symptoms at the time of diagnosis. When present, symptoms include recurrent nephrolithiasis, peptic ulcers, dehydration, constipation, and altered mental status. Distinctive bone manifestations include osteitis fibrosa cystica, which histologically results from an increase in the giant multinucleated osteoclasts in scalloped areas on the surface of the bone and a replacement of the normal cellular and marrow elements by fibrous tissue. On x-ray, this will appear as resorption of the phalangeal tufts and replacement of the usually sharp cortical outline of the bone in the digits by an irregular outline. Historically, this finding was present on presentation in 10–25% of cases, but is rare today due to earlier diagnosis of disease. Laboratory studies show elevated serum calcium with decreased serum phosphate. Diagnosis can be confirmed with measurement of parathyroid hormone levels. The optimal management of asymptomatic primary hyperparathyroidism has been debated as surgical removal of autonomous adenomas is generally curative. However, it was unclear whether all patients need to be treated surgically. The most recent recommendations suggest that the more aggressive surgical approach be considered in most patients due to concerns of subtle neuropsychiatric symptoms, long-term skeletal effects, and potential for cardiovascular deterioration. The current guidelines recommend surgery for individuals less than 50 years in age, creatinine clearance <60 mL/min, osteoporosis on bone density scanning, or serum calcium >1 mg/mL above normal. There is no indication for surgery based upon 24-hour urine calcium levels or presence of nephrolithiasis. Likewise, presence of cardiovascular disease is not in the guidelines for recommendation of surgical intervention.

95. The answer is A.

(Chap. 34) Granulomatous disorders including sarcoidosis, tuberculosis, and fungal infections can be associated with hypercalcemia caused increased conversion of 25-hydroxy-vitamin D to 1,25-hydroxy vitamin D by macrophages within the granulomas. This process bypasses the normal feedback mechanisms, and elevated levels of both 25-hydroxy- and 1,25-hydroxy vitamin can be seen. This does not normally occur as 1,25-hydroxy-vitamin D levels are normally tightly controlled through feedback mechanisms on renal 1-hydroxylase, the primary producer of activated vitamin D in normal circumstances. In addition, the normal feedback provided by parathyroid hormone concentrations is also bypassed and the PTH level may be low.

96. The answer is D.

(Chap. 34) This patient demonstrates evidence of tertiary hyperparathyroidism, with inappropriate

elevations in parathyroid hormone despite increases in calcium and phosphate. In addition, the patient is demonstrating clinical evidence of disease including bony pain and ectopic calcification. Tertiary hyperparathyroidism most commonly develops in individuals with long-standing renal failure who have been nonadherent to therapy. In this case scenario, the hypoxemia and ground glass infiltrates on chest CT represent ectopic calcification of the lungs. This can be difficult to identify with typical imaging, and a technetium-99 bone scan will show increased uptake in the lungs. Treatment of tertiary hyperparathyroidism with severe clinical manifestations requires parathyroidectomy. Pathologically, these individuals demonstrate the emergence of monoclonal growth in one or more previously hyperplastic parathyroid glands with subsequent autonomous parathyroid function.

97. The answer is B.
(Chap. 34) Hypocalcemia can be a life-threatening consequence of thyroidectomy if the parathyroid glands are inadvertently removed during the surgery, as the four parathyroid glands are located immediately posterior to the thyroid gland. This is an infrequent occurrence currently as the parathyroid glands are better able to be identified both before and during surgery. However, hypoparathyroidism may occur even if the parathyroid glands are not removed by thyroidectomy due to devascularization or trauma to the parathyroid glands. Hypocalcemia following removal of the parathyroid glands may begin any time during the first 24–72 hours, and monitoring of serial calcium levels is recommended for the first 72 hours. The earliest symptoms of hypocalcemia are typically circumoral paresthesias and paresthesias with a "pins-and- needles" sensation in the fingers and toes. The development of carpal spasms upon inflation of the blood pressure cuff is a classic sign of hypocalcemia and is known as Trousseau sign. Chvostek sign is the other classic sign of hypocalcemia and is elicited by tapping the facial nerve in the preauricular area causing spasm of the facial muscles. A prolongation of the QT interval on the ECG suggests life-threatening hypocalcemia that may progress to fatal arrhythmia, and treatment should not be delayed for serum testing to occur in a patient with a known cause of hypocalcemia. Immediate treatment with IV calcium should be initiated. Maintenance therapy with calcitriol and vitamin D is necessary for ongoing treatment of acquired hypoparathyroidism. Alternatively, surgeons may implant parathyroid tissue into the soft tissue of the forearm, if it is thought that the parathyroid glands will be removed. Hypomagnesemia can cause hypocalcemia by suppressing parathyroid hormone release despite the presence of hypocalcemia. However, in this patient, hypomagnesemia is not suspected after thyroidectomy, and magnesium administration is not indicated. Benztropine is a centrally acting anticholinergic medication that is used in the treatment of dystonic reactions that can occur after taking centrally acting antiemetic medications with dopaminergic activity, such as metoclopramide or compazine. Dystonic reactions involve focal spasms of the face, neck, and extremities. While this patient has taken medications that can cause a dystonic reaction, the spasms that she is experiencing are more consistent with tetanic contractions of hypocalcemia than dystonic reaction. Finally, measurement of forced vital capacity is most commonly used as a measurement of disease severity in myasthenia gravis or Guillain-Barré syndrome. Muscle weakness is a typical presenting feature but not paresthesias.

98. The answer is E.
(Chap. 34) Malignancy can cause hypercalcemia by several different mechanisms, including metastasis to bone, cytokine stimulation of bone turnover, and production of a protein structurally similar to parathyroid hormone by the tumor. This protein is called parathyroid hormone-related peptide (PTHrp) and acts at the same receptors as parathyroid hormone (PTH). Squamous cell carcinoma of the lung is the most common tumor associated with the production of PTHrp. Serum calcium levels can become quite high in malignancy because of unregulated production of PTHrp that is outside of the negative feedback control that normally results in the setting of hypercalcemia. PTH hormone levels should be quite low or undetectable in this setting. When hypercalcemia is severe (>15 mg/dL), symptoms frequently include dehydration and altered mental status. The electrocardiogram may show a shortened QTc interval. Initial therapy includes large-volume fluid administration to reverse the dehydration that results from hypercalciuria. In addition, furosemide is also added to promote further calciuria. If the calcium remains elevated, as in this patient, additional measures should be undertaken to decrease the serum calcium. Calcitonin has a rapid onset of action with a decrease in serum calcium seen within hours. However, tachyphylaxis develops, and the duration of benefit is limited. Pamidronate is a bisphosphonate that is useful for the hypercalcemia of malignancy. It decreases serum calcium by preventing

bone resorption and release of calcium from the bone. After IV administration, the onset of action of pamidronate is 1–2 days with a duration of action of several weeks. Thus, in this patient with ongoing severe symptomatic hypercalcemia, addition of both calcitonin and pamidronate is the best treatment. The patient should continue to receive IV fluids and furosemide. The addition of a thiazide diuretic is contraindicated because thiazides cause increased calcium resorption in the kidney and would worsen hypercalcemia.

99. The answer is B.

(Chap. 35) Osteoporosis refers to a chronic condition characterized by decreased bone strength and frequently manifests as vertebral and hip fractures. In the United States, about 8 million women have osteoporosis compared to about 2 million men for a ratio between men and women of 4 to 1. An additional 48 million individuals are estimated to have osteopenia. The risk of osteoporosis increases with advancing age and rapidly worsens following menopause in women. Most women meet the diagnostic criteria for osteoporosis between the ages of 70 and 80. Caucasian women have an increased risk for osteoporosis when compared to African-American women. The epidemiology for bone fractures follows the epidemiology for osteoporosis. Fractures of the distal radius (Colles' fracture) increases up to age 50, plateaus by age 60, and there is only a modest increase in risk thereafter. This is contrasted with the risk of hip fractures. Incidence rates for hip fractures double every 5 years after the age of 70. This change in fracture pattern is not entirely due to osteoporosis, but also related to the fact that fewer falls in the elderly occur onto an outstretched arm and are more likely to occur directly onto the hip. Black women experience hip fractures at approximately half the rate as white women. The mortality rate in the year following a hip fracture is 5–20%. Vertebral fractures are also common manifestations of osteoporosis. While most are found incidentally on chest radiograph, severe cases can lead to height loss, pulmonary restriction, and respiratory morbidity.

100. The answer is C.

(Chap. 35) There are multiple risks for osteoporotic bone fractures that can be either modifiable or non-modifiable. These are outlined in **Table 35-1**. Non-modifiable risk factors include a previous history of fracture as an adult, female sex, white race, dementia, advanced age, and history of fracture (but not osteoporosis) in a first degree relative. Risk factors that are potentially modifiable include low calcium intake, alcoholism, impaired eyesight, recurrent falls, inadequate physical activity, poor health and estrogen deficiency including menopause prior to age 45 or prolonged premenstrual amenorrhea. Excessive thinness and low body weight are also risk factors for osteoporosis although the osteoporosis guidelines do not clearly delineate what is considered excessive thinness. Current cigarette smoking is a risk factor for osteoporosis-related fracture while a prior history of cigarette use is not.

101. The answer is B.

(Chap. 35) Osteoporosis is a common disease affecting 8 million women and 2 million men in the United States. It is most common in postmenopausal women, but the incidence is also increasing in men. Estrogen loss probably causes bone loss by activation of bone remodeling sites and exaggeration of the imbalance between bone formation and resorption. Osteoporosis is diagnosed by bone mineral density scan. Dual-energy x-ray absorptiometry (DXA) is the most accurate test for measuring bone mineral density. Clinical determinations of bone density are most commonly measured at the lumbar spine and hip. In the DXA technique, two x-ray energies are used to measure the area of the mineralized tissues and compared to gender- and race-matched normative values. The T-score compares an individual's results to a young population, whereas the Z-score compared the individual's results to an age-matched population. Osteoporosis is diagnosed when the T-score is −2.5 SD in the lumbar spine, femoral neck, or total hip. An evaluation for secondary causes of osteoporosis should be considered in individuals presenting with osteoporotic fractures at a young age and those who have very low Z-scores. Initial evaluation should include serum and 24-hour urine calcium levels, renal function panel, hepatic function panel, serum phosphorous level, and vitamin D levels. Other endocrine abnormalities including hyperthyroidism and hyperparathyroidism should be evaluated, and urinary cortisol levels should be checked if there is a clinical suspicion for Cushing's syndrome. Follicle-stimulating hormone and luteinizing hormone levels would be elevated but are not useful in this individual as she presents with a known perimenopausal state.

102. The answer is C.

(Chap. 35) Determination of when to initiate screening for osteoporosis with bone densitometry testing can be complicated by multiple factors. In general, most women do not require screening for

osteoporosis until after completion of menopause unless there have been unexplained fractures or other risk factors that would suggest osteoporosis. There is no benefit to initiating screening for osteoporosis in the perimenopausal period. Indeed most expert recommendations do not recommend routine screening for osteoporosis until age 65 or older unless risk factors are present. Risk factors for osteoporosis include advanced age, current cigarette smoking, low body weight (<57.7 kg), family history of hip fracture, and long-term glucocorticoid use. Inhaled glucocorticoids may cause increased loss of bone density, but as this patient is on a low dose of inhaled fluticasone and is not estrogen-deficient, bone mineral densitometry cannot be recommended at this time. The risk of osteoporosis related to inhaled glucocorticoids is not well-defined, but most studies suggest that the risk is relatively low. Delaying childbearing until the fourth and fifth decades does increase the risk of osteoporosis but does not cause early onset of osteoporosis prior to completion of menopause. The patient's family history of osteoporosis likewise does not require early screening for osteoporosis.

103–107. Answers: 103-B; 104-E; 105-D; 106-A; 107-C.

(Chap. 35) In the past 20 years, multiple pharmacologic options have become available for the treatment of osteoporosis. Prior to the 1990s, estrogen either alone or in combination with a progestin was the primary treatment for osteoporosis. Since that time, many new agents have been introduced although estrogen is effective at preventing bone loss, reducing bone turnover, and yields small increases in bone mass of the spine, hip, and total body. The selective estrogen receptor modulator raloxifene binds to the estrogen receptor and is approved for the prevention and treatment of osteoporosis as well as the prevention of breast cancer. Tamoxifen is another well-known SERM, but it is only approved for the treatment and prevention of breast cancer. Both drugs have a favorable effect on bone turnover and bone mass. Raloxifene has been demonstrated in clinical trials to reduce the occurrence of vertebral fracture by 30–50% although the effect on nonvertebral fracture is not known. Bisphosphonates are the most widely used category of medications for the prevention and treatment of osteoporosis. Alendronate, risedronate, ibandronate, and zoledronic acids are approved medications in this class. Bisphosphonates act to impair osteoclast function and reduce osteoclast number by inducing apoptosis. Zoledronic acid is retained in the bone for a very long time and is dosed intravenously only once yearly. Exogenous administration of calcitonin, a polypeptide hormone produced by the thyroid gland, is sometimes administered as a nasal spray in the treatment of osteoporosis. It acts to suppress osteoclast activity by direct action on the osteoclast calcitonin receptor. In clinical studies, the effect on bone mass and vertebral fracture risk is small and has no effect on nonvertebral fractures. Denosumab is a fully human monoclonal antibody to RANKL, the final common effector of osteoclast formation, activity, and survival. When denosumab binds to RANKL, osteoclast maturation is significantly impaired. It is administered by subcutaneous injection twice yearly and has been demonstrated to decrease fracture risk in the spine, hip, and forearm over a 3-year period from 20–70%. Teriparatide is a recombinant parathyroid hormone (1-34hPTH) that is approved for the treatment of osteoporosis. It is administered by daily subcutaneous injection and has been shown to decrease both vertebral and nonvertebral fracture risk. As teriparatide is an analogue of PTH, the drug acts like PTH with direct actions on osteoblast to stimulate new bone formation, which is unique among the treatments for osteoporosis.

108. The answer is B.

(Chap. 35) This individual with cystic fibrosis has malabsorption of vitamin D and chronic inflammation, placing them at increased risk of osteoporosis. Upon diagnosis of osteoporosis with a T-score <–2.5, the patient was appropriately initiated on therapy with a bisphosphonate, vitamin D3, and calcium. The appropriate interval for following osteoporosis with bone densitometry after initiating treatment is not clearly established as most treatments yield only small or moderate bone mass increments. Thus, the changes need to be greater than ~4% in the spine and ~6% in the hip to be considered significant in any given individual. Medication-induced changes in BMD take several years to produce significant changes, and BMD should be repeated at intervals >2 years. Only further declines in BMD should prompt a change in regimen.

INDEX

Bold page number indicates the start of the main discussion of the topic; page numbers with "*f*" and "*t*" refer to figures and tables, respectively.

B